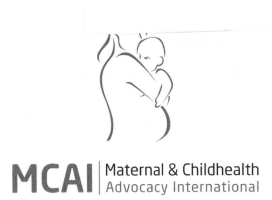

MCAI | Maternal & Childhealth
Advocacy International

International Maternal & Child Health Care

A practical manual for hospitals worldwide

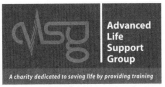

Advanced
Life
Support
Group

A charity dedicated to saving life by providing training

Radcliffe Publishing
London • New York

Radcliffe Publishing Ltd
St Mark's House
Shepherdess Walk
London N1 7BQ
United Kingdom

www.radcliffehealth.com

Editor: David Southall
Associate Editors: Alice Clack, Johan Creemers, Angela Gorman, Assad Hafeez, Brigid Hayden, Ejaz Khan, Grace Kodindo, Rhona MacDonald, Yawar Najam, Barbara Phillips, Diane Watson, Dave Woods, Ann Wright

British Library Cataloguing in Publication Data

A catalogue record for this book is available from the British Library.

ISBN-13: 978 184619 992 9

The paper used for the text pages of this book is FSC® certified. FSC (The Forest Stewardship Council®) is an international network to promote responsible management of the world's forests.

Typeset by Darkriver Design, Auckland, New Zealand
Manufacturing managed by 21six

Contents

Section 1: General issues regarding hospital care

Contents

Section 2: Pregnancy-related problems

Authors are Katie Christie, Alice Clack, Johan Creemers, Brigid Hayden, Grace Kodindo, Shamsunnisa Sadia, David Southall, Diane Watson and Ann Wright. (Unless otherwise stated)

Section 3: Neonatal care

Section 4: Children in hospital

Section 5: The child presenting with a system or organ dysfunction

Contents

Section 6: Infections in children

Contents

Foreword

Professor David Southall and the expert contributors to this textbook must be commended. They have delivered a consolidated, practical guide on maternal and child health with an understanding that care should not be compromised even in the face of conflict, material shortage, or human resource limitations.

Maternal and child health has made great strides in recent decades, but requires continued work. This textbook tackles the challenge by taking a uniquely holistic perspective and will help to push forward this public health agenda. This book is enriched by in-depth clinical questions, in addition to a sympathetic and exceptional understanding of the challenges facing health systems worldwide.

The segment on respectful and compassionate care caught my attention in particular. It is a crucial aspect of quality medical service and a patient's continued engagement in the healthcare system. This goes hand-in-hand with grief management, medical and nursing ethics, and the realisation that healthcare moves well beyond the clinical setting alone. Comfort and communication go a long way, and I applaud the authors for their promotion of complete care.

I am particularly grateful to the authors for providing this textbook free of charge in resource-limited clinical settings. I am excited to see literature that understands the importance of continued education for a strong health workforce.

It is with the help of textbooks like this that we can move towards increased access to evidence-based, comprehensive healthcare for women and children. It is my hope that this textbook will become an essential part of a holistic, systems-based approach to maternal and child healthcare.

Dr Bernice Dahn MD MPH FLCP
Deputy Minister of Health/
Chief Medical Officer, Republic of Liberia
July 2014

Preface

This textbook is written to help health workers treating pregnant women and adolescents, their newborn infants, and children admitted to hospitals in countries all over the world. It is especially aimed at those working in settings in which material and human resources are limited, where borders and infrastructures are insecure, and in rural areas where health workers may find it particularly difficult to work. Building on existing global efforts, dedicated doctors, nurses and midwives in these settings are already providing life-saving healthcare, but often find their work hard and sometimes overwhelming. Access to up-to-date evidence-based guidelines in such settings is often extremely difficult. The Internet is often too slow, printing from computers is often too expensive, and so, in our experience, books remain essential.

This textbook has been written and peer-reviewed by over 100 experts from around the world, with experience in hospital settings in which there are poor resources, who have freely given their time and expertise. Covering all aspects of hospital care for pregnant women and adolescents, newborn infants and children, this textbook addresses a full range of possible illnesses, conditions, and injuries and includes complications of pregnancy and delivery. Based on the latest evidence and guidelines available, including Cochrane reviews and World Health Organization (WHO) guidelines, this textbook builds on existing efforts and identifies an internationally applicable minimum standard of healthcare in poorly resourced hospitals and reflects the management of problems often inherent in resource-limited countries. The textbook proposes minimum standards, both in the treatments given and also in the medical ethics and professional standards, which should be practised in caring for the particularly vulnerable patients attending hospitals in resource-limited settings.

MCAI is funding the costs of publishing, printing and distributing this textbook on a 'not for profit' basis. Following requests from health workers in resource-limited settings, the aim of the editors and authors is to provide this textbook free of charge (on condition that health workers agree to use and look after the textbook; see inside cover). The textbook is particularly targeted at frontline health workers in the most disadvantaged hospitals in the world, particularly those in rural areas of low-income countries, especially those treating all women and children regardless of their or their family's ability to pay. In all other countries, the textbook will be charged at above cost price with all profit from these sales going to help fund the provision of further copies of the textbook for health workers in low income countries and the work of MCAI in strengthening the emergency healthcare systems of hospitals in the world's poorest countries.

The aim of all authors and editors is to provide a useful, comprehensive reference for all health workers in all settings to help them provide the best possible clinical care and management for pregnant women and adolescents, their newborn infants, and children.

Contributors

Professor Miriam Adhikari
Research Co-ordinator Postgraduate & Research, Nelson R Mandela School of Medicine, University of KwaZulu Natal, 2nd Floor Medical School, 719 Umbilo Road, Durban 4001

Dr Michele Afif
MBBS BSc MSc FRCPCH. Consultant Paediatrician, North West London Hospitals NHS Trust, UK

Dr Anita Aijaz
Consultant Psychiatrist, Psychosocial Centre, Hilal-e-Ahmer Clifton Karachi Project Director, SHAMIL community mental health project, Pakistan, Association for Mental Health, Karachi, Pakistan. Consultancy and volunteer work for ROZAN NGO working on issues of emotional health, gender and violence against women and children

Dr Katherine Ajdukiewicz
MD, MBChB, FRCP, DTMH, MFTM RCPS (Glasg). Consultant in Infectious Diseases & Tropical Medicine; Honorary Senior Lecturer, The University of Manchester, Manchester Academic Health Science Centre, Pennine Acute Hospitals NHS Trust, North Manchester General Hospital, UK

Dr Jamshed Akhtar
MBBS, FCPS (Paediatric Surgery), Masters in Bioethics. PGD Biomedical Ethics Associate Professor & Head, Department of Paediatric Surgery, National Institute of Child Health, Karachi 75510, Pakistan

Professor Savvas Andronikou
MMBCh (Wits), FCRad (diag), FRCR (Lond) and PhD (UCT). Paediatric radiologist and Professor of Radiology at the University of the Witwatersrand, South Africa

Dr Ramandeep Arora
Paediatric Oncology Registrar, Alder Hey Children's NHS Foundation Trust, Liverpool, UK

Professor Theunis Avenant
M Med (Paed). Infectious Diseases Specialist, Department of Paediatrics and Child Health, University of Pretoria, Head, Department of Paediatrics, Kalafong Hospital and University of Pretoria, University of Pretoria, Private Bag x396, Pretoria 0001, South Africa

Dr Wendi Bailey
BSc, MSc, PhD. Senior Principal Experimental Officer, in charge of Clinical Diagnostic Parasitology, Liverpool School of Tropical Medicine, UK

Dr Alastair Baker
MB ChB MBA FRCP FRCPCH. Consultant Paediatric Hepatologist, Paediatric Liver Centre, King's College Hospital, London, SE5 9RS, UK

Dr Gillian Barber
RM RN MA (Education) PhD. Advisor in international midwifery and nursing education, and social anthropologist, UK

Professor Zulfiqar A Bhutta
Noordin Noormahomed Sharief Professor & Founding Chair, Division of Women and Child Health, The Aga Khan University, Pakistan

Dr June Brady
Clinical Professor of Pediatrics, University of California, San Francisco, USA. Previously Visiting Professor, University of Zimbabwe

Dr James Bunn
Consultant paediatrician, Alder Hey Children's Hospital, Liverpool, UK

Dr Mary Bunn
MB BChir, MRCGP, M Phil Pall Medicine. Queenscourt Hospice, Southport, Formerly Umodzi Palliative Care for Children, Queen Elizabeth Central Hospital, Blantyre, Malawi

Dr Su Bunn
MB ChB MRCPCH MD. Consultant Paediatric Gastroenterologist, Dept of Paediatric Gastroenterology, Great North Children's Hospital, Newcastle upon Tyne NE1 4LP, UK

Dr Pornthep Chanthavanich
Associate Professor, Faculty of Tropical Medicine, Mahidol University, Thailand

Dr Tsitsi Chawatama
Specialist registrar in paediatrics, St Mary's Hospital, London, UK, Previously VSO/RCPCH fellow, Ethiopia

Ms Katie Christie
Founder and Director of Midwifery, The Maternity Unit at the Aberdeen Women's Centre, Aberdeen, UK

Dr Gavin Cho
BHB, MBChB, MRCP (UK), FRACP, FRCPA. Consultant Haematologist at Central Middlesex Hospital and Medical Director for the Brent Sickle Cell and Thalassaemia Centre, London, UK

Dr Alice Clack
MBChB, BSc, MRCOG. Consultant obstetrician, Maternal and Childhealth Advocacy International, Liberia

Andrew Clarke
RN RHV MPH. Technical Advisor, Kidasha, UK/Nepal. Clinical Lead Health Visitor, Lancashire Care NHS Foundation Trust, UK. Director: Child Friendly Healthcare Initiative, Maternal & Childhealth Advocacy International

Dr Ed Cooper
Paediatrician and clinical consultant to the Partnership for Child Development, Department of Infectious Disease Epidemiology, Imperial College Faculty of Medicine, London, UK

Dr Brian Coulter
MD, FRCP(I), FRCPCH. Honorary Clinical Lecturer, Liverpool School of Tropical Medicine, UK, Editor-in-Chief, Paediatrics and International Child Health

Dr Johan Creemers
Consultant Obstetrician and Perinatologist, University Medical Centre, Groningen, The Netherlands

Dr David Cundall
MA MB BS MRCP FRCPCH DTM&H. Retired Consultant Paediatrician, UK, Coordinator Nigeria Health Care Project

Dr Paul Dienye
MBBS, FWACP(Fam. Med), FMCGP. Chief Consultant, Family Physician and Coordinator of Residency Training (Family Medicine), University of Port Harcourt Teaching Hospital and Braithwaite Memorial Specialist Hospital, Port Harcourt, Nigeria

Dr Peter Driscoll
BSC MBChB, MD, FRCS, FCEM. Senior clinical teaching fellow, St Andrew's University, Scotland

Dr Abdul Karim Duke
Consultant in Congenital Heart Disease, Glenfield Hospital, Leicester LE3 9QP, UK

Professor Tim Eden
Professor of Paediatric and Adolescent Oncology, University of Manchester, UK

Professor Wagih El Masri
Consultant Surgeon in Spinal Injuries at Robert Jones & Agnes Hunt Orthopaedic & District Hospital NHS Trust, UK. Former President of the International Spinal Cord Society, Keele University

Professor Gamal Gabra
Consultant Haematologist, Regional Blood Transfusion Centre – National Blood Service, Edgbaston B15 2SG, Birmingham, UK

Dr Sapthagiri Gantasala
Specialist Registrar in Paediatrics, Oxford Children's Hospital, Oxford OX3 9DU, UK

Angela Gorman
Chief Executive Officer, Life for African Mothers, Llanishen, Cardiff CF14 5DZ, UK

Professor John W Gregory
MBChB, DCH, MD, FRCP, FRCPCH. Professor in Paediatric Endocrinology & Honorary Consultant, Department of Child Health, School of Medicine, Cardiff University, Heath Park, Cardiff CF14 4XN, UK

Dr Assad Hafeez
MBBS, FCPS, MRCP, FRCPCH, MSc Epidemiology, PhD. Dean and Executive Director, Health Services Academy, Ministry of National Health Services, Regulations and Coordination, Islamabad, Pakistan

Dr Jay Halbert
MBBS BSc DTMH MRCPCH. Founder and Director, Maternal and Child Healthcare in Myanmar

Dr Prudence Hamade
MB CHB MRCPCH. Senior Technical Advisor, Malaria Consortium, International Malaria Consortium Head Quarters, Development House, 56–64 Leonard Street, London, UK

Professor Roderick Hay
DM, FRCP, FRCPath, FMedSci. Chairman, International Foundation for Dermatology, Willan House, 4 Fitzroy Square, London, W1P 5HQ, UK

Dr Brigid Hayden
MB ChB FRCOG Cert. Med. Ed. Consultant in Obstetrics and Gynaecology and Honorary Senior Lecturer, Bolton Hospital NHS Trust, UK, Convenor Maternal and Childhealth Advocacy International, UK

Dr Lynne Jones MD, OBE. Early Child Development Adviser, Aga Khan Foundation, Mozambique, Honorary Research Associate in Developmental Psychiatry, University of Cambridge, UK

Associate Professor Ejaz Khan
Diplomate, American Board of Paediatrics and Paediatric Infectious Diseases, Shifa International Hospital, Islamabad, Pakistan

Dr Grace Kodindo
MD/Ob-Gyn. Consultant Obstetrician, Chagoua and Farcha hospitals, N'djamena, Chad

Dr Ike Lagunju
Consultant Paediatric Neurologist and Senior Lecturer, University College Hospital, Ibadan, Nigeria

Professor David Lalloo
Professor of Tropical Medicine, Dean of Clinical Sciences and International Public Health, Liverpool School of Tropical Medicine, UK

Dr Heather Lambert
Consultant paediatric nephrologist, Newcastle Hospitals NHS Foundation Trust, UK

Dr Camille Lazaro
OBE, MBBS, DCH, FRCP, FRCPCH. Emeritus Consultant Paediatrician, Newcastle University Hospitals Trust, UK

Dr Rhona MacDonald
MB ChB, MRCGP, MPH, DCH, DRCOG. Honorary Executive Director, Maternal and Childhealth Advocacy International, UK. Senior Editor *PLOS Medicine* and Editor at Large, *WHO Bulletin*

Mr Ian Mackie
Consultant Orthopaedic Surgeon, Nevill Hall Hospital, Abergavenny, UK

Qudrat Ullah Malik
MBBS, MRCPI, FCPS. Consultant Paediatrician and Head of Paediatric Department, Quetta Institute of Medical Sciences, Quetta, Pakistan

Dr Sarah Malleson
MB.BS. Family Practice Resident, University of British Columbia, Canada

Dr Maha Mansour
Consultant Neonatologist, Singleton Hospital – Abertawe Bro Morgannwg University, Health Board, Swansea, SA2 8QA, UK

Wendy Martin
RN, RM, BMedSci, LLM, MSc. Head of Clinical Quality & Patient Safety & Supervisor of Midwives, NHS Midlands & East, UK

Dr Kieran McHugh
FRCR FRCPI DCH. Consultant Paediatric Radiologist, Great Ormond Street Hospital for Children, London WC1N 3JH, UK

Dr Paddy McMaster
MD FRCPCH. Consultant in Paediatric Infectious Diseases, North Manchester General Hospital, Manchester M8 5RB, Past Chair, Children's HIV Association, UK

Professor Anne Merriman
MBE, FRCPI, FRCP (Edin), MCommH. Palliative Care Consultant to Institute of Hospice and Palliative Care in Africa, Founder and Director of Policy and International Programmes Hospice Africa (Uganda), PO Box 7757, Kampala, Uganda

Dr Muhammad Saeed Minhas
Associate Professor of Trauma and Orthopedic Surgery, Jinnah Postgraduate Medical Centre, Karachi, Pakistan

Professor Elizabeth Molyneux
Professor of Paediatrics, College of Medicine, Box 360, Blantyre 3, Malawi

Dr Comfort Momoh
MD, MBE. FGM/Public Health Specialist, Founder of the African Well Woman's Clinic at Guy's and St Thomas Foundation Trust in London, UK

Dr Mary Montgomery
FRCPCH. Consultant Paediatric Intensivist Children's Acute Transport Service, UK

Professor Allie Moosa
MD FRCPCH FAAP. Professor and visiting consultant pediatric neurologist, Adan Hospital, Kuwait

Dr Sarah Morley
FRCPCH FFICM PhD. Consultant in Paediatric Intensive Care, Cambridge University Hospitals NHS Trust, Consultant in Paediatric Transfusion – NHS Blood and Transplant Service, UK

Dr Alli Morrison
Consultant Paediatrician, Darlington Memorial Hospital, Darlington DL3 6HX, UK

Dr Rob Moy
MD MSc FRCPCH. Retired Senior Lecturer in Child Health, University of Birmingham, UK

Dr Victor Musiime
MB ChB, MMED. Head of Paediatrics, Joint Clinical Research Centre Kampala, Uganda

Dr Yawar Najam
MRCPI DCH. Consultant Paediatrician/Neonatologist, Shifa International University Hospital, Shifa College of Medicine, Islamabad, Pakistan

Mr Yogesh Nathdwarawala
Consultant Orthopaedic Surgeon, Nevill Hall Hospital, Abergavenny, UK

Dr Anne Nesbitt
Consultant Paediatrician, Royal College of Paediatrics and Child Health (RCPCH) Global Links Programme, Ola Children's Hospital, Freetown, Sierra Leone

Professor Charles Newton
Professor of Paediatrics, Centre for Geographical Medicine, KEMRI/Wellcome Trust Collaborative Programme, PO Box 230 Kilifi, 80108, Kenya

Dr Tim O'Dempsey
DCH, DTCH, DTM&H, FRCP. Senior Lecturer in Clinical Tropical Medicine, Liverpool School of Tropical Medicine, UK

Dr Bernhards Ogutu
MD. Consultant Paediatrician, University of Nairobi, Kenya

Dr Susan O'Halloran
MBBS FRCPCH. Consultant paediatrician, Maternal and Childhealth Advocacy International, The Gambia

Dr Bernadette O'Hare
FRCPCH MPH. Senior Lecturer, Paediatrics and Child Health, College of Medicine – University of Malawi, Private Bag 360, Chichiri, Blantyre 3, Malawi

Dr Simon Parke
FRCPCH. Consultant paediatrician, Royal Devon and Exeter Hospital, EX2 5DW, UK

Dr Barbara M Phillips
MB ChB, MRCP (UK), Hon FRCPCH, FFAEM. Retired Consultant in Paediatric Emergency Medicine, UK

Professor Barry Pizer
Consultant Paediatric Oncologist, Alder Hey Children's NHS Foundation Trust, Liverpool, UK

Professor Shakeel A Qureshi
MBChB, FRCP, FRCPCH. Consultant Paediatric Cardiologist, Evelina Children's Hospital, London SE1 7EH, UK

Dr Zdenka Reinhardt
Consultant in Congenital Heart Disease, Freeman's Hospital, Newcastle upon Tyne NE7 7DN, Department of Paediatric Cardiology, Guy's Hospital, London SE1, UK

Professor Anthony Roberts
OBE MA BSc BM BChFRCS. President of Restore – Burn and Wound Research, UK

Dr Joan Robson
FRCS FRCPCH FCEM. Consultant in Emergency Paediatrics (retired). Formerly at Alder Hey Children's Hospital, Liverpool L12 2AP and College of Medicine, Box 360, Blantyre 3, Malawi

Dr Oliver Ross
MB ChB, FRCA. Consultant Paediatric Anaesthetist, University Hospital, Southampton, UK

Professor Terence Ryan
Emeritus Professor of Dermatology, University of Oxford and Oxford Brookes University, Honorary President International Society of Dermatology, UK

Dr Saraswathy Sabanathan
MRCPCH. Clinical Research Fellow, Oxford University Clinical Research Unit, Hospital for Tropical Diseases, Ho Chi Minh City, Vietnam

Dr Shamsunnisa Sadia
MBBS, MCPS, FCPS, PGD-PETM. Associate Professor Obstetrics & Gynaecology, Islamic International Medical College Trust, Pakistan Railways Hospital, Rawalpindi, Pakistan

Professor Chaudhry Aqeel Safdar
FRCS AMC. Paediatric Surgeon, National University of Sciences and Technology, NUST Campus H-12, Islamabad, Pakistan

Wandifa Samateh
RN, SCM, MSc. Principal Nursing Officer, Bansang Hospital, Department of State for Health, Banjul, The Gambia

Dr Martin Samuels
MB BS BSc MD FRCPCH. Consultant Paediatrician, University Hospital of North Staffordshire, UK, and Great Ormond Street Hospital, London, Chair of the APLS course and Trustee, ALSG, UK

Dr Christiaan Scott
MBChB, FCPaed (SA), Grad Cert Paed Rheum (UWA). Senior Specialist Paediatric Rheumatology, Red Cross War Memorial Children's Hospital, Cape Town, South Africa

Dr Massimo Serventi
Paediatrician, Box 1498, Dodoma, Tanzania

Dr Neela Shabde
Clinical Director – Children & Families, Cumbria, Clinical Commissioning Group, Lonsdale Unit, Penrith CA11 8 HX, UK

Professor Surjit Singh
MD; DCH (London); FRCPCH (Lon), FRCP (Lon) FAMS. Professor of Pediatrics, Advanced Pediatrics Centre, Post Graduate Institute of Medical Education and Research (PGIMER), Chandigarh, India 160012

Anita Smith
MBE, MRG. Director, Bansang Hospital Appeal, Kettering, UK

Dr John Sandford Smith
Retired Consultant Ophthalmologist, Leicester Royal Infirmary, UK, Formerly Senior Lecturer, Ahmadu Bello University Hospital, Kaduna, Nigeria

Dr Susan Smith
Consultant Psychiatrist, University of Wales Hospital, Cardiff, UK

Professor Alan Smyth
FRCPCH. Consultant Paediatrician and Professor of Child Health, University of Nottingham, UK

Dr Anthony Solomon
PhD, MRCP, DTM&H. Senior Lecturer and Wellcome Trust Intermediate Clinical Fellow, Clinical Research Department, London School of Hygiene & Tropical Medicine, UK

Professor David Southall
OBE, MD, FRCPCH. Honorary Medical Director Maternal and Childhealth Advocacy International, MCAI

Professor Taunton Southwood
FRCPCH. Professor of Paediatric Rheumatology,
Birmingham Children's Hospital, UK

Professor Shoba Srinath
DPM, MD (Psychiatry). Professor and Head
Department of Child and Adolescent Psychiatry,
National Institute of Mental Health and
Neurosciences, Bangalore, India

Dr Francis Ssali
MBChB, MSc, DTM&H, MMED. Head Clinical
Services Joint Clinical Research Centre, Kampala,
Uganda

Dr Peter B Sullivan
MA MD FRCP FRCPCH. Reader in Paediatric
Gastroenterology, Head of the University Department
of Paediatrics, Oxford Children's Hospital, Oxford, UK

Professor James Tumwine
Professor, Paediatrics and Child Health School of
Medicine, College of Health Sciences, Makerere
University, Mulago Hospital, Kampala, Uganda

Dr Sirijitt Vasanawathana
Chief of Pediatrics, Khon Kaen Regional Public
Hospital, Thailand

Dr Jerry KH Wales DM, MA, BM BCh, MRCP,
FRCPCH (Hon), DCH (Hon). Senior Lecturer in
Paediatric Endocrinology, Academic Unit of Child
Health, Sheffield Children's Hospital, Sheffield, UK

Mary J Warrell
MB BS, FRCP, FRCP(E), FRCPath. Oxford Vaccine
Group, University of Oxford, UK

Dr Diane Watson
MB ChB, FRCA. Consultant Anaesthetist, Royal
Gwent Hospital, Newport, UK

Dr Douglas Wilkinson
Founder, Primary Trauma Care Foundation,
Consultant Anaesthetist in Intensive Care, John
Radcliffe Hospital, Oxford, UK

Dr Bridget Wills
FRCPCH, DM. Senior Clinical Research Fellow,
Oxford University Clinical Research Unit Hospital for
Tropical Diseases, Ho Chi Minh City, Vietnam

Dr Geoffrey Woodruff
FRCSEd FRCOphth. Consultant Paediatric
Ophthalmologist Emeritus, Leicester Royal Infirmary,
UK

Professor Dave Woods
MD FRCP. Emeritus Professor in Neonatal Medicine,
School of Child and Adolescent Health, University of
Cape Town, South Africa

Dr Ann Wright
Consultant Obstetrician, Royal Gwent Hospital,
Newport, UK, Associate Professor UITM, Specialist
Obstetrics and Gynaecology, Hospital Selayang,
Malaysia

Dr Pamela Yerassimou
Consultant Psychiatrist, Whitchurch Hospital, Cardiff,
UK

Introduction

This in-depth manual has been written for doctors, midwives and nurses caring for pregnant women and adolescent girls, newborn infants and children in the poorest, most disadvantaged, countries of the world, particularly concentrated in sub-Saharan Africa and South Asia. It is primarily designed to develop a minimum standard of care in hospitals for every woman, baby and child, regardless of the resources available for the country as a whole.

The startling numbers in the Tables below illustrate the unethical and unacceptable mortality rates for pregnant women, newborn infants and children in resource-poor countries. The continued presence of armed conflict and, in many cases, the associated and deliberate targeting of healthcare (see www.ihpi.org) has contributed to a worsening situation in many countries.

ARTICLE 25 of the Universal Declaration of Human Rights adopted in 1948 states the following: 'Everyone has the right to a standard of living adequate for the health and well-being of himself and of his family, including food, clothing, housing and medical care and necessary social services, and the right to security in the event of unemployment, sickness, disability, widowhood, old age or other lack of livelihood in circumstances beyond his control. Motherhood and childhood are entitled to special care and assistance. All children, whether born in or out of wedlock, shall enjoy the same social protection'.

There is no question that a considerable burden of unnecessary suffering is endured by women and children in hospitals; not only those in poorly-resourced settings. This situation is not all related to a lack of funds; much also relates to deficiencies in the training of health workers. Often, the training and continuous professional development of doctors, midwives and nurses is a low priority and even after training they are often not provided with adequate salaries, professional recognition or up to date evidence-based teaching and clinical materials. Standard medical textbooks for health workers in disadvantaged countries are usually too expensive and out-of-date, hampering their continuing medical education.

TABLE 1 Comparison of maternal and child mortality rates in rich versus poor countries in the world

	47 high income countries defined as those with GNI ≥ 12,616 USD per capita per annum[†]		33 low income countries defined as those with GNI ≤ 1035 USD per capita per annum[†]	
	Range	Median	Range	Median
Under 5 year mortality rate per 1000 live births: 2012 data	2–21	5	40–182	90
Maternal mortality ratio (MMR)* per 100,000 live births: 2010 data 'adjusted'	2–47	8	70–1100	460

Data from State of the World's Children (2014) by UNICEF.

*MMR is the number of deaths of women from pregnancy-related causes per 100,000 live births during the same period. The data that are 'adjusted' refer to 2010 United Nations inter-agency maternal mortality estimates released in May 2012.

[†]GNI = Gross National Income from World Bank data; USD = United States Dollars

TABLE 2 Details of individual numbers of maternal and under 5 year deaths comparing low and high income countries

	Total number of births 2012	Total number of maternal deaths 2010 adjusted*	Total number of child deaths under 5 years 2012	Number of live births resulting in 1 maternal death	Number of live births resulting in 1 child death
Low income countries (N = 33, 32 with data on maternal deaths and 33 with data on under 5 year child deaths)	26,007,000	110,376 (median number for individual countries = 2049)	2,197,982 (median number for individual countries = 43,228)	**236**	**12**
High income countries (N = 47, 45 with data on maternal deaths and 47 with data on under 5 year child deaths)	14,149,000	2190 (median number for individual countries =7)	84,479 (median number for individual countries = 420)	**6461**	**167**

Data from State of the World's Children (2014) by UNICEF.

Editing and writing this book has been challenging for the editors and authors. We have identified what we regard as the acceptable minimum standards of treatment for all major diseases and injuries that affect the pregnant woman, newborn baby, infant and child, wherever they are cared for. But we also wanted to offer a set of ideal standards for care where resources are adequate. Therefore, we have incorporated the essential minimum standard of care alongside some of the best standards currently available. However, readers will notice that for most of the treatments recommended, the minimum and gold standards are identical because there are certain treatments that should be provided as essential hospital care, whatever the pressures. This manual should ideally be supplemented by scenario- and skill-based short training courses, combined with apprenticeship and small group teaching on the wards and in the operating theatre.

We believe in the continuing value of printed books to the practical application of healthcare, recognising that with time and improved access to high-speed internet in low resource settings, electronic materials, particularly videos and an easily accessed internet, will introduce major benefits. In the meantime books should be available for all health workers regardless of their ability to pay for them. We hope that you will find this in-depth manual helpful.

Acknowledgements

The editors are extremely grateful to the following people, without whom, producing this textbook would not have been possible:

- All of our authors (see contributor list)
- Radcliffe Publishers, with particular thanks to Tanya Dean, Jamie Etherington and Gillian Nineham
- Jo Hargreaves (freelance copyeditor)
- Vivianne Douglas from Darkriver Design
- Alison Grove, Janette Latta and Mairi Stephen (all three MCAI staff), Bethany Jones (manuscript work), Rachel Drummond and Laura Ella-Kirk (artists) and Dr Joan Robson (fundraising) for their invaluable contributions
- Dr Alison Earley Trustee of MCAI for her review of the HIV in children proof and Professor Helen Foster, Professor of Paediatric Rheumatology, Newcastle University for her input on pGALS to the chapter on Rheumatology disorders
- Dr Maurice King and Professor Glen Mola for allowing us to use copyright-free a large number of figures (some of which we have modified) from their book *Safe Motherhood in Developing Countries*
- The paediatric section of this textbook is partially based on an earlier book published in 2002 by BMJ Books on behalf of MCAI and entitled *International Child Health Care: a practical manual for hospitals worldwide*. We thank all of the Editors and authors of this previous book. In particular, we dedicate this new book in memory of Dr Christiane Ronald, a paediatrician who worked for MCAI for many years.

Permissions

The authors are grateful to the following organisations for permission to reproduce source material:

- **Wiley and Advanced Life Support Group** for Figures 1.12.3–1.12.12, 1.12.14, 1.12.18–1.12.22, 1.13.1–1.13.4, 1.13.11–1.13.13, 1.13.16, 1.13.19, 3.2.2–3.2.4, 7.3.A.1, 7.3.B.1–7.3.B.7, 8.2.1–8.2.6; 8.2.10–8.2.11 8.3.1–8.3.2, 8.4.B.7, 8.4.B.13 and 8.5.2–8.5.4.
  From: Samuels M, Wieteska S (eds) *Advanced Paediatric Life Support: the practical approach*, Fifth Edition. Manchester: Advanced Life Support Group. © 2005 Blackwell Publishing Ltd.*
- **World Health Organization** for Figures 1.2.1, 1.13.8, 2.3.7, 2.3.8, 2.3.13, 2.3.15, 2.5.D.ii.2, 2.5.D.ii.3, 2.5.D.iv.13–2.5.D.iv.16, 2.5.F.4–2.5.F.6, 2.5.F.11, 2.5.F.12, 2.5.G.1, 2.5.G.2, 2.6.E.8, 2.13.7, 2.13.8, 2.13.11, 2.13.17–2.13.25, 2.13.27, 2.13.38–2.13.40, 6.1.L.1, 8.1.1, 8.1.2, 8.4.B1–8.4.B6, 8.3.A.1–8.3.A.3, 8.5.5, 8.5.6, 8.6.4–8.6.11, 9.10 and 9.11.
  From:
  - *WHO Guidelines on Hand Hygiene in Health Care*
  - *Managing Complications in Pregnancy and Childbirth: a guide for midwives and doctors*
  - *WHO/UNICEF Child Growth Standards (2009) and the identification of severe acute malnutrition in infants and children under 5 years of age*
  - *UNICEF/WHO Progress Towards Global Immunization Goals – 2012 – Summary presentation of key indicators – Updated July 2013*
- **BMJ Group** for Figures 2.10.1–2.10.5, 7.6.8
  - Simpson J, Robinson K, Creighton SM, Hodes D. Female genital mutilation: the role of health professionals in prevention, assessment and management. *BMJ*. 2012; **344**: e1361.
  - Hobbs CJ, Wynne JM. The sexually abused battered child. *Arch Dis Child*. 1990; **65**(4): 423–7.
- **Maurice King Knowledge Engineer**, use of copyright-free material in King M, Mola G *et al.* (2012) *Primary Mother Care and Population* for Figures 2.1.2, 2.1.2, 2.3.1–2.3.6, 2.3.9, 2.3.10, 2.3.12–2.3.14, 2.3.16, 2.3.17, 2.3.19–2.3.21, 2.3.24, 2.5.D.i.1, 2.5.D.iv.2–2.5.D.iv.4, 2.5.D.iv.12, 2.5.E.1–2.5.E.3, 2.5.F.1–2.5.F.3, 2.5.F.8, 2.5.F.9, 2.5.F.18, 2.6.D.1–2.6.D.5, 2.6.E.1–2.6.E.3, 2.6.E.8, 2.6.E.10, 2.6.E.11, 2.6.G 1, 2.6.G.3, 2.7.A.1, 2.13.1, 2.13.4, 2.13.6, 2.13.8–2.13.10, 2.13.12, 2.13.13, 2.13.15, 2.13.17, 2.13.21, 2.13.26, 2.13.28–2.13.37
- Thanks also to Hesperian, *Disabled Village Children*, hesperian.org/books-and-resources, for Figures 4.2.D.1 and 4.2.E.1.

Disclaimers

1. The authors and editors have done all they can to ensure that drug doses and other facts in this book are accurate. While every effort has been made to ensure the accuracy of the information, as publishers we can give no guarantee on information about drug dosages or the applications of the drugs or procedures described in this textbook. In every individual case the user must check current indications and accuracy by consulting relevant pharmaceutical literature and following the guidelines laid down by manufacturers of specific medical devices. Users must also follow the guidelines of relevant authorities in the countries in which they are practising. The publishers cannot accept responsibility or legal liability for any errors in or misuse of material in this textbook.

2. The Advanced Life Support Group (ALSG) is very pleased to be a partner in this landmark text which presents up-to-date and practical information in an accessible form to clinicians working in low resource settings. ALSG clinicians have made a significant contribution to the textbook but the organisation must make it clear that their contribution has been confined to emergency topics as this is the organisation's field of experience and expertise in both high and low resource settings.

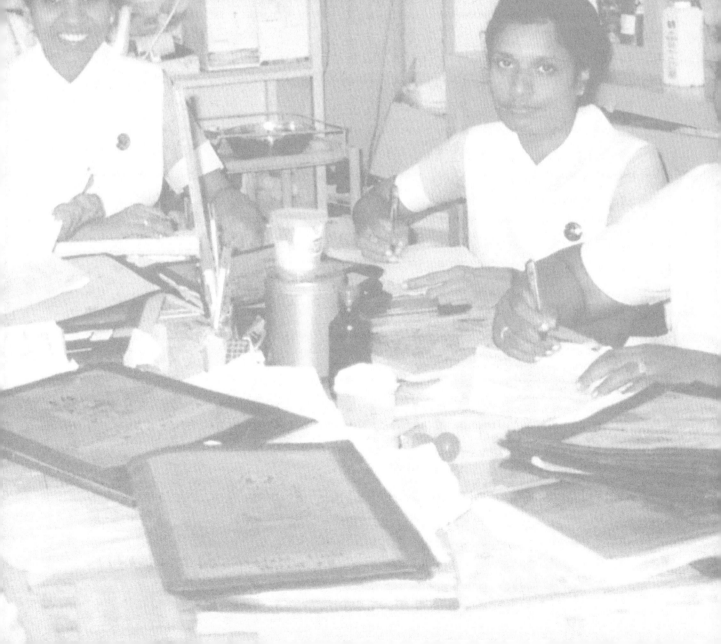

Section 1

General issues regarding hospital care

1.1 Hospital management: non-clinical support and facilities

Introduction

For effective delivery of healthcare, a secure financial strategy with robust financial and manpower controls, a properly maintained technical infrastructure, clear lines of accountability, and good management and communication lines all need to be in place. Ideally there should be clearly defined written personnel procedures, good training systems, and written policies and guidelines for all staff functions. The facilities and functions described in this section need to be in place, and are as important as the quality of medical care given. The services and facilities discussed in this text are basic, not comprehensive; well-resourced countries may have many additional ones. **If these services and facilities are in place, and are managed efficiently, supported and maintained, mainline healthcare delivery will be effective.**

Giving advice on generic hospital management is difficult, since the ability to deliver a minimum standard of care depends on the political, social and economic context in which the hospital is situated. Ideally there should be a named person responsible for each facility and service, in addition to an overall hospital manager or management team. The hospital manager or management team should have overall responsibility for finances, estates and facilities, human resources, direct clinical patient care and support services (laboratories, radiology, therapies, pharmacy, etc.), training for all staff and the administrative services necessary to support all of these activities. There should always be a head nurse, a head of support services and a senior doctor within the management team.

Staff management

Staff motivation and retention (human resource management) is an essential component of hospital management.

In order to provide good-quality essential health services to the people whom they serve, hospitals must put in place strategies and mechanisms to retain staff and help them to provide the best possible care for patients. The reasons for the healthcare worker crisis in hospitals in resource-limited countries include inadequate numbers of healthcare professionals, who are poorly distributed due to an unplanned 'brain drain' both regionally and internationally (attrition). According to the World Health Organization (2006), this phenomenon is caused by workers experiencing **low salaries, poor, unsafe work environments, a lack of defined career paths, and poor-quality education and training.**

Another most important issue is the support of every healthcare worker's family. Ministries of Health must not disrupt such vital bonds by moving staff away from their families, without their full and freely given agreement.

In the light of the above factors that face health services and compromise hospital-based care, managers must endeavour to motivate the limited human resources available to ensure retention.

A systematic review of six papers evaluating the management and leadership strategies that promote healthcare worker retention in resource-limited countries has identified a number of key lessons, which can be summarised as follows.

Payment of financial incentives to healthcare professionals

This particularly refers to professionals working in unpopular rural areas. Hospitals are run by boards which, as such, should be able to autonomously initiate better financial incentives for their staff. The above-mentioned review found that 86% of the studies showed payment of an attractive salary and allowances was a key motivational strategy for maintaining healthcare workers in their posts. Often what made most healthcare workers leave their jobs, particularly in the public health sector, was being unable to provide basic support for their families on the meagre salaries provided. According to a study conducted in South Africa, an increase in salary of healthcare workers has resulted in many health professionals who had previously left the public health sector, to work in private facilities, returning to the public sector.

Appreciation of healthcare workers

The community loyalty, personal commitment and willingness to make personal sacrifices that are shown by healthcare workers must be recognised and encouraged. This means that both the hospital management and the communities that they serve must demonstrate their appreciation of these attitudes.

Staff must be respected for and thanked for the work they do. Personal appraisal followed by periodic awards is a motivating factor for staff retention. The views of all staff should be listened to, and they must be involved in decision making to enable the best problem-solving approaches to be identified and implemented – it is their hospital and their community.

Orderlies, porters and cleaners are just as important in patient care as doctors and nurses, and this needs to be made clear to all staff. It can be helpful for doctors, nurses and hospital managers to participate and help the cleaners during, for example, the monthly deep cleaning of a ward.

An annual awards ceremony can be very helpful. For example, each department could be awarded certificates for:
- the most punctual member of staff
- the most improved member of staff
- the best dressed member of staff
- an award of excellence for the best all-round member of staff.

The awards could also include special categories, such as:
- the most long-serving member of staff (e.g. the refuse collector)
- an award for providing services above and beyond the 'call of duty'.

This allows awards to be made to staff who might not be in a position to further their education and to receive a certificate.

Receiving such recognition in front of management and invited guests who are prominent in the hospital's catchment area is a huge honour and boost to morale.

Training and supervision

Studies conducted on human resource management for health services in Africa indicate healthcare workers' frustration at having to be assigned to responsibilities and functions for which they have limited or no training. This can be effectively managed by providing 'on-the-job' support through the provision of simple and clear guidelines on clinical procedures. Although resources may be limited for specialised advanced training, priority should be given to locally conducted ongoing training that is cost-effective and sustainable, aimed at equipping healthcare staff with the knowledge necessary to provide efficient and good-quality patient care.

Providing a programme, space and encouragement for healthcare workers to take turns to train and update their peers (e.g. an internal continuing medical education programme) can also be a low-cost and effective way for healthcare workers to share new or updated practice, as well as to develop their own teaching skills.

Similarly, provision of basic information technology, computers and an Internet connection where possible is an important way of reducing professional isolation, helping healthcare workers to remain updated in their practice and to connect with the wider health community.

Some hospitals have benefited greatly by training the locally recruited nurse attendants (healthcare assistants) to second level (state-enrolled nurses) at the local nurse training school. Such nurses are usually born locally and their families live nearby, which often ties them to continuing to serve the community in which they live. In one site that has used this approach, the hospital has been able to train over 30 nurse attendants to the second level.

The introduction of an on-call support service to nurses working out of hours can be valuable. Senior nursing staff who are knowledgeable and experienced have volunteered to help with difficult health or social problems that arise. This provides a link between management and the nursing and clinical staff, facilitating resource mobilisation and ensuring that staff are on duty at the right time and filling gaps where necessary. Many social problems for both staff and patients can be heard and addressed appropriately.

Similarly, it is important to have a suggestions box that allows any member of staff to air their views anonymously if they wish to do so.

Provision of essential equipment and supplies

The lack of or inadequate provision of medical supplies, drugs and equipment in hospitals is one of the most difficult situations that healthcare workers have to cope with. Research has shown the demotivating situation that healthcare workers face when trying to treat patients without the necessary drugs and equipment. The provision of adequate and regular medical supplies, drugs and equipment is part of the answer to the ongoing question of how health systems in developing countries can best retain their health workforces. Such provision should be a management priority.

Provision of social and family amenities

Provision of basic facilities such as housing and good accommodation for healthcare staff is found to have contributed immensely to retention in many parts of the resource-limited countries where such projects have been implemented as part of a retention package.

For example, this is evident in Bansang Hospital, Gambia, West Africa, where staff retention for the past 5 years has been well recognised by authorities. Healthcare workers in Bansang Hospital are given fully furnished accommodation with water and electricity at no cost to the staff. This helps staff to increase their savings and thus boost their income, as they do not have to pay rent or utility bills. This initiative has not only enabled the hospital to retain its staff, but has also served to attract other healthcare workers to come and work there.

A particular challenge for recruiting and retaining experienced healthcare professionals in remote regions is the provision of education for their children, particularly at secondary level. Arrangements for children to be educated and looked after elsewhere are offered in some countries, but this remains a barrier to retention.

Nutrition is an important aspect of medical care for inpatients, particularly those whose relatives cannot provide the nutritious or special diets required. Encouraging all staff to grow their own vegetables and fruit for both patients and staff gives staff a sense of belonging, and extends their care for patients. In Bansang Hospital, Gambia, staff have for the past 3 years formed their own 'Charitable Farming Association'. They pay to become a member, and in return for this they can sustain the feeding of the patients with couscous and beans. Farming activities are to increase in 2014, as the hospital has been given 20 hectares of land, and will now grow rice.

A social centre for staff (with a television, sports facilities, etc.), particularly those who are not living close to or with their families, can be very helpful.

In conclusion, financial incentives can contribute to retention, but other non-financial incentives are equally likely to lead to sustainable retention. Given the economic situation in most resource-limited countries, the wages paid to healthcare workers in prosperous economies might not be realistic in low-income countries. However, the implementation of cost-effective human resource strategies is a more realisable step forward.

Furthermore, the implementation of one strategy at the expense of others is unlikely to result in the long-term aim of achieving healthcare worker retention. Therefore there is a need to adopt both financial and non-financial strategies to retain healthcare staff. Strategies might differ between low-income countries, due to socio-cultural and economic differences.

Essential services and facilities
Hospital security and access

The security and accessibility of the hospital are of paramount importance, especially given the relative lack of police resources in many resource-limited countries. There is also a need for governmental and international agencies to ensure that hospitals are protected and do not become targeted during armed conflict.

At the local level, the hospital should have a perimeter fence with secure entrances where all persons attending have to demonstrate a legitimate reason for entry. No weapons should be allowed into the hospital, and in some countries it may be necessary to have a metal detector to screen all visitors.

A well-organised car parking system is required, with strictly policed access areas for emergency vehicles and for parents or relatives bringing very sick patients to and from the hospital.

Safety and cleanliness
There should be clear written evacuation and fire policies, together with appropriate equipment (e.g. fire extinguishers). The perimeter fence should be of a construction that will keep out animals.

Communication systems
Good communication systems for staff, visitors and patients are essential. Ideally both outside and internal telephone systems should be available. If telephone systems are not feasible, alternative effective reliable systems of communication should be used. A hospital paging system for doctors, senior nurses and managers aids communication in emergency situations.

Internet access is invaluable for information sharing and education, both within a country and globally. Provision can be sought via governmental or non-governmental donor sources. A nominated person with overall responsibility for hospital computer systems predisposes to a cohesive service both internally and externally, avoiding duplication and ensuring appropriate usage.

Effective communication between groups of staff improves the effectiveness and efficiency of care. Regular meetings should discuss individual patients, debrief following deaths and clinical incidents, and audit specific aspects of clinical and unit management, such as infection control. The outcome of audit, particularly any changes in practice, needs to be available to those staff it affects, but such meetings should be educational and not used for apportioning blame.

Utilities
Water and sanitation
Hygiene within the hospital is paramount, and is dependent on a constant and high-quality water supply and adequate sanitation and washing facilities (i.e. bathrooms, showers, toilets and accessible sinks with an effective, functioning drainage system), all of which are vital if hospital-related infection (see Section 1.2) is to be minimised.

Electricity
An electricity supply within the hospital, which functions independently of any power losses to the rest of the area, is mandatory. Therefore a generator of sufficient power should be an essential item of equipment (the generator size is calculated from bed dependency and operating theatre requirements). In resource-limited countries where an erratic power supply is common due to high fuel costs, solar back-ups are needed for hospitals to function efficiently and effectively. There should be special emergency circuits. Power-cut simulations should be carried out regularly to test the system.

Heating and ventilation
Ideally there should be a functioning central heating system within the hospital. For this to work, there will also need to be a continuous water supply. If either of these cannot be ensured, electric heaters should be installed in all areas where there are patients.

In hot weather, there should be sufficient windows (that can be opened) to allow a comfortable temperature to be maintained during the hottest part of the day. An air-conditioning system or fans, either electric or manual (to be operated by relatives), should be available in areas of the hospital that become particularly hot, and for patients who must be kept cool (e.g. children with high fevers or head injuries).

Laundry service
Bedding and other items must be frequently washed. Therefore the hospital must have a staffed laundry service, ideally with a sufficient number of industrial washing machines and drying facilities. Where hand washing is the only option, staff should wear protective clothing and high-quality thick gloves. Clean bedding, towels and nappies must be available. A small supply of nightwear and other clothing may be needed on the wards for families who do not have a change of clothes with them.

Cleaning services
Patients who are being cared for in hospital are particularly vulnerable to nosocomial (hospital-acquired) infection (see Section 1.2). To reduce this risk, sufficient staff should be employed on a rota over the 24-hour period to keep all areas of the hospital and grounds clean at all times. Written cleaning policies and training for cleaners should be in place, and a supply of appropriate cleaning materials and disinfectants readily available.

Clean hospital grounds, pathways and entrances reduce the risk of dirt being transmitted to the ward and other patient areas by staff, relatives and other visitors. Stray animals must be kept away from the hospital premises.

Vermin must be kept away from the hospital buildings. Professional advice must be sought as soon as any signs of vermin are found.

Toilets, bathrooms and other facilities needed for personal hygiene and for equipment cleaning are of particular importance, and these areas should always be kept scrupulously clean.

Certain areas, such as operating theatres, as well as certain items of equipment, must always be aseptic (see Section 1.5). Ideally there should be a central sterilising service. If this is not possible there should be suitable sterilisers and a supply of appropriate disinfectants at a range of dilutions. Wherever possible the manufacturers' instructions for specific items of equipment should be followed.

Waste disposal system
A powerful incinerator that operates 24 hours a day is essential for the safe disposal of clinical waste. A system for handling and disposal of all clinical and non-clinical waste, including 'sharps', is also needed. Written policies for various types of waste disposal, and appropriate training, should be available to all staff.

Facility and utility maintenance services

Buildings, utilities and equipment

It is essential for these to be maintained to as high a standard as possible. Suitably trained engineers, builders and other maintenance staff are necessary. **There is no point in having expensive medical and surgical equipment if it cannot be maintained or used.** A sufficient number of trained bioengineers are therefore essential. All equipment that is used in the hospital should be robust, compatible if at all possible, suitable for the conditions and level of expertise available, and, when new, should be purchased with accompanying staff training and servicing arrangements.

Porters

For the functional relationships between different departments (e.g. the movement of patients to and from the operating theatres), a well-organised, trained and sympathetic team of porters is essential.

Caterers

Hospital food must be prepared under scrupulously hygienic conditions, and by staff who do not have gastroenteritis or superficial skin infections. Ideally, nutritious food should be provided free of charge. Special diets for malnourished children should be available (see Section 5.10.B).

Administrative support

Rather than diverting away the skills of a trained nurse, dedicated reception and other administrative support staff need to be employed to aid facility managers and other non-clinical and clinical staff. There must be a staffed system for storing and processing medical and nursing records. There should be strict rules about who has access to these records, where they are stored and for how many years they are kept.

Human resource issues

Hiring and dismissing staff

There should be transparent procedures for advertising for, interviewing and employing staff. These must include non-discriminatory policies, in particular with regard to gender, age, and ethnic and religious status.

Employment and financial issues

It is essential that the medical and nursing professions in all countries are highly regarded and respected, so it is important that the salaries for doctors and nurses in the national health services reflect this. If not, the staff may have to undertake other jobs during the day, and will not feel valued for their work. A lack of funding for salaries also increases the risk of corrupt practices, with some doctors taking supplies and equipment from their hospital to use in private clinics, thus depriving the poorest and most needy in the community.

Individual job descriptions and responsibilities should be agreed between healthcare professionals, their professional organisations and hospital management.

Arbitrary and compulsory transfer of staff from one place to another, at short notice and without consultation, is damaging both to morale and to the effectiveness of health services, and should be avoided.

There should be systems for ensuring the regular and secure recording of the time spent at work and the appropriate payment arrangements based on the contracted number of hours worked (part- or full-time). On-call emergency work and its payment should also be part of the contract.

There should be a professional registration system for each country, which ensures a basic level of training, as well as a system that validates experience and ability at specific intervals after initial registration.

Concern about individual performance should be addressed by a senior staff member on a one-to-one basis. Written guidelines should be used in a transparent way. Sometimes a period of supervised practice or retraining is appropriate.

Training and continuing staff education (see also Section 1.3)

Induction training concerning hospital policies should be mandatory for all staff.

Governments in well-resourced countries could encourage a support system of education for those working in less well-resourced regions.

New teaching techniques, such as skill- and scenario-based teaching (e.g. EMNCH courses) (see Section 1.3), should be introduced.

Professional registration requirements for healthcare workers

These will vary from one country to another. However, some form of governmental registration is essential. There should also be procedures governing the employment of expatriate staff in the health service.

Vetting of healthcare workers

All staff who are working with patients, whether they are local or from abroad, should be checked to ensure that they are suitably trained and have not been involved in the abuse of children. This is also important with regard to expatriate staff.

Staff health (see also Section 1.17)

There needs to be a system to advise the hospital management about staff health problems that may affect patient care. Staff with health-related problems that are affecting their performance need access to a supportive **occupational healthcare system**. There should be systems in place to protect patients from staff who are ill. This is a difficult but extremely important issue, particularly with regard to illnesses such as TB, HIV and hepatitis. Sometimes other support is necessary so that a healthcare worker's performance can be restored in the interests of all.

Needlestick injury

Although the risk of infection is very small, a policy should be in place to deal with this issue urgently, especially in hospitals where there are many patients with HIV infection and hepatitis.

Needlestick injuries are the commonest type of sharps injury, although other contaminated sharp instruments may also cause injuries. All healthcare workers must be educated about the potential exposure that can occur during their duties, and should have appropriate vaccinations. The risk of hepatitis B, hepatitis C and HIV infection should be assessed and appropriate immunisation or chemoprophylactic steps taken after an incident. Immediate treatment of such injuries should encourage washing thoroughly with running water and an antiseptic solution. Consult the infection control team for further advice, and follow their basic protocol. An incident-reporting system should be in place. This should not be seen as punitive; active support by managers should encourage prompt and accurate reporting.

Exposure to human immunodeficiency virus (HIV)

The route of transmission of HIV is from person to person via sexual contact, sharing of needles contaminated with HIV, infusions that are contaminated with HIV, or transplantation of organs or tissues that are infected with HIV. The risk of a healthcare worker acquiring HIV after a needlestick or other 'sharps' injury is less than 0.5%. Risk reduction must be undertaken for all bloodborne pathogens, including adherence to standard precautions using personal protective equipment, appropriate safety devices, and a needle disposal system to limit sharps exposure. Training for healthcare workers in safe sharps practice should be ongoing.

Information on preventive measures must be provided to all staff who may potentially be exposed to blood and blood products. Policies that are in line with the local and national guidelines must include screening of patients, disposal of sharps and wastes, use of protective clothing, management of inoculation accidents, and sterilisation and disinfection procedures. Hospital policy must include measures to obtain serological testing of source patients promptly where necessary, usually with the patient's informed consent. Post-exposure prophylaxis should be started as per local or national guidelines.

A suggested strategy for use when a healthcare worker has been potentially exposed to HIV

1 Discuss with the patient (or in the case of a child, the family) what has happened, and ask whether the patient's HIV status is known. If it is not, discuss the possibility of testing, if the injury occurred during normal working hours. Remember that anyone undergoing an HIV test has the right to counselling. If the injury occurred out of hours, or the family decline testing, proceed to Step 3.

2 If the patient has negative HIV ELISA and is over 18 months of age, infection is extremely unlikely. If they are under 18 months of age, a positive ELISA may reflect maternal antibodies. However, any positive test result should lead to Step 3. If the result is negative, the healthcare worker is not at risk of HIV infection. However, further testing of both the child and the healthcare worker for hepatitis B and C may be warranted.

3 Arrange a baseline HIV ELISA for the healthcare worker after appropriate counselling. If the result is positive, they will need to discuss further treatment with their own doctor.

4 If the healthcare worker's baseline serology is negative and the patient is HIV positive, antiretroviral prophylaxis should be started urgently. Current recommendations advise 1 month of treatment. The healthcare worker will need a repeat ELISA after 3 to 6 months to check their status.

Exposure to hepatitis B virus

The route of transmission of hepatitis B virus is through body fluids such as blood, saliva, cerebrospinal fluid, peritoneal, pleural, pericardial and synovial fluid, amniotic fluid, semen,

vaginal secretions and any other body fluid containing blood, **and also through blood products**. It is important to follow standard precautions, but immunisation is the best way of preventing transmission to healthcare staff. All healthcare workers who are in contact with patients or body fluids must be vaccinated against hepatitis B.

Staff who are infected with bloodborne pathogens may transmit these infections to patients, and therefore require careful evaluation with regard to their duties. This status should not be used to discriminate against them.

Exposure to hepatitis C virus

The route of infection is mainly parenteral. Sexual transmission does occur, but is far less frequent. No post-exposure therapy is available for hepatitis C, but seroconversion (if any) must be documented. As for hepatitis B viral infection, the source person must be tested for hepatitis C virus infection. For any occupational exposure to bloodborne pathogens, counselling and appropriate clinical and serological follow-up must be provided.

Confidentiality

Systems need to be in place to ensure that patient' records and the personal files of employed staff are kept confidential.

Other services for patients and their relatives

Health information should be available (see the Maternal and Child Healthcare Initiative (MCHI) manual).

Toilets should be available for visitors, as well as facilities for those visitors with a disability. If possible, telephones should also be available for visitors.

Ideally there should be written policies concerning the rights and responsibilities of patients, resident parents/carers and visitors. These policies should be prominently displayed around the hospital, and should include issues such as the prevention of smoking, the effects of alcohol, violence (verbal and physical) and weapons in the hospital. Smoking is particularly important in relation to children's health, but in the case of stressed parents it may be inappropriate to ban it altogether. Instead it should be limited to defined areas.

Family-centred care

The role of families in caring for patients alongside and in partnership with professional staff is vital, but must be handled extremely carefully. Families must not be exploited, but equally in resource-limited countries hospital care would not be possible without their assistance. Good understanding of roles and effective communication are of paramount importance (see also Section 1.20 and the MCHI manual).

Play, sensory stimulation and support for children's wards

The importance of play and developmental support cannot be overemphasised. A friendly and stimulating environment helps the child to understand and cope with their hospitalisation and to get better far more quickly (as advocated in the World Health Organization recommendations for the recovery management of children with malnutrition). It also helps to support the parents, and can provide them with additional skills that they can continue to use at home once the patient has been discharged. Many mothers cannot afford to stay at the hospital for long periods because there is strong pressure to return to their village, where they are pivotal to the daily routine, farming, etc. Mothers can be supported by passing on the knowledge of play as taught by a play worker. Giving the sick child access to play and information facilities in hospital also helps to reduce loneliness and fear.

Some well-resourced countries have training programmes and qualifications for play specialists. These are not available in most low-income countries. However, much can be achieved by recruiting suitable people to support therapeutic, informational and recreational play with children in hospital. It is effective, as both an adjunct and core part of treatment, in the hands of a skilled play worker, and any resources can be made of local and low-cost materials.

Play workers need to have good communication and empathy skills with children and families. They also need to have a good understanding of child development and the particular needs of children in hospital (especially children who are alone and/or who have disabilities or other additional needs). In addition, play workers need to be trained in how to deal with some specific situations, such as the comatose child (the fact that these children can hear and have feelings when touched, and how to encourage the parents to talk and play with the child).

Conclusion

The provision, organisation and financing of these services, facilities and functions, and the management of the human resources needed to service them, are as important as those needed to provide the clinical and clinical support services. A sound hospital infrastructure and management are of paramount importance for the provision of good-quality care.

Further information on other work-related issues concerning healthcare staff can be found in Sections 1.17 and 1.20.

1.2 Prevention of hospital-acquired infection

Introduction

Nosocomial or hospital-acquired infection is a major problem not only in terms of cost but also, more importantly, because it increases morbidity and mortality in patients. Such infections may affect up to 10% of all patients. Nosocomial infection requires a source of microorganisms and a chain of transmission. It is essential that all healthcare staff scrutinise their own practice to ensure that they are not part of this chain of transmission.

Please see the *Maternal and Child Healthcare Initiative Manual* **for more information on standards of care relating to the prevention of hospital-acquired infection (http://media.wix.com/ugd/dd2ba4_ef4f40edd 7a8993a8621a2caea7e4338.pdf).**

The combination of use of powerful antibiotics and poor hygiene also predisposes to the development of antibiotic-resistant microorganisms, which are difficult both to eradicate from the environment and to treat.

Pregnant women and girls, as well as children with chronic and debilitating illness, are particularly at risk of infection. However, not all infections are related to their particular disease process, but rather they may be caused by failure of both hospital management and individual healthcare workers to introduce and adhere to strict infection control policies.

Every research study relating to the prevention of infection and cross-infection in hospitals during the last 100 years has emphasised the importance of hygienic conditions **in the entire hospital**.

Requirements and procedures

The following measures are essential in order to minimise the risks of infection and cross-infection.

A clean and adequate water supply

Just as water and sanitation are of central importance in the prevention of cross-infection in emergency refugee camps, they are also of vital importance in hospitals, particularly where there are vulnerable patients. Running water (both hot and cold) is preferable. Hot water should be stored at 65°C, distributed at 60°C, and the temperature then reduced to 43°C to be used from the taps. This process helps to ensure that water-borne infections such as Legionnaire's disease are not passed on to staff or patients.

Accessible sinks in all areas

These should preferably be equipped with elbow-operated taps, and there should be **adequate washing and toilet facilities for staff and patients**.

Effective cleaning policies

The whole of the hospital, including the grounds, should be kept clean. Entrances should screen visitors' shoes for dirt, and corridors need to be cleaned at least twice a day with a disinfectant (see below). **Ward areas, floors, window-sills, light fittings and curtains need to be kept scrupulously clean, but the priority is the adequacy and cleanliness of the toilets and bathrooms.** These should be kept scrupulously hygienic by frequent cleaning and disinfection. **Staff appointed as cleaners should be given adequate status and salaries to reflect the importance of the work they are doing, as well as training in how to keep the hospital clean and why this is so important.**

Effective services for disposal of human and other waste

Human and other waste should be disposed of and collected separately. Foot-operated bins are preferable, and frequent rubbish collections are essential. Ideally the hospital should have its own incinerator.

Laundry service

All bedding, towels, flannels and curtains must be regularly washed with a detergent and disinfectant. Industrial washing machines are essential.

Strict hand-washing policies

Viruses and bacteria can survive on the hands for 2 to 3 hours. **Correct hand-washing technique for all staff, visitors and patients is the most important factor in the prevention of cross-infection.** It is easily taught, and frequently an improvement in practice is demonstrated in the short term. However, when examined over a longer period of time, old habits and short cuts reappear.

Good hand-washing techniques are dependent on adequate supplies of clean water, ideally elbow-operated taps, a liquid soap supply and an effective method of hand drying (*see* Figure 1.2.1). Where it is impossible to provide liquid soap and paper towels, some ingenious solutions have been attempted. Bar soap suspended in a net bag over the sink area and individual cloth towels for each patient, changed every 24 hours or at the discharge of the patient and kept within their bed space, can be effective. Added emollient protects the hands from chafing. Antiseptics can be added to liquid soap to improve antimicrobial activity, and chlorhexidine is a cheap and effective antiseptic that is widely available throughout the world. However, there is no good evidence that this increases the effectiveness of hand washing substantially. Antiseptics should be used before invasive procedures and where there is heavy soiling with potentially contaminated body fluids or other human waste. Povidone iodine should be reserved for use as a surgical scrub.

When running water is not available or hand washing is difficult, a 70% alcohol gel is useful. This is a new but fairly expensive product that has a significant part to play in the prevention of introduction of cross-infection in high-risk areas. When rubbed on and allowed to dry, it is effective in disinfecting the hands. After initial conventional hand washing it can be used between each patient contact, but further hand washing is still recommended after every five to six rubs.

All of the above-mentioned items may be regarded as a considerable extra cost for a health service, but are cost saving when balanced against an increased length of hospital stay due to infection, the additional medications required and sometimes unnecessary deaths caused.

All staff should have a personal responsibility for hygiene, but every ward should also identify an individual (ideally a nurse with the support of a microbiologist, if available) to be responsible for the education of all staff in techniques that will prevent the spread of infection, particularly effective hand washing and drying. This education programme will need to be ongoing, as even in the best centres these programmes are only effective for relatively short periods of time. The organisation needs to support the identified staff member in reinforcing that all grades and members of staff have responsibility for their practice (especially doctors,

who should act as role models). In addition, it needs to become the norm for this identified staff member, no matter how junior they are, to be recognised as the expert in their unit, and anyone who is asked to carry out hand washing must immediately and unquestioningly comply with this request.

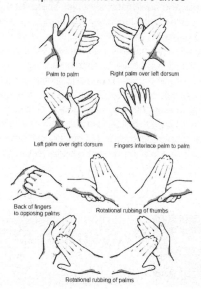

Repeat each movement 5 times

Palm to palm

Right palm over left dorsum

Left palm over right dorsum

Fingers interlace palm to palm

Back of fingers to opposing palms

Rotational rubbing of thumbs

Rotational rubbing of palms

FIGURE 1.2.1 Effective hand washing.

Disposal of body fluids

Each ward or unit must have an area set aside for this purpose. It and all the equipment that it contains must be kept scrupulously clean and body fluids disposed of quickly, with any spillage removed immediately. If there is likely to be a risk of body fluids being contaminated with life-threatening organisms, additional precautions should be taken. After hand washing, disposable clean gloves should be used by all staff and family members who will be assisting with the toileting of patients. Care must be taken with sharp objects such as hypodermic needles, in order to protect the patient, their family, other unit visitors and staff. An empathetic approach is necessary to ensure that the patient and their family do not feel stigmatised and undeserving of normal care and attention.

Cleaning, disinfection and sterilisation of equipment and furniture

The manufacturer's instructions for individual items of equipment must always be followed. These will usually clearly state which items need to be sterilised and where disinfection will be sufficient. They will also indicate appropriate dilutions for disinfectants. All equipment should be cleaned before being sterilised or disinfected.

Sterilisation

This is the complete elimination and destruction of all forms of microbial life. This is frequently achieved by steam under pressure, dry heat, gas or liquid chemicals. Such a sterilisation system must be available in every ward where invasive procedures are undertaken, and such systems are also required for instruments and towels used in the operating theatre.

Disinfection

This is a process that eliminates the majority of microorganisms, with the exception of the most resistant endospores. It is usually accomplished using liquid chemicals called disinfectants. Hypochlorites are inexpensive and effective disinfectants. They are active against most microorganisms, including HIV and hepatitis B. However, they do have a corrosive effect on metals, and if used on fabric or carpet can bleach out colours. Hypochlorites in a diluted form (usually 0.1% solution) for domestic use are contained in household cleaners available worldwide. These household cleaners can be used in the hospital environment for general cleaning, but stronger solutions (0.5% chlorine solution) must also be available, particularly for the disposal of body fluids, for initial cleaning of bloodstained instruments, and following outbreaks of notifiable infections. A 0.5–1% solution is recommended for the treatment of blood and body fluid spills, and 0.05–0.1% solution can be used for all surfaces. Hypochlorites are available as tablets, which makes the process of dilution easier.

How to prepare high-level disinfectant solutions

The best compound for the preparation of chlorine solutions for disinfection is household bleach (also known by other names such as Chlorox® and Eau de Javel). Household bleach is a solution of sodium hypochlorite which generally contains 5% (50 g/litre or 50 000 ppm) available chlorine.

Thick bleach solutions should never be used for disinfection purposes (other than in toilet bowls), as they contain potentially poisonous additives.

When preparing chlorine solutions for use, the following points should be noted:

- Chlorine solutions gradually lose strength, and freshly diluted solutions must therefore be prepared daily.
- Clear water should be used, because organic matter destroys chlorine.
- A 1:10 bleach solution (0.5%) is caustic. Avoid direct contact with the skin and eyes.
- Bleach solutions give off chlorine gas, so must be prepared in a well-ventilated area.
- Use plastic containers for mixing and storing bleach solutions, as metal containers are corroded rapidly and also affect the bleach.

Two different dilutions of bleach are used for disinfection.

1:10 bleach solution (containing 0.5% chlorine)

This is a strong disinfectant, which is used to disinfect the following:

- excreta
- bodies
- spills of blood or body fluids
- medical equipment (e.g. delivery sets, kidney dishes, suture instruments, catheters, speculum).

To prepare a 1:10 bleach solution, add one volume (e.g. 1 litre) of household bleach to nine volumes (e.g. 9 litres) of clean water.

Always wear gloves. Immediately after delivery or examination, clean the instruments below the level of solution in the plastic bucket using a brush. Leave for 10 minutes and then place them in soapy water, wash with a brush, and flush every catheter with a 10–20 mL syringe. Next rinse with clean water and air dry, and then sterilise or boil for 20–30 minutes. Store dry in a metal bowl.

Change the solution after 24 hours or when it becomes bloodstained.

Label buckets with tape indicating the date and time when the solution was prepared and when it needs to be changed.

0.5% solution is also used to prepare 1:100 bleach solution.

1:100 bleach solution (containing 0.05% chlorine)

This is used for the following:

- disinfecting surfaces
- disinfecting bedding
- disinfecting reusable protective clothing before it is laundered
- rinsing gloves between contact with different patients (if new gloves are not available)
- rinsing gloves, aprons and boots before leaving a patient's room
- disinfecting contaminated waste before disposal.

To prepare 1:100 bleach solution, add one volume (e.g. 1 litre) of 1:10 bleach solution to nine volumes (e.g. 9 litres) of clean water.

Note that 1:100 bleach solution can also be prepared directly from household bleach by adding 1 volume of household bleach to 99 volumes of clean water (e.g. 100 mL of bleach to 9.9 litres of clean water), but making it up from 1:10 bleach solution is easier.

Cleaning

This is often the most neglected of the three processes, and it must precede sterilisation and disinfection. When undertaken using a disinfectant detergent, cleaning alone will effectively reduce the number of microorganisms and make safe those items that come into contact with the intact skin (e.g. blood pressure cuffs, bed rails, intravenous poles).

Isolation of patients with specific infections

For isolation procedures to be effective they need to be instituted early. Two or more patients with the same infection can be isolated together. Different isolation techniques will be needed, and the use of gowns, gloves and masks will be necessary if the infection is very contagious and/or very serious. In some cases, nursing the patient in a cubicle or single room until medical tests are complete is all that is necessary. When there is a need for gowns, gloves and masks, these will require frequent changing or washing to ensure their efficacy, and must be used by everyone who comes into contact with the patient, including medical staff and carers. Ideally, they should be used only once and then removed and discarded or sent for laundering on leaving the isolation area. An area will need to be set aside for changing, with supplies of gowns, gloves, aprons and masks. Gowns made of cotton material will need to be worn with plastic aprons. Children's compliance with isolation techniques will improve if the element of fear is removed. This can be achieved by all medical staff allowing the child to see their face (through a window) before donning a mask. It is also essential that when children are in hospital, infection control policies do not interfere with the child's contacts with their parents.

Infection control measures following the death of a patient

When a patient dies, the amount of time that the parents

and other family members are able to spend with them will vary according to the facilities that are available. Rituals and beliefs concerning the death of an individual, and the management of the body, usually involve religious or cultural observance. There are many beliefs surrounding the distinction between physical and spiritual life, in particular the belief that something of the individual survives death, either to be reborn through reincarnation or to fulfil their spiritual destiny in the afterlife. It is important that the correct funerary procedures, if any, are followed in order to ensure that the bereaved are not distressed by any omission which they consider important.

All societies, whether religious or not, have to deal with the problem of the death of their patients and the bereavement of parents and other close family members. Like other transitions in an individual's life, death is usually marked by a rite of passage in which central values are restated and important social bonds re-emphasised. Precise customs vary in different religions and traditions, but common features include the washing and laying out of the corpse (which may be embalmed), and the wake, or watching over the dead body. These customs may need to be modified to prevent the spread of infection to other members of the community, or because of the need to perform post-mortem examinations to establish an exact cause of death. Effective hand-washing procedures remain of paramount importance.

In countries where the climate is characterised by extremes of temperature, refrigeration of dead bodies until they can be returned to the family is essential. Each hospital should have a mortuary building adjacent to, but separate from, the hospital. To prevent the spread of infection, staff working in the mortuary will need to be provided with separate clothing for use in that department. The use of two pairs of gloves, or thick rubber gloves and protective clothing, will be necessary for the post-mortem examination if there is suspected infection of the body with life-threatening bacteria or viruses.

The mortuary department will need to have facilities for families to see and spend time with their dead relative, and a separate comfortable area where documentation can be completed and any necessary interviews with local government officials can be conducted. The mortuary department not only provides facilities for post-mortem examination, but also, in large centres, it can be part of the government facilities for forensic post-mortems, which may provide additional resources for the hospital. Having these centres within a hospital may improve services for families, but care needs to be taken that there is a culture of openness that involves families in the consent procedures for all examinations performed after the patient's death.

Conclusion

Each member of the hospital has a role to play in the prevention of hospital-acquired infections. The greatest responsibility lies with the healthcare professionals, particularly nurses and doctors, who in the hospital setting are in contact with patients and their families 24 hours a day, and because of this are the main perpetrators of cross-infection. However, they can also demonstrate good practice by, for example, being the catalysts for change, and improving the education of other hospital staff and families.

Further reading

Alvarado CJ (1999) Sterilization vs disinfection vs clean. *Nursing Clinics of North America*, **34**, 483–91.

Purssell E (1996) Preventing nosocomial infection in paediatric wards. *Journal of Advanced Nursing*, **5**, 313–18.

Wilson J (1995) *Infection Control in Clinical Practice*. London: Bailliere Tindall.

Yost AJ and Serkey JM (1999) Rule-makers who establish infection control standards. *Nursing Clinics of North America*, **34**, 527–53.

World Health Organization (2002) *Prevention of Hospital-Acquired Infections: a practical guide*, 2nd edition. www.who.int/csr/resources/publications/whocdscsreph200212.pdf

World Health Organization (2009) *WHO Guidelines on Hand Hygiene in Health Care. First global patient safety challenge: clean care is safer care*. http://whqlibdoc.who.int/publications/2009/9789241597906_eng.pdf

World Health Organization (2010) *Guide to Local Production: WHO-recommended Handrub Formulations*. www.who.int/gpsc/5may/Guide_to_Local_Production.pdf

1.3　Continuing medical education for healthcare professionals

Continuing medical education takes many forms, including the following:
- on-the-wards training
- short courses on the management of emergencies
- use of a readily available pocketbook
- the availability of a postgraduate education centre with library and Internet facilities
- departmental meetings
- online websites and organisations
- local (Ministry of Health) guidelines and publications
- courses and conferences
- Internet-based membership organisations (e.g. HIFA 2015 and CHILD 2015).

Every healthcare professional needs to engage in continuing medical education in order to keep up with the pace of change. They may be a long way away from a university. They may have no library within reach. They may not be sent any journals to read. They may not be able to go away for further education. In resource-limited countries they may not be able to afford a computer or Internet access, or to print out the myriad of teaching materials available on the web.

On-the-wards training

This is probably the most effective way of keeping frontline staff up to date, especially with regard to the management of emergencies such as eclampsia or the newborn infant who does not breathe at birth. For these mini-teaching sessions, as little as 1 to 2 hours a week can be very effective, and ideally a senior staff member who has been trained in medical education (e.g. through the Generic Instructor Course of the Advanced Life Support Group, ALSG) should lead. Manikins (e.g. of the newborn infant), in which the lungs expand only when the airway is positioned correctly and the face mask is properly applied, can be helpful. It can also be useful to include refreshments and to make the teaching sessions friendly and socially supportive so that staff look forward to them and are keen to participate and learn.

Short courses on the management of emergencies

The ALSG in collaboration with Maternal and Childhealth Advocacy International (MCAI) has designed and made available for low-income countries 3- to 5-day courses in the emergency management of obstetric, neonatal and paediatric emergencies (see www.alsg.org and www.mcai.org.uk). These courses, which are certified, consist of a combination of lectures, workshops, skill stations and clinical scenarios, undertaken by volunteer instructors who have been through a Generic Instructor Course (GIC) on medical education, and who are skilled in the clinical components of the course.

Pocketbook

A pocketbook that is available at all times is one of the best ways of accessing up-to-date evidence-based information, and is particularly valuable for the management of emergencies when there is no time to go and look for a textbook.

The new edition of the WHO *Pocket Book of Hospital Care for Children* (www.who.int/maternal_child_adolescent/documents/child_hospital_care/en/index.html) is a valuable adjunct to the ward care of sick children in low-resource situations. A useful supplement to this pocketbook is the 2012 WHO publication 'Recommendations for management of common childhood conditions: Newborn conditions, dysentery, pneumonia, oxygen use and delivery, common causes of fever, severe acute malnutrition and supportive care' (http://whqlibdoc.who.int/publications/2012/9789241502825_eng.pdf).

Postgraduate education centre with library and Internet facilities

A postgraduate medical education centre that can be accessed by all healthcare staff is a good way of providing continuing medical education support. This education centre could, at the very minimum, consist of a reasonably sized, comfortable room containing a library and if possible at least one computer. This could function as the area where regular departmental meetings are held. All non-governmental organisations (NGOs) are concerned with sustainable development, and most of them regard education as a priority that requires major investment. If you are unable to obtain funding from your health service, cultivate a relationship with an NGO or similar organisation, and try to gain investment from them or other sources.

- The library should contain the basic textbooks, in editions that are as up to date as possible.

- If possible, subscriptions for the major obstetric and paediatric journals should be obtained or accessed online.
- It may be that none of the standard textbooks are published in your language. English is the major international scientific language, so it seems reasonable to focus on English language texts.
- If your centre has an electricity supply, if you are able to obtain a computer with CD-ROM, and if it is possible to install a telephone line or mobile Internet sticks are available, this will allow you to communicate by email with specialists in other countries, and to access the Internet in order to obtain up-to-date information on diseases and their treatment. The organisation Teaching-aids At Low Cost (TALC) (www.talcuk.org) is useful in this regard. Computers are now being designed solely for Internet use, and these are less expensive than the standard personal computer (PC). This investment, for the price of perhaps six good books, can make available a vast amount of up-to-date information. In most countries a subscription is required for access to the Internet, and there will be telephone line usage charges, for which funding will be needed. Again, English is likely to be the language of choice for your global communication.
- Security may be a problem. The postgraduate education centre will need to be designed with this in mind, so that books and computers are not stolen.

Departmental meetings

Many departments will need to hold regular meetings. Cases can be presented and discussed, and a journal club can be organised. Morbidity and mortality audit meetings are very useful for identifying areas where practice can be improved by the team. However, it is very important that this kind of meeting is supportive, non-judgemental, and does not to assign blame. It is a good idea for each department to hold one of their weekly meetings in English.

Online websites and organisations

The Internet has many millions of pages. A number of websites are listed below, which will give you an introduction to online obstetric and paediatric information.

- **World Health Organization (www.who.int).** It is important to remember the WHO when working in low-resource settings. It is tempting to compare standards of care with those in the UK and other well-resourced countries. However, the WHO has produced numerous publications and guidelines on minimum standards of care and is a very valid resource.
- UNICEF: www.unicef.org
- UNFPA: www.unfpa.org

UNICEF and UNFPA, like the WHO, can be an invaluable resource.

- Paediatric Information Education Resource (PIER): http://pediatriceducation.org
- International Paediatric Association (IPA): www.ipa-world.org
- Hong Kong College of Paediatrics: www.paediatrician.org.hk
- American Academy of Pediatrics: www.aap.org/en-us/Pages/Default.aspx
- Canadian Paediatric Society: www.cps.ca/en
- Regional and General Paediatric Society (RGPS), Royal

Australasian College of Physicians: www.racp.edu.au/page/educational-and-professional-development
- British Paediatric Surveillance Unit: www.rcpch.ac.uk/what-we-do/bpsu/british-paediatric-surveillance-unit
- *Archives of Disease of Childhood* (journal): http://adc.bmj.com
- *Developmental Medicine and Child Neurology* (journal): www.cambridge.org
- *Ambulatory Child Health* (journal): http://onlinelibrary.wiley.com/journal/10.1111/(ISSN)1467-0658
- *Pediatrics* (journal): http://pediatrics.aappublications.org
- European Society for Paediatric Research: www.espr.info
- Neonatal and Paediatric Pharmacists Group (NPPG): www.networks.nhs.uk/nhs-networks/nppg-neonatal-and-paediatric-pharmacists-group
- Institute of Child Health of London: www.ich.ucl.ac.uk
- *British Medical Journal* (journal): www.bmj.com
- Systematic Review Training Unit: www.ucl.ac.uk/ich/homepage
- OMIM (genetics syndromes): www.ncbi.nlm.nih.gov/omim
- Bibliography of online texts: www.drsref.com.au/books.html
- Children's Hospital of Philadelphia: www.chop.edu
- Paediatric X-rays: http://radiologyeducations.com
- American Academy of Pediatrics: www.aap.org
- Facts for families: www.aacap.org/info_families/index.htm
- British Society of Paediatric Endocrinology: www.bsped.org.uk
- International Society for Paediatric and Adolescent Diabetes: www.ispad.org
- Johns Hopkins Program for International Education in Gynecology and Obstetrics (Jhpiego): www.jhpiego.org
- Videos on maternal and child healthcare for low-resource settings: www.glowm.com
- http://globalhealthmedia.org
- http://www.healthynewbornnetwork.org/multimedia/video/born-too-soon-kangaroo
- http://medicalaidfilms.org

Local (Ministry of Health) guidelines and publications

Some countries are beginning to develop professional bodies (e.g. paediatric societies, obstetric societies, groups for nurses and midwives). Some of these professional bodies are developing guidelines and have access to resources which will be useful.

In addition, some Ministries of Health are working with organisations such as the WHO, UNICEF, the Johns Hopkins Program for International Education in Gynecology and Obstetrics (Jhpiego) and Save the Children to develop programmes and guidelines to improve local healthcare. It is important for those working in low-resource countries to be aware of the activities of the relevant government.

Courses and conferences

These will differ from one country to another, and will be linked with the Ministry of Health and professional bodies.

Web-based membership organisations: HIFA 2015 and CHILD 2015

- HIFA 2015: www.hifa2015.org and https://dgroups.org/groups/child2015/
- CHILD 2015: www.hifa2015.org/child2015-forum

The goal of these organisations is that, by 2015, every person worldwide will have access to an informed healthcare provider.

HIFA 2015 is a campaign and knowledge network with more than 5000 members representing 2000 organisations in 167 countries worldwide. Members include healthcare workers, publishers, librarians, information technologists, researchers, social scientists, journalists, policy makers and others – all working together towards the HIFA 2015 goal.

HIFA 2015 contributes to the broader goal of the Global Health Workforce Alliance: 'All people everywhere will have access to a skilled, motivated and supported healthcare worker, within a robust health system.'

Members interact via two email discussion forums: HIFA2015 and CHILD2015. Together these organisations are building the HIFA2015 Knowledge Base, a picture of information needs and how to meet them. Membership is free and open to all.

1.4 Essential imaging facilities

Introduction

Despite the fact that the use of ionising radiation ('X-rays') for diagnostic purposes was discovered more than 100 years ago, up to two-thirds of the world's population still have no access to primary care diagnostic imaging services. Some rural clinics may be located in remote impoverished areas such that imaging equipment is impossible for the population to access. However, clinics in larger towns, and certainly **every institution that merits the title of 'hospital'** should have, at the very least, **simple radiographic and ultrasound equipment available**. This will necessitate the training of healthcare workers to use the equipment appropriately and safely. Local healthcare workers will also interpret most of the examinations performed, and therefore need training in radiographic interpretation. Many African countries, for example, do not have a single radiologist. As most radiographic equipment is now digital, in the absence of a specialist opinion, teleradiology services are an option in a few areas. Various teleradiology solutions exist in different regions and are expanding, but they are not widespread. For the under-resourced setting, charitable specialist opinions would need, of necessity, to be provided free of charge.

A basic service

In the context of severely limited resources, health planners have to be selective in their choice of imaging technology. Some radiographic equipment can be so expensive that its purchase might be to the detriment of other important components of a basic health service. The radiographic equipment should nevertheless reflect the standard of care in each clinic or hospital. Albeit suboptimal, very basic orthopaedics can be carried out utilising plain radiographs alone. Proper fracture reduction necessitates that a C-arm fluoroscopy unit should ideally be available. A CT scanner should be on site at a regional centre where there are surgeons available with basic neurosurgical skills (e.g. capable of making burr holes for extradural haematoma evacuation).

- The majority of radiographic studies in hospitals everywhere are plain radiographic examinations. In a small rural or suburban hospital, plain radiography will account for approximately 90% of all the necessary examinations and, where available, ultrasound will meet the needs of much of the remaining 10%.
- Good diagnostic imaging frequently leads to less hospitalisation, allows for quicker and more accurate diagnosis, and results in less suffering and pain. The WHO recommends that even small hospitals and clinics with only one doctor should have imaging equipment.
- Access to most of the equipment described below should be available to all sick and injured children.

Diagnostic radiographic equipment

- Radiographic equipment that is easy to operate and maintain, such as the World Health Imaging System for Radiography (WHIS-RAD). This is based on much practical experience, and is ideally suited to radiology departments in disadvantaged countries.
- WHIS-RAD was fully specified in 1995. A WHIS-RAD unit is easily applicable to children and small infants, is relatively inexpensive, is safe for patients and operators, and produces high-quality images.
- In recent years the cost of obtaining and processing X-ray film has become problematic, particularly in developing countries. Fortunately, WHIS-RAD is now available in digital format or retrofit. The use of computed radiography (CR) with reasonably priced liquid crystal display (LCD) monitors allows for easy data storage, archiving and retrieval, as well as the potential for utilising teleradiology resources.
- A CR plate has the added advantage of a large dynamic range such that repeat X-rays are seldom necessary.
- Radiation doses from a WHIS-RAD unit are typically lower than those from many conventional radiographic machines, which is particularly appealing where standards of radiation protection, the use of cones, lead protection and dosimetry may be variable and often non-existent.
- The X-ray generator specified for WHIS-RAD may be used with almost any power supply, however variable. WHIS-RAD batteries can operate for up to 3 weeks before they need to be recharged.

- Patients can be examined in a standing, sitting or recumbent position.
- The WHO has produced a range of radiology manuals for the developing world setting. The *WHO Manual of Diagnostic Imaging: Radiographic Techniques and Projections* provides a very clear explanation of how to use the equipment, even for those with no formal training in radiography. Operators can be trained in a matter of months. This and other useful information is available from the Diagnostic Imaging for Clinics and Small Hospitals website (www.dicsh.info).
- The proposed publication of the *WHO Manual of Diagnostic Imaging: Paediatric Examinations* has unfortunately been severely delayed.
- Donations of old but functional radiographic equipment by well-resourced countries, although laudable, are often worthless. Bulky outdated equipment often cannot be installed, operated or maintained locally. The service manuals are often missing, obtaining spare parts is a major problem, and many of these machines break down irreparably.
- Portable X-ray equipment typically requires reliable power sources and expert radiography, such that its use is only practicable in larger centres.

A comprehensive list of the indications for diagnostic radiography is too long to include here. Suffice it to say that all children with a serious pneumonia, suspected tuberculosis or fractured limbs, to name a few examples, merit radiography. In practice, chest and skeletal examinations are the most frequent indications for diagnostic imaging worldwide. Where resources are less stretched, radiographic machines with slit-beam technology could be considered. These units, such as the LODOX Statscan, are also fully digital, have sufficiently low radiation doses to permit their use within a ward without special protective barriers, and offer flexibility for those with little radiographic positioning skill. In addition, they provide rudimentary CT information which is useful for head trauma patients, at a fraction of the price of CT scanners.

Diagnostic ultrasound scanning equipment

The wide range of applications of ultrasound in children and pregnant women, its versatility and its safety probably make it better suited to disadvantaged countries than any other imaging modality. Sonography is harmless – it does not generate ionising radiation, and is thus particularly suitable for imaging children, adolescent girls in particular, and pregnant women.

- Ultrasound machines are simple to operate, but the images are also easy to misinterpret. It is therefore critically important that the person performing and interpreting an ultrasound study is suitably trained and competent. **Sonography must be taught on a supervised practical basis in a local environment.** The WHO recommends a 6-month minimum training period for diagnostic sonography.
- Initiatives such as that by Imaging the World (http://imagingtheworld.org) allow for alternative basic sonographic training to be shortened to as little as a few days. Reliance instead is placed on transmission of images over the Internet to a secure server, from which the images can be accessed and read anywhere in the world.

The WHO recommends minimum specifications for a general-purpose ultrasound scanner.

- The scanner should be able to operate from the local electrical power supply.
- Servicing should be available locally.
- It must be possible to store the unit safely under adverse conditions.
- When scanning children, at least two different MHz transducers (sector and linear array) are desirable.
- Doppler techniques are included on all modern ultrasound equipment, such that exclusion of a deep venous thrombosis, for example, should be possible.
- Some form of archived permanent hard-copy record is recommended for patient follow-up, and in the interests of teaching and training in general.

Additional points

- Mobile ultrasound scanners can be operated at the bedside or in the Emergency Department.
- Abdominal and pelvic ultrasound has a well-established role in the assessment of adolescent gynaecological conditions and paediatric emergencies.
- Sonography plays a major role in the management of pregnancy, from dating the age of the fetus to identifying multiple pregnancies, ascertaining the position of the placenta and generally identifying potential problems, thus allowing the clinician to plan safe delivery.
- Sonography can quite simply resolve mass lesions from organomegaly.
- It is noteworthy that hydronephrosis is the commonest abdominal mass in the neonate and infant, and this is easily diagnosed with ultrasound scanning.
- Evaluation and drainage of pleural effusions or ascites is relatively straightforward, particularly with ultrasound guidance.
- Ultrasound scanning can be a useful tool for guiding other interventions, such as drainage of larger abscesses or an image-guided biopsy of a solid mass.
- Alternatively, evaluation of solid mass lesions and cysts should at least be possible, to aid patient referral to larger regional centres.
- Sonography of the infant brain is easily performed at the bedside, and can provide useful information in the infant who is febrile, unconscious or has seizures.
- In trauma patients, abdominal ultrasound scanning can prevent unnecessary surgery.
- Finally, ultrasound studies frequently reduce the need for plain abdominal radiographs and yield more diagnostic information.

1.5 Essential operating-theatre resources

Design of the operating theatre (OT)

- Ideally it should be located next to the labour ward.
- It should be of adequate size (minimum 7 m × 7 m) for the placement of essential equipment and the unobstructed movement of staff.
- It should not be used for storing purposes, for which a separate side room should be available which can also be used for hand washing.

Essential equipment

- Ordinary OT table with a facility for the lithotomy position and lowering and raising the height of the table, preferably mechanically operated.
- A good focusing OT light is very important.
- A simple anaesthetic machine suitable for the resources available in the country (e.g. Diamedica-Glostavent, for resource-limited countries), with an uninterrupted oxygen and nitrous oxide supply, is the most essential item of equipment for the anaesthetist. Reserve cylinders for both oxygen and nitrous oxide should always be available. If nitrous oxide is not available, the patient can be maintained on ether or halothane, but the level of anaesthesia has to be deep, requiring more intensive post-operative monitoring.
- The suction machine (which should have both electrical and manual functions, in case of electrical failure) should be periodically emptied and cleaned with antiseptic solution after every individual patient. It must be constantly checked.
- A fumigation machine is essential for the sterilisation of the OT.
- Anaesthetic equipment and supplies (see Section 1.22 for a list of essentials).
- All emergency drugs (e.g. lignocaine, adrenaline, atropine, sodium bicarbonate, 25% dextrose, morphine, etc.), with syringes, should be readily available in the OT (see Section 1.22).
- A boiler is essential for sterilisation if an autoclaving facility is not available. A heater of some kind is also essential for warming up crystalloid infusions to be used during surgery to prevent hypothermia.
- Monitoring equipment (see Section 1.22 for a list of essentials).
- Room heaters are essential, especially for surgery on infants. The OT temperature should be in the range 28–32°C to prevent hypothermia in babies. Hot-water bottles can provide heat for infants and are inexpensive, but it is essential to be vigilant about safety. Radiant warmers, incubators and electric blankets are helpful if they are available. Equally, air conditioning is also required in hot countries to ensure appropriate working temperatures for patient and OT staff.
- A cautery machine is useful for reducing blood loss

during surgery. An ordinary unipolar cautery will suffice for most procedures. A probe that has been heated with a Bunsen burner until it is red hot can provide thermocoagulation on touching the bleeding sites. This is a low-cost and effective method when a cautery machine is not available.

- Adequate supply of linen, towels, gowns and gloves.
- The minimum instruments required for minor surgery are as follows:

Artery forceps:
Mosquito	6
Kelly's	6

Towel clips:
Bulldog	6

Scissors:
Metzenbaum	1
Mayo's	1

Thumb forceps:
Tooth	1
Non-tooth	1

Intestinal clamps:
Non-crushing	2 (4)
Martin artery forceps	2
Right-angled forceps	1
Needle holders (paediatric) which can hold 3.5 to 5.0 sutures	2

Retractors:
Right-angled	2
Zerneys	2
Devers	2
Malleable	2
Suction tip	1
Eye goggles for protection of staff from splashing	3

Durbin (formally ECHO) (www.durbin.co.uk) provides complete instrument kits, which are particularly relevant for Caesarean section and laparotomy.

- A whiteboard and pens with which to document the use of swabs and needles, aiming to ensure that none are left in the patient when surgery ends.

Operating-theatre staff

Apart from the surgeon, an adequately trained doctor or nurse anaesthetist is essential.

- **Nursing staff** should be adequately trained in the care and handling of instruments and equipment in the OT. They should be made responsible for the proper functioning of all equipment, and trained in the sterilisation of the OT and the instruments used.
- **OT assistants** are important for transporting patients to and from the ward. They should be aware of the function of the equipment in the OT. They should also be counselled about the hazards of contact with blood and other patient body fluids, and especially made aware of the risks of infection with HIV and hepatitis B and C.
- **OT cleaners** should also be aware of the threat of these communicable diseases. It is essential to clean the OT between one case and the next to prevent nosocomial infections.

Practices and procedures to reduce the risk of infection in the OT

- The floors, walls, table and all equipment in the OT should be cleaned and disinfected at least once a day, and also after every case involving infection.
- Autoclaving is the standard method of sterilisation, but if it is not available, boiling for 1 hour should be used instead.
- Spirit flaming of all the instruments (whereby the instruments are placed in a kidney tray, spirit is poured into the tray and a matchstick is used to flame it) can be undertaken where minimal equipment is available.
- There must be restricted entry to the OT, and this should only be permitted after a complete change of clean clothes (except for underwear) and shoes, and with the wearing of a proper clean head covering and mask (these items should be used once only before discarding or washing). Hand and forearm washing for at least 5 minutes before gowning and gloving up, using an antiseptic soap solution, will reduce the incidence of infection.
- The OT should be situated in the most inaccessible part of the hospital so that there is minimum encroachment by the general hospital patients.
- Ideally there should be an air-purifying/air-conditioning system in the OT.
- All tubing (suction, oxygen, anaesthetic) should be regularly cleaned and disinfected according to the individual manufacturer's instructions, in order to reduce the risk of nosocomial infection.
- Proper waste disposal bins for clinical and non-clinical waste from the OT are essential.

Set-up of the recovery room

- The recovery room should be adjacent to the OT so that the surgeon and the anaesthetist have immediate access to the patient.
- Nursing care, oxygen, suction and emergency medicines should be available, as should resuscitation and monitoring equipment (*see* Sections 1.12 and 1.13).
- **An adequately trained doctor or nurse anaesthetist, who is proficient in resuscitative measures and critical care management, should be present whenever patients are in the recovery room.** Frequent evaluation and monitoring of surgical patients should be undertaken during the first 24 hours following a major operation. This should include observations/measurements of hydration, urine output, output from drains, soakage from the wound, pulse, respiratory rate and blood pressure. Post-operative pain management is most important, and a relatively 'pain-free' patient has a better outcome (*see* Section 1.15).

Further reading

Integrated Management for Emergency and Essential Surgical Care (IMEESC) toolkit: www.who.int/surgery/publications/imeesc/en/index.html

World Federation of Societies of Anaesthesiologists (WFSA) *Guide to Infrastructure, Supplies and Anesthesia Standards at Three Levels of Health Care Facility Infrastructure and Supplies*: www.ncbi.nlm.nih.gov/pmc/articles/PMC2957572/table/Tab1

Lifebox: www.lifebox.org

1.6 Drug and fluid administration

Enteral fluids

- The best method of maintaining caloric intake is through enteral feeding.
- If the patient is unable to drink then pass a gastric tube (see Section 8.5).

When commencing feed by naso- or orogastric tube:
1. Fill the syringe to the required amount with feed.
2. Draw the plunger back as far as possible.
3. Attach the syringe to the tube.
4. Kink the tube and remove the plunger.
5. Allow feed to pass into the stomach using gravity.
6. Observe the patient's colour and respiratory rate for any signs of aspiration.

- Breast milk is the best food for infants. It is always available at the correct temperature, no preparation is required, and no sterilising equipment is involved. If the infant is too ill to suck and is fed through a gastric tube, encourage the mother to express milk into a sterile receptacle.
   1. To encourage the release of milk and ease of expression, it may help if the mother expresses milk while holding the baby.
   2. Store excess milk in a in a refrigerator (<5°C) for up to 5 days or freezer (minus 20°C) for up to 6 months.
   3. Defrost the quantity needed for 4 hours of feeding at a time.
- Oral rehydration solutions are used in gastroenteritis to maintain electrolyte balance. Prepare by **adding 1 sachet to 210 mL (7 oz) of clean water**. (One ounce = 30 mL.)

Intravenous fluids

Intravenous (IV) fluids must only be used when essential and enteral feeds are not available or not absorbed. Always check the container before use, to ensure that the seal is not broken, the expiry date has not been passed, and the solution is clear and free of visible particles.

Choice of crystalloid fluid
Dextrose/gluose-only fluids

It is clear that although glucose or dextrose is necessary to prevent or manage hypoglycaemia, fluids containing only dextrose which are hypotonic should never be used for IV fluid replacement or maintenance, or for the emergency management of shock.

This is because the dextrose is rapidly metabolised, so the effect of a dextrose-only IV fluid on the child's body in shock may produce hyponatraemia, which could lead to brain damage or death. In addition, this solution is rapidly moved out of the circulation and into the cells, and the state of shock will not be resolved.

Sodium-containing fluids

The fluid traditionally infused into the circulation for the management of shock has been normal saline (0.9% NaCl). This fluid has increasingly been shown to be dangerous, especially in the sick patient. An infusion of normal saline causes a hyperchloraemic acidosis (a high chloride concentration leading to acidosis) which, in the shocked patient, who is already acidotic, causes a deterioration in the health of cells in vital organs even though perfusion of the cells has been improved by the increased circulating volume.

There are sodium-containing alternatives to normal saline which are safer because they approximate more closely to human serum/plasma in content (see Table 1.6.1), although they are slightly more expensive. We recommend the use of either of these alternatives – **Ringer-lactate and Hartmann's solution**, which are widely available – for all fluid replacement. Hospitals are advised to change their standard crystalloid from 0.9% ('normal') saline to Ringer-lactate or Hartmann's solution as soon as possible. Not all hospitals will have access to these solutions immediately, so there may sometimes be no alternative but to start fluid replacement with normal saline. However, if more than 20 mL/kg needs to be given, one of the safer alternatives should be used in very sick children if at all possible.

Putting dextrose into Ringer-lactate or Hartmann's solution

A crystalloid containing approximately 5% dextrose can be obtained by adding 50 mL of 50% dextrose to a 500-mL bag of Ringer-lactate or Hartmann's solution.

A crystalloid containing approximately 10% dextrose can be obtained by adding 100 mL of 50% dextrose to a 500-mL bag of Ringer-lactate or Hartmann's solution.

(It will therefore be necessary to remove 50–100 mL of fluid from the 500-mL bag first.)

Ensure that the above process is performed with a

TABLE 1.6.1 Comparison of electrolytes, osmolality and pH levels in IV fluids with those in human serum

Fluid	Na$^+$ (mmol/L)	K$^+$ (mmol/L)	Cl$^-$ (mmol/L)	Ca^{2+} (mmol/L)	Lactate or bicarbonate (mmol/L)	Osmolarity (mOsmol/L)	pH
Human serum	135–145	3.5–5.5	98–106	2.2–2.6	22–30	276–295	7.35–7.45
Ringer-lactate/ Hartmann's solution	131	5.0	111	2.0	29	279	6.0
0.9% normal saline	154	0	154	0	0	310	5.4

sterile no-touch technique, swabbing the entry point to the bag with an alcohol swab.

Dextrose/glucose solutions that are not in Ringer-lactate or Hartmann's solution are dangerous for replacing fluid losses.

Never infuse plain water IV: this causes haemolysis and will be fatal.

Always specify the concentrations of dextrose and saline solution to be infused.

Maintenance requirement of electrolytes

Daily sodium and potassium requirements in IV fluids:

- sodium (Na^+): 3–4 mmol/kg/24 hours in children; 150 mmol/24 hours in pregnancy
- potassium (K^+): 2–3 mmol/kg/24 hours in children; 100 mmol/24 hours in pregnancy.

Crystalloids containing a similar concentration of sodium to plasma (Ringer-lactate or Hartmann's solution) are used to replace vascular compartment losses. When infused IV, only around 25% remains inside the vascular compartment; the rest passes into the extracellular space.

All fluids should be prepared and administered using an aseptic technique. It is important to observe the cannula site directly (by removing the dressing) for redness and swelling before each IV injection. Observe the patient for pain or discomfort at the IV site. If there are any signs of inflammation, stop all fluids, reassess the need for continuing IV fluid drugs, and resite the cannula if necessary.

The rate of administration of fluids can be calculated in drops per minute as follows:

In a standard giving set with a drop factor of 20 drops = 1 mL, then mL/hour divided by 3 = drops/minute.

- Record that rate of fluid intake per hour on a fluid balance chart.
- Ensure that the IV site is kept clean.
- Flush the cannula with 0.9% saline or Ringer-lactate or Hartmann's solution 4-hourly if continuous fluids are not being given.

Prescribing practice and minimising drug errors

Introduction

- Oral administration is safer and less expensive, if it is tolerated and if the condition is not life-threatening.
- The following antibiotics are as effective when given orally as when administered intravenously, although initial IV doses will increase the blood levels more quickly:
  - amoxicillin, ampicillin, chloramphenicol, ciprofloxacin, co-trimoxazole, erythromycin, flucloxacillin, fluconazole, metronidazole, sodium fusidate.
- If a drug is given down an orogastric or nasogastric tube, flush the tube through afterwards so that the drug does not remain in the tube.
- Rectally administered drugs are less reliably absorbed than those given orally.
- Liquid formulations are better than suppositories for rectal administration of drugs in infants.

Prescribing

- Use approved names.
- Dosages should be in grams (g), milligrams (mg) or

micrograms. **Always write micrograms in full.** Volumes should be in millilitres (mL).

- Avoid using numbers with decimal points if at all possible (e.g. write 500 mg, not 0.5 g). If decimal points are used, they should be preceded by a zero (e.g. write 0.5 mL, not .5 mL).
- Write times using the 24-hour clock.
- Routes of administration can be abbreviated to IV (intravenous), IM (intramuscular), PO (orally), SC (subcutaneous), NEB (nebuliser) and PR (rectally).
- 'As-required' prescriptions must be specific with regard to how much, how often and for what purpose the drug is being given (also indicate the maximum 24-hour dose).
- 'Stop dates' for short-course treatments should be recorded when the drug is first prescribed.

Measuring drug doses

- Multiple sampling from drug vials increases the risk of introducing infection, as the vials do not contain preservatives or antiseptic.
- Dilute drugs so that volumes can accurately be measured. For example do not use doses of less than 0.1 mL for a 1-mL syringe without diluting sufficiently for you to be able to give an accurate amount of the drug.
- Do not forget to consider the dead space in the hub of the syringe for small volumes.
- For dilutions of more than 10-fold, use a small syringe to inject the active drug, connected by a sterile three-way tap to a larger syringe, and then add diluent to the large syringe to obtain the desired volume.

Delivery

- All IV solutions, including drugs, must be given aseptically.
- Give IV drugs slowly in all cases.
- After injecting into the line (e.g. through a three-way tap), use the usual rate of the IV infusion to drive the drug slowly into the patient.
- If there is no ongoing infusion, give sufficient follow-up (flush) of 0.9% saline, Ringer-lactate or Hartmann's solution or 5% dextrose to clear the drug from the cannula or T-piece.
- Repeat flushes of 0.9% saline can result in excess sodium intake in infants, so use Ringer-lactate or Hartmann's solution if possible.
- Flush over a period of 2 minutes to avoid a sudden surge of drug (remember the hub).

Infusions

- These must be given aseptically.
- Adjust the total 24-hour IV fluid intake so that additional infusions for drugs do not alter the total fluid volume.
- Never put more drug or background IV into the syringe or burette than is needed over a defined period of time.
- Check and chart the rate of infusion, and confirm this by examining the amount left every hour.
- Use a cannula, **not butterfly needles**, for infusions if available.
- **Do not mix incompatible fluids IV.**
- Do not add drugs to any line containing blood or blood products.
- Infusions of glucose higher than 10%, calcium salts and adrenaline, can cause tissue damage if they leak outside the vein.
- Most IV drugs can be given into an infusion containing

0.9% saline, Ringer-lactate or Hartmann's solution or up to 10% glucose (the exceptions include phenytoin and erythromycin).

- If you are using only one line, wait 10 minutes between each drug infused, or separate the drugs by infusing 1 mL of 0.9% saline or Ringer-lactate or Hartmann's solution.

Safe IV infusions when no burettes are available

Mark the infusion bottle with tape for each hour of fluid to be given, and label each hour.

> or

Empty the infusion bottle until only the exact amount of fluid to be given is left in the bottle.

Intravenous lines

Placement of the line

- Always place the cannula aseptically and keep the site clean.
- Use sterile bungs, *not* syringes, for closing off cannula/butterfly needles between IV injections.

Care of the line

- Change the giving set every 3 or 4 days.
- Change the giving set after blood transfusion, or if a column of blood has entered the infusion tubing from the vein, as this will be a site of potential bacterial colonisation.
- Always inspect the site of the cannula tip before and during drug injection. Never give a drug into a drip that has started to tissue. Severe scarring can occur, for example, from calcium solutions.
- Always use luer lock connections to minimise extravasation.

Sampling from the line

- Clear the dead space first (by three times its volume).
- Glucose levels cannot be accurately measured from any line through which a glucose solution is infused.
- Blood cultures should always be taken from a separate fresh venous needle or stab sample.
- After sampling, flush the line. **Remember that repeat flushes of 0.9% saline can result in excess sodium intake in infants.**

Complications

Infection

- Local infection can become systemic, especially in neonates or the immunosuppressed (e.g. HIV-infected patients).
- If there is erythema in the tissue, remove the cannula.
- If lymphangitis is present, remove the cannula, take a blood culture from a separate vein and start IV antibiotics.

Air embolism

- Umbilical or other central venous lines are particularly high risk.
- Another source of air embolus is through the giving set, especially when infusion pumps are used. **Infusion pumps must not be used if there are not enough nurses to closely monitor the infusion.**
- Always use a tap or syringe on the catheter, especially during insertion.

- If air reaches the heart it can block the circulation and cause death.

Haemorrhage

- In neonates this can occur from the umbilical stump.
- All connections must be luer locked.
- The connections to the cannula and its entry must be visualised at all times.

Minimising errors with IV infusions

- Prescribe or change infusion rates as infrequently as possible.
- Always have the minimum possible number of IV infusions running at the same time.
- Use a burette in which no more than the prescribed volume is present (especially in infants and young children, or with drugs such as quinine or magnesium sulphate in pregnancy).
- Record hourly the amount given (from the burette, syringe or infusion bag) and the amount left.
- Check the infusion site hourly to ensure that fluid has not leaked outside the vein.
- Ensure that flushes are only used if they are essential, and are given slowly over a period of at least 2 minutes.
- Be careful with potassium solutions given IV (use the enteral route when possible).
- Check and double check the following:
  - Is it the right drug? Check the ampoule as well as the box.
  - Is it at the right concentration?
  - Is the shelf life within the expiry date?
  - Has the drug been constituted and diluted correctly?
  - Is it being given to the right patient?
  - Is the dose correct? (Ideally two healthcare workers should check the prescription chart.)
  - Is it the correct syringe? (Deal with one patient at a time.)
  - Is the IV line patent?
  - Is a separate flush needed? If so, has the flush been checked?
  - Are sharps disposed of (including glass ampoules)?
  - Has it been signed off as completed (ideally countersigned)?
  - If the drug has not been received, is the reason stated?

Intramuscular (IM) injections

- **IM injections are unsafe for patients in shock**, especially opiates, where a high dose can be released once recovery of the circulation occurs.
- To avoid nerve damage, only the anterior aspect of the quadriceps muscle in the thigh is safe in infants.
- Use alternate legs if multiple injections are needed.
- Do not give IM injections if a bleeding tendency is present.
- **Draw back the plunger to ensure that the needle is not in a vein before injecting** (especially if administering adrenaline or lidocaine).

In very resource-limited situations, the IM route might be preferred because the drug may reach the patient sooner than if the patient had to wait in a queue to have an IV line sited. It also requires less nursing time and is less expensive;

venous cannulae are often in short supply. The IM route is as effective as the IV route in many situations.

Storage of drugs

Hospitals have struggled for many years to ensure that appropriate medicines are available when needed, while at the same time avoiding the problems of controlling the abuse and illegal use of these substances. Medicines that are of most concern in this respect are narcotics and sedatives. Supplies of these drugs must be available for the treatment of acutely ill patients, at the point of admission, in high-dependency care and post-surgical areas, and in all areas involved in the care of patients with terminal illness. Tragically, many care settings have solved the problem of storage by refusing to have stocks of these drugs readily available, either in the belief that patients, especially children, due to their physiological immaturity, do not feel pain, or due to fear of abuse by the patients and their families or healthcare staff.

The responsibility for the safe custody and storage of all medicines and drugs on a ward or department is that of the nurse in charge at any one time. Designated cupboards for the different types of drugs should be available. All cupboards, which should be permanently fixed to an inside wall, should have secure locks that make them inaccessible to unauthorised staff and visitors. Drug cupboards should be kept locked at all times, the keys being the responsibility of the nurse in charge.

Correct storage of drugs is paramount for prolonging the shelf life of the drug, as well as for complying with safety and legal requirements.

Due to the shelf life of some drugs, they need to be stored in a refrigerator, with the temperature set to store the drugs at between 2°C and 8°C. Drugs that need to be stored under these conditions include the following:

- reconstituted oral antibiotics
- eye drops
- rectal paracetamol
- some vaccines
- insulin (although this can be stored for up to 1 month at room temperature)
- oral midazolam
- pancuronium/vancuronium
- ergometrine
- oxytocin.

Calculating and giving the correct dose

Children should be weighed naked and their weight (in kg) recorded on the prescription chart. The use of a drug formulary should be considered when calculating the therapeutic dose. To ensure that the correct amount of drug is given from the stock bottle or vial, the following calculation should be used:

(prescribed dose divided by concentration of the stock solution) × (volume of stock dose).

For example, 125 mg (the amount prescribed) divided by 250 mg/5 mL (concentration of the stock solution) × 5 mL (volume of stock dose)
= 125/250 × 5 mL = 2.5 mL.

So the amount given would be 2.5 mL.

Medical staff should change the prescribed dose if after using the above calculation the dose is not easily measurable (e.g. 1.33 mL, 2.46 mL). To ensure that the calculated dose is given accurately, a pre-marked syringe should be used. The smaller the required dose, the smaller the syringe that should be used, as it will give a more accurate measurement (i.e. a 1- or 2-mL syringe should be used, not a 10-mL syringe).

Other forms of measurement can be used for larger doses, such as 5 or 10 mL. These include a pre-measured medicine pot or a 5-mL pre-measured medicine spoon. For safety, the calculation should ideally be done by two trained nurses, and the amount dispensed checked by the same two nurses. Although it is recognised in some hospitals that one trained nurse can check oral medication on their own, ideally IV and IM drugs should be checked by two trained nurses or a nurse and a doctor.

Safe use of morphine in hospital

Narcotic drugs, which may be controlled by law within the country concerned, should have a separate cupboard permanently fixed to the wall and locked. The keys to drug cupboards should be kept separately to all other keys and be carried by a qualified nurse for the period of each shift, and then handed over to the nurse taking over the next shift.

A logbook is necessary for recording the ordering and use of narcotic drugs. It is completed to order stocks, using one page for each order. It also records the use of each ampoule, tablet or dose of liquid. The name of the patient, hospital identification, date and time when the drug was given, and whether or not any portion of the drug was discarded is entered in the register (see Figure 1.6.1). Then each entry is signed by two staff members. Ideally, both must hold a nursing, medical or pharmacology qualification, and one must be a member of the ward or unit staff.

In addition, two members of unit staff must check the stock levels once in every 24-hour period and sign to confirm that the stocks are correct. Any discrepancy must be reported immediately to the senior nurse manager for the hospital.

Each hospital should have a policy for dealing with unauthorised use of narcotic drugs, and in some countries this will involve national law enforcement agencies.

When new drug stocks are required, the order book is sent to the central pharmacy, ideally in a container with a tamper-proof seal. Once the pharmacist has placed the order in the container, it is sealed and must not be opened until its arrival in the receiving ward or department.

When the stock arrives in the unit, the seal is broken in the presence of the messenger and the contents are checked against the order book, which is then signed by both. Drugs are then entered in the drug register, with two staff members checking and signing. The drugs are placed in the appropriate cupboard, which is then relocked.

In most hospital wards and units, these precautions will both ensure that adequate narcotic drugs are available when they are needed by patients, and prevent provision of supplies to those who may abuse them.

Use of morphine

- Morphine is a safe drug if administered by doctors and nurses who know how to use it and how to monitor patients who have been given it. It is not addictive if used only in the short term for severe pain.

AMOUNT(S) OBTAINED					NAME, FORM OF PREPARATION AND STRENGTH.. AMOUNT(S) ADMINISTERED					
Amount	Date received	Serial no. of requisition	Date	Time	Patient's name	Amount Given	Given by (signature)	Witnessed by (signature)	Stock balance

FIGURE 1.6.1 Page of a controlled drugs record book.

- It is not difficult to use, but because it is a controlled drug it requires special procedures to ensure its security.
- It is relatively inexpensive.
- It is a powerful and effective drug that is recommended by the WHO as the first-line medication for the treatment and prevention of severe pain.

Special procedures required to ensure the secure and appropriate use of morphine

1 Morphine must be stored in a secure locked box attached to the wall of each ward/area where it might be needed.
2 The box must always contain sufficient quantities for any anticipated clinical need.
3 The keys to the box must be readily available to staff who are caring for patients, and held by the senior person on the ward 24 hours a day.
4 A logbook recording every individual dose given and the name of the patient to whom it was administered must be signed by two members of staff.
5 Any unused morphine must be safely disposed of.
6 Every vial must be accounted for and the vials counted to check that the number tallies with the logbook at the beginning of each shift.

Morphine is usually available in 1- or 2-mL ampoules at a concentration of 10 mg/mL. **Always check the strength.**

The dose is 10 mg IV for pregnant women (5 mg initially and then another 5 mg after 5 minutes if necessary).

The dose is 200 micrograms/kg IV for children (100 micrograms/kg initially and then another 100 micrograms/kg after 15 minutes if necessary). **Two people must check the calculation.**

The volume is small, so dilute with 0.9% saline or 5% dextrose up to 10 mL.

Check the dilution.

The prescription of morphine must be clearly written, dated and signed (do not use fractions for doses).

The antidote, naloxone, must also be kept in the secure box.

The patient's notes must record the prescription and use of morphine.

All patients who are receiving morphine need regular monitoring and charting of ABC in particular:

- respiratory rate
- blood pressure
- oxygen saturation
- AVPU score.

Oxygen and a bag-valve-mask system of appropriate size must be available near to every patient who is receiving morphine.

An example of a page of a controlled drugs record book, such as would be used for morphine, is shown in Figure 1.6.1.

Summary

- Morphine is an essential drug that must be used when severe pain is present or likely to occur.
- To ensure its safe use, attention to the logistics of secure storage is of paramount importance.
- Close monitoring of ABC and D (disability) is essential, and naloxone must be available at all times.
- The prescribing and recording of doses of morphine and naloxone must be carefully undertaken.

1.7 Safe blood transfusion practice

Introduction

Blood or blood products should be transfused only when they are needed to save life or to prevent major morbidity.

The risk of transmission of infection is a major concern in countries with limited resources and poorly organised blood transfusion services.

Blood must be stored safely, or a bank of adequately screened donors must be available 24 hours a day, especially for obstetric emergencies or major trauma.

When giving a blood transfusion, care must be taken to ensure that the blood is compatible with that of the recipient, is infection free and is given safely.

Clinical situations that require blood transfusion

Normal haemoglobin (Hb) levels (after the neonatal period) are around 129 g/L (12.9 g/dL). Children with severe anaemia have Hb levels of 50 g/L or less. An Hb level of 50 g/L is widely accepted as the level at which transfusion might be indicated, and less than 40 g/L if there is severe malnutrition. Note: g/L divided by 10 = g/dL.

The WHO defines anaemia as any Hb level below 110 g/L. However, in pregnancy, normal haemodilution means that a cut-off value of less than 10 g/dL is more appropriate. In a pregnant woman, transfusion may be considered at an Hb level of 60–70 g/L, taking into account other factors.

In addition to Hb level, the following factors must be taken into account when considering transfusion.

- **Heart rate.** If it is rapid, this will favour the decision to transfuse. Remember that normal values for heart rate and respiratory rate vary with the age of the child.
- **Respiration rate.** If it is rapid, this will favour the decision to transfuse.
- **Is the patient grunting?** If so, this will favour the decision to transfuse.
- **Is the patient already in circulatory collapse (shock)?** If so **the need for transfusion is very urgent**.

Some patients will not show any of these features, and it might then be justifiable to delay transfusion and use haematinics (i.e. iron and folic acid). Some patients may show the above features and have an Hb level higher than 50 g/L. It will also be necessary to transfuse such patients if their symptoms are caused or significantly worsened by the anaemia and not an alternative pathology only (e.g. heart failure).

After birth, the haemoglobin level drops to less than 100 g/L in term infants at 8–12 weeks of age, but in premature infants it can drop to 70–100 g/L even earlier, at 6 weeks. (Oxygen delivery is well maintained because of rising levels of haemoglobin A, which releases oxygen more freely than haemoglobin F, which is found in the fetus.)

Causes of anaemia in neonates

- Hypovolaemic shock can result from acute blood loss, as for example in premature separation of the placenta or feto–maternal haemorrhage, twin-to-twin transfusion, and other causes of fetal or neonatal haemorrhage.
- Neonates may lose a considerable blood volume as a result of sampling for laboratory tests. Therefore samples should be minimised.
- Reduce the need for transfusion in neonates by providing adequate antenatal care, to reduce the risks of premature delivery and when possible prevent nutritional anaemia in the mother.
- Encourage breastfeeding.
- Ensure that there is early provision of vitamin K prophylaxis, iron, vitamins and other haematinics, especially in premature babies.

Causes of anaemia in children

These include the following:

- surgery
- haematological malignancies
- malaria
- sickle-cell disease
- congenital haemolytic anaemias (thalassaemia, glucose-6-phosphate dehydrogenase deficiency)
- burns
- major trauma.
- malnutrition (*see* Section 5.10.B).

Causes of anaemia in pregnancy

These include the following:

- obstetric emergencies such as antepartum and postpartum haemorrhage
- severe anaemia that is untreated or unresponsive to haematinics
- major trauma.

Transfusion policies and guidelines

- In hypovolaemic shock, erythrocyte-free volume expanders may be used to maintain tissue **perfusion**. Oxygen and top-up blood transfusion (10–20 mL/kg. over 5–10 minutes) may be required when tissue **oxygenation** is compromised.
- Transfuse for anaemia only when there are clinical signs, such as tachycardia, tachypnoea, recurrent apnoea, failure to thrive or early signs of anaemia-induced heart failure.
- When possible, provide malaria prophylaxis, particularly in pregnant women and children (*see* Sections 2.8.D and 6.3.A.d) with sickle-cell disease. Early treatment of clinical malaria reduces the profound haemolysis that is a major reason for transfusion in endemic areas.
- Anaemia due to malaria responds to treatment with antimalarial drugs and folic acid.
- Blood transfusion is not required for sickle-cell disease in the steady state. It may be indicated in severe anaemia with incipient or established cardiac failure,

acute splenic enlargement, sequestration crisis with rapidly falling haemoglobin levels, aplastic crisis, acute chest syndrome, stroke, and sometimes as exchange transfusion for severe priapism (*see* Section 5.11.B on sickle-cell disease).

- National programmes for thalassaemia and other congenital haemolytic disorders, such as glucose-6-phosphate dehydrogenase deficiency, help to reduce transfusion requirements.

In situations where blood transfusion is unavailable or potentially unsafe, the following recommendations have been made:

- Transfusion is not necessary if the Hb level is more than 50 g/L.
- Transfusion may be necessary if the Hb level is less than 50 g/L and there is incipient cardiorespiratory distress (air hunger, hypotension, tachycardia and oedema).
- Transfusion may be necessary if the Hb level is less than 40 g/L and complicated by malaria or bacterial infection, even without incipient cardiac failure.
- Transfusion may be necessary if the Hb level is less than 30 g/L, with no apparent complications.

In situations where blood transfusion is safe and available, recommendations for its use are as follows.

Neonates and infants less than 4 months old
- Blood loss of more than 15% over 2 days.
- Haemoglobin level of less than 70 g/L with clinical manifestations of anaemia.

Infants aged 4 months or older
- Acute blood loss that is unresponsive to crystalloid and colloid infusions.
- Intra-operative blood loss of more than 15% of total blood volume and post-operative haemoglobin level of less than 80 g/L with clinical symptoms.
- Haemoglobin level of less than 110 g/L with severe pulmonary disease.
- Acute haemolysis with haemoglobin level of less than 80 g/L with signs of anaemia.
- To suppress endogenous haemoglobin in sickle-cell disease crises and thalassaemic syndrome.

Red-cell-free components
- Fresh frozen plasma (FFP) is only recommended when a specific haemostatic defect has been identified. In the absence of specific testing, consider administering FFP to a patient with signs of disseminated intravascular coagulation who is acutely unwell, as it may be life-saving.
- Freeze-dried plasma is now available, and its advantages include a long shelf life and the lack of need for refrigeration.
- Platelets are prepared from fresh blood using a special, simple centrifugation method, and the remaining blood can be given back to the donor. Once extracted by this method, platelets can last for up to 5 days at room temperature (around 23°C). Platelets should not be stored in a refrigerator. Transfused platelets survive only briefly, and repeated infusion may be required for active bleeding, or before essential procedures such as a lumbar puncture in a child with severe thrombocytopenia.

Blood donation and provision
- Ideally blood is obtained by routine whole blood collection from an established panel of blood donors with quality standards for testing, processing and distribution.
- Most transfusions are required and given as an emergency procedure. Ideally, emergency collection of blood for paediatric use should not be necessary (see below).
- Safe transfusion is enhanced by the following measures:
  - collection of blood from repeat regular donors screened using a standard health-check questionnaire, and who are found negative for all markers for transfusion-transmissible infection
  - collection in a multi-pack which allows each donation to be divided into small volumes, in a closed sterile system to reduce wastage and donor exposure
  - multiple, small-volume packs can be used for multiple transfusions in one child or neonate without having to repeat the pre-transfusion tests.
- Group O rhesus-negative small-volume packs facilitate transfusion across the ABO barrier. They must be checked for high-titre anti-A or anti-B by a suitable antiglobulin method.
- Establish a routine procedure for collection, testing and processing which should cover routine and emergency transfusions.
- Maternal blood is not recommended for transfusing into the newborn infant, even in an emergency, although theoretically it can be used after compatibility testing with the recipient's serum.

Pre-transfusion testing
Minimum acceptable tests on blood prior to transfusion
1 ABO and Rhesus D grouping.
2 Screening for hepatitis B antigen and antibodies to HIV-1 and -2, hepatitis C virus and syphilis.
3 Additional tests for locally prevalent infections, such as malaria and Chagas disease.
   - 0.1–0.2 mL blood in an EDTA bottle is required for grouping, and 2 mL of clotted blood in a plain bottle for compatibility testing.
   - In infants under 4 months of age, maternal blood testing for compatibility is always required: 4 mL of EDTA plus 5 mL of clotted blood.
   - Blood group the neonate using a cord, capillary or small venous sample (2–3 drops and specific standard reagents Anti-A, Anti-B, Anti-A+B and Anti-RhD). Red cells only are used, because antibody levels in the sera of neonates are too low to be of significant value.
   - The inclusion of control A, B, O, RhD-positive and RhD-negative cells in the procedure is part of good laboratory practice, and should be part of the testing method.
   - If possible, two methods should be used for grouping, to ensure reliability.
   - For neonates and infants up to 4 months of age, compatibility testing is not required if the mother's serum is negative for allo-antibodies. Compatibility between the mother's serum and red cells to be transfused is required only if the mother has antibodies or if there is a previous history of haemolytic disease of the newborn.

The most suitable method for compatibility is the anti-human globulin technique at 37°C for 1 hour. Agglutination should be read before and after the addition of the anti-human globulin reagent.

Blood groups

There are four major blood groups: A, B, AB and O. To avoid ABO incompatibility, the blood group of both the donor and the receiver must be known. Blood can only be donated in the direction of the arrows shown in Figure 1.7.1.

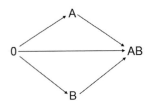

FIGURE 1.7.1 Safe transfusion of ABO blood groups.

- Donors with blood group O can donate to patients (receivers) with blood group A, B, AB or O.
- Donors with blood group A can donate to patients with blood group A or AB.
- Donors with blood group B can donate to patients with blood group B or AB.
- Donors with blood group AB can donate only to patients with blood group AB.

Blood is also categorised according to its rhesus status. Therefore:
- Rhesus-negative donors can give to Rhesus-positive and Rhesus-negative patients.
- Rhesus-positive donors can only give to Rhesus-positive patients.

If the blood group is unknown and blood is required before a cross-match can be performed, give O-Rhesus-negative blood if this is available.

Exchange transfusion

- This is used for haemolytic disease of the newborn with severe anaemia and/or severe hyperbilirubinaemia (*see* Section 3.4). Exchange of double the neonate's blood volume is often required using 160–180 mL/kg of whole blood and/or plasma reduced red cells. The latter are prepared by removing approximately 100 mL of plasma to create a haematocrit of 0.5–0.6.
- Patients with sickle-cell anaemia and acute chest syndrome or impending cerebrovascular episodes may benefit from exchange transfusion (*see* Section 2.5.B).
- Blood should be fresh (less than 5 days old), and also screened for HbS if it is issued for sickle-cell disease.

Use Rhesus-negative blood, group O or the same ABO group as the infant compatible with maternal and infant serum.

The blood should be warmed with a heating coil or stood for 1 hour at room temperature or under the mother's clothing.

Exchange transfusion: indications and technique
Indications
- Severe haemolytic anaemia: use double volume exchange.
- Severe hyperbilirubinaemia: use double volume exchange.
- Polycythaemia: use partial exchange with Ringer-lactate or Hartmann's or 0.9% saline (*see* Section 3.4).

$$\text{Double volume exchange (mL)} = 2 \times 80 \times \text{weight (kg)}.$$

$$\frac{80 \times \text{weight (kg)} \times (\text{actual haematocrit} - \text{desired haematocrit})}{\text{actual haematocrit}}$$

Technique
1 Exchange transfusion should preferably be through umbilical or peripheral venous and arterial catheters so that simultaneous withdrawal and transfusion of blood/volume occurs. If this is not possible, a single large-bore venous cannula may be used with a three-way tap to allow alternate withdrawing and transfusing of aliquots. An aseptic technique must be maintained.
2 Use a 5- or 10-mL syringe to draw 5- or 10-mL aliquots (depending on the baby's weight) from the baby via the arterial line over a 3-minute cycle, and discard them. Simultaneously infuse 5- or 10-mL aliquots through the venous line over a 3-minute cycle.
3 The baby's temperature, pulse, respiratory rate and blood pressure must be monitored as for transfusions, and in addition blood glucose levels must be monitored every 30 minutes.
4 Use a nasogastric tube to evacuate the stomach contents, and keep the patient nil by mouth.
5 Use a separate IV line to administer dextrose solution to maintain blood glucose levels and hydration.
6 Check the baby's haemoglobin, bilirubin, glucose and calcium levels at the beginning and end of the procedure.
7 Check a blood film, Coombs' test, and if possible coagulation and arterial or capillary blood gas at the beginning of the procedure.

Potential complications include hypoglycaemia, electrolyte disturbance, thrombocytopenia, coagulopathy, sepsis, air embolus, circulatory overload and gastrointestinal complications (e.g. acute dilation of stomach, intestinal ischaemia).

Bedside transfusion
A child's body contains 80 mL of blood for every kg of body weight. For example, a 3-year-old weighing 12 kg will have 960 mL of blood in their body.

A pregnant mother's body contains 100 mL of blood for every kg of body weight.
- Venous access for bedside transfusion should be chosen with no smaller than a 22- to 24-gauge vascular catheter, and a much larger one in pregnant mothers.
- Blood is usually cleaned and filtered in the lab, so when transfusing it to a patient the only filter that needs to be used is the usual on-line filter in a standard giving set.
- Blood should be treated like any other IV fluid, and given using an accurate measurement of rate and time. **A burette should be used for infants or in children for whom**

too rapid an input could be dangerous (e.g. in incipient or actual heart failure).

Blood transfusion reactions

Blood transfusion can be life-saving and provides great clinical benefit to many patients. However, it is not without risks, which include the following:

- immunological complications
- errors and 'wrong blood' episodes
- infections (bacterial and viral).

Causes of acute complications of transfusion

Acute haemolytic transfusion reaction

- Incompatible transfused red cells react with the patient's own anti-A or anti-B antibodies or other alloantibodies (e.g. anti-rhesus (Rh) D) to red cell antigens. Complement can be activated and may lead to **disseminated intravascular coagulation (DIC)**.
- Infusion of ABO-incompatible blood is almost always a result of errors in labelling sample tubes and/or request forms, or inadequate checks at the time of transfusion. When red cells are mistakenly administered, there is about a 1 in 3 risk of ABO incompatibility and a 10% risk of mortality, with the most severe reaction seen in a group O individual receiving group A red cells.
- Non-ABO red cell antibody haemolytic reactions tend to be less severe.

Infective shock

- Bacterial contamination can be fatal.
- Acute onset of tachycardia, low pulse pressure, hypotension, rigors and collapse rapidly follows the transfusion.

Transfusion-related acute lung injury (TRALI)

- TRALI is a form of acute respiratory distress due to donor plasma containing antibodies against the patient's leukocytes.
- Transfusion is followed within 6 hours of transfusion by the development of a prominent non-productive cough, breathlessness, hypoxia and frothy sputum. Fever and rigors may be present.
- Chest X-ray if available shows multiple perihilar nodules with infiltration of the lower lung fields.

Fluid overload

- This occurs when too much fluid is transfused or it is transfused too quickly, leading to **pulmonary oedema** and **acute respiratory failure**.
- Patients at particularly high risk are those with severe or chronic anaemia, or severe malnutrition and who have normal blood volumes (i.e. who are not bleeding), and those with symptoms of **cardiac failure** prior to transfusion.
- These patients should receive packed cells rather than whole blood via slow transfusion, with diuretics if required.

Non-haemolytic febrile reactions to transfusion of platelets and red cells

- Fevers (more than 1°C above baseline) and rigors may develop during transfusion due to the patient's antibodies to transfused white cells.

- This type of reaction affects 1–2% of patients.
- Multiparous women and those who have received multiple previous transfusions are most at risk. Reactions are unpleasant but not life-threatening. Usually symptoms develop towards the end of a transfusion or in the subsequent 2 hours. Most febrile reactions can be managed by slowing or stopping the transfusion and giving paracetamol.

Severe allergic reaction or anaphylaxis

- Allergic reactions occur when patients have antibodies that react with proteins in transfused blood components.
- Anaphylaxis occurs when an individual has previously been sensitised to an allergen present in the blood, and subsequently, on re-exposure, releases immunoglobulin E (IgE) or IgG antibodies. Patients with anaphylaxis become acutely dyspnoeic due to bronchospasm and laryngeal oedema, and may complain of chest pain, abdominal pain and nausea.
- Urticaria and itching are common within minutes of starting a transfusion.
- These symptoms are usually controlled by slowing the transfusion and giving antihistamine, and the transfusion may be continued if there is no progression at 30 minutes.
- Pre-treatment with an antihistamine should be given if the patient has experienced repeated allergic reactions to transfusion.
- For treatment of anaphylaxis, *see* Sections 2.7.C and 5.1.B.

Presentation

Symptoms or signs may occur after only 5–10 mL of transfusion of incompatible blood, so **patients should be observed very closely at the start of each blood unit transfused**.

Symptoms

These include the following:

- a feeling of apprehension or that 'something is wrong'
- flushing
- chills
- pain at the venepuncture site
- muscle aches
- nausea
- pain in the abdomen, loins or chest
- shortness of breath.

Signs

These include the following:

- fever (a rise in temperature of 1.5°C or more) and rigors
- hypotension or hypertension
- tachycardia
- respiratory distress
- oozing from wounds or puncture sites
- **haemoglobinaemia**
- **haemoglobinuria**.

Investigations and management

- If a serious acute transfusion reaction is suspected, **stop the transfusion**, take down the donor blood bag and giving set, and send the donor bag back to the blood bank with notification of the event. Set up a new giving set with Ringer Lactate, Hartmann's or 0.9% saline solution.
- To detect a haemolytic reaction, send post-transfusion

blood (for full blood count and clotting, repeat typing and cross-matching, antibody screen and direct Coombs' test) and a urine specimen (if available, for detection of urinary haemoglobinuria) from the transfusion recipient.

- Where bacterial contamination is suspected, send blood cultures from the patient and also bag remnants.
- If the patient is dyspnoeic, obtain a chest X-ray if possible and check for fluid overload and pulmonary oedema.

TABLE 1.7.1 Investigations for blood transfusion reactions

Type of reaction	Investigation findings
Acute haemolytic reactions	• Visual inspection of centrifuged plasma: pink-red discoloration (haemoglobinaemia) indicates significant intravascular haemolysis • Visual inspection of centrifuged urine: red discoloration indicates haemoglobinuria • Retyping of donor and recipient red blood cells (RBCs): any discrepancy suggests that the transfusion has been mismatched and blood samples have been mixed up • Direct antiglobulin ('Coombs') test (DAT): ABO related acute transfusion reactions usually cause a positive DAT test • Evidence of increased RBC destruction (e.g. a fall in haemoglobin and/or rise in bilirubin levels) • There may be evidence of DIC • Negative blood cultures
Febrile non-haemolytic reactions	• Visual inspection of the recipient's plasma and urine is normal • Retyping shows no incompatibility • DAT test is negative
Allergic and anaphylactic reactions	• Urticaria, itching and dyspnoea (for symptoms and signs of anaphylaxis, see Section 2.7.C)
TRALI	• Pulse oximeter shows hypoxaemia • Chest X-ray (if available) shows bilateral lung infiltrates • Full blood count frequently shows low white blood cell count and high eosinophil count
Transfusion-transmitted bacterial infection	• Blood cultures are positive and congruent for both donor and recipient blood

Management

- Where the only feature is a rise in temperature of less than 1.5°C from baseline, or urticaria, recheck that the correct blood is being transfused, give paracetamol and antihistamine, reset the transfusion at a slower rate and observe the patient more frequently.
- Although fever or rigors are not uncommon in response to a transfusion and may represent a non-haemolytic febrile reaction, they may also be the first sign of a severe adverse reaction.
- Where the reaction is more severe:
  - Stop the transfusion and call a doctor urgently to review the patient.
  - Vital signs (temperature, blood pressure, pulse, respiratory rate and oxygen saturation levels) and respiratory status (dyspnoea, tachypnoea, wheeze and cyanosis) should be checked and recorded. Look for signs of heart failure (basal lung crepitations and enlarged liver).
  - Check the patient's identity and recheck against details on the blood unit and compatibility label or tag.
- Initial management if **ABO incompatibility** is suspected is as follows:
  - Take down the blood bag **and** the giving set with blood in it.
  - Keep the IV line open with Ringer-lactate or Hartmann's solution.
  - Give oxygen and fluid support.
  - Monitor urine output, usually following catheterisation, and maintain it at more than 2 mL/kg/hour in infants, > 1 mL/kg/hour in children and > 30 mL/hour in pregnancy, giving furosemide if it falls below this.
  - Consider inotropic support if hypotension is prolonged.

- Treat DIC by giving fresh new blood fully matched to the recipient.
  - Inform the hospital transfusion department immediately.
- If **another haemolytic reaction or bacterial infection of blood unit** is suspected:
  - Send haematological and microbiological samples for investigations as outlined above.
  - General supportive management is as for ABO incompatibility.
  - Start broad-spectrum IV antibiotics if bacterial infection is considered likely.
- If **anaphylaxis or severe allergic reaction** is suspected:
  - Follow the anaphylaxis protocols for women and children (see Section 2.7.C and Section 5.1.B).
- If **TRALI** is suspected:
  - Give high-concentration oxygen, IV fluids and inotropes (as for acute respiratory distress syndrome).
  - Ventilation may be urgently required; discuss this with an anaesthetist.

TRALI improves within 2–4 days in over 80% of cases if there is adequate management and respiratory support.

- If **fluid overload** is suspected:
  - Give IV furosemide and high-concentration oxygen.

Delayed complications of transfusion
Delayed haemolysis of transfused red cells

- In those who have previously been immunised to a red cell antigen during pregnancy or by transfusion, the level of antibody to the blood group antigen may be so low as to be undetectable in the pre-transfusion sample.
- However, after transfusion of red cells bearing that antigen, a rapid secondary immune response raises the

antibody level dramatically, leading to the rapid destruction of transfused cells.

- At 5–10 days post-transfusion, patients present with fever, falling haemoglobin levels (or an unexpectedly poor rise in haemoglobin levels), jaundice and haemoglobinuria.
- A rise in bilirubin levels and positive direct antiglobulin test (DAT) will also be present.

Development of antibodies to red cells in the patient's plasma (alloimmunisation)

- Transfusion of red cells of a different phenotype to that of the patient will cause alloimmunisation (e.g. development of anti-RhD in RhD-negative patients who have received RhD-positive cells).
- This is dangerous if the patient later receives a red cell transfusion, and can cause **haemolytic disease of the newborn (HDN)**.

Iron overload

- Each unit of blood contains 250 mg of iron, and those receiving red cells over a long period of time may develop iron accumulation in cardiac and liver tissues.
- Chelation therapy (with **desferrioxamine**) is used to minimise iron accumulation in those most at risk.

Infection

- The risk of becoming infected with HIV, hepatitis B or hepatitis C from transfusion is now small. However, since there is always the potential for unrecognised or unknown infection to be spread via transfusion, **all non-essential transfusions should be avoided.**
- Blood must be stored at the correct temperature at all times (at 1–6°C for up to 35 days if using citrate-phosphate-dextrose adenine anticoagulant *or* up to 21 days if using citrate-phosphate-double dextrose). Ideally each blood bag should be labelled with a temperature-sensitive strip that changes colour when the correct temperature for storage has been exceeded for a clinically significant period of time.

Improving safety
Reducing transfusion errors

- Introduce robust hospital transfusion protocols.
- Provide training for all staff involved in blood administration/taking samples for cross-matching.
- An understanding of transfusion medicine should be a core curricular component for all doctors in training.
- Improved information technology, such as use of a unique barcode on the patient's wristband/blood sample and prepared blood, is important.
- Appoint specialist transfusion practitioners.

Reducing unnecessary transfusion

- Transfusion risks related to the use of allogeneic blood can be eliminated by the use of autologous blood (whereby patients collect and store their own blood for use in planned surgery). However, this practice is not risk-free.
- Ensure that blood products are only used when the patient is judged more likely to benefit from than be harmed by a transfusion.
- Always record in the patient's notes the indication for giving blood.
- Adopt procedures such as checking for and correcting anaemia prior to planned surgery, stopping anticoagulants and antiplatelet drugs before surgery, minimising the amount of blood taken for laboratory samples, and using a simple protocol to guide when haemoglobin should be checked and when red cells should be transfused.
- Accept a lower haemoglobin concentration as a trigger for transfusion.
- Accept a lower post-transfusion target haemoglobin level.

1.8 Essential laboratory services

Basic services provided in the laboratory and on the ward

Whenever possible, the regional or central laboratory should procure the chemicals, prepare the reagents and standards, and distribute them with the necessary controls and approved testing procedure to district laboratories. Details on how to prepare the required reagents, standards and controls can be found in the 1995 WHO publication *Production of Basic Diagnostic Laboratory Reagents*.[1]

For all small hospitals, the WHO recommends six basic investigations as an absolute minimum:

- haemoglobin or packed cell volume
- blood smear for malaria
- blood glucose levels
- microscopy of cerebrospinal fluid (CSF) and urine
- blood grouping and cross-matching
- for newborn care, blood bilirubin levels.

Tests that can be performed on the wards

These include the following:

- blood grouping
- rapid diagnostic test for *Plasmodium falciparum* (or urgent thick blood film for malarial parasites)
- urine microscopy (*see* Sections 5.6.A and 8.5)
- HIV rapid screening test
- HBsAg screening test
- 'hot stool' examination (for *Entamoeba histolytica*)
- rapid haemoglobin (WHO paper-based method)

- CSF/gland/chancre aspirate/wet preparation for trypanosomes.

Tests to be performed in the laboratory

These include the following:

- thick and thin blood films for malaria and/or rapid diagnostic test for *Plasmodium falciparum*
- smears for *Leishmania amastigotes*
- rapid rk39 Ab test for *Leishmania* antibodies
- Ziehl–Neelsen sputum smears for TB
- Ziehl–Neelsen slit skin smears for leprosy
- Gram-stained smears
- haemoglobin estimation and platelets
- total and differential white cell count
- erythrocyte sedimentation rate (ESR)
- sickle-cell test
- HIV and hepatitis screening tests
- blood grouping and cross-matching
- urine deposits
- formol-ethyl acetate concentration and Kato-Katz thick smears for stool parasites.

Essential equipment

A functioning **microscope** is essential, and also saves time and therefore salary costs. Ideally a binocular instrument should be available, with × 10 eyepieces and × 10, × 40 and × 100 (oil immersion) objectives with integral illumination. LED light sources and options for using solar-powered batteries are now available.

A robust **bench-top centrifuge** is also needed. Ensure that lidded conical tubes (15 mL) can be used, and that there is an inner safety lid. A built-in timer and variable rotor speed are also desirable.

Haematological investigations
Haemoglobin

- **Haemoglobin colour scale** (WHO) filter paper 'matching method' (visual comparative technique): simple, cheap and portable, but is not suitable for use with artificial light. Available from WHO, Geneva.
- **Haemoglobinometer (BMS)** visual comparator method: a useful method for testing small numbers of sample. No dilution or measurement of sample is required, and standard is included. Available from Cascade HealthCare Products Inc., USA (www.1cascade.com).
- **DHT Hb523 haemoglobinometer:** portable, battery-operated and requires 0.04% ammonia. Suitable when multiple investigations are required (www.haemoglobinometer.co.uk).
- **Microhaematocrit centrifugation:** if no other method is available this can be used for estimation. Note that there may be raised values caused by plasma loss (e.g. due to burns or dehydration).

White blood cell count

- **Improved Neubauer haemocytometer:** spare cover glasses, Turk's solution (white blood cell diluent), 20-µl micropipette and hand tally counter are required.

Erythrocyte sedimentation rate (ESR)

- The **Westergren method** is recommended.

Differential white cell counts

- Thin blood film stained with Leishman's/Rapyd Giemsa (pH 6.8). Tally counters are required.
- **Film may also be used to examine red cell morphology for cases of suspected nutritional anaemia (e.g. iron deficiency).**

Sickle-cell test

- A simple slide test using 2% sodium metabisulphite (prepared daily) will enable the morphology of sickled red blood cells to be seen, but cannot differentiate between sickle-cell disease and trait. The HbS solubility filtration test can differentiate sickle-cell anaemia from sickle-cell disease.

HIV test

- Rapid antibody tests are easy to use for blood transfusion screening purposes and for diagnostic screening. Many brands are available, their sensitivities and specificities vary, and brand use may depend on local availability.

Hepatitis B and C testing

- Rapid tests are available to detect HBsAg and anti-HCV antibody (refer to **WHO Blood Safety Unit** for details of appropriate tests).

Blood groups

- **Blood grouping/cross-matching sera should be available.**

Biochemical investigations

Low-cost, easily maintained equipment is urgently required in low-resource settings to measure plasma sodium and potassium levels. Hyponatraemia and hypokalaemia are common and dangerous conditions that need early detection and management.

Important biochemical investigations include the following:

- Tests on whole blood, serum or plasma:
  - urea, creatinine and electrolytes
  - glucose
  - albumin
  - bilirubin
  - amylase
  - AST (aspartate aminotransferase).
- In specialised hospitals, the following can be measured:
  - alkaline phosphatase
  - ALT (alanine aminotransferase)
  - calcium
  - cholesterol
  - cholinesterase
  - iron
  - triglycerides.
- Urine clinical chemistry tests:
  - protein
  - glucose
  - bilirubin and urobilinogen
  - ketones
  - haemoglobin
  - nitrite
  - specific gravity.

- Faecal clinical chemistry tests:
  - occult blood
  - lactose
  - excess fat.
- Cerebrospinal fluid clinical chemistry tests:
  - protein (c. 1 mL of CSF)
  - glucose (0.5 mL into a fluorite oxalate bottle).

Investigations for specific diseases
Malaria
- Thick blood film stained with Field's/Giemsa) stain; use finger prick or venous blood.
- Using Field's the film can be stained within 20 seconds (compound stain powders 'A' and 'B' are available to mix with water).
- To confirm diagnosis of the species, a methanol-fixed thin blood film (hand stained at pH 7.2) using Rapyd Giemsa/Leishman's or reverse Field's stain may be useful.
- Thick blood films may also reveal *Borrelia*, microfilariae and trypanosomes.
- The WHO has recommended the use of rapid diagnostic tests (RDTs) as a parasite-based diagnosis **where good-quality microscopy cannot be maintained** (for guidance on choosing the most appropriate RDT, visit www.who.int/tdr).

African trypanosomiasis
- Immediate examination of a wet preparation and/or thick blood film stained as described above is the simplest way of diagnosing *Trypanosoma brucei rhodesiense* (if a chancre is present, a sample may be taken from between the edge and the centre of the lesion and examined as for blood).
- Gland fluid from a swollen posterior cervical gland may be examined (this is particularly useful in *T.b. gambiense*), with immediate examination for motile trypanosomes or stained as for blood.
- If these tests are negative, up to four microhaematocrit (MHCT) tubes of blood should be taken. These are centrifuged for 5 minutes, stuck to microscope slides and the buffy coat area examined for motile trypanosomes (Woo test).
- All samples must be examined as soon as possible to avoid parasite lysis.
- If the blood is positive for trypanosomes, or it is suspected that the patient has late-stage (stage II) CNS disease, a lumbar puncture must be taken and CSF examined microscopically **within 30 minutes of the procedure in order to visualise trypanosomes**. The number of white blood cells should be counted using a haemocytometer.

Leishmaniasis
- For cutaneous leishmaniasis, a smear taken from the raised red edge of a lesion may be taken and stained with rapid Giemsa/Leishman's (diluted with buffered water at pH 7.2) to demonstrate amastigotes.
- For suspected visceral leishmaniasis, haematological investigations plus an antibody detection test such as the Rapyd Leishman's which utilises rk39 antigen are the most useful and safe investigations. Note that in HIV-positive individuals false-negative antibody test results are common.

TB and leprosy
For suspected TB
- If possible, up to three consecutive morning sputum samples should be examined.
- The Ziehl–Neelsen (ZN) method of staining should be used.
- The addition of bleach to liquefy the sample may improve sensitivity, and lowers the risk of laboratory infection.

For suspected leprosy
- The ZN method of staining should be used on slit skin smears.

Diarrhoeal diseases
For suspected parasitic cause
- Direct microscopy using saline smears (plus iodine to aid identification of cysts) should be used. A concentration technique such as formol-ether (or ethyl-acetate/petrol) concentration or the Kato–Katz cellophane technique (WHO) is particularly useful when looking for parasites such as *Schistosoma mansoni*, where the female worm only produces around 200 eggs per day.

For suspected bacteriological cause
- Ideally the specimen should be sent for culture and sensitivity testing.
- Culture may not be possible due to the need for sterile facilities and supplies of media.
- If possible, samples should be sent to a reference laboratory for culture.
- Supplies of the following transport media and sterile swabs should be available:
  - Stuart's medium or Amies medium for suspected *Salmonella typhi* and *Shigella*
  - alkaline peptone water and Cary-Blair medium for *Vibrio cholerae*.
- If microscopy of a fluid stool containing blood shows red blood cells, white blood cells/macrophages and numerous bacteria, **bacterial dysentery** is likely.
- If the sample is loose with blood and mucus, then a 'hot stool' (examined within 30 minutes of voiding) should be examined for motile *Entamoeba histolytica* trophozoites.

Urinary infections and renal diseases
Urine examination
- Urine 'dipstick' tests are useful for detecting blood, protein, glucose, bilirubin, urobilinogen, infection, nitrites and white blood cells.
- A midstream urine (MSU) sample may be examined microscopically for the following:
  - *Schistosoma haematobium* ova (or terminal urine)
  - pus (white blood cells)
  - erythrocytes
  - casts
  - bacteria (suspected urinary tract infection).
- The addition of a drop of 1% methylene blue in physiological saline may aid microscopical examination.
- If urine is to be sent for culture, 20 mL of an MSU sample should be mixed with 3 mg of boric acid (a preservative).
- It is important to give instructions to ward staff on how to obtain an MSU sample, bag urine and suprapubic aspirate.

Ulcers and exudates

- For suspected bacterial (and fungal) infections, a smear of the pus or exudate should be stained with Gram stain.

Meningitis

- A Gram-stained CSF deposit may be useful in cases of suspected meningitis.
- The India ink stain is used for cryptococcal meningitis.

References

1 World Health Organization (1995) *Production of Basic Diagnostic Laboratory Reagents.* Can be obtained from WHO Regional Office, PO Box 1517, Alexandria.
2 Cheesbrough M (2005) *District Laboratory Practice in Tropical Countries. Part 1*, 2nd edn. Cambridge, UK: Cambridge University Press.

1.9 Records, history taking and examination

Records

- Records can be held by patients or parents, or by the hospital, or both.
- If they are patient or parent held, they can be developed into health booklets containing advice on how to manage illnesses (possibly in the form of pictures for illiterate parents). Immunisation information, if included, should comply with national immunisation programmes.
- Hospital records need to be kept confidentially in a logical system for audit purposes, with easy access to previous notes.
- Discharge information and advice should be entered in the patient- or parent-held booklet.
- If possible, diagnoses should be coded and entered according to the International Classification of Diseases (ICD) or in accordance with local policy and coding.

History taking

- The medical history should, when age appropriate, include the child's own input. The source of the information may be the mother, the father or the child him- or herself, and the source should be documented.
- It is important to listen, especially to the mother's worries about her child, taking into account her general frame of mind, her experience with previous children and her ability to communicate.
- Time can be a restricting factor due to the workload, but it is important to ask about the following:
  - pregnancy and previous deliveries (including stillbirths)
  - infant or young child feeding history
  - the immunisation record (best kept by the parents)
  - previous admissions or visits to hospital
  - existing medical problems
  - social circumstances at home, and the family history
  - the family's cultural beliefs and their religion and/ or tribe
  - medication taken by the patient, and any allergies
  - the patient's presenting complaints and current treatment, if any.
- Most patients and their families are anxious. They need reassurance, kindness and understanding.

Examination

The following basic equipment is required:

- stethoscope
- otoscope (if available)
- ophthalmoscope (if available)
- tendon hammer
- bright torch light (or mobile phone light)
- thermometer
- Pinard's stethoscope or Sonicaid (a hand-held Doppler)
- microscope (if available).

Conducting the examination

- A triage nurse (*see* Section 1.10) can be helpful for making a preliminary assessment of patients. They can assess each patient and use the recorded body temperature, weight, general condition and pain score of the patient to decide how urgently he or she should be seen by the doctor.
- Do not rush the examination. A thorough examination is often needed, and taking time can help to gain the confidence of the patient and their family.
- If the patient is critically ill, quick action is required and questions can be asked later.
- Try to be gentle and avoid palpating a painful body part before everything else has been done. You want to avoid having a crying patient whom you cannot examine or auscultate.
- Small children and infants are best examined on the parent's lap; older ones can be asked to lie down.
- In general, the examination of a child will follow the same systematic approach as in adults. However, you may need to be more opportunistic.

Essential emergency examination checklist

Always check the following in the order shown:

- **A**irway
- **B**reathing
- **C**irculation
- **D**isability
- **E**xposure.

In the case of a critically ill patient, proceed to basic and/or advanced life support using the structured approach (*see* Section 1.11).

Patients who are not in need of immediate resuscitation

- **Introduce yourself to the patient and parent, if present.**
- **Interact with any child throughout the examination.**
- **General inspection:** document dysmorphism, skin rashes or bruises, nutritional status, weight and height for age, jaundice, pallor, clubbing, (for child) relationship with parent, and state of consciousness.
- **Respiratory system:** document chest wall expansion (is it symmetrical? is there recession?), respiratory rate, cyanosis, palpation, percussion, and auscultation.
- **Cardiovascular system:** remember to feel all of the pulses, particularly the femoral pulses. Measure the blood pressure (the cuff **must** cover two-thirds of the upper arm circumference), examine the jugular venous pressure, palpate the cardiac impulses (i.e. for left and right ventricles), and auscultate the apex, left sternal edge, pulmonary and aortic areas and carotids and over the back.
- **Abdominal system:** if the patient is pregnant, assess the size of the uterus, the presentation of the fetus and listen for the fetal heart. In an infant check the genitals for cryptoorchidism, hernias and gender. Rectal examinations are occasionally necessary but need to

be explained to the patient, parent and child (where appropriate). Inspect the mouth and teeth.

- **Neurological system:** use the AVPU or Glasgow Coma Scale score (*see* Section 1.11). Observe infants for their degree of responsiveness and rapport appropriate for age, social and motor skills, and look for neurocutaneous stigmata. Test for age-appropriate reflexes and saving reactions when assessing developmental delay. Leave sensation testing until last. Ideally, fundoscopy needs mydriatics, a dark room and (occasionally) sedation.
- **Motor system:** Always examine infants for dislocated/dislocatable hips. Check the gait.
- **Urine:** Test for protein, glucose and blood, and ideally for infection using a microscope or appropriate stick tests.

Patients and parents have the right to be told any abnormal findings, and the actual process of the examination should be explained to the patient in age-appropriate language.

The history and examination findings, including the patient's weight and height, should be recorded, with daily entries on management and progress. (Be aware of the local guidelines on nutritional assessments, especially in settings where malnutrition is common.) When the patient is discharged they should be given discharge information about the admission and any further treatment and advice that needs to be shared with their primary care healthcare workers.

See Section 9 (Appendix) for examples of various charts, including those for vital signs, fluid balance, growth and body mass index (BMI).

1.10 Triage: seeing the sickest first

Triage involves **determining the priority of a patient's treatment based on the severity of their condition, not on when they arrived or their place in a queue.**

Introduction

The word 'triage' comes from the French word 'trier' (meaning 'to sort'). It is the process by which patients presenting to a health facility with an illness or injury are assigned a clinical priority. It is an essential step in clinical risk management, as it means that, if done correctly, those patients who are most in need of care receive it first. Triage should have a robust mechanism to ensure that patients at imminent risk of death or who are seriously ill or injured, requiring immediate resuscitation or emergency management, are provided with treatment before patients with conditions that are less critical, who can wait for further assessment and treatment.

Triage divides patients into the following three categories:
1 those who are at imminent risk of death, and require immediate resuscitation
2 those who are seriously ill or injured, and who need timely emergency management
3 those who have conditions which can wait before further assessment and possible treatment.

Of course, it is not always immediately apparent which category a patient is in, so most methodologies are based on a rapid physiological assessment of vital functions (airway and breathing, circulatory status and conscious level).

The models of decision making, of which there are many, require three steps:
1 rapid initial assessment
2 determination of the appropriate categories
3 selection of the most appropriate category.

Triage scheme for children and pregnant women
Rapid initial assessment

When a woman or girl who is or might be pregnant presents to a health facility she is of immediate concern and should be given priority through triage without disadvantaging seriously affected men or older women. Infants and children can also become dangerously ill quickly, and therefore need urgent triage.

This process requires the ability to recognise, first, those patients who need resuscitation (**immediate management, group 1, 'red'**), and, second, those who need **urgent treatment (group 2, 'orange')** (*see* Table 1.10.1). This process must take only a few seconds, as any delay can be fatal.

TABLE 1.10.1 A possible triage scale (adapted from the Advanced Life Support Group)

Triage number	Type of action	Colour	Maximum target time to action (minutes)
Category 1	Immediate	Red	0
Category 2	Urgent	Orange	15
Category 3	Non-urgent	Green	60 (1 hour)

From the moment of arrival at the health facility (some information may be given before arrival, by contact between the ambulance crew and the facility), a decision on those who need resuscitation must be made. The decision making is based on the clinical signs listed in the second column of Tables 1.10.2 and 1.10.3.

Once a triage category has been identified, the patient should have observations of respiration rate and characteristics (e.g. wheeze, stridor, recession), pulse rate, blood pressure, temperature and a rapid measure of conscious level, such as AVPU score (Alert, responds to Voice, responds to Pain, Unconscious; *see* Sections 1.11 and 1.12), measured and recorded.

Table 1.10.2 (for pregnant women) and Table 1.10.3 (for infants and children) show those features which, on rapid examination, determine that immediate resuscitation is required.

TABLE 1.10.2 Clinical signs on simple observation or from the history which indicate the need for immediate resuscitation in pregnant mothers

Underlying mechanism	What does the healthcare worker undertaking triage see in the patient or hear from the relatives?
A problem that is obstructing, or might obstruct, the upper airway A: AIRWAY	The patient is unconscious The patient is fitting or has been fitting There is major trauma to the face or head, including burns There is severe stridor or gurgling in the throat
Any problem producing apnoea, severe respiratory distress or cyanosis B: BREATHING	The patient is not breathing The patient is gasping The patient is cyanosed The patient is having so much difficulty breathing that they cannot speak
Any problem producing cardiac arrest, shock or heart failure C: CIRCULATION	The patient has heavy vaginal bleeding The patient has suffered major trauma The patient appears shocked (very pale/white, cannot sit up, has a reduced conscious level)

TABLE 1.10.3 Clinical signs on simple observation or from the history which indicate the need for immediate resuscitation in infancy and childhood

Underlying mechanism	What does the healthcare worker undertaking triage see in the patient or hear from the parents?
A problem that is obstructing, or might obstruct, the upper airway A: AIRWAY	The patient is unconscious The patient is fitting or has been fitting There is major trauma to the face or head, including burns There is severe stridor or gurgling in the throat The child has inhaled a foreign body which is still in the throat
Any problem producing apnoea, severe respiratory distress or cyanosis B: BREATHING	The patient is not breathing The patient is gasping The patient is cyanosed The patient is having so much difficulty breathing that they cannot speak or vocalise (cry)
Any problem producing cardiac arrest, shock or heart failure C: CIRCULATION	The patient has suffered major trauma The patient appears shocked (very pale/white, cannot sit up, weak, very rapid or absent pulse, and has a reduced conscious level)

Tables 1.10.4 and 1.10.5 list those features which indicate the need for urgent management (orange) within 15 minutes.

TABLE 1.10.4 Clinical signs on simple observation or from the history in a pregnant mother which indicate the need for urgent management but not resuscitation

Underlying mechanism	What does the healthcare worker undertaking triage see or hear from the patient or the relatives?
A problem that might obstruct the upper airway in the future A: AIRWAY	There is trauma to the face or head, or burns to this area, but the patient is conscious and able to speak
	Ingestion or accidental overdose of drugs which may alter the conscious level?
A problem producing respiratory distress B: BREATHING	The patient has difficulty breathing but can speak, and there is no cyanosis
Any problem that might, unless rapidly treated, lead to shock or heart failure C: CIRCULATION	The patient has vaginal bleeding which is heavy*, but is not yet shocked (they are able to stand or sit up and speak normally)
	The patient has suffered major trauma and is not yet shocked, but may have internal bleeding (they are able to stand or sit up and speak normally)
	Any burns covering more than 10% of the body
	The patient has fainted and has abdominal pain (this includes possible ruptured ectopic pregnancy) but they are now able to stand or sit up and speak normally
	The patient has passed products of conception and is still bleeding, but is not shocked (they are able to stand or sit up and speak normally)
	The patient has severe abdominal pain, but is not shocked (they are able to stand or sit up and speak normally)
	The patient is extremely pale, but is not shocked (severe anaemia) (they are able to stand or sit up and speak normally)
Possible severe pre-eclampsia and impending eclampsia	The patient is complaining of a headache and/or visual disturbance
Severe dehydration	The patient is complaining of severe diarrhoea/vomiting and is feeling very weak, but is not shocked (they are able to stand or sit up and speak normally)
Possible complication of pregnancy	The patient has abdominal pain not due to uterine contractions of normal labour
Possible premature labour	The patient is not yet due to deliver, but has had ruptured membranes (with or without contractions)
Infection that might become dangerous	The patient has a high fever > 38°C (they are hot to touch or shivering, but are able to stand or sit up and speak normally)
Possible intrauterine death	After 24 weeks of pregnancy the patient has not felt fetal movements for 24 hours or more
Prolapsed cord	The patient says that her membranes have ruptured and she can feel the umbilical cord

*Heavy bleeding is defined as a clean pad or cloth becoming soaked within less than 5 minutes.

Note that a low blood pressure in a pregnant woman or a child is a late and ominous sign.

Helping to ensure that triage works well

The following actions will help to prevent life-threatening delays:

1 Train all staff (including clerks, guards, door keepers and switchboard operators) to recognise those who need resuscitation.
2 Practise triage and the structured approach to emergencies with all staff in the facility.
3 Ensure that access to care is never blocked. Emergency equipment must always be available (not locked away) and in working order. This requires daily checks and the keeping of logbooks. Essential emergency drugs must be constantly available.
4 Give proper training of appropriate staff in the use of the equipment and drugs required.
5 A special trolley containing equipment and drugs for emergencies must be available at all times.

6 Protocols on the structured approach to emergencies (see below) must be available. Pathways of emergency care should be prominently displayed on the walls in areas where emergencies are managed.
7 Implement systems by which patients with emergencies can be exempted from payment, at least temporarily. These include local insurance schemes and health committee emergency funds. This exemption must be made known to all gatekeepers and security staff.

Special priority signs
Haemorrhage

Haemorrhage is a feature of many presentations, particularly in pregnancy and following trauma.

Category 1 patients (red) are those who are exsanguinating. Death will occur quickly if the bleeding is not arrested.

A haemorrhage that is not rapidly controlled by the application of sustained direct pressure, and which continues to bleed heavily or soak through large dressings quickly, should also be treated **immediately (Category 1, red).**

TABLE 1.10.5 Clinical signs on simple observation or from the history in an infant or child which indicate the need for urgent management but not resuscitation

Underlying mechanism	What does the healthcare worker undertaking triage see or hear from the patient or relatives?
A problem that might obstruct the upper airway in the future A: AIRWAY	There is trauma to the face or head, or burns to this area, but the patient is conscious and able to speak/cry
	An overdose of respiratory depressant substance has or may have been taken
A problem producing respiratory distress B: BREATHING	The patient has difficulty in breathing but can speak/cry and there is no cyanosis
Any problem that might, unless rapidly treated, lead to shock or heart failure C: CIRCULATION	The patient has suffered major trauma and is not yet shocked, but may have internal bleeding (they are able to stand or sit up and speak/cry normally)
	Any burns covering more than 10% of the body
	The patient has fainted and has abdominal pain (a post-pubertal girl might have a ruptured ectopic pregnancy) but they are able to stand or sit up and speak/cry normally
	The patient has severe abdominal pain but is not shocked (they are able to stand or sit up and speak/cry normally)
	The patient is extremely pale but not shocked (severe anaemia) (they are able to stand or sit up and speak/cry normally)
Severe dehydration	The patient has severe diarrhoea/vomiting and is feeling very weak, but is not shocked (they are able to stand or sit up and speak/cry normally); the eyes may be sunken and a prolonged skin retraction time will be present
Infection that might become dangerous	The patient has a high fever > 38°C (they are hot to touch or shivering, but are able to stand or sit up and speak/cry normally)
The child shows evidence of severe malnutrition	Any child with visible severe wasting (especially of the buttocks), and swelling (oedema) of both feet, who is unwell or considered unwell by their parents, but is able to stand or sit up
Any neonate or young infant (less than 2 months old) who is unwell	**This indicates a possibility of dangerous sepsis**

Conscious level

Category 1 or immediate priority (red) includes all unconscious patients (U or P on the AVPU scale).

In patients with a history of unconsciousness or fitting, further dangerous events are possible. Those who respond to voice are categorised as **Category 2 urgent (orange).**

Pain

Patients with severe pain should be allocated to **Category 1 immediate (red)**, and those with any lesser degree of pain should be allocated to **Category 2 urgent (orange)**.

For patients who have sustained **significant trauma or other surgical problems**, anaesthetic and surgical help is required **urgently**.

If there is an **urgent referral** from another healthcare facility or organisation, the patient must be seen **immediately** or **urgently**, depending on the circumstances.

Importance of regular reassessment

Triage categories may change as the patient deteriorates or gets better. It is important, therefore, that the process of triage (clinical prioritisation) is dynamic rather than static.

To achieve this, all clinicians involved in the pathway of care should rapidly assess priority whenever they encounter the patient. Changes in priority must be noted, and the appropriate actions taken.

All patients with symptoms or signs in the **immediate (red)** or **urgent (orange)** categories represent emergencies or potential emergencies, and need to undergo the structured approach to emergencies as outlined in Section 1.11.

Non-urgent cases

Proceed with assessment and further treatment according to the patient's needs once the immediate and urgent patients have been stabilised.

1.11 Structured approach to managing emergencies in pregnancy and childhood

Approach to emergencies

Training

Members of the clinical team must know their roles. They will ideally have trained together in:

- clinical situations and their diagnoses and treatments
- drugs and their use, administration and side effects
- emergency equipment and how it functions.

The ability of a facility to deal with emergencies should be assessed and reinforced by the frequent practice of emergency drills.

Initial management

- Stay calm.
- **Do not leave the patient unattended.**
- Have a team leader in charge to avoid confusion.
- **Shout for help.** Ask one person to go for help and another to get emergency equipment and supplies (e.g. oxygen cylinder and emergency kit). Ideally resuscitation equipment and drugs should be available on one dedicated trolley.
- Assess and resuscitate in sequence using the structured approach – **Airway, Breathing, Circulation, Disability (Neurological Status)** (see below).
- If the patient is conscious, ask what happened and what symptoms they have.
- **Constantly reassess the patient**, particularly after any intervention.

Structured approach to any pregnant woman, infant or child presenting as an emergency

Approach emergencies using the structured ABCD (Airway, Breathing, Circulation, Disability) approach, which ensures that all patients with a life-threatening or potentially life-threatening problem are identified and managed in an effective and efficient way whatever their diagnosis or pathology.

The structured approach to the seriously ill patient, which is outlined here, allows the health worker to focus on the appropriate level of diagnosis and treatment during the first hours of care. Primary assessment and resuscitation are concerned with the maintenance of vital functions and the administration of life-saving treatments, whereas secondary assessment and emergency treatment allow more specific urgent therapies to be started.

Secondary assessment and emergency care require a system-by-system approach in order to minimise the risk of significant conditions being missed.

Following cardiac and/or respiratory arrest, the outcome both for pregnant women and for children is poor. Earlier recognition and management of potential respiratory, circulatory or central neurological failure which may progress rapidly to cardiac and/or respiratory arrest will reduce mortality and secondary morbidity. The following

section outlines the physical signs that should be used for the rapid primary assessment, resuscitation, secondary assessment and emergency treatment of pregnant women, and of babies and children.

Primary assessment and resuscitation involves sequential assessment and resuscitation of vital functions – Airway, Breathing and Circulation.

If there are no life-threatening signs, the primary assessment can be completed within about 1 minute. If life-threatening signs are identified, resuscitation procedures are required.

If you are working on your own and have been unable to summon help, you must resuscitate Airway before Breathing, and Breathing before Circulation. This is because oxygen cannot be carried around in the blood to the vital organs if the blood is not oxygenated first, and the lungs cannot oxygenate the blood if there is no airway to allow air containing oxygen to enter the lungs.

If assistance is available, one person can deal with Airway, another with Breathing and a third with Circulation, all working simultaneously, but there must be a 'team leader' to take overall control.

During resuscitation, interventions that are either life-saving or designed to prevent the patient reaching a near-death situation are performed (see below). These include such procedures as basic airway opening procedures, suction, oropharyngeal airway insertion, intubation, assisted ventilation, venous cannulation and fluid resuscitation (when safe and appropriate). At the same time, oxygen is provided to all patients with life-threatening Airway, Breathing or Circulatory problems, vital signs are recorded, and essential monitoring is established.

This sequential primary assessment and any necessary resuscitation occur **before** any illness-specific diagnostic assessment or treatment takes place. Once the patient's vital functions are working safely, secondary assessment and emergency treatment can begin.

After each intervention, its effects should be tested by reassessment. Regular reassessments are a key component of the structured approach.

During **secondary assessment**, illness-specific pathophysiology is sought and emergency treatments are instituted. Before embarking on this phase, it is important that the resuscitative measures are fully under way. During the secondary assessment, vital signs should be checked frequently to detect any change in the patient's condition. If there is deterioration, primary assessment and resuscitation should be repeated in the in the 'Airway, Breathing, Circulation' sequence.

Primary assessment and resuscitation

Assessment and resuscitation occur at the same time. The order of assessment and resuscitation enables identification of immediately life-threatening problems, which are treated as they are found.

A rapid examination of vital ABC functions is required. **If at any stage a life-threatening A, B, or C problem is identified: CALL FOR HELP.**

After ABC, always assess for neurological problems, and resuscitate their components (sometimes referred to as 'D' for disability of the ABC approach).

Primary assessment and resuscitation of airway

The first priority is establishment or maintenance of airway opening. If there is a need for resuscitation in a patient who is bleeding (e.g. in cases of massive postpartum haemorrhage or trauma), try to stop this at the same time as you are opening the airway.

PRIMARY ASSESSMENT

LOOK – for chest or abdominal movement.
LISTEN – for breath sounds.
FEEL – for breath.
Talk to the patient.
A patient who can speak or cry has a clear airway.

Signs associated with airway obstruction may include any of the following:

- an absence of breathing
- stridor, snoring, or gurgling in the throat
- cyanosis
- chest wall recession
- agitation, reduced consciousness, or coma.

Be alert for foreign bodies (*see* Section 1.12 on choking).

Airway obstruction is most commonly due to obstruction by the tongue in an unconscious patient.

Resuscitation

Open the airway and keep it open.

If there is no evidence of air movement, open the airway using the following:

- a head tilt, chin lift or jaw thrust manoeuvre (*see* Section 1.12 on basic life support). If this opens the airway and breathing starts, keep the airway open manually until it can be secured. Be careful when using head tilt if the cervical spine is at risk, but **opening the airway is always the priority**
- suction/removal of blood, vomit or a foreign body.

If there is no improvement after adjusting the airway manually and trying different techniques, place **an oropharyngeal airway**, which may be helpful **if the patient is unconscious and has no gag reflex**. Avoid using a nasopharyngeal airway if there is any suspicion of base of skull injury.

If the airway is still obstructed, a definitive airway by intubation or surgical airway may be needed.

Give oxygen to all patients.

Be careful not to distress young children with partial upper airway obstruction due to infections such as epiglottitis and severe croup, as this may precipitate acute worsening of their airway obstruction. Having a parent or other known adult present will help to keep the child calm.

Identify the 'at-risk' airway

Reassess the airway after any airway-opening manoeuvres. If there continues to be no evidence of air movement, then airway opening can be assessed by performing an airway-opening manoeuvre while giving rescue breaths. Proceed to Breathing (see below).

Advanced airway management

Advanced airway management techniques for securing the airway by **intubation** may be required in patients with any of the following:

- persistent airway obstruction
- altered level of consciousness, with failure to protect the airway, especially from vomiting
- facial trauma, including burns, penetrating neck trauma with expanding haematoma, and severe head injury (*see* Section 7).

This should be performed by skilled professionals such as an anaesthetist (if available) (*see* Section 1.24 for details). The following sequence should be followed:

1 pre-oxygenation with 100% oxygen with manual lung inflation if required
2 administration of a carefully judged, reduced dose of an anaesthetic induction agent
3 application of cricoid pressure
4 suxamethonium 1–2 mg/kg
5 intubation with a correctly sized tracheal tube.

Confirmation of correct placement of the tube

Signs such as chest movement and auscultation remain helpful, but are occasionally misleading, especially in inexperienced hands. The most important point is to see the tube pass through the vocal cords. The correct size is a tube that can be placed easily through the cords with only a small leak. Intubation of the right main bronchus is best avoided by carefully placing the tube only 2–3 cm below the cords and noting the length at the teeth before checking by auscultation (best in the left and right lower axillae). Capnography, if available, is a useful adjunct for helping to confirm correct tube placement.

If it is not possible to provide an airway using intubation, a **surgical airway** may be required.

NOTE: It is extremely risky to proceed to Circulation (and IV/IO cannulation) when partial upper airway obstruction is present in young children (e.g. due to epiglottitis, severe croup or a foreign body), as invasive procedures can precipitate complete airway closure. Stabilise the airway first. This will require help from an anaesthetist.

Emergency treatment situations

1 For **severe croup**, nebulised adrenaline can be helpful (5 mL of 1 in 1000). Always give oral steroid as soon as possible (150 micrograms/kg of dexamethasone or 1 mg/kg of prednisolone).
2 For upper airway obstruction due to **anaphylaxis**, nebulised adrenaline (5 mL of 1 in 1000) and IM adrenaline (1 mg IM in pregnancy and 10 micrograms/kg in children).
3 **Inhaled foreign body** (*see* Section 1.12).
4 For **severe bronchiolitis**, clear the nasal airways by using gentle suction.

If the patient has major trauma or postpartum haemorrhage and is obviously bleeding rapidly, to the point of exsanguination (*see* Section 7.3.A), measures to stop the exsanguination must be instituted at the same time as Airway resuscitation.

Throughout primary assessment and resuscitation, protect the cervical spine with a collar, sand bags and tape if the patient is likely to have an unstable cervical spine and if subsequent surgical stabilisation is possible (*see* Section 7.3.A.).

Primary assessment and resuscitation of breathing

An open airway does not guarantee adequate ventilation. The latter requires an intact respiratory centre and adequate pulmonary function augmented by coordinated movement of the diaphragm and chest wall.

Primary assessment

Assess whether breathing is adequate by:
- assessing **effort:**
  - recession
  - rate
  - added noises
  - accessory muscles
  - alar flaring
- assessing **efficacy:**
  - listening for reduced or absent **breath sounds**, or any wheezing, with a stethoscope or ear on chest wall
  - **chest and/or abdominal expansion** (symmetrical or asymmetrical)
  - abdominal excursion
  - SaO_2 if available
- assessing effects on **heart rate**
- assessing effects on **skin colour** (check the possibility of cyanosis)
- assessing effects on **mental status**.

Evidence of life-threatening respiratory difficulty

This includes the following:
1. absence of breathing (apnoea)
2. very high or very low respiratory rates
3. gasping, which is a sign of severe hypoxaemia, and may indicate impending respiratory arrest and death
4. severe chest wall recession, usually with increased respiratory rate, but pre-terminally with a fall in rate
5. severe hypoxaemia (cyanosis)
6. signs of tension pneumothorax (respiratory distress with hyper-resonant percussion) (*see* Section 7.3.A)
7. major trauma to the chest (e.g. tension pneumothorax, haemothorax, flail chest) (*see* Section 7.3.A)
8. signs of severe asthma (severe respiratory distress with wheezing, but a silent chest in severe asthma can be a near-fatal situation).

Evidence of respiratory difficulty which can progress if not treated

This includes the following:
1. increased respiratory rate
2. inspiratory stridor
3. reduced or absent breath sounds on auscultation
4. expiratory wheezing
5. chest expansion (most important), and reduced abdominal excursion

6. pulse oximetry showing oxygen saturation (SaO_2) of less than 94% (normal SaO_2 in a patient at sea level is 94–100% in air).

Fast breathing is caused by either an airway problem, lung disease or metabolic acidosis.

TABLE 1.11.1 Respiratory rates 'at rest' for different age groups

Age (years)	Respiratory rate (breaths/minute)
< 1	30–40
1–2	25–35
2–5	25–30
5–12	20–25
> 12	15–20
In pregnancy	15–20*

* In pregnancy, respiratory rate does not change although tidal volume increases resulting in approximately 50% increase in minute ventilation.

The WHO suggests a breathing rate of 30 per minute or more in pregnancy as evidence of shock.

Care should be taken when interpreting single measurements. Infants can show rates of between 30 and 90 breaths/minute depending on their state of activity. It is more useful to use trends in measurements as an indicator of improvement or deterioration.

WHO definitions of fast breathing in young children are as follows:
- < 2 months: ≥ 60 breaths/minute
- 2–12 months: ≥ 50 breaths/minute
- 12 months to 5 years: ≥ 40 breaths/minute

Slow breathing rates may result from fatigue or raised intracranial pressure, or may immediately precede a respiratory arrest due to severe hypoxaemia.

Other signs of breathing difficulty
Chest wall recession
- Intercostal, subcostal or sternal recession reflects increased effort of breathing, which is seen in particular in infants, who have more compliant chest walls.
- The degree of recession indicates the severity of respiratory difficulty.
- In the patient with exhaustion, chest movement and recession will decrease.

Inspiratory or expiratory noises
- Stridor, usually inspiratory, indicates laryngeal or tracheal obstruction.
- Wheeze, predominantly expiratory, indicates lower airway obstruction.
- Volume of noise is not an indicator of severity.

Grunting
- This is observed in infants and children with stiff lungs to prevent airway collapse (it represents the noise made by closure of the larynx during expiration, which is the body's attempt to increase lung volume).
- It is a sign of severe respiratory distress.

Accessory muscle use

- In infants, the use of the sternocleidomastoid muscle creates 'head bobbing' and does not help ventilation.
- Flaring of the alae nasi is also seen in infants with respiratory distress.

Exceptions
Increased effort of breathing does not occur in three circumstances:

1 exhaustion
2 central respiratory depression (e.g. from raised intracranial pressure, poisoning or encephalopathy)
3 neuromuscular disease (e.g. poliomyelitis).

Effects of breathing failure on other physiology
Heart rate: this is increased with hypoxia, but decreases when hypoxia is severe, when bradycardia is a sign of impending cardiorespiratory arrest.

Skin colour: hypoxia first causes vasoconstriction and pallor. Cyanosis is a late sign and may indicate impending cardiorespiratory arrest. In an anaemic patient it may never be seen, however hypoxic the patient is.

Mental status: hypoxia causes initial agitation, then drowsiness, followed by loss of consciousness.

Resuscitation of breathing
In the patient with absent or inadequate breathing, it is essential to breathe for the patient using:

- mouth-to-mouth or mouth-to-mouth-and-nose ventilation, *or*
- bag-valve-mask ventilation: if using oxygen, add a reservoir to increase the oxygen concentration.

Intubate (if skilled professionals are available) and provide assisted ventilation through the tube if long-term ventilation is needed or bag–mask ventilation is ineffective.

However, do not persist with intubation attempts without ventilating the patient intermittently with a bag and mask as necessary to prevent hypoxaemia during the intubation process.

Give high-flow oxygen to all patients with respiratory difficulty.

Give as much oxygen as possible through a mask with a reservoir bag to any patient who is breathing but has respiratory difficulty or the other signs of hypoxia (e.g. cyanosis).

Situations in which emergency treatment is given

1 Perform **needle thoracocentesis** if the diagnosis is tension pneumothorax (*see* Figure 8.3.1). This should be followed by a chest drain.
2 Consider inserting a chest drain if there is major trauma to the chest (*see* Figure 8.3.2).
3 Give **nebulised salbutamol** if the patient has severe, life-threatening asthma (2.5 mg for children < 5 years of age, or 5 mg for children > 5 years of age and pregnant mothers). If a nebuliser is not available, use a spacer and metered-dose inhaler (100 micrograms/puff; 10 puffs initially for all age groups).
4 Give **nasal continuous positive airway pressure (CPAP)** if a neonate has severe respiratory distress (*see* Section 8.3).
5 Give **IM adrenaline** (1 mg in pregnancy and 10 micrograms/kg in children) and **nebulised salbutamol** (see above) if wheezing is due to anaphylaxis.
6 Give **anticoagulant** (IV unfractionated heparin) if pulmonary embolus is diagnosed in pregnancy or post delivery (*see* Section 2.5.H).
7 Give **calcium gluconate** (10 mL 10% IV over 10 minutes) if respiratory arrest is due to magnesium toxicity in a patient treated for eclampsia with magnesium sulphate.

Primary assessment and resuscitation of circulation
Primary assessment
The circulatory system is more difficult to assess than airway and breathing, and individual measurements must not be over-interpreted.

If there is no palpable pulse, a very slow heart rate (< 60 beats/minute in an infant, or < 40 beats/minute in a child or pregnant woman) or no 'signs of life' (e.g. movements, coughing, normal breathing), cardiac arrest or near-cardiac arrest is likely, and basic life support must be started (*see* Section 1.12).

Agonal gasps (irregular, infrequent breaths) do not provide adequate oxygenation and are not for these purposes a 'sign of life'.

In addition to cardiac arrest or near-arrest, shock and heart failure are additional life-threatening issues that it is important to identify.

Shock
The following clinical signs can help to identify shock (inadequate circulation) (*see* Sections 2.5.A and 5.5.A).

TABLE 1.11.2 Heart rates 'at rest' at different ages

Age (years)	Heart rate (beats/minute)
< 1	110–160
1–2	100–150
2–5	95–140
5–12	80–120
> 12	60–100
Pregnancy	70–115*

* The heart rate in pregnancy increases by 10–15 beats per minute.

Heart rate

- Heart rate increases in shock and heart failure.
- Severe bradycardia due to hypoxaemia may be a sign of near cardiorespiratory arrest.

The **WHO definition of tachycardia** is a heart rate of > 160 beats/min in children aged under 1 year, and > 120 beats/minute in those aged 1–5 years.

The WHO defines a heart rate in pregnancy of 110 beats per minute or more as evidence of shock.

Pulse volume

Absent peripheral pulses or reduced strength of central pulses can signify shock.

Capillary refill time (CRT)

- Pressure on the centre of the sternum or fingernail for 5 seconds should be followed by return of the circulation to the skin within 3 seconds or less. CRT may be prolonged by shock, cold environment, or the vasoconstriction that occurs as a fever develops.
- Prolonged CRT is not a specific or sensitive sign of shock, and should not be used alone as a guide to the need for or the response to treatment.

Blood pressure

- The cuff should cover at least 80% of the length of the upper arm, and the bladder should be more than two-thirds of the arm's circumference. In pregnant mothers, the largest possible cuff should be used to avoid missing a raised blood pressure.
- Korotkoff phase 5 (K5, disappearance of sound) should be used to measure diastolic pressure. Korotkoff phase 5 (K5A, muffling or softening of sound) should only be used if the sound does not disappear until near to zero cuff pressure.
- In pregnancy the patient should ideally be sitting or lying in the lateral tilt positions when pressure is measured. In both of these positions, the cuff must be level with the heart.
- Hypotension is a late sign of circulatory failure in both children and pregnant mothers, and will be rapidly followed by cardiorespiratory arrest unless it is treated urgently.

TABLE 1.11.3 Systolic and diastolic blood pressure in children

Age (years)	Systolic blood pressure (mmHg) 5th centile	Systolic blood pressure (mmHg) 50th centile
< 1	65–75	80–90
1–2	70–75	85–95
2–5	70–80	85–100
5–12	80–90	90–110
> 12	90–105	100–120

Blood pressure may be difficult to measure and interpret, especially in infants and children under 5 years of age. The following formula can be used to calculate average systolic blood pressure in children (50th centile):

$$85 + (2 \times \text{age in years})$$

WHO defines normal adult BP as 120/80 mmHg. Blood pressure falls early in pregnancy due to a decrease in systemic vascular resistance. It is usually 10 mmHg below baseline and reaches a lowest mean value of 105/60 mmHg in the second trimester. During the third trimester it gradually returns to the pre-pregnancy level at term.

The normal systolic blood pressure in pregnancy is in the range 95–135 mmHg. The normal diastolic blood pressure is in the range 60–85 mmHg.

The WHO suggests a systolic BP of < 90 mmHg in pregnancy as evidence of shock. A systolic BP < 95 mmHg should prompt a search for other possible indicators of developing shock.

The cardiovascular system in children and pregnant mothers compensates well initially in shock.

Hypotension is a late and often sudden sign of decompensation and, if not reversed, will be rapidly followed by death. Serial measurements of blood pressure should be performed frequently.

Effects of circulatory failure on other organs

Respiratory system: tachypnoea and hyperventilation occur as a result of the acidosis caused by poor tissue perfusion.

Skin: pale or mottled skin indicates poor perfusion.

Mental status: circulatory failure causes initial agitation, then drowsiness, followed by unconsciousness.

Urine output: a reduction in urine output to < 2 mL/kg/hour in infants, < 1 mL/kg/hour in children or < 30 mL/hour in pregnant mothers indicates inadequate renal perfusion.

In pregnancy: fetal compromise can be the first sign of shock in the mother.

The **WHO definition of shock** is cold hands, *plus* CRT of > 3 seconds, *plus* a weak and rapid pulse.

Life-threatening shock is usually associated with:

- severe tachycardia
- a weak-volume pulse (ideally assess centrally: brachial, femoral or carotid)
- low blood pressure (this is a late sign, and very difficult to measure in young children)
- extreme central pallor (if due to severe anaemia)
- raised respiratory rate (due to acidosis)
- poor skin circulation, with a CRT of > 3 seconds
- reduced conscious level.

Remember that anaphylaxis is one cause of shock, and typically there is a relevant history and other signs such as angio-oedema and urticaria.

Remember that if shock is due to heart failure, fluid overload will be fatal (for information on how to recognise and manage shock caused by heart failure, *see* Section 2.7.A).

Resuscitation in shock

For cardiac arrest or near arrest, **chest compressions** should be undertaken (for information on basic and advanced life support, *see* Sections 1.12 and 1.13).

Ensure that there is an open and secure airway.

Give **high-flow oxygen** to any patient who has an inadequate circulation (whether due to shock or to heart failure). This should be administered via a face mask with a reservoir bag (or an endotracheal tube if intubation has been necessary).

Venous or intra-osseous access should be obtained and blood for essential tests taken (haemoglobin, cross-matching, blood clotting factors, and urea and electrolytes if possible).

Lateral tilt

In pregnancy and after 20 weeks' gestation (whenever the uterus can be palpated abdominally), place the patient in the left lateral tilt position to prevent uterine pressure on the abdominal and pelvic veins stopping blood return to the heart.

In all patients with shock, lie them flat (or tilted) and **elevate the legs**.

Fluids in shock

In most cases of shock, if obvious bleeding is the cause then the first priority must be to stop this. IV or IO fluids are then required as the immediate resuscitation treatment, once the airway has been opened and secured and oxygen is being given. However, different causes of shock require different approaches to treatment, as described below.

- If loss of fluid causing **hypovolaemia** is the cause of shock: for infants and children give an immediate **IV/IO bolus of 10–20 mL/kg of crystalloid (usually Ringer-lactate or Hartmann's solution)** as appropriate for weight (see below), provided that heart failure is not present (see above). For pregnant women and girls, give an IV bolus **of 500–1000 mL of crystalloid**.

  For a child, weight can be estimated on the basis that birth weight doubles by 5 months, triples by 1 year, and quadruples by 2 years.

  After 12 months of age, the following formula can be applied, but it needs to be modified according to whether the child is small or large compared with the average:

  $$\text{weight (kg)} = 2 \times (\text{age in years} + 4)$$

- If the loss of fluid causing shock is due to **severe gastroenteritis**, there will usually be evidence of severe dehydration and a history of profound or long-standing diarrhoea. Give **20 mL/kg of Ringer-lactate or Hartmann's solution as an initial IV or IO bolus** as rapidly as possible, reassess, and then repeat if necessary. In cases of cholera, up to 60 mL/kg might be required in children, and 3 litres in pregnant mothers. Additional potassium will usually be required (see Section 5.12.A).

- If the loss of fluid causing shock is due to **bleeding**, which is **one of the commonest causes in pregnancy**, give crystalloid immediately and then try to obtain blood for transfusion as rapidly as possible, ideally fresh blood. Give O-negative blood if this is available.

  The concept of **targeted crystalloid fluid resuscitation** is important and requires urgent research into management if the cause of hypovolaemic shock is haemorrhage due to penetrating injury in trauma or to obstetric haemorrhage such as ruptured ectopic pregnancy. Here the initial boluses of IV crystalloids required to treat shock would only be given to keep the vital organs (especially the brain, heart and kidneys) perfused before surgery and/or specific medical treatments to stop the bleeding have started to take effect. Fresh blood is particularly useful to combat the coagulopathy that occurs in major blood loss if specific coagulation components such as platelets are unavailable.

  Giving too much IV crystalloid can increase the blood pressure and theoretically increase bleeding by disrupting early clot formation. IV crystalloid also dilutes the red cells (and coagulation factors) in the circulation, but whether or not this could reduce oxygen-carrying capacity requires further research.

  We suggest that when giving boluses of crystalloid in **shock due to bleeding (before blood is available and before procedures undertaken to stop haemorrhage are effective)** in patients with penetrating major trauma or obstetric haemorrhage, only the amount needed to maintain the blood pressure at a level sufficient to perfuse the vital organs is given. There is no clear evidence to indicate the precise blood pressure that should be achieved in pregnant women or in children who are in

shock due to haemorrhage. **Adequate perfusion of vital organs may best be indicated by a radial pulse that can be palpated and a conscious level of A or V on the AVPU scale (i.e. the woman or child is either awake or will respond by opening their eyes when spoken to). During pregnancy, the adequacy of the fetal heart rate may also be helpful.**

In children under 2–3 years of age, the radial pulse may be difficult to feel and the presence of a palpable brachial pulse may be the best available indicator at present.

In this situation, therefore, and to maintain a palpable radial pulse in pregnancy, start with IV boluses of 500 mL of crystalloid or ideally blood, and reassess after each bolus.

In children, in order to maintain a radial or brachial pulse give 10 mL/kg IV boluses of crystalloid or ideally blood, and reassess after each bolus.

In situations where there is brisk active blood loss and delay in obtaining blood or effective intervention to halt the bleeding, several boluses of crystalloids may be required. The importance of undertaking measures to halt the bleeding and obtaining blood for transfusion rapidly cannot be overstated.

- If shock is due to **septicaemia with purpura** (meningococcus or dengue), give IV or IO boluses of Ringer-lactate or Hartmann's or 0.9% saline as fast as possible, 20 mL/kg in children and 1 litre in pregnant mothers, and then reassess. Usually at least 40 mL/kg in children and 2–3 litres in pregnant mothers will be required to overcome shock (see Section 2.5.A). In this situation, **inotropes may be valuable if they are available and safe to use** (see Section 2.5.A).

- If shock is due to **anaphylaxis**, give **adrenaline**, 10 micrograms/kg (0.1 mL/kg of 1 in 10 000) IM in children and 1 mg (1 mL of 1 in 1000) IM in pregnant mothers, in addition to IV or IO fluid.

- If shock is due to **diabetic ketoacidosis**, there will usually be evidence of severe dehydration and coma. Give **10 mL/kg of 0.9% saline (or Ringer-lactate or Hartmann's solution) as an initial IV bolus** as rapidly as possible, reassess, and then repeat if necessary. Once shock has been initially managed, give fluid more cautiously, as overloading can cause cerebral oedema and death in patients with this condition.

- If shock is due to **severe anaemia**, IV crystalloid boluses such as Ringer-lactate or Hartmann's solution must be given with extreme care (due to the risk of heart failure). As soon as possible, give blood carefully (10 mL/kg in children and 50 mL in pregnant mothers, over 15 minutes) and then reassess and repeat if it is safe to do so.

Partial exchange transfusion may be helpful in this situation, especially if it is possible to access a large superficial vein in the antecubital fossa. Successively remove 20-mL aliquots of the patient's blood and replace each 20 mL with 40 mL of packed donor red blood cells until shock has resolved.

Heart failure

This life-threatening situation can be seen in severe anaemia, after fluid overload, in the presence of structural heart disease and with severe hypertension (usually in pregnancy). It is important to distinguish heart failure from

International Maternal & Child Health Care

shock, as the resuscitation required is different. Some of the following signs will be present in heart failure:

- tachycardia out of proportion to respiratory difficulty
- severe palmar pallor (if anaemia is the cause)
- raised jugular venous pressure
- gallop rhythm on auscultation of the heart
- some heart murmurs (if structural heart defect is responsible)
- an enlarged, sometimes tender, liver
- crepitations on listening to the lung bases
- cyanosis that does not respond to oxygen in the case of infants with cyanotic congenital heart disease.

In pregnancy, **severe hypertension** can cause heart failure (check the blood pressure; patients with values above 170/110 mmHg can present with heart failure).

Resuscitation for heart failure
1 **Sit the patient up.**
2 Give **oxygen**.
3 Give **furosemide** 1–2 mg/kg by IV/IO injection in children and 40 mg IV in pregnant mothers.
4 Consider giving **morphine** (50 micrograms/kg in children and 3 mg in pregnant mothers), and reassess. Morphine should be used with caution, especially in patients with altered mental status and impaired respiratory drive.
5 If the patient has severe anaemia, consider **exchange transfusion**.

Situations where emergency treatment is given in heart failure with shock
1 **Supraventricular tachycardia (usually in a child)** can cause both shock and heart failure. The heart rate will be > 180 beats/minute, and in infants can reach > 220 beats/minute. If available, ECG will confirm tachycardia. Treat by **vagal manoeuvres**, defibrillation if available, or adenosine if rapid IV access is available (*see* Section 5.4.C).
2 In **ventricular tachycardia**, defibrillation is needed if shock is present (*see* Section 1.13).
3 If **congenital** or **rheumatic heart disease** or **cardiomyopathy** is the cause of heart failure, inotropes or digoxin may be appropriate, but specialist advice will be needed.
4 If cyanotic congenital heart disease in the newborn is the cause of shock, give prostaglandin E2, but specialist paediatric advice will be necessary (*see* Section 5.4.A).

Primary assessment and resuscitation of neurological failure (disability)
Always assess and treat Airway, Breathing and Circulation problems before undertaking neurological assessment.

Primary assessment
Conscious level: AVPU

Alert is the normal state for an awake person. If the patient does not respond to **Voice** (i.e. being spoken to and asked 'Are you all right?'), it is important that assessment of the response to **Pain** is undertaken next. A painful central stimulus can be delivered by sternal pressure, by supraorbital ridge pressure or by pulling frontal hair. A patient who is **Unresponsive** or who only responds to pain has a significant degree of coma which can seriously interfere with vital Airway and Breathing functions.

Fits
Generalised convulsions, also known as 'fits' or 'seizures', can seriously interfere with vital Airway and Breathing functions, both during the fit itself and immediately afterwards, when lowered levels of consciousness may be present.

Posture
Many patients who have a serious illness in any system are hypotonic. Stiff posturing, such as that shown by decorticate (flexed arms, extended legs) or decerebrate (extended arms, extended legs) posturing, is a sign of serious brain dysfunction. **These postures can be mistaken for the tonic phase of a convulsion.** Alternatively, a painful stimulus may be necessary to elicit these postures.

Severe extension of the neck due to upper airway obstruction can mimic the opisthotonus that occurs with meningeal irritation. In infants, a stiff neck and full fontanelle are signs that suggest meningitis.

Pupils
Many drugs and cerebral lesions have effects on pupil size and reactions. However, the most important pupillary signs to seek are dilatation, unreactivity and inequality, which suggest possible serious brain disorders.

Always check blood glucose levels or suspect hypoglycaemia in any unwell infant or young child, especially if they have impaired consciousness.

Hypoglycaemia with a blood glucose level of less than 2.5 mmol/L (45 mg/dL) can cause impaired consciousness, coma or fits.

Respiratory effects of central neurological failure
The presence of any abnormal respiratory pattern in a patient with coma suggests mid- or hindbrain dysfunction.

Circulatory effects of central neurological failure
Systemic hypertension with sinus bradycardia (Cushing's response) indicates compression of the medulla oblongata caused by herniation of the cerebellar tonsils through the foramen magnum. **This is a late and pre-terminal sign.**
Raised intracranial pressure (ICP) may cause:
- hyperventilation
- slow sighing respirations
- apnoea
- hypertension
- bradycardia.

Resuscitation
1 If the patient is unconscious (P or U on the AVPU scale) but their airway and breathing are adequate, place them in the **recovery position**, so that if they vomit there is less likelihood of aspiration because when unconscious, the gag reflex may not be operative.
2 If the patient is unconscious or fitting, **always give oxygen**.
3 If **hypoglycaemia** is a cause of reduced consciousness (or a suspected cause, but immediate blood glucose measurements are not possible), treatment with glucose is urgently required. Give 2–5 mL/kg of 10% glucose IV or IO in children (*see* Section 5.8.B) and 100 mL of 25% glucose IV or IO in pregnant mothers. (Make 100 mL of 25% glucose by adding 50 mL of 50% glucose to 50 mL of Ringer-lactate or Hartmann's solution).
If IV or IO access is not immediately available in a

40

child, give sublingual sugar, 1 teaspoonful moistened with 1 to 2 drops of water. **Children should be monitored for early swallowing which leads to delayed absorption, and in this case another dose of sugar should be given.** Continue to attempt IV or IO access, as parenteral glucose is a more reliable method of treating hypoglycaemia.

If sublingual sugar is given, repeat the doses at 20-minute intervals.

Recheck the blood glucose level after 20 minutes, and if the level is low (< 2.5 mmol/litre or < 45 mg/dL), repeat the IV/IO glucose (5 mL/kg) or repeat the sublingual sugar.

4 If fitting occurs in pregnancy, give **magnesium sulphate** (*see* Section 2.5.E).

5 If fitting occurs in an infant or child and continues in your presence for more than 5 minutes and there is no hypoglycaemia, give **IV or rectal anticonvulsants**. Always make sure that a bag and mask are available in case the patient stops breathing, which is a possibility. Commonly used anticonvulsants in this situation are diazepam or, if there is no IV access, rectal diazepam, rectal paraldehyde or buccal midazolam (*see* Section 5.16.E).

   ● IV or IO diazepam: 250 micrograms/kg IV over 5 minutes
   ● rectal diazepam: 500 micrograms/kg
   ● rectal paraldehyde: 0.4 mL/kg
   ● buccal midazolam: 300 micrograms/kg.

6 To gain time in **acutely raised intracranial pressure** (e.g. in cases of head injury), consider the use of IV **mannitol**, 250 –500 mg/kg, which will draw fluid out of the brain for a short while, thereby temporarily reducing the ICP. Because the effect of mannitol is only short-lived (a matter of hours), it is used to gain time while definitive care is being set up (e.g. surgical intervention to drain an extradural or subdural haematoma).

7 In any case where **meningitis** or **encephalitis** is suspected, it is vital that suitable antibiotics and/or antiviral drugs are started IV or IO as soon as the condition is suspected (*see* Sections 2.7.E, 3.4, 5.16.B and 5.16.C). Antibiotic choices might include **cefotaxime** or **chloramphenicol**, **penicillin**, **amoxicillin** and **gentamicin** in the newborn. Consider adjunctive treatment with dexamethasone 150 micrograms/kg every 6 hours for 4 days starting before or with the first antibiotic dose. Do not use dexamethasone in cases where there is also septic shock (e.g. in meningococcal disease).

Secondary assessment and emergency treatments

The secondary assessment takes place once vital functions have been assessed and the initial resuscitation of those vital functions has been started. Primary assessment and resuscitation can usually be undertaken in less than 1 minute if the patient does not have a life-threatening airway, breathing, circulation or neurological problem.

Secondary assessment includes a focused medical history, a focused clinical examination and specific investigations. It differs from a standard medical history and examination in that it is designed to establish which emergency treatments might benefit the patient. Time is limited, and a focused approach is essential. At the end of secondary assessment, the practitioner should have a better understanding of the illness or component of injury likely to be affecting the patient, and may have formulated a differential diagnosis. Emergency treatments will be appropriate at this stage – to treat either specific disorders (e.g. asthma) or conditions (e.g. raised intracranial pressure). Emergency treatments will be undertaken at this stage in addition to those given as part of resuscitation/life-saving treatments, in order to manage specific components of serious illnesses or injuries (e.g. steroids for asthma, Caesarean section for antepartum haemorrhage). The establishment of a definite diagnosis is part of definitive care.

The history often provides the vital clues. In the case of infants and children, the history is often obtained from an accompanying parent, although a history should be sought from the child if possible. Do not forget to ask any health worker who has seen the patient about the initial condition and about treatments and the response to treatments that have already been given.

Some patients will present with an **acute exacerbation/complication of a known condition**, such as pregnancy, asthma or epilepsy. Such information is helpful in focusing attention on the appropriate system, but the practitioner should be wary of dismissing new pathologies in such patients. The structured approach avoids this problem. Unlike trauma (*see* Section 7), illness affects systems rather than anatomical areas. The secondary assessment must reflect this, and the history of the complaint should be sought with special attention to the presenting system or systems involved. After the presenting system has been dealt with, all of the other systems should be assessed and any additional emergency treatments commenced as appropriate.

The secondary assessment is not intended to complete the diagnostic process, but rather it aims to identify any problems that require emergency treatment.

An outline of a structured approach in the first hour of emergency management is given below. It is not exhaustive, but addresses the majority of emergency conditions that are amenable to specific emergency treatments in this time period.

The symptoms, signs and treatments relevant to each emergency condition are elaborated further in the relevant sections of the textbook.

Secondary assessment of airway and breathing

TABLE 1.11.4 Airway and breathing: signs and symptoms

Common symptoms	Clinical signs	Emergency investigations
Breathlessness	Bubbly noises in throat	Oxygen saturation
Coryza	Cyanosis	Blood culture (if infection is suspected)
Tachypnoea	Recession	
Choking	Noisy breathing – stridor	Chest X-ray (selective)
Cough	Drooling and inability to drink	
Abdominal pain		
Chest pain	Wheeze	
Apnoea	Tracheal shift	
Feeding difficulties	Abnormal percussion note	

(continued)

Common symptoms	Clinical signs	Emergency investigations
Hoarseness Chest pain	Crepitations on auscultation Acidotic breathing Grunting	ECG (if pulmonary embolus is suspected) (selected and if available)

Examples of emergency treatment for airway and breathing

- If in a young child there is a harsh stridor associated with a barking cough and severe respiratory distress, upper airway obstruction due to **severe croup** should be suspected. **Nebulised adrenaline** will already have been given as resuscitation, but now give **oral prednisolone** as emergency treatment (*see* Section 5.1.A).
- If there is a quiet stridor and drooling in a sick-looking child, consider **epiglottitis** or **bacterial tracheitis**. **Intubation** is likely to be urgently required, preferably by an anaesthetist, and is initial resuscitation if the airway is completely closed. Do not put the airway at risk by performing unpleasant or frightening interventions. **Give intravenous antibiotics as emergency treatment, but only after the airway has been secured** (*see* Section 5.1.A). A surgical airway may also be needed as emergency treatment or as resuscitation if intubation is not possible, so contact a surgeon.
- With a sudden onset and significant history of inhalation, consider a laryngeal foreign body. If the 'choking' protocol has been unsuccessful, the patient may require laryngoscopy (*see* Section 1.12). Do not put the airway at risk by performing unpleasant or frightening interventions, but contact an anaesthetist/ENT surgeon urgently. However, in extreme, life-threatening cases, immediate direct laryngoscopy as part of resuscitation to remove a visible foreign body with Magill's forceps may be necessary.
- Stridor following ingestion or injection of a known allergen suggests **anaphylaxis** (*see* Section 5.1.B). Patients in whom this is likely should have received IM and nebulised adrenaline (**10 micrograms/kg for a child** and 1 mg for an adult) as resuscitation treatment. IV or oral **steroids** would then be part of emergency treatment.
- Patients with a history of asthma or with wheeze, significant respiratory distress and/or hypoxia should receive inhaled salbutamol and oxygen as resuscitation, but then need **oral steroids and further inhaled bronchodilators** as emergency treatment (*see* Section 5.2.B).
- Infants with wheeze and respiratory distress are likely to have bronchiolitis, and require oxygen, as well as clearing of nasal secretions as resuscitation, and **IV or NG fluids** as emergency treatment (*see* Section 5.2.A).
- In acidotic breathing, measure blood glucose levels to confirm diabetic ketoacidosis. A bolus of IV Ringer-lactate or Hartmann's solution will already have been given as resuscitation for any shock due to dehydration, and **insulin** can now be given as emergency treatment (*see* Section 5.8.A).
- In clinically suspected pulmonary embolus in pregnancy, IV **unfractionated heparin** should be given as resuscitation, and subcutaneous **low-molecular-weight heparin** should be given as emergency treatment (*see* Section 2.5.H).

Secondary assessment of circulation

TABLE 1.11.5 Circulation: signs and symptoms

Common symptoms	Signs	Emergency investigations
Haemorrhage Breathlessness Palpitations Feeding difficulties Abdominal pain Chest pain Apnoea Feeding difficulties Hoarseness Drowsiness	Tachycardia or bradycardia Abnormal pulse volume or rhythm Abnormal skin perfusion or colour Haemorrhage or hidden haemorrhage Severe malnutrition Fever Hypotension or hypertension Cyanosis Pallor Enlarged liver Lung crepitations Reduced urine output Cardiac murmur Peripheral oedema Raised jugular venous pressure Gallop rhythm on auscultation of the heart Dehydration Purpuric rash	Oxygen saturation Blood culture (if infection is suspected) Chest X-ray (selective) ECG (selective and if available) Haemoglobin Urea and electrolytes (if available) Clotting studies (if available) Malarial parasites

Examples of emergency treatment for circulation

- Further IV/IO **boluses of fluid** should be considered in shocked patients with hypovolaemia from gastroenteritis or with sepsis who have not shown a sustained improvement in response to the first bolus given at resuscitation (*see* Sections 2.5.A, 5.5.B and 5.5.C).
- However, in trauma, if there is uncontrolled internal bleeding, **early surgical intervention** has priority, and too much IV fluid may be harmful. **Continued blood transfusion** is an emergency treatment after the initial resuscitation (*see* Section 7.3.A).
- Consider **inotropes, intubation and central venous pressure monitoring**, if available, as emergency treatment for shock (*see* Section 2.5.A).
- Consider **IV broad-spectrum antibiotics** as emergency treatment for shock in patients with no obvious fluid loss, as sepsis is likely. Antibiotics are essential if purpura is present, as a diagnosis of meningococcal infection is likely (*see* Section 6.1.G).
- If a patient has a cardiac arrhythmia, the appropriate protocol should be followed after initial resuscitation (*see* Section 5.4.C).
- If anaphylaxis is suspected, IM adrenaline 10 micrograms/kg in children, or 1 mg in pregnant mothers, in addition to fluid boluses, should be given as resuscitation treatment, and **steroids and antihistamines** should be given as emergency treatment (*see* Sections 5.1.B and 2.7.C).
- Targeted treatment is needed for obstetric emergencies

that are known to cause shock. These include sepsis (for which **antibiotics** are needed), and antepartum or postpartum haemorrhage (for which specific treatment including **medication** and **urgent surgery** is needed together with **replacement of lost blood** (*see* Sections 2.5.D.i, iii and iv).

- Surgical advice and interventions for certain gastrointestinal emergencies such as volvulus would constitute emergency treatment. The following symptoms and signs may suggest intra-abdominal emergencies: vomiting, abdominal pain, abdominal tenderness and/or rigidity, lack of bowel sounds, rectal bleeding, abdominal mass (*see* Section 5.19).

Secondary assessment of neurological failure (disability)

TABLE 1.11.6 Neurological failure: signs and symptoms

Common symptoms	Signs	Emergency investigations
Headache Drowsiness Vomiting Behavioural changes Visual disturbance	Altered conscious level Convulsions Bradycardia Altered pupil size and reactivity Abnormal postures Meningism Fever Papilloedema or retinal haemorrhage Altered deep tendon reflexes Hypertension	Blood glucose Oxygen saturation Blood culture (if infection is suspected) Haemoglobin Urea and electrolytes (if available) Malarial parasites

Examples of emergency treatment for neurological failure

- If hypoglycaemia with a blood glucose level of less than 2.5 mmol/L (45 mg/dL) is a possible diagnosis, it will have been treated as part of resuscitation, but the prevention of further hypoglycaemia by IV glucose infusion represents emergency treatment. Remember that there will be a reason for the hypoglycaemia, so further monitoring and treatment are needed until the child is drinking appropriate fluids or has an IV infusion in place through which dextrose can be given.

- If convulsions persist after initial anticonvulsant drugs, treatment with further doses of anticonvulsants (*see* Sections 2.5.E, 2.7.E and 5.16.E) represents emergency treatment.
- If there is evidence of raised intracranial pressure (i.e. decreased conscious level, abnormal posturing and/or abnormal ocular motor reflexes), the patient should receive oxygen and bag-valve-mask ventilation as resuscitation, if they have apnoea or slow or poor breathing. Emergency treatment could include:
  - nursing with head in-line and 20–30 degrees head-up position (to aid cerebral venous drainage)
  - repeat IV infusion with mannitol 250–500 mg/kg over 15 minutes; however, the treatment becomes less effective with each dose (*see* Section 7.3.C)
  - in more long-standing raised ICP, caused by tumours in the brain, dexamethasone will help to reduce raised ICP for a few days while specialist neurosurgical intervention is sought, or as palliation (*see* Section 5.14). The initial dose is 25 mg for patients over 35 kg and 20 mg for patients less than 35 kg, followed by a sliding scale of 4 mg every 3 hours for 3 days, then every 6 hours for 1 day, and continuing to decrease by 1–2 mg per day.
- In patients with a depressed conscious level or convulsions, antibiotics are urgently required, but then consider encephalitis and give acyclovir as appropriate, as emergency treatment (*see* Sections 2.7.E and 5.16.C).
- In unconscious patients with pinpoint pupils, consider the possibility of opiate poisoning. After supporting breathing if necessary, a trial of naloxone should be given as emergency treatment (*see* Section 1.15).

Developmental and family history

Particularly in a small child or infant, knowledge of the child's developmental progress and immunisation status may be useful. The family circumstances may also be helpful, and asking about these may sometimes prompt parents to remember other details of the family's medical history.

Drugs and allergies

Any medication that the patient is currently taking, or has taken, should be recorded. In addition, if poisoning is a possibility, ask about any medication in the home that a child might have had access to. A history of allergies should be sought.

1.12 Basic life support for children and pregnant mothers

Introduction

Basic life support (BLS) is a technique that can be employed by one or more rescuers to support the respiratory and circulatory functions of a collapsed patient using no or minimum equipment.

Resuscitation from cardiac arrest in pregnant women and in children

The international guidelines for resuscitation from cardiac arrest (European Resuscitation Council, 2010) detail two approaches to basic life support. One is for adults and the other for children.

The 'adult' programme is predicated on resuscitation from a sudden cardiac event (e.g. ventricular fibrillation from a coronary occlusion) in a patient who was ventilating before the event and therefore has oxygen in their blood. In this group, chest compressions to move the oxygenated blood into the coronary and cerebral arteries are of prime importance, and therefore the rescuer's sequence of actions after assessment starts with chest compressions, not rescue breaths.

The sequence of actions in the 'child' programme is predicated on a hypoxic event (including any respiratory failure or obstruction, or hypoxia at a cellular level as seen in shock). In this type, re-establishing oxygenation is of prime importance, and moving the oxygenated blood to the coronary and cerebral arteries is the second step. Therefore the rescuer's sequence of actions after assessment starts with rescue breaths and then moves on to chest compressions.

The 'child'-type cardiac arrest is seen in almost all children (excluding those rare arrhythmic events in children with congenital or acquired heart disease and those in whom sudden, unexpected collapse is preceded by apparent normal respiratory and circulatory function), and in adults who have a terminal acute illness involving respiratory or circulatory pathology. This includes patients who have had convulsions, trauma (including drowning), poisoning, bleeding, sepsis, etc.

In addition, international guidelines on resuscitation from cardiac arrest agree that, where possible, guidelines should be simplified as there is evidence that complex guidelines cause 'provider paralysis', resulting in no or poor life-saving effort being made.

In view of the above, the Advanced Life Support Group

(ALSG)/Maternal Childhealth Advocacy International (MCAI) programme for resource-limited countries teaches a programme of basic life support for infants, children and pregnant mothers which reflects the known pathologies in these groups (i.e. respiratory and circulatory causes of cardiac arrest) and recognises that the clinicians who provide resuscitation attend patients of all ages.

The sequence taught therefore includes five preliminary rescue breaths and a subsequent ratio of 15:2.

Because of minor differences in technique based on anatomical differences between the groups, children are classified into two groups:

- infants (< 1 year of age)
- children between 1 year of age and puberty.

Basic life support for infants, children and pregnant mothers (see Figures 1.12.1 and 1.12.2)

The initial approach: the three S's

Safety: it is essential that the rescuer does not become a second victim. Therefore they should approach the patient with care, and remove the patient from any continuing source of danger if necessary.

Stimulate: ask the question 'Are you all right?' in order to establish the state of consciousness of the patient.

Shout: this is essential because help will be needed.

If more than one rescuer is present, one person should start basic life support. The second person should activate the Emergency Medical Services (EMS) system and then returns to assist in the basic life support effort.

If the patient is an infant or pre-pubertal child, and there

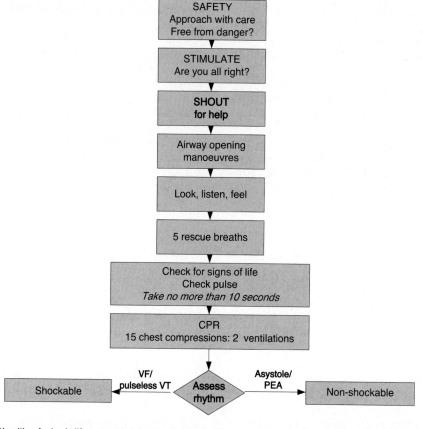

FIGURE 1.12.1 Algorithm for basic life support in infants and children. CPR, cardiopulmonary resuscitation; VF, ventricular fibrillation; VT, ventricular tachycardia; PEA, pulseless electrical activity.

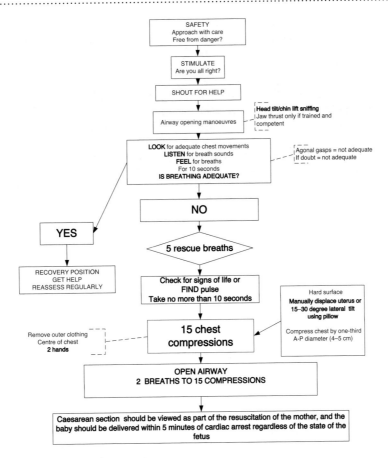

FIGURE 1.12.2 Algorithm for basic life support in pregnant women.

is only one rescuer and no help has arrived, the rescuer should open the airway, deliver the five rescue breaths and give 1 minute of cardiopulmonary resuscitation (CPR), and then activate the EMS system (if one is available) using a mobile phone if available so as to continue CPR. If a mobile is not available and the patient is a baby, the rescuer will probably be able to carry them to a telephone while continuing CPR.

Similarly, if the patient is a pregnant mother, and there is only one rescuer, they should activate the EMS system, where one is available, if no help has arrived in response to the initial shout for help after opening the airway, delivering the five rescue breaths and giving 1 minute of CPR.

'Are you all right?'

An initial simple assessment of responsiveness consists of asking the patient 'Are you all right?' and gently shaking them by the shoulder. Infants may make some noise or open their eyes.

In cases associated with trauma, or possible trauma, the cervical spine should be immobilised during this procedure by placing one hand firmly on the forehead while one of the patient's shoulders is shaken.

Airway-opening actions

An obstructed airway may be the primary problem, and correction of the obstruction can result in recovery without the need for further intervention. If the patient is unconscious but breathing, the recovery position should be used. For pregnant mothers the left lateral position must be adopted (see Section 2.5).

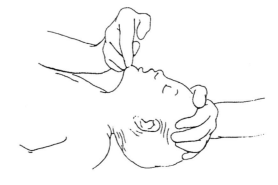

FIGURE 1.12.3 Head tilt with chin lift in neutral position for the infant.

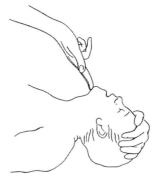

FIGURE 1.12.4 Head tilt with chin lift in 'sniffing' position for the child and mother.

If the patient is not breathing, this may be because the airway is blocked by the tongue falling back and obstructing the pharynx. Attempt to open the airway using the **head tilt/chin lift manoeuvre**. The rescuer places their nearest hand on the patient's forehead, and applies pressure to tilt the head back gently. The correct positions are **'neutral' in the infant (0–1 year of age)** (see Figure 1.12.3) or **'sniffing' (nose up in the air) in the child or pregnant mother** (see Figure 1.12.4).

The fingers of the other hand should then be placed under the chin, and the chin of the supine patient should be lifted upwards. As this action may close the patient's mouth, it may be necessary to use the thumb of the same hand to part the lips slightly.

As an alternative to the head tilt/chin lift, the **jaw thrust manoeuvre** can be very effective, but requires more training and experience.

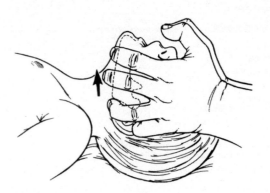

FIGURE 1.12.5 Jaw thrust to open airway.

Jaw thrust is achieved by placing two or three fingers under the angle of the mandible bilaterally, and lifting the jaw upward (see Figure 1.12.5). This is potentially safer than the head tilt/chin lift if there is a history of major trauma, as the latter manoeuvre may exacerbate a cervical spine injury.

BUT airway opening is always the most important action which must be achieved, and should always take precedence over concerns about a possible cervical spine injury.

Patency of the airway should then be assessed by:

- **looking** for adequate chest movements
- **listening** for breath sounds
- **feeling** for breaths.

This is best achieved by the rescuer placing their face above that of the patient, with the ear over the nose, the cheek over the mouth, and the eyes looking along the line of the chest. They should take no longer than 10 seconds to assess breathing.

If there is anything obvious in the mouth and it is easy to reach, remove it.

Do not perform a blind finger sweep in the mouth. A blind finger sweep can damage the soft palate, and foreign bodies may be forced further down the airway and become lodged below the vocal cords.

Breathing actions

If airway-opening techniques do not result in the resumption of adequate breathing within 10 seconds, and a self-inflating bag–mask system is not available, then the rescuer should commence mouth-to-mouth or mouth-to-mouth-and-nose exhaled air resuscitation.

Definition of adequate breathing

A patient may have very slow or shallow breathing, or take infrequent, noisy, agonal gasps. Do not confuse this with normal breathing.

Rescue breaths

If in doubt about the adequacy of breathing, five initial rescue breaths should be given. While the airway is held open, the rescuer breathes in and seals their mouth around the patient's mouth or mouth and nose (in the case of infants) (see Figures 1.12.6 and 1.12.7). If the mouth alone is used, the nose should be pinched using the thumb and index finger of the hand maintaining head tilt. Slow exhalation, 1–2 seconds, by the rescuer should result in the patient's chest rising. The rescuer should take a further breath him- or herself before the next rescue breath.

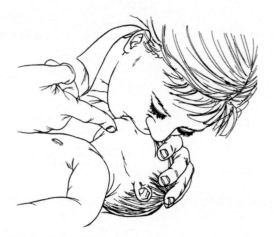

FIGURE 1.12.6 Mouth-to-mouth and nose breaths in neutral position for an infant.

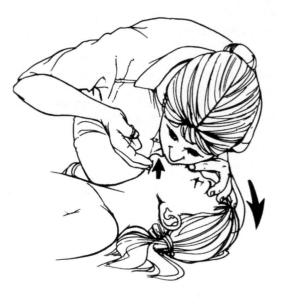

FIGURE 1.12.7 Mouth-to-mouth breaths with pinched nose in sniffing position for a child or mother.

As children and mothers vary in size, only general guidance can be given regarding the volume and pressure of inflation (see Box 1.12.1).

If the chest does not rise, the airway is not clear. The usual cause is failure to correctly apply the airway-opening techniques discussed earlier. The first step is to readjust the head tilt/chin lift position and try again. If this is not successful, jaw thrust should be tried. If two rescuers are present, one should maintain the airway while the other breathes for the patient.

Failure of both head tilt/chin lift and jaw thrust should lead to suspicion that a foreign body is causing the obstruction (see below).

While performing rescue breaths, the presence of a gag reflex or coughing is a positive sign of life (see below).

Circulation actions

Once the initial five breaths have been given successfully, circulation should be assessed and managed.

Check signs of life and/or pulse (take no more than 10 seconds)

Even experienced health professionals can find it difficult to be certain that the pulse is absent within 10 seconds, so the absence of **'signs of life'** is the best indication for starting chest compressions. 'Signs of life' include movement, coughing, gagging or normal breathing (but not agonal gasps, which are irregular, infrequent breaths). Thus the absence of evidence of normal breathing, coughing or gagging (which may be noticed during rescue breaths) or any spontaneous movement is an indication for chest compressions.

Inadequacy of circulation is also indicated by the absence of a central pulse for up to 10 seconds, but it can be difficult and therefore time wasting to be certain about this – hence the current emphasis on assessing the presence of 'signs of life'.

In babies and young children, if a slow pulse (less than 60 beats/minute) is felt, this is still an indication for chest compressions. In children and pregnant mothers, the carotid pulse in the neck can be palpated. However, infants generally have a short fat neck, so the carotid pulse may be difficult to identify. The brachial artery in the medial aspect of the antecubital fossa or the femoral artery in the groin should be felt in infants. If there are no signs of life and/or a pulse is absent for up to 10 seconds, **start chest compressions**. Compressions should also be started if in an infant or young child there is an inadequate heart rate (less than 60 beats/minute), **but only if this is accompanied by signs of poor perfusion**, which include pallor, lack of responsiveness and poor muscle tone.

Start chest compressions if:
- there are no signs of life *or*
- there is no pulse *or*
- there is a slow pulse (less than 60 beats/minute in an unconscious infant or young child with poor perfusion).

'Unnecessary' chest compressions are almost never damaging. It is important not to waste vital seconds before starting chest compressions after oxygenating the patient with the rescue breaths. If there are signs of life and the pulse is present (and has an adequate rate, with good perfusion), but apnoea persists, exhaled air resuscitation must be continued until spontaneous breathing resumes.

Chest compressions

For the best output, the patient must be placed on their back, on a hard surface. The chest should be compressed by a third of its depth. Children vary in size, and the exact nature of the compressions given should reflect this. In general, infants (less than 1 year of age) require a different technique from pre-pubertal children, in whom the method used in adults can be applied with appropriate modifications for their size.

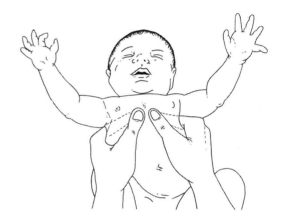

FIGURE 1.12.8 Two-thumb method for chest compressions in an infant (two rescuers).

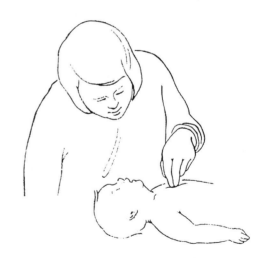

FIGURE 1.12.9 Two-finger method for chest compressions in an infant (one rescuer).

Position for chest compressions

Chest compressions should compress the lower half of the sternum.

Infants: Infant chest compression can be more effectively achieved using the hand-encircling technique: the infant is held with both the rescuer's hands encircling or

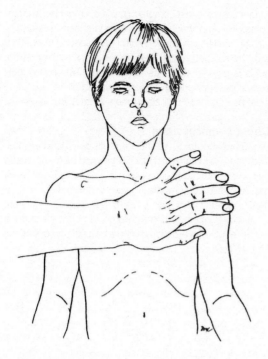

FIGURE 1.12.10 Chest compressions using one hand in a child.

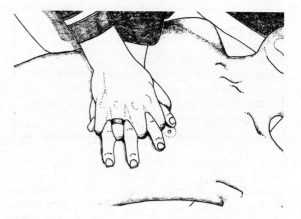

FIGURE 1.12.11 Chest compressions using two hands in a larger child or mother.

partially encircling the chest. The thumbs are placed over the lower half of the sternum and compression is carried out as shown in Figure 1.12.8. This method is only possible when there are two rescuers, as the time needed to reposition the airway precludes the use of the technique by a single rescuer if the recommended rates of compression and ventilation are to be achieved. The single rescuer should use the two-finger method as shown in Figure 1.12.9, employing the other hand to maintain the airway position.

Small children: Place the heel of one hand over the lower half of the sternum. Lift the fingers to ensure that pressure is not applied over the child's ribs. Position yourself vertically above the child's chest and, with your arm straight, compress the sternum to depress it by approximately one third of the depth of the chest (Figure 1.12.10).

For *larger children or pregnant mothers*, or for small rescuers, compressions may be achieved most easily by using both hands with the fingers interlocked (Figure 1.12.11). The rescuer may choose one or two hands to achieve the desired compression of one third of the depth of the chest.

Once the correct technique has been chosen and the area for compression identified, **15 compressions should be given to 2 ventilations.**

Technique for giving chest compressions in larger children and pregnant mothers

- Kneel by the side of the patient, who must be positioned on a firm surface, the uterus having been displaced if appropriate (see below).
- Place the heel of one hand in the centre of the patient's chest.
- Place the heel of your other hand on top of the first hand.
- Interlock the fingers of your hands and ensure that pressure is not applied over the patient's ribs. Do not apply any pressure over the upper abdomen or the bottom end of the bony sternum (breastbone).
- Position yourself vertically above the patient's chest and,

with your arms straight, press down on the sternum to a depth of 5–6 cm.
- After each compression, release all the pressure on the chest without losing contact between your hands and the sternum.
- Repeat at a rate of about 100–120 times a minute (a little less than 2 compressions a second).
- Compression and release should take an equal amount of time.

Technique for giving breaths in larger children and pregnant mothers (see Figure 1.12.12)

- After 15 compressions, open the airway again using the head tilt and chin lift (use the jaw thrust if you are experienced and capable of doing it properly and there are two rescuers).
- Pinch the soft part of the patient's nose closed, using the index finger and thumb of your hand on their forehead.
- Allow the patient's mouth to open, but maintain chin lift.
- Take a normal breath and place your lips around the patient's mouth, making sure that you have a good seal. If you have a bag-valve-mask, this can be used instead of mouth-to-mouth basic life support in all age groups.
- Blow steadily into the patient's mouth while watching for their chest to rise; take about 1 second to make their chest rise, as in normal breathing; this is an effective rescue breath.
- Maintaining the head tilt and chin lift, take your mouth away from the patient and watch for their chest to fall as air is exhaled.
- Take another normal breath and blow into the patient's mouth once more to give a total of two effective rescue breaths. Then return your hands without delay to the correct position on the sternum and give a further 15 chest compressions.
- Continue with chest compressions and rescue breaths in a ratio of 15:2.
- Stop to recheck the patient only if they start breathing **normally**; otherwise **do not interrupt resuscitation**.
- If your rescue breaths do not make the chest rise as in normal breathing, then before your next attempt:
  - check the patient's mouth and remove any visible obstruction
  - recheck that there is adequate head tilt and chin lift
  - try the jaw thrust if you are able to do this effectively.

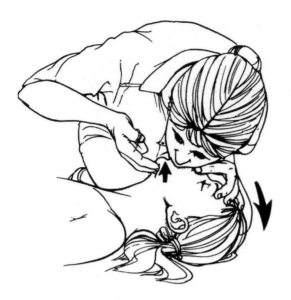

FIGURE 1.12.12 Giving breaths for a larger child or a mother.

- Do not attempt more than two breaths each time before returning to chest compressions.
- **If there is more than one rescuer present, a different person should take over CPR about every 2 minutes to prevent fatigue. Ensure that there is minimal delay during the changeover between rescuers.**

Continuing cardiopulmonary resuscitation

The compression rate for all age groups is 100–120 compressions per minute. A ratio of 15 compressions to 2 ventilations is maintained irrespective of the number of rescuers. With pauses for ventilation there will be less than 100–120 compressions per minute, although the **rate** is 100–120 per minute. Compressions can be recommenced at the end of inspiration and may augment exhalation.

If no help has arrived, the emergency services must be contacted after 1 minute of cardiopulmonary resuscitation. **Apart from this interruption to summon help, basic life support must not be interrupted unless the patient moves or takes a breath.**

Effective chest compressions are tiring for the rescuer. Continually check that the compressions and ventilations are satisfactory (they should be performed 'hard and fast') and, if possible, alternate the rescuers involved in this task.

Any time spent readjusting the airway or re-establishing the correct position for compressions will seriously decrease the number of cycles given per minute. This can be a real problem for the solo rescuer, and there is no easy solution. In infants and small children, the free hand can maintain the head position. The correct position for compressions does not need to be measured after each set of ventilations.

The cardiopulmonary resuscitation manoeuvres recommended for infants and children are summarised in Table 1.12.1.

TABLE 1.12.1 Summary of basic life support techniques in infants and children

	Infants (< 1 year)	Children (1 year to puberty) and pregnant mothers
Airway		
Head-tilt position	Neutral	Sniffing
Breathing		
Initial slow breaths	Five	Five
Circulation		
Pulse check	Brachial or femoral	Carotid
Landmark	Lower half of sternum	Lower half of sternum
Technique	Two fingers or two thumbs	One or two hands
CPR ratio	15:2	15:2

Call emergency services (if available)

If no help has arrived, the emergency services must be contacted after 1 minute of resuscitation has been delivered. A mobile phone can be used or an infant or small child may be carried to a static telephone or to get help while attempts are continued. Apart from any necessary interruption to summon help, basic life support must not be interrupted unless the patient moves or takes a breath, or you are exhausted.

If recovery occurs and signs of life return, place the patient in the recovery position and continue to reassess them and ensure that specialist help arrives.

Special circulation actions in the pregnant mother (*see* Figures 1.12.13 and 1.12.14)

Place the patient on a hard surface in the left lateral tilt position to overcome vena caval compression. This can be achieved with a wedge placed under the right hip to displace the gravid uterus to the left, or it is possible to improvise with a pillow or coat. If an assistant is available, they can displace the uterus to the left side of the vena cava. Effective chest compressions can be accomplished at a 15–30-degree tilt to the left, but displacement of the uterus is the more effective method.

Chest-compression-only CPR.

- If you either unable or unwilling to give rescue breaths, give chest compressions only. This is particularly relevant in countries where there is a high prevalence of HIV, hepatitis or TB (see below).
- If chest compressions only are given, these should be continuous at a rate of 100 compressions per minute.
- Stop to recheck the patient only if they start to breathe **normally**; otherwise do not interrupt resuscitation.

Continue resuscitation until:

- qualified help arrives and takes over *or*
- the patient starts breathing normally *or*
- you become exhausted.

Pregnant at more than 20 weeks lying supine

Pregnant and showing a lateral tilt position

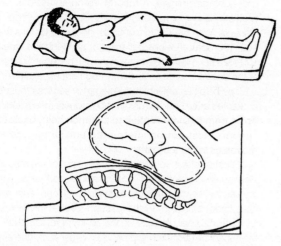

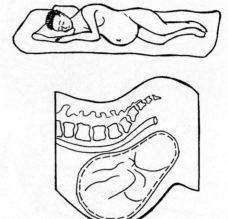

The inferior vena cava is compressed against the vertebral column

Looking from above the inferior vena cava is not compressed

FIGURE 1.12.13 The supine hypotensive syndrome. On the left the mother is lying on her back, her uterus is occluding her inferior vena cava. On the right the mother is lying in a lateral position (the recovery position here) and the inferior vena cava is no longer compressed.

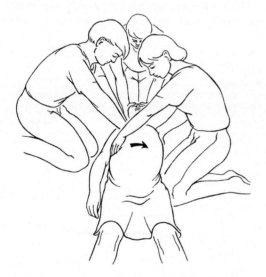

FIGURE 1.12.14 Displacing the gravid uterus manually.

Basic life support and infection risk

Few cases have been reported. The most serious concerns are meningococcus and TB. In the case of meningococcus, rescuers involved in the resuscitation of the airway in such patients should take standard prophylactic antibiotics.

There have been no reported cases of transmission of either hepatitis B or human immunodeficiency virus (HIV) through mouth-to-mouth ventilation. Blood-to-blood contact is the single most important route of transmission of these viruses, and in non-trauma resuscitation the risks are negligible. Sputum, saliva, sweat, tears, urine and vomit are low-risk fluids. Precautions should be taken, if possible, in cases where there might be contact with blood, semen, vaginal secretions, cerebrospinal fluid, pleural and peritoneal fluids, or amniotic fluid. Precautions are also recommended if any bodily secretion contains visible blood. Devices that prevent direct contact between the rescuer and the patient (such as resuscitation masks)

can be used to lower the risk. Gauze swabs or any other porous material placed over the patient's mouth is of no benefit in this regard.

Infection rates vary from country to country, and rescuers must be aware of the local risk. In countries where HIV/AIDS is more prevalent, the risk to the rescuer will be greater.

If available, bag-valve-mask ventilation is preferable to mouth-to-mouth ventilation.

The recovery position

The patient should be placed in a stable, lateral position that ensures maintenance of an open airway with free drainage of fluid from the mouth, ability to monitor and gain access to the patient, security of the cervical spine and attention to pressure points (*see* Figure 1.12.15). The Resuscitation Council (UK) recommends the following sequence of actions when placing a patient in the recovery position:

- Remove the patient's spectacles (if present).
- Kneel beside the patient and make sure that both of their legs are straight.
- Place the arm nearest to you out at right angles to their body, elbow bent with the hand palm uppermost.
- Bring the far arm across the chest, and hold the back of the hand against the patient's cheek nearest to you.
- With your other hand, grasp the far leg just above the knee and pull it up, keeping the foot on the ground.
- Keeping their hand pressed against their cheek, pull on the far leg to roll the patient towards you on to their side.
- Adjust the upper leg so that both the hip and knee are bent at right angles.
- Tilt the head back to make sure the airway remains open.
- Adjust the hand under the cheek, if necessary, to keep the head tilted.
- Check the patient's breathing regularly.

If the patient has to be kept in the recovery position for **more than 30 minutes**, turn them to the opposite side in order to relieve the pressure on the lower arm.

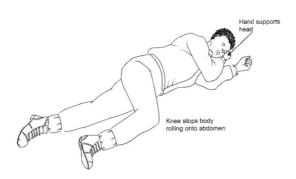

FIGURE 1.12.15 The semi-prone or recovery position.

Automatic external defibrillators (AEDs)

The use of the AED is now included in basic life support teaching for adults because early defibrillation is the most effective intervention for the large majority of unpredicted cardiac arrests in adults. As has already been stated, in children and young people and in pregnant and puerperal women, circulatory or respiratory causes of cardiac arrest predominate. However, in certain circumstances, in children and pregnant mothers there may be a primary cardiac cause of cardiac arrest, and the use of an AED may be life-saving.

An algorithm for AED use is shown in Figure 1.12.16. The standard AED can be used in children over the age of 8 years and in adults. For children aged 1–8 years, an AED can be used, but paediatric paddles are essential. An AED cannot currently be used for infants under 1 year old, as the devices are not accurate enough in this age group.

These devices are becoming much more widely available and are relatively inexpensive. They are life-saving in cases where there is a shockable rhythm, and are included in the training for basic rather than advanced life support, as they were designed for community use. If defibrillation is to be successful, it must be performed within 15 minutes of the onset of fibrillation (and the earlier it is performed, the greater the likelihood of success), so for cases of collapse that might produce fibrillation in the community, waiting until arrival at hospital would be too late.

However, AEDs are also now widely used in treatment of hospital cardiac arrests by first responders, and are therefore included here.

Attach AED pads

Expose the chest and place one adhesive defibrillator pad on the patient's chest to the right of the sternum below the right clavicle, and one in the mid-axillary line, taking care to avoid breast tissue. Keep the axillary electrode vertical to maximise efficiency.

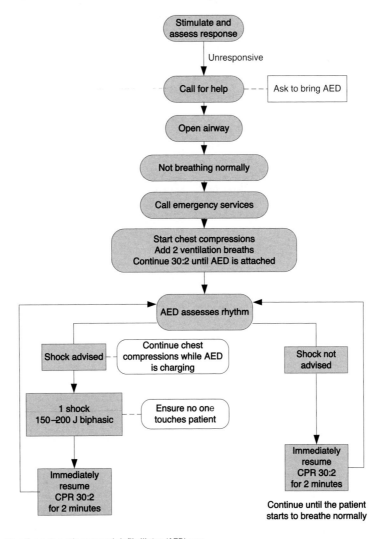

FIGURE 1.12.16 Algorithm for automatic external defibrillator (AED) use.

If a shock is indicated, most AED devices will do this automatically, but some will ask the operator to deliver the shock by pressing a button. Immediately after the shock, resume compressions for 2 minutes, after which there will be a further prompt for a rhythm analysis.

If defibrillation is **not** indicated, CPR should be continued for 2 minutes, at which stage the AED will prompt further analysis of the rhythm.

Perimortem Caesarean section

The UK Resuscitation Council considers that prompt Caesarean delivery should be seen as part of resuscitation in cardiac arrest in advanced pregnancy. Delivery of the fetus will obviate the effects of aortocaval compression and significantly increase the likelihood of successful resuscitation. It will reduce maternal oxygen consumption, increase venous return, make ventilation easier and allow CPR in the supine position.

When to perform it

All the evidence suggests that a Caesarean delivery should begin within 4 minutes of cardiac arrest and be accomplished by 5 minutes. In practice this means that preparations for surgical evacuation of the uterus should begin almost at the same time as CPR following cardiac arrest. Pregnant women develop anoxia faster than non-pregnant women, and can suffer irreversible brain damage within 4–6 minutes of cardiac arrest. CPR should be continued throughout the Caesarean section and afterwards, as this increases the likelihood of a successful neonatal and maternal outcome.

Where to perform it

The woman should **not** be transferred to an operating theatre as this will merely waste time. She should be delivered at the site of collapse unless this is physically impossible. Diathermy will not be needed, as blood loss is minimal in patients with no cardiac output. If the mother is successfully resuscitated, she can be moved to theatre to be anaesthetised and to complete the operation.

How to perform it

A minimal amount of equipment is required in this situation. Sterile preparation and drapes are unlikely to improve survival. A surgical knife is sufficient.

No one surgical approach in particular is recommended, and the choice of approach should be based on operator preference. The classical midline abdominal approach is aided by the natural diastasis of recti abdomini that occurs in late pregnancy and the relatively bloodless field in this situation. However, many obstetricians are more familiar with a lower transverse abdominal incision and can deliver a baby in less than 1 minute.

Open cardiac massage during surgery is a possibility when the abdomen is already open and the heart can be reached relatively easily through the diaphragm (if a midline approach has been used).

An anaesthetist should attend at the earliest opportunity to provide a protected airway, ensure continuity of effective chest compressions and adequate ventilation breaths, and help to determine and treat any underlying cause (4 Hs and 4 Ts, *see* Section 1.13).

If resuscitation is successful and the mother regains a cardiac output, appropriate anaesthesia and pain relief will be required and the woman should be moved to a theatre to complete the operation.

Fetal outcome

It must be emphasised that Caesarean section is part of resuscitation and is performed to improve maternal survival, and it is worthwhile performing this procedure once the uterus has reached the level of the umbilicus (i.e. around 20 weeks' gestation). If done promptly, it can also improve fetal survival, although gestational age at the time of delivery also clearly influences the fetal outcome. In the UK, the 2006–2008 National Audit Report on maternal mortality (*'Saving Mothers' Lives': The Eighth Report of the Confidential Enquiries into Maternal Deaths in the United Kingdom*) there were no neonatal survivors among those delivered at less than 28 weeks. However, 47% of those delivered at more than 36 weeks did survive; all but one of the cases in this group involved CPR commenced in hospital, demonstrating the advantage of early evacuation of the uterus for the neonate as well as the mother.

Although uterine evacuation is a well-validated step in maternal resuscitation, there is still reluctance among some obstetricians to perform peri-arrest Caesarean section, due to concerns about neonatal neurological damage. However, in a comprehensive review of postmortem Caesarean deliveries between 1900 and 1985 by Katz and colleagues, 70% (42/61) of infants delivered within 5 minutes survived, and all of them developed normally. Only 13% (8/61) of those delivered at 10 minutes and 12% (7/61) of those delivered at 15 minutes survived. One infant in each of the groups of later survivors had neurological damage. Later series confirm the advantage of early delivery for intact fetal survival, although there are a few case reports of intact infant survival more than 20 minutes after maternal cardiac arrest.

The evidence suggests that if the fetus survives the neonatal period, the probability of normal development is high.

The decision to abandon CPR if it is unsuccessful

CPR should be continued if the rhythm continues as ventricular fibrillation (VF)/ventricular tachycardia (VT). The decision to abandon CPR should only be made after discussion with senior clinicians.

Medico-legal issues

No doctor has been found liable for performing a postmortem Caesarean section in the UK jurisdiction.

Choking
Introduction

The vast majority of deaths from foreign body airway obstruction (FBAO) occur in preschool children. Virtually anything may be inhaled, but foodstuffs predominate. The diagnosis may not be clear-cut, but should be suspected if the onset of respiratory compromise is sudden and associated with coughing, gagging and stridor.

Airway obstruction also occurs with infections such as acute epiglottitis and croup. In these cases, attempts to relieve the obstruction using the methods described below are dangerous. Children with known or suspected infectious causes of obstruction, and those who are still breathing and in whom the cause of obstruction is unclear, should be taken to hospital urgently. The treatment of these children is dealt with in Section 4.

If a foreign body is easily visible and accessible in the mouth, remove it, but while attempting this take great care not to push it further into the airway. Do not perform blind finger sweeps of the mouth or upper airway, as these may further impact a foreign body and damage tissues without removing the object.

The physical methods of clearing the airway, described below, should therefore only be performed if:

1 the diagnosis of FBAO is clear-cut (witnessed or strongly suspected) and ineffective coughing and increasing dyspnoea, loss of consciousness or apnoea have occurred.

2 head tilt/chin lift and jaw thrust manoeuvres have failed to open the airway of an apnoeic child.

If the child is coughing, this should be encouraged. A spontaneous cough is more effective in relieving an obstruction than any externally imposed manoeuvre. An effective cough is recognised by the patient's ability to speak or cry and to take a breath between coughs. The child should be continually assessed and not left alone at this stage. No intervention should be made unless the cough becomes ineffective (i.e. quieter or silent), and the patient cannot cry, speak or take a breath, or becomes cyanosed or starts to lose consciousness. Then call for help and start the intervention.

These manoeuvres are then alternated with each other, and with examination of the mouth and attempted breaths as shown in Figure 1.12.17.

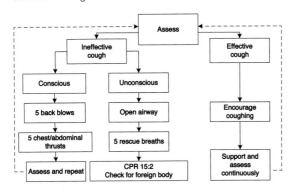

FIGURE 1.12.17 Algorithm for the management of choking.

Infants

Abdominal thrusts may cause intra-abdominal injury in infants. Therefore a combination of back blows and chest thrusts is recommended for the relief of foreign body obstruction in this age group (see Figures 1.12.18 and 1.12.19).

The baby is placed along one of the rescuer's arms in a head-down position, with the rescuer's hand supporting the infant's jaw in such a way as to keep it open, in the neutral position. The rescuer then rests his or her arm along the thigh, and delivers five back blows with the heel of the free hand.

If the obstruction is not relieved, the baby is turned over and laid along the rescuer's thigh, still in a head-down position. Five chest thrusts are given using the same landmarks as for cardiac compression, but at a rate of one per second. If an infant is too large to allow use of the single-arm technique described above, then the same manoeuvres can be performed by lying the baby across the rescuer's lap.

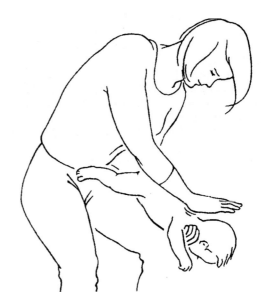

FIGURE 1.12.18 Back blows in an infant.

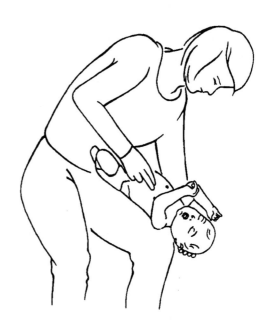

FIGURE 1.12.19 Chest thrusts in an infant.

Children

Back blows can be used as described for infants or, in the case of a larger child, with the child supported in a forward-leaning position (see Figure 1.12.20). In children the abdominal thrust (Heimlich manoeuvre) can also be used (see Figures 1.12.21 and 1.12.22). This can be performed with the patient either standing or lying down, but the former is usually more appropriate.

If this manoeuvre is to be attempted with the child standing, the rescuer moves behind the patient and passes his or her arms around the patient's body. Owing to the short height of children, it may be necessary for an adult to raise the child or kneel behind them to carry out the standing manoeuvre effectively. One hand is formed into a fist and placed against the child's abdomen above the umbilicus and below the xiphisternum. The other hand is placed over the fist, and both hands are thrust sharply upwards into the abdomen. This procedure is repeated five times unless the object that is causing the obstruction is expelled before then.

To perform the Heimlich manoeuvre in a supine child, the rescuer kneels at the child's feet. If the child is large, it may be necessary to kneel astride him or her. The heel of one hand is placed against the child's abdomen above the umbilicus and below the xiphisternum. The other hand is placed on top of the first, and both hands are thrust sharply upwards into the abdomen, with care being taken to direct the thrust in the midline. This procedure is repeated five times unless the object that is causing the obstruction is expelled before then.

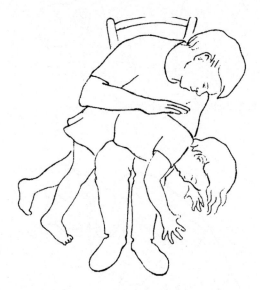

FIGURE 1.12.20 Back blows in a small child.

Following successful relief of the obstructed airway, the child should be assessed clinically. There may still be some foreign material present in the respiratory tract. If abdominal thrusts have been performed, the child should be assessed for possible abdominal injuries.

Each time breaths are attempted, look in the mouth for the foreign body and remove it if it is visible. Take care not to push the object further down, and avoid damaging the tissues. If the obstruction is relieved the patient may still require either continued ventilations if they are not breathing,

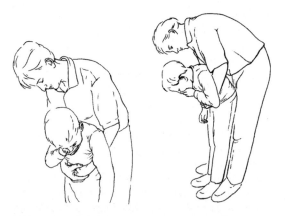

FIGURE 1.12.21 Heimlich manoeuvre in a standing child.

or chest compressions if there are no signs of a circulation. Advanced life support may also be needed.

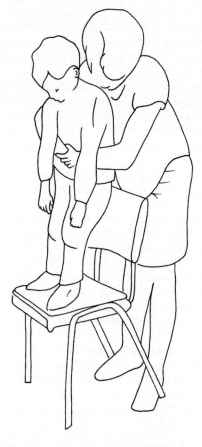

FIGURE 1.12.22 Heimlich manoeuvre using a chair.

If the child is breathing effectively, place them in the recovery position and continue to monitor them.

Unconscious infant or child with foreign body airway obstruction

- Call for help.
- Place the child in a supine position on a flat surface.
- Open the mouth and attempt to remove any visible object.
- Open the airway and attempt five rescue breaths, repositioning the airway with each breath if the chest does not rise.
- Start chest compressions even if the rescue breaths were ineffective.
- Continue the sequence for single-rescuer CPR for about 1 minute, then summon help again if none is forthcoming.
- Each time breaths are attempted, look in the mouth for the foreign body and remove it if it is visible. Take care not to push the object further down, and avoid damaging the tissues.
- If the obstruction is relieved, the patient may still require either continued ventilations if they are not breathing but are moving or gagging, or both ventilations and chest compressions if there are no signs of a circulation. Advanced life support may also be needed.
- If the child is breathing effectively, place them in the recovery position and continue to reassess them.

1.13 Advanced life support for children and pregnant mothers

Introduction

As described in Section 1.12 on basic life support, the pregnant mother in cardiac arrest has usually suffered from the same deranged pathophysiology as the arrested child (i.e. respiratory or circulatory collapse rather than a primarily cardiac event).

The 'child' type of cardiac arrest is seen in almost all children (excluding those rare arrhythmic events in children with congenital or acquired heart disease, and those in whom sudden, unexpected collapse is preceded by apparent normal respiratory and circulatory function), and in adults who have a terminal acute illness involving respiratory or circulatory pathology. This includes patients who have had convulsions, trauma (including drowning), poisoning, bleeding, sepsis, etc.

In addition, there is international agreement that, where possible, guidelines on resuscitation of patients with cardiac arrest should be simplified, as there is evidence that complex guidelines cause 'provider paralysis', resulting in no or poor life-saving effort being made.

In view of this, the Advanced Life Support Group (ALSG)/Maternal Childhealth Advocacy International (MCAI) programme for resource-limited countries teaches a programme of basic life support (BLS) and advanced life support (ALS) for infants, children and pregnant mothers which reflects the known pathologies in these groups (i.e. respiratory and circulatory causes of cardiac arrest) and recognises that the clinicians who provide resuscitation attend patients of all ages.

Airway and breathing

Management of the airway (A) and breathing (B) components of the ABC must take priority in all situations. Resuscitation will fail if effective ventilation does not occur.

Before effective resuscitation techniques can be applied, it is essential that the operator is able to:

1 understand the airway equipment available and how to use it
2 recognise respiratory failure and when it may occur
3 perform a systematic and prioritised approach (the structured ABC approach) to the management of the infant, child or mother who has a problem of the airway or breathing (see Section 1.11).

Airway: equipment and skills for opening and maintaining the airway

Essential airway and breathing equipment includes the following:

- face masks (ideally with reservoirs)
- airways, including laryngeal mask airways (LMAs) if anaesthetic skills are available
- self-inflating bag-valve-mask devices
- tracheal tubes, introducers and connectors
- laryngoscopes

- Magill's forceps
- suction devices
- surgical airway packs for performing an emergency surgical airway.

This equipment should be available in all resuscitation areas, ideally on a resuscitation trolley. It is crucial to gain familiarity with it before an emergency situation occurs.

Pharyngeal airways

There are two main types of pharyngeal airway, namely **oropharyngeal** (see Figures 1.13.1 and 1.13.2) and **nasopharyngeal**.

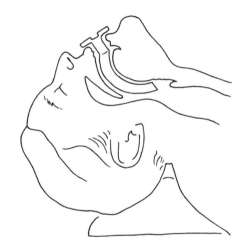

FIGURE 1.13.1 Oropharyngeal airway, showing position when inserted.

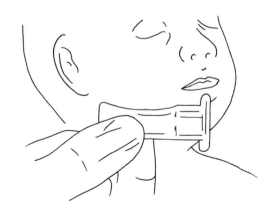

FIGURE 1.13.2 Oropharyngeal airway, showing sizing technique.

Oropharyngeal airways

The oropharyngeal or Guedel airway is used in the unconscious or obtunded patient to provide an open airway channel between the tongue and the posterior pharyngeal wall.

In the awake patient with an intact gag reflex, it may not be tolerated and may induce vomiting.

The oropharyngeal airway is available in a variety of sizes. A correctly sized airway when placed with its flange at the centre of the incisors, then curved around the face, will reach the angle of the mandible. Too small an airway may be ineffective, and too large an airway may cause laryngospasm. Either may cause mucosal trauma or may worsen airway obstruction. Reassessment following placement is therefore a vital part of safe insertion of an airway device.

There are two methods for inserting an oropharyngeal airway in children, depending on whether the child is small or large. However, there is no specific age of transition from one to the other – the choice of method depends on practicality and the skills of the operator. The important point is not to push the tongue back by inserting the airway carelessly.

The twist technique is used for larger children and in pregnant mothers. With this technique the convex side of the airway is used to depress the tongue as the airway is pushed into the mouth. The airway should be inserted upside down until the tip has passed the soft palate, and then rotated through 180 degrees so that the natural curve of the Guedel airway follows the curve of the tongue and pharynx (see Figure 1.13.3).

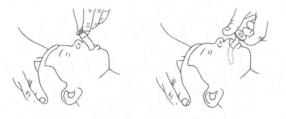

FIGURE 1.13.3 Oropharyngeal airway shown being inserted concave side up, then in place concave side down.

However, in infants and small children, as the tongue is larger relative to the size of the mouth, the airway cannot be rotated in the mouth without causing trauma. Therefore the tongue is depressed with a spatula and not by the convex side of the airway (see Figure 1.13.4).

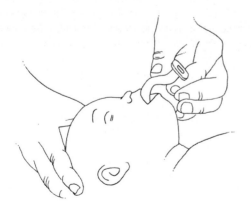

FIGURE 1.13.4 When inserting the airway without rotation, a tongue depressor can be helpful (not shown).

Nasopharyngeal airways
The nasopharyngeal airway is often better tolerated than the Guedel airway. **It is contraindicated in fractures of the base of the skull.** It may also cause significant haemorrhage from the vascular nasal mucosa if it is not inserted with care, preferably with lubrication. A suitable length can be estimated by measuring from the lateral edge of the nostril to the tragus of the ear. An appropriate diameter is one that just fits into the nostril without causing sustained blanching of the alae nasi. If small-sized nasopharyngeal airways are not available, shortened endotracheal tubes may be used.

Ensure that insertion of one or other of these devices results in an improvement in the patient's airway and breathing. It if does not improve the airway as shown by improved breathing, then a reappraisal of the choice or size of airway is urgently required.

In pregnant mothers, the nasopharyngeal tube is not commonly used, because of the tendency for nasal mucosal bleeding to occur in pregnancy.

Laryngoscopes
There are two principal designs of laryngoscope, namely **straight bladed** and **curved bladed**.

The straight-bladed laryngoscope is usually employed to directly lift the epiglottis, thereby uncovering the vocal folds. The advantage of this approach is that the epiglottis is moved sufficiently so that it does not obscure the cords. The potential disadvantage is that vagal stimulation may cause laryngospasm or bradycardia.

The curved-bladed laryngoscope is designed to move the epiglottis forward by lifting it from in front. The tip of the blade is inserted into the mucosal pocket, known as the vallecula, anterior to the epiglottis, and the epiglottis is then moved forward by pressure in the vallecula. This may be equally effective for obtaining a view of the cords, and it has the advantage that less vagal stimulation ensues, as the mucosa of the vallecula is innervated by the glossopharyngeal nerve instead.

A laryngoscope blade appropriate for the age of the patient should be chosen. It is possible to intubate with a blade that is too long, but not with one that is too short.

Laryngoscopes are notoriously unreliable pieces of equipment which may develop flat batteries and unserviceable bulbs very quickly between uses. Therefore it is vital that a spare is available at all times, and equipment must be regularly checked to ensure that it is in good working order.

Tracheal tubes
Uncuffed tubes should be used during resuscitation, by operators who do not have paediatric anaesthetic experience, for children up to approximately 10 years of age. If the operator is familiar with cuffed tube placement, both cuffed and uncuffed tubes are acceptable for infants and children undergoing emergency intubation, but not for neonates. Up until the age of around 10 years, the larynx is circular in cross section and the narrowest part of it is at the cricoid ring, rather than the vocal cords. An appropriately sized tube should give a relatively gas-tight fit in the larynx, but the fit should not be so tight that no leak is audible when the bag is compressed. Failure to observe this condition may lead to damage to the mucosa at the level of the cricoid ring, and to subsequent oedema following extubation.

The appropriate size of an uncuffed tracheal tube is estimated as follows:

internal diameter (mm) = (age in years/4) + 4
length (cm) = (age in years/2) + 12 for an oral tube
length (cm) = (age in years/2) + 15 for nasal tube.

These formulae are appropriate for ages over 1 year. Neonates usually require a tube of internal diameter 3–3.5 mm, although preterm infants may need one of diameter 2.5 mm. Cuffed tubes should not be used in neonates.

For cuffed tracheal tubes, the appropriate internal diameter for children aged 2 years or older is estimated as follows:

$$\text{internal diameter (mm)} = (\text{age in years}/4) + 3.5.$$

For infants of weight over 3 kg and up to 1 year in age a size 3 cuffed tube is usually acceptable, and for those aged 1–2 years a size 3.5 cuffed tube can generally be used.

The size of tracheal tubes is measured in terms of their internal diameter in millimetres. They are available in whole- and half-millimetre sizes. The clinician should select a tube of appropriate size, but also prepare one a size smaller and one a size larger.

In the case of resuscitation in a young child where the lungs are very 'stiff' (e.g. in a cardiac arrest from severe bronchiolitis), a cuffed tube rather than an uncuffed tube may be used by a non-expert, but the risk of airway damage from the cuff must be balanced against the risk of failure to inflate the lungs.

In pregnant mothers, cuffed tubes must be used because of the high risk of gastric reflux in the pregnant patient causing aspiration of acidic gastric material and severe respiratory problems.

Tracheal tube introducers

Intubation can be facilitated by the use of a stylet or introducer, which is placed through the lumen of the tracheal tube. There are two types – either **soft and flexible** or **firm and malleable**.

The soft and flexible type can be allowed to project beyond the tip of the tube, so long as it is handled very gently. The firm and malleable type is used to alter the shape of the tube, but can easily damage the tissues if allowed to protrude from the end of the tracheal tube. Tracheal tube introducers should not be used to force a tracheal tube into position.

Bougies, which are flexible, deformable, blunt-ended gum elastic rods of different sizes, can be used to help to introduce a tracheal tube when access is difficult. A Seldinger-type technique is used. The bougie is introduced into the trachea using the laryngoscope, the endotracheal tube is then passed over it into the trachea, and finally the bougie is removed.

In pregnant mothers:

1 A 15 French bougie should be used for endotracheal tube sizes 6.0–11.0.
2 Lubricate the bougie with KY jelly.
3 Perform laryngoscopy. If the cords are not visible, identify landmarks to aid intubation.
4 Place the bougie into the pharynx and direct it into the larynx. If necessary, bend the bougie to negotiate the corner. Correct placement may be confirmed by detection of tracheal 'clicks' and 'hold-up' of the bougie (the absence of hold-up indicates oesophageal placement).
5 Hold the tube firmly in place and gently withdraw the bougie.
6 Remove the laryngoscope and confirm tube placement as usual.

Tracheal tube connectors

In pregnant mothers, the proximal end of the tube connectors is of standard size, based on the 15-mm/22-mm system, which means that they can be connected to a standard self-inflating bag.

The same standard system exists for children, including neonates.

Magill's forceps

Magill's forceps (*see* Figure 1.13.5) are angled to allow a view around the forceps when they are in the mouth. They may be useful to help to position a tube through the cords by lifting it anteriorly, or to remove pharyngeal or supraglottic foreign bodies.

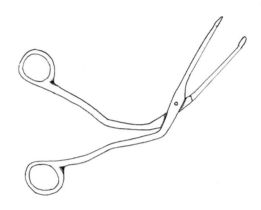

FIGURE 1.13.5 Magill's forceps.

Suction devices

These are used to remove blood, vomit and secretions from the mouth and throat, usually with a rigid suction tube (Yankauer suction tube; see below). In resuscitation areas, ideally the suction device should be connected to a central vacuum unit. This consists of a suction hose inserted into a wall terminal outlet, a controller (to adjust the vacuum pressure), a reservoir jar, suction tubing and a suitable sucker nozzle or catheter. In order to aspirate vomit effectively, it should be capable of producing a high negative pressure and a high flow rate, although these can be reduced in non-urgent situations, so as not to cause mucosal injury.

Portable suction devices are required for resuscitation when central suction is not available (as is the case in most resource-limited hospitals), and for transport to and from the resuscitation room. These are either manual, mains electrical or battery powered. A manual or battery-operated suction system must be available at all sites where resuscitation may be needed.

To clear the oropharynx of debris (e.g. vomit), a rigid sucker (e.g. Yankauer sucker) should be used with care not to damage delicate tissue or induce vomiting. The Yankauer sucker is available in both adult and paediatric sizes. It may have a side hole, which can be occluded by a finger, allowing greater control over vacuum pressure.

Tracheal suction catheters (see *Figure 1.13.6*)

These may be required after intubation to remove bronchial secretions or aspirated fluids. In general, the appropriate size in French gauge is numerically twice the internal diameter in millimetres (e.g. for a 3-mm tube the correct suction catheter is a French gauge 6).

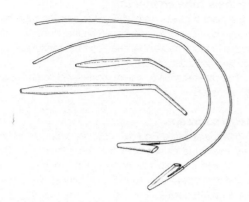

FIGURE 1.13.6 Tracheal and oral or nasal suction catheters.

Advanced airway techniques

Advanced airway techniques are used when the above techniques fail to maintain and protect an airway over the longer term, particularly if there is potential for it to become obstructed and thus prevent accurate control of oxygenation and ventilation. Advanced airway techniques (tracheal intubation, surgical cricothyroidotomy and surgical tracheostomy) are described in Section 8.2.

Breathing: equipment and skills for helping the patient to breathe

The following equipment for oxygenation and ventilation should be readily available:

- an oxygen source
- masks for those who are spontaneously breathing
- close-fitting face masks (for artificial ventilation)
- self-inflating bag-valve systems to be used with close-fitting face masks
- T-piece and open-ended bag systems (only to be used by those with anaesthetic skills)
- mechanical ventilators
- chest tubes
- gastric tubes.

Oxygen treatment
Indications
Give oxygen to patients:

- with respiratory distress (severe indrawing of the lower chest wall, also known as recessions, raised respiratory rate, gasping, grunting with each breath, nasal flaring, head bobbing, etc.)
- with cyanosis (blueness) that is central (around the lips and tongue, or inside the mouth in children with dark skin)
- who are shocked
- who are fitting
- who are unconscious, with abnormal oxygen saturation (SaO_2) on a pulse oximeter.

Ideally, where the resources for this are available, oxygen therapy should be guided by pulse oximetry (see below). Give oxygen to children with an SaO_2 of < 94%, and aim to keep SaO_2 at 94–98% (except at high altitude, where normal oxygen saturation levels are lower). If pulse oximeters are not available, the need for oxygen therapy has to be guided by clinical signs, which are less reliable.

Provision of oxygen
Oxygen must be available at all times. The two main sources of oxygen are cylinders and oxygen concentrators.

Oxygen cylinders contain compressed gas. A flow meter needs to be fitted to regulate flow. A hissing noise can be heard if gas is being delivered.

Flow meters are used to ascertain how much oxygen is being delivered. Take the reading of flow rate from the middle of the ball. Always switch off the flow when the source is not in use (ensure that the indicator ball is at the bottom of the flow meter and not moving).

Do not leave anything inflammable near to the oxygen supply. Do not allow smoking near to the oxygen supply.

At least once a day, check that an adequate oxygen supply is available (use a signed logbook). If a gauge indicating the amount left in the cylinder is not available, switch on the flow and listen for a hissing noise. Replace empty cylinders promptly. Ensure that cylinders are stored and secured in an upright position in suitable containers so that they cannot fall over and cause injury. Cylinder keys to permit changes of regulator should be tied to each cylinder.

Oxygen concentrators may be available. They produce more than 95% oxygen with a flow of 1–8 litres/minute but, unlike cylinders, they require a continuous electricity supply. For this reason, all areas where patients might need oxygen must have both cylinders and concentrators.

There are now small oxygen plants available that can provide oxygen for a defined area or even for the whole of a hospital or health facility. Some of them can be used to fill oxygen cylinders as well, thus providing a constant back-up (www.ogsi.com).

Oxygen delivery
A mask with a reservoir bag (*see* Figure 1.13.7) allows up to 100% oxygen to be delivered. Without a reservoir, it is only possible to deliver around 40% oxygen. If only low flow rates of oxygen are available, do not use a reservoir bag.

If an oxygen mask is being used, ensure that the mask is large enough to cover the mouth and nose. Both low- and high-flow oxygen (with a delivery rate of up to 15 litres/minute) can be given. Hold the mask in place using the

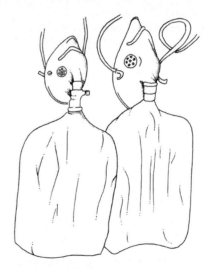

FIGURE 1.13.7 Reservoir bags.

elastic strap around the back of the head or, in the case of a young child, ask the mother to hold it as close as possible to the child's face.

Nasal cannulae (also known as nasal prongs) (*see* Figure 1.13.8) are the preferred method of delivery in most circumstances, as they are safe, non-invasive, reliable and do **not** obstruct the nasal airway. Head boxes are not recommended, as they use up too much oxygen and deliver a low concentration. Face masks can be used for resuscitation purposes, ideally with a reservoir attached to deliver 100% oxygen.

Monitoring

Nursing staff must know how to place and secure the nasal cannulae correctly. Check regularly that the equipment is working properly, and remove and clean the cannulae at least twice a day.

Monitor the patient at least every 3 hours to identify and correct any problems, including:

- SaO_2 values measured by pulse oximeter
- nasal cannulae out of position
- leaks in the oxygen delivery system
- incorrect oxygen flow rate
- airway obstructed by mucus (clear the nose with a moist wick or by gentle suction).

Pulse oximetry

Normal oxygen saturation at sea level in a child is 95–100%. Oxygen is ideally given to maintain oxygen saturation at 94–98%. Different cut-off values might be used at high altitude or if oxygen is scarce. The response to oxygen

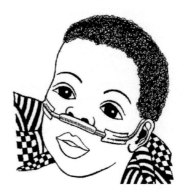

FIGURE 1.13.8 Nasal cannulae delivering oxygen and taped in place.

therapy in lung disease can be measured with the pulse oximeter, as the patient's SaO_2 should increase (in patients with cyanotic heart disease, SaO_2 does not change when oxygen is given). The oxygen flow can be titrated using the pulse oximeter as a monitor to obtain a stable SaO_2 of 94–98% without giving too much oxygen. This is especially important in pre-term babies with respiratory disease (*see* Section 3.4).

Assessment of oxygenation at and above sea level

A systematic review in 2009 found an SpO_2 of 90% is the 2.5th centile for a population of healthy children living at an altitude of approximately 2500 m above sea level. This decreases to 85% at an altitude of approximately 3200 m.

TABLE 1.13.1 SpO_2 levels at different altitudes[a]

Altitude	Location	n	Age	SpO₂ (%)	Author	Year
Sea level	UK	70	2–16 (mean, 8) years	Range, 95.8–100 Median, 99.5	Poets *et al.*	1993
Sea level	Peru	189	2 months to 5 years	Range, 96–100 Mean, 98.7	Reuland *et al.*	1991
1610 m	Colorado	150	< 48 hours 3 months	95% CI, 88–97 Mean, 93 95% CI, 86–97 Mean, 92.2	Thilo *et al.*	1991
1670 m	Nairobi	87	7 days to 3 years	Range, 89.3–99.3 Mean, 95.7	Onyango *et al.*	1993
2640	Bogota	189	5 days to 2 years	Range, 84–100 Mean, 93.3	Lozano *et al.*	1992
2800	Colorado	72	3–670 days	Range, 88–97 Mean, 91.7	Nicholas *et al.*	1993
3100	Colorado	14	6 hours to 4 months 1 week to 4 months	Range, 81–91 Mean, 80.6±5.3 Mean, 86.1±4.6	Niemeyer *et al.*	1993
3658	Tibet[b]	15	6 hours to 4 months	Immigrant, 76–90 Indigenous, 86–94	Niemeyer *et al.*	1995
3750	Peru	153	2–60 months	Range, 81–97 Mean, 88.9	Reuland *et al.*	1991

[a]Values given are those in quiet sleep.

[b]Ranges refer to those born to immigrant Chinese mothers and to those indigenous babies whose families have lived at that altitude for innumerable generations.

Duration of oxygen therapy

Continue giving oxygen continuously until the patient is able to maintain an SaO_2 of 94% or higher in room air. When the patient is stable and improving, take them off oxygen for a few minutes. If the SaO_2 remains in the range 94–98%, discontinue oxygen, but check again 30 minutes later, and 3-hourly thereafter on the first day off oxygen to ensure that the patient is stable. Where pulse oximetry is not available, the duration of oxygen therapy has to be guided by clinical signs, which are less sensitive.

Breathing for the patient
Face masks with seal over nose and mouth for positive pressure ventilation (see Figure 1.13.9)

These face masks are used for either mouth-to-mask or, more commonly, bag–mask ventilation. Masks are available in various sizes, and the appropriate size to cover the mouth and nose should be chosen.

Face masks for mouth-to-mouth or bag-valve-mask ventilation in infants are of two main designs. Some masks conform to the anatomy of the patient's face and have a low dead space. Circular soft plastic masks give an excellent seal and are often preferred. Children's masks should be clear so that the child's colour or the presence of vomit can be seen.

A pocket mask is a single-size clear plastic mask with an air-filled cushion rim designed for mouth-to-mask resuscitation. It can be supplied with a port for attaching it to an oxygen supply, and can be used in adults and children. It can be used upside down to ventilate infants.

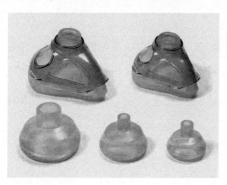

FIGURE 1.13.9 Face masks with cushioned rim for a leak-proof fit, and round shape for infants.

Self-inflating bags (see Figure 1.13.10)

This is one of the most important pieces of equipment, allowing hand ventilation by face mask without a supply of gas. The two appropriate sizes are **500 mL** and **1600 mL (the smaller size for infants under 1 year of age, and the larger size for children and mothers)**. There is also a 250-mL version for small premature babies. These bags have pressure-limiting valves that operate at 30–45 cm H_2O. Test the valve by placing the mask on a surface and pressing the bag and ensuring that the valve opens. It can be overridden if necessary for stiff, poorly compliant lungs by loosening the screw at the top.

The bag connects to the patient through a one-way valve to direct exhaled air to the atmosphere. The other end connects to the oxygen supply and can attach to a reservoir bag which allows high concentrations (up to 98%) of oxygen to be delivered. Without the reservoir bag, only

concentrations of up to 40% can be delivered. The bag itself is easily dismantled and reassembled. It is important to realise that this system **will operate without an attached oxygen supply**, allowing resuscitation to be initiated before oxygen is available. However, if resuscitation is failing, check that oxygen is being delivered into the bag and to the patient and that the oxygen supply has not been disconnected.

Always use high-flow oxygen (if available) and a reservoir bag during resuscitation apart from at birth where room air is satisfactory for almost all babies (see Section 3.2).

It is also important to clean the system after each patient.

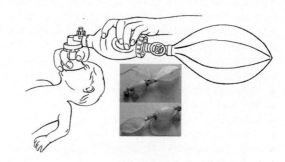

FIGURE 1.13.10 Two sizes of self-inflating bags and masks.

It is essential that the mask is properly sized and correctly placed over the mouth and nose of the patient (see Figures 1.13.11 and 1.13.12).

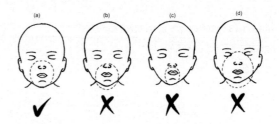

FIGURE 1.13.11 (a) Correct placement of infant mask. (b), (c) and (d) Incorrect placement of infant mask.

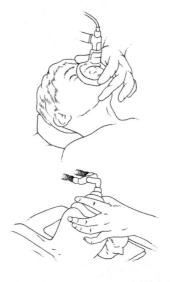

FIGURE 1.13.12 Two views of single-handed grip on mask.

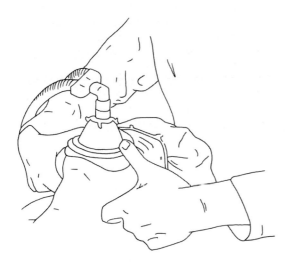

FIGURE 1.13.13 Two-handed grip on mask incorporating jaw thrust.

If the chest does not rise, the airway is not clear. The usual cause is failure to correctly apply the airway-opening techniques discussed previously. The first step to try is to readjust the head-tilt/chin-lift position and try again. If this is not successful, the jaw-thrust manoeuvre should be tried (*see* Figure 1.13.13). Failure of both the head-tilt/chin-lift and jaw-thrust manoeuvres should lead to suspicion that a foreign body is causing the obstruction.

Once breathing has restarted, replace the bag-valve-mask system with a simple face mask and reservoir. Because of the internal valves it is not possible to spontaneously breathe through the bag-valve-mask system.

Chest tubes
In cases with a significant haemothorax or pneumothorax (particularly tension pneumothorax), ventilation may be compromised and insertion of a chest drain is mandatory (*see* Section 8.3).

Gastric tubes
Insertion of a gastric tube is essential after intubation, and may also relieve respiratory distress in spontaneously breathing patients with abdominal emergencies or gastric stasis. It allows decompression of a stomach full of air from both bag and mask ventilation as well as air swallowed by a distressed patient. Without a gastric tube, the patient may vomit or there may be aspiration of stomach contents. In addition, venting of stomach gas will avoid diaphragmatic splinting. A nasogastric tube will increase airway resistance through the nose, which in a spontaneously breathing infant with respiratory failure can be significant. An orogastric tube has less effect on ventilation, but is less readily tolerated and less easily fixed in position.

Further information
Additional breathing procedures are described in Section 5.2.B (on spacers and nebulisers), Section 8.3

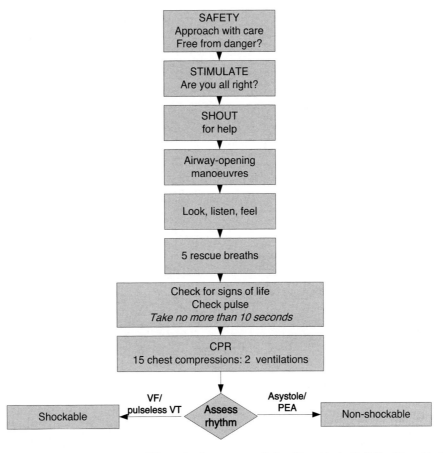

FIGURE 1.13.14 Initial approach to cardiac arrest. CPR, cardiopulmonary resuscitation; VF, ventricular fibrillation; VT, ventricular tachycardia; PEA, pulseless electrical activity.

(on needle thoracocentesis) and Section 8.3 (on chest drain insertion).

Circulation: equipment and skills for maintaining the circulation

Details of how to undertake the following procedures are covered in Section 8.4:

- peripheral venous cannulation
- blood sampling from an IV cannula
- intraosseous cannulation and infusion
- cutdown long saphenous venous cannulation
- insertion of central venous catheters
- needle pericardiocentesis.

Management of cardiac arrest

Cardiac arrest occurs when there is no effective cardiac output. Before any specific therapy is started, effective basic life support must be established (*see* Figure 1.13.14).

Four cardiac arrest rhythms can occur:

1 asystole
2 pulseless electrical activity (including electromechanical dissociation)
3 ventricular fibrillation
4 pulseless ventricular tachycardia.

These are divided into two groups. Asystole and pulseless electrical activity, which do not require defibrillation, are called 'non-shockable' rhythms. Ventricular fibrillation and pulseless ventricular tachycardia, which do require defibrillation, are called 'shockable' rhythms.

Non-shockable cardiac arrest
Asystole

This is the most common cardiac arrest rhythm in infants and children, and in pregnant mothers. The response of the heart to prolonged severe hypoxia and shock (which are the usual pathologies in these groups) is progressive bradycardia leading to asystole.

The ECG will distinguish asystole from ventricular fibrillation, ventricular tachycardia and pulseless electrical activity. The ECG appearance of ventricular asystole is an almost straight line; occasionally P-waves are seen (*see* Figure 1.13.15). Check that the appearance is not caused by an artefact (e.g. a loose wire or disconnected electrode). Turn up the gain on the ECG monitor.

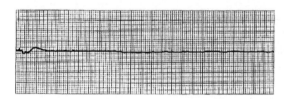

FIGURE 1.13.15 ECG appearance of asystole.

Pulseless electrical activity (PEA)

This is the absence of a palpable pulse or other signs of life despite the presence on the ECG monitor of recognisable complexes that normally produce a pulse (*see* Figure 1.13.16). PEA is treated in the same way as asystole, and is often a pre-asystolic state.

PEA in children and pregnant mothers is often due to

major trauma, often with an identifiable and reversible cause such as severe hypovolaemia, tension pneumothorax or pericardial tamponade. PEA is also seen in hypothermic patients and in those with electrolyte abnormalities. It may be seen after massive pulmonary thromboembolus.

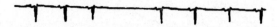

FIGURE 1.13.16 Pulseless electrical activity (PEA) in a child with no pulse or signs of life.

Management of asystole/PEA in children and pregnant mothers

The first essential step is to establish ventilations and chest compressions effectively. Ensure a patent airway, initially using an airway manoeuvre to open the airway and stabilising it with an airway adjunct. Ventilations are provided initially by bag and mask with high-concentration oxygen.

Provide effective chest compressions at a rate of 100–120 per minute with a compression:ventilation ratio of 15:2. The depth of compression should be at least one-third of the antero-posterior diameter of the chest, and compressions should be given in the middle of the lower half of the sternum. Ideally a cardiac monitor is attached. Properly performed basic life support is key to any chance of successful resuscitation from cardiac arrest. Ensure that the person performing chest compressions is keeping the correct rate and depth of compression, and if possible change operator every 2 to 3 minutes, to avoid fatigue causing poor performance.

If asystole or PEA is identified, give **adrenaline 10 micrograms/kilogram** (0.1 mL of 1:10 000 solution/kg) **intravenously or intra-osseously in children and 1 mg IV in pregnant mothers**. Adrenaline increases coronary artery perfusion, enhances the contractile state of the heart and stimulates spontaneous contractions. The drug is best given through a central line, but if one is not in place it may be given through a peripheral line. Where there is no existing IV access, the IO route is recommended as the route of choice, as it is rapid and effective. In each case, the adrenaline is followed by a normal crystalloid flush (2–5 mL).

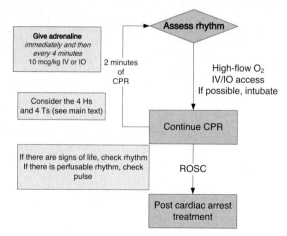

FIGURE 1.13.17 Algorithm for the treatment of non-shockable (asystole and PEA) rhythms in children. Doses of drugs used in pregnancy are given in the text above. CPR, cardiopulmonary resuscitation; IV, intravenous; IO, intra-osseous; ROSC, return of spontaneous circulation.

If available, and as soon as is feasible, a skilled and experienced operator should **intubate the patient's airway**. This will both control and protect the airway and enable chest compressions to be given continuously, thus improving coronary perfusion. Once the patient has been intubated and compressions are uninterrupted, the ventilation rate should be 10–12 breaths per minute. It is important for the team leader to check that the ventilations remain adequate when chest compressions are continuous. An algorithm for non-shockable rhythms is shown in Figure 1.13.17.

During and following adrenaline treatment, chest compressions and ventilation should continue. It is vital that chest compressions and ventilations continue uninterrupted during advanced life support, as they form the basis of the resuscitative effort. The only reason for interrupting compressions and ventilation is to shock the patient if necessary (see below), and to check the rhythm. A brief interruption may be necessary during difficult intubation. Giving chest compressions is tiring for the operator, so if enough personnel are available, change the operator frequently and ensure that they are achieving the recommended rate of 100–120 compressions per minute together with a depression of the chest wall by at least one-third of the antero-posterior diameter of the chest.

At intervals of about 2 minutes during the delivery of chest compressions, pause briefly to assess the rhythm on the monitor. If asystole persists, continue CPR while again checking the electrode position and contact.

- If there is an organised rhythm, check for a pulse and signs of life.
- If there is a return of spontaneous circulation (ROSC), continue post-resuscitation care, increasing the ventilation rate to 12–20 breaths per minute.
- If there is no pulse and no signs of life, continue the protocol.
- Give adrenaline about every 4 minutes at a dose of 10 micrograms/kg IV/IO in children and 1 mg IV in pregnant mothers.

In pregnant mothers, if there is asystole or a slow heart rate (< 60 beats/minute), give atropine 3 mg IV just once to counteract any excessive vagal tone.

Reversible causes of cardiac arrest

The causes of cardiac arrest in childhood and pregnancy are multifactorial, but the two commonest final pathways are through hypoxia and hypovolaemia.

All reversible factors are conveniently remembered as the **4Hs and 4Ts** (see below). Sometimes cardiac arrest is due to an identifiable and reversible cause, such as shock due to massive haemorrhage. In the trauma setting, cardiac arrest may be caused by severe hypovolaemia, tension pneumothorax or pericardial tamponade.

It is often appropriate to give an early IV bolus of Ringer-lactate or Hartmann's solution (10 mL/kg in a child and 500 mL to 1 litre in a mother, depending on her weight), as this will be supportive in cases related to severe hypovolaemia. In addition, however, a tension pneumothorax and/or pericardial tamponade require definitive treatment. Continuing blood replacement and the prevention of haemorrhage may also be required.

Rapid identification and treatment of reversible causes such as hypovolaemic shock, hypothermia, electrolyte and acid–base disturbance, tension pneumothorax and pericardial tamponade are vital.

During CPR it is important to continually consider and correct reversible causes of the cardiac arrest based on the history of the event and any clues that are found during resuscitation.

The 4Hs and 4Ts

1 **Hypoxia** is a prime cause of cardiac arrest in childhood, and its reversal is key to successful resuscitation.
2 **Hypovolaemia** may be significant in arrests associated with trauma, gastroenteritis, pregnancy-related haemorrhage, anaphylaxis and sepsis. It requires infusion of crystalloid, and in the case of haemorrhage, blood should be given.
3 **Hyperkalaemia, hypokalaemia, hypocalcaemia, acidaemia, hypermagnesaemia** (following excess magnesium sulphate in eclampsia) and other metabolic abnormalities may be suggested by the patient's underlying condition (e.g. renal failure, eclampsia), tests taken during the resuscitation or clues from the ECG. Intravenous calcium (0.2 mL/kg of 10% calcium gluconate in children and 10 mL of 10% calcium gluconate in pregnant mothers) is indicated in cases of magnesium overdose, hyperkalaemia and hypocalcaemia.
4 **Hypothermia** is associated with drowning incidents and requires particular care. A low-reading thermometer must be used to detect it (see Section 7.3.E).
5 **Tension pneumothorax** and **cardiac Tamponade** are especially associated with PEA and are often found in trauma cases.
6 **Toxic** substances, resulting either from accidental or deliberate overdose or from an iatrogenic mistake, may require specific antidotes.
7 **Thromboembolic** phenomena (pulmonary or amniotic fluid) in pregnancy.

Shockable cardiac arrest

These arrhythmias are less common in children and in pregnant mothers, but either of them may be expected in patients with sudden collapse, hypothermia, poisoning by tricyclic antidepressants, or cardiac disease. The protocol for ventricular fibrillation (VF) (see Figure 1.13.18) and pulseless ventricular tachycardia (pVT) (see Figure 1.13.19) is the same, and is shown in Figure 1.13.20.

A sudden witnessed collapse is also suggestive of a VF/pVT episode.

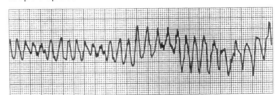

FIGURE 1.13.18 An episode of ventricular fibrillation.

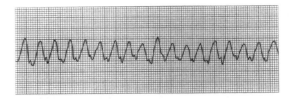

FIGURE 1.13.19 Ventricular tachycardia.

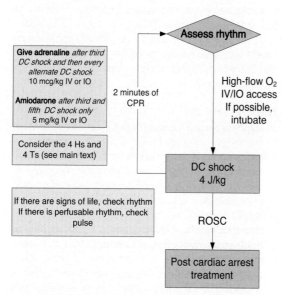

Give adrenaline *after third DC shock and then every alternate DC shock* 10 mcg/kg IV or IO

Amiodarone *after third and fifth DC shock only* 5 mg/kg IV or IO

Consider the 4 Hs and 4 Ts (see main text)

If there are signs of life, check rhythm
If there is perfusable rhythm, check pulse

Assess rhythm

2 minutes of CPR

High-flow O₂
IV/IO access
If possible, intubate

DC shock
4 J/kg

ROSC

Post cardiac arrest treatment

FIGURE 1.13.20 Algorithm for the treatment of shockable (VF and pVT) rhythms in children. Doses of drugs and size of shock used in pregnancy are given in the text below. CPR, cardiopulmonary resuscitation; IV, intravenous; IO, intra-osseous; ROSC, return of spontaneous circulation.

If the patient is being monitored, the rhythm can be identified before significant deterioration occurs. With immediate identification of VF/pVT, asynchronous electrical defibrillation of 4 joules/kg in children and 200 joules in pregnant mothers should be undertaken immediately and the protocol continued as described below.

In unmonitored patients, basic life support will have been started in response to the collapse, and VF/pVT will be identified when the cardiac monitor is put in place.

An **asynchronous shock of 4 joules/kg in children and 200 joules in pregnant mothers** should be given immediately and **CPR immediately resumed** without reassessing the rhythm or feeling for a pulse. Immediate resumption of CPR is vital because there is a pause between successful defibrillation and the appearance of a rhythm on the monitor. Cessation of chest compressions will reduce the likelihood of a successful outcome if a further shock is needed. However, no harm accrues from 'unnecessary' compressions.

Paediatric paddles (4.5 cm) should be used for children under 10 kg.

One electrode is placed over the apex in the mid-axillary line, while the other is placed immediately below the clavicle just to the right of the sternum. If the paddles are too large, one should be placed on the upper back, below the left scapula, and the other should be placed on the front, to the left of the sternum.

Automated external defibrillators (AEDs) are now commonplace in well-resourced countries. The standard adult shock is used for children over 8 years of age. For children under 8 years, attenuated paediatric paddles should be used with the AED (if available).

For infants under 1 year of age, a manual defibrillator which can be adjusted to give the correct shock is recommended. However, if an AED is the only defibrillator available, its use should be considered, preferably with paediatric attenuation pads. The choice of defibrillation for infants in decreasing order of preference is as follows:

1 manual defibrillator
2 AED with dose attenuator
3 AED without dose attenuator.

Many AEDs can detect VF/VT in children of all ages, and differentiate between 'shockable' and 'non-shockable' rhythms with a high degree of sensitivity and specificity.

If the shock fails to defibrillate, attention must revert to supporting coronary and cerebral perfusion as in asystole. Although the procedures for stabilising the airway and obtaining circulatory access are now described sequentially, they should be undertaken simultaneously under the direction of a resuscitation team leader.

The airway should be secured, the patient **ventilated** with high-flow oxygen, and **effective chest compressions** continued at a rate of 100–120 per minute, with a compression depth of at least one-third of the antero-posterior diameter of the chest, and a ratio of 15 compressions to 2 ventilations. As soon as is feasible, a skilled and experienced operator should **intubate the child's airway.** This will both control and protect the airway and enable chest compressions to be given continuously, thus improving coronary perfusion. Once the patient has been intubated and compressions are uninterrupted, the ventilation rate should be 10–12 breaths per minute. It is important for the team leader to check that the ventilations remain adequate when chest compressions are continuous. **Obtain circulatory access.** Whenever venous access is not readily obtainable, intra-osseous access should be considered early on in children, as it is rapid and effective. Central venous lines provide more secure long-term access, but they offer no advantages compared with IO or peripheral IV access. In each case any drug is followed by a crystalloid flush (2–5 mL).

Two minutes after the first shock, pause the chest compressions briefly to check the monitor. If VF/VT is still present, give a **second shock of 4 joules/kg** and **immediately resume CPR**, commencing with chest compressions.

Consider and correct reversible causes (the 4Hs and 4Ts) while continuing CPR for a further 2 minutes.

Pause briefly to check the monitor.

If the rhythm is still VF/VT, give a **third shock of 4 joules/kg**.

Once chest compressions have resumed, give **adrenaline 10 micrograms/kg in children and 1 mg in pregnant mothers IV** and **amiodarone 5 mg/kg in children and 300 mg in pregnant mothers** intravenously or intra-osseously, flushing after each drug.

After completion of the 2 minutes of CPR, pause briefly to check the monitor, and if the rhythm is still VF/VT give an immediate **fourth shock of 4 joules/kg** and **resume CPR.**

After a further 2 minutes of CPR, pause briefly to check the monitor and if the rhythm is still shockable, give an immediate **fifth shock of 4 joules/kg**.

Once chest compressions have resumed, give a second dose of **adrenaline 10 micrograms/kg** and a second dose of **amiodarone 5 mg/kg** intravenously or intra-osseously in children and **1 mg of adrenaline IV** and **150 mg amiodarone in pregnant mothers**. An amiodarone infusion can be continued if there is refractory VF/pVT of 900 mg over 24 hours in adults and 15 mg/kg over 24 hours in children.

After completion of the 2 minutes of CPR, pause briefly before the next shock to check the monitor. Continue giving shocks every 2 minutes, minimising the pauses in CPR as much as possible. Give adrenaline after every **alternate** shock (i.e. every 4 minutes) and continue to seek and treat reversible causes.

Note: After each 2 minutes of uninterrupted CPR, pause briefly to assess the rhythm on the monitor.

In addition, if at any stage there are signs of life, such as regular respiratory effort, coughing or eye opening, stop CPR and check the monitor.

- If the rhythm is still VF/VT, continue with the sequence as described above.
- If the rhythm is asystole, change to the asystole/PEA sequence.
- If organised electrical activity is seen, check for signs of life and a pulse. If there is ROSC, continue post-resuscitation care. If there is no pulse (or a pulse of < 60 beats/minute) and no other signs of life, continue the asystole/PEA sequence.

In VT or VF that does not respond to the above sequence, and where there is no evidence of previous administration of magnesium for eclampsia, consider giving magnesium sulphate 25–50 mg/kg up to a maximum of 2 grams in children and an **8 mmol IV bolus (4 mL of 50% magnesium sulphate) in pregnant mothers**.

Sodium bicarbonate

If VF/VT is due to tricyclic antidepressant overdose or hyperkalaemia, sodium bicarbonate may be helpful. Give 1 mmol/kg (1 mL/kg of an 8.4% solution or 2 mL/kg of a 4.2% solution) in children, and give 50 mmol in pregnant mothers.

Amiodarone

Amiodarone is the treatment of choice in shock-resistant ventricular fibrillation and pulseless ventricular tachycardia. The dose of amiodarone for VF/pulseless VT is 5 mg/kg via rapid IV/IO bolus in children, and **300 mg IV in pregnant mothers**.

Lidocaine is an alternative to amiodarone if the latter is unavailable. The dose is 1 mg/kg IV or IO in children and **100 mg** as an IV bolus **in pregnant mothers**.

It is DC shock that converts the heart back to a perfusing rhythm, not the drug. The purpose of the anti-arrhythmic drug is to stabilise the converted rhythm, and the purpose of adrenaline is to improve myocardial oxygenation by increasing coronary perfusion pressure. Adrenaline also increases the vigour and intensity of ventricular fibrillation, which increases the success rate of defibrillation.

Precordial thump

A precordial thump may be given in monitored patients in whom the onset of VT or VF is witnessed, if there are several clinicians present and if the defibrillator is not immediately to hand. However, it is rarely effective, and early activation of emergency services and obtaining an AED are more appropriate. Start CPR as soon as possible.

Drugs used in non-shockable and shockable cardiac arrest
Oxygen

Although 100% oxygen must be used during the resuscitation process, once there is return of spontaneous circulation (ROSC) this can be detrimental to tissues that are recovering from hyperoxia. Pulse oximetry should be used to monitor and adjust for oxygen requirement after a successful resuscitation. Saturations should be maintained in the range 94–98%. **Always ensure that oxygen delivery is discontinued during defibrillation shocks, to avoid the risks of explosions and fire.**

Adrenaline

Adrenaline is the first-line drug for treatment of cardiac arrest. Its effect is to increase blood flow to the brain and myocardium by constricting alternative arterioles. It renders the myocardium more susceptible to defibrillation.

The initial IV or IO dose is 10 micrograms/kg (0.1 mL/kg of 1 in 10 000 solution) in children and 1 mg (1 mL of 1 in 1000 solution) in pregnant mothers. In children with no existing IV access, the intra-osseous route is recommended as the route of choice, as it is rapid and effective. In each case, adrenaline is followed by a 0.9% saline flush (2–5 mL).

Sodium bicarbonate

Good basic life support is more effective than alkalising agents, which may be considered if spontaneous circulation has not returned after the first or second dose of adrenaline. Sodium bicarbonate is recommended in the treatment of patients with VT/VF due to hyperkalaemia and tricyclic antidepressant overdose (see above).

The dose is 1 mmol/kg in children (1 mL/kg of an 8.4% solution or 2 mL/kg of 4.2% solution), and 50 mmol in pregnant mothers.

- Sodium bicarbonate must not be given in the same intravenous line as calcium, otherwise precipitation will occur.
- Sodium bicarbonate inactivates adrenaline and dopamine, so the line must be flushed with Ringer-lactate or Hartmann's solution if these drugs are subsequently given.
- **Sodium bicarbonate must not be given via the intra-tracheal route.**

Glucose

Hypoglycaemia is defined as a glucose concentration of less than 2.5 mmol/litre (45 mg/dL).

All patients, but especially infants and preschool children, can become hypoglycaemic when seriously ill. Blood glucose levels should therefore be checked frequently, and **hypoglycaemia must be corrected**. If it is suspected and blood glucose levels cannot be measured, always give 2–5 mL/kg of 10% glucose in children or 100 mL of 25% glucose in pregnant mothers, preferably IV if not enterally (via a gastric tube). Make 100 mL of 25% glucose by adding 50 mL of 50% glucose to 50 mL of Ringer-lactate or Hartmann's solution. If blood glucose levels can be measured, avoid hyperglycaemia (maintain blood glucose concentration below 12 mmol/litre).

Cardiac arrest and cardiopulmonary resuscitation in the obstetric patient
Background

Cardiac arrest in late pregnancy or during delivery is rare, and maternal survival rates are very low (3–33% in published series). The cause of the arrest is not often reversed, and the physiological changes present in late pregnancy hinder effective CPR.

Cardiac arrest in the mother results in absent uterine

perfusion, and the fetus will also die. Even when CPR is ideal, it is not possible to generate a cardiac output of more than 30%.

Causes

These include the following:

- massive haemorrhage
- pulmonary embolism
- trauma
- amniotic fluid embolism
- severe infection
- local anaesthetic toxicity.

Physiological changes of pregnancy that relate to cardiopulmonary resuscitation

- Pregnant mothers more easily develop hypoxaemia.
- The enlarged uterus along with the resultant upward displacement of the abdominal viscera decreases lung compliance.
- The most serious physiological change is aorto-caval compression in the supine position. **It is essential that CPR is performed in the left lateral position in any pregnant woman where the uterus is a significant intra-abdominal mass (usually after 20 weeks' gestation).** During closed-chest cardiac compression the best cardiac output that can be achieved is between one-fourth and one-third of normal. Although many factors contribute to this, poor venous return to the heart is of paramount importance. At term the vena cava is completely occluded in 90% of supine pregnant patients. This results in a decrease in cardiac stroke volume of as much as 70%. **It is helpful to manually displace the uterus to the left in advanced pregnancy** (*see* Figure 1.13.21).
- Caesarean section performed early in resuscitation greatly improves the effectiveness of maternal resuscitation.

Perimortem Caesarean section

- Caesarean section should be performed as soon as possible, as described in Section 1.12 on basic life support. This will immediately relieve the vena caval obstruction and increase the likelihood of survival for both infant and mother. CPR must be continued throughout the procedure until spontaneous and effective cardiac activity occurs.
- Assisted ventilation may have to be continued for a longer period of time. Some infants have survived when delivered after 20 minutes of maternal resuscitation.
- Without Caesarean section, less than 10% of mothers who arrest in hospital will survive to discharge. Removal of the infant improves maternal circulation during resuscitation, and cardiac output immediately increases by 20–25%.

Perform the Caesarean section with a midline vertical incision, or whatever method the operator is most

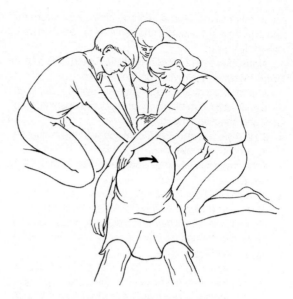

FIGURE 1.13.21 Displacing the gravid uterus to the left.

familiar with, and remove the baby as fast as possible. Remove lateral tilt when the baby is delivered.

When to stop resuscitation

Local guidelines should be in place. Resuscitation efforts are unlikely to be successful, and cessation can be considered, if there is no return of spontaneous circulation at any time after 20 minutes of life support and in the absence of recurring or refractory VF/VT. The exceptions are patients with a history of poisoning or a primary hypothermic insult, in whom prolonged attempts may occasionally be successful. Prolonged external cardiac compressions during which central (femoral or arterial) pulses were felt have successfully resuscitated patients with tricyclic antidepressant overdose.

The presence of the parents at the child's side during resuscitation enables them to gain a realistic understanding of the efforts made to save their child's life. In general, family members should be offered the opportunity to be present during the resuscitation of their child.

The most important points can be summarised as follows:

- A staff member (if available) must be designated as the parents' support and interpreter of events at all times.
- The team leader, not the parents, decides when it is appropriate to stop the resuscitation.
- If the presence of the parents is impeding the progress of the resuscitation, they should be sensitively asked to leave.
- The team needs a debriefing session to support staff and reflect on practice.

1.14 High-dependency care in pregnancy and childhood

> High-dependency care is a service provided for patients with potentially recoverable pathological processes who can benefit from more detailed observation and treatment than is generally available on the standard hospital ward.
>
> High-dependency care is usually provided for patients with threatened or established organ failure, which may have arisen as a result of:
> - an acute illness
> - a complication of pregnancy or delivery
> - trauma
> - a predictable phase in a planned treatment programme (e.g. after major surgery).

Introduction

Health needs are best met through an integrated approach involving several agencies, including primary and secondary healthcare, education and social services. **Together such services may help to prevent some of the conditions that lead to patients requiring intensive care.** For example, vaccination programmes will decrease the number of children who develop respiratory failure due to preventable diseases such as pertussis and measles. Education and legislation are important for reducing the number of individuals who are seriously injured in road traffic accidents and in accidents in the home.

High-dependency care is a low-volume, high-demand specialty. Women and girls with complications of pregnancy and children under 2 years of age account for most of those who require high-dependency care. There also may be seasonal variation, with a peak in the winter months associated with respiratory-related illness, or a peak in the rainy season associated with malaria.

Dedicated intensive care units in large tertiary care centres have been shown to have the best outcomes. Ideally, every country in the world should have units that provide this service. **However, the majority of patients who require high-dependency or intensive care will present to smaller peripheral hospitals rather than to large tertiary centres.** Therefore it is absolutely essential that staff in smaller district hospitals are able to recognise and appropriately treat sick children and pregnant women in the early stages of their illness (*see* EESS-EMNCH programme – Essential and Emergency Surgical Skills – *Emergency Maternal, Neonatal and Child Healthcare Manual and Pocket Book*, which can be found on the MCAI website: www.mcai.org.uk).

All medical and nursing staff who undertake high-dependency care should be well trained in emergency care so as to be able to stabilise critically ill or injured patients, and initiate appropriate medical therapy, which may involve intubation and ventilation. A proportion of such patients may then be safely transferred to an intensive care unit if this is still appropriate and a bed is available. Often, with good initial resuscitation and early diagnosis and treatment, the need for intensive care can be avoided. In a patient who requires intensive care, there should be early consultation with the regional/national intensive-care unit, usually by telephone or radio, so that further management can be jointly decided until a retrieval team, if available, arrives to collect the patient.

Transportation of critically ill patients (*see* Section 1.19), particularly those receiving assisted ventilation, requires appropriately trained staff and equipment. Transportation is best thought of as 'a high-dependency care bed on wheels', and the aim should be that the patient does not deteriorate during transport. Before the patient is moved, proper resuscitation and stabilisation are essential.

Children and pregnant mothers exhibit fundamental differences that influence the training of staff and the type and size of equipment available. These differences extend across anatomy, physiology, pharmacology and behaviour. However, both of these patient groups have less reserve and tend to decompensate early and quickly. They also have a greater capacity to make a full recovery.

Provision of high-dependency care is not just about equipment and facilities. The surrounding environment and contact with their family is crucial to the promotion of a patient's recovery.

Levels of high-dependency/intensive care

There are three levels of care that are designed to make the most appropriate use of staff and equipment resources (*see* Table 1.14.1). In most resource-limited countries, only Level 1 care is likely to be available, and then only in the most well-funded hospitals, such as those in the capital cities or where medical students are trained.

The majority of patients can be managed at Level 1 with close monitoring, good nursing care and appropriate medical therapy. By providing optimal therapy it is often possible to prevent the deterioration of the patient (e.g. through good fluid management, early but appropriate treatment with antibiotics, and the use of oxygen).

Many hospitals will have poor outcomes if patients have to be ventilated in sites where there is a lack of maintained ventilators, and no reliable oxygen source or blood gas analyser. As far as possible in countries with limited resources, intubation and ventilation should be avoided until they are absolutely necessary. Many patients can tolerate high pCO_2 levels with a compensated pH – it is hypoxia that is potentially fatal. It may be appropriate to develop and have available non-invasive modes of ventilatory support, such as nasal mask or cannula **continuous positive airways pressure (CPAP)**, nasal or face mask **intermittent positive pressure ventilation (IPPV)**, **bilevel positive airways pressure (BiPAP)**, or **negative pressure ventilation (CNEP or INPV)**. Similarly, the more invasive a procedure or monitoring process is, the greater the risk of complications.

Finally, it is essential that hospitals which provide high-dependency care have an on-site biomedical engineer to keep all of the equipment serviced and safe.

TABLE 1.14.1 Levels of high dependency and intensive care

Level 3 (intensive care)		
Multi-organ failure		
Ideally one or more nurses per patient		
Invasive monitoring		
Examples: ventilation, haemofiltration		
Optimise medical therapy	↓ ↑	
Level 2 (intensive care)		
Single-organ failure		
Ideally one nurse per patient		
Non-invasive or invasive monitoring		
Example: ventilation		
Intubate ↑		
Optimise medical therapy	↓ ↑	Extubate ↓
Level 1 (high-dependency care)		
Requirement for closer observation and monitoring than is available on the standard ward		
Ideally one nurse for every two patients		
Non-invasive monitoring		
Examples: after major surgery, non-intubated child with severe croup, pregnant woman with severe pre-eclampsia or eclampsia		

Minimum standards for a lead centre providing intensive care

Medical staff

- Senior doctors or physician assistants with appropriate training in high-dependency care medicine.
- Training programme for junior medical staff specialising in high-dependency care.
- Provision of 24-hour cover at both senior and junior level.
- Resident junior cover for 24 hours by staff with skills in emergency care and resuscitation, whose only clinical responsibility is to the high-dependency care unit.
- Access on site to other specialist consultants (e.g. obstetrician, paediatrician, ENT surgeon, anaesthetist).

Nursing staff

- Nursing staff with training in high-dependency care and resuscitation.
- Ongoing training and support for nursing staff.
- Continuous 24-hour observation of each patient at all times by a nurse qualified in high-dependency care, with observations documented.

Support staff

- Availability of a physiotherapist.
- Availability of a pharmacist 24 hours a day.
- Availability of a dietitian.
- Availability of a biomedical engineer 24 hours a day.

Equipment and drugs

- Medical staff and nursing staff with training in how to use all equipment.
- Equipment maintained on a regular basis and according to manufacturer's guidelines by a biomedical engineer.
- Controlled drugs, especially morphine, available immediately and for 24 hours a day.

Retrieval service

- Available 24 hours a day from the community or other health facilities without high-dependency care (e.g. via an emergency ambulance service; see www.reproductive-health-journal.com/content/pdf/1742-4755-7-21.pdf).
- Does not take staff from the high-dependency unit, leaving it uncovered.
- Usually an experienced doctor, midwife or nurse.
- Able to provide phone or radio advice.
- Equipped with portable battery-operated monitors (ECG, heart rate, respiratory rate, oxygen saturation) and suction. Possible to provide hand bag ventilation by face mask or endotracheal tube rather than have a transport ventilator.

Clinical effectiveness and management

- Protocols for admissions, discharges, retrievals, resuscitation and stabilisation, and for treating major conditions.
- Data collection and regular audit of deaths and near-miss cases to improve care provided.

Facilities for families

- Access for carers of children and partners of pregnant mothers at all times.
- Accommodation and food for families.
- Maternal and Child Health Initiative (MCHI) environment (see MCHI manual).

Essential equipment for the high-dependency care of children and pregnant mothers

1 Beds that are manually operated to tilt the head up or feet down.
2 Wedges for lateral tilt for pregnant mothers.

3 Suction systems and suction catheters, both electrical and manual (ideally wall suction).

4 Pulse oximeters and ECG monitors (one for each bed).

5 Resuscitation trolley containing drugs and equipment (particularly oropharyngeal airways, laryngoscopes with spare bulbs, endotracheal tubes and introducers, bag-valve-masks (child and adult), masks with reservoir bags.

6 Mobile screens.

7 Mobile oxygen cylinders and one oxygen concentrator for each bed, with face masks and nasal cannulae (infant, child and adult).

8 Wall sockets (six per bed).

9 One basic infant ventilator and one child/adult ventilator.

10 Nasal or mask CPAP systems (neonatal, child and adult).

11 Two automatic external defibrillators (AEDs).

12 Infusion pumps (if there are sufficient staff).

13 IV drip stands.

14 Basic CVP monitoring system.

15 Blood warmer (ideally).

16 Fridge for pharmacy drugs.

17 Fridge for blood for transfusion.

18 Lockable cupboard for drugs not needing refrigeration.

19 Metal lockable cupboard for controlled drugs.

20 Cupboard for storing IV fluids.

21 End-of-bed chart tables and specially designed high-dependency care charts.

22 One portable ultrasound scanner.

23 One portable fetal heart monitor.

24 Burette giving sets.

25 Portable examination light.

26 Portable fans.

27 Suitable storage boxes (preferably easy to clean and label).

28 Blackboard for documenting priority issues for each patient.

29 Wall-mounted pathways of care.

30 Hand wash facilities × 3/4.

31 Separate sluice and patient and staff toilet and washing facilities.

32 Steriliser.

For details of procedures that are likely to be used in high-dependency care, *see* Section 2.13 (on obstetrics) and Section 7 (on children and all-age trauma).

1.15 Pain control in pregnancy and childhood

Introduction

It is ethically wrong and a failure of professional duties for any patient to suffer uncontrolled pain.

- Uncontrolled pain has adverse cardiovascular, respiratory, immunological and metabolic consequences, as well as long-term psychological effects.

- Both pharmacological and non-pharmacological approaches are valuable in both acute and chronic pain.

- **Attempts should be made to anticipate and prevent pain rather than trying to relieve it when it is established.** This method usually results in less analgesia being needed. 'As-required' regimens should be avoided. Analgesics should be used in regular and adequate doses.

- There is little place for IM pain relief, particularly as a repeated treatment. Many patients would rather suffer and hide their pain than receive IM analgesia.

- If a **conscious** child has to be restrained for a procedure, this must be done kindly but firmly by a person or persons (ideally a parent or caregiver) and not by contraptions such as straitjackets or the tying down of limbs.

- It is vital to ask for and value the patient's own judgement concerning the adequacy of pain relief provided.

- When beginning a course of treatment for pain it is important to realise that such treatment may continue for a long time. **Pain must be controlled quickly from the onset to ensure confidence in treatment, with an emphasis on preventative measures.**

Assessment of pain

- Establish the severity of pain that is being experienced.
- Help to select the right amount and type of pain relief.
- Indicate the success of pain management.

Methods for assessing pain

- Description by the patient (self-reporting), possibly involving the use of a self-report scale (*see* Figures 1.15.1 and 1.15.2)

- Observation of behavioural changes (e.g. crying, guarding of the injured part, facial grimacing). This method is best for children in collaboration with carers. The Alder Hey Triage Pain Score may be useful in this context (*see* Appendix on p. 80).

- Physiological changes (e.g. vasoconstriction, tachycardia, tachypnoea). However, these can also be due to serious medical causes.

- Expectation of pain because of the pathophysiology involved (e.g. obstructed labour, placental abruption, fracture, burn or other significant trauma).

- Keeping a diary of long-term pain.

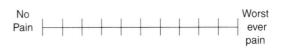

FIGURE 1.15.1 Visual scale for assessing the severity of pain.

| Too much pain | A lot of pain | Medium pain | A little pain | No pain |

FIGURE 1.15.2 A commonly used faces pain scale for assessing the severity of pain in children.

Problems with assessing pain

- Suffering being hidden by a frightened patient, especially a child.
- Difficulty in differentiating anxiety from pain.
- Family members (and healthcare professionals) may underestimate or overestimate pain.
- Pre-verbal and non-verbal children (and any older patient with learning difficulties or with sensory handicap) may not be able to adequately express their need for pain control.
- Cultural factors (beliefs, perceptions and behaviour).

Treatment of pain

Many patients, particularly babies and children, are under-treated for pain because of:

- fear of the harmful side effects of medications
- failure to accept that children feel pain in the same way that adults do
- fear of receiving IM injections
- limited availability of the required spectrum of pain medications.

Methods for reducing pain without drugs
Environmental factors

Negative aspects of the environment should be minimised or removed. These include an overly 'clinical' appearance, and evidence of invasive instrumentation. Needles should be kept out of sight. An attractive, decorated environment with toys, mobiles and pictures may help the child to feel more relaxed.

- Privacy is important.
- Pain caused by fractures can be reduced by splinting to immobilise them.
- Pain from burns can be reduced by applying a light covering.
- Parents should be present with their child during invasive procedures, unless there are very good medical reasons why they should be excluded, or they choose not to be present.

Supportive and distractive techniques for children

Age-appropriate distraction strategies include:

- the presence of familiar objects (comforters) (e.g. pillow, soft cuddly toy)
- singing, concentrating on nice things, jokes, games and puzzles
- imaginary journeys
- blowing soap bubbles
- breathing out (but not hyperventilation, which may increase anxiety)

- a mirror that allows the child to see the view through a nearby window
- listening to stories or music.

Drug treatment for pain using local anaesthetic drugs
Infiltration (the most widely used method)
Lidocaine 0.5–2%

- Used for rapid and intense sensory nerve block.
- Onset of action is within 2 minutes; the procedure must not be started until an anaesthetic effect is evident.
- Effective for up to 2 hours.
- Doses:
  - neonates to 12 years: maximum dose given locally 3 mg/kg – 0.3 mL/kg of 1% solution or 0.6 mL/kg of 0.5% solution (7 mg/kg with 1 in 200 000 adrenaline)
  - children over 12 years and pregnant mothers: up to a maximum of 200 mg (500 mg if used with adrenaline) not more than 4-hourly.
- Adrenaline is rarely added in children and never for digits.
- Strength: 1% or 0.5%.
- Preparation of lidocaine 0.5% solution. Combine:
  - lidocaine 1%, 1 part
  - Ringer-lactate or Hartmann's solution or sterile distilled water, 1 part.

Do not use local anaesthetic containing adrenaline in areas served by an end artery or with a poor blood supply (e.g. finger, toe, penis), as tissue necrosis will occur.

Advantages of adding adrenaline include the following:
- less blood loss
- longer effect of anaesthetic (usually 1–2 hours)
- lower risk of toxicity because of slower absorption into the general circulation.

The concentration of adrenaline to use is 1:200 000 (5 micrograms/mL). In children, the maximum dose of adrenaline is 5 micrograms/kg.

Note: It is critical to measure adrenaline carefully and accurately using a 1-mL or, at the most, 2-mL syringe. (An insulin syringe may be used if a regular 1-mL syringe is not available.) Mixtures must be prepared observing strict infection prevention practices.

TABLE 1.15.1 Formulas for preparing 0.5% lidocaine solutions containing 1:200 000 adrenaline

Desired amount of local anaesthetic needed (mL)	Ringer-lactate or Hartmann's solution (mL)	Lidocaine 1% (mL)	Adrenaline 1:1000 (mL)
20	10	10	0.1
40	20	20	0.2
100	50	50	0.5
200	100	100	1.0

Local infiltration into an abscess is not recommended, because local anaesthetics are ineffective in inflamed tissues.

Complications of local anaesthesia
Prevention of complications

- If more than 40 mL of 0.5% lidocaine are to be used, add adrenaline as described above. Procedures that may require more than 40 mL of 0.5% lidocaine are Caesarean section and repair of extensive perineal tears.
- Use the lowest effective dose.
- Inject slowly.
- Avoid accidental injection into a vessel. There are three ways of doing this:
  - the **moving needle technique** (preferred for tissue infiltration): the needle is constantly in motion while injecting, which makes it impossible for a substantial amount of solution to enter a vessel
  - the **plunger withdrawal technique** (preferred when considerable amounts are injected into one site): the syringe plunger is withdrawn before injecting, and if blood appears the needle is repositioned and another attempt is made
  - the **syringe withdrawal technique**: the needle is inserted and the anaesthetic is injected as the syringe is being withdrawn.

Symptoms and signs of lidocaine allergy and toxicity
Lidocaine can be absorbed through mucous membranes in a large enough dose to be toxic.

Symptoms of allergy: shock, redness of skin, skin rash/hives, bronchospasm, vomiting, serum sickness (*see* Sections 2.7.C and 5.1.B on anaphylaxis in mothers and children, respectively).

TABLE 1.15.2 Lidocaine toxicity

Mild toxicity	Severe toxicity	Life-threatening toxicity (very rare)
Numbness of lips and tongue	Sleepiness	Tonic–clonic convulsions
Metallic taste in mouth	Disorientation	Respiratory depression or arrest
Dizziness/lightheadedness	Muscle twitching and shivering	Cardiac depression or arrest
Ringing in ears	Slurred speech	
Difficulty in focusing eyes		

- Direct intra-arterial or IV injection of even a small amount may result in cardiac arrhythmias and convulsions (see above).
- Resuscitative facilities and healthcare professionals with resuscitative skills should be present.
- Lidocaine can be absorbed through mucous membranes in sufficient concentration to be toxic.

Immediately stop injecting and prepare to treat severe and life-threatening side effects.

If symptoms and signs of mild toxicity are observed wait a few minutes to see if the symptoms subside. Check vital signs and talk to the patient. Delay the procedure for at least 4 hours if possible.

Adrenaline toxicity
This is caused by excessive amounts or inadvertent IV administration, and results in:

- restlessness
- sweating
- hypertension
- cerebral haemorrhage
- rapid heart rate
- cardiac arrest.

Bupivacaine 0.25%
- This is used to provide longer-lasting local anaesthesia.
- Onset of action is up to 30 minutes.
- It is effective for up to 8 hours.
- Maximum dosage is 2 mg/kg (in mothers the pre-pregnant weight is used for calculations).

For uses of other preparations of bupivacaine, *see* Section 1.24.

Local anaesthetics given through the surface of the skin or mucous membranes
1 **Lidocaine:** apply on gauze to painful mouth ulcers before feeds (apply with gloves, unless both the family member and the patient are HIV-positive, in which case the family member does not need protection from infection). It acts within 2–5 minutes.
2 **TAC (tetracaine–adrenaline–cocaine):** apply to a gauze pad and place over open wounds; it is particularly useful when suturing. Care needs to be taken close to mucous membranes to avoid toxicity from absorption of cocaine. If available, other topical anaesthetic agents such as lidocaine–adrenaline–tetracaine seem to be equally effective and avoid the potential toxicity associated with cocaine.

Systemic drug treatment for pain
The World Health Organization (WHO) has altered the previous three-step approach to the treatment of pain, removing the use of codeine between Step 1 and Step 2 (*see* Figure 1.15.3). Although widely available, codeine is unpredictable in its effects, due to its very variable metabolism between individuals, with the potential for both toxicity and inadequate analgesia. It is now recommended that if Step 1 drugs do not control pain, morphine should be used next.

Non-opiate analgesics
Paracetamol
- This is the most widely used analgesic and anti-pyretic.
- It does not cause respiratory depression.
- It is dangerous in overdose but a very safe and effective drug if used in recommended doses.
- It is given by mouth, rectally or intravenously.
  - The maximum daily dose should not be given for more than 3 days.
  - Caution is needed in patients with liver impairment.
  - There are no anti-inflammatory effects.
  - Paracetamol can be combined with NSAIDs and both have a morphine-sparing effect, lowering the dose, and therefore severity of side effects of morphine.

| Paracetamol ±
Aspirin ±
Non-steroidal anti-inflammatory drugs (NSAIDs) |
| :---: |

STEP 1

| Morphine for moderate to severe pain
± Paracetamol or NSAIDs or both
± Adjuvants * |
| :---: |

STEP 2

*An adjuvant is another drug (e.g. steroid or anxiolytic) or type of treatment (e.g. TENS or radiotherapy) that can prevent and relieve pain.

FIGURE 1.15.3 WHO two-step analgesic ladder.

Non-steroidal anti-inflammatory drugs (NSAIDs) (e.g. ibuprofen, diclofenac)

- These are anti-inflammatory, anti-pyretic drugs with moderate analgesic properties.
- They are less well tolerated than paracetamol, causing gastric irritation, platelet disorders and bronchospasm.
- They should be avoided in patients with gastric ulceration, platelet abnormalities or significant asthma.
- NSAIDs are especially useful for post-traumatic and bone pain because of their anti-inflammatory effect.
- They are given by the oral or rectal route (e.g. diclofenac).

Caution: do not give NSAIDs in the third trimester of pregnancy, as they may close the ductus arteriosus and predispose to pulmonary hypertension of the newborn. They may also delay the onset and progress of labour.

There is a risk of gastric haemorrhage through whichever route the NSAIDs are given.

Opiate analgesics

For a discussion of the importance of properly storing, handling and monitoring the use of morphine, *see* Section 1.6.

Morphine

- Morphine is the most important drug in the world for pain control, and the WHO recommends that it should be universally available.
- **In resource-limited countries it is mostly administered orally, which is useful for chronic or anticipated pain but less effective for acute pain. The latter requires IV administration of morphine.**
- At an appropriate dose, analgesia occurs without impaired consciousness.
- Nausea and vomiting are rare with oral treatment, but when morphine is given intravenously for the first time it may produce this side effect.

Intravenous use of morphine

- In single doses it has minimal haemodynamic effects in a supine patient with normal circulating blood volume.
- In hypovolaemic patients it can contribute to hypotension. Therefore:
  - monitor the patient's cardiovascular status
  - have an IV fluid bolus of Ringer-lactate or Hartmann's solution ready (20 mL/kg for a child and 500 mL to 1 litre for pregnant mothers).
- In excessive dosage it can produce a dose-dependent depression of ventilation and decreased respiratory rate, leading to apnoea.
- Patients who are receiving morphine in hospital (where it is often intravenously administered) need observation and/or monitoring of respiratory rate and sedation.
- Morphine is better controlled by the IV than the IM route. If using the IV route, give a small dose initially and repeat every 3–5 minutes until the patient is comfortable. Individuals vary widely with regard to the dose needed to provide pain relief. **It is rarely appropriate to give morphine intramuscularly, and for patients who are in shock, giving morphine IM is dangerous, as it can be initially poorly absorbed, and then quickly absorbed when perfusion improves, potentially leading to too high a blood level of the drug.**
- Morphine can also be given by subcutaneous infusion in hospital (e.g. as a post-operative analgesic), especially if small battery-operated syringe drivers are available.
- Intravenous morphine can be dangerous in situations of raised intracranial pressure without the means to provide respiratory support.
- During late pregnancy or delivery, morphine can cause respiratory depression in the neonate.

TABLE 1.15.3 Orally administered drugs for mild or moderate pain

Medicine	Neonate 0–29 days	Infant 30 days to 3 months	3 months to 12 years	Maximum daily dose	In pregnancy
Paracetamol	10 mg/kg every 6–8 hours
Maximum 4 doses in 24 hours
5 mg/kg if jaundiced	10 mg/kg every 4–6 hours	15 mg/kg up to 1 g every 4–6 hours
Maximum 4 doses/4 g in 24 hours	4 doses in 24 hours	500 mg to 1 g 6-hourly
Ibuprofen	Not recommended	Not recommended	5–10 mg/kg every 6 hours	40 mg/kg/day	Do not use in pregnancy
Diclofenac	Not recommended	Not recommended	**Over 6 months**, 0.3–1 mg/kg 3 times daily	3 mg/kg/day	Do not use in pregnancy

Naloxone

Naloxone is an opiate antagonist that reverses the sedative, respiratory-depressive and analgesic effects of morphine, and so should be given to treat morphine overdose.

Preparations of non-opioid drugs:

Doses can be obtained from the *British National Formulary* and the newly published *PCF4 Palliative Care Formulary*, available at www.palliativedrugs.com/palliative-care-formulary.html (accessed July 2014).

Paracetamol: oral suspension, 120 mg/5 mL, 250 mg/5 mL; tablets, 500 mg.

Ibuprofen: oral suspension, 100 mg/5 mL; tablets, 200 mg, 400 mg.

Diclofenac: tablets, 25 mg, 50 mg; dispersible tablets, 10 mg.

Notes on ibuprofen and diclofenac

- Do not use in patients less than 1 year old, or in pregnancy.
- Caution is needed in patients with asthma, liver or renal failure.
- Contraindications include dehydration, shock, bleeding disorders and hypersensitivity to aspirin.
- NSAIDs and paracetamol can be used in combination.

If rectal drugs are available, the doses are similar to oral doses.

TABLE 1.15.4 Intravenous paracetamol for mild or moderate pain

Age/weight	Dose	Maximum dose in 24 hours
Preterm over 32 weeks	7.5 mg/kg every 8 hours	25 mg/kg
Term neonate	10 mg/kg every 4–6 hours	30 mg/kg
Pregnant woman or child less than 50 kg body weight	15 mg/kg every 4–6 hours	60 mg/kg
Pregnant woman or child more than 50 kg body weight	1 g every 4–6 hours	4 g

Intravenous paracetamol

- Paracetamol IV is formulated as a 10 mg/mL aqueous solution (in ready-to-use 50-mL and 100-mL vials for infusion over 15 minutes).
- It is useful, effective and safe.
- The peak analgesic effect of IV paracetamol occurs within 1 hour, with a duration of approximately 4–6 hours.
- Ensure that the correct dose is given, as serious liver toxicity can occur in overdose.

- Side effects are rare. They include rashes, blood disorders and hypotension on infusion.
- Caution is needed in patients with severe renal impairment, severe malnutrition (and thus low reserves of hepatic glutathione) or dehydration.
- Paracetamol helps to reduce the amount of narcotics required when used in combination with them.

TABLE 1.15.5 WHO advice: oral and rectal morphine for severe pain in hospital

Age	Dose	Interval
1 month to 1 year	80–200 micrograms/kg	Every 4 hours
1–2 years	200–400 micrograms/kg	Every 4 hours
2–12 years	200–500 micrograms/kg	Every 4 hours
Over 12 years and in pregnancy	5–10 mg	Every 4 hours

Note: the upper doses seem quite high – if a child weighs 20 kg, they would be receiving 10 mg – the same as an adult.

We suggest that you start with the lower dose and give more frequently, e.g. every hour if needed, until the patient is comfortable, then increase the dose if morphine needs to be given every hour. The Table immediately below (Table 1.15.6) already has lower doses.

Almost all patients with chronic pain can be managed with oral morphine when this is given in the doses shown in Tables 1.15.6 and 1.15.7 in combination with non-opioid analgesics

These are starting doses and can be increased as necessary on an individual patient basis if pain is not controlled

TABLE 1.15.6 *British National Formulary (BNF)* and *BNF for Children (BNFc)* recommended doses for oral and rectal morphine

Age	Initial dose (adjust according to response)	Interval
1–3 months	50–100 micrograms/kg	Every 4 hours
3–6 months	100–150 micrograms/kg	Every 4 hours
6–12 months	200 micrograms/kg	Every 4 hours
1–2 years	200–300 micrograms/kg	Every 4 hours
2–12 years	200–300 micrograms/kg	Every 4 hours
12–18 years	5–10 mg	Every 4 hours
Adults/pregnant mothers	5–10 mg	Every 4 hours

Preparations of morphine

1 Prepared mixture:
- 10 mg/5 mL
- 30 mg/5 mL
- 100 mg/5 mL.

2 Morphine oral solutions can be made by dissolving powder in clean water, and are available in Africa at concentrations of 5 mg/5 mL, 50 mg/5 mL and 100 mg/5 mL.

3 Tablets: 10 mg, 20 mg and 50 mg.

4 Suppositories: 15 mg and 30 mg.

5 Slow-release tablets: 10 mg, 30 mg, 60 mg and 100 mg.

6 Slow-release suspension sachets: 5 mg, 20 mg, 30 mg, 60 mg, 100 mg and 200 mg.

Note: See Section 1.16 on palliative care for use of morphine at home.

Parenteral morphine

IV morphine is only needed if oral or rectal preparations are not going to be absorbed (e.g. in shock) or where rapid emergency onset is needed. IV morphine is potentially less safe, especially if staff shortages mean that the correctly calculated dose is not given.

TABLE 1.15.7 Intermittent IV (bolus) morphine dosage*

Age	Dose	Interval	Maximum dose
Neonate	25–50 micrograms/kg	Every 6 hours	
1–6 months	100 micrograms/kg	Every 6 hours	2.5 mg/dose
6 months to 2 years	100 micrograms/kg	Every 4 hours	2.5 mg/dose
2–12 years	100–200 micrograms/kg	Every 4 hours	
Over 12 years and in pregnancy	10 mg	Every 4 hours	

* We suggest that the total dose recommended is drawn up in 10 mL 0.9% saline and that 2 mL boluses of this solution are given every 3–5 minutes until the patient is comfortable. Also, if pain returns despite regular paracetamol/nonsteroidal analgesia, further dose of oral/IV morphine can be given within 6 hours if the respiratory rate is normal and the patient is not sedated.

Intravenous infusion of morphine requires continuous monitoring including oxygen saturation and respiratory rate and sedation score every 5 minutes for the first 15 minutes after start of the infusion and every 15 minutes subsequently for one hour and at least every 30 minutes after that. It should only be undertaken in a high dependency care situation. In resource limited situations, intermittent IV boluses as in Table 1.15.7 are safer.

Monitoring during morphine administration:

Side effects occur only in overdose and should not be seen at the doses stated here. They include the following:

1 Respiratory depression. **If the respiratory rate is:**
- < 20 breaths/minute in patients aged less than 6 months
- < 16 breaths/minute in those aged less than 2 years
- < 14 breaths/minute in those aged 2–10 years
- < 12 breaths/minute in those aged 10–18 years and in pregnant mothers

alert medical staff and ensure that bag-valve-mask and naloxone are available.

Monitor SaO$_2$ as appropriate (it should be higher than 94% in air).

2 Constipation. Use prophylactic laxatives.

3 Monitor for urinary retention.

4 Patients with liver and renal impairment may need lower doses and longer time interval between doses. Caution in patients with head injuries

Always ventilate with bag-valve-mask first if patient is unresponsive before giving naloxone. This is because arrhythmias and pulmonary oedema can be caused if naloxone is given to a patient with high blood carbon dioxide concentrations.

Naloxone doses to reverse opioid induced respiratory depression

1 Neonate to 1 month of age: 5–10 microgram/kg repeated every 2–3 minutes until adequate response

2 1 month to 12 years of age: 5–10 microgram/kg, subsequently 100 mcg/kg

3 12 to 18 years and in pregnancy: – 0.2–2.0 mg/kg. Repeat at intervals of 2–3 minutes to a maximum of 10 mg.

If respiratory rate is low, but the patient's oxygen saturation is acceptable (>94%) with facemask oxygen, in order to avoid complete reversal of analgesia draw up 400 microgram naloxone into 20 mL and give 1–2 mLs every 2 minutes until the patient is rousable and the respiratory rate increased to an appropriate rate for age.

Preparations of naloxone: Ampoule 20 microgram/mL

Give IV or IM if IV is not possible. Repeat after 2–3 minutes if there is no response; the second dose may need to be much higher (up to 100 micrograms/kg). An IV infusion may be needed if protracted or recurrent depression of respiration occurs because naloxone is short acting compared with most opioids.

Starting dose for naloxone infusion: 60% of the dose that maintained adequate respiration for 15 minutes.

Alternatively: Neonate – 5 to 20 microgram/kg/hour, adjusted according to response; 1 month to 18 years and in pregnancy – 5 to 20 microgram/kg/hour.

(For the newborn, to treat respiratory depression due to maternal opioid administration during labour or delivery 200 microgram as a single IM dose is recommended or 60 microgram/kg.)

Prevention and treatment of nausea and vomiting due to initial high-dose morphine

1 Cyclizine. This covers the widest range of causes of nausea and vomiting with the least side effects. It is not recommended orally in children < 2 years and rectally < 6 years.

The IV doses are:

- 1 month to 6 years: 500 microgram to 1 mg/kg 8 hourly
- 6 to 12 years: 25 mg 8 hourly
- 12 to 18 years and in pregnancy: 50 mg 8 hourly

2 Domperidone – where gastric emptying is a problem, then as in Table 1.15.8 for doses.

TABLE 1.15.8 Domperidone for prevention and treatment of nausea and vomiting

Domperidone	
Oral	**Rectal**

From 1 month up to 35 kg in a child:
 	
  250–500 micrograms/ kg 3–4 times daily, up to a maximum of 2.4 mg/kg in 24 hours
 	
Over 35 kg and in pregnant mothers:
 	
  10–20 mg 3–4 times daily, up to a maximum of 80 mg daily
 	
Tablets, 10 mg
 	
Suspension, 5 mg/5 mL
	Not recommended for children weighing < 15 kg
	
	Children weighing 15–35 kg, 30 mg twice daily
	
	Children weighing > 35 kg or in pregnant mothers, 60 mg twice daily
	
	Suppositories, 30 mg

Both of the above can cause extrapyramidal side effects, including acute dystonia, which can be treated with diazepam IV 100 microgram/kg, or, if over 12 years and in pregnancy, 5–10 mg IV.

Specific clinical situations in which analgesia may be required
Invasive procedures

- These are often painful, undignified, or both. Ideally they should be undertaken in a treatment room so that other patients are not frightened by the procedures, and so that the patient's bed-space remains a safe place that is not associated with such events.
- Such procedures often have to be repeated. Therefore provide optimal treatment on the first occasion in order to reduce the likelihood of dread of future procedures.
- Fear is often the main emotion that needs to be addressed, so explain each step.
- Both pharmacological and non-pharmacological methods should be used.
- For major procedures that require powerful analgesia/ sedation, two healthcare workers should be present – one to perform the procedure and the other to administer analgesia and sedation and ensure that the airway is maintained.
- Major procedures include chest drain insertion and repeated lumbar puncture. **Such procedures may be best undertaken under general anaesthesia or ketamine if this can be given safely (which may not be the case in resource-limited countries).**
- For venous cannulation, size-appropriate catheters must

be available. For example, it is not appropriate to use an 18- or 20-gauge cannula in a neonate. Although the use of local anaesthetic creams (e.g. EMLA) prior to cannulation represents best practice, they are expensive. In some circumstances, the urgency of the situation will not allow use of local anaesthetic creams.

- Give analgesics at an appropriate time before the procedure (30 minutes beforehand for IM and 30–60 minutes beforehand for oral medication depending on the drug used) aiming for maximal effect during the procedure.
- Check the level of anaesthesia by pinching the area with forceps. If the patient feels the pinch, wait 2 minutes and then retest.
- Wait a few seconds after performing each step or task for the patient to prepare for the next one.
- Handle tissue gently and avoid undue retraction, pulling or pressure.
- Talk to the patient throughout the procedure.

Analgesia during labour

For severe pain, give morphine bolus 2.5–5 mg and repeat once after 5 minutes if the pain is not controlled. Then wait 2–4 hours before repeating.

Nitrous oxide plus oxygen can be effective in reducing pain during labour (*see* Section 2.3).

Barbiturates and sedatives should never be used to relieve anxiety in labour.

Severe pain

- Severe pain is likely to occur in obstetric emergencies, post-operatively, and in patients with major trauma, significant burns, or displaced or comminuted fractures.
- Give IV morphine as described in Table 1.15.6.
- A further dose can be given after 5–10 minutes if sufficient analgesia is not achieved.
- Monitor ABC (heart rate, respiratory rate, chest wall expansions, blood pressure, SaO$_2$).
- Have IV Ringer-lactate or Hartmann's solution available (20 mL/kg for children and 500 mL to 1 litre for pregnant mothers as a bolus if hypotension occurs following IV morphine injection: this is unusual).
- Ketamine could be used as an alternative.

Head injuries

- An analgesic dose does not necessarily cause sedation.
- If the patient is conscious and in pain, the presence of a potential deteriorating head injury is **not** a contraindication to giving morphine. Give IV up to a maximum dose of 100 micrograms/kg for a child or 5 mg for a pregnant mother.
- If the patient's conscious level does deteriorate, assess ABC. If hypoventilation occurs, ventilate with a bag-valve-mask.
- If necessary, a dose of naloxone will help to distinguish whether reduced conscious level is due to morphine or increasing intracranial pressure, as it will reverse the effects of the morphine, including the analgesic effect.

Pre-operative management

This should include patient assessment, including a history of previous painful experiences from the patient and family (the parents of a child). The following questions should be asked.

- What sort of painful things have happened in the past?

- How does the patient usually react to sudden pain? And to chronic pain?
- Does the patient tell you (or others) if he or she is in pain?
- What does the patient do to get relief from pain?
- Which actions appear to be most effective?

Pain management during surgery

- Morphine/NSAIDs can reduce post-operative pain (but do not give NSAIDs to pregnant patients).
- Consider wound infiltration with bupivacaine or lidocaine.
- Use local or regional anaesthetic as part of the overall strategy (see Section 1.24).

Prophylactic anti-emetics for children aged 4 years or older and in pregnancy when morphine is part of the post-operative pain control plan can be very effective (see Table 1.15.10).

Post-operative pain management

- Provide analgesia before the pain becomes established; the amount of pain can often be anticipated depending on procedure.
- Use safe and effective doses of morphine along with other analgesics to reduce the amount of morphine required.
- Avoid intramuscular injections.
- **Assess, give analgesia, and then reassess.**
- Those most at risk of poor pain control are children with limited or no verbal ability.
- If the pain seems to be out of proportion to surgical trauma, consider the possibility of surgical complications and arranged reassessment by surgeons.
- If the patient is asleep, assume that the pain level is acceptable. Don't wake them up to make an assessment, count the respiratory rate and check regularly whether they are still asleep. If they are awake and lying quietly do not assume that they are comfortable without asking them.

Special issues with regard to pain in the newborn infant

- Most studies (some of them controlled) have shown that neonates (both premature and full term) react to pain.
- Infants can easily be forced to put up with suffering.
- Small doses should be measured and given with an oral syringe.
- Adequate general anaesthesia, using morphine when needed, should be given for all surgical procedures on neonates.
- Local anaesthetics must be used when they would be used in an older child undergoing the same procedure.

Pain control during procedures in neonates

- A sugar-dipped dummy, coated with 2 mL of 25–50% sucrose 2 minutes before the procedure, can be helpful.
- Breastfeeding during procedures may be equally helpful.
- In all cases, comfort and containment (swaddling) should be provided by a parent or nurse.

Pain management in high-dependency care

- Where possible, all invasive procedures should be elective. Every effort should be made to avoid unexpected emergency procedures, such as intubation, by adequate monitoring of airway, oxygenation and chest movement.
- **Emergency procedures are frequently extremely painful, dangerous to the patient, and often can**

be avoided by early recognition of a deteriorating condition (see Section 1.11).

- Muscle relaxants should be avoided if possible and **never** be used unless the patient is pain free, sedated and being ventilated.
- Provide a day/night cycle (uninterrupted natural sleep can reduce the need for analgesia/sedation).
- Ensure that there is minimal noise and low lighting from 8 pm to 8 am.
- Emergency admissions at night should take place away from sleeping patients.
- Monitors should be set to alarm audibly only when this is essential.
- Consider the use of ear plugs, especially when the patient is paralysed.
- Provide human input through voice, touch, music, cuddling, rocking, holding and pacifying.
- Consider the use of distraction, play therapy, relaxation, behavioural techniques, hypnosis and aromatherapy, particularly for patients who are undergoing long-term intensive/high-dependency care.
- Provide privacy whenever possible.
- Be alert for depression after prolonged intensive care.
- Consider the use of methadone and clonidine for the control of morphine and sedation withdrawal after prolonged treatment.

Sedation

Sedation is not recommended for use in pregnancy after the first trimester, because of the risks of re-gurgitation and aspiration if the airway is not protected.

A health worker skilled in anaesthesia should be asked for advice and help with managing conditions where sedation is being considered.

Sedation in children

- This may be useful when added to analgesics for lengthy or repeated procedures. The aim of sedation is to make the procedure more comfortable while allowing verbal contact with the patient to be maintained.
- Start with a small dose IV, wait for 2–3 minutes, observe the response, and repeat the dose if necessary.
- Sedation relieves anxiety but not pain.
- Sedation may reduce a patient's ability to communicate discomfort, and therefore should **not** be given without concomitant analgesia if there is pain.
- Side effects include hyper-excitability or prolonged sedation, delaying discharge after the procedure.

Sedation and anaesthesia form a spectrum. If you give enough 'sedation' you can induce anaesthesia (i.e. loss of consciousness and the inability to feel pain). This is why it is not recommended in pregnancy, because of the increased risk of aspiration of stomach contents into the lungs, causing life-threatening pneumonia.

The fine distinction lies in the ability of the patient to maintain vital functions without assistance, and to respond to being roused (see Table 1.15.9).

Any healthcare worker who is administering a sedative, especially a benzodiazepine, must stay with the patient and have available a bag-valve-mask of suitable size and be able to use it to ventilate the patient if they develop abnormally slow breathing.

TABLE 1.15.9 The differences between sedation and anaesthesia

Vital function	Sedation	General anaesthesia
Response to being roused	Present	Absent
Respiration	Rate and depth may be slightly reduced	Rate and depth are markedly reduced or absent
Swallowing reflex	Present	Absent
Gag reflex	Present	Absent
Cough reflex	May be reduced	Absent
Cardiovascular stability	Mild hypotension may occur	Hypotension should be anticipated

Loss of any of the above reflexes is routine in anaesthetic environments, but should **not** occur when sedation is being provided.

Minimum information required to prescribe sedation

Anyone who is giving intravenous sedation could inadvertently produce anaesthesia, and must therefore be able to deal with the possible consequences. This means that they must be able to:

- **support respiration**
- **manage and maintain the airway**
- **use suction appropriately**
- **intubate if necessary.**

High-dependency nursing (*see* Section 1.14) or perioperative nursing care in the recovery room after surgery is required.

A combination of drugs may give better effects with fewer side effects than continually repeating doses of the same drug (e.g. morphine or ketamine combined with benzodiazepine). Each of the drugs should be given separately and the doses adjusted.

Some patients are difficult to sedate for predictable reasons (e.g. treatment for epilepsy may make the dose required much higher than normal).

Some patients are very resistant to sedation, possibly due to excessive anxiety, so the first dose of sedation may not succeed, and a higher dose may be needed.

Patients who need sedation should have their oral intake restricted as for anaesthesia.

Some children are more vulnerable to the effects of sedation, particularly those with respiratory or upper airway problems, causing complete upper airway obstruction and should not be sedated unless a health worker skilled in anaesthesia/airway management is present.

Sedation in children is difficult and potentially dangerous, and this practice is increasingly being abandoned.

- Children may refuse to take sedatives.
- The effects of sedatives in children are unpredictable.
- The interval between taking the medicine and becoming sedated, and also the time taken to recover, are difficult to predict in children.
- Some children, especially those who are very young, can take large doses of sedatives with no apparent effect.
- Some children become paradoxically over-excited as a result of taking sedatives.
- There is a danger that the dose needed to sedate a child will compromise the reflexes that protect the airway.

Wherever possible, procedures in children should be done without sedation. Instead ensure that, if possible, a parent or other familiar caregiver can stay with the child to reassure and comfort them. Give good analgesia with ketamine, oral morphine and local anaesthesia, and use skilful restraint to keep the child still. Explain carefully to the child, if they are old enough to understand, what you are doing at each stage of the procedure, to reduce their anxiety and encourage their cooperation.

The minimum information required to prescribe sedation includes the following:

- age and weight if the patient is a child
- the procedure for which sedation is required
- the patient's previous sedation history
- any other drugs that are being taken
- **other major illnesses that affect respiratory function and upper airway competence**
- current health status, including coughs, colds and pyrexia
- oral intake status.

TABLE 1.15.10 Patients at risk of airway obstruction/respiratory depression from the effects of sedation

Risk factor	Underlying cause
Impaired upper airway Obstruction	Croup
	Foreign body
	Congenital stridor (e.g. Pierre–Robin syndrome, cleft palate)
	Baby with very blocked nose
Impaired reflexes	Pre-existing neuromuscular problems
	Swallowing difficulties
	Known bulbar problems, especially if combined with reflux
Impaired central respiratory drive	Head injury
	Drug effects (opiates)
	Raised intracranial pressure
	Impaired level of consciousness
	Encephalopathy (hypoxic, metabolic, infective)
Impaired respiratory muscle function	Neuropathy and myopathy
	Chronic illness and weakness
	Malnutrition
	Prematurity
	Infancy
Impaired lung function	Chest infection
	Pleural effusions
	Chronic lung disease
Impaired cardiovascular function	Haemorrhage
	Sepsis
	Drugs

Sedative drugs commonly used for children
Promethazine (Phenergan)
Give 0.5 mg/kg deep IM or IV or 1–2 mg/kg orally, up to a maximum of 50 mg.

Chloral hydrate
Chloral hydrate is more suitable for younger babies (less than 18 months of age or less than 15 kg), but may paradoxically worsen agitation (e.g. in Down's syndrome).

TABLE 1.15.11 Sedative drugs

Drug	Route	Onset	Duration	Dose
Promethazine Tablets: 10 mg	Oral	30 minutes to 1 hour	Up to 12 hours	Not recommended for patients under 2 years of age Children: 2–5 years, 15–20 mg 5–10 years, 20–25 mg 10–18 years, 25–50 mg
Promethazine Liquid injection: 25 mg/mL	Slow IV or deep IM injection	30 minutes to 1 hour	Up to 12 hours	1 month to 12 years: 0.5–1 mg/kg (up to a maximum of 25 mg) 12–18 years: 25–50 mg
Chloral hydrate Liquid: 100 mg/mL Suppositories: 100 mg and 500 mg	Oral or rectal	30 minutes to 1 hour	1–2 hours	Neonates to 12 years old: 30–50 mg/kg 12–18 years: 45–60 mg Maximum dose 1 g

Management of long-term pain and pain during terminal care
This is discussed in Section 1.16.

Appendix: Alder Hey Triage Pain Score
Cry/voice
Score 0: Child is not crying and, although they may be quiet, they are vocalising appropriately with carer or taking notice of surroundings.

Score 1: Child is crying but consolable/distractible or is excessively quiet and responding negatively to carer. On direct questioning the child says it is painful.

Score 2: Child is inconsolable, crying and/or complaining persistently about pain.

Facial expression
Score 0: Normal expression and affect.

Score 1: Some transient expressions that suggest pain/distress are witnessed, but less than 50% of the time.

Score 2: Persistent facial expressions suggesting pain/distress more than 50% of the time.

Posture
This relates to the child's behaviour towards the affected body area.

Score 0: Normal.

Score 1: Exhibiting increased awareness of the affected area (e.g. by touching, rubbing, pointing, sparing or limping).

Score 2: Affected area is held tense and defended so that touching it is deterred; non-weight-bearing.

Movement
This relates to how the child moves their whole body.

Score 0: Normal.

Score 1: Movement is reduced or the child is noted to be restless/uncomfortable.

Score 2: Movement is abnormal, either very still/rigid or writhing in agony/shaking.

Colour (applicable only to children with paler skins)
Score 0: Normal.

Score 1: Pale.

Score 2: Very pale 'green', the colour that can sometimes be seen with nausea or fainting – extreme pallor.

Further reading
British National Formulary and British National Formulary for Children. www.bnf.org/bnf/index.htm (accessed 9 December 2012).

WHO Guidelines on the Pharmacological Management of Persisting Pain in Children with Medical Illnesses. http://whqlibdoc.who.int/publications/2012/9789241548120_Guidelines.pdf (accessed 9 December 2012).

Freedom from Pain. Pharmacists working with doctors and nurses to secure this human right in Africa. A publication of Hospice Africa Uganda, PO Box 7757, Kampala. Email: info@hospiceafrica.org.ug

1.16 Palliative care for children in resource-limited countries

Introduction

Most children who need palliative care in resource-limited countries will require identification and treatment in the community rather than in hospital. Moreover, in the presence of effective care and support networks, **home has frequently been demonstrated to be the best setting for palliative care for both the child and the family**.

A high proportion of children do not reach hospitals in Africa. This percentage ranges from approximately 57% in Uganda to 85% in Ethiopia. Also, hospitals need to be aware that most families would wish for their child to die at home, where they can look after them and they can be buried with their ancestors near to the home. The cost of transporting a body is very high, so economic factors also play a part.

Therefore any treatment that is given in the hospital must be of a kind that can be continued at home, otherwise the child will never be able to leave the hospital. Healthcare workers in hospital, with the support of Ministries of Health and community leaders, must set up systems to help community health workers to provide care in the community, including the safe management of morphine treatment when it is required.

Allowing the family and child to choose the setting for palliative care is of great importance. However, it is recognised that the necessary resources may be minimal or absent in many locations, and local conditions will determine what options are available.

This section describes the use of affordable medications that have been proven to work in resource poor settings. In resource limited situations, it is vital that government funds are spent carefully on measures which work and are not too expensive thus ensuring that the poorest families can also receive their right to palliative care for their children.

Although palliative care actually means relief of symptoms in all care, the term is usually associated with relieving symptoms when the emphasis is no longer on curative treatment. The decision to stop or withdraw curative treatment will never be easy for parents or healthcare professionals, and may evolve over a period of time. **It is important, however, to state that even when we cannot cure the body, it is never true that nothing more can be done.**

Like all of us, children have personal needs, and careful attention must be given to the physical, social, emotional and spiritual needs of the child and their family. Staff, too, should be receiving support through what can be a distressing time.

Essential healthcare for the dying child

- Include parents or familiar caregivers.
  - This matters at all times.
  - Their familiar presence will comfort the child.
  - Even apparently unconscious children may still know their parents' or caregivers' voices.
  - Parents invariably want to be able to provide care for their child. This is a natural wish and can aid their own coping strategies.
- Set realistic goals.
  - The art of terminal care is to know when both goal and treatment must change.
  - The goal is to help the child to enjoy and cope with what is left of their life.
  - It should be clearly and well communicated that resuscitation measures are not to be a feature of terminal care.

BOX 1.16.1 WHO definition of palliative care

Palliative care is an approach that improves the quality of life of patients and their families facing the problem associated with life-threatening illness, through the prevention and relief of suffering by means of early identification and impeccable assessment and treatment of pain and other problems, physical, psychosocial and spiritual.

Palliative care:

- provides relief from pain and other distressing symptoms
- affirms life and regards dying as a normal process
- intends neither to hasten nor to postpone death
- integrates the psychological and spiritual aspects of patient care
- offers a support system to help patients live as actively as possible until death
- offers a support system to help the family cope during the patient's illness and in their own bereavement
- uses a team approach to address the needs of patients and their families, including bereavement counselling, if indicated
- will enhance quality of life, and may also positively influence the course of illness
- is applicable early in the course of illness, in conjunction with other therapies that are intended to prolong life, such as chemotherapy or radiation therapy, and includes those investigations needed to better understand and manage distressing clinical complications.

WHO definition of palliative care for children

- Palliative care for children is the active total care of the child's body, mind and spirit, and also involves giving support to the family.
- It begins when illness is diagnosed, and continues regardless of whether or not a child receives treatment directed at the disease.
- Health providers must evaluate and alleviate a child's physical, psychological, and social distress.
- Effective palliative care requires a broad multidisciplinary approach that includes the family and makes use of available community resources; it can be successfully implemented even if resources are limited.
- It can be provided in tertiary care facilities, in community health centres and even in children's homes.

— Our aim is now not to cure, and never to kill, but always to comfort.

— The social needs and goals of a dying child include access to siblings and friends to play with and talk to. They should be made welcome.

- Listen and explain.

  — It should be clear from the child's deteriorating condition that the goals are changing and death is imminent. This must be gently explained and the parents' and child's questions answered. It is wise, especially with children, to clarify the real question that is being asked. Replies must be honest, but the truth should be shared sensitively, a little at a time.

  — Explanations are very important for both parents and children, and appropriate, understandable terms should be used.

  — Forewarning of procedures, with hugs and praise afterwards, will reduce fears and fantasies.

  — Honesty results in greater trust and cooperation than saying something won't hurt when it will.

  — All of those involved, from a young child to an elderly grandparent, will harbour fears and anxieties. Active listening is a major part of caring for a dying child and their family. Great comfort can be derived from the acknowledgement and expression of anxiety, and this helps to dissipate the feelings of isolation that are frequently experienced.

  — Adolescents will also have particular concerns and worries, and often have spiritual needs as well. Spirituality is a major aspect of life even for younger children in Africa. All members of the team must be aware of this and ready to discuss it with them.

- List and treat the child's symptoms.

  — In palliative care, symptom intervention and practical care are paramount.

  — Even with limited resources, symptoms can often be helped. Problem lists are a useful key to active needs.

  — The availability of drugs does not guarantee their skilful use, but when medication is used effectively it will make both life and death more bearable. It can be helpful to give the family a treatment chart showing times or relationship to sunrise and sunset (see Figure 1.16.1).

— The child and carer together should make a list of all the symptoms. This can guide palliation even when the cause is incurable.

— Ask the carer to chart extra doses required and any medication-related problems that arise.

The duration and nature of palliative care will be unique to each child and their particular disease. **For those children who cannot be cured (sadly they are the majority in resource-limited settings), highly effective symptom control is paramount to enable a good quality of life for the time that is remaining.**

It is essential to approach the management of any symptom systematically.

For palliative care issues concerning HIV infection, *see* Section 6.2.D.

Common symptoms
Pain
For pain assessment, *see* Section 1.15.

Principles of pain control
Pain is probably the most common symptom in palliative care, and is frequently seen in both malignant and non-malignant disease. It is a complex sensation related to the physiological insult to the tissues, but is also influenced by psychological, social and cultural factors.

It is helpful to think of severe pain in terms of response to opioids.

- **Opioid-responsive** pain is relieved by opioids.
- **Opioid-semi-responsive** pain is relieved by the concurrent use of an opioid and an adjuvant drug.
- **Opioid-resistant** pain is not relieved by opioids.

Neuropathic or nerve pain is more likely to fall into the semi-responsive or unresponsive groups. Bone pain falls into the semi-responsive group.

Analgesic approaches to pain relief
The optimal approach to pain management in children includes drug therapy, with analgesics usually being the mainstay of treatment. Correct use of analgesic drugs

Medicine	Reason	Morning		Afternoon		Evening		Night
		On Waking	10 am	12 noon	2 pm	6 pm	10 pm	Bedtime
Morphine 5 mg in 5 mL	Pain	2.5 mL	2.5 mL		2.5 mL	2.5 mL		5 mL
Senna	Constipation						2	
Ibuprofen 200 mg	Pain	2		2		2		2

Medication chart for... Date....................

FIGURE 1.16.1 Example of treatment chart for family use in the community.

will relieve pain in most children, and should be based on the four key concepts recommended by the WHO:

- by the **ladder**
- by the **clock** (or by the sun if there is no clock!)
- by **mouth**. Injections are not given at home because there are too few community health workers. Subcutaneous infusion pumps are not always acceptable, and also need close monitoring, which is often not possible
- by the **child or carer**.

By the ladder

Use the 'two-step' approach to analgesia, non-opioids and opioids. The second step in the three-step ladder that was proposed in 1986 by the WHO is now widely being omitted, and a two-step ladder is used instead (*see* Figure 1.16.2). This is because the middle step, namely codeine, is expensive and causes severe constipation, and if the child has cancer they will need morphine, so can commence with a small dose that can then be titrated to the pain. Pain is classified as mild, moderate or severe, and the analgesic choices are adjusted accordingly. The ladder approach is based on drugs that are widely available in most countries. The sequential use of analgesic drugs is based on the child's level of pain, with a non-opioid analgesic usually being the first step.

Importantly, however, assessment of a child's pain may indicate the need for immediate use of a strong opioid. Morphine is the safest and most effective opioid, and the only affordable one in resource-limited settings.

There should be no hesitation in moving on to Step 2 of the analgesic ladder if pain control is inadequate.

Only one drug from each pharmacological group should be used at the same time but remember that paracetamol plus a non-steroidal drug can be used together if there is no contraindication. Strong opioids can be increased until pain is relieved. Occasionally an alternative strong opioid (rarely affordable in resource-limited countries) may be substituted if side effects from the first opioid tried are intolerable.

The aim is for the child to be:

- pain free on movement
- pain free at rest
- pain free at night.

Paracetamol ±
Aspirin ±
Non-steroidal anti-inflammatory drugs (NSAIDs)

STEP 1

Morphine for moderate to severe pain
± Paracetamol or NSAIDs or both

± Adjuvants *

STEP 2

FIGURE 1.16.2 WHO two-step analgesic ladder. *An adjuvant is another drug (e.g. steroid or anxiolytic) or type of treatment (e.g. TENS or radiotherapy) that prevents but can also relieve pain.

By the clock (or by sunrise/sunset)

Analgesia should be given regularly (e.g. every 4 hours or according to the half-life).

There is no place for 'when-requested' prescribing of

analgesics in palliative care. The dose must be titrated against that needed to control the pain of the individual patient.

Paracetamol and ibuprofen should be given at the recommended doses (*see* Section 1.15), but the dose of morphine needed must be titrated against that needed to control the pain.

The dosing interval should be determined according to the severity of the child's pain and the duration of action of the drug being used. Additional 'rescue' doses for intermittent and breakthrough pain should be prescribed and explained to the family, so that these can be given as soon as breakthrough pain occurs.

The effectiveness of analgesia should be regularly reviewed, so that it can be titrated effectively against pain.

By the appropriate route

Children should receive drugs by the simplest, most effective and least painful route. For this reason the oral route is the preferred route.

IM injections should not be used. They are painful, and there is a risk of abscess and/or haematoma formation, particularly in children who may have low platelet counts or other blood-clotting problems. Also, use of the parenteral route means that the patient must be in hospital or a clinic and cannot go home. Children who are afraid of injections may deny that they are in pain and therefore suffer unnecessarily.

When selecting the best route of analgesic administration it is important to consider the nature and severity of the pain, the potency of the drug, the required dosing interval and the compliance of the child.

By the child

The doses of any analgesic must be based on the individual child's symptoms and circumstances. There is no single dose that will be appropriate for all children.

Regular reassessment of the child's pain and of the effectiveness of the analgesia is essential, so that the drug doses can be adjusted accordingly to keep the child pain free.

For some children, particularly those with cancer-induced pain, very large doses of opioids may be required in order to achieve satisfactory pain control.

Therefore it should be noted that some of the suggested dosage recommendations included in this section differ from those specified elsewhere in the manual. This is appropriate in palliative care, and it reflects the differences in goals and priorities between the acute setting and the palliative setting.

CASE EXAMPLE: Haji, aged 3 years, presented with a clinical diagnosis of retinoblastoma. He was in severe pain. The lesion was too friable for a biopsy. Morphine was commenced immediately, based on weight, according to the WHO recommendation for children. This was titrated against the pain, and Haji's pain was controlled on 100 mg 4-hourly and 100 mg at night. The radiologists allowed him to receive radiotherapy without a biopsy. The tumour disappeared. The morphine was reduced until he was pain free and well.

Today Haji is well, aged 9 years, and is attending school.

Analgesics
Non-opioid analgesics

Non-opioid analgesics are used to relieve mild pain or, in combination with opioids, to relieve moderate and severe pain. **Paracetamol** is the drug of choice because it has a very high therapeutic ratio for children and can be given orally or rectally. It is available in an elixir, tablet and suppository form, and can be given 4- to 6-hourly. Non-steroidal anti-inflammatory drugs (NSAIDs) such as **ibuprofen** and **diclofenac** are also helpful (for doses, see Section 1.15).

It is now recommended that one should progress straight from paracetamol and NSAIDs to morphine.

Strong opioid analgesics (morphine)

Morphine is required either alone, or in combination with non-opioid analgesics and/or adjuvant drugs, to provide effective pain relief. Morphine does not have an analgesic 'ceiling affect' (i.e. there is no maximum dose), and children may require extremely large doses to obtain pain relief, but start at the recommended dose for severe pain (as described in Section 1.15).

The strong opioid of choice internationally is oral morphine.

The oral route is preferred for morphine, but if the subcutaneous or IV route is required, it can be given by a slow continuous infusion, which will give a steady level of analgesia and is preferred to intermittent subcutaneous or IV administration. Although a continuous infusion is commonly used in well-resourced countries, it is possible to achieve complete pain control with oral or rectal paracetamol or morphine in the palliative care setting. In resource-limited settings, children and their families may be alarmed by infusions.

Children have been found to rapidly eliminate morphine metabolites, and this is most marked in younger children (under 9 years). This group of children may require more frequent dosing and relatively higher doses to achieve pain relief. However, if oral doses are given at regular intervals, the most potent metabolite of morphine, M6G, accumulates and leads to smooth pain control.

Morphine must be available in all countries. However, this is not the case at present. In Africa, only 15 out of 56 countries have oral morphine available for use at home, which is where most terminally ill patients want to die. Oral morphine that is made up in the country or within a district of the country is the affordable ideal. The drug is then immediately available, so pain can easily be controlled with it.

More complicated formulae and preparations may be available as immediate- or sustained-release preparations, including immediate-release suppositories. Once-daily preparations are commercially available, but there is little experience of their use in children, and they are too expensive for most resource-limited countries. Ideally, morphine should be free to all in need, and prescribed by a recognised prescriber. Usually only doctors can prescribe. However, in Uganda, nurses can now prescribe after completing a Diploma in Palliative Care and clinical officers after a 9 week special training that emphasises prescribing methods and controls. Clinical officers have been trained for 4 years and can do more than nurses in most countries. In some African countries they are allowed to prescribe class A drugs after qualification.

Immediate-release morphine (from the list of essential medicines for children published by the WHO in 2010)

- Morphine tablets (Sevredol): 10 mg, 20 mg and 50 mg.
- Morphine sulphate mixture (Oramorph): 10 mg/5 mL.
- Morphine sulphate mixture (Oramorph concentrate): 100 mg/5 mL.

The most affordable preparation is a morphine solution made from morphine powder in a pharmacy without the exorbitant profit taken by the 'middle man' (see Section 1.15).

The oral morphine starting dose is 150–300 microgram/kg every 4 hours.

Immediate-release morphine should be given regularly every 4 hours. It may be useful to increase the night-time dose by 50–100% to eliminate night-time waking. Immediate-release oral morphine is the best choice in children because it is easier to titrate exactly against the pain. Sustained-release morphine tablets (MST Continus) (5 mg, 10 mg, 15 mg, 30 mg, 60 mg, 100 mg and 200 mg) and morphine granules for suspension (MST Continus) (20 mg, 30 mg, 60 mg, 100 mg and 200 mg), although available, are very expensive and therefore inappropriate for most situations in resource-limited countries. Those planning for a service must keep in mind the needs of the poor and spend the money available for morphine wisely so that there is enough for all in need.

Breakthrough pain

Immediate-release morphine should be prescribed at a dose equivalent to the 4-hourly doses as soon as pain breaks through (i.e. 16–17% of the total daily dose). The WHO recommends that it should be 5–10% of the total daily dose. This can be given up to hourly for breakthrough pain, and the parents should be advised to keep a record of all extra doses given so that the regular dose of morphine can be titrated accurately, and more supplied as necessary.

Titration of the morphine dose

Pain relief should be reviewed regularly. The morphine dose should be titrated against the level of pain. If frequent breakthrough analgesia is required, the total dose of morphine taken during the day (regular doses plus 'breakthrough' doses) must be assessed. Usually increments of 20–50% of the previous total daily dose are required. Regular review allows the regular dose of morphine to be adjusted according to the level of breakthrough pain. **Remember to**

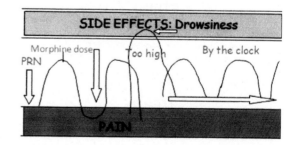

FIGURE 1.16.3 'As needed' (PRN) versus 'by the clock' versus 'high dose'. Initially, to the left, the PRN dosage regime results in episodes of unrelieved pain. In the middle, too high a dose produces drowsiness. To the right, the by-the-clock dosage regime results in constant relief of pain without drowsiness. (Diagram supplied by Dr Anne Merriman.)

increase the dose of breakthrough morphine accordingly, when the regular dose is increased.

Alternatives to oral route of administration

Indications for these include:

- persistent vomiting
- non-compliance with oral medication
- dysphagia
- bowel obstruction
- physical deterioration that prevents oral intake
- unsatisfactory response to oral medication.

Rectal route

This route may be acceptable for some children who are unable to take oral medication. Any oral preparation can be given rectally with similar effects:

- Paracetamol can be given as a suppository.
- Morphine solution (see above) can be easily given rectally and is very effective.
- Morphine suppositories (10 mg, 15 mg, 20 mg or 30 mg) can be given if available.

Although one can use the same dose and interval as for the oral route (i.e. 4-hourly), this is traumatic for the child, and generally a larger dose given in tablet suppository form as half the daily dose 12-hourly is more acceptable.

Subcutaneous route

Many drugs are well absorbed subcutaneously and can be easily established in those children who do not have established venous access. However, many resource-limited countries will not be able to use syringe drivers, and buccal and rectal administration may be just as effective, especially if human resources for managing the syringe driver/infusion pumps safely are not available, although some parents may be able to manage them.

Changing from oral morphine to subcutaneous morphine

The potency of morphine administered by injection is approximately twice that of oral morphine. Therefore use **half of the total daily oral morphine dose** as the equivalent 24-hour morphine dose for subcutaneous infusion.

If syringe drivers are not available, parents can be trained to give regular boluses of morphine subcutaneously or IV at home. The total daily dose of either morphine or diamorphine is divided by a practical number that coincides with the number of individual doses to be given (usually 1- to 2-hourly during the day, and 4-hourly at night).

Intravenous route

- This will usually only be indicated where a child has an established venous access, such as a Hickman line (unlikely to be available in most resource-limited countries), or when death is likely to occur within 7 days, when community health workers may place a peripheral venous cannula.
- Divide the total daily dose of oral morphine by two to obtain the equivalent daily dose of morphine given IV or subcutaneously.

As approximately 80% of children will die at home in resource-limited countries, oral or rectal morphine is likely to be the mainstay of treatment, with IV morphine only available to a small proportion of these patients.

Although diamorphine is the drug of choice for subcutaneous infusion, because it is more soluble, it is not available in most countries of the world. Divide the total daily dose of oral morphine by 3 to obtain the equivalent daily dose of diamorphine given IV or subcutaneously. The starting dose in opioid-naive patients is 12.5–25 micrograms/kg/hour by continuous infusion. For both subcutaneous and IV routes, the diamorphine should be titrated according to breakthrough pain in increments of 20–50%.

Side effects of opioids

All opioid drugs cause similar side effects. These problems are well known, and should be anticipated and treated whenever children are given opioids, so that pain control is not accompanied by unacceptable side effects. When appropriate, parents and children should be informed about the possible side effects and their management. Children on strong opioids should be assessed regularly.

Constipation

This is a common side effect, and laxatives such as bisacodyl (dulcolax) or senna or sodium docusate must always be prescribed with strong opioids (see below). Advice should be given to increase intake of fluids and fibre (vegetables, fruit and cereals) in the child's diet where appropriate.

Nausea and vomiting

Routine anti-emetics are not commonly needed, but should be prescribed if required in case of opioid-induced nausea and vomiting. When such symptoms do occur, they normally resolve within 3 to 4 days.

Drowsiness and confusion

Daytime drowsiness, dizziness and mental clouding can occur at the start of treatment and sometimes following a dose increase. They almost always resolve within a few days. Cognitive and psychomotor disturbances are minimal once the patient is receiving a stable dose of opioid.

Pruritus

Itching is a not uncommon side effect of opioid treatment in children. Simple skin care alone may be effective. Also consider the following:

- Avoid hot baths
- Avoid using soap. Add Oilatum to the bath water and use aqueous cream as a soap substitute.
- Pat the skin dry rather than rubbing it.
- Avoid overheating and sweating.
- Use cool cotton clothing and bedding.
- Keep the fingernails short to reduce damage caused by scratching.

If itching is persistent, review the medication. If itching is opioid related and the drug cannot be changed, the addition of a systemic antihistamine such as chlorpheniramine may be beneficial.

Pruritus associated with obstructive jaundice will require good skin care plus systemic medication such as stanozolol, ondansetron or levomepromazine, if available.

Respiratory depression

Respiratory depression is uncommon in the conscious patient with severe pain. If it does occur, management will be dictated by the child's overall condition and the place of care.

Nightmares and hallucinations

Both can occur. If they are distressing and not resolved by reassurance or resolution of other anxieties, try giving haloperidol at night (50–100 micrograms/kg).

Urinary retention

Urine retention may be a problem, particularly after rapid dose escalation. Most children respond to simple measures such as a warm bath, warm packs or relief of constipation. Catheterisation may be required, but is usually only needed for a short period.

Morphine toxicity

This can occur as a result of:
- too high a dose
- too rapid dose escalation
- pain that is not morphine responsive
- renal impairment
- previous therapeutic intervention to relieve pain (e.g. radiotherapy or nerve block).

Warning signs include:
- drowsiness
- confusion
- pinpoint pupils
- myoclonic jerks
- hallucinations (auditory and visual)
- vomiting
- nightmares.

If toxicity occurs, consider reducing the morphine dose (several doses may need to be missed), then restart at a lower dose or stop morphine altogether.

Toxicity is rare when morphine is titrated against the pain. Constipation is the worst complication, and can be prevented by introducing a laxative when morphine is started, unless the child has diarrhoea already, in which case the constipation would be beneficial for a few days, but the laxative needs to be introduced as soon as it ceases.

Watch carefully for breakthrough pain. Address any side effects as discussed above. Escalating doses of opioids and metabolic disorders can exacerbate myoclonic jerks. Oral diazepam can be useful. If the child is unable to swallow, rectal diazepam or subcutaneous midazolam are effective.

Consultation with healthcare professionals who are experienced in palliative care is recommended.

Addiction and tolerance

Fear of addiction is not relevant when using opiates in palliative care, provided that a permanent source of opiates is available, **which must be the case**. In Uganda, in 2012, around 20 000 patients had been treated with affordable oral liquid morphine, without any abuse or addiction. Approximately 30% of these cases were children.

Prescribing opioids in patients with renal impairment

The active morphine metabolites are excreted by the kidney and accumulate in renal impairment, causing toxicity. When prescribing any opioid analgesics in children with renal failure, caution must be exercised, as patients with renal failure are extremely sensitive to opioids. Renal failure is part of the dying process, and the team must be aware of this and reduce doses or increase time intervals as the child approaches death.

Suggested management strategies are as follows:
- Prescribe smaller doses of opioid analgesic.
- If problems with toxicity continue, consider giving smaller doses less frequently (i.e. 6- to 8-hourly).

Alternatives to oral morphine for severe pain

For information on approaches that can be used in well-resourced settings, see the Further reading section on p. 91.

Adjuvant therapy

Few children are truly morphine intolerant, and if the pain is not responding to morphine, always consider the aetiology of the pain and review the use of adjuvant therapy.

Neuropathic pain

Co-analgesics such as an anticonvulsant or tricyclic antidepressants are essential, because this pain is only semi-responsive to opioids. The possibility of neuropathic pain should be considered if the pain has a burning or stabbing/shooting component. According to the WHO, there is no evidence on which to make recommendations for or against antidepressants and anticonvulsants. However, the WHO does agree that there is wide experience of the use of amitriptyline in children, and doctors are familiar with the use of the carbamazepine in children who have seizures. However phenytoin is more available, affordable and therefore of choice in less resourced countries. However some anti-retroviral drugs (ARVs) may interact with phenytoin so there is a need to check this out for children with HIV on ARVs.

Nerve compression pain

This may arise from compression of a nerve root, and morphine plus a trial of oral steroids should be tried. The steroid should relieve pain within 48 hours, probably by reducing oedema around the tumour. If there is no improvement, steroid treatment should be discontinued.

Nerve injury pain

This may arise either from tumour invasion of a nerve or as a side effect of radiotherapy.

Anticonvulsants

These drugs are useful for pain that is shooting or stabbing. Carbamazepine and sodium valproate are commonly used. Clonazepam and gabapentin are more recent additions that are not widely available in resource-limited countries. The cheapest, most effective drug with the fewest side effects is phenytoin.

Start at a low dose and gradually increase the dose to avoid sedation and toxicity. Low doses are usually the most effective, and this therapy should stop if the pain does not respond to low doses.

Carbamazepine

This drug is expensive, has side effects, and needs to be monitored, so is not so useful in the community setting.
- Starting dose: 2.5 mg/kg twice daily, increasing by 2.5–5 mg/kg/day at weekly intervals.

- Maintenance dose: 10–20 mg/kg/day in two to three divided doses, increasing gradually as above.

This corresponds to the *British National Formulary for Children (BNFC)* dose for epilepsy and trigeminal neuralgia.

Sodium valproate (often not available)
- Starting dose: 20/mg/day in two divided doses, increasing if required by increments of 5 mg/kg at weekly intervals.
- Maintenance dose: 20–30 mg/kg/24 hours in divided doses.

The *BNFC* doses for epilepsy are:
- Age < 12 years: initially 10–15 mg/kg/day in one to two divided doses, increasing to 25–30 mg/kg/day in two divided doses.
- Age ≥ 12 years: initially 600 mg/day in one to two divided doses, increasing by 150–300 mg every 3 days to 1–2 g/day (maximum of 2.5 g/day) in two divided doses.

Phenytoin
- Age < 12 years: (1.5–2.5 mg/kg starting dose to target) and then 2.5–5 mg/kg twice daily (maximum 7.5 mg/kg twice daily or 300 mg once daily).
- Age 12–18 years: 75–150 mg adjusted according to response up to 150–200 mg twice daily (maximum 300 mg twice daily).

The *BNFC* doses for epilepsy are:
- Age < 12 years: 1.5–2.5 mg/kg twice daily, increasing to 2.5–5 mg/kg twice daily (usual maximum 7.5 mg/kg twice daily).
- Age ≥ 12 years: 75–150 mg twice daily, increasing to 150–200 mg twice daily (maximum 300 mg twice daily).

Tricyclic antidepressants
- These drugs are useful for pain that is burning in nature.
- Give at night to avoid excessive sedation during the day. They can cause constipation.
- The analgesic effect begins after about 3–7 days of treatment, but may take longer than this.
- Starting dose: amitriptyline 0.5 mg/kg at night increasing, if needed, to 1 mg/kg/day. Increase carefully to avoid excessive drowsiness. Lower doses are the most effective.

The *BNFC* doses for neuropathic pain are:
- Age 2–12 years: 0.2–0.5 mg/kg (maximum 10 mg), increasing gradually to a maximum of 1 mg/kg twice daily.
- Age > 12 years: 10 mg at night, increasing gradually up to 75 mg at night if needed.

For difficult cases, consider referral to or discussion with a pain control team if one is available.

Bone pain
Non-steroidal anti-inflammatory drugs (NSAIDs)
- NSAIDs have analgesic, anti-pyretic and anti-inflammatory properties. They are often effective in relieving musculoskeletal pain that is associated with bone metastases or soft tissue inflammation.

- Regular dosing is required for their full effect, but the maximum effect is usually seen within 2 weeks.
- It is worth trying another NSAID if there is no response to the first type.
- Damage to the gastrointestinal mucosa is the most frequent side effect. Gastric erosion and bleeding can be severe and difficult to control. If possible, ensure that NSAIDs are taken after food.
- NSAIDs are not usually appropriate for children with thrombocytopaenia, because of their potential to cause gastric erosions and so increased tendency to bleed.
- According to the WHO there is no evidence for recommending the use of bisphosphonates in children. In adults, modest improvements in pain have been observed, but also serious side effects such as osteonecrosis of the jaw.

For common dosages of NSAIDs, *see* Section 1.15.

Steroids
Steroids have specific benefits in palliative care because of their ability to produce euphoria, improve appetite and increase weight gain. They also have an anti-inflammatory effect, which may be helpful in patients with nerve compression and raised intracranial pressure.

However, steroids should be used with caution in children, as the side effects of long-term steroid treatment can far outweigh its benefits. They include rapid weight gain, change in appearance, mood swings, behaviour changes and insomnia, which can be distressing for both the child and the parents, and the risk of gastric erosions. Most children experience symptom relief after short intensive courses, and if the prognosis is long, steroids should be withdrawn. If there is no improvement in symptoms within a short period of time (e.g. 5–7 days), steroids should be discontinued. If the initial symptom relief is not maintained, long-term use of these drugs should be avoided.

Dexamethasone
Dexamethasone should be taken before 6 pm, and ideally in the morning, in order to minimise insomnia.

High-dose dexamethasone is normally used to relieve pain associated with raised intracranial pressure, or spinal cord or nerve compression. Give steroids in the morning to avoid sleepless nights and to copy the normal diurnal rhythm of cortisol.

The initial dose is given in the morning as 25 mg for patients over 35 kg and 20 mg for patients less than 35 kg, followed by a sliding scale of reducing by 4 mg every 3 days until down to 10 mg per day, then continuing to decrease by 1–2 mg per day.

IM or IV in an emergency or until can swallow (usually once only):
- Age 1 month to 12 years: 100–400 micrograms/kg, once daily in the morning.
- Age 12–18 years: 8–24 mg daily.

Low-dose dexamethasone is normally used to improve appetite and well-being.
- Age 2–8 years: 0.5–1 mg, once daily in the morning.
- Age > 8 years: 1–2 mg, once daily in the morning.
- Radiotherapy.

This therapy is only available in just over half the countries in Africa.

Radiotherapy can be particularly useful for treating isolated sites of a disease if a tumour is radiosensitive. This may include bony metastases, spinal cord compression, and relief of nerve compression from a solid tumour and isolated cerebral metastases. Radiotherapy can also be used in the management of fungating tumours. Single treatments or short courses are often appropriate and effective in palliative care, if radiotherapy is available.

Non-pharmacological approaches

Non-drug therapies must be an integral part of the management of children's pain, complementing but not replacing appropriate drug therapy.

A combination of non-pharmacological approaches, used in conjunction with analgesics, may be extremely effective. These approaches include:

- progressive relaxation
- diversional therapy with music, art or traditional games, according to the age of the child
- hypnosis and guided imagery
- massage and reflexology
- heat pads or cold packs
- transcutaneous electrical nerve stimulation (TENS).

Management of other symptoms
Nausea and vomiting

These are common symptoms in palliative care. The causes may be multifactorial, and it is important to try to determine the cause(s) in order to implement an effective treatment plan.

Common causes

Cancer-related causes include:

- raised intracranial pressure
- the presence of an abdominal mass
- irritation of the upper gastrointestinal tract
- gastric outflow obstruction
- anxiety
- uraemia
- pain
- blood in the stomach.

Treatment-related causes mainly involve the side effects of drugs, especially:

- opioids
- chemotherapy
- NSAIDs
- carbamazepine
- antibiotics.

Management

- Identify the cause(s) as described above (e.g. constipation, raised intracranial pressure) and implement appropriate management.
- Consider stopping gastric irritants such as antibiotics, NSAIDs and steroids if possible.
- Prescribe an H_2-receptor antagonist (ranitidine, 2–4 mg/kg 12-hourly, or cimetidine, 5–10 mg/kg 6-hourly).
- Or the proton pump inhibitor omeprazole (age < 2 years, 700 micrograms/kg once daily increased to 3 mg/kg once daily, maximum dose of 20 mg once daily; body weight 10–20 kg, 10 mg once daily, increased to 20 mg if needed; body weight over 20 kg, 20 mg daily increased to 40 mg once daily if needed. Give the higher dose for 12 weeks only).

- Prescribe an appropriate anti-emetic according to cause.
- Review the therapy regularly and adjust it as required.
- IV fluids may be needed to counteract dehydration, but nasogastric tube insertion should be avoided where possible.
- If treatment is unsuccessful, consider the following:
  - Was the cause of the vomiting correctly identified and the appropriate anti-emetic prescribed?
  - Has the anti-emetic had time to work at maximum dose?
  - Is the route of administration appropriate for the child?

Anti-emetic therapy

Severe nausea and vomiting may require initial management by subcutaneous or IV infusion and then switching to oral medication when control is gained. The choice of anti-emetic depends on the cause of vomiting and the site of the anti-emetic action, so combinations of drugs with different sites of action are sometimes required, but to avoid side effects, avoid combining drugs of the same class. Extra-pyramidal side effects can occur with cyclizine, metoclopramide and domperidone (see Section 1.15).

Haloperidol is the anti-emetic of choice for opioid-induced vomiting. It acts on the chemoreceptor trigger zone.

Dosage: 12.5–25 micrograms/kg twice daily by mouth, subcutaneously or IV. Haloperidol can be given orally at night.

Cyclizine is used for nausea and vomiting caused by raised intracranial pressure or intestinal obstruction.

Dosage: all ages, by mouth, 1 mg/kg three times daily up to a maximum of 50 mg per dose.

The *BNFC* doses are as follows:

Oral or rectal route:

- Age < 6 years: 500 microgram–1 mg/kg (rectal 12.5 mg) up to three times daily
- Age 6–12 years: 25 mg up to three times daily
- Age > 12 years: 50 mg up to three times daily.

IV or subcutaneous route:

- All ages, 1 mg/kg 8-hourly or

Continuous IV/subcutaneous infusion:

- Age < 2 years: 3 mg/kg over 24 hours
- Age 2–5 years: 50 mg over 24 hours
- Age 6–12 years: 75 mg over 24 hours
- Age > 12 years: 150 mg over 24 hours.

Dexamethasone

Dosage: use moderate doses (e.g. 100 micrograms/kg 12-hourly).

Metoclopramide

This acts on both the upper gastrointestinal tract and the chemoreceptor trigger zone, and speeds up gastric emptying. The extrapyramidal side effects are more common in children. It is useful for oesophageal reflux, gastric stasis, gastric irritation, gastric outflow and high bowel obstruction.

Its use should be avoided in patients where there is complete bowel obstruction.

Dosage:
Oral route:
- Age 1–12 years: 100 micrograms/kg, two to three times a day
- Age > 12 years: 5–10 mg, two to three times a day.

Subcutaneous/IV route:
- Age 1–12 years: 500 micrograms/kg over 24 hours
- Age > 12 years: 15–30 mg over 24 hours.

Domperidone acts on both the upper gastrointestinal tract and the chemoreceptor trigger zone, and speeds up gastric emptying.

Dosage:
Oral route:
- Age 1–12 years: 200–400 micrograms/kg, three to four times a day
- Age > 12 years: 10–20 mg, three to four times a day.

Rectal route:
- Age 1–12 years: 15–30 mg, two to three times a day
- Age > 12 years: 30–60 mg, two to three times a day.

Constipation

Constipation is common in paediatric palliative care, and the causes may be multi-factorial. The prevention and relief of constipation in the terminally ill child is very important, as if left unresolved it can cause abdominal pain and discomfort, and nausea and vomiting.

Consider the following causes:
- drug induced (e.g. opioids, anticholinergics, antidepressants)
- reduced physical activity
- poor oral intake and general debility
- dehydration
- bowel obstruction
- spinal cord compression.

Management
- Treat the underlying cause where this is appropriate and possible.
- Constipation should be anticipated when opioid, anticholinergic or antidepressant drugs are being used, and laxatives should be prescribed prophylactically.
- Use laxatives appropriately and at the right doses, and avoid mixing two drugs from the same group (e.g. two stimulants).
- A good first choice is the combination of a stimulant laxative and a softening agent (e.g. senna plus sodium docusate).
- Titrate doses up as required, rather than adding a new laxative.
- If oral therapy fails, consider rectal measures such as suppositories/enemas.

Bowel obstruction

Bowel obstruction may be mechanical or functional, or both. The aim is to control pain and nausea. In children with advanced disease, surgical management is not usually indicated. The aim of treatment is the palliation of symptoms. Nasogastric tubes and IV fluids are rarely appropriate,

although for persistent vomiting due to obstruction a nasogastric tube may be helpful.

Management
Elimination of pain and colic:
- For constant background pain, administer buccal morphine solution or morphine by continuous IV or subcutaneous infusion, using a portable syringe driver.
- If colic is present, avoid prokinetic anti-emetics (e.g. metoclopramide, domperidone).
- Discontinue bulk-forming, osmotic and stimulant laxatives.
- Relieve associated constipation, continue to use softening agents if possible, and use rectal measures to relieve faecal impaction.
- If colic persists, add hyoscine butylbromide (Buscopan), 10–20 mg orally 8-hourly or give IV as a single dose over at least 1 minute (age 2–5 years, 5 mg IV; 6–10 years, 10 mg IV; 11–15 years, 15 mg IV; 15–18 years, 20 mg IV). Repeat 8-hourly as required.

Elimination of nausea and reduction of vomiting
- The choice of anti-emetic depends on whether colic is present.
- If colic is present, cyclizine is the first-line drug. Add haloperidol if nausea persists.
- If colic is absent and flatus is present, a trial of subcutaneous or IV metoclopramide is indicated. If this is ineffective, instigate management as described above.
- Dexamethasone may be of benefit in second-line management.

Dyspnoea

Shortness of breath associated with pulmonary complications in advanced paediatric cancer can be very distressing for both the child and the parents, and requires effective management. The underlying pathophysiology needs to be considered when deciding on the management.

Common causes of dyspnoea include:
- metastases
- effusions
- pulmonary fibrosis
- anaemia
- infection
- superior vena cava (SVC) obstruction
- anxiety/fear
- increased secretions
- cardiac failure
- chest wall pain or constriction
- pulmonary embolus
- gross ascites.

Management
- Identify the cause.
- Give a clear explanation to the parents and the child.
- Treat the specific cause(s) or modify the pathological process (e.g. high-dose steroids and radiotherapy for superior vena caval obstruction).
- Non-drug measures are also important and include:
  - a calm approach
  - breathing exercises
  - an appropriate position
  - providing cool air (e.g. with a fan)
  - play therapy.

Drug treatment

Morphine has a complex effect on respiration, which is not fully understood. It can reduce the respiratory rate to a more comfortable level. This drug should be prescribed regularly in children with continuous breathlessness at standard analgesic starting doses. If the child is already on morphine, increase the dose by 30–50%.

The anxiolytic and sedative effects of **benzodiazepines** also cause relaxation of the respiratory muscles. This may be helpful if the child or teenager is very anxious, and these drugs should be administered as a single dose and then at night or twice daily. The long half-life of benzodiazepines (around 36 hours) means that they should be avoided if possible.

Diazepam (oral route):
Dosage:
- Age 4 weeks to 1 year: 200 micrograms/kg, two to three times daily
- Age 1–12 years: 2 mg, two to three times daily
- Age > 12 years: 5–10 mg, two to three times daily.

Lorazepam is not always available, but is well absorbed sublingually (so is useful for panic attacks), short acting, with a rapid onset of relief and a shorter half-life.
Dosage:
- Age 1–12 years: 50–100 micrograms/kg (maximum of 4 mg per dose) (*BNFC*).
- Age > 12 years: 1–4 mg per dose. The dose may be repeated after 12 hours.

Corticosteroids may be useful, particularly in patients with superior vena caval obstruction and multiple lung metastases. Moderate doses of dexamethasone should be used and the benefit should be apparent within 5 days. The dose should then be reduced to the lowest effective dose.

Oxygen will be of benefit for hypoxic patients, but is rarely available for home use. It may also be helpful if a child is very anxious.

Nebulised saline or **salbutamol** may provide subjective relief, especially if wheezing is present.

Cough

Consider the following causes:
- respiratory infection
- airways disease
- malignant obstruction
- drug induced
- oesophageal reflux
- aspiration of saliva.

Wherever possible, the cause of the cough should be treated. Symptomatic management should follow the guidelines for the management of dyspnoea.

Drug management may include the following:
- simple linctus
- codeine linctus (this will cause constipation, so add a stool softener)
- opioids (as above)
- nebulised saline
- oral antibiotics (these are indicated if symptomatic chest infection with a productive cough is affecting quality of life).

Anxiety

Anxiety is not uncommon in palliative care. Talk to the child and give enough time to both the child and the parents or carers to discover the cause, and give reassurance. Try to identify the cause of the child's anxiety (e.g. whether it is related to symptoms or fears about what is happening). Simple explanations, reassurance and a calm environment are important. Physical therapies such as relaxation and massage may be helpful, or anxiolytics such as diazepam or lorazepam as required or regularly may be of benefit if other measures fail.

Anxiety and discomfort go together, so reassess the child's pain.

Bleeding
Massive external bleeding
Death from massive external bleeding is uncommon in children, but the risk of this is frightening and distressing for both the child and the parents, and prevention of such bleeding should be the aim of management, although this may not always be possible.

Causes of external bleeding include the following:
- a low platelet count
- clotting deficiencies
- primary or secondary liver disease
- disease progression
- initial treatment (e.g. radiotherapy, chemotherapy).

Management
If there is a risk of massive haemorrhage, it is extremely valuable to have IV or subcutaneous morphine and an appropriate sedative (e.g. rectal diazepam, buccal midazolam) readily available at home.

Persistent surface bleeding
This is not uncommon in children with leukaemia, and can be alarming to both the child and their family, but can be managed in the home environment.

Management
- Topical treatment soaking gauze in adrenaline 1 in 1000 solution and applying it directly to the bleeding point.
- Other haemostatic dressings can be used for persistent surface bleeding (e.g. in fungating tumours). These include crushed metronidazole sprinkled on to the area, or an alginate dressing such as Kaltostat if this is available.
- Tranexamic acid can be useful if it is available, and can be used topically undiluted, applied directly to bleeding gums or nostrils, or used as a mouthwash. It can also be given systemically or parenterally as prophylaxis.
- The use of a dark-coloured handkerchief or towel at home to mop up the blood may help to reduce anxiety.

Spinal cord compression
Consider spinal cord compression if the following signs and symptoms are present:
- localised pain in the spine, radiating around the chest
- sudden onset of weakness (e.g. of the legs)
- sensory disturbance
- sphincter dysfunction.

This is usually a clinical diagnosis, and action needs to be taken immediately.

Investigations such as computerised tomography (CT) and magnetic resonance imaging (MRI) are not usually available.

Management

- Patients with paraparesis have a better prognosis than those who are totally paraplegic.
- Loss of sphincter function is a poor prognostic sign.
- Rapid onset of complete paraplegia has a poor prognosis.
- The main therapeutic options are:
  - corticosteroids that can shrink the tumour and relieve spinal cord compression
  - radiotherapy.
- Steroids should be given in high doses initially and then reduced according to the response. These drugs often bring about an early improvement and relief of pain by reducing the peri-tumour inflammation. Give steroids in the morning to avoid insomnia and to copy the normal diurnal rhythm of cortisol.
- High-dose **dexamethasone**: The initial dose is given in the morning as 25 mg for patients over 35 kg and 20 mg for patients less than 35 kg, followed by a sliding scale of reducing by 4 mg every 3 days until down to 10 mgs per day, then continuing to decrease by 1–2 mg per day. The intial dose can be given IV if urgency required but oral doses should then follow. However, if symptoms recur revert to a higher maintenance dose.
- Referral for concurrent radiotherapy should be considered if the prognosis is not very poor. This therapy is not available in around 30% of African countries, and unless the parents have enough financial resources to take their child to another country, palliative support is the best option.
- Surgery, such as laminectomy, is only rarely indicated.
- Consider using a pressure-relieving mattress, and give pressure area care.
- Pay attention to bowel function.
- Start physiotherapy to prevent contractures.
- Perform catheterisation.
- Avoid danthron-containing laxatives if the child is catheterised or incontinent, because of the risk of danthron burns.

Psychological support

Children experience significant psychological suffering as a result of loss of their ability to walk or run, as well as their inability to play and go to school. They therefore need understanding and sympathetic advice from their healthcare provider and carer at this time.

Convulsions

Convulsions may be a potential or existing problem for children with brain tumours or other neurological and metabolic disorders.

For emergency management of seizures in palliative and terminal care, **diazepam** given rectally is the drug of choice.
Dosage:
- Age < 1 year: 2.5 mg (half of a 5 mg rectal tube/rectal solution)
- Age 1–4 years: one 5 mg rectal tube/rectal solution
- Age 5–12 years: 5 mg or 10 mg rectal tube/rectal solution
- Age > 12 years: 10 mg rectal tube/rectal solution.

For continuing severe seizures, consider giving midazolam by the buccal route, subcutaneously or by IV infusion if the child is in hospital (*see* Section 5.16.E). Care is required with midazolam as it may give permanent anaesthesia so that communication becomes impossible.

Muscle spasm

Muscle spasm can be severe in children with neurological and neurodegenerative disorders. It may occur alone or be triggered by pain elsewhere (e.g. due to constipation).

Useful drugs for muscle spasm

Diazepam orally (initial doses are shown):
- Age 1 month to 1 year: 250 microgram/kg twice daily
- Age 1–5 years: 2.5 mg twice daily
- Age 5–12 years: 5 mg twice daily
- Age > 12 years: 10 mg twice daily up to a maximum dose of 40 mg/day (*BNFC*).

Baclofen orally
- Age 1–10 years: initial dose 300 microgram/kg/day in four divided doses, increasing to usual dose of 0.75–2 mg/kg/day in divided doses
- Age > 10 years: 5 mg three times daily, increasing to 20 mg three times daily (up to a maximum dose of 100 mg/day).

Incontinence

Incontinence can be the source of much discomfort and anxiety for both children and their families, as well as presenting difficulties in keeping the child clean and protecting their skin.

Children with some degenerative conditions may have had faecal or urinary incontinence for a long time, whereas for others this may become a feature during the end stage of their disease (e.g. due to local tumour, neurological/spinal cord damage to bladder control, laxative imbalance).

For children with long-standing difficulties, intermittent catheterisation or the use of an indwelling catheter may be a well-established, successful and accepted method (*see* Section 4.2.D).

Some useful suggestions include the following:
- Review laxatives where appropriate.
- Consider giving intranasal **desmopressin**, 20–40 micrograms at bedtime, if nights are disturbed by urinary incontinence. Alternatively, desmopressin tablets, 200–400 micrograms, or sublingual tablets, 120–240 micrograms, can be used (*BNFC* doses for enuresis). Care is needed as desmopressin can cause water retention and hyponatraemia, so start with lower doses.
- Keep a urinal or bedpan close to the bedside.
- Use cotton pads or towels (with plastic underneath) on top of the bed sheet. This will avoid the need to change all the sheets, and thus minimise disturbance to the child.
- Keep the area well ventilated (or keep a window open if appropriate).
- Try to ensure that the skin is kept clean, and use dimethicone, zinc and castor oil or other barrier creams if these are available.
- Help the child to wash regularly.
- Try to preserve and maintain the child's dignity at all times. Give reassurance and support to both the child and the parents.

Fungating wounds

Fungating wounds are rare in paediatric palliative care, but in resource-limited settings they are not infrequently encountered. They may occur with soft tissue sarcomas, often of the head and neck, which can be very distressing for the child and their family.

Useful tips for management (where available) include the following:

- Soak any dressings with saline or Ringer-lactate or Hartmann's solution to ease removal, as these tumours may be friable and prone to bleeding.
- If possible, have available topical adrenaline 1 in 1000, or an alginate dressing (e.g. Kaltostat, or tranexamic acid), to apply topically to the tumour if it bleeds profusely (e.g. during a dressing change).

These tumours can cause offensive smells due to anaerobic microorganisms, which can be distressing to the child and their family. Sprinkle crushed metronidazole tablets on the fungating area. Oral metronidazole does not penetrate the fungating area, as the blood supply to it is poor. Metronidazole is cheap and readily available in all resource-limited countries, and it is very effective. Charcoal dressings, if available, may help to absorb the odour. The use of honey for dressings is also of benefit in controlling bacteria and odour. Simple measures such as the use of aromatherapy oils around the home may be helpful, too.

The final days and hours of life
Terminal restlessness and agitation

These symptoms are not uncommon in the final stages of life. Useful drugs include buccal midazolam, and oral or rectal diazepam.

Midazolam is the sedative of choice, as it can be given via the buccal mucosa.

Dosage:

The initial regime is 30–100 micrograms/kg given as required. Titrate upwards as required (the upper dose may be limited by volume).

Rectal diazepam may also be useful.

Dosage:

5–10 mg rectal tube as required. The dose may be repeated if child remains very agitated and restless.

Increased secretions

- Increased secretions (the 'death rattle') can be more distressing for the parents and carers than for the child. It is important to explain this to those caring for the child.
- Good mouth care is essential.
- Anti-secretory agents are useful, but can cause drowsiness and anti-cholinergic side effects.
- Start drug treatment early in order to avoid build-up of excessive secretions.

Hyoscine hydrobromide (scopolamine)

- This drug is anticholinergic.
- It reduces pharyngeal secretions.
- It should be used prophylactically at the first sign of excess secretions.
- It mixes with other commonly used drugs.
- Potential routes for administration: oral, as a sublingual tablet, IV or subcutaneous.

Dosage:

Oral/sublingual route:
- Age 1–12 years: 10 micrograms/kg/dose, four times a day
- Age > 12 years: 300 micrograms/dose, four times a day.

Subcutaneous or IV infusion:
- All ages: 10–50 micrograms/kg/24 hours.

Loss of the oral route for food and medication

As a child's condition deteriorates it may become difficult to use the oral route for medication. Buccal and rectal routes are the best options in this situation, and work well. As discussed earlier, other routes that can be used at this point are the rectal, subcutaneous and (where already established) IV routes. Children who have been treated for cancer in well-resourced hospitals may have central IV access, which can be used effectively in palliative care, but usually only in hospital.

Drugs that can be given via the subcutaneous or IV route include analgesics, anti-emetics, sedatives, anxiolytics and anticholinergic drugs. These can be combined together in an infusion, provided that they are compatible with each other.

If they are available, it is possible to use small portable infusion pumps (e.g. Graseby MS 26, WalkMed) to deliver combinations of medication over 24 hours. However, these devices are unlikely to be available for home use in most resource-limited countries, and home palliative care teams would not generally be able to provide this form of treatment. Sometimes individual carers may be able to manage this form of treatment.

Additional notes

- Avoid administering high concentrations of drugs in combination, especially when using cyclizine.
- Avoid mixing dexamethasone with other drugs if possible.
- Never give chlorpromazine, prochlorperazine or diazepam subcutaneously.
- More than two drugs can be combined in portable syringe drivers, although there is little supporting evidence in the form of clinical data. Always consult your local pharmacist before using any unusual combinations.

Psychological support for the child, parents and siblings

Care that is child and family centred is an essential principle of palliative care. The availability of an experienced key worker to coordinate the child's care with community healthcare professionals is essential, with good communication both between professionals and between professionals and the family being of paramount importance.

Initially, parents may need a lot of support when deciding whether to withdraw curative treatment and where to care for their child. Whether the care setting is in hospital or at home, the parents will have many questions, fears and anxieties at this time, and if possible the opportunity to discuss their worries, changes in the child's condition and symptom management should be available 24 hours a day. Commonly asked questions include 'How long will it be?' and 'How will my child die?' These questions are not easy to answer, and will also depend on the nature of the child's illness. For example, a child with leukaemia may have a very short period of palliative care, whereas a child with a brain tumour or neurodegenerative disease may live for several months. It is probably best to give an indication of time span, but to emphasise that every child is different, and to guide the parents as the disease progresses. 'Days or weeks', 'weeks or months' or even 'hours rather than days' give adequate warning without being too precise.

Parents may worry about their child being in pain, but also have anxieties about the use of strong medication such as morphine. A clear explanation of the use of analgesics is essential in this situation.

Many parents will want advice on talking to the dying child and their siblings. How to prepare the child's brothers and sisters will depend very much on their age and level of understanding, and on parental beliefs. For older children and teenagers it is probably best to be honest, to prepare them gradually for what is happening and allow them to ask questions and participate in their sibling's care if appropriate. With younger children, the language used must be very simple and clear. For example, it is important to avoid using the phrase 'going to sleep' as the analogy for death. It is probably more appropriate to prepare younger children for a sibling's death when the end is obviously very close. Cultural preferences also need to be taken into account.

Talking to the child who is dying is a very personal matter for parents, and will also be influenced by the child's age and understanding of the illness. For example, a teenager with cystic fibrosis may have anticipated death in adolescence or young adulthood, and a teenager who has had multiple relapses of cancer for many years may now realise that the treatment is no longer working. Where possible and appropriate, it is important that children and teenagers are given the opportunity to express their wishes and anxieties. When children are not allowed to express themselves they can become very anxious and agitated, or even withdrawn. Healthcare professionals can only try to encourage the parents to have an open and honest approach to their child's questions and wishes at this time.

Preparation for death

Parents commonly have many questions about the time and nature of death, and what happens afterwards. It can be very helpful to try to prepare them for what may happen at the time of death if they wish to have this information. Changes in breathing are commonly distressing, and simple explanations of, for example, Cheyne–Stokes respiration or the 'death rattle' can avoid unnecessary distress. A single expiratory breath after death if the child is moved is not uncommon, and it should be explained to the parents that this does not mean that their child is still alive. Explanations of the changes in colour and very cold feel of the skin are important for parents and siblings. If they are not warned in advance, parents may become distressed that their child was incontinent at the time of death. In the case of some diseases (e.g. leukaemia), the parents will need to be warned that their child may bleed from the nose or mouth at the time of or after death, and given simple practical measures for managing this situation.

Some families will require professional support around the time of the child's death, and it is essential that this is available.

After their child has died, the parents must be reassured that they need not rush to do anything, but may spend some time with their child. However, it is also important that any specific cultural or religious requirements are acknowledged and attended to. The parents should be encouraged, if they wish to do so, to hold, wash and dress their child. Some parents may want to take photographs, locks of hair, or hand and foot prints, or organise favourite toys, photographs, letters or other items for the child 'to take with them'. The participation of siblings in these activities can be very helpful.

In countries where it is usually necessary for a child's death to be confirmed by a medical practitioner it is very rare for a post-mortem to be required. The death certificate then gives the authority for the death to be registered (according to each country's prevailing law) and the funeral arrangements to be made.

The specific cultural and religious beliefs of the family and the country in which they live will play an important role in the child's funeral. However, the parents may need advice about the choice between burial or cremation, or about the funeral service itself.

Support after death

Support for parents, siblings and the extended family around the time of the child's death and in the weeks and months afterwards will be very much influenced by the family's culture and family network, and by the support provided during the child's terminal care. Bereavement contact from the professionals involved with the family should be offered wherever possible.

Clinicians need to be aware of the cultural support and customs that affect bereavement, and refrain from imposing their own personal needs and values on others.

Ongoing bereavement support should be based on the family's specific needs and requests, and the availability of appropriate bereavement support for both parents and siblings. Bereavement literature and parent support groups may be helpful where available.

Recognition of the child's birthday and the anniversary of their death provide an opportunity for healthcare professionals and friends to show the family that their child has not been forgotten.

Acknowledgement

We are extremely grateful to Dr Janet Goodall for her help with writing this section.

Further reading

Goldman A, Hain R and Liben S (2006) *Oxford Textbook of Palliative Care for Children*. Oxford: Oxford University Press.

Amery J (ed.) *Children's Palliative Care in Africa*. International Children's Palliative Care Network www.icpcn.org (accessed July 2014).

International Children's Palliative Care Network (ICPCN). www.icpcn.org.uk (accessed 9 December 2012).

World Health Organization. *Cancer Pain Relief and Palliative Care in Children*. www.who.int/cancer/palliative/en/ (accessed July 2014).

Palliative Care Formulary for Children (available on the Internet and as a hard-copy publication). www.palliativedrugs.com/palliative-care-formulary.html (accessed July 2014).

Merriman A (2012) *Freedom from Pain*, 2nd edition. Uganda: Hospice Africa. www.hospiceafrica.or.ug (accessed 9 December 2012).

Jassal S (2008) *Basic Symptom Control in Paediatric Palliative Care: the Rainbows Children's Hospice Guidelines*.

www.rainbows.co.uk/wp-content/uploads/2011/06/
Rainbows-Hospice-Basic-Symptom-Control-In-Paediatric-
Palliative-Care-8th-Ed-2011-protected.pdf (accessed
9 December 2012 but now requires a password).

Hain R and Jassal S (2010) *Paediatric Palliative Medicine*.
Oxford Specialist Handbooks in Paediatrics. Oxford: Oxford
University Press.

Jassal S and Hain RD (2011) *Association for Paediatric*

Palliative Medicine Master Formulary. www.appm.org.
uk/10.html.

World Health Organization. *Guidelines on the*
Pharmacological Treatment of Persisting Pain in Children
with Medical Illnesses. http://whqlibdoc.who.int/publica
tions/2012/9789241548120_Guidelines.pdf (accessed
July 2014).

British National Formulary for Children. www.medicinescom
plete.com/mc/ (accessed July 2014).

1.17 Hospital issues regarding immunisation

Introduction

Immunisation is one of the most effective disease prevention strategies in children. In this process, an antigen is introduced into the body, where it stimulates immunity against the specific antigen by priming the specific memory cells. Subsequent natural infection produces an effective and vigorous response by the body, and the patient is thus protected from the disease and its effects and complications.

In 1974, the World Health Organization (WHO) initiated the Expanded Programme on Immunisation (EPI). This aims to develop widespread national commitment to achieve high vaccination coverage in mostly low-income countries. The choice of the original six EPI vaccines was based on the importance of the disease and the availability of safe, efficacious and low-cost vaccines.

The WHO recommended vaccination schedule is widely used in almost all countries, with newer vaccines being added as some programmes evolved (*see* Table 1.17.1).

TABLE 1.17.1 Current EPI vaccination schedule recommended by the WHO, May 2014

Age	Vaccine
Birth	BCG*, OPV#0, HBV#1
6 weeks	DTP#1, HiB#1, OPV#1, HBV# 2 PCV#1 RV#1
10 weeks	DTP#2, HiB#2, OPV#2, HBV#3 IPV#1 PCV#2 RV#2
14 weeks	DTP#3, HiB#3, OPV#3, IPV#2 PCV#3
9 months	MCV/RCV #1 Yellow fever (in countries where it poses a risk)
12–15 months	MCV/RCV#2
9 years girls	HPV#1 plus HPV# 2 after at least 6/12

BCG, bacillus Calmette-Guérin; OPV, oral poliovirus vaccine; IPV, inactivated polio vaccine HBV, hepatitis B vaccine; DTP, diphtheria, tetanus and pertussis; HiB, Haemophilus influenzae type B; Pneumococcus PCV; Rotavirus RV; Measles/Rubella MCV/RCV; Human papilloma virus HPV

*BCG must not be given if HIV infection is present or clinically suspected

See these links for further information:

www.who.int/immunization/policy/immunization_tables/en/

www.who.int/immunization/policy/Immunization_routine_table2.
pdf?ua=1

Vaccine schedules are a continuously changing phenomenon. It is recommended that regional variations on programmes are followed.

Polio

Live oral poliovirus vaccine (OPV) and inactivated poliovirus vaccine (IPV) are the two effective vaccines that are available, but there are important differences between them.

- WHO no longer recommends an OPV only vaccination schedule, at least 1 dose of IPV should be added to the schedule.

- In polio-endemic countries and in countries at high risk for importation and subsequent spread, WHO recommends an OPV birth dose (a zero dose) followed by a primary series of 3 OPV and at least 1 IPV doses.

- The WHO target to eradicate poliomyelitis within the next 10 years is dependent on high infant immunisation coverage and national immunisation days (NIDs), which aim to eradicate the circulation of wild virus. NIDs are designed to complement routine immunisation by targeting the most vulnerable individuals in as short a time period as possible. OPV is given over a 2-day period, 1 month apart, and the NIDs are repeated annually for at least 3 years.

Pertussis

Fever and mild local reactions are common. Consider a two-dose schedule for those areas where services can be provided only twice a year.

Measles

Accelerated implementation of strategies to reduce the burden of measles is required. Targeting children under 5 years of age in major cities is a priority. Strategies to reduce the impact of infant measles include:

- increasing coverage to the 9–23 months age group

- a two-dose schedule at 6 months and 15 months is most appropriate for epidemic situations, and a two-dose schedule at 9 months and 15 months is currently recommended routinely.

Tetanus

All healthcare workers at antenatal clinics should guarantee that no women attending will have a child who dies of neonatal tetanus, by giving immunisation and advice about umbilical cord care. Vaccination of young adolescent girls is recommended in areas with poor antenatal coverage. Mothers who were not seen antenatally should be vaccinated when they bring their infants to clinic.

BCG

This offers good protection against disseminated tuberculosis and also affords some protection from leprosy. Where the risk of tuberculosis is high, BCG is recommended at birth or as soon as possible thereafter.

It is recommended for children living in countries with a high-disease burden for HIV and for high-risk children living in countries with low-disease burden.

Children who are HIV positive or have unknown HIV status with symptoms consistent with HIV should not be vaccinated.

New vaccines and EPI

Hepatitis B and yellow fever vaccines have been recommended since 1992. The HiB vaccine is also a priority, and is given as combination now in EPI programmes with the DPT and HBV as three doses. Newly introduced vaccines are the pneumococcal conjugate vaccine (PCV) and the rotavirus vaccines. Unfortunately there is no vaccine yet available against HIV or hepatitis C.

Other vaccines to consider based upon local epidemiology and resource limitations would be:

- MMR (Measles, Mumps and Rubella) vaccine instead of MCV/RCV as at present recommended
- Typhoid vaccine
- Varicella vaccine
- Meningococcal (Conjugate) vaccine.

Contraindications to immunisation

All vaccines

- Anaphylactic reaction.
- Moderate to severe acute illnesses with or without fever.
- Evolving neurological disease.

Specific vaccines

- Encephalopathy (DPT/DaPT).
- Immunodeficiency (OPV, BCG, MMR).
- Anaphylactic reaction to egg and neomycin (MMR, VZV).
- Pregnancy (MMR, OPV, IPV).
- Precautions for DPT:
  - fever > 105 °F
  - collapse or shock-like state
  - seizures
  - persistent inconsolable crying.

Conditions that are not contraindications to immunisation

- Minor illnesses, such as upper respiratory infections or diarrhoea, with fever < 38.5 °C.
- Allergy, asthma or other atopic manifestations (e.g. hay fever, 'snuffles').
- Prematurity, small-for-date infants.
- Malnutrition.
- Child being breastfed.
- Family history of convulsions.
- Convalescent phase of illness.
- Penicillin or other allergies.
- Treatment with antibiotics, low-dose corticosteroids or locally acting (e.g. topical or inhaled) steroids.
- Dermatoses, eczema or localised skin infection.
- Chronic diseases of the heart, lung, kidney or liver.
- Stable neurological conditions (e.g. cerebral palsy, Down's syndrome).
- History of jaundice after birth.

HIV infection and vaccination

Individuals with known or suspected asymptomatic HIV infection should receive all EPI vaccines (including against rotavirus) as early in life as possible according to nationally recommended schedules. Because of the risk of early and severe measles, infants should receive a standard dose at 6 months, with a second dose as soon after age 9 months as possible.

Children who are HIV positive or have unknown HIV status with symptoms consistent with HIV should not be vaccinated with BCG.

Also *see* Sections 2.8.C and 6.2.D HIV Infection.

TABLE 1.17.2 WHO/UNICEF recommendations for the immunisation of HIV-infected children and women of childbearing age

Vaccine	HIV positive without symptoms	HIV positive with symptoms	Optimal timing of immunisation
BCG	No	No	
DPT	Yes	Yes	6, 10 and 14 weeks
OPV	Yes	Yes	0, 6, 10 and 14 weeks
Measles	Yes	Yes	6 and 9 months
Hepatitis B	Yes	Yes	As for uninfected children
Rotavirus	Yes	Yes	6, 10 weeks
Yellow fever	Yes	(No pending further studies)	–
Tetanus toxoid	Yes	Yes	5 doses

Additional vaccines that should be seriously considered in HIV-infected children include the following:

- Varicella vaccine:
  - recommended in asymptomatic/mildly symptomatic children
  - two doses should be given with a 3-month interval

— strongly recommended for HIV-negative siblings and other children in the household

— contraindicated in moderately and severely immuno-compromised children.

- Other vaccines:

— influenza virus vaccine annually, specific strain only

— hepatitis A

— parenteral typhoid vaccine (oral administration is contraindicated).

TABLE 1.17.3 Recommended vaccine storage time and temperature

Vaccines	Shelf life	Transport state-district	State/district	Transport to PHC	PHC
DTT/TT and typhoid	1–1.5 years (4–8°C)	+4 to +8°C	3 months (4–8°C)	4–8°C	1 month (4–8°C)
BCG	8 months (4–8°C)	+4 to +8°C	3 months (4–8°C)	4–8°C	1 month (4–8°C)
Measles and OPV	2 years at −20°C	−20°C to +8°C	3 months (−20°C)	−20°C to + 8°C	1 month (4–8°C)

Logistic actions to avoid unnecessary risk, vaccine wastage and missed opportunities are essential.

Immunisation instruments recommended by EPI

Disposable single-use plastic syringes are safe and economical, but it is important to correctly destroy and dispose of the syringes and sharps after use. Used needles and syringes should be placed in a hard container, sealed, autoclaved, and ideally incinerated for disposal.

- Opened vials of OPV, DPT and hepatitis B vaccines may be used in subsequent immunisation sessions until a new shipment arrives (provided the expiry date has not passed, vaccines are kept in the cold chain and the vials have not been used outside the health centre).
- Opened vials of measles, yellow fever and BCG vaccines must be discarded at the end of each immunisation session.
- Vaccine vial monitors (VVMs) will enable field staff to reject vials of vaccine that are heat damaged.
- Screen and immunise at every contact. The rate of non-immunisation of eligible children at clinics may be as high as 30%.
- Reduce wastage by choosing the correct vial size.
- Ensure appropriate use of the vaccine cold box. Cold boxes only work if they are kept cold with the lid tightly shut. Ice packs are placed in the bottom and around the sides of the box and on the top of the vaccines. Newspaper should be placed between the vaccines and the icepacks to protect DPT and tetanus vaccines from the ice. A thermometer should be placed with the vaccines to record the temperature of the vaccines when they are removed from the cold box. The diluent that is used to reconstitute measles and BCG vaccine must also be kept cold.
- Effective supervision requires focus on the essentials.
- Evaluate and monitor the programme.

Care of refrigerators

A constant supply of electricity, gas or kerosene is required. The electric plug can be taped to its socket to ensure that it is not inadvertently removed. For gas and kerosene fridges, a reserve full bottle of gas or can of fuel should always be present. A regulator valve should be used with the gas bottle. Kerosene tanks should be filled daily using a funnel and filter to remove dirt. The refrigerator should be positioned in a completely upright position with a draught blowing on the temperature exchanger to keep it cool. A fan can be used for this if there is no wind and the ambient temperature is high.

Summary

- Vaccines are the best form of prevention, especially for children under 5 years of age.
- They are safe, effective, generally economical, and easily available.
- Immunisation of a child should start at birth and continue until they are old enough to attend college.
- Standards must be maintained with regard to procurement, delivery, storage and administration of all vaccines.
- In the event of missed doses, in most cases the vaccination schedule can be completed from the time when the dose was missed.
- Mild fever and upper respiratory tract infections are not contraindications to giving vaccination.
- Do take every opportunity to recommend vaccination for children.

Immunisation issues in pregnancy
Vaccination against tetanus

The most important vaccination that should be given to all pregnant women and girls is to prevent tetanus in women and in the newborn infant. After two doses, protective antibodies are present in more than 80% of recipients. The vaccine is safe in pregnancy, and two doses of vaccination last for at least 3 years.

If the woman or girl has a tetanus-susceptible wound, including following an unsafe abortion, protect against future tetanus risks by immunising her immediately if she is not already protected. In addition, provide prophylaxis with tetanus immunoglobulin if the wound is large and possibly infected with soil or instruments contaminated with animal excreta.

In the antenatal setting, check the immunisation status of the pregnant woman (either by a history or from the record card), regardless of whether she intends to continue the pregnancy.

If the woman has not previously been vaccinated, or her immunisation status is unknown, give two doses of TT/Td 1 month apart as soon as possible before delivery, TT1 and TT2 (one dose is not enough to give protection to the mother or newborn baby). Two doses protect for 1 to 3 years. If there is time in the remainder of the pregnancy, give another dose, TT3, 6 months after the second initial dose; otherwise give the third dose, TT3, in the next pregnancy. Three doses protect for at least 5 years. A fourth dose can be given at least 1 year after TT3, and protects for at least 10 years.

If the woman can prove her previous vaccination history, and provided she has had between 1 and 4 doses in the past, give one additional dose before delivery.

Before giving the vaccine, shake the vial and make sure that the material in the base of the vial is completely mixed with the liquid. If it is suspected that the vaccine has been frozen and thawed, this mixing may not occur and the vial should not be used.

If neonatal tetanus occurs, give the mother one dose of TT as soon as possible, and repeat the dose 4 weeks later and then again 6 months after the second dose.

Record the doses given on a central hospital/clinic register. However, it is of paramount importance to record them on a card or maternal health record kept by the mother.

Immunisation against hepatitis B virus (HBV)

All pregnant women and girls should ideally be offered screening for HBV.

They may have become infected at their birth (vertical transmission) or by sexual contact or through infected blood transfusion or use of dirty needles. Hepatitis B can be passed from a mother to her baby during or shortly after delivery. Having a Caesarean section does not prevent the virus from being transferred to the baby. If a ventouse delivery is undertaken a soft cap is preferred to the metal cup. Breastfeeding is safe.

During pregnancy, all women should have a blood test for a marker of hepatitis B virus, which is called hepatitis B surface antigen (HBsAg). Normally the HBsAg should be negative.

If a pregnant woman's HBsAg test or hepatitis B e-antigen (HBeAg) test are positive, the infant must be given hepatitis B immunoglobulin (HBIG) as soon as possible after birth to reduce the transmission rate from 70–90% to 5–10%.

Similarly, if a woman develops HBV infection during pregnancy, HBIG prophylaxis (400 IU given intramuscularly), which is safe, should be administered urgently within 24 hours of infection if possible. Acute HBV infection may be asymptomatic or present with signs of acute hepatitis. If available, antiviral therapy can be given to pregnant women who have high viral loads.

HBIG provides immediate protection for the woman or infant, but the effect only lasts a few months. Women or their babies should then be given a course of HBV vaccination (the initial dose being given at the time of HBIG, and then two further doses at 1 and 6 months after the initial dose).

The newborn infant, in addition to receiving the HBIG described above, should receive the hepatitis B vaccine at birth, again at 1–2 months, and finally at 6 months of age.

It is important to complete all three doses for long-term protection. The infant should have a blood test for hepatitis B infection and for hepatitis B antibody at 9–18 months of age. If the antibody test is negative, a fourth dose of the vaccine should be given at that time.

Women who are HBsAg-positive must not donate breast milk.

Vaccinations that should not be given during pregnancy
Live vaccines
- BCG (live attenuated strain).
- Oral typhoid vaccine.
- Measles–mumps–rubella (MMR).
- Rotavirus.
- Varicella.
- Yellow fever (unless travelling to areas in which yellow fever is endemic).

Inactivated vaccines
- Oral cholera.
- 7-Valent pneumococcal conjugate.

WHO recommendations for Immunisation of Health Care Workers:

Hepatitis B. Immunisation is suggested for groups at risk of acquiring infection who have not been vaccinated previously (for example HCWs who may be exposed to blood and blood products at work).

Polio. All HCWs should have completed a full course of primary vaccination against polio.

Diphtheria. Particular attention should be given to revaccination of HCWs with diphtheria boosters every 10 years. Special attention should be paid to immunising HCWs who may have occupational exposure to *C. diphtheria*.

Measles. All HCWs should be immune to measles and proof/documentation of immunity or immunization should be required as a condition of enrolment into training and employment.

Rubella. If rubella vaccine has been introduced into the national programme, all HCWs should be immune to rubella and proof/documentation of immunity or immunisation should be required as a condition of enrolment into training and employment.

Meningococcal disease. One booster dose 3–5 years after the primary dose may be given to persons considered to be at continued risk of exposure, including HCWs.

Further reading
Vaccines and vaccination against yellow fever. WHO Position Paper – June 2013 www.who.int/wer/2013/wer8827.pdf

1.18 Recognition by hospital workers of the abuse and exploitation of pregnant women and children

For health workers in hospitals, the two most important issues are:

1 that abusive injuries are recognised and diagnosed
2 that future abuse is where possible prevented by the involvement of agencies such as social services, the police and legal teams working together.

Child abuse and family violence against pregnant women represent a worldwide problem.

Categories of ill treatment and abuse

A new way of looking at this subject divides the ill treatment or abuse into three categories based on the intention of the perpetrators.

Ill treatment resulting from human weakness

This occurs at some time in every family, often without realisation.

It is best addressed through education, religious or other community initiatives.

Ill treatment resulting from stress

This can involve violence, which is sometimes very severe. Perpetrators are often unhappy, are suffering from an undiagnosed or untreated mental illness, dependent on drugs or alcohol, unsupported, and were often inadequately parented in their own childhood. After violent acts, the perpetrator usually becomes distressed. They do love and care for their victim.

This problem needs professional support that is appropriately led by local social services staff, not punitive legislation.

Abuse that is undertaken for gain

This often involves the most serious and prolonged forms of violence, resulting in great suffering. The perpetrator usually has a psychopathic personality disorder and is immune or insensitive to the suffering of others. Indeed, they may even enjoy inflicting emotional or physical pain. Mental illness is not responsible for this form of abuse. Although the perpetrators are aware that what they are doing is wrong, they are gaining from doing it. They will do all that they can to avoid being detected, by employing elaborate and plausible lies, characteristically weaving objects of truth into a latticework of deceit. The perpetrators are usually dangerous and frighten local social workers, health visitors, doctors and teachers, who need to be involved in a protected manner. The perpetrators may work in groups such as the criminal gangs involved in human trafficking.

The kinds of abuse undertaken in this third category include:

- trafficking of women and children as slaves or for prostitution
- sadistic injuries (e.g. deliberate burns from cigarettes, scalding, holding the person against hot objects, etc.)
- multiple fractures, often inflicted at different times, reflecting the severity of violence

- excessive ritual punishments (e.g. regular and savage beatings, usually with implements)
- deliberate starvation, as distinct from neglect as in the second category
- the fabrication or inducement of illness
- sexual abuse.

The most difficult issue is to distinguish this form of abuse from perpetrator stress-related ill treatment (the second category above).

The possibility of ill treatment or abuse must be considered in the differential diagnosis of all children or pregnant women or girls who have suffered an injury and present to hospital.

All professionals who are working with children and pregnant women or girls need to be aware of the clinical manifestations of abuse and do everything that they can to protect their patients from further harm.

Some cultural practices are abusive. For example, female genital cutting (*see* Section 2.10) not only causes great suffering at the time, but can interfere with future childbirth and sexual relationships.

Abuse and ill treatment occurs across all social classes.

Features of family members known to be associated with ill treatment or abuse

Observe the relationship between the family and the patient.

- Is it loving and caring?
- Were any family members themselves abused as children?
- Are the parent(s) of a child young and/or unsupported?
- Are the parent(s) of a child single or substitutive?
- Does the parent of a child have learning difficulties?
- Do the parents of a child have a poor or unstable relationship?
- Is there existing domestic violence, drug or alcohol abuse in the family?
- Does the parent of a child have a mental illness (e.g. postnatal depression)?

Critical threshold for concern

Arriving at the critical threshold may be immediate and straightforward (e.g. the finding of bruising on a small infant, or a direct disclosure of abuse from a child or pregnant girl). In some circumstances the situation is less clear (e.g. if there are a number of non-specific signs or indicators, or in cases of neglect). At some point a balanced assessment is required between the provision of family support for a patient who is judged to be 'in need', and taking action directly to protect them.

The 'critical threshold' is that point beyond which behaviour(s) towards a patient can be considered to be ill treatment or abuse, and beyond which it becomes necessary to take action. That is the time to raise concerns with the parents, carers and/or family and the time to refer to the statutory agencies (either social services or the police, depending on the local legislative system).

1.19 Transport of ill patients

The transport of patients who are ill should follow the same principles whether the distance is long or short, and whether the journey is within or between healthcare facilities.

All transfers pose a potential risk, and should only be undertaken if safe treatment cannot be given within the facility where the patient is at present.

Preparation and planning allow mitigation of risks to both the patient and healthcare staff.

Staff who are trained in transport provide better-quality transfers.

Stabilisation prior to transport is preferable, as better-quality transport is of benefit to patient outcomes. However, time-critical pathologies may change the balance of risk and benefit between time spent on stabilisation and the need for rapid transfer for definitive treatment.

Never assume that resources and equipment will be available in transport vehicles. Prepare beforehand to be self-sufficient.

Use the principles of ABCD to guide management of the patient for transport.

Use a checklist (*see* Table 1.19).

Pregnancy-related emergencies involve two patients – the mother and the baby.

Many obstetric emergencies require urgent, rapid and safe transport from home to the nearest facility where there is comprehensive emergency obstetric care (EmOC). This is particularly relevant for emergencies such as massive obstetric haemorrhage, eclampsia, obstructed labour, shoulder dystocia and complicated breech delivery.

Ideally, every pregnant woman or girl should have a local transport plan ready in advance for an unexpected

Think ahead
Plan ahead
Anticipate problems
Be prepared

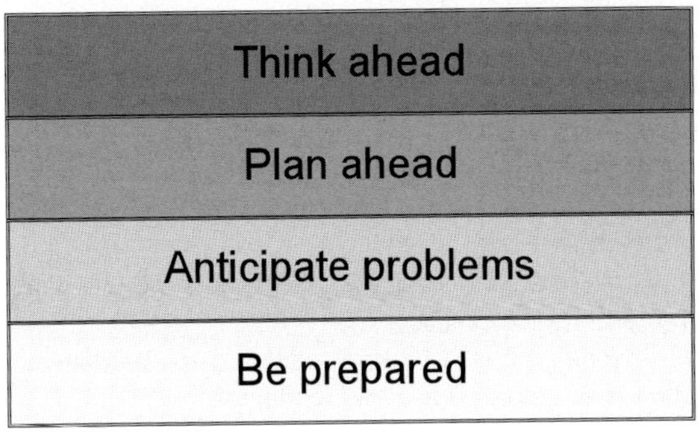

FIGURE 1.19.1 Safe transport rules.

emergency. This could consist of a village taxi, a relative's car, or some other form of transport, the fuel for which needs to be secured in advance.

Ideally, there should also be an emergency transport system based in the nearest health facility with comprehensive EmOC and having a midwife on call 24 hours a day who can go out with an ambulance containing suitable emergency equipment and drugs to the home of a mother with a life-threatening emergency, stabilise her and transport her back to the health facility.

The following paper describes a system of this type: www.reproductive-health-journal.com/content/pdf/1742-4755-7-21.pdf.

Motor cycle and side-car ambulances (e.g. www.eranger.com) can be extremely effective for transporting pregnant women and girls along difficult roads in rural areas to a hospital or clinic.

TABLE 1.19 Transport checklist

Airway/Breathing		Yes/No
Is the airway safe?	Is there anything that can be done to improve the airway?	Yes/No
Is oxygen required?	Pulse oximeter (battery operated with additional power from the ambulance cigarette lighter) can help to guide the need for oxygen	Yes/No
Is oxygen available?	Oxygen cylinders full and working – enough for the return expected journey	Yes/No
Is ventilatory support required?	Bag-valve-mask of the correct size available and working	Yes/No
Suction	Manual system and catheters available	Yes/No
Circulation		Yes/No
IV access	Working and secured	Yes/No
Volume	Ringer-lactate or Hartmann's solution bags and delivery kits	Yes/No
D Neurology		Yes/No
Temperature	Sufficient blankets available	Yes/No
Blood sugar level	Glucose for IV or gastric tube administration available	Yes/No
Other		Yes/No
Birthing needs	Delivery kit, bag-valve-mask for neonate, towels, oxytocin, misoprostol, magnesium sulphate and condom catheter	
Documentation	All relevant documentation with the patient	Yes/No
Family members	Family members know what the plan is	Yes/No
Healthcare communication	Receiving site is aware of the patient and their expected time of arrival	Yes/No

1.20 Ethics in healthcare

Introduction

Ethics is the study of morality. Morality is defined as the values used in human behaviour and decision making.

Medical ethics

Medical ethics is the branch of ethics that deals with moral issues in medical practice.

Anyone who is involved in patient care uses ethics, whether or not they have had formal teaching in medical ethics (most people have not).

Usually law and ethics are closely related, but there are some differences:

- Laws differ between countries, whereas ethics are applicable to all countries.
- Ethical obligations take priority over legal duties.
- When law conflicts with medical ethics, healthcare workers should advocate for changing the law.

There are four basic principles of ethics in healthcare which apply to most moral issues that arise in healthcare:

1 **Autonomy:** this means self-determination. If a patient is fully informed and competent (i.e. is able to understand the implications of having treatment or no treatment), they have the right to refuse or accept treatment. Such decisions must be respected, even if they are not thought by health workers to be in the patient's best interests.

2 **Beneficence:** this means doing good and promoting well-being. This has to be considered for the individual patient, and may conflict with autonomy.

3 **Non-maleficence:** this means doing no harm. In healthcare, it is recognised that there is a risk of harm whenever investigations or treatment are carried out to benefit the patient. Maleficence refers to harm inflicted with no intended benefit to the patient.

4 **Justice:** this means equality before the law or fairness. It refers to the fair allocation of scarce resources to patients, and the justification for money spent in the health service. This may mean equal access to healthcare, maximum benefit of resources available, or allowing people choice in their healthcare. This decision may not be able to be taken by an individual. In a society where justice prevails, the aim is for all citizens to have equal access to healthcare.

Medical ethics in different countries

Different cultures and societies have different expectations about the relative values of the individual ethical principles. Some societies expect a beneficent or non-maleficent approach, whereas others expect an overriding respect for autonomy. It is essential that, as well as working within professional ethics, health workers respect the law in the countries where they practise, provided that the law does not harm the patient.

If a law or laws do harm patients or fail to protect them from harm, the healthcare workers should advocate for appropriate change in those law(s).

Some cultures put less weight on individualism, and involve the family and/or community in decision making.

Gender may also affect decision making. In some societies, decision making is the man's responsibility and the woman has no autonomy.

In some countries, health workers will not be forced to do anything unethical, whereas in others, there may be pressure from the police or the army to participate in torture or reveal the names of patients and their injuries and so break confidentiality.

In 2001 in South Africa, the Treatment Action Campaign (TAC) launched legal action to demand more widespread access to nevirapine to reduce mother-to-child transmission of HIV/AIDS. The High Court issued an order to the government to make nevirapine available to pregnant women with HIV.

In the USA, the emphasis is on the individual's autonomy, whereas in Africa the community may be more important, so the principles of beneficence and distributive justice may predominate.

Codes of ethics

The nursing and medical professions have their own international codes of ethics, adopted by the International Council of Nurses (ICN) and the World Medical Association (WMA), respectively.

There are more similarities than differences in medical ethics worldwide, and the World Medical Association has the role of setting standards in medical ethics that are applicable worldwide. The association was set up in 1947 to prevent a repetition of the unethical conduct of physicians in Nazi Germany and elsewhere. The WMA has developed an *International Code of Medical Ethics*, which was last revised in 2006.

The International Council of Nurses developed a code of ethics for the nursing profession in 1953, which was last revised in 2005.

WMA International Code of Medical Ethics

- This was adopted by the 3rd General Assembly of the World Medical Association, London, England, in October 1949.
- It was amended by the 22nd World Medical Assembly, Sydney, Australia, in August 1968.
- It was next amended by the 35th World Medical Assembly, Venice, Italy, in October 1983.
- It was most recently amended by the 57th World Medical Association General Assembly, Pilanesberg, South Africa, in October 2006.

Duties of physicians in general

A physician shall:

- always exercise their independent professional judgement and maintain the highest standards of professional conduct
- respect a competent patient's right to accept or refuse treatment
- not allow their judgement to be influenced by personal profit or unfair discrimination
- be dedicated to providing competent medical service in full professional and moral independence, with compassion and respect for human dignity
- deal honestly with patients and colleagues, and report to the appropriate authorities those physicians who practice unethically or incompetently or who engage in fraud or deception
- not receive any financial benefits or other incentives solely for referring patients or prescribing specific products
- respect the rights and preferences of patients, colleagues, and other health professionals
- recognise their important role in educating the public, but use due caution in divulging discoveries or new techniques or treatment through non-professional channels
- certify only that which they have personally verified
- strive to use healthcare resources in the best way to benefit patients and their community
- seek appropriate care and attention if they suffer from mental or physical illness
- respect the local and national codes of ethics.

Duties of physicians to patients

A physician shall:

- always bear in mind the obligation to respect human life
- act in the patient's best interest when providing medical care
- owe his or her patients complete loyalty and all the scientific resources available to him or her. Whenever an examination or treatment is beyond the physician's capacity, he or she should consult with or refer to another physician who has the necessary ability
- ensure that he/she remains competent to provide medical care in his/her field by continual professional development
- submit him/herself to assessment of health, probity, knowledge and competence by peers when appropriate
- respect a patient's right to confidentiality. It is ethical to disclose confidential information when the patient consents to it or when there is a real and imminent threat of harm to the patient or to others and this threat can be only removed by a breach of confidentiality
- give emergency care as a humanitarian duty unless they are assured that others are willing and able to give such care
- in situations when they are acting for a third party, ensure that the patient has full knowledge of that situation
- not enter into a sexual relationship with their current patient, or into any other abusive or exploitative relationship.

Duties of physicians to colleagues

A physician shall:

- behave towards colleagues as he or she would have them behave towards him or her

- not undermine the patient–physician relationship of colleagues in order to attract patients
- when medically necessary, communicate with colleagues who are involved in the care of the same patient. This communication should respect patient confidentiality and be confined to necessary information.

The ICN Code of Ethics for Nurses

This code has four principal elements that outline the standards of ethical conduct.

Elements of the code

1 **Nurses and people**
- The nurse's primary professional responsibility is to people requiring nursing care. In providing care, the nurse promotes an environment in which the human rights, values, customs, spiritual beliefs of the individual, family and community are respected.
- The nurse ensures that the individual receives sufficient information on which to base consent for care and related treatment.
- The nurse holds in confidence personal information, and uses judgement in sharing this information.
- The nurse shares with society the responsibility for initiating and supporting action to meet the health and social needs of the public, in particular those of vulnerable populations.
- The nurse also shares responsibility to sustain and protect the natural environment from depletion, pollution, degradation and destruction.

2 **Nurses and practice**
- The nurse carries personal responsibility and accountability for nursing practice, and for maintaining competence by continual learning.
- The nurse maintains a standard of personal health such that the ability to provide care is not compromised.
- The nurse at all times maintains standards of personal conduct which reflect well on the profession and enhance public confidence.
- The nurse, in providing care, ensures that use of technology and scientific advances is compatible with the safety, dignity and rights of people.

3 **Nurses and the profession**
- The nurse assumes the major role in determining and implementing acceptable standards of clinical nursing practice, management, research and education.
- The nurse is active in developing a core of research-based professional knowledge.
- The nurse, acting through the professional organisation, participates in creating and maintaining safe, equitable social and economic working conditions in nursing.

4 **Nurses and co-workers**
- The nurse sustains a cooperative relationship with co-workers in nursing and other fields.
- The nurse takes appropriate action to safeguard individuals, families and communities when their health is endangered by a co-worker or any other person.

Ethics in different situations, namely consent, confidentiality, end-of-life decisions and research, will be discussed below.

The ethics of consent

Informed consent is the process of a 'competent' patient receiving information needed to make a choice. It has five elements:

1 **Disclosure of information:** The patient has the right to the information necessary to make his or her decisions and to be informed of the consequences of his or her decisions.

2 **Comprehension:** The patient should understand the purpose of any test or treatment, the implications of the results, and the implications of not having the test or treatment.

3 **Voluntariness** (freedom from control by others): The patient has the right to self-determination, which includes making free decisions regarding him- or herself.

4 **Competence:** A mentally competent adult patient has the right to give or withhold consent to any diagnostic procedure or therapy.

5 **Choice:** Children may be able to consent to some procedures, but not to other more complex procedures.

Article 12 of the United Nations Convention on the Rights of the Child (1989) states:

> 'A child who is capable of forming his/her view has the right to express those views freely on all matters affecting the child, the views of the child being given due weight in accordance with the age and maturity of the child.'

The child's competence and parental involvement: respect for autonomy

Where a child is not competent to give or withhold consent to treatment, a person with parental responsibility must act as an advocate for the child to authorise investigations or treatment which are in the child's best interests. Parents have the right to be involved in the decision-making process, and this right is protected by law in most countries.

It is the doctor's responsibility to assess a child's capacity to decide whether he or she can consent to, or refuse, a proposed investigation or treatment before providing it. A competent child must be able to understand the nature, purpose and possible consequences of the proposed investigation or treatment, as well as the consequence of non-treatment. Competence is presumed at different ages in different countries. Children's competence is related to experience as well as to age, and young children can often clearly demonstrate that they have the competence to make decisions about treatment. Such competence has a legal standing in some countries (such as the so-called 'Gillick' competence in English law).

Providing the information: an essential component of consent

In some societies, disease and pain are interpreted in terms of sin and retribution. This may make it difficult for health workers to explain diagnostic and management options in medical terms.

Information should include details of the possible diagnoses and prognosis, possible management options, the purpose of a proposed investigation or treatment, and the likely benefits and probabilities of success, and discussion about any serious or frequently occurring risks. Wherever possible the information should be given in a way that is clearly understood and remembered.

All this information may be overwhelming for patients and their families. The principles of beneficence and non-maleficence might suggest that a more paternalistic and less forthright doctor might be behaving more ethically. However, it is important that personal views about how much to disclose are not imposed on the patient when explaining an illness or treatment to them.

When providing information, it is essential that professionals do their utmost to find out about the patient's (and family's) needs and priorities. This is often the most difficult part of the communication process, and involves responding honestly to any questions the patient or family raise and, as far as possible, answering these as fully as possible. It is for the competent patient, not the doctor, to determine what is in the patient's own best interests.

Finally, information for decision making should not be withheld from the patient and their family, unless it is judged that disclosure would cause the patient or family serious harm (the principle of non-maleficence). It may also be inappropriate to discuss treatments that are not available.

Emergency situations

If the patient is unconscious or otherwise unable to consent to, or decline, treatment and there is no one legally able to consent for them (this varies between countries, and may be the patient's child, brother, sister, etc.), urgent investigation and treatment may be carried out. This is sometimes called presumed consent, where the healthcare worker does what they think is in the best interests of the patient.

The UK General Medical Council (1998) advice on consent for emergencies includes the following:

> 'In an emergency, where consent cannot be obtained, you may provide medical treatment to anyone, provided the treatment is limited to what is immediately necessary to save life or avoid significant deterioration in the patient's health.'

Summary of consent

- Practise within the limits of the law of the country (unless this is harmful to the patient).
- Assess the level of competence of the patient before deciding how much and how to tell them.
- The patient and their family can tell you how much information they need to make a decision.
- All decisions must be free from coercion.

Confidentiality

This is not an ethical principle, but it involves a respect for autonomy, beneficence towards the patient, and a desire to act with non-maleficence.

Confidentiality respects an individual's autonomy and their right to control information relating to their own health. In keeping information confidential, the doctor is acting beneficently.

Most countries have laws to enable the breaking of confidentiality in some circumstances – for example, to protect the safety of a third person, or:

1 to prevent a serious crime, as information may need to be disclosed to the police

2 to report suspected child abuse

3 to report someone who is HIV positive who is unwilling

to inform their sexual partner(s) about this and does not consent to the healthcare worker telling the partner(s). The healthcare worker should inform the patient of his or her intention to inform the partner(s).

Information should only be disclosed without the patient's consent by health workers to individuals who need to know, and the recipient(s) of such information should keep it confidential.

Patient rights (family rights in the case of young children)
These are as follows:
1 to participate in developing a plan of treatment
2 to receive an explanation of how components of treatment will be provided
3 only to have confidentiality broken under certain conditions (e.g. knowledge or suspicion of child abuse, intent of the patient to harm him- or herself or others, or the presence of a communicable disease that may harm others)
4 to receive clinically appropriate care and treatment
5 to be treated in a manner that is free from abuse, discrimination and/or exploitation
6 to be treated by staff who are sensitive to the family's cultural background
7 to be given privacy.

End-of-life issues
These include the following:
- attempts to prolong the life of a dying patient
- euthanasia and medically assisted suicide
- care of terminally ill patients.

Attempts to prolong the life of a dying patient
Where there is no benefit to the patient these attempts are unethical. Futile treatments are those that are assessed as bound to fail and which are prolonging the dying phase. Withholding or withdrawing treatment is not the same as participating in assisted suicide or assisted euthanasia. This does not include palliative treatment, which must always be offered (*see* Section 1.16).

The patient may decide to discontinue treatment for a life-threatening illness while able to understand the information needed to make an informed choice, and prefer to die with dignity, being treated palliatively. Alternatively, they may wish to continue treatment even if they understand that it can provide little benefit. They must always be offered palliative treatment, whatever their choice.

> Euthanasia and assisted suicide are illegal in most countries and prohibited in most medical codes of ethics, and the WMA states that assisted suicide is unethical.

Euthanasia
Euthanasia (also known as 'assisted dying') means intentionally performing an act that is intended to end another person's life and:
- the patient has voluntarily asked for their life to be ended and is competent, informed and has an incurable illness

- the agent knows about the patient's condition and their desire to die, and commits the act with the intention of ending life
- the act is undertaken with compassion and without personal gain.

Assisted suicide
This is knowingly and intentionally providing a person with the knowledge or means to commit suicide, including counselling about lethal doses of drugs, prescribing or supplying the drugs.

This does not mean that healthcare workers should abandon dying patients, but rather they should provide compassionate end-of-life care, including relief of pain and suffering (*see* Section 1.16).

This includes patients who have refused potentially life-saving treatment while competent to do so. For example, if a patient refuses potentially life-saving surgery for a ruptured ectopic pregnancy, they should still receive nursing and medical care and symptomatic relief of suffering.

Withholding or withdrawing medical care
If the patient is a child, the healthcare team and the parents must enter a partnership of care whose function is to serve the best interests of the child.
1 Although there is no significant ethical difference between withdrawing and withholding treatment, there are significant practical differences.
2 Optimal ethical decision making concerning patients requires open and timely communication between members of the healthcare team, the patient and the family.
3 Parents must decide on behalf of a child who is unable to express preferences, unless they are clearly acting against the child's best interests. Cultural practices and religious beliefs may have an impact on this.
4 The wishes (antecedent, if known) of a child who has sufficient understanding and experience should be given substantial consideration.
5 Resolution of disagreement should be by discussion, consultation and consensus.
6 The duty of care is not an absolute duty to preserve life by all means.
7 A shift from life-sustaining treatment to palliation represents a change in aims and objectives, and does not constitute a withdrawal of care.
8 Health workers should never withdraw treatments that alleviate pain or promote comfort.
9 There is a difference between treatment of the dying patient and euthanasia. When a dying patient is receiving palliative care, the underlying cause of death is the disease process. Treatments that may incidentally hasten death are justified, if their primary aim is to relieve suffering.

Hospital ethics committees
Despite the growth of medical ethics and the publication of many professional codes of practice in recent years, it is still difficult for individuals to obtain guidance in resolving specific ethical dilemmas they face. Some hospitals have set up a hospital ethics committee or clinical ethics forum to discuss these dilemmas.

The jurisdiction of the ethics committee includes clinical

situations involving all patients, including infants and children under 18 years of age.

Function of hospital ethics committees

1 **Education:** The committee should provide members of the hospital/medical staff with access to the language, concepts, principles and knowledge of ethics.
2 **Policy review and development:** the committee can assist the hospital and healthcare staff in the development of polices and guidelines regarding recurrent ethical issues and questions which arise in the care of individual patients.
3 **Case review:** the committee should be a forum for analysis of ethical questions that arise in the care of individual patients.

Appointment and membership

The committee is multidisciplinary, and should include doctors, nurses, midwives, social worker, pastoral care, hospital director and chief of medical staff. A 30% membership from the general community has been suggested to ensure breadth of perspective and clarity of output.

Research ethics

Each year £35–40 billion is spent on healthcare research worldwide, but only 10% of this is aimed at the health problems of 90% of the world's population.

Under-resourced countries need research to help to prevent and treat diseases such as tuberculosis and malaria, but lack funds and trained personnel, and therefore need expertise and financial support from public and private sectors in wealthy countries. This can lead to exploitation of the people in the country where research is needed and undertaken.

The principles that should be followed by anyone who is designing or conducting healthcare research in under-resourced countries are as follows:

- to alleviate suffering
- to show respect for people
- to be sensitive to cultural differences
- not to exploit those who are vulnerable
- the scientific and social importance of the research should outweigh the risks and burdens to the study subjects
- all research should have social as well as scientific value
- the populations involved in the research should benefit from the results
- staff working in the public sector where there are insufficient staff to provide proper care for patients (e.g. in most of sub-Saharan Africa) should not be taken from their work in order to undertake research.

It is important that there are national guidelines in every country which set priorities for healthcare research, and if external sponsors propose research outside these priorities, it must be justified to the appropriate research ethics committees.

There should be three levels of review for each research proposal:

1 relevance to healthcare priorities in the country
2 scientific validity
3 ethical acceptability.

There are a number of national and international guidelines and regulations with regard to research (e.g. WMA, Council for International Organizations of Medical Science in collaboration with WHO, European Council and European Parliament), but these are often inappropriate for under-resourced countries.

Consent to research

For this to be valid, it should be given freely after full disclosure of all relevant information in a manner understandable by the research subject. Consent for the research may be withdrawn by the subject at any time without there being any adverse effects on the subject. However, in some communities it is usual for male members of the family or a community to make decisions on behalf of women and children.

Level of care

The level of care provided to the control group (i.e. the group that is not having the active potential treatment) is controversial. Some argue that, if the research is externally sponsored, the people in the control group should receive the same standard of care as would be received in the sponsor's country. Others argue that this prevents some research from being conducted. For example, if two treatments are being compared in the under-resourced country, it is more appropriate for the new treatment to be compared with the one currently available in that country, not one that is inaccessible there.

Post-research considerations

If an intervention is effective, should it be made available to the research participants and the community? The country concerned may not be able to afford this, particularly if it is a new and expensive drug, but a decision should be made with the national government via its research ethics committee about what will happen after the trial period is over.

Healthcare worker relationships

As well as having an ethical duty towards patients, healthcare workers have an ethical duty towards other healthcare workers, to the healthcare system and to society.

The health worker–patient relationship

1 The healthcare worker's primary role is to be an advocate for each patient's care and well-being. They should always place the interests of their patients first. The healthcare worker also has a duty to accept responsibility for his or her clinical decisions.
2 The healthcare worker must treat each patient with honesty, compassion, dignity and respect. They should not exclude or discriminate against any patient because of ethnic origin, race, sex, creed, age, socio-economic status, diagnosis, physical or mental disability, or sexual orientation.
3 The healthcare worker's commitment to patients includes health education and continuity of care by good communication with subsequent health workers.

The healthcare worker–healthcare worker relationship

Traditionally, healthcare workers have been part of a hierarchical system, both within and between professions.

Doctors have been at the top of the caregiving hierarchy, above nurses and other healthcare workers. This situation is gradually changing, with other healthcare professionals increasingly questioning the reasoning behind a doctor's decision.

1 Healthcare workers have a responsibility to maintain moral integrity, intellectual honesty and clinical competence. They should be aware of the limitations of their expertise and seek consultation or assistance in clinical situations in which they are not expert.

2 Healthcare workers should work as a team, supporting each other and working together for the benefit of the patient.

3 Healthcare workers have an obligation to educate and share information with colleagues, including trainee healthcare workers. They should be committed to life-long learning and continuously improve their knowledge and clinical skills relevant to their practice.

4 There is an ethical obligation to report impairment or misconduct of colleagues in order to prevent potential harm to patients.

The relationship between the healthcare worker and the system of care

1 The healthcare worker's duty of patient advocacy should not be altered by the system of healthcare delivery in which they practise.

2 If there are conflicts of interest, the patient's interests should take priority over those of others.

3 Healthcare professionals should campaign against unethical practices.

4 Healthcare professionals should not be influenced by commercial enterprises (e.g. companies that manufacture drugs, diagnostic tools or equipment). The duty of the physician is to evaluate objectively what is best for the patient. Gifts designed to influence clinical practice are not acceptable.

5 Healthcare professionals should advocate to their departments of health for improved medical facilities and treatments for patients where acceptable basic facilities and treatments are lacking (e.g. oxygen, effective pain relief, blood transfusion services, access to vital skills such as surgery, basic life-saving drugs).

In many countries, there are huge divisions between the rich minority and the poor, exploited and disadvantaged majority. Healthcare professionals should be aware of this and acknowledge how their actions support such divisions, and aim to provide high standards of care independent of a patient's or family's ability to pay.

The relationship of the healthcare worker to society

Healthcare workers have a responsibility to society as well as to patients, and sometimes society's best interests may take precedence over those of the patient (e.g. mandatory reporting of patients with a designated disease, those who are unfit to drive and those suspected of child abuse).

In other circumstances there may be requests from the police or the military to take part in practices that violate human rights (e.g. torture). Healthcare workers should report unjustified interference in the care of their patients, especially if fundamental human rights are being denied. If the authorities are unhelpful, contact with a national medical or nursing association, the WMA or World Nursing Federation, or a human rights organisation may be needed.

The increasing mobility of society means that healthcare workers have a responsibility for global health, including preventing the spread of infectious diseases between societies and countries.

Another effect of globalisation is the mobility of healthcare professionals, and their migration from low-income to high-income countries. The shortage of healthcare workers is one of the biggest health problems facing low-income countries today.

The governments of low-income countries invest in the education and training of healthcare professionals, and therefore lose these resources and the contribution of these workers when graduates migrate. The factors considered by the migrant may be economic, social and/or family related. Often in low-income countries there are low wages, poor working conditions, lack of leadership and very few incentives, as well as limited opportunities for their children. High-income governments encourage migration when there is a need, often with no compensation for the government where the migrant was trained.

This presents an ethical dilemma whereby if emigration was prevented it would restrict the autonomy of the individual, but on the other hand the health of a society suffers if there is mass migration of healthcare professionals.

Further reading

World Organization Against Torture http://kofiannanfoundation. org/newsroom/speeches/2010/06/world-organisation-against-torture (accessed 9 December 2012).

Medical Foundation for the Care of Victims of Torture www. freedomfromtorture.org (accessed 9 December 2012).

Ethics – World Medical Association. www.wma.net/ en/20activities/10ethics (accessed 9 December 2012).

The ICN Code of Ethics for Nurses – International Council of Nurses. www.icn.ch/about-icn/code-of-ethics-for-nurses (accessed 9 December 2012).

General Medical Council. GMC List of ethical guidance – General Medical Council. www.gmc-uk.org/guidance/ ethical_guidance.asp

Nuffield Foundation. The Ethics of Clinical Research in Developing Countries. http://nuffieldbioethics.org/project/ research-developing-countries-follow/

Naicker S, Plange-Rhule J, Tutt J *et al.* (2009) Shortage of healthcare workers in developing countries – Africa. *Ethnicity and Disease*, **19**, S1 60–4. http://txfvzgw.ishib. org/journal/19-1s1/ethn-19-01s1-60.pdf

Global Health Workforce Alliance (2011) *Progress Report on Kampala Declaration and Agenda for Global Action*. www.who.int/workforcealliance/knowledge/resources/ kdagaprogressreport/en/

1.21 Traditional medicine and its relevance to hospital care

BOX 1.21.1 Minimum standards
- Consider traditional medicine as a possible cause of any child presenting with symptoms suggesting poisoning.
- ABCD structured approach.
- Hypoglycaemia and electrolyte disturbance management.
- Antibiotics.
- Wound management.
- Tetanus immunisation promotion.

Introduction

Traditional medicine encompasses diverse health practices, remedies, approaches, knowledge and beliefs incorporating plant, animal and mineral products, spiritual therapies, charms, manual techniques, exercises, and in fact any kind of salutary method applied singly or in combination to diagnose, treat and prevent illnesses or maintain well-being, which has been handed down by the tradition of a community or ethnic group. In contrast with conventional medicine, which focuses on experiment and disease-causing pathogens, traditional medicine postulates that the human being is both a somatic and spiritual entity, and that disease can be due to supernatural causes arising from the anger of ancestral or evil spirits, the result of witchcraft, or the entry of an object into the body. It is therefore not only the symptoms of the disease that are taken into account, but also psychological and sociological factors. Thus the holistic nature and culture-based approach to traditional healthcare is an important aspect of the practice, and sets it apart from conventional western approaches. Traditional medicine is culturally treasured by various communities around the world. It thus plays an almost inestimable role in healthcare delivery to the people.

In many parts of sub-Saharan Africa, it is estimated that about 80% of the population use traditional health services. Most rural and urban dwellers often supplement treatment by orthodox medical practitioners with treatment by traditional healers. In Ghana, Mali, Nigeria and Zambia, it has been found that the first-line treatment for 60% of children with high fever from malaria is the use of herbal medicines at home. Traditional medicine is extensively used in Latin America and Asia. In China, 40% of all healthcare is delivered by traditional health practitioners. In 2007, there were an estimated 190 000 traditional health practitioners in South Africa. They treat an array of health-related problems as well as culture-bound syndromes or ailments considered to be non-responsive to western medicine. In 2002, the World Health Organization (WHO) estimated that traditional medicine provided 80–90% of healthcare in Africa.

For example, among Nigerians, there are powerful cultural and religious beliefs and practices relating to health. Approximately 85% of the population use traditional medicine and consult its practitioners for healthcare. The majority

(70%) of Nigeria's population is rural and relies almost exclusively on traditional medicine for its healthcare needs.

The popularity of traditional medicine has been attributed to poverty, limited or no access to good-quality orthodox medicine, illiteracy and ignorance. Other factors include affordability, availability, efficacy, costly or inefficient orthodox medical facilities, unfriendliness of hospital staff, poor communication (e.g. patients not being told the nature and cause of their illness), inadequate technical services leading to poor-quality care, treatment that is divorced from the patient's culture, family and community, and the treatment only addressing biological aspects of the illness rather than also addressing spiritual aspects.

The traditional healer, as defined by the WHO (1976), is a person who is recognised by the community in which they live as being competent to provide healthcare by using vegetable, animal and mineral substances and certain other methods based on the social, cultural and religious background, as well as the knowledge, attributes and beliefs that are prevalent in the community, regarding physical, mental and social well-being and the causation of disease and disability. They rely exclusively on practical experience and observations handed down from one generation to the next, whether verbally or in writing. For most countries of the world, a traditional healer may be able to perform many functions, thus being more versatile as a healer.

The elements of traditional medicine include, among others, herbal medicine, massage, homeopathy, mud baths, music therapy, wax baths, reflexology, dance therapy, hydrotherapy, mind and spirit therapies, self-exercise therapies, radiation and vibration, osteopathy, chiropractic medicine, aromatherapy, preventive medicine, radiant heat therapy, therapeutic fasting and dieting, spinal manipulation and psychotherapy.

Traditional healers

There are various categories of traditional healers. Some of them may have areas of special interest.

Herbalists

A herbalist is a person who specialises in the economic or medicinal uses of plants. The whole plant may be used or parts of the plant, including the whole root, root bark, whole stem, stem bark, leaves, flowers, fruits and seeds, which may be administered to the patient in the following forms:

1 a powder that can be swallowed or taken with pap/traditional porridge (cold or hot) or any drink
2 a powder that is rubbed into cuts made on any part of the body with a sharp knife
3 a preparation that is soaked for some time in water or local gin, and decanted as required before drinking; the materials could also be boiled in water, cooled and strained
4 a preparation that is pounded with native soap and used

for bathing; such 'medicated soaps' are commonly used to treat skin diseases

5 pastes or ointments, in a medium of palm oil or shea butter

6 soup which is consumed by the patient

7 herbal preparations may also be administered as an enema.

The plants are gathered from the environment, and are therefore part of every cultural tradition and have helped the development and growth of herbalism. Some of the plants that are facing extinction due to drought, bush burning, rapid growth of communities, farming or other factors are specially cultivated by some herbalists to maintain a steady source of supply.

Traditional birth attendants (TBAs)

A traditional birth attendant assists the mother at childbirth, and initially acquired her skills delivering babies by herself or by working with other birth attendants. TBAs are predominantly female. For example, around 60–85% of childbirth in Nigeria is overseen by TBAs, especially in the rural communities. They therefore occupy a prominent position in the healthcare system. Their skills are wide ranging, including diagnosis of pregnancy, antenatal care, conduct of labour and postnatal care. They are quite acceptable to those living in rural communities because their practice is linked to socio-cultural practices. For this reason, some governments have started to train TBAs in an attempt to reduce maternal and child morbidity and mortality.

Traditional bone setters

Traditional bone setters are knowledgeable in the art and skill of setting broken bones in the traditional way, using their skill to ensure that the bones unite and heal properly. They are involved in setting various types of fractures using wooden splints made from bamboo plants, and they use dry fibre from banana stems as bandaging. Wounds resulting from such fractures are usually cleaned and bleeding stopped by the application of plant extracts. Some practitioners fracture similar bones in a bird and treat it alongside the fractured limb of the patient. This is used to determine the time that it will take for the patient's fracture to heal, and the correct time for removing the wrapped splints and clay cast. Importantly, some bone setters collaborate with orthodox medical practitioners who treat the open wounds, offer radiological services and give advice on cases that require referral. This may help to reduce the number of complications occurring in their practices.

Traditional surgeons

These practitioners undertake minor surgery. The procedures that they perform include the cutting of tribal marks, male circumcision and female genital mutilation (see Section 2.10), ear piercing, and incision and drainage of abscesses, to name just a few. Complications such as haemorrhage, tetanus and sepsis have been reported in their practices.

Traditional psychiatrists

The traditional psychiatrist specialises mainly in the treatment of patients with mental disorders. Psychotics who are violent are usually restrained by chaining them with iron or by clamping them down with wooden shackles. Those who are diagnosed as demon possessed are usually caned or beaten into submission and then given herbal hypnotics or highly sedative herbal potions to calm them. Such herbal preparations include extracts of the African Rauwolfia species. Treatment and rehabilitation of people with mental disorders usually take place over a long period of time. Incantations and various forms of occultism are often employed.

Practitioners of therapeutic occultism

These are traditional practitioners who use supernatural or mysterious forces, incantations, or prescribed rituals associated with the community's religious worship, and they adopt various inexplicable methods to treat a range of diseases. They are usually respected within the community because of their ability to deal with unseen and supernatural forces. They are regarded as witches and wizards.

Traditional medicine ingredient dealers

These dealers are involved in the buying and selling of plants, animals (including insects) and minerals used to make herbal preparations. Some of them also cultivate certain medicinal plants. Although they are not traditional healers, they have knowledge of products that cure different disease conditions, and can therefore prescribe and administer these. Due to this fact, some of them are referred to as traditional healers.

Relevance of traditional medicine

Many communities have developed various traditional systems using locally available resources for the alleviation of their health problems. This has resulted in the appearance of a number of different categories of healers, and a variety of healing methods, strategies and medicines or remedies.

Most people who live in rural communities do not have access to orthodox medicine. For example, in Nigeria it is estimated that about 75% of the population still prefer to solve their health problems by consulting traditional healers. Furthermore, many rural communities have great faith in traditional medicine, particularly its inexplicable aspects, as they believe that it represents the wisdom of their forefathers which also incorporates their socio-cultural and religious background, which orthodox medicine seems to neglect.

There is some justification for the use of herbs by the various traditional healers. A range of herbs have been used in the treatment of various disease conditions, including the African Rauwolfia species (used to treat cardiovascular diseases such as hypertension), rose periwinkle (used to treat diabetes), the Chinese herb Artemisia annua (used to treat malaria) and lemon grass (used to treat diseases of the respiratory system). Although herbal medicines may have beneficial active ingredients, the dosage cannot be controlled as there is no assay system for defining potency, and this increases the risk to patients who receive such treatment.

In environments where illness is believed to have a magical/spiritual origin, people become involved in intense prayers and sacrifices to compensate for their frailty and powerlessness. Western explanations of illness are rarely taken seriously. Local people may embrace traditional medicine to the exclusion of all other approaches, or combine it with orthodox medicine. Adverse drug interactions may result from such combinations of approach. Medical practitioners working in places where traditional medicine is practised must be patient and respectful in their encounter with patients who are using traditional approaches. With health education and therapy that bring real health benefits, local people will become persuaded to accept effective evidence-based treatment.

Although the disadvantages of traditional medicine are numerous, it does also have a few advantages. The traditional healers and their drugs are available in these communities and their drugs are relatively easy to obtain compared with those of orthodox medicine. The healing system cares for the body, mind and soul of the patient in the context of the family, community, God or gods. The relationship between the practitioner and the patient can be close, encouraging and intense, with active participation of the family and neighbours. The practitioners are well known, trusted and respected in the community, and their methods fit very well with the culture and customs of the people. The drugs are cheap and readily available, and the healers accept payments either as a whole, in part or in kind, which also makes their treatments much more accessible for the people.

Complications of traditional medicine

Contrary to popular opinion that traditional medicine, especially herbal medicine, is natural or safe, it can be hazardous to health if these preparations are taken in recommended or larger amounts, injected or combined with prescription drugs. Some Asian herbal products have been found to contain potentially dangerous concentrations of harmful substances such as arsenic, mercury and lead, many of which cause liver failure, haemorrhage or heart failure.

Where confidence in conventional medical care is low, there is a tendency to resort to more risky traditional remedies which may be more toxic. Conversely, when confidence in conventional medical care improves, there is an increasing movement towards the use of less toxic remedies, even though the use of some traditional remedies may continue to satisfy cultural and social needs.

In many low-income countries, patients are subjected to traditional treatment as first aid therapy in emergency conditions at home. Caregivers may apply interventions that are ineffective, harmful, and have no pathophysiological basis.

The application of traditional medical care that is ineffective may also lead to delayed presentation of potentially curable conditions to conventional care, resulting in unnecessary deaths and morbidity.

Some cultural practices are harmful to the health and survival of the newborn infant, and it is often young 'first-time' mothers who are most likely to follow these practices. Giving newborn infants cold baths, discarding colostrum, and providing food other than breast milk soon after birth is common practice. The application of butter, ash or other substances, such as cow dung, to the umbilical stump increase the risk of life-threatening infection.

Examples of problems resulting from traditional medicine practices
Experience of the use of traditional medicine in Nigeria
In Nigeria, as in most other developing countries, children are subjected to unorthodox treatment as first aid therapy in emergency conditions at home. Caregivers may apply

interventions that are ineffective, harmful, and have no pathophysiological basis. The use of traditional medicine is largely ethnocentric.

Crude oil
In the Niger Delta region of Nigeria, crude oil is available in large amounts. It is highly regarded locally as a remedy for a variety of ailments, including febrile convulsions, gastrointestinal disorders, burns, 'foot rot' and leg ulcers, and poisoning. It is also used in witchcraft. The oil is applied to the skin, mixed with alcohol or water as a drink, and instilled into body orifices such as the nostrils, ears, anus, vagina and urethra. The use of crude oil as traditional medicine in Nigeria has been reported to have an analgesic effect comparable to that of aspirin. Complications associated with its use have been reported in children with febrile convulsions.

Complications caused by crude oil have been reported to affect a number of organs, including the skin, lungs, liver and kidneys. Skin exposure may result in the formation of vesicles, blisters and even extensive epidermolysis. Ingestion of crude oil may result in nausea, vomiting and diarrhoea, and the aspiration of crude oil during vomiting results in chemical pneumonitis. Central nervous system symptoms range from vertigo and headache caused by ingestion of small doses, to lethargy, convulsions, coma and death with larger doses. Renal failure has been described as another toxic effect.

Cow's urine concoction
'Cow's urine' concoction (CUC) is a traditional medicine used in the management of convulsive disorders in childhood among the Yoruba-speaking people of south-western Nigeria. It is prepared from leaves of tobacco, garlic and basil, lemon juice, rock salt and onion bulbs, which are soaked in cow urine, which acts as the vehicle in which the active principles of these constituents dissolve. Over 50 chemical compounds have been identified in CUC, the major ones being benzoic acid, phenylacetic acid, p-cresol, thymol and nicotine. These components are toxic, and have harmful effects on the different systems of the body. The main effects are severe respiratory depression, effects on the cardiovascular system and the central nervous system, and hypoglycaemia. These toxic effects acting singly or in combination are believed to be the cause(s) of death from CUC.

Cow dung
It is estimated that 30–40% of infections resulting in deaths from neonatal sepsis are transmitted at the time of childbirth and have early onset of symptoms (developing during the first 72 hours after birth). Worldwide, 60 million births occur outside healthcare facilities, and even within such facilities, hygienic practices may be suboptimal.

The unhealed umbilical cord is an important portal for local and invasive infections during the neonatal period. It is rapidly colonised by bacteria from the maternal genital tract and then from the environment. Infection can emanate from the bamboo stick that is used to cut the umbilicus, and from the cow dung (believed to have desiccating properties) that is used to dress the umbilical stump. Localised umbilical infection (omphalitis) emanating from these sources can spread to the abdominal wall, the peritoneum, or through the umbilical or portal vessels leading to systemic sepsis, which if untreated has a high fatality rate. Neonatal tetanus is a very important complication resulting from these practices, which are common among the Yorubas of south-western Nigeria and the Maasai people of Kenya. Cow dung is also used to anoint the heads of the sick among the Maasai people.

Traditional eye medications

In one study, complications occurred in 55% of the individuals studied, and included corneal opacities, staphyloma and corneal ulcers. Other complications were panophthalmitis, endophthalmitis, uveitis, cataract and bullous keratopathy. Eleven individuals in one study underwent enucleation of the affected eye.

Traditional healers tend to prefer to use substances that cause irritation and pain, as these are perceived by both healers and patients to be more potent. Such substances may be acidic or alkaline, resulting in ocular burns. No particular attention is paid to concentration and sterility, as most of these concoctions (mixture of various substances, which may be plant or animal extracts) are prepared without regard for hygiene, including the use of contaminated water, local gin, saliva and even urine.

Most of these ocular conditions could have been adequately treated using standard medicines, which were sometimes available.

Experience of the use of traditional medicine in pregnancy in South Africa

A recently published review showed that a large percentage of pregnant women still use herbal remedies during pregnancy and childbirth, and in one study the use of at least 56 botanical species was documented.

Such herbal treatments are known collectively as *Isihlambezo*, which is taken as an antenatal tonic during the last trimester of pregnancy in the belief that it promotes a favourable pregnancy and a quick and uncomplicated labour. It is also used to treat common pregnancy-related ailments such as oedema, indigestion, constipation, infection and high blood pressure. It is even believed by some that such traditional medicines may be able to turn a breech baby.

Many different plants are ingredients of *Isihlambezo*, and the recipes for this tonic vary depending on factors such as the traditional healer consulted, the general state of health of the woman, the geographical area and the tribal community. The ingredients are boiled or infused in water and the 'tea' is then taken by the spoonful or cupful. The concentration of the mixture may be increased at the end of pregnancy in order to speed up labour.

Isihlambezo mixtures can be purchased from and dispensed by traditional healers and herbalists or 'muti' shops, and individual ingredients can be obtained from open herbal medicine markets throughout the country. In the rural areas, the ingredients for *Isihlambezo* are often harvested from the local countryside by senior women in the tribal community or by traditional birth attendants.

Imbelekisane and *Inembe* are more specific remedies used as uterotonic drugs in cases of prolonged and difficult labour. However, interviews conducted with traditional healers in KwaZulu-Natal revealed that *Imbelekisane* and *Inembe* are regarded by them as dangerous medicines.

Teratogenicity can be largely ruled out, as these remedies are usually only used in the last trimester. However, the potential for maternal and fetal toxicity remains. Sixteen of the species used in these remedies are known to be poisonous, and one of these, *Callilepis laureola* (*Impila*), is extremely poisonous and has been responsible for many fatalities resulting from hepato-renal failure. Other toxic effects that have been linked to the use of these medicines in pregnancy include low neonatal birth weights, fetal meconium staining of amniotic fluid, and fatal uterine rupture.

All of the plants investigated in the above-mentioned study were able to directly stimulate uterine contraction to varying degrees. *Clivia*, *Agapanthus* and *Rhoicissus* significantly augmented the initial response of the uterus to oxytocin, and were able to produce initial phasic contractions followed by tonic contractions at higher doses. Herbal remedies containing these plants must therefore be considered to have the potential to cause uterine hyperstimulation and its associated adverse effects, including uterine rupture.

Experience of traditional medicine in the Eastern Cape area of South Africa

In another publication, traditional remedies were found to be regularly used in the home management of children in the Eastern Cape, and probably in the great majority of cases these remedies do little harm beyond delaying presentation to the healthcare system. However, serious effects were occasionally identified. Most often the traditional remedy was given to treat a symptom of an underlying disease, rather than being the cause of the condition or symptoms.

- **iYeza lo moya:** commonly given to infants by mouth, with few problems reported. However, a traditional enema may also be given, which may have more toxic effects.
- **Senecio extracts:** infusions of this weed with yellow flowers have been reported to cause veno-occlusive disease in a small number of children.
- **Impila:** extracts from this root may cause fatal hepato-renal failure, often presenting with hypoglycaemia.
- **River onion:** this is used both orally and rectally, and causes hepato-renal failure in a significant number of children.
- **Jeyes fluid:** this is sometimes added to rectal and oral remedies, and causes local and systemic effects.

Surgical complications of traditional medicine in East Africa

A series of case histories in 2007 included a 6-year-old girl sustaining a spiral fracture of the humerus during a road traffic accident. The parents refused hospital treatment and took her to a traditional bone setter. Two weeks later she was brought back to the hospital with a gangrenous upper limb, which was the result of placing a tourniquet around the axilla. Debridement was undertaken but the child lost the whole of the skin of the forearm and most of the hand.

A second case involved an 18-month-old boy who underwent circumcision by a traditional practitioner. On subsequent admission to hospital he was found to have partial amputation of the glans penis.

Traditional medicine used in pregnancy in Malaysia

In one study, 108 mothers (51% of those studied) used at least one type of herbal medicine during pregnancy. The type most commonly used (by 64%) was coconut oil ingested only during the third trimester. The most common indication (90% of cases) was to facilitate labour.

The older generation, parents and in-laws were those who most strongly encouraged the use of herbal medicines. The main reasons for using these medicines were to facilitate labour, to promote the baby's physical health and intelligence, to prevent a retained placenta or to promote abortion.

Management of suspected adverse effects of traditional medicine

These include a rapid assessment of:

- Airway
- Breathing
- Circulation
- Disability.

Regular assessment and treatment of these essential systems will ensure that management keeps abreast with progress and with the prevention of deterioration.

However, when treating patients who have been given traditional medicines, first look for a medical cause of the symptoms and signs before assuming that the illness is due to the traditional remedy.

TABLE 1.21.1 Serious complications caused by traditional medicines, and their management

System affected	Symptoms and signs	Treatment
Cardiovascular	Increased cholinergic actions such as lacrimation, salivation, rhinorrhoea, diarrhoea, vomiting and miosis, severe bradycardia or heart block	IV atropine may help
	Anticholinergic actions such as hyperthermia, tachycardia or tachyarrhythmias, mydriasis, constipation or acute urinary retention	Anticholinesterase drugs may help
Neurological	Weakness, epileptic fits, coma and intracranial bleeding	Check blood clotting Anticonvulsants
Pulmonary	Anaphylaxis, bronchoconstriction Severe interstitial pneumonitis, non-cardiac pulmonary oedema, acute eosinophilic pneumonia	Specific treatment for anaphylaxis and bronchoconstriction (*see* Section 5.1.B) Corticosteroids
Liver toxicity	Nausea, anorexia, vomiting, jaundice with elevated liver transaminases	Supportive (*see* Section 5.7.A)
Nephrotoxicity	Acute renal failure and tubular dysfunction	Supportive (*see* Section 5.6.C)
Heavy metal contamination with lead, arsenic, thallium or uranium	Gastrointestinal disorders, hepatitis, polyarthritis, encephalopathy (including ataxia and severe psychiatric disturbances)	(*see* Section 7.4)

- Clean any areas that are visibly affected with a topical application of sterile water, and apply a non-adhesive dressing if necessary.
- If available, laboratory investigations can be helpful for identifying organ systems that may be affected by a toxic traditional medicine. Take blood for a biochemical profile (urea and electrolytes, liver function tests, amylase and glucose) and a full blood count with indices. If there is any significant abnormality, refer the patient to the relevant specialist team.
- Symptoms and signs such as convulsions should be treated with diazepam injection, hypoglycaemia should be corrected with glucose infusion, and fluid and electrolyte disturbances should be corrected with appropriate oral administration or intravenous infusion.
- Appropriate antibiotics should be administered to patients with infective conditions.

Conclusion

Traditional medicine continues to represent a very large component of community healthcare, especially in resource-limited regions. Efforts to make traditional medicine safer are urgently required, and might include official regulation to monitor the activities of traditional practitioners, standardise their practices and undertake toxicity studies on their products, in collaboration with scientists and recognised institutions. However, this will also require the traditional healers to be willing to work with such control of their practice, which could be a problem if the healers see this as an attempt to limit their practice, or to steal their secrets and remedies.

1.22 Emergency equipment and drugs for obstetric and paediatric care

Introduction

Wherever healthcare is offered, people who consider that they need emergency care will arrive unexpectedly. All healthcare facilities should be prepared to receive and treat such patients as quickly, effectively and compassionately as possible.

Preparation, **training** and **practice** are the keys to success in emergency care.

Preparation involves considering and having available the necessary equipment and drugs for all of the possible pathologies requiring emergency care that are likely to present to the facility.

Training involves ensuring that healthcare workers in the emergency area have been trained to assess life-threatening and urgent care needs and to respond to these in a recognised and structured way so that no essential steps are omitted.

Practice involves the emergency team rehearsing their response to emergencies together so that they become competent when presented with real situations.

Hospitals should have a dedicated 'Emergency Room' where patients of all ages and with all conditions can present. However, patients will often attend the ward where they have previously been seen, and of course emergencies can arise within any ward, especially if that ward is understaffed.

Therefore it is vital that every ward, as well as the emergency room, is prepared with the drugs and equipment necessary to respond successfully to any emergency in that area.

This section describes the drugs and equipment necessary to treat emergencies in women and girls during pregnancy, labour and the postpartum period, as well as in infants and children.

The emergency room should be staffed at all times. The number of staff will depend on the size of the facility and the expected number of patients. In a large city hospital where hundreds of patients attend every day, there may be 10 to 20 nurses and 6 to 8 doctors on duty at any one time. However, in a small peripheral clinic, with only one or two inpatient wards and three or four labour-room beds, there may not be enough staff for one of them to spend all of his or her time awaiting an emergency. In that case, a simple and reliable means of calling for assistance must be put in place for emergency cases arriving at the facility. Again, **preparation** is key, and the immediate availability of the necessary emergency equipment and drugs, together with a **trained** and **practised** healthcare worker, is paramount.

Training in the structured approach to recognition and treatment of life-threatening illness and injury should be available to all healthcare workers who may be called upon to treat emergency patients. There are a number of training programmes available, including the World Health Organization's Integrated Management of Neonatal and Childhood Illnesses (IMNCI), the Emergency Triage Assessment and Treatment (ETAT) course, the Emergency Maternal and Neonatal Health (ESS-EMNH) and Emergency Child and Trauma Health (ESS-ECTH) courses of Maternal Childhealth Advocacy International (mcai.org.uk), and the Advanced Life Support Group (ALSG) courses (alsg.org).

Wherever there are unexpected emergencies, decisions have to be made about which patient is the most urgent one. Emergency healthcare is not offered on a 'first come, first served' basis. Those with the greatest need are treated first. This sorting system is called **triage** (for a detailed explanation, *see* Section 1.10).

Throughout this textbook, details of diagnoses and treatments, including practical procedures, for improving the care of patients with emergency healthcare needs can be found. In this section we now list the emergency equipment and drugs that are essential for providing this care.

Resuscitation equipment for the emergency room

Airway and breathing

- Suction apparatus:
  - wall, electrical or manual suction
  - Yankauer (adult and paediatric) and soft suction catheters
  - a manual suction device, for use by midwives.
- Face masks – adult, child, infant non re-breathing with reservoir bags (for delivering 100% oxygen).
- Self-inflating resuscitation bag with 500-mL (for infants and young children) and 1600-mL (for older children and adults) reservoir bags and face masks in a range of sizes (masks that are too large may be used inverted).
- Nasal cannulae for prolonged lower level oxygen delivery.
- Airway devices:
  - oropharyngeal airways in a range of sizes (000, 00, 0, 1, 2 and 3)
  - endotracheal tubes in a range of sizes (2.5–7.5 mm), and connectors.*
- Laryngeal masks (e.g. I-Gel Size 1, 1.5, 2, 2.5, 3 and 4).
- Laryngoscopes:*
  - adult curved and paediatric straight-bladed
  - spare bulbs and batteries.
- Magill's forceps.*
- Cannulae for cricothyroidotomy.*

Circulatory access and bleeding control

- Peripheral vascular cannulae in a range of sizes (18–25G).
- Intraosseous needles (16–18G) or EZ-IO drill with adult and paediatric needles.
- Sterile catheters 4, 5, 6.5, 8 Fr gauge 40 90 cm long (for suction, feeding, etc.) for umbilical access (for newborn), umbilical vessel dilator, and artery forceps.
- Central venous catheters.*
- Syringes, including a 50-mL syringe for fluid boluses, plus a three-way tap.
- Intravenous giving sets and graduated burettes.
- Condom catheter (*see* Section 2.5.D.iv).
- Cut-down instruments, scalpel and forceps.

*These items are to be used only if facilities exist for intubation and assisted ventilation (e.g. on a high-dependency or intensive-care unit).

Trauma

- Hard cervical collars (adult short and regular, paediatric) and sandbags/foam blocks.
- Peripheral vascular cannulae, (18–25G) three-way taps and syringes.
- Scalpels, sutures, needle holders and scissors.
- Splints.
- Chest drains in a range of sizes (12, 18, 20, 22, 28, 32 Ch).
- Dissecting forceps.
- Underwater drainage system, or flap valves.
- Nasogastric tubes in a range of sizes (4, 5, 6.5, 8, 10 Fr).

Drugs, fluids, etc.

- Oxygen supply.
- Ringer-lactate or Hartmann's solution or 0.9% saline, vials and bags or bottles.
- Colloid (e.g. 4.5% albumin, gelatine, hetastarch).
- Adrenaline, 100 micrograms/mL (1 in 10 000) and 1 mg/mL (1 in 1000).
- Amiodarone, 30 mg/mL.
- Glucose, 10%, 25% and 50%.
- Water for injection.
- Normal saline for injection.
- Mannitol, 20% and/or saline, 2.7% (or 3%).
- Diazepam, rectal solution.
- Lorazepam, diazepam or midazolam (can be used as buccal or IV treatment).
- Phenytoin.
- Phenobarbitone.
- Atropine.
- Sodium bicarbonate.
- Calcium chloride.
- Magnesium sulphate.

- Broad-spectrum antibiotic (e.g. cefotaxime, ceftriaxone, gentamicin).
- Penicillins: penicillin G, amoxicillin, flucloxacillin.
- Metronidazole.
- Hydralazine.
- Misoprostol.
- Quinine.
- Morphine/diamorphine.
- Naloxone.
- Insulin.
- Local anaesthetic (e.g. lignocaine) and general (e.g. ketamine) anaesthetic agents.*
- Paralysing agents.*
- Skin cleansing solution (e.g. chlorhexidine, alcohol, iodine).
- Vaginal antiseptic lotion (Hibitane).
- Steroids (prednisolone, hydrocortisone).
- Salbutamol nebules, inhaler and IV solution.
- Aminophylline.
- Furosemide.

Monitoring and other equipment

- Pulse oximeters.
- ECG monitors including one with with defibrillator with paediatric pads or an automatic external defibrillator (AED).
- Sphygmomanometer or blood pressure oscillometer.
- Thermometers (including low-reading thermometer).
- Nebuliser.
- Large-volume spacers.
- Blood/urine glucose testing kits.
- Urine protein testing sticks.
- Urinary catheters (silicon, rubber or soft feeding tubes) of various sizes (12–30 Fr).

*These items are to be used only if facilities and skills exist for intubation and assisted ventilation.

1.23 Grief and loss in societies affected by conflict and disaster

Introduction

Why do we grieve? Wouldn't life be much simpler if we did not experience all those painful emotions that occur when someone we love dies? Perhaps so – no weeping and wailing, no stoical silence, no anger and irritation, no smiling and carrying on as usual, no sudden flood of pain and memories to overwhelm and paralyse us, no rush of tears when we hear a familiar tune. That sounds much easier. The trouble is that grief is actually the price tag on another emotional experience, without which human life would be quite unbearable. We grieve because we love. Love is the essential emotion that keeps us connected and attached to family and friends and allows us to survive as rather puny animals in a hostile world. If we did not love we could not suffer loss, but neither could we survive in selfish isolation.

This section provides a brief introduction to understanding grief and loss in families living in societies affected by disaster and conflict, and offers some guidance on how to support these families. It will address the following questions:

- What is the impact of loss on individuals and groups in conflict and disaster settings?
- What is grief and how is it related to attachment?
- Is grief an illness?
- How does grief affect our health?
- When is grief abnormal?
- What is mourning and why does it matter?

- What happens when large numbers of people die at one time?
- How do we distinguish between the effects of traumatic events and the effects of loss?
- What is cultural bereavement?
- What are the effects of grief in childhood?
- What can we do to help grieving families and children?

In a society affected by conflict or disaster, most children will be seen in the company of their surviving adult relatives, whose own mental state will have a profound effect on the child. The family doctor must therefore be responsive to, and able to assess and support, the whole family. For this reason, this section looks at grief in both adults and children, and it outlines a general approach to supporting families and children. However, it does not give detailed management advice on the wide variety of specific symptomatic problems that can occur in grief (e.g. bedwetting, sleep disturbance), as there are a number of excellent manuals available on this topic.[1]

What is the impact of loss on individuals and groups in conflict and disaster settings?

The central experience for almost all of those living in communities affected by conflict or disaster is loss. Even if no one in your family dies, something will be lost. You may be injured or lose your health. Your home or your school may be destroyed, or the neighbourhood may be swept away. Your friends or work colleagues may be killed or flee. If you flee yourself you will lose everything that made up your world and kept you rooted and connected. As well as these external losses, you may lose aspects that are central to your internal sense of self, such as feelings of being safe and in control, and your sense of identity as, for example, a mother, father, schoolchild, farmer or shopkeeper. Some of the possible losses that can be experienced are listed in Table 1.23.1. Their effect can be overwhelming. Understanding how people react to such losses, how to distinguish between normal and abnormal grief, and how to assist in appropriate mourning will be some of the key tasks for healthcare workers in these contexts. It is also essential to understand other psychological reactions, such as post-traumatic stress disorder (PTSD), and set them in context.

TABLE 1.23.1 Some of the losses that can be experienced by those exposed to conflict, disaster, or life as a refugee

Internal losses	External losses
Control	Family members
Autonomy	Friends
Security	Home
Identity	Community/country
Self-respect	Work/school
Belief in the future	Money and other material possessions
Sense of belonging	Physical health
Trust	Religion
The past	Language
Meaning of life	Familiar life

What is grief and how is it related to attachment?

The ability to form strong relationships with others is necessary for our survival as human beings. We call this ability **attachment**. The sense of loss that we feel when a loved one is absent leads us to search them out. Attachment is the glue that keeps families and groups connected together. Human beings could not have survived in previous eras if they had not lived in groups that enabled them to feed and shelter themselves. Loss is the sense of sadness, fear and insecurity that we feel when a loved person is absent. It can also be felt in relation to objects and places.

In the 1950s, the World Health Organization (WHO) commissioned John Bowlby to observe what happened to small children when they were separated from their mothers. In Britain in those days, if a child went to hospital for an operation, the parent was not allowed to remain with them. John Bowlby sat watching the infant to see how they reacted, how they adapted to the separation, and how they behaved when the parent returned. He defined a cycle of behaviours that can be observed in any infant who is separated from their mother and then reunited with her.

First there would be a period of loud and angry protest. The child would hope that their cries would bring their mother running back. When this did not happen, a period of despair and withdrawal followed in which the child would cry, not wish to engage with others, and refuse to eat or play. Later the child might appear to 'adapt'. They would start to eat again, play with other children, make friends with the nurses and appear detached and indifferent to the loss of their mother. Indeed if the parent reappeared at this stage, the child's first response might be to ignore her, and then if they did engage with her, to be naughty and angry. Only after some time would the original relationship reform and re-engagement occur. Bowlby noted that this attachment/separation behaviour is most visible in children between 6 months and 3 years of age. However, these behaviours can reappear in any individual throughout the life cycle when they are faced with separation from someone they love.

Attachment behaviour is any form of behaviour that results in a person attaining or maintaining proximity to some clearly identified individual who is conceived as better able to cope with the world. It is most obvious whenever a person is frightened, fatigued or sick, and is assuaged by comforting and caregiving. At other times, the behaviour is less in evidence. Nevertheless, for a person to know that an attachment figure is available and responsive gives him a strong and pervasive feeling of security and so encourages him to value and continue the relationship. Whilst attachment behaviour is at its most obvious early in childhood, it can be observed throughout the life cycle, especially in emergencies. Since it is seen in virtually all human beings (though in varying patterns), it is regarded as an integral part of human nature and one we share (to a varying extent) with members of other species. The biological function attributed to it is protection. To remain within easy access of a familiar individual known to be ready and willing to come to our aid in an emergency is clearly a good insurance policy – whatever our age.

Bowlby, 1988[2]

Many writers have noted the similarity between a child's behaviour after separation from a parent and our reactions to the loss of a loved person who has died. Death reactivates attachment behaviour. Faced with the permanent loss that death represents, we may find ourselves angrily protesting, searching and yearning, trying our best to maintain and hang on to the connection. Or we may experience periods of indifference and denial as a way of avoiding the pain. Many people alternate between periods of acute grieving and yearning and periods of avoidance or detachment. In the past, some authors have argued that these feelings occur in stages. Elisabeth Kubler-Ross constructed a model of bereavement in which the individual was said to progress through the following periods, often cyclically:[2]

1 denial
2 anger
3 bargaining
4 depression
5 acceptance.

It was suggested that people could become stuck at different stages, and that 'grief work' was necessary to progress through all the stages to recovery. There is now a growing understanding of the enormous variability in our responses to bereavement. How people grieve and how they cope will depend on individual factors such as their temperament and personality. What were their experiences as a child? Were they loved and securely attached to those who cared for them or were they abused or insecure? This will affect the way that they form relationships with other people, and the way that they experience loss, as will their age, gender, and experience of previous losses. The way that people grieve will also depend on the nature of the loss and how it occurred. Was it sudden or expected? Was it violent, unjust, or part of a massive loss, or did it occur after a prolonged illness? What did the loss mean to the person? Were they thrust into isolation and poverty, or were they possibly liberated from an abusive relationship? In all cases, social factors such as cultural and religious beliefs and community and family dynamics will play a role in determining how grief is experienced and expressed. The current social situation will also influence this. Is the family in danger or in flight? What material resources do they have? Do they face legal difficulties because of the loss? Is social support available or are they isolated? The case examples below and the vignettes in the Appendix all illustrate these variations.

Table 1.23.2 lists the wide variety of emotional, cognitive, behavioural and physiological changes that can occur in response to bereavement. An individual may experience some, all or none of these. The reactions may occur in many different patterns and combinations depending on the factors described above. Some individuals experience few reactions, others more. Some people find that their reactions change over time or occur in varying combinations.

People may feel anger and sadness at the same time. An anniversary or a particular place may trigger a memory, which reactivates the feelings of grief again, perhaps years after the event, possibly interrupting a long period of acceptance. Some have described grief as a 'relapsing illness'. Stroebe and her colleagues have created a model to show how many people may fluctuate between a 'loss orientation' of yearning and sadness and a 'restoration orientation' of

more avoidant states of denial and getting on with things (see Figure 1.23.1).

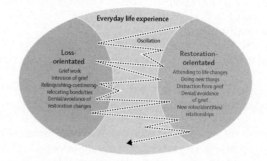

FIGURE 1.23.1 The dual process model of coping with bereavement. Thanks to Stroebe M, Schut H. *Death Studies* 1999; **23**: 197–224.

Which feelings and behaviours occur, which state dominates and what is regarded as normal for both children and adults will depend very much on how grief is expressed in that culture, by that family and in that individual, as well as on the religious values, temperament and personality of the individual. For example, in Bosnia it is regarded as appropriate for Serbian women to attend the funeral and to display their emotions visibly, keening and weeping. In Bosnia, Muslim culture values a more stoical approach and sees the open display of emotions as inappropriate. In some cultures, for example in parts of South-East Asia, vivid dreams may be regarded as appropriate messages from the dead. In western culture, dreams may be seen as an upsetting form of sleep disturbance. In Kosovar families with whom I have worked, there was often one individual (usually an older adolescent girl), who might cry a great deal, hyperventilate and faint, while the rest of the family remained stoical. The fainting girl might cause concern, but also seemed to play a role in vividly expressing grief for the rest of the family, whose concern for her also acted as a form of distraction from the loss (see Appendix, Vignette 2).

> Near the end of his life, Sigmund Freud was consulted by a woman who had become depressed following the death of her husband. After listening to her, Freud quietly stated, 'Madam, you do not have a neurosis, you have a misfortune.'

Is grief an illness?

Acute grief may be painful and feel like an illness, but it should be understood, in all its variety, as a normal reaction to loss. Some combinations of reactions do appear to mimic certain acute mental illnesses. For example, loss of appetite combined with sleep disturbance, sadness, ruminations and various somatic complaints appears similar to clinical depression. However, that diagnosis should not be made if someone has suffered an acute loss. Some individuals may adopt the behaviours of the deceased, dress in their clothes, act strangely or hear their voice, see them and talk to them. Again this should not be regarded as psychotic behaviour, but rather as a possible manifestation of acute grief. Or there may be flashbacks, vivid intrusive thoughts and dreams of the deceased, and the individual may be anxious and aroused, similar to those with PTSD. None of these reactions are necessarily pathological.

TABLE 1.23.2 Reactions to bereavement[3]

Affective	Cognitive	Behavioural	Physiological-somatic
Depression, despair, dejection, distress	Preoccupation with thoughts of the deceased, intrusive ruminations	Agitation, tenseness, restlessness	Loss of appetite
Anxiety, fear, dread	Vivid memories	Fatigue, apathy	Sleep disturbances
Guilt, self-blame, self-accusation	Sense of the presence of the deceased	Overactivity	Energy loss, exhaustion
Anger, hostility, irritability	Lowered self-esteem, self-reproach	Searching	Somatic complaints
Anhedonia (loss of pleasure)	Helplessness, hopelessness, pessimism about the future	Weeping, sobbing, crying	Physical complaints similar to those of the deceased
Loneliness	Suicidal ideation	Social withdrawal	*Endocrine and immunological changes*
Yearning, longing, pining	Sense of unreality	Normal behaviour and continuation of normal activities	Susceptibility to illness, disease, mortality
Shock, numbness	Memory and concentration difficulties	*In children*	
No reaction	Suppression, avoidance, disbelief	Acting out	
	Fantasies	Regressive behaviour	
		School difficulties	
		Rapid maturing	

How does grief affect our health?

That is not to say that bereavement does not have physical and mental health consequences.[4] Bereaved people experience more physical complaints, have more health consultations, use more medication and experience more hospitalisations than those who are not bereaved. Paradoxically, those who are grieving intensely actually have fewer health consultations than the normal population, and high-intensity grief is a predictor of more severe physical disorders 1 year later. Perhaps this is because early warning signs are missed. Regarding the impact of bereavement on mental health, the majority of people recover but there is a greater vulnerability to depression, anxiety and PTSD. Bereavement is associated with increased mortality from many causes. People who have suffered a recent bereavement are more likely to die of alcohol-related disorders, coronary artery disease, unnatural deaths and suicide. It is thought that this additional risk may be due to a number of factors, including loneliness, changes in social circumstances, a reduction in material resources, and lack of care. The mortality risk is higher in the earliest months and in specific groups, namely mothers who have lost a child and widowers. Therefore there is some basis for the saying that you can die of a 'broken heart'.

When is grief abnormal?

The decision as to what is abnormal and inappropriate grief will depend on an understanding of the individual, the family, the culture and the wider context. You cannot decide what is abnormal without this cultural and personal knowledge. The community and family may be able to tell when they feel that the grief is too intense, too long or unusual in its manifestations. The new diagnostic formulations,[5] *DSM-V* and *ICD-11*, that psychiatrists are using to categorise mental disorders are considering formulations for prolonged or complicated grief. For example, the suggested definition of prolonged grief disorder in *ICD-11* is as follows:

'Prolonged grief disorder is a disturbance in which, following the death of a person close to the bereaved, there is persistent and pervasive yearning or longing for the deceased, or a persistent preoccupation with the deceased that extends beyond 6 months after the loss and that is sufficiently severe to cause significant impairment in the person's functioning. The response can also be characterised by difficulty accepting the death, feeling one has lost a part of one's self, anger about the loss, guilt, or difficulty in engaging with social or other activities. The persistent grief response goes far beyond expected social or cultural norms, and depends on cultural and contextual factors.'

What is mourning and why does it matter?

Mourning refers to the culturally appropriate processes that help people to pass through grief. All societies and cultures mourn, but they do so in different ways. Mourning processes usually include acknowledgement and acceptance of the death, saying farewell, time periods for grieving, processes for continuing to focus attention on the dead, and processes for moving beyond the loss and forming new attachments. It might be helpful to take a moment to jot down on a sheet of paper the ways in which you mourn the dead in your own culture. Try to answer the following questions:

- How do other people know that someone has died or that you are bereaved?
- What happens at a funeral?
- What are the burial customs?
- What happens to the body?
- Who visits the bereaved?
- What are the different roles, if any, for men and women?
- What do younger and older children do?
- Are there different ceremonies at different time periods after the death to mark different stages of mourning?
- What ways do you use to remember the dead?
- What is the role of the dead person in continuing family life?

Different societies have different time periods set aside for mourning, and different ideas about what is appropriate behaviour for different family members. They may also have different views on the appropriate role of children in these rituals. Sometimes families may be in conflict over what is appropriate to communicate to children and what is the appropriate way to mourn. This is particularly the case in societies that are in a state of upheaval (see Appendix, Vignette 1).

What happens in situations of massive loss?

Conflict, disaster and displacement disrupt the possibility of appropriate mourning. There may be uncertainty about missing relatives. The body may have been lost, abandoned, treated inappropriately, or buried in a mass grave. During flight it is impossible to carry out the normal mourning rituals. Other processes also occur in large-scale upheavals. For example, in Aceh, Indonesia, after the 2004 Tsunami, people found themselves living in a landscape that had been swept completely clean by the Wave, where every familiar marker had disappeared along with their communities, families and livelihoods. There were no bodies and no places to go to remember the dead. In Haiti, after the earthquake, people camped out among crushed houses that entombed their families. Massive losses that affect whole communities may remove entire social networks of support. Moreover, even in functioning communities, they have the effect of depriving each individual of the normal support that they would have received if their loss had been a singular occurrence. Because everyone is affected, few are in the position to play the role of visitor and comforter. There is no one to come round, help the bereaved widow with the childcare and household tasks, arrange the funeral and cook a meal, because everyone who survived is in the same situation. Everyone struggles alone. And the bereaved may become more reticent than usual about their own feelings, not wishing to burden similarly affected neighbours. At the same time, the pain of the loss is amplified by the knowledge that the bereaved person's loss is one of many in a community. The outside world is focused on the scale of the event: '300 000 dead', 'half a million killed'. Lost within these figures, the individual bereavement becomes insignificant, just one of many thousands, adding to the pain of the survivor.

CASE EXAMPLE: Giving significance to loss

In early 2005 I was working on the East Coast of Sri Lanka after the tsunami. On one occasion, when I was walking along a completely deserted, devastated street, a man came running up to me. I was holding my camera and assumed I might have offended him by taking pictures. 'No, no,' he said, 'please take a picture of *this house*.' I looked at the gutted empty building and did as he requested, then turned back. He was near to tears. 'My mother died here,' he said. So we sat on the ground and he talked for some time about his mother. I suddenly realised that for this man I was more than just a sympathetic ear, I was the outside world witnessing and memorialising his individual loss. Not just 10 000 dead, but his mother. I was making her significant.

Traumatic experiences, grief and mourning

Traumatic experiences can interfere with mourning. Avoidance that may be protective in helping the bereaved to cope with the memories of a traumatic event may make it difficult for them to mourn their loss because the memories

of the lost person are always accompanied by painful memories of the circumstances of the loss, so 'remembering' is too painful. In such circumstances, the traumatic symptoms may need treatment before the bereaved person is able to mourn. Table 1.23.3 lists the differences in emotional, cognitive and behavioural reactions that may occur.

Cultural bereavement

The Australian anthropologist and child psychiatrist Maurice Eisenbruch has pulled some of these experiences together in the term 'cultural bereavement' to describe the massive losses experienced by refugees and all those displaced by war:

> 'Cultural bereavement is the experience of the uprooted person – or group – resulting from loss of social structures, cultural values and self-identity: the person – or group – continues to live in the past, is visited by supernatural forces from the past while asleep or awake, suffers feelings of guilt over abandoning culture or homeland, feels pain if memories of the past begin to fade, but finds constant images of the past (including traumatic images) intruding into daily life, yearns to complete obligations to the dead and feels stricken by anxieties, morbid thoughts and anger that mar the ability to get on with daily life. It is not in itself a disease but an understandable response to catastrophic loss of social structure and culture.'[7]

In his work with Cambodian adolescents, Eisenbruch found that those refugee children who had been encouraged to assimilate rapidly into a new culture suffered more cultural bereavement than those who were encouraged to participate in traditional ceremonies and cultural practices. He believes that the concept allows for a more integrated and culturally sensitive approach to the experience of loss than attempting to classify any disabling symptoms only in terms of pathological categories according to western diagnostic criteria such as PTSD or traumatic bereavement. Disabling symptoms may be best addressed by a combination of restoring appropriate cultural practices and, if necessary, symptomatic relief.

Grief in childhood

The following are some frequently asked questions about children who have suffered a bereavement:

- Do children grieve?
- Are they too young to understand?
- Should we protect them from unpleasantness and distress?
- Will loss in childhood cause later mental illness?

Children's understanding of and reactions to death

Children's reactions to death are as variable as those of adults, and any or all of the reactions listed in Table 1.23.2 may occur. The most important point to note is that their understanding of death changes according to their development and life experiences. The following notes are based on western experience, and should be taken as a guide only. Working with victims of conflict and disaster in many low-resource settings has taught me that in many societies, particularly rural ones, children understand death at

TABLE 1.23.3 Distinguishing between the effects of traumatic events and loss[6]

Reactions to loss	Reactions to traumatic event
Separation anxiety	Anxiety about threat presented by traumatic event
Sadness more than anxiety	Anxiety more than sadness
Yearning and preoccupation with loss	Fearful, anxious and preoccupied with traumatic event
Sense of security intact	Personal sense of safety challenged
Primary relationships disrupted	Primary relationships intact
Intrusive memories are images and thoughts of the deceased	Intrusive memories of traumatic event plus re-experiencing accompanying emotions
Memories are positive and comforting	Uncontrollable intrusions are negative and distressing
Dream of the dead person is comforting	Nightmares of event are terrifying
Seeking out reminders of the loved one	Hypervigilant, scanning environment for threat
Avoidance of reminders of the absence of the loved one (denial)	Avoidance of reminders of threat
Anger at loss	Irritable, diffuse, unfocused anger and rage
Guilt about not doing enough	Guilt about surviving
Mourning as a tribute to the dead person	
Sleep EEG is normal	Increased REM sleep intensity
Coping involves reconstructing life without the loved one	Coping involves re-establishing a sense of safety
Recovery: Resolves attachment issues	*Recovery:* Habituates to fearful responses

an earlier age. In other respects the categorisation below holds true.

Children under 5 years

There is little understanding that death is final. For example, a 4-year-old child in England, having helped to formally bury his dead pet rabbit in the garden, asked if he could now dig it up so that he could have the rabbit back again. Magical thinking results in misconceptions about cause and effect. An egocentric view of the world can lead to feelings of responsibility (e.g. 'Mummy won't come back because I was naughty'). Reactions are similar to those following any separation – the longer the absence, the greater the distress. The death may be followed by detachment, so that the surviving family may think the child does not care about the loss. Regressive behaviour, soiling, bed wetting, clingy behaviour, sleeplessness and minor illnesses can all occur.

Children over 5 years

Children begin to understand that death is irreversible, that certain physical changes occur, and that there is permanent separation. They may still not regard it as something that can affect them. They may continue to have some magical, concrete and egocentric thinking. At this age, children more commonly use concepts of good and bad, they are curious about cause and effect, and are able to articulate concern for others.

There is a desire to stay connected to the dead parent. Many children dream about and talk with the dead parent frequently, feel that the dead parent is watching them, and keep physical objects associated with them. One study found that 43% of children in a large community sample thought about their dead parent on a daily basis 1 year after the death.[8] The reactions were variable. Boys were already learning to suppress their feelings, 91% of the children in the same study cried on the first day, and 50% had transient emotional and behavioural problems. Concentration and school work are also affected, and repetitive play is very common.

Children from 10 years to adolescence

There is a growing understanding of abstract concepts – for example, that death is universal and inevitable and can affect the child or adolescent personally. There is a growing concern with justice and injustice, and an awareness of inconsistencies. The conflict between the desire for autonomy and the need for closeness can be resolved by 'indifference and detachment', or by identification and nostalgia. In a group for adolescent refugee boys who had been 'ethnically cleansed' from Northern Bosnia (all of them had lost their homes, and some had also lost their family), all of the boys spoke passionately and with great longing about their home towns, describing them as the 'most beautiful place to live'.[9] Revenge fantasies are not unusual. There are fewer somatic and behavioural problems, and a depressed mood is common. Poor concentration and lack of interest occur at school. The oldest child in the family who has lost a same-sex parent is at greatest risk.

CASE EXAMPLE: The surviving brother

G is a 13-year-old boy. During a long and brutal war his older brother was killed on the front line. G had always been very close to his brother. Three years later he continued to think about him on a daily basis. He visited the grave frequently and watched the video of the funeral once a week. He did not like to sleep alone, and he felt sad much of the time, although he was doing well at school. He talked about his brother a great deal. He wanted to be as much like his brother as possible, whom he believed was one of the bravest and most incorruptible people. He was angry about the peace agreement. He felt that it was unjust and made a mockery of the aims for which his brother fought.

As in adults, the reactions of children to bereavement are enormously variable. Age, personality, culture and family values, and especially the way the parents or surviving caregivers react, will all affect the expression of grief.

Children within one family exposed to the same losses may all handle grief in different ways (*see* 'Case example: When to tell the story', p. 118). And the experience of grief may wax and wane. When discussing grief feelings with children, I sometimes use the image of a wave. (This is obviously inappropriate with children who have either never seen the sea or who have experienced the Tsunami.) I ask them to imagine that they are standing at the edge of the sea and that a big wave comes along and knocks them over. They feel terrible, but manage to struggle to their feet. Then there is a period of calm water before the next wave. This time they are more prepared, so that when the next wave comes it does not knock them over. What will happen over time is that, although the waves never go away completely, the periods of calm sea will grow longer, the waves will get smaller and the child will grow stronger (*see* Figure 1.23.2).

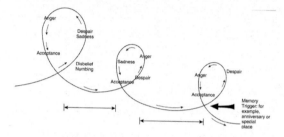

FIGURE 1.23.2 Waves of grief. The time intervals between waves get longer, and the waves get smaller.

Long-term effects

Many people worry that if children experience the loss of someone significant early in life this will have long-term effects on their mental health. Research evidence suggests that children who suffer an early bereavement do have a higher incidence of psychiatric disorder in later childhood, and that adults who lost a parent in childhood are more vulnerable to psychiatric disorder than the general population, and are particularly vulnerable to depression and anxiety precipitated by further losses.

Research has shown that the following life events are most likely to be associated with later mental illness:

- those that require people to undertake a major revision of assumptions about the world
- those that are lasting in their implications
- those that take place over a short period of time without preparation.

A traumatic death can have all of these features. However, there are significant factors that can modify the impact of a bereavement. The child's long-term mental health also depends on the following:

- the response of the surviving parent or relatives
- the availability of other support
- subsequent life circumstances
- the degree of continuity in the child's life
- how the loss is viewed by others
- what resources are available.

This list provides an immediate guide to what needs to be done to enhance a child's resilience and coping in the face of loss. The 'Case example: Different girls' from Pakistan illustrates how important these aspects are and what a great difference the behaviour of the surviving relatives can make.

CASE EXAMPLE: Different girls

After the Pakistan Earthquake in December 2005, I worked with children who had lost their parents. Contrast the experiences of two young teenage girls from the same rural Islamic society, affected by the same terrible event, but living in somewhat different settings with quite different responses from those caring for them. Shamsa was 14 and living with her aunt and uncle and her six younger brothers and sisters in one tent in a displaced persons camp near the town of Balakot. Her village had been completely destroyed and her mother and father had been killed. Shamsa acted as mother to her siblings and helped her aunt to care for her cousins. The aunt and uncle had told the children 'Your mother is in the village and will come soon.' Shamsa and her smaller sisters looked ill-kempt and neglected. They cried constantly, which suggested that the comforting lie was not working. They knew that their house had been turned to rubble, so where was their mother now? When I asked Shamsa what she thought, she told me in a whisper that her mother was dead. The aunt and uncle gave me permission to explain to all the children what had actually happened. Their calm reaction suggested that I was confirming something they already knew. Shamsa also told me she would like to get out of the tent. As she was the oldest girl, she carried the burden of household tasks and childcare, and her aunt was very reluctant to let her go to the camp school or any of the other activities arranged for children. However, she let the younger ones go and the improvement in their mood was very apparent. Shamsa continued to weep and grieve. Finally, when the aunt herself became involved in a livelihood programme with other camp women, she gave Shamsa permission to go to school. This had the immediate effect of alleviating some of Shamsa's sadness. In contrast, 12-year-old Sadia still lived in her village higher up in the mountains above the town. She too had lost her mother when their house was destroyed. She moved in with her grandmother but stayed in her village. When I met her she was laughing and playing with the other village children. She had just had her hands hennaed in beautiful flower patterns. She had been told that her mother was dead and said she still felt very sad. But she liked living with her grandmother and she did not cry all the time. When playing with the other village children she was able to be happy, and she had many relatives and friends who cared about her.

NOTE: names changed for reasons of confidentiality

How do we assist grieving families?

TABLE 1.23.4 Key actions to support grieving families

• Attend to their basic needs
• Access resources
• Assist mourning in a culturally appropriate manner
• Answer questions and provide information
• Accompany them
• Be available
• Focus attention on their individual loss: give it significance
• Altruism opportunities
• Avoidance as required
• Advice as needed

Not all grieving families require a health worker's intervention. But in situations of conflict, disaster and displacement the natural sources of social support are absent for the reasons listed above. In this case, the healthcare worker is the supportive community if unaffected him- or herself. Some key activities are listed in Table 1.23.4. Your role may be to accompany and support the bereaved as any neighbour might do in normal times. Obviously if a family lacks basic resources or is not safe, helping to address these basic needs is a priority. Help may be needed to trace missing bodies or identify them. Outsiders may have a significant role to play simply by encouraging and taking part in the normal processes of mourning. This may involve assisting an individual to organise a funeral, or it may involve helping a community. Vignette 3 provides an illustration of how one non-governmental organisation (NGO) assisted mourning in a disaster-affected community. If any individual has such severe symptoms of distress that they cannot function or carry out necessary tasks, providing symptomatic relief will help.

Regarding discussion of the loss, you should follow the lead of the bereaved. This usually means being available and able to listen without forcing them to talk. There is no evidence that 'grief work' (i.e. the experiencing, confronting and working through of negative emotions) is helpful, and there is some evidence that it may have long-term negative consequences. Contrary to some popular western stereotypes, positive emotions in the early period after loss are indicative of good outcomes, not pathology. Individuals who choose the more avoidant orientation (see Figure 1.23.1) are not in harmful denial, and this does not have to be challenged.[10]

On the other hand, it is not necessary to 'break down' continuing attachment to the deceased. Good memories assist mourning and give pleasure and comfort. This connection may be maintained throughout a bereaved person's life without pathological effect. Depending on the culture, it may involve regular visits to the grave, talking actively or praying to the dead, frequent dreams or visions. Indeed, ritualised celebrations of connection with the dead in some societies actually strengthen living family bonds as they bring families together.[11,12] A continuing connection should only cause concern if continuing yearning, searching and longing cause misery and dysfunction, dominate life in the long term and prevent the bereaved from forming any new attachments.

If the loss has occurred as a result of some form of political injustice or abuse, unresolved issues of reparation and justice may prolong grief and make mourning difficult. Helping the victims to access justice may be another part of your role (see 'Case example: When to tell the story' on p. 118).

How do we help grieving children?

Many families present to healthcare workers because they have concerns about the long-term impact of events on the child, and want advice on how to talk about such abnormal events with their children. The healthcare worker's role should be to facilitate the process of normal grieving, and to help to sustain and support the protective aspects mentioned in this section. While treating pathology where it is evident, you should take care to avoid pathologising where it is not.

A particularly important role may be to facilitate clear communication between family members. As some of the case studies and vignettes in this section illustrate, many families are concerned that telling the child what happened will cause unnecessary distress, and that as the child is 'too young to understand', it is better to lie or avoid the subject when it comes up. Children are very protective of surviving parents, and are quick to sense when a question is causing distress. They may avoid asking for information because the questions make their parent cry. False information leads to confusion and a lack of trust. The following case example illustrates this.

CASE EXAMPLE: Telling the truth

The father of this family was a member of a 'Liberation Army', and was killed in the fighting. His 32-year-old wife had two surviving children aged 8 and 9 years, and continued to live with her husband's relatives. She told the children that their father was working in another country. The children would frequently ask her why he did not phone and if he would bring them presents. They were confused because other children in the village told them their father was dead. When they questioned their mother she would start to cry, so they became nervous about asking her. The mother and her brother-in-law asked for advice about what to do, and accepted my suggestion that they should sit with the children and explain in simple terms what had happened, answering all the children's questions as they came up, and sharing the experience of grief. The mother told me that the relief of not having to lie to the children had slightly eased her own distress and made it easier to respond to them. Moreover, rather than being bewildered by their father's silent absence, the children now talked about him in the village with pride.

The following is a list of pointers specifically for supporting grieving children:

1 **Provide consistent, enduring, appropriate care.**
   - Reunite children with their families or extended families as soon as possible.
   - In the absence of family, create enduring family-type networks with a low ratio of caretaker to children.
   - Consistent caregiving by one or two caregivers, not a number of different volunteers (however well intentioned), is essential to prevent attachment problems, particularly in younger children.

2 **The more continuity that there is with the child's previous life the better.** Children may wish to avoid traumatic reminders, especially at the outset, but removing them completely from a familiar environment will cause more pain and problems in the long term.

3 **Support the carers by attending to their basic needs and their own mental states.** Help them to access the appropriate agencies to solve the practical problems that they will encounter. Attention to basic needs is essential. Engaging in the process of rebuilding their lives helps families to come to terms with their losses (see Appendix, Vignette 1).

4 **Facilitate normal grieving and mourning** with memorials for absent bodies, and appropriate religious ceremonies.

5 **Don't hide the truth.**
- Children need clear, honest, consistent explanations appropriate to their level of development.
- They need to accept the reality of the loss, not be protected from it.
- Magical thinking should be explored and corrected. What is imagined may be worse than reality, and children may be blaming themselves for events beyond their control.

6 **Grief work and debriefing may not be therapeutic or appropriate.** The insistence on getting a child to 'debrief' or tell the story of their loss may not be therapeutic or appropriate. Not all cultures put as high a value on the ventilation of individual feelings as western culture does. The therapist's goal should be to encourage a supportive atmosphere for the children, where open communication is possible, difficult questions are answered, and distressing feelings are tolerated. This means that the child will be free to express their grief in the manner that they find appropriate to the person they most trust, and at a time of their own choosing.

7 **Provide symptomatic relief.** Help the family to cope with traumatic symptoms such as bedwetting, nightmares and regressive behaviour, if they occur. Give the parents information about what to expect and straightforward management advice.

8 **Restart normal educational and play activities as soon as possible.**

9 **Help the child to maintain connection with the lost parent.** Encourage the surviving parent to allow the child to choose a memento to keep, to give them access to photographs, or to let the child draw a picture, make objects, or create a memory box. Answer the child's questions about the dead parent.

10 **The question of justice** will be important for families in situations of political violence. Many will state that they cannot come to terms with their losses while the fate of loved ones is unknown, bodies remain unidentified, or perpetrators are still at large. These issues will affect the children, and older children may bring them up spontaneously and wish to discuss them. Healthcare workers may be asked for their own views. Stating a willingness to learn and understand, along with an acknowledgement of one's own biases and subjectivity, is the most helpful position. Political and cultural literacy are essential. The family should be put in touch with the appropriate human rights or justice agencies if they wish to give formal evidence, so that the therapeutic and confidential nature of your own work remains clear and the family are not confused about the purpose of the interview. Giving testimony to such agencies should always be at their own request. In this case it may prove therapeutic (*see* 'Case example: When to tell the story', below).

CASE EXAMPLE: When to tell the story

The family consisted of three surviving children (two girls and a boy) who had witnessed the death of their mother and aunt and 15 other members of their extended family. They had been physically injured in the attack and spent some time in hospital. At our first meeting, 4 months after the event, two of the children did not believe their mother was dead. They hoped she had survived as they had. We

---

sat together with the children's father, who told them gently that he thought that in all probability she was dead. The children cried and we did not discuss it further that day. The following week the bodies had been identified, funeral notices posted and the funeral arranged. The family had returned to the house where the massacre had occurred and appeared to be functioning well. The boy had no symptoms, although the younger girl was sad and quiet. When asked if they wanted to talk about what happened, she said no. Her brother said that he had already talked with journalists and did not feel a need to go over it again. The older girl (aged 14 years) had some intrusive thoughts and memories, and poor sleep and appetite. She wanted to walk me around the site and retell the events in detail.

The other children did not wish to join in. During the walk the older girl told me that she now knew her mother was dead. All the children then wanted to show me all their old photographs, and they participated in identifying their dead relatives and telling me stories about their life before the war. After the funeral (which only the older girl attended, at her own request) the children appeared more cheerful, and all of them were looking forward to school. The surviving family provided an extremely loving and supportive network, and although the father was extremely sad, he allowed the children to talk about their mother whenever they wanted. Later the whole family was sent to another country for medical treatment for the children. They attended local schools where they learned English, and appeared to be adjusting well.

One year after the events the International Criminal Tribunal wished to interview the family about the massacre, and the three children insisted that they would like to give their accounts. All the children made statements that were recorded on video, and gave similar detailed stories about the events surrounding the massacre. Although they found it distressing, they each obviously regarded it as significant and important, and were pleased to have had the chance to contribute in this way. This example demonstrates that children in the same family will not all deal with their grief in the same way. If given the opportunity they will find the most appropriate time to tell their own stories in the way that will give their loss significance and meaning for themselves.

Appendix

The following three examples are drawn from fieldwork in various conflict and disaster situations. They illustrate the variability of responses and provide examples of practical ways to support grieving families and communities.

Vignette 1: Complex needs and conflict in a grieving family

A is an 18-year-old high-school student, living in a rural area in the heart of a conflict region, the second oldest of seven children (four girls and three boys). She wanted to study medicine. Her life and health were normal until the shelling began and her family fled to the forest, where they spent 3 months. The local police, who were of a different ethnic origin, found them and separated the men from the women and elderly men and sent the latter home. They got home to find their village full of soldiers and police and themselves under siege at their home, where they were harassed and sometimes beaten. Meanwhile their invalid pensioner father was shot in a massacre of 10 men from the village. He was buried while they were under siege. A was referred to me 1 month after this by a local doctor who was concerned about her mental state. When I first saw her she was extremely sad and frightened. She was crying all the time, and ruminating about her father being captured. She found everywhere frightening, and was too afraid to go to sleep. When she did fall asleep, she woke early. She had no appetite, and a diurnal mood swing.

I first assessed her at the doctor's home, where we had a long talk, at her instigation, about everything that had happened to her. I felt that the severity of her depressive symptoms might necessitate use of an antidepressant, but delayed making a decision until I was able to assess her at home with her family. I visited them a week later and found all seven members of the family living in one restored room of their fire-damaged home. To my surprise, A was a great deal better, her sleep and appetite having returned to normal over the course of the week. She informed me that she felt this was because she felt she had someone to talk to, and who 'wanted to come and visit'. However, all the female members of the family were preoccupied with the father's death, tearful when discussing it, and had conflicting views about how to manage the grief. The mother and one sister no longer wanted to wear the symbolic mourning clothes, but to move on. The other three sisters were wearing black mourning bands in their hair and wanted to do so for the appropriate period of 1 year. One of these sisters complained of having some panic attacks. They also all felt angry and concerned about their material circumstances. They had no access to their father's pension, as this would have meant going to a police station run by the ethnic group in power to get new identity papers (all of theirs had been burnt), and identifying themselves as from a conflict area and as being members of a family with a massacre victim. Anxiety made sleep difficult.

Interestingly, the boys in the family (aged 7, 8 and 14 years) appeared cheerful, busy and well, insisting that they were symptom free, although they missed their father. All the boys attended school regularly. The girls did not go, as there was no money for books. They therefore sat around at home with little to do.

We agreed to have family meetings to help them to resolve their conflicting views about how to grieve, and relaxation therapy to provide some symptomatic relief. We did this as a group and they practised themselves on a daily basis, with the mother running the group. Over the next weeks there was a marked improvement in the whole family. The three girls continued to wear their mourning bands, and the mother was more tolerant of this. A began to press me to help her to get an ID card so that she could go to a nearby town, get a job and earn some money. However, the security situation deteriorated too much for this to be possible. My last visit before evacuation was distressing, as there was fighting on the nearest main road and the sound of shelling of nearby villages. We all knew that they might have to flee again in the near future.

I returned to see the family 3 months later. They had spent these months internally displaced, being pushed from one village to another, and with very little to eat. During this time, the 14-year-old son, who had separated himself from the family because he believed that he endangered them, had been killed along with another male relative. The family had returned to their home to find it completely burnt to the ground except for an outhouse. They had nothing left and were using an ammunition box as a table, and sleeping under a small piece of plastic in the garden, because the outhouse attracted snakes. As before, the healthiest members of the family appeared to be the smallest boys, who denied any symptoms except some tearfulness now and then. They appeared active and cheerful except when witnessing their mother's distress. The mother was devastated, and could not stop crying. She could not sleep, eat or function, and expressed suicidal ideas. A had moved away to live with an aunt in a nearby town, and had a number of somatic symptoms. We provided clothes for the family and basic material equipment for the house. The mother was started on antidepressant therapy.

The family then lost contact with our service for 6 months. They had been provided with materials to build a warm room, but the aid agency had failed to realise that with no adult males left in the family there was no one to build it. The family therefore moved into a grim damp refugee flat in town. The mother had found the antidepressants helpful but had run out of medication. Two daughters had escaped the situation by marriage. The boys were well and attending school. The other daughters remain trapped within the prison of their mother's unremitting grief. They spent all day in the flat with their mother talking and crying. She did not wish to be left alone. They wanted to show her how much they cared for her and insisted on doing every household task, which added to her feeling of being a useless burden. We began 'family work' again, encouraging the girls to join the free local youth club and to allow the mother to re-establish her maternal role in the family, supporting her by restarting the antidepressant medication at her request, and getting in touch with the aid agency about the family's house.

Some reflections on this case: For most families of this particular ethnic group, the immediate and respectful burial of the dead is crucial. This is followed by 7 days of visiting by friends and family, who sit all day with the bereaved and discuss the dead. These normal mourning processes had not been possible either for the father or for the son. It seems likely that the surprisingly sudden symptomatic relief that A gained from my initial intervention was a result of my contributing to some of this normal mourning by being an outsider who visited and listened. A family approach meant that differences could be brought out in the open in a respectful way. The family also formed a natural group so could encourage and support each other in doing relaxation work. Attending to human rights concerns such as identity papers and security was also important. However, all this was undone by the second round of conflict and loss. There is something particularly devastating about loss coming again immediately a family has begun to work its way towards recovery. Being made homeless and not being given support to rebuild their house have contributed to their sense of bereavement and powerlessness, and prolonged the period of grief. The mother told me repeatedly that if she could start rebuilding her house she would feel better.

Some families are strongly patriarchal. There are different coping strategies available to boys and girls. All the women in this family came across as strong and capable, but all of them felt that the loss, first of an invalid father and then of the oldest son, had completely destroyed the family's capacity to function. Much of the work with grieving female survivors has to address their insecurity and lack of confidence in their own self-worth. This family required a complex approach, including participation in normal mourning, attention to basic needs, help with family communication, symptomatic relief, help with re-establishing normal family roles, and adapting to new roles in the absence of male support.

Vignette 2: Supporting the whole family

Family B had lost more than 20 members, mostly female and children, in a massacre. I was asked to visit because of concerns about the mental health of the surviving children who had witnessed the attack and were all under 6 years of age. At the first session, most of the remaining extended family, including the children, had gathered to meet me in the only intact room in the house. I already knew the outline of what had happened, and used this first meeting to draw a genogram. I have found that in situations of mass violence, in a culture where the extended family is of central importance, this simple technique has a number of useful functions.

- It is a collective act, with everyone joining in, introducing themselves and explaining their connection to others.
- It is interesting for the children, who join in the actual drawing on a large sheet of paper in the centre of the room.
- By asking the family to include those who have died, it allows for a collective naming of the dead. In this family my symbolically putting a simple black line through these names took on a ritual significance, and the children were quick to point out when I missed someone out.
- The naming allows the person who has died to be identified, but how much is said about that person or what happened is up to the family. Thus it provides the opportunity for storytelling without forcing the issue.
- What is said about the dead is said in front of the whole family, so there is a collective narrative from which the children are not excluded.

Once the genogram had been drawn, the family told me their concerns about the children and their own fears about letting the children talk, as it seemed to upset them. At this meeting, I gave the simple advice about communication outlined above, and arranged to meet the family regularly and to have play therapy with the children. At the next meeting, the family informed me that they were concerned about the oldest teenage girl, who fainted regularly at the same time every afternoon, and was the most nervous and sensitive member of the family. Her sister was one of the dead, and her mother was particularly concerned about her health, but never cried herself. They wanted reassurance that the girl was not seriously ill. Having provided this, I wondered aloud if the teenage daughter was in some way grieving for the whole family and that this exhausting work might be causing her to faint. It also meant that the mother did not have time to think about her own sadness. The daughter said that she wished her mother would cry a little and not worry about her so much, in which case she could look after her.

By the next meeting, the daughter was no longer fainting and the mother was now actively grieving. I continued with family meetings and play therapy over the next 6 months. During this time the oldest child (5 years of age) of another section of the family, in which the mother had died, began to tell his father fragments of what he had seen and to ask

questions about his mother. The father had taken out photographs of his wife to show to all the children. At no point did the children tell the story to me, nor did I insist upon it, seeing my role as facilitating and supporting communication within the family. Over the following year the children became much less tearful and withdrawn, and increasingly outgoing, cheerful, communicative and energetic. They all attended the formal reburial of their family. Their father remarried and their new stepmother was well accepted. The father began on the process of rebuilding his house. They remained well at our last contact, and the oldest child had begun school without problems.

Vignette 3: Assisting communal mourning

The South-East Asian tsunami that occurred on 26 December 2004 destroyed an area along the coast of Northern Sumatra 300 miles long and 6 miles wide. At least 130 000 people were killed in that country alone, and 400 000 were left homeless. In some villages more than 70% of the community were killed. One issue was the problem created by large mass graves. For example, outside the provincial capital Banda Aceh, approximately 20 000 people were buried in a small piece of land next to the main road, with no identification and no acknowledgement of their lives. Nothing grew there. Driving from the airport, one might witness a lone figure standing or sitting on the ground in quiet meditation or prayer. Our non-governmental organisation (NGO) psychosocial team talked with local community leaders in an effort to understand how to assist the Acehnese people in their mourning at this site, and took up their suggestion to collaborate in building a Quiet House. The house was built by local people in less than 10 days with NGO supervision. It overlooked the grave site and provided shelter, privacy and beauty for the relatives of the dead, without the traffic of the main road intruding. The house was designed to emphasise traditional culture, and was landscaped with flowering plants and trees. To provide comfort for the bereaved, the Imam wrote a well-known Muslim prayer: 'From him (Allah) we come and to him (Allah) we return.'

One of the local workers became tearful, explaining 'I think my family are buried here but I don't know. This is why I don't come here … but now I can come and talk to them. It is very important for the people of Aceh to have a place where they can come and feel a sense of loss and family again.' The project led to requests for further Quiet Houses at other sites.[13]

Note: Dr Jones is a members of the WHO ICD-11 Working Group on the Classification of Disorders Specifically Associated with Stress, reporting to the WHO International Advisory Group for the Revision of ICD-10 Mental and Behavioural Disorders. The views expressed in this article are those of the author and, except as specifically noted, do not represent the official policies or positions of the International Advisory Group or the World Health Organization.

References

1 Macksoud M (1993) *Helping Children Cope with the Stresses of War: a manual for parents and teachers*. New York: UNICEF.
2 Kubler-Ross E (1969) *On Death and Dying*. London: Routledge.

3 Adapted from Stroebe M, Schut H and Stroebe W (2007) Health outcomes of bereavement. *Lancet*, **370**, 11960–73.

4 Stroebe M, Schut H and Stroebe W (2007) Health outcomes of bereavement. *Lancet*, **370**, 11960–73.

5 Maercker A, Brewin CR, Bryant RA *et al.* (2013) Proposals for mental disorders specifically associated with stress in the International Classification of Diseases-11. *Lancet*, **381**, 1683–5.

6 Adapted from Hendricks JH, Black D and Kaplan T (2000) *When Father Killed Mother: guiding children through trauma and grief.* London: Routledge.

7 Eisenbruch M (1991) From post-traumatic stress disorder to cultural bereavement: diagnosis of South East Asian refugees. *Social Science and Medicine*, **33**, 673–80.

8 Worden JW and Silverman PR (1993) Children's reactions to the death of a parent. In: Stroebe MS, Stroebe W and Hanson RO (eds) *Handbook of Bereavement.* Cambridge, UK: Cambridge University Press.

9 Jones L (1998) Adolescent groups for encamped Bosnian refugees: some problems and solutions. *Clinical Child Psychology and Psychiatry*, **3**, 541–51.

10 Currier JM, Neimeyer RA and Berman JS (2008) The effectiveness of psychotherapeutic interventions for bereaved persons: a comprehensive quantitative review. *Psychological Bulletin*, **134**, 648–61.

11 Bonanno GA, Papa A and O'Neill K (2002) Loss and human resilience. *Applied and Preventive Psychology*, **10**, 193–206.

12 Bonnano GA, Brewin CR, Krzysztof K *et al.* (2010) Weighing the cost of disaster: consequences, risks and resilience in individuals, families and communities. *Psychological Science in the Public Interest*, **11**, 1–49.

13 Jones L, Ghani H, Mohanraj A *et al.* (2007) Crisis into opportunity: setting up community mental health services in post-tsunami Aceh. *Asia-Pacific Journal of Public Health*, **19**, 60–68.

1.24 Obstetric and paediatric anaesthesia in low resource settings

The Safe Anaesthesia Working Group of the World Health Organization's 'Safe Surgery Saves Lives' global initiative updated the 1992 International Standards for the Safe Practice of Anaesthesia in 2010. The aim of these Standards is to contribute to decreased patient morbidity and mortality worldwide, particularly in lesser resourced countries where regions have not adopted their own standards.

The fundamental principle of these Standards is the continuous presence of an appropriately trained, vigilant anaesthesia professional. The Standards also highly recommend pulse oximetry during anaesthesia, which means it is mandatory, although compromise may be unavoidable in emergencies.

Compliance with these International Standards should be advocated by health care workers in all facilities where anaesthetics are given.

Obstetric anaesthesia

The limiting factor is often the availability of doctors and nurses trained in anaesthesia; women, babies and children die because of the lack of trained staff.

Remember that there are two patients – the mother and the baby. The condition of the mother affects the condition of the baby. Therefore maintaining adequate oxygenation and resuscitation of the mother is the best initial way of treating and preventing fetal distress.

All pregnant mothers after 20 weeks' gestation who are lying down must be put in the left lateral tilt position to avoid aorto-caval compression and supine hypotension.

Conduct of anaesthesia

Considerations in the obstetric patient in addition to routine anasthesia include those listed below.

1 Physiological

Hypoxaemia

Pregnant women are at risk of hypoxia. They use oxygen faster than non-pregnant women, and because of the pregnancy it is more difficult for them to breathe deeply.

Hypovolaemia

Signs of hypovolaemia e.g. due to bleeding occur later than in the non-pregnant, because blood volume increases during pregnancy. This means that blood pressure, a late sign of blood loss, may be maintained in the hypovolaemic patient until induction of anaesthesia, when there may be catastrophic hypotension. Estimation of blood loss is difficult and it may be concealed e.g. placental abruption with retroplacental bleeding. Placental perfusion is compromised before blood pressure, so fetal distress may be a warning of possible maternal circulatory compromise.

Acid regurgitation

Hormonal effects cause relaxation of the lower oesophageal sphincter, and pressure effects from the gravid uterus contribute to an increased risk of regurgitation and aspiration if laryngeal reflexes are impaired (e.g. during anaesthesia or eclamptic fits). An H_2 receptor antagonist and sodium citrate or other appropriate non-particulate antacid should be given to all pregnant women beyond the first trimester before general anaesthesia, which should involve a rapid sequence induction with cricoid pressure.

2 Pregnancy-related disease

- Pre-eclampsia/eclampsia
  - blood pressure control
    » Blood pressure should be controlled prior to anaesthesia if possible. Spinal anaesthesia is recommended for Caesarean section if there are no contraindications (signs of coagulopathy or raised intracranial pressure). If general anaesthesia

is needed, attempts should be made to obtund the hypertensive response to intubation (see general anaesthesia for Caesarean section).
— Treatment with magnesium
» Magnesium potentiates the effect of non-depolarising muscle relaxants, so smaller doses of muscle relaxant are needed if general anaesthesia is necessary.
— HELLP (Haemolysis, elevated liver enzymes, low platelets)
» If platelet count is less than $100\,000 \times 10^9$/L, a coagulation profile is indicated prior to spinal anaesthesia. If platelet count is less than $75\,000 \times 10^9$/L, there is a risk of a spinal haematoma and so spinal anaesthesia is contraindicated. This has to be considered against the risks to the patient of alternative anaesthesia (general or local infiltration).
— Oedema of tissues
» This includes facial and airway oedema. The larynx and vocal cords may be involved and a smaller than usual diameter endotracheal tube may be required e.g. 6.5 mm, 6.0 mm.

- Risk of increased intra-operative blood loss e.g. if there has been antepartum haemorrhage, placenta praevia, long labour, maternal dehydration and ketosis or blood clotting abnormality (due to pre-eclampsia and HELLP syndrome, or anticoagulant medication). Ensure IV access with 2 wide bore patent cannulae prior to induction of anaesthesia.
- Sepsis (due to ascending genital tract infection or intrauterine infection). Early recognition of sepsis may be difficult, so it is important to suspect it from the patient's history (e.g. prolonged rupture of membranes).

3 Underlying medical conditions

- Examples include known cardiac abnormalities, previous cardiac surgery, and diabetes, all of which may be affected by pregnancy.
- Symptoms of chest pain or dyspnoea may indicate an undiagnosed heart valve abnormality, which may be either congenital or acquired (e.g. from rheumatic fever). unmasked by the circulatory changes in pregnancy and labour.

4 Drugs

Ketamine: This causes an increase in blood pressure, so should not be given to women with hypertension, but it can be used for induction of anaesthesia for women needing general anaesthesia for Caesarean section. It may increase uterine tone, which may cause fetal distress, or difficulty delivering the baby at Caesarean section.

Opioids: These drugs cross the placenta, so ideally should not be given until the cord is clamped, otherwise the baby may be slow to establish regular breathing.

5 Equipment

It is vital to ensure that all resuscitation equipment is available and working, in order to prevent avoidable delays if there is an emergency. Check the bag-valve-mask, airway equipment, oxygen, IV fluids, suction, saturation monitor and blood pressure machine before every operation. Ensure that difficult airway equipment (e.g. stylets, bougies) is readily available.

Choice of anaesthesia for Caesarean section

The choice of anaesthesia for major surgical procedures such as Caesarean section depends on the clinical condition of the patient, the anaesthetist's experience, and the equipment and drugs available. It should be decided after a balance of risks and benefits has been considered.
1 Most Caesarean sections are performed with spinal anaesthesia unless there are contraindications (see below).
2 General anaesthesia is used when spinal anaesthesia is contraindicated. Intubation as part of a rapid sequence induction is needed to minimise the increased risk of regurgitation and aspiration in a pregnant woman.
3 Local anaesthetic infiltration can be used in situations where there is no trained anaesthetist, or if the patient is moribund.

Spinal (sub-arachnoid) anaesthesia for Caesarean section

A spinal injection gives a dense block of rapid onset (within 5–15 minutes) that lasts for about 2 hours, and can be ideal for Caesarean section. The mother remains conscious. Spinal anaesthesia can also be used perinatally for
- evacuation of residual products of conception
- manual removal of placenta
- repair of third- and fourth-degree tears.

Spinal anaesthesia causes vasodilatation with consequent hypotension. This can be prevented with fluid loading before spinal insertion, and treated with IV fluid boluses and a vasoconstrictor (e.g. ephedrine).

Uses of spinal anaesthesia

It can be used for:
- Caesarean section
- laparotomy (not optimal)
- evacuation of residual products of conception
- manual removal of placenta
- repair of third- and fourth-degree tears.

Precautions

- Correct hypovolaemia first.
- Be aware of the presence of a coagulation disorder (e.g. with severe pre-eclampsia, eclampsia or placental abruption), which can lead to a dangerous bleed around the spinal cord. Spinal anaesthesia should not be used in these circumstances.

Contraindications

These include the following:
- maternal refusal
- inadequate resuscitation facilities
- uncorrected hypovolaemia
- coagulopathy (e.g. if there is spontaneous bruising)
- fixed cardiac output (e.g. aortic valve stenosis)
- allergy to local anaesthetics
- local infection around the spinal area.

Giving a spinal anaesthetic
Preparation

- Explain to the patient the type of anaesthesia.
- Do not give a pre-operative sedative, as it may reduce the baby's respiration and conscious level at birth.

- Give an antacid (e.g. sodium citrate 30 mL) immediately prior to anaesthesia.

Procedure

- Ensure that there is a **large-bore IV cannula (14 or 16G) and IV infusion running**.
- Infuse 500–1000 mL of IV fluids (Ringer-lactate or Hartmann's solution) to preload the mother and avoid hypotension. Also ensure that atropine 0.6 mg and ephedrine 30 or 50 mg diluted to 10 mL with Ringer-lactate or Hartmann's solution are immediately available.
- Check the patient's blood pressure.
- Sterility is critical. Use antiseptic skin solution to clean the patient's back over a wide area. Use sterile gloves and ideally a sterile apron. Do not touch the point or shaft of the spinal needle with your hand. Hold the needle only by its hub.
- Prepare the spinal anaesthetic (heavy bupivacaine 0.5%, 2–2.5 mL).
- Inject 1% lidocaine solution using a fine 25G needle to anaesthetise the skin over the site (L3/4 or L4/5). Do not use a space above L2/3 because the spinal cord ends at around L1/2.
- Introduce the finest spinal needle available (24G) (ideally using an introducer needle if available) in the midline through the anaesthetised skin, at a right angle to the skin in the vertical plane. Fine spinal needles greatly reduce the risk of post-dural puncture headache.
- If the **needle hits bone** it may not be in the midline. Withdraw the needle and reinsert it, directing it slightly upwards while aiming in the direction of the umbilicus. It is important to have two correct planes (i.e. midline and also not too near to the spinous processes above or below).
- Advance the spinal needle towards the sub-arachnoid space. A loss of resistance may be felt as the needle pierces the ligamentum flavum.
- Once the needle has passed through the ligamentum flavum, push the needle slowly through the dura. You may feel another slight loss of resistance as the dura is pierced.
- Remove the stylet. Cerebrospinal fluid (CSF) should flow out of the needle.
- If CSF does not come out, reinsert the stylet and rotate the needle gently. Remove the stylet to see if fluid is flowing out. If you continue to fail, try another space.
- Once CSF flows out of the needle, inject 2–2.5 mL of the local anaesthetic solution described above.

Never proceed with the injection if the patient complains of pain on injection.

- All patients should have their head and shoulders raised on a pillow to prevent high spread of the anaesthetic. When using 'heavy' (i.e. heavier than CSF) bupivacaine, as is used in a spinal anaesthetic, the position of the patient affects where the local anaesthetic collects, and can be used to influence the height of the block. The position of the block can be brought higher by placing the table head down. Gravity can be made to influence the level of the block for up to 20 minutes after the injection.
- Lie the mother on her back. Have the operating table tilted at least 15 degrees to the left, or place a pillow or folded linen under the mother's right lower back to decrease the risk of supine hypotensive syndrome.
- Recheck the blood pressure every 5 minutes after the spinal needle is inserted until the end of the procedure. A fall in blood pressure is likely.
- If there is significant hypotension (i.e. systolic blood pressure < 100 mmHg or a fall in blood pressure of more than 20%), or if the mother has nausea or vomiting:
  - Give the IV infusion as fast as possible.
  - Give ephedrine in 3–6 mg increments or an alternative available vasopressor until there is a response.
  - Give high-flow oxygen via face mask.
- After the spinal injection wait 5 minutes and check for weakness of the legs, then pinch the skin with forceps. Start below the umbilicus and work up on both sides of the body until pain is felt. Wait 5 minutes, and then retest the level of the spinal block until there is no pain with pinch up to the level of the nipples. Anaesthesia should now be adequate for Caesarean section.
- After surgery the mother does not have to lie flat, but may not be able to move her legs for 2 to 4 hours. The first time she mobilises after a spinal anaesthetic she should be accompanied in case she has residual weakness.

Complications of spinal anaesthesia

1 Hypotension.
2 Sensory block: if the bladder is full it will be unnoticed by the patient.
3 Headache can occur following a spinal anaesthetic, but is uncommon if small gauge spinal needles are used. Headache occurs because of leakage of CSF, which causes traction on intracranial structures. A typical headache is frontal and/or occipital, and worse on sitting or standing, but better when lying down. It can be immediate or delayed. Management consists of analgesia as per the WHO pain ladder (see Section 1.15) and keeping the patient well hydrated.
4 If there is bradycardia, tingling or weakness in the hands, or difficulty breathing, the block is likely to be too high. Give the mother atropine 0.6 mg if she is bradycardic, increase the IV infusion rate and give ephedrine.
5 Rarely, intracranial spread can also occur. It produces loss of consciousness and apnoea, and is termed a total spinal block. Resuscitation is required.

Management of spinal blocks which are too high or total

Call for help.

Airway:

- Assess and maintain patency.
- Give oxygen 15 litres/minute via face mask, and measure SpO$_2$ using a pulse oximeter (which should already be attached).

Breathing

- Assess and give chest inflations with a bag-valve-mask if there is apnoea or inadequate breathing.
- Ideally protect the airway by intubation if the patient is unconscious (P or U on the AVPU scale).

Circulation

- High or total spinal blocks can cause cardiac arrest.
- Assess pulse and blood pressure.

- Give chest compressions if the patient is in cardiac arrest or has an inadequate central pulse (the blood pressure may be unrecordable).
- Tilt the patient to the left if this has not already been done.
- Treat hypotension with IV Ringer-lactate or Hartmann's solution and ephedrine.
- Treat bradycardia < 50 beats/minute in the mother with atropine 0.6 mg IV, repeated after 3 minutes as necessary.

Check the fetal heart after maternal resuscitation and consider the timing and method of delivery.

Consider and exclude other causes of unconsciousness (e.g. eclampsia, hypoglycaemia, epilepsy, opioid drugs, intracranial bleed).

Keep a chart of pulse, blood pressure, respiratory rate, SaO_2, fetal heart rate and treatments given.

For management of anaphylaxis, see Section 2.7.C.

General anaesthesia

If spinal anaesthesia is contraindicated, rapid sequence induction and intubation is the recommended anaesthetic if expertise and equipment are available. See in Paediatric anaesthesia section of this section for the '10 golden rules of anaesthesia', essential monitoring, essential drugs, essential equipment, and how to intubate steps 1–6.

General anaesthesia is indicated
1 If spinal fails or is refused by the patient
2 If there is a medical contraindication for spinal anaesthesia:
   - suspected coagulopathy,
   - raised intracranial pressure (impaired consciousness following eclamptic fits)
   - fixed cardiac output (e.g. aortic stenosis)
3 If there is no time for a spinal anaesthetic to be given.

Conduct of General Anaesthesia
1 Minimise aspiration risk by the following:
   - restrict oral intake, especially solids for women in labour
   - give H2 receptor antagonist e.g. ranitidine 150 mg orally if time, or 50 mg IV if emergency
   - give sodium citrate 30 mL orally just prior to induction of anaesthesia
   - assess patient, with particular attention to airway.
2 Check drugs available:
   - Induction agents
     — Thiopentone 3–5 mg/kg or
     — Ketamine 1.5–2 mg/kg – causes less hypotension than thiopentone, useful if patient hypovolaemic e.g. if antepartum haemorrhage. Contraindicated if pre-eclampsia or eclampsia or suspected raised intracranial pressure.
   - Muscle relaxant – Suxamethonium 1–2 mg/kg
   - Other drugs – to reduce hypertensive response to intubation, given if the patient has severe pre-eclampsia/eclampsia, magnesium 4 g (2 g if already receiving magnesium) or lidocaine 1.5 mg/kg, and/or rapid onset opioids if available. If opioids are used, the baby may need naloxone after initial resuscitation if not breathing adequately.
3 Check equipment – laryngoscopes, endotracheal tubes and ensure difficult airway equipment, including stylets,

bougies, laryngeal mask and cricothyroidotomy kit are available.
4 Lie patient on theatre table with left lateral tilt and ensure suction is on and under pillow. Connect monitoring.
5 Start an IV infusion of Hartmann's solution via a large gauge (14 or 16G) cannula.
6 Explain to the patient and anaesthetic assistant about cricoid pressure and pre-oxygenate the patient for 3 minutes.
7 Give predetermined dose of induction agent and suxamethonium and support jaw until relaxed, or until fasciculations subside.
8 Intubate patient and inflate cuff. Check position of endotracheal tube before allowing cricoid pressure to be released.
9 Maintain anaesthetic with a volatile agent or intermittent boluses of ketamine.
10 After the baby is delivered, oxytocin is given, as requested by the surgeon, usually 5 units as a bolus, followed by an infusion. Oxytocin may cause tachycardia and hypotension, so care must be given to patients with hypovolaemia or other patients for whom tachycardia would cause cardiovascular compromise e.g. stenotic cardiac valve disease. In these patients, the oxytocin bolus can be drawn up into 20 mL 0.9% saline and given slowly over 5–10 minutes. After delivery the mother can be given opioid analgesia for post-operative pain relief.

Failed intubation

This is more likely to occur at emergency Caesarean sections, when it is often unexpected and leads to rapid oxygen desaturation. An early decision should be made to abandon repeated attempts at intubation.

The priority is to OXYGENATE the patient.
1 Maintain cricoid pressure. This should not interfere with bag-valve-mask ventilation if correctly placed, and may need to be adjusted.
2 Inform surgeon and scrub nurse to help.
3 Ventilate the patient with 100% O2, initially with mask.
4 If mask ventilation not successful,
   a. insert oropharyngeal airway
   b. consider using 2 hands to maintain airway with assistant squeezing bag
   c. insert laryngeal mask.
5 If ventilation is still inadequate, a percutaneous cricothyrotomy should be performed.
6 If this is unsuccessful, either surgeon or anaesthetist should perform surgical cricothyrotomy or tracheostomy.

If ventilation and oxygenation is possible at any of the steps before cricothyroidotomy, and the Caesarean section is elective, the patient should be woken up and a spinal or local infiltration should be used.

If the Caesarean section is an emergency, you should consider whether to wake the patient up and give spinal anaesthesia, or proceed with the patient breathing spontaneously and give volatile anaesthesia or intermittent ketamine IV.

If spinal anaesthesia is not possible, intubation fails, or expertise and/or equipment is unavailable, and Caesarean section is urgently needed, the priority is to maintain oxygenation with bag-valve-mask and anaesthetise with either a volatile agent or ketamine depending on the experience of the practitioner.

Ketamine in early pregnancy

Ketamine causes a trance-like state where patients become mentally removed from their surroundings. It causes sleep, analgesia and short-term memory loss (amnesia). The patient is unconscious, pain-free and has no memory of the time under anaesthesia. The airway protective reflexes are usually present but cannot be guaranteed. Therefore it is important that the patient is **starved and anaesthetised on a tipping table with suction available**. It can only be used as a sole anaesthetic agent in the first trimester and if there is no increased risk of regurgitation. Patients should be fasted for 6 hours prior to ketamine anaesthesia.

Ketamine is contraindicated in patients with high blood pressure (including pregnancy-induced hypertension), eclampsia or heart disease.

Effects of ketamine:

Central nervous system: Ketamine causes sympathetic nervous system stimulation. The additional use of diazepam (after delivery if ketamine is used for a Caesarean section) will reduce the amount of sympathetic stimulation. Ketamine also raises intracranial pressure, which makes it unsuitable for patients with eclampsia.

The effects start 10–15 seconds after IV injection. Ketamine produces a 'dissociative state'. The eyes may remain open and may make quick side-to-side movements (nystagmus), and the patient may move during surgery if ketamine is the only drug used. The patient can be quite agitated, crying and distressed on waking up. This can be minimised by using diazepam with ketamine and avoiding stimulation while emerging from anaesthesia. This can also be helped by including diazepam (see below) as part of the premedication.

Cardiovascular system: Ketamine causes mild stimulation of the cardiovascular system. The blood pressure rises by about 25% and heart rate increases by about 20%. This increases the workload of the heart.

Respiratory system: If given too quickly, IV ketamine can cause the patient to stop breathing for up to a minute. If this happens, ventilate the patient until the effect wears off. The airway is usually maintained, but still needs to be monitored closely. The oxygen saturation may decrease, so give oxygen.

Ketamine causes bronchodilatation. Laryngeal spasm may occur, and may be partly caused by increased secretions resulting from ketamine use (see below for the importance of an atropine premedication in helping to prevent this). If it occurs, continuous positive airways pressure by mask with oxygen or manual ventilation with a bag and mask should relieve this potentially dangerous problem. If it doesn't relieve the obstruction and oxygen saturations are falling, or the patient is cyanosed, give a short acting muscle relaxant (suxamethonium 1 mg/kg IV) and continue bag valve mask ventilation until adequate breathing returns (usually about 5 minutes later).

Muscle: Ketamine increases muscle tone. This makes it an unsuitable drug for major abdominal surgery where abdominal relaxation is necessary. Some body movements can occur.

Uterus and placenta: Ketamine may increase the tone of the uterus. It readily crosses the placenta, so the fetus receives some of the drug.

Premedication before ketamine

- Atropine 10–20 micrograms/kg (up to a maximum of 600 micrograms) IM 30 minutes before or IV at the time of induction of anaesthetic.
- Diazepam 100 micrograms/kg (up to a maximum of 10 mg in pregnancy) can be given IV at the time of induction to prevent hallucinations. When performing a Caesarean section after ketamine induction, give diazepam only **after** the baby has been delivered as diazepam can cross through the placenta and prevent the newborn baby from breathing.
- Give oxygen at 6–8 litres/minute by mask or nasal cannulae.

Administration of ketamine in pregnancy

1 Should only be used without intubation in the first trimester.
2 Can be used as an induction agent as part of rapid sequence induction in 2nd and 3rd trimester if there are no contraindications, e.g. pre-eclampsia, eclampsia.

Start an IV infusion of crystalloid and ensure that a reliable IV cannula is in place.

Ketamine may be given by IV injection or by IV infusion. At doses of **250–500 micrograms/kg IV** ketamine is a good **analgesic**. At doses of **1–2 mg/kg IV** ketamine is an **anaesthetic**.

Giving IV diazepam 100 microgram/kg will reduce nightmares and hallucinations, but respiratory depression is more likely than with ketamine alone.

Ketamine injection

- Check vital signs (pulse, blood pressure, respiration and temperature).
- Oxygen should be given to ensure that SaO_2 remains above 94%, ideally near 100%.

Induction of anaesthesia is achieved by slowly administering ketamine 2 mg/kg body weight IV slowly over 2 minutes. For short procedures lasting less than 15 minutes, this will provide adequate anaesthesia.

- Check the adequacy of anaesthesia at the operation site before proceeding with the surgery. Pinch the incision site with forceps. **If the pregnant woman feels the pinch, wait 2 minutes and then retest.**
- Monitor vital signs (pulse, blood pressure and respiration) every 5 minutes during the procedure.

Give additional IV boluses of ketamine 1 mg/kg body weight as needed.

Ketamine infusion

- For longer procedures, infuse ketamine 200 mg in 100 mL of 5% dextrose at 2 mg/minute (i.e. 20 drops per minute with a standard giving set with a drop factor of 20) and titrate to response. More or less may be needed. Stop the infusion 10 minutes before the end of the operation. If the patient needs a blood transfusion, give it through a different IV line.
- Monitor vital signs (pulse, blood pressure and respiration) every 5 minutes during the procedure.

Post-procedure care

Discontinue ketamine infusion and administer a post-operative analgesic appropriate to the type of surgery performed. The patient takes about 2 hours to wake up, and needs to be in a quiet area. Let her wake up naturally without stimulation. Maintain observations every 30 minutes until the patient is fully awake.

Local anaesthesia for Caesarean section

In extreme situations, Caesarean section can be undertaken under infiltration with local anaesthetic. Although not ideal, this can be necessary in an extremely ill patient (e.g. if unconscious and/or eclamptic), where general anaesthetic/intubation is not available and spinal anaesthetic is inadvisable.

Up to 100 mL of lidocaine 0.5% with adrenaline 1:200 000 is used to infiltrate the layers of the abdominal wall either side of the midline from the symphysis pubis to 5 cm above the umbilicus.

Paediatric anaesthesia

This must only be undertaken by anaesthetic practitioners with adequate experience, preparation and equipment. If these skills and equipment are not available, the child should be referred to a more experienced hospital if at all possible.

Ketamine anaesthesia is commonly used in children and is usually safe, but it must still be undertaken with care.

The '**10 golden rules of anaesthesia**' (originally defined by Maurice King in his manual *Primary Anaesthesia*) form the basis of essential safe anaesthetic practice for all cases, and are listed below.

1 Do an adequate pre-operative assessment.
2 Ensure that the patient has been nil by mouth for an appropriate time.
3 Use a tipping table.
4 Check all equipment and drugs.
5 Have suction ready.
6 Keep the airway open.
7 Be prepared to ventilate the patient (with oxygen).
8 Check the pulse, blood pressure and oxygen saturation (SpO$_2$).
9 Have a vein open with a reliable venous cannula.
10 Have an assistant ready to apply cricoid pressure.

In addition:
- Create a non-frightening environment. If possible and appropriate, the parents should be present up to the time of induction of anaesthesia.
- Be aware of anatomical, physiological and pharmacological concepts relevant to infancy and childhood.
- Know the normal values of the main physiological variables.
- For all emergencies, remember ABC for assessment and treatment, and call for help early.
- Know the hourly fluid and blood requirements for every patient (for children these are based on their weight).
- Ensure that all equipment and drugs are available for the child.

Pre-operative assessment
- Past medical history (including anaesthetic history), in particular any cardiorespiratory illness, and the presence of respiratory tract infection, which increases the risk of adverse respiratory events during anaesthesia.
- Medication and allergies.
- Nil-by-mouth guidelines (if unsure, ensure 6 hours nil by mouth for all oral intake)
  - clear fluids: 2 hours
  - breast milk: 4 hours
  - food: 6 hours.
- Weigh the child.
- Note the physiological status: airway, oxygenation and ventilation, cardiovascular stability, hydration.
- Assess airway and ease of intubation. Burns, facial deformity, small chin and reduced mouth opening are all signs of a potentially difficult airway. If any problems with airway or intubation are anticipated, consider referring the child to a more experienced hospital.
- If the child is sick, consider whether the procedure is really necessary, and if it is, ensure adequate resuscitation prior to any procedure.
- Plan the fluid requirements. **Do not give hypotonic solutions such as 0.18% saline in 5% dextrose. Give Ringer's lactate or Hartmann's solution, which are best and essential intra-operatively.** Neonates, infants and sick children need glucose (dextrose) intra-operatively, and therefore a 5% or 10% solution of glucose in Ringer-lactate or Hartmann's solution is ideal. Check the blood glucose levels regularly, and give additional glucose (10%) 2 mL/kg as required.
- **Basic maintenance fluids in children:**
  - Give 4 mL/kg/hour for the first 10 kg of body weight.
  - Then add 2 mL/kg/hour for the next 10 kg of body weight.
  - Then add 1 mL/kg/hour for each kg thereafter.
- **Additional fluids:** Judge these clinically: cardiovascular status and urine output (> 0.5–1 mL/kg body weight/hour for a child).
- **Premedication:** give oral paracetamol. Avoid sedative premedications unless you are experienced in their use.
- **Explain what is to happen to the child and their family.**

Intra-operative considerations
Planning the anaesthetic
- Maintenance of normal physiological status is part of balanced anaesthesia.
- **General anaesthesia** involves a reduced conscious level (sleep), muscle relaxation and analgesia. Anaesthetic drugs rarely provide all three of these (e.g. ketamine is a poor muscle relaxant, ether is not analgesic, local anaesthetics provide no fall in conscious level). Therefore modern anaesthesia uses combinations of drugs to provide balanced anaesthesia.
- **Avoid general anaesthesia wherever possible.** Most operations can be performed using one or all of the following: sedation, local anaesthesia and ketamine. These techniques should be the basis of anaesthesia for the non-specialist anaesthetist.
- **General anaesthesia is indicated** where other methods are precluded due to lack of knowledge, lack of drug, the nature of the surgical procedure (abdominal surgery) or contraindication for ketamine/local anaesthetic drug.
- Inhalation anaesthesia with or without muscle relaxant

and local anaesthetic/opioid as analgesia is the standard combination.

- Intravenous ketamine is an excellent induction agent unless it is contraindicated. Thiopentone is a useful alternative if inhalational anaesthesia is planned and intravenous induction is required.
- Induction can be achieved by inhalation of anaesthetic gases, provided that there is adequate expertise and equipment. This is not safe for patients with a full stomach, but in those with acute upper airway obstruction it must be used (intravenous induction often leads to apnoea or a worsening of airway obstruction).
- **Neonates and infants form a special group. Do not undertake anaesthesia without concern in this age group, and it should be administered only by an experienced practitioner.** Sedation and ketamine anaesthesia are more difficult to perform safely. Under general anaesthesia, neonates and infants do not breathe well (due to difficult airway maintenance, unfavourable chest wall/lung mechanics and limited reserve in the face of hypoxaemia). Therefore, in general, ventilation must be controlled. Caution must be exercised with regard to drug doses (opioids and local anaesthetics due to side effects, suxamethonium is required at a higher dose), and post-operative risks are increased. Ketamine or inhalational anaesthesia with controlled ventilation is the technique of choice.

For all anaesthesia:

- Remember the '10 golden rules'.
- Give oxygen if it is available (especially at altitude).
- Use all monitoring that is available. The best monitor is the anaesthesia provider closely watching the patient at all times. A pulse oximeter is the most essential basic monitor.
- Maintain normothermia (using warm fluids and high ambient temperature).
- Give fluids for maintenance with additional fluid as indicated clinically.
- The optimal haemoglobin level depends on age, but preferably should always be higher than 8 g/dL. Correction of chronic anaemia is not necessary unless major blood loss is expected.
- Analgesia: paracetamol, non-steroidal anti-inflammatory drugs, local anaesthetic infiltrations and blocks, and opioids (morphine and pentazocine).
- Plan to maintain spontaneous ventilation wherever possible. Never use muscle relaxants without knowledge of and experience in how to intubate.

When to intubate

- **To protect the airway/lungs:** All acutely ill children and pregnant women have poor gastric emptying. If in doubt, or if there is a strong indication of a 'full stomach' (acute abdomen) you must protect the lungs with an endotracheal tube. Intravenous induction with the application of cricoid pressure prior to intubation is the technique of choice. Prolong nil by mouth times post trauma to minimise the risk of regurgitation.
- **To ensure a safe maintained airway:** In the case of a difficult airway or potentially difficult intubation, **never** give muscle relaxant until the airway is secured with an endotracheal tube (i.e. keep breathing!). Upper airway obstruction is a contraindication to intravenous anaesthesia, including ketamine.
- **To provide positive pressure ventilation:** Prolonged surgery, where muscle relaxant is essential (abdominal surgery).
- **To improve oxygenation in neonates and infants:** You can administer 100% oxygen and maintain better lung volumes with positive end-expiratory pressure (PEEP).

Post-operative care

- **Basic recovery care:** attention to ABC, maintenance of normothermia, continued fluid therapy, and provision of safe and effective analgesia.
- Commence oral fluids as soon as possible.
- If intravenous fluids are required (due to ongoing losses or nil by mouth), give at 70% maintenance with additional fluids matched to losses.
- Regular oral/rectal analgesia (paracetamol, non-steroidal anti-inflammatory drugs) with opioid as rescue analgesia. Consider opioid infusion (*see* Section 1.6 and Section 1.15).
- Pain assessment scores to titrate analgesia (*see* Section 1.16).
- Family care and communication.

Techniques
Sedation

In pregnancy and in children should only be administered by experienced health workers; usually an anaesthetist.

- Conscious sedation through to general anaesthesia: based on loss of airway self-maintenance, gradual loss of protective reflexes and decreased responsiveness.
- All drugs can have unpredictable and prolonged effects.
- Cardiorespiratory compromise is the greatest danger.
- **Avoid sedation altogether in patients with upper airway obstruction.**
- Prepare as for general anaesthesia.
- Drugs: chloral hydrate, midazolam or diazepam.
  - chloral hydrate: 25–50 mg/kg orally (infants)
  - midazolam: 200 micrograms/kg intranasally, orally or sublingually
  - diazepam: 200 micrograms/kg IV (500 micrograms/kg rectally).

Local anaesthetic

- Advantages:
  - It is cheap, and minimal equipment is required.
  - Its use can avoid the need for general anaesthesia.
  - The procedures are simple and brief.
  - It can be used for post-trauma analgesia and post-operative analgesia.
- Disadvantages:
  - Slow onset, and prolonged effect.
  - Each block can have major complications.
  - Toxicity: central nervous system (seizures) and cardiovascular (arrhythmias).
  - All techniques can be lethal.
  - It is not sedative!
- Safety:
  - Always ensure sterility.
  - **Never exceed the maximum doses of local anaesthetics: lignocaine 3 mg/kg (7 mg/kg with adrenaline), and bupivacaine 2 mg/kg (with or without adrenaline).**

- Be very cautious with doses in neonates.
- Know the **anatomy**.
- Use blunted needles (easier to identify layers), ideally 25–29 gauge.
- Always **aspirate** before any injection (this is not a 100% guarantee of avoiding intravascular injection).
- All injections should be **easy** (i.e. there should be no resistance to injection; resistance indicates intra-neural injection).
- Be aware of the possibility of toxicity, and assess for it during and after administration of local anaesthesia (an early symptom of toxicity is tingling of the lips, which are a highly vascular area).

Applications

This can be administered topically, by infiltration or by regional blocks.

Do not combine local anaesthetic with adrenaline in digital or penile blocks.

- **Topical application:** easy to do and can be very effective (e.g. Ametop or EMLA skin anaesthesia, local anaesthetic soaked dressings, eye drops).
- **Infiltration:** use a small needle, and slow injection.

Nerve blocks

For all blocks, first consider whether ketamine anaesthesia would be safer and more tolerable for the child.

- Explain this type of anaesthesia to the patient and carers, and gain their consent.
- Warn the patient about motor blockade and the sensation of sensory blockade.
- Apply the principles of safe use of local anaesthetics.
- The onset of effect can be slow (30–60 minutes).
- The effect can be prolonged (up to 24 hours).
- Be aware of the distribution of analgesia for each block.

Femoral block/'3 in1'

- Femoral shaft fractures, burns, grafts from anterior thigh.
- Medial calf only blocked below the knee.
- Lie the patient in a supine position. The femoral nerve lies lateral to the vascular sheath just below the inguinal ligament (the nerve, artery and vein lie laterally to medially, respectively).
- Sterilise the skin, and provide skin analgesia.
- Identify the artery. The injection point is 0.5–1 cm lateral to the artery.
- Advance a 21G blunted needle at 45 degrees to the skin until two 'pops' are felt (the fascia lata and fascia iliaca).
- Aspirate, inject lignocaine 1% with adrenaline (1 in 200000), 0.5– 0.7mL/kg.
- Larger volume blocks obturator and lateral cutaneous nerves in addition, hence '3 in 1'.

Brachial plexus block (axillary approach)

- This is the easiest and safest approach.
- It blocks the whole arm except for the upper arm and shoulder.
- Lie the patient supine, abduct the arm to 90 degrees, rotate it externally, forearm to 90 degrees.
- Identify the artery, sterilise the skin, and provide skin analgesia.
- Advance 1 inch with a 22 G needle, aiming for the apex of the axilla, over and parallel to the artery.

- After one pop is felt, let go of the needle. It will bounce with arterial pulsation if correctly sited.
- Support the needle, then carefully aspirate and inject 0.5mL/kg lignocaine 1% with adrenaline 1 in 200000. Intravascular injection is a significant risk.

Intercostal block

- This is useful for fractured ribs and upper abdominal surgery.
- The risk of complications is high, but it is an effective block.
- Identify the postero-medial curve of the rib.
- Sterilise the skin and provide skin analgesia.
- Advance a 22–24G needle perpendicular to the skin until you hit the rib.
- 'Walk' the needle just under the rib, aspirate and inject.
- Repeat at each rib.
- Beware of the maximum dose, 0.5mL/kg of 1% lignocaine with adrenaline 1 in 200000, as intravascular uptake from this site is high.

Intravenous regional anaesthetic (IVRA)/Bier's block

- This is used for distal limb excisions and fracture manipulations.
- It involves intravenous injection of local anaesthetic into an arm with a tourniquet blocking off the arterial and venous supply. It is therefore dangerous and must only be performed with the appropriate equipment.
- Exsanguinate the arm by elevation.
- Apply the tourniquet (a double one if available).
- Insert two IV cannulae – one in the limb to be blocked as distal as possible, and the other for safety in another limb.
- Inflate the tourniquet (to twice the arterial pressure).
- **Inject lignocaine 1% (10mL at 1 year, 20mL at 5 years, 30mL at 10 years) into the cannula in the limb to be blocked (but not with adrenaline and not with bupivacaine).**
- There is a 10-minute onset, and it is safe to release the tourniquet after 30 minutes.

Ilioinguinal/iliohypogastric block (field block)

- This is used for hernia repair and orchidopexy.
- Lie the patient supine and identify the anterior superior iliac spine.
- This is 1 cm medial and 1 cm caudal.
- Sterilise the skin and provide skin analgesia.
- Advance a 22 G blunted needle perpendicular to the skin until one pop is felt (after the skin). Then aspirate and inject.
- Two pops are acceptable. Three pops or 'feels too far' runs the risk of femoral nerve block.
- Infiltrate 0.5mL/kg 1% lignocaine with 1 in 200000 adrenaline after aspiration.
- Withdraw to skin and infiltrate.

Central blocks

Central neural blockade should only be used by experienced anaesthetic practitioners in older children. It is not appropriate to discuss central blocks for children in this textbook. Please refer to a specialist anaesthetic textbook.

Ketamine

Ketamine anaesthesia is not always safe, and must only

ever be undertaken with great care. Remember the 10 Golden Rules of anaesthesia and ensure that adequate preparation has taken place.

Ketamine is an analgesic, dissociative anaesthetic that induces a trance-like cataleptic state dissociated from the environment.

- **Advantages:**
  - airway maintenance
  - cardiovascular stability
  - useful for short procedures, and limb and extra-cavity surgery.
- **Disadvantages:**
  - airway is not guaranteed, and interference risks laryngospasm and bronchospasm; cardiovascular stability is no alternative to good resuscitation
  - **hypoxaemia and apnoea**, especially after bolus administration
  - hypertonus, especially with prolonged anaesthesia (greater than 1 hour)
  - resistance is unpredictable except in developmentally delayed children
  - it raises the intracranial and intraocular pressure
  - emergence phenomena (e.g. hallucinations), although these are perhaps less common in children, and can be minimised with benzodiazepines.
- Use as low a dose as possible.
- Recovery may be prolonged.
- Use only with great caution in neonates (apnoea is very likely to occur).

Ketamine doses
- 1 mg/kg slow IV bolus.
- Repeat half the first dose (500 micrograms/kg) after 15 minutes.
- 7 mg/kg IM induction dose.

For IV infusion:
- Make up a solution of 1 mg/mL by placing 500 mg in a 500-mL bag of 5% glucose or 0.9% saline.
- Maintenance after the initial bolus.
- Aim for 2–4 mg/kg/hour for general anaesthesia.
- Aim for a lower dose, of 500 micrograms to 1 mg/kg/hour, for analgesia.

Marked tachyphylaxis can occur with infusions that last for more than 30–60 minutes.

Inhalational anaesthesia
Do not undertake this unless you are trained in anaesthesia.
- **Airway maintenance skills and the ability to recognise an appropriately anaesthetised patient are the absolute minimum requirements for safe practice.**
- The best simple guide to depth of anaesthesia is the level of sympathetic nervous system arousal.
- The equipment for this type of anaesthesia is generally more specialised.
- Spontaneous ventilation via mask or endotracheal tube and breathing system is the safest application.

Ether is a relatively safe drug to use, although it is no longer widely available. It can be given by an open method or by a breathing system and vaporiser, usually of the draw-over type. Induction of anaesthesia is slow and relatively predictable. Respiratory depression is late, and cardiovascular stability is well maintained. Recovery can be prolonged. Ether has **no analgesic effect**.

Halothane is a potent but highly effective inhalational anaesthetic agent. It can only safely be given via a vaporiser. It is easy and dangerous to use too much.

Trichloroethylene (trilene) has the advantages of slow onset, high potency and an analgesic effect. Tachypnoea and post-operative nausea are seen. It is rarely if ever used alone.

Essential equipment
This should follow the World Health Organization (WHO) or World Federation of Societies of Anaesthesiologists (WFSA) standards. The minimum is Level 1 facility.

Minimum equipment required for ketamine and local anaesthesia provision
- Equipment to support the airway and ventilation (bag-valve-mask).
- Suction (foot operated or electric).
- Intravenous cannulae.
- Syringes.
- Needles.
- Pulse oximeter.

Preferred equipment for ketamine, inhalational anaesthesia and resuscitation
- Oxygen masks: with and without reservoir bags (paediatric and adult sizes).
- Oxygen supply: cylinders with oxygen flow meter or oxygen concentrator.
- Intravenous fluids (isotonic solutions such as Hartmann's, Ringers-lactate or 0.9% saline) not dextrose solutions without electrolytes, except in the first 2 days of life.
- Intravenous administration sets (ideally burettes).
- Paediatric anaesthetic face masks (ideally clear masks with inflatable rims that provide an airtight seal and have minimal dead space).
- Oropharyngeal airways (Guedel), sizes 0–4.
- Bag-valve-mask incorporating non-rebreathing valve (paediatric), reservoir tubing/bag and self-inflating bag (preterm neonatal (250 mL) and full term neonatal and child (500 mL) sizes.
- Ayre's T-piece, with Jackson–Rees modification (open-ended 500-mL bag).
- Endotracheal tubes: 2.0–9.0 mm internal diameter, cuffed and uncuffed, PVC.
- Laryngoscopes: straight-bladed and curved-bladed.
- Magill's forceps (adult and paediatric sizes).
- Fixation tape.
- Suction apparatus (manual, foot/hand pump).
- Suction catheters.
- Yankauer suckers, paediatric and adult.
- A means of administering inhalational anaesthetic agents: continuous-flow (Boyles type) require a continuous oxygen supply; simple draw-over (OMV, EMO based, triservice); or new hybrid machines, such as the Universal Anaesthesia Machine (www.gradianhealth.org) or the Glostavent (www.diamedica.co.uk) (please refer to specialist anaesthetic textbooks).

Essential monitoring
- This improves patient safety, reducing morbidity and mortality.

- Use in any location and for any technique, including sedation.
- Use from induction through to recovery.
- Documentation is essential.

The best and only universally available monitor is the presence and vigilance of the person administering the anaesthetic.

Minimum monitoring includes colour, pulse rate and volume, chest wall movements, capillary refill time, respiratory rate and auscultatory findings, and pupil size. This monitoring can and should be performed repeatedly by the anaesthetist.

Always remember to check:
- equipment prior to use
- whether there is enough oxygen
- whether oxygen is flowing into the patient
- the patient's arterial oxygen saturation (SpO$_2$), electrocardiogram, non-invasive blood pressure (this is extremely valuable), temperature (ideally core temperature), blood glucose levels, urine output, and capnography (expensive but useful).

Essential drugs
- Oxygen.
- Intravenous fluids.
- Local anaesthetics (lignocaine and bupivacaine).
- Ketamine.
- Atropine.
- Diazepam.
- Midazolam.
- Paracetamol.
- Morphine or another opiate.
- Suxamethonium bromide (if no refrigeration facilities are available), (lasts 5 minutes, higher dose is needed in neonates, salivation, hyperkalaemia, masseter spasm, anaphylaxis).
- Pancuronium (or atracurium or vecuronium); neostigmine.
- Adrenaline (resuscitation doses: 1 in 10 000 = 100 micrograms/mL; 1 in 1000 = 1 mg/mL).
- Thiopentone (apnoea, hypotension).
- Inhalational agents.

Intubation
This is used:
- to secure the airway
- to protect the airway
- for prolonged ventilation
- for intra-operative ventilation
- for tracheo-bronchial toilet
- for the application of high airway pressures and positive end-expiratory pressure (PEEP)
- for cardiopulmonary resuscitation (all of the above)
- in patients with raised intracranial pressure to maintain normal oxygenation and normocapnia.

Choice of tube
- Uncuffed under 25 kg: the larynx is narrowest below the glottis at the circular non-distensible cricoid ring (modern cuffed tubes are increasingly available for infants and young children).
- The correct tube is that which passes easily through the glottis and subglottic area with a small air leak detectable at 20 cmH$_2$O (i.e. sustained gentle positive pressure).
- Size of uncuffed tubes: measure the tube internal diameter against the diameter of the little finger of the child:
  - preterm neonates: 2.5–3.5 mm internal diameter
  - full-term neonates: 3.0–4.0 mm internal diameter
  - infants under 1 year of age and after the neonatal period: 3.5–4.5 mm internal diameter
  - children over 1 year: internal diameter in mm = age/4 + 4

    length of tube in cm = age/2 + 12 for oral tube
    = age/2 + 15 for nasal tube.

Aids to intubation
- Laryngoscope: blade (straight for neonates and infants because of their long, floppy epiglottis; curved for older children and pregnant mothers), bulb and handle.
- Magill's forceps.
- Introducer (not further than the end of the tube itself).
- Gum elastic bougie (over which the tube can pass).
- Cricoid pressure (can aid visualisation of the larynx).
- Suction apparatus must be available, plus Yankauer and other catheters.
- Syringe (cuffed tube).

Predictors of difficulty
- Difficulty in opening mouth
- Reduced neck mobility
- Laryngeal/pharyngeal lesions
- Congenital: Pierre-Robin syndrome, mucopolysaccharidoses.
- Acquired: burns, trauma.
- **Look from the side: a small chin is a predictor of difficulty.**

Complications
- Displacement: oesophageal, endo-bronchial, out of larynx.
- Obstruction: kinking, secretions.
- Trauma: from the lips to larynx.
- Hypertensive response.
- Vagal response.
- Laryngeal or pharyngeal spasm.
- Aspiration of gastric contents.

How to intubate
1 Prepare and check the equipment.
   - Choose an appropriate tube size, with one size above and one size below available.
   - Get the tape ready to fix the tube.
   - Suction must be available.
   - Induce anaesthesia and give muscle relaxant unless completely obtunded. **Do not attempt this in a semi-conscious patient.**
2 Position:
   - Children over 3–4 years of age and pregnant mothers: 'sniffing morning air' position (head extended on shoulders and flexed at neck).
   - Children under 3 years (especially neonates and infants): neutral position (large occiput).
   - Keep in a neutral position with in-line immobilisation if there is an unstable cervical spine (e.g. due to trauma or Down's syndrome).

3 Pre-oxygenate every child prior to intubation.
4 Introduce the laryngoscope into the right side of the mouth, sweep the tongue to the left, and advance the blade until the epiglottis is seen.
- Curved blade: advance the blade anterior to the epiglottis, and lift the epiglottis forward by moving the blade away from your own body.
- Straight blade: advance the blade beneath the epiglottis into the oesophagus, pull back, and the glottis will 'flop' into view.
- Recognise the glottis.
- Insert the endotracheal tube gently through the vocal cords.
- Stop at a predetermined length.
5 Confirm that placement is correct.
- The chest moves up and down with ventilation and equally on both sides.
- Listen to breath sounds in the axillae and anterior chest wall.
- Confirm that there are no breath sounds in the stomach.
- Oxygen saturations do not go down.
6 Secure the tube.

If you are skilled, proceed to nasal intubation. This is **best for long-term ventilation, but is contraindicated in base of skull fracture.**

- Fresh gas flow through T-piece circuit to prevent re-breathing CO_2.
- Minute ventilation (MV) is 1000 mL plus 100 mL/kg.
- For spontaneous ventilation: 3 × MV.
- For positive pressure ventilation: 1.5 × MV.
- Minute ventilation = rate × tidal volume.
- Ventilator rates and tidal volumes (by hand or mechanical).
- Tidal volume is that which is **enough to see the chest expand adequately**, or 5–10 mL/kg.
- Rates:
  - neonates: 30–40 breaths/minute
  - infants: 25–30 breaths/minute
  - children: 20 breaths/minute
  - adolescents: 15 breaths/minute.

Further reading

Merry AF, Cooper JB, Soyannwo O *et al.* (2010) International Standards for a Safe Practice of Anesthesia 2010. *Canadian Journal of Anesthesia*, **57**, 1027–34.

Bartholomeusz L. (2007) *Safe anaesthesia: a training manual where facilities are limited.* Available as a DVD from TALC – Teaching-aids At Low Cost. ISBN: 9780955258770

King M. (2003) *Primary anaesthesia.* Oxford Medical Publications. ISBN: 019261592-0

1.25 Non-invasive respiratory support

Introduction

Respiratory support is needed when the patient fails to sustain an adequate airway, oxygenation or ventilation, despite treatment of the condition leading to respiratory failure. Respiratory failure may result from:
- respiratory illnesses
- severe shock
- coma
- convulsions
- meningo-encephalitis
- neuromuscular disorders
- raised intracranial pressure (e.g. from trauma).

Infants and young children are more likely to progress to respiratory failure because:
- they are more susceptible to infection
- their airway is smaller
- their thoracic cage is more compliant
- their ribs are (nearer) horizontal
- their respiratory muscles are more prone to fatigue.

Pregnant women and girls are also more susceptible to respiratory failure. They have reduced immune function, an expanding abdominal mass which impairs lung expansion, and are more prone to gastro-oesophageal reflux and aspiration of gastric contents.

As respiratory failure progresses, it will ultimately lead to cardiorespiratory arrest and death. Thus recognition of the severity of the conditions that lead to respiratory failure, followed by appropriate treatment, will reduce morbidity and mortality.

Use of respiratory support

The following **clinical signs** should be observed when assessing the adequacy or inadequacy of breathing:
- intercostal, sub-costal and supra-sternal recession
- respiratory rate
- inspiratory and expiratory noises
- use of accessory muscles
- adequacy of breath sounds and chest expansion
- heart rate
- skin colour
- mental status.

To help to assess the development of respiratory failure, it is necessary to assess **changes** in the clinical signs listed above. In the following situations, however, these signs are less useful because there is absent or decreased work of breathing:
- in patients with fatigue or exhaustion (e.g. after prolonged respiratory effort)

- in those with cerebral depression due to raised intracranial pressure, poisoning or encephalopathy
- in children with neuromuscular disease.

In these cases, pay more attention to the chest expansion and air entry on auscultation of the chest, heart rate, skin colour, mental status and, if available, SaO$_2$ measurement.

Pulse oximetry measures the arterial oxygen saturation through the skin (SpO$_2$ or SaO$_2$). Values of SpO$_2$ lower than 94% in air at sea level (for values at high altitude, *see* Section 5.1.D) are abnormal and would warrant at least initial treatment with additional inspired oxygen. Values

of less than 85% in oxygen are very low, but even values greater than 95% in oxygen may be associated with significant hypoventilation. **It is essential to remember that, in respiratory failure, even a normal SaO$_2$ while receiving additional inspired oxygen is likely to be associated with significant hypoventilation or intrapulmonary shunting.** Measurement of transcutaneous, end-expired or blood carbon dioxide levels will confirm this.

When respiratory fatigue is severe, oxygenation is poor or deteriorating, or carbon dioxide levels are raised, respiratory support should be used, if available. The various forms of respiratory support are outlined in Table 1.25.1, along with their indications.

TABLE 1.25.1 The various forms of respiratory support, with nursing care and medical treatment required, and examples of relevant conditions treated

Mode of respiratory support	Interface with patient	Level of nursing care	Associated medical treatment	Clinical use	Examples of relevant conditions treated
High-flow high-humidity oxygen	Nasal cannulae	Home, ward, HD	Nil	To provide a flow above the patient's needs, that helps to wash out dead space, and improves comfort and clearance of the airways. It may provide mild CPAP	Bronchiolitis, post-operative, chronic lung disease of prematurity
Continuous positive airways pressure (CPAP)	Nasal cannulae or nasopharyngeal tube	HD	Sedation or analgesia may be needed	To keep the upper and lower airways patent and maintain adequate lung volume (oxygenation)	Neonatal respiratory distress syndrome, **bronchiolitis***
	Nasal mask or face mask	Home, ward, HD	Nil		Sleep-related upper airway obstruction
		Intensive care (IC)	Sedation or analgesia may be needed		Acute upper airway obstruction before, **instead of*** or after extubation
Intermittent positive pressure ventilation (IPPV)	Nasal mask or pillows, face mask (NIPPV)	Home to IC	Nil	To treat hypoventilation (raised CO_2) when airway control and clearance are adequate	Chronic (e.g. central, neuromuscular)
					Acute (e.g. after surgery)
	Endotracheal tube	IC	Anaesthesia for intubation. Sedation or analgesia will be needed	To treat hypoventilation when clearance/support of airway(s), or when close control of ventilation is needed	Procedures or surgery requiring anaesthesia
					Severe respiratory illnesses, raised intracranial pressure
	Tracheostomy	Home to IC	ENT surgical procedure	Long-term ventilation where day and night support is needed	Brainstem/high spinal injury or neuromuscular disease
Continuous negative extrathoracic pressure (CNEP)	Chamber or jacket	Home to IC	Nil	To keep the lower airways patent and maintain adequate lung volume	Bronchiolitis and other severe lower respiratory infections, especially where the nose is blocked by secretions
Intermittent negative pressure ventilation (INEP or INPV)				To treat hypoventilation where airway control and clearance are adequate or maintained by CPAP	Central hypoventilation (e.g. apnoea of prematurity or neuromuscular disease)

HD, high dependency; IC, intensive care.

Shaded areas are those that require a lower dependency of care (e.g. they have been used in the home setting), but may be useful in acute conditions.

* High-risk situation, in which CPAP may be ineffective and intubation may be required.

Notes on the use of positive pressure ventilation

1 Monitoring of patient status and either airway or extra-thoracic pressures is necessary when undertaking any form of respiratory support except for high-flow, high-humidity oxygen (see below).

2 Positive airway pressure involves a flow of air or other gas mixture to the patient's airways. This flow may be continuous (as in CPAP) or intermittent (as in IPPV). It may vary with inspiration and expiration (as in BiPAP), or to accommodate the leaks or variable compliance of ventilator tubing, airways or lung units.

3 Mask ventilation can be well tolerated by children, but it may be more difficult for infants and young children to tolerate appliances on their face.

4 In the presence of excess airway secretions or an open mouth, nasal masks and nasal cannulae may not produce as effective airway pressures as ventilation with tracheal intubation (or relatively higher pressures may be needed to achieve the same effect).

5 The pressures used with masks and cannulae may be higher than those used with tracheal intubation, because of the greater potential for air leaks and other volume loss in compliant upper airway structures.

6 Infants and young children will sometimes only tolerate masks and cannulae if sedation is used, in which case close monitoring of respiratory failure must be undertaken in case full intubation and ventilation are needed.

7 Endotracheal intubation should be undertaken with rapid-sequence drug or gaseous induction, and subsequent analgesia, anxiolysis and sedation must be provided.

8 Positive pressure ventilation administered through an endotracheal tube must be accompanied by adequate humidity of the inspired gases.

9 Oxygen may be administered either using a built-in mixer in the ventilator, or by entraining a supply in the ventilator tubing nearer to the patient.

10 Positive pressure ventilators should be able to provide manipulation of either the pressure or volume administered, and the time intervals for inspiration and expiration. There should be alarms for failure to cycle, and for excessive pressure/volume administered.

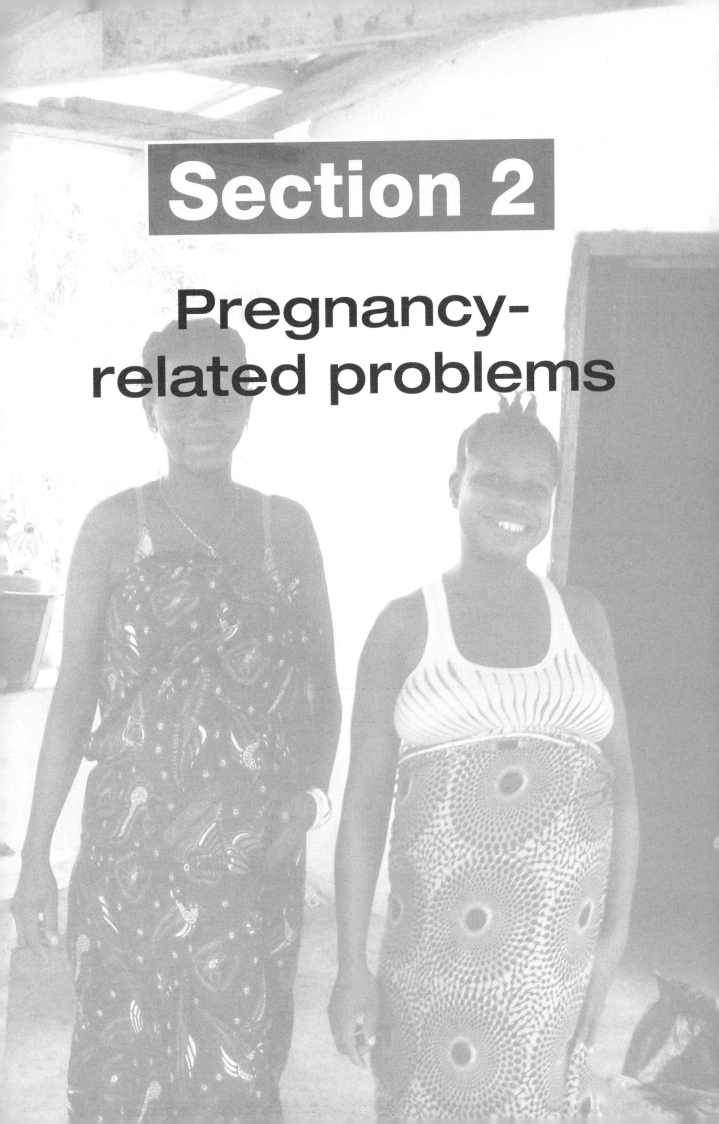

Section 2

Pregnancy-related problems

2.1 Antenatal care and the hospital

Introduction

For a variety of logistic and cultural reasons in resource-limited countries, the first time a woman attends a health facility during pregnancy may be because of a medical problem or because she is in labour. This often means that she is medically compromised even before giving birth, and at high risk of morbidity and mortality.

Antenatal care in such settings tends to be opportunistic, and the ways in which care is delivered must be innovative and optimised to ensure that comprehensive care reaches as many pregnant women and girls as possible. This might mean outreach teams going out to the rural areas ('trekking'), rather than the women having to make the long journey to the healthcare facility, often on foot. Usually the staff who undertake such visits are midwives and nurses, rarely doctors.

Such problems particularly affect rural areas at long distances from the nearest facility and where roads are poor. Hospital workers have a duty to ensure that they work with the community health teams to facilitate antenatal care.

Definitions of pregnancy-related events

Maternal mortality is the death of any woman or girl, from any cause, while pregnant or within 42 days of the end of pregnancy.

Gravidity is the number of times that a woman or girl has been pregnant. **Parity** is the number of times that she has given birth to a fetus with a gestational age of 24 weeks or more, regardless of whether the child was born alive or was stillborn.

For example, in gravida 2:para 2 (G2 + P2) the woman or girl has had two pregnancies and two deliveries after 24 weeks, and in gravida 2:para 0 (G2 + P0) the woman or girl has had two pregnancies, neither of which survived to a gestational age of 24 weeks. If these individuals are both currently pregnant again, they can be referred to as G3 + P2 and G3 + P0, respectively.

- A **nulliparous** woman or girl has not given birth previously (regardless of outcome).
- A **primigravid** woman or girl (a primigravida) is in her first pregnancy.
- A **primiparous** woman or girl has given birth once.
- A **multigravid** woman or girl (a multigravido) has been pregnant more than once.
- A **multiparous** woman has given birth more than once.
- A **grand multipara** is a woman who has already delivered four or more infants who have achieved a gestational age of 24 weeks or more. Such women are considered to be at higher than average risk in subsequent pregnancies.
- A **grand multigravida** has been pregnant four times or more.

Multiple pregnancies present a problem with regard to terminology. A multiple gestation counts as a single event, and a multiple birth, should be interpreted as a single parous event.

Rationale for antenatal care

Antenatal care is primarily a means of screening for, diagnosing, and treating conditions which could cause problems during the pregnancy, at delivery and after birth. These conditions may be pre-existing maternal medical disorders or obstetric or fetal complications which arise during the pregnancy itself.

Basic antenatal care

Two conditions are of particular importance to detect and manage antenatally, namely **pre-eclampsia** and **anaemia**, as they contribute to a large proportion of maternal and perinatal deaths.

Pre-eclampsia may vary in severity, but commonly presents with mildly raised blood pressure and proteinuria, and may progress to full-blown pre-eclampsia with dangerously high blood pressures, heavy proteinuria and generalised oedema (see Section 2.5.E). Mild and moderate pre-eclampsia is usually asymptomatic, and therefore routine testing of blood pressure and urine in pregnancy is crucial to its detection.

Severe pre-eclampsia can be associated with symptoms such as headache, visual disturbance and epigastric pain, and commonly leads to eclamptic fits, cerebrovascular accidents or HELLP syndrome (Haemolysis, Elevated Liver enzymes and Low Platelets), all of which carry a very high mortality. Timely intervention, by lowering the blood pressure, delivering the baby and treating fits if they occur, may be life-saving.

It is also vitally important to detect and treat anaemia antenatally, to reduce the woman's risk of dying should she experience a postpartum haemorrhage (see Sections 2.5.B and 2.8.D).

As far as possible there should be a structured approach to antenatal care. (A card or booklet designed and implemented by individual Ministries of Health for pregnant women or girls to keep and bring to clinics is helpful.) At the first encounter, an attempt should be made to obtain as full a history as possible, time permitting. This should include the following details:

- the date of the last menstrual period (LMP), regularity of the menstrual cycle, any contraceptive usage, the date of the positive pregnancy test (if available), and any particular complaints in pregnancy to date
- the previous obstetric history, including complications, mode of delivery and outcome
- the previous medical history
- the family history, especially with regard to hypertension, diabetes mellitus, multiple births and congenital abnormalities
- use of drugs, smoking, and alcohol consumption
- allergies.

The patient must always be examined.

- Look for signs of anaemia (pallor, leuconychia or white

nails, koilonychia or spoon-shaped nails, and angular stomatitis), malnutrition, oedema and other medical conditions unrelated to the pregnancy.

- The blood pressure must be measured, and ideally the woman should be weighed.
- The chest should be examined for cardiac and respiratory signs.
- Abdominal inspection and palpation should be done, looking for scars and checking for signs of pregnancy, including measurement of the symphysio-fundal height and feeling for the number of fetuses, fetal lie and presentation, and engagement of the presenting part (*see* Figures 2.1.1 and 2.1.2).
- An attempt should be made to auscultate the fetal heart with a Pinard's stethoscope, if the uterus is palpable abdominally.

Accurate dating of the pregnancy is important, as it influences decision making during the antenatal period, particularly around the timing of delivery and whether this is by Caesarean section (CS) or induction of labour. It also aids assessment of the maturity of the fetus if the mother goes into spontaneous labour early.

Bimanual examination, which must be undertaken in an aseptic and careful way (especially if there could be an ectopic pregnancy), is a useful diagnostic tool for dating an early pregnancy (in conjunction with the menstrual date), and in the absence of scanning facilities might be the only available means of calculating the estimated date of delivery (EDD).

At around 4 weeks' gestation, the cervix starts to change in colour and texture, feels soft and acquires a bluish tinge which may be visualised on speculum examination. The uterus first becomes palpable abdominally at around 12 weeks' gestation.

Prior to this an estimation of gestational age can be obtained from vaginal examination by assessing uterine size with the following comparisons:

- 6 weeks is equivalent to a plum or golf ball
- 8 weeks is equivalent to a tennis ball
- 10 weeks is equivalent to an orange
- 12 weeks is equivalent to a grapefruit
- 14 weeks is equivalent to a small melon (palpable abdominally).

The accuracy of clinical assessment may be reduced by obesity, fibroids, and if the uterus is retroverted.

Multiple pregnancy and molar change can also lead to a pregnancy larger than dates. At follow-up visits, the history and examination can be more focused on pregnancy events since the last visit. Examination should look for signs of intercurrent problems, anaemia and oedema. At every visit, the blood pressure must be measured and the abdomen palpated to check on the progress of pregnancy.

At all visits after 20 weeks there should be direct questioning for symptoms of pre-eclampsia. If the blood pressure is elevated or rapidly progressive oedema is present, a urine sample **must** be tested for protein.

Prior to the due date, there should be a discussion about the mode and place of delivery for women with a previous Caesarean section scar. Birth attendants and family members must be informed that there is a high risk of scar rupture, and the woman must deliver in a healthcare site where emergency facilities are available if needed.

They should also be informed of any concerns you may have which might put them at risk of needing intervention at delivery (e.g. twins, a high fetal head at term). These would indicate that they must deliver at an appropriate healthcare facility.

Ideally, there should be waiting homes near the healthcare facility where comprehensive emergency obstetric care (EmOC) is available, set up by the regional health teams, to which they and their attendants can move near to the time of delivery so that they do not have to make a long and potentially dangerous journey while in labour.

All of these details, along with the results of any investigations, should be noted on a small hand-held record (http://eepd.org.uk/wiki/index.php?title=Hand_Held_Records) which the pregnant woman or girl is encouraged to carry with her at all times throughout the pregnancy.

As the pregnancy progresses, the uterus continues to grow and has usually reached the level of the umbilicus by 20–24 weeks (*see* Figure 2.1.1). Measuring the height of the fundus above the symphysis pubis can also provide a good indication of the growth and gestation of the fetus. The woman should first empty her bladder. The measurement is then made by placing the zero point of the tape measure on the upper border of the symphysis and taking the tape along the uterus in a longitudinal direction to the upper border of the fundus, with the mother lying in the left lateral tilt position.

Between 20 and 34 weeks' gestation, the length of this measurement (in centimetres) should correspond to the gestational age in weeks of a well-grown fetus (*see* Figure 2.1.2).

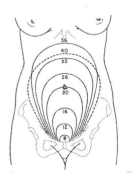

FIGURE 2.1.1 Average size of normal gravid uterus at different gestations.

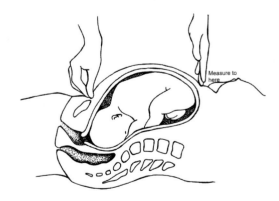

FIGURE 2.1.2 Measuring fundal height.

A difference of more than 2 cm too long or too short can indicate complications such as multiple pregnancy (too long), intrauterine growth retardation (too short), or inaccurate measurements of the estimated date of delivery.

It should be recognised that fundal height is not an accurate assessment of gestation or fetal size. Even in the absence of confounding factors such as multiple gestation and poly/oligohydramnios, it varies widely depending on the height and weight of the mother and lie of the fetus. In addition, the 'normal' fetal size also varies widely depending on patient build and ethnic origin.

Antenatal investigations and interventions

- Ideally a full blood count should be done at least once during the pregnancy, to check the haemoglobin level and, if possible, the red cell indices. Portable systems for measuring haemoglobin include the haemocue and WHO colour card from a finger prick sample, or perhaps, in the future, percutaneous measurement using a transcutaneous haemoglobinometer (currently under development by Masimo).
- Urinalysis must be performed at every visit, to check for protein and glucose.
- Screening for bloodborne viruses (hepatitis B and C and HIV) is not always available (see Section 1.8). All mothers should be advised of the risks involved, and of the precautions they can take to reduce the risk of transmission. Healthcare professionals also need to be made aware of universal precautions and adhere to them at all times.
- Serum samples should be taken for blood grouping and Rhesus status.
- All women should be tested for and when appropriate treated for syphilis (see Section 2.8.H).

ABO and Rhesus incompatibility

At a mother's first visit to the healthcare site, blood should be taken for ABO typing, determination of Rhesus (Rh) status and detecting the presence of harmful antibodies.

The main antibodies of concern are anti-D (usually acquired following feto-maternal haemorrhage), anti-c and anti-kell (which usually follow blood transfusion), all of which can cause severe haemolytic disease of the newborn. ABO incompatibility can also cause neonatal jaundice in one in 30 cases.

Potential Rh-D sensitising events for a Rhesus-negative mother include miscarriage, termination of pregnancy, ectopic pregnancy, antepartum haemorrhage, and invasive procedures such as external cephalic version. If the mother is not given anti-D immunoglobulin after such events, a second challenge will lead to a massive rise in anti-D antibodies in the mother's circulation, which can then cross the placenta and destroy Rhesus-positive fetal cells, causing fetal anaemia. The anti-D immunoglobulin should ideally be given within 3 days of the sensitising challenge, but may be effective when given up to 13 days after the challenge. The WHO recommends 125 IU per mL of fetal red blood cells found in the maternal circulation. A Kleihauer test can be performed to identify the presence and quantity of feto-maternal haemorrhage. In well-resourced countries, a dose of 250 IU of anti-D immunoglobulin is given before 20 weeks' gestation, and 500 IU after 20 weeks. (This is almost always adequate but additional units are given if the Kleihauer test indicates a larger feto-maternal haemorrhage.)

Due to limited infrastructure, blood bank facilities will not be available at all healthcare sites, but staffed laboratories should be available in district hospitals where the serum sample, taken at the healthcare site, adequately labelled and batched, can be sent for processing.

Immunisation and antimalarial prophylaxis

Routine administration of anti-tetanus toxoid should be offered to all women to reduce the risk of neonatal and maternal tetanus. For women who have never received tetanus toxoid vaccine, or who have no documentation of such immunisation, a total of five doses is recommended – two doses given 1 month apart in the first pregnancy, then one dose in each subsequent pregnancy (or at intervals of at least 1 year), up to a total of five doses.

A single dose does not offer adequate protection, and as the highest level of antibody occurs 24 weeks following the second dose, ideally this should be given around 16 weeks' gestation, with the first dose being given at least 4–8 weeks earlier in the first trimester, if early attendance allows this.

Intermittent antimalarial prophylaxis should also be offered. Among its other advantages, this may reduce the burden of severe anaemia (see Section 2.8.D).

Ultrasound scanning

Facilities for ultrasound scanning in this setting are usually limited. There may be no funding for a machine. If there is a machine, the staff need to be adequately trained and have the time to use it. Scanning can be useful for assessing the site of pregnancy, the period of gestation, viability, the number of fetuses, presentation and the progress of the pregnancy. If the image quality is good enough, it may also allow the detection of abnormalities, and although intervention might not be possible, this would mean that problems could be anticipated, delivery planned and the mother counselled appropriately.

Specific antenatal problems

It is not possible to discuss the management of every antenatal condition here. Conditions such as anaemia, hypertension and diabetes, which are common complications of pregnancy and becoming increasingly so, are discussed in detail elsewhere in this textbook.

Hyperemesis

Some nausea and vomiting is common in early pregnancy. However, in a small proportion of patients, severe vomiting (hyperemesis) can occur. This condition is more common where there is a larger than normal placental mass (e.g. in multiple pregnancy and molar pregnancy).

Signs of dehydration such as tachycardia, dry mucous membranes and a slow skin pinch can develop. The patient often develops ketoacidosis, which makes the nausea and vomiting worse. For details on managing this condition, see Section 2.6.I.

Organising an effective antenatal care system

Blood bank facilities

A functional and effective blood transfusion service (see Section 1.7) is a vital component of a national health system.

The WHO expects all countries to have national policies and a legislative framework for blood safety, with a centrally coordinated and quality system in place. Ideally, all donors should be unpaid volunteers, and unnecessary transfusion should be avoided. Currently there are large discrepancies between wealthy and resource-limited countries in the availability of this service.

Antenatal care networks

One important factor in the delivery of an effective antenatal service is establishing good networks between the community and the healthcare facilities in which births occur.

As was mentioned in the introduction to this section, 'trekking' is the setting up of an outreach service by which healthcare providers go to the women, rather than vice versa. This serves to offset the problems of distance and lack of transportation, and may be the first step in facilitating these linkages, as the staff have an opportunity to offer education to the mothers, birth attendants, family and community members on the potential benefits for women of delivering in a healthcare facility. The staff can also advise on warning signs to look out for, and on emergency measures that can be taken before professional help arrives.

Patients and their attendants need to know that they will receive the care they need regardless of whether or not they can afford it.

Perhaps most importantly, hospital staff need to reiterate the vital role that community members can have in averting a tragedy. This will hopefully reduce suspicion and encourage early communication when help is needed, so that critical delays in getting help to a mother can be avoided. A local emergency taxi service set up in each village, and ideally funded by the community and available at all times for women to be taken to the healthcare facility, is one way of addressing this.

One of the responsibilities of the regional health teams is to provide **waiting homes** near to a health facility, providing comprehensive EmOC, as mentioned earlier, where the high-risk expectant mother and her family members can stay for a short period prior to the birth in case an emergency arises.

If help is summoned following an emergency in the community, an emergency ambulance system, manned by personnel who have been trained in resuscitation and stabilisation, can be used for retrieval, further reducing the delay before the mother first receives skilled care (e.g. wheelbarrow ambulances, http://niaje.com/blog/kiberas-wheelbarrow-ambulance-innovation-out-of-necessity/).

Conclusion

The main keys to providing effective antenatal care are education on the role that it plays and emphasis on the importance of teamwork by all of the parties involved, to ensure the best possible outcome for both mother and baby.

2.2 Nursing pregnant women and girls in hospital (midwifery)

Introduction

Irrespective of where midwifery care is provided, there are universal requirements that should govern the provision of care:

1 provision of a safe healthcare environment for patients and staff
2 respectful and compassionate care for women, the neonate(s) and the family
3 skilled and competent staff to provide a good standard of evidence-based care
4 health education and promotion.

These areas of critical importance are further considered and described concisely in the subsections below. More detailed information on each area can be found in the references listed at the end of this section.

The global human resources target for effective delivery of obstetric care is one skilled birth attendant (SBA) for every 100 expected births. SBAs are defined as midwives, nurses, health officers, medical doctors and obstetricians/gynaecologists.

Definition of maternal death

In every action that is undertaken as part of midwifery, the prevention of maternal death must be the first priority.

According to the WHO, pregnancy-related death is defined as the death of a woman or girl while pregnant or within 42 days of the termination of pregnancy, irrespective of the cause of death.

Safe environment
WHO checklist

The WHO has recently produced a helpful checklist for patient safety with regard to childbirth (www.who.int/patientsafety/implementation/checklists/en/index.html).

Infection control

The microorganisms that cause infection can be transmitted to patients and staff by several routes. These include aerosol, droplet (e.g. coughing and sneezing) and faecal–oral routes, direct contact (person to person), indirect contact (through contaminated food or water, contaminated surfaces or objects), via blood and body fluids, and via insects and parasites. It is vital that basic infection control practices

TABLE 2.2.1 Elements of the WHO Safe Childbirth Checklist

Checklist item		Qualifying caption
On admission of the mother to the birth facility		
Does the mother need referral?	☐ Yes, organised	According to the facility's criteria
	☐ No	
Partograph started?	☐ Yes	Start plotting when cervix is ≥ 4 cm, then cervix should dilate ≥ 1 cm/hour. Every 30 minutes, plot heart rate, contractions and fetal heart rate. Every 2 hours, plot temperature. Every 4 hours, plot blood pressure
	☐ No, will start when ≥ 4 cm	
Does the mother need to start antibiotics?	☐ Yes, given	Give if temperature is ≥ 38°C, or if there is a foul-smelling vaginal discharge, rupture of membranes longer than 18 hours, *or* labour longer than 24 hours
	☐ No	
Does the mother need to start magnesium sulphate?	☐ Yes, given	Give if (1) diastolic blood pressure is ≥ 110 mmHg and 3+ proteinuria, *or* (2) diastolic blood pressure is ≥ 90 mmHg and 2+ proteinuria, and any of the following: severe headache, visual disturbance *or* epigastric pain
	☐ No	
Does the mother need to start antiretroviral medicine?	☐ Yes, given	Give if the mother is HIV positive and in labour
	☐ No	
☐ Supplies are available for cleaning hands and wearing gloves for each vaginal examination		
☐ Birth companion encouraged to be present at birth		
☐ Confirm that the mother and/or companion will call for help during labour if the mother has a danger sign		Call for help if the mother has bleeding, severe abdominal pain, severe headache, visual disturbance, urge to push, *or* difficulty emptying bladder
Just before pushing (or before Caesarean section)		
Does the mother need to start antibiotics?	☐ Yes, given	Give if temperature is ≥ 38°C, or if there is a foul-smelling vaginal discharge, rupture of membranes longer than 18 hours now, labour longer than 24 hours, *or* Caesarean section
	☐ No	
Does the mother need to start magnesium sulphate?	☐ Yes, given	Give if (1) diastolic blood pressure is ≥ 110 mmHg and 3+ proteinuria, *or* (2) diastolic blood pressure is ≥ 90 mmHg and 2+ proteinuria, and any of the following: severe headache, visual disturbance *or* epigastric pain
	☐ No	
Are essential supplies at the bedside for the mother?	☐ Gloves	Prepare to care for the mother immediately after birth: (1) Exclude the possibility of a second baby, (2) Give oxytocin within 1 minute, (3) Use controlled cord traction to deliver the placenta, (4) Massage the uterus after the placenta has been delivered
	☐ Soap and clean water	
	☐ Oxytocin 10 IU in syringe	
Are essential supplies at the bedside for the baby?	☐ Clean towel	Prepare to care for the baby immediately after birth: (1) Dry the baby and keep them warm, (2) If the baby is not breathing, stimulate and clear the airway, (3) If they are still not breathing, cut the cord, ventilate with bag and mask, and (4) shout for help
	☐ Sterile blade to cut cord	
	☐ Suction device	
	☐ Bag and mask	

Checklist item		Qualifying caption
☐ Has an assistant been identified and informed to be ready to help at birth if needed?		
Soon after birth (within 1 hour)		
Is the mother bleeding too much?	☐ Yes, shout for help	If blood loss is ≥ 500 mL, or if blood loss is ≥ 250 mL and the mother is severely anaemic, massage the uterus, consider additional uterotonic drugs, start an intravenous line, and treat the cause
	☐ No	
Does the mother need to start antibiotics?	☐ Yes, given	Give antibiotics if the placenta is manually removed, or if the temperature is ≥ 38°C and any of the following are present: foul-smelling vaginal discharge, lower abdominal tenderness, rupture of membranes longer than 18 hours at time of delivery, *or* labour longer than 24 hours at time of delivery
	☐ No	
Does the mother need to start magnesium sulphate?	☐ Yes, given	Give if (1) diastolic blood pressure is ≥ 110 mmHg and 3+ proteinuria, *or* (2) diastolic blood pressure is ≥ 90 mmHg and 2+ proteinuria, and any of the following: severe headache, visual disturbance *or* epigastric pain
	☐ No	
Does the baby need a referral?	☐ Yes, organised	According to the healthcare facility's criteria
	☐ No	
Does the baby need to start antibiotics?	☐ Yes, given	Give these if antibiotics were given to the mother, or if the baby has any of the following: breathing too fast (> 60 breaths/minute) or too slow (< 30 breaths/minute), chest in-drawing, grunting, convulsions, no movement on stimulation, *or* too cold (temperature < 35°C and not rising after warming) or too hot (temperature > 38°C)
	☐ No	
☐ Does the baby need special care and monitoring?		Recommended if more than 1 month early, birth weight < 2500 grams, needs antibiotics, *or* required resuscitation
Does the baby need to start an antiretroviral drug?	☐ Yes, given	Give antiretroviral drug if the mother is HIV positive
	☐ No	
☐ Started breastfeeding and skin-to-skin contact (if mother and baby are well)?		
☐ Confirm that the mother or companion will call for help if:		The mother has bleeding, severe abdominal pain, severe headache, visual disturbance, breathing difficulty, fever/chills, *or* difficulty emptying bladder
		The baby has fast breathing or difficulty breathing, fever or is unusually cold, stops feeding well, is less active than normal, *or* the whole body becomes yellow
Before discharge		
Is the mother's bleeding controlled?	☐ Yes	
	☐ No, treat and delay discharge	
Does the mother need to start antibiotics?	☐ Yes, given	Give if the temperature is > 38°C and any of the following: chills, foul-smelling vaginal discharge, *or* lower abdominal tenderness
	☐ No	
Does the baby need to start antibiotics?	☐ Yes, give antibiotics, delay discharge, and give special care or refer	Give if the baby is breathing too fast (> 60 breaths/minute) or too slow (< 30 breaths/minute), or if there is chest in-drawing, grunting, convulsions, no movement on stimulation, too cold (temperature < 35°C and not rising after warming) or too hot (temperature > 38°C), has stopped breastfeeding well, *or* there is umbilical redness extending to the skin or draining pus
	☐ No	
Is the baby feeding well?	☐ Yes	

Checklist item		Qualifying caption
	☐ No, help and delay discharge	
☐ Family planning options discussed and offered to mother		
☐ Confirm that the mother or companion will call for help after discharge if:		The mother has bleeding, severe abdominal pain, severe headache, visual disturbance, breathing difficulty, fever/chills, *or* difficulty emptying bladder
		The baby has fast breathing or difficulty breathing, fever or is unusually cold, stops feeding well, is less active than normal, *or* the whole body becomes yellow
☐ Follow-up arranged for mother and baby		

are adhered to in order to reduce or eliminate the sources and spread of infection (*see* Section 1.2).

Situations in which equipment, treatment rooms and delivery beds are covered in dirt, old blood and rat droppings, with goats and pigs wandering freely through the grounds and rats nesting in incubators and other equipment (all of which can be seen in resource-limited settings in public health facilities) are unacceptable and a source of infection. It is important to understand the reasons why women are developing serious wound infections post Caesarean section, which include, for example, overcrowded recovery rooms, with beds and surroundings not cleaned properly for months.

Washing hands between patients and after all invasive procedures is one of the infection control procedures that is of paramount importance, as dirty hands play a large part in spreading infection. Facilities for handwashing (i.e. a basin and clean towels), plus the availability of soap and water, are essential within any ward or healthcare facility.

It is also extremely important to ensure that any equipment used for the care of patients is cleaned after every use, with anything broken being replaced or mended. It is also necessary for the equipment to be stored in a clean and tidy area, so that it does not become contaminated when not in use. This will ensure that vital equipment is kept clean and in working order, ready to be used safely at any time.

An example of a situation where the above basic minimum standards are not met is the absence of clean oxygen tubing with nasal cannulae to help a baby to survive, and only dirty equipment available, with nothing to thoroughly clean it. There is then the dilemma of whether to use the unclean equipment with the associated severe risk of infection to the sick infant.

The environment in which women and babies are cared for also needs to be regularly cleaned. This includes regular cleaning of trolleys, bedding and sanitation facilities. Omission of these tasks will lead to the harbouring of infection, whether this is through direct or indirect contact or by the attraction of flies and mosquitoes to dirty surfaces or pools of fluid.

It is appreciated that, in some healthcare facilities, cleaning solutions (e.g. disinfectant) can be difficult to obtain because of lack of supplies or their cost making them unavailable. Using basic soap and water or even just cooled boiled water is better than not cleaning at all, and will remove microorganisms and the organic matter on which they thrive.

Instruments and other equipment that penetrates skin or mucous membranes or enters the vascular system or sterile spaces needs to be free of viable microorganisms, including viruses and bacterial spores. This is achieved by sterilising the equipment, usually in a hot oven or autoclave. It is important that the healthcare staff maintain the ovens and/or autoclaves in working order. They also need to fully appreciate how the process of sterilisation works. It is not appropriate for instruments to be placed in hot ovens or autoclaves without first cleaning them to remove visible blood and organic debris. Another common mistake is for healthcare staff to remove sterilised instruments and then proceed to cool them off using unsterilised water from the roof or tap.

Healthcare staff should wear protective clothing when indicated, if it is available. This includes new sterile gloves for every invasive procedure, and disposable or cleanable plastic aprons to avoid contamination of uniforms with bodily fluids during messy or potentially messy procedures.

Another extremely important element of infection control is to ensure that healthcare staff have received appropriate training in the disposal of used sharps (e.g. needles) into sharps boxes. The process for removal of these full sharps boxes from the health facility, and their incineration, also needs to be clear and robust, to prevent contaminated sharps from ending up on the local village dump, where children often scavenge and play.

Physical safety

The safety of the physical environment in which women and their babies are cared for is also very important, and staff need to give this full consideration. Broken beds and equipment can be dangerous. The former may collapse, and the latter may have sharp edges that can cause a wound. Babies can fall off high surfaces if these are not guarded.

Respectful and compassionate care

A good midwife or healthcare worker will treat every woman, irrespective of her personal circumstances, with compassion and respect. Pregnancy, labour, delivery and the postnatal period can all be anxious times for a woman. It is at these times that guiding, supportive and empathetic care is required. It is completely unacceptable within any society for women to be verbally and physically assaulted by their carers. Fellow staff should never tolerate this type of behaviour from colleagues towards women.

Good care will involve providing full, understandable explanations of any required interventions to the woman and her family, with the woman giving her consent to those interventions.

When in labour, women often find the intense pain of contractions easier to bear if they can be upright and moving about. This position is also better physiologically, as it promotes the progress of labour and promotes the well-being of the fetus. In most cases this is the position which should be encouraged until delivery is imminent. The position for delivery should, where possible, be the one that the woman prefers (e.g. upright or squatting), but this will also be dictated by the type of delivery and the degree of observation of the mother and her baby that is required. Women should not be instructed by their carers to lie flat on a hard trolley for almost their entire labour, as there is no necessity for them to do so, and this position is detrimental to the progress of labour and to the well-being of the fetus.

It is also important during labour and delivery to ensure that the basic care needs of women for a comfortable, safe environment are met. Light food and drinking water need to be available, with intake of water encouraged throughout labour to prevent dehydration. Ideally a relative or friend should be able to stay with the woman during labour and delivery to provide emotional support throughout. However, this may not always be possible in the very cramped, busy delivery wards that exist in some countries. If this is the case, there is all the more need for caring, empathetic staff. Strong analgesics for pain relief during labour may be unavailable in developing countries, and therefore these women often require greater resilience and coping skills, so encouragement and support from healthcare staff and the family is crucial throughout this time.

Skilled and competent staff
Management of emergencies
All midwives, traditional birth attendants and healthcare staff who provide maternity care need training to recognise what is normal and what is abnormal for both the mother and the fetus/neonate. Healthcare workers should know how to manage emergency situations relevant to their level of knowledge, and when and who to call for help.

In many areas within resource-limited countries there is no accessible surgical or anaesthetic care, and the nurse-midwife may well be the last point of referral. The nurse-midwife therefore needs to be trained and competent in all emergency procedures that may need to be performed within the environment in which they work. These emergency procedures are described in more detail within the relevant sections of this book.

General care
In the antenatal period, it will be the midwives' responsibility to ensure through physical examination, fetal heart auscultation, blood pressure monitoring, urinalysis, and screening for and treatment of anaemia that the pregnancy is progressing satisfactorily (see Section 2.1). WHO recommends 4 routine antenatal visits: <16, 24–28, 30–32 and 36–38 weeks gestation, and more frequently if at any stage it is identified as a high-risk pregnancy. During the pregnancy it may be necessary for the midwife to initiate treatment and follow up any problems that are discovered (e.g. anaemia, hypertension, infections).

When a woman goes into established labour her well-being and progress should be regularly monitored by either the traditional birth attendant or ideally a skilled birth attendant. This monitoring should include a 4-hourly check of the blood pressure and body temperature, a half-hourly check of the maternal pulse and fetal heart rate, and vaginal examination 4-hourly in the first stage of labour to check that the labour is progressing appropriately. During labour, the woman should be encouraged to void urine at regular intervals and as a minimum every 4 hours to avoid having an overfull bladder which could impede descent of the fetus through the birth canal. For poor progress in labour, amniotomy and/or careful augmentation with oxytocin may be indicated.

All observations that are recorded in labour should be recorded on a WHO partograph. Use of the partograph will help healthcare staff to recognise poor labour progress and/or observations of concern.

Fetal heart auscultation with a Pinard's stethoscope or portable Doppler ultrasound device (e.g. a Sonicaid) also needs to occur regularly, although the required frequency of the latter in the first stage of labour will be determined by the availability of facilities for performing an urgent Caesarean section for fetal distress. Once the second stage of labour has been reached the woman will usually start to experience the urge to push, and the midwife should encourage pushing in normal labour once this urge is sufficiently intense. Vaginal examinations should then occur at least hourly to assess progress if delivery is not imminent. At this stage it can be possible to deliver the fetus more rapidly (if the fetal heart rate is indicating signs of distress) by using episiotomy, forceps or ventouse. The second stage of labour can be particularly stressful for the fetus and therefore in the second stage the fetal heart should be auscultated at least every 15 minutes to determine signs of distress that would necessitate an accelerated delivery.

During delivery, the nurse-midwife needs to assist the woman in having a controlled delivery in order to avoid perineal trauma and/or harm to the newborn child. Active management of the third stage of labour by a skilled birth attendant with oxytocin is essential. Sterile delivery equipment needs to be available. At the very least in the community for the traditional birth attendant this should include a sterile instrument to cut the cord, with a sterile cord clamp and/or ties.

As previously stated, the healthcare worker needs to be constantly alert for any deviation of labour and delivery away from the normal (e.g. premature delivery, twin delivery, haemorrhage, hypertension, etc.), so that care can be adapted accordingly and emergency assistance sought if it is required and available.

The healthcare worker needs to be able to perform basic resuscitation of the newborn if this is required at delivery. Therefore bag-valve-mask resuscitation equipment needs to be readily available to healthcare staff trained in its use, including traditional birth attendants.

In addition, during the postnatal period the healthcare worker will need to ensure that they have the skills and knowledge necessary to provide appropriate care for the mother and child. This will include monitoring the progress of both mother and child, again being able to recognise the abnormal and initiate and/or provide the appropriate care to address any problems. The healthcare worker will need to be able to give all necessary advice to the mother and her family on her postnatal recovery and childcare, including advice and support with infant feeding.

Health education and promotion

The midwife or healthcare worker should use every interaction she has with the woman and her family throughout pregnancy, labour and the postnatal period as an opportunity to provide health advice, promote good health and deliver education. This should include antenatal education and information on the recognition of danger signs occurring at any stage during the pregnancy and in the postnatal period, including haemorrhage, abdominal pain, reduced fetal movements, severe headache and any other signs and symptoms of pre-eclampsia, and the immediate action to take when these signs occur. The healthcare worker also needs to provide education on parenting and childcare, again with advice on recognising abnormalities in the child, in order to seek appropriate medical advice. There will also be an ideal opportunity to give family planning advice and advice on the necessary immunisations,

prophylactic treatments and available health screening for the whole family.

Critical incident audit and feedback to improve perinatal and maternal mortality and morbidity

There is little doubt that this is a vital activity that should be undertaken on a regular basis, and that resources and time must be made available for this. Effective methods of preventing maternal and perinatal mortality are available, but the systems of care that should ensure they are put in place are frequently impaired. Critical incident reviews are potentially a simple cost-effective way of defining the local problems and pointing the way to local solutions.

Further reading

Pattinson RC, Say L, Makin JD *et al.* (2005) Critical incident audit and feedback to improve perinatal and maternal mortality and morbidity. *Cochrane Database of Systematic Reviews*, Issue 4. Art. No.: CD002961. DOI: 10.1002/14651858. CD002961.pub2.

2.3 Managing normal labour and delivery

> **BOX 2.3.1 Minimum standards**
> - WHO partograph
> - Disinfectant cream for vaginal examinations
> - Sterile gloves
> - Fetal heart monitor (Pinard's or Doppler)
> - Oxytocin and a safe way of giving it
> - Amniotic hook
> - Sterile vaginal speculums
> - Postnatal care programmes for mother and baby

Positions for assisting with delivery of the baby

All mothers in labour should be sitting upright or in a lateral or semi-recumbent position (*see* Figure 2.3.3). They should not lie flat on their back, as this causes compression of the inferior vena cava and aorta, with reduced cardiac output, as well as limited ability to push. They should be encouraged to stand and be mobile for as long as is comfortably possible.

Basic anatomy to aid understanding of the birthing process

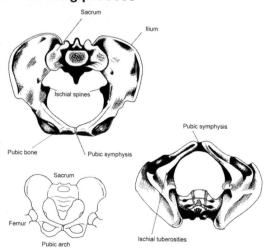

FIGURE 2.3.1 Basic anatomy of the pelvis.

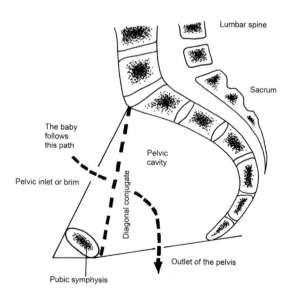

FIGURE 2.3.2 The baby's birth path.

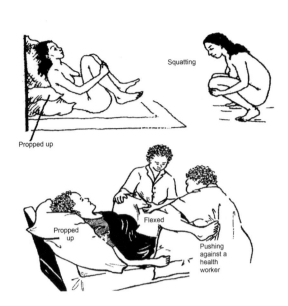

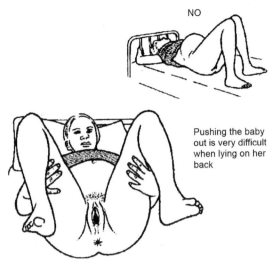

FIGURE 2.3.6 Pushing in the wrong position.

FIGURE 2.3.3 Good positions during the second stage.

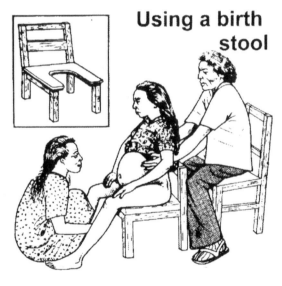

FIGURE 2.3.4 Using a birthing stool.

Figure 2.3.4 shows delivery on a birth stool. A TBA is delivering this mother's baby, and the husband is helping. Sitting up like this helps the uterus to contract, and it also makes it easier for the mother to bear down. In addition, when the mother opens her legs they act as pivots to help to increase the diameter of the pelvis.

The WHO partograph

See World Health Organization (2008) *Managing Prolonged and Obstructed Labour* (http://whqlibdoc.who.int/publications/2008/9789241546669_4_eng.pdf).

The partograph is a graphic record of the progress of labour and relevant details of the mother and fetus. It was initially introduced as an early warning system to detect labour that was not progressing normally. This would allow for timely transfer to occur to a referral centre, for augmentation or Caesarean section as required. The partograph indicates when augmentation is needed, and can point to possible cephalopelvic disproportion before labour becomes obstructed.

It increases the quality and regularity of observations made on the mother and fetus, and it also serves as a one-page visual summary of the relevant details of labour.

The partograph has been used in a number of countries, and has been shown to be effective in preventing prolonged labour, in reducing operative intervention, and in improving the neonatal outcome.

It is important to ensure that adequate supplies of the form are always available.

The WHO partograph begins only in the active phase of labour, when the cervix is 4 cm or more dilated (see below).

However, it is a tool which is only as good as the healthcare professional who is using it. The observations that are recorded will document the following:

- **Maternal well-being:** record pulse rate every 30 minutes, blood pressure and temperature 4-hourly, urine output and dipstick testing for protein, ketones (if available) and glucose after voiding, **and** record all fluids and drugs administered. If the findings become abnormal, increased frequency of observation and testing will be required, and intervention may be implemented.

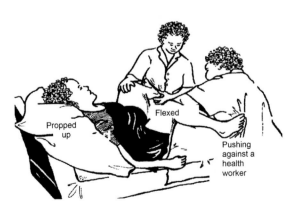

FIGURE 2.3.5 The pushing position, pushing with healthcare worker support.

- **Fetal well-being:** record fetal heart rate for 1 minute every 15–30 minutes after a contraction in the first stage, and every 5 minutes in the second stage. If abnormalities are noted, urgent delivery can be considered.
- **Liquor:** clear, meconium stained (thick or thin), bloody or absent. Thick meconium suggests fetal distress, and closer monitoring of the fetus is indicated. Check every 30 minutes.
- **Frequency, duration and strength of uterine contractions (assessed by palpation):** record every 30 minutes.
- **Abdominal examination:** to assess descent of the fetal head.

- **Vaginal examination:** this should be done no less than every 4 hours to assess cervical dilatation, descent of the fetal head, and moulding of skull bones. More frequent examination is only undertaken if indicated.

There must be a team approach, and senior staff must oversee the care of high-risk patients. Ideally there should be one-to one care.

Key to partogram
- **Amniotic fluid:** I = membranes intact, C = membranes ruptured, clear fluid, M = meconium-stained fluid, B = bloodstained fluid.

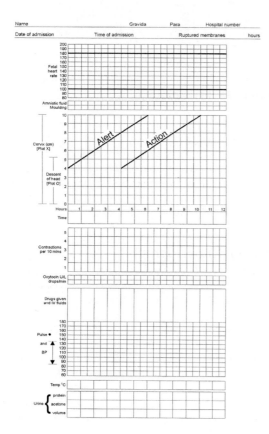

FIGURE 2.3.7 The modified WHO partogram without latent phase.

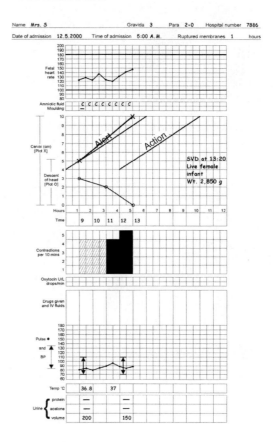

FIGURE 2.3.8 Sample partogram showing normal progression of labour.

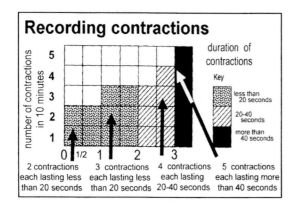

FIGURE 2.3.9 How to record contraction frequency and length. The number of squares filled in records the number of contractions in 10 minutes. The shading shows the length of contractions.

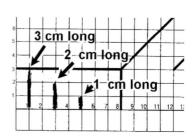

FIGURE 2.3.10 Recording effacement: the length of the cervix. Effacement can be recorded by thickening a line with a pen as shown in the diagram, or 'percentage' effacement can be written in the squares.

- **Moulding:** 0 = bones are separated and sutures can be easily felt; + 1 = bones are just touching each other; + 2 = bones are overlapping but can be reduced; + 3 = bones are severely overlapping and irreducible.
- **Cervical dilatation:** assess at each VE and mark with a cross ×. Begin at 4 cm.
- **Alert line:** starting at 4 cm of cervical dilatation, up to the point of expected full dilatation at the rate of 1 cm per hour.
- **Action line:** parallel and 4 hours to the right of the alert line.
- **Descent assessed by abdominal palpation:** this refers to the part of the head (which is divided into five parts) palpable above the symphysis pubis; recorded as a circle (O) at every vaginal examination. At 0/5, the sinciput (S) is at the level of the symphysis pubis.
- **Hours:** this refers to the time elapsed since the onset of the active phase of labour (observed or extrapolated).
- **Time:** record the actual time at 30-minute intervals.
- **Contractions:** chart every 30 minutes; palpate the number of contractions in 10 minutes and their duration in seconds (< 20 seconds, 20–40 seconds, > 40 seconds).
- **Oxytocin:** record the amount (in units) of oxytocin per volume of IV fluids, and the number of drops per minute, every 30 minutes when used.
- **Drugs given:** record any additional drugs given.
- **Pulse:** record every 30 minutes and mark with a dot (•).
- **Blood pressure:** record every 4 hours and mark with arrows, unless the patient has a hypertensive disorder or pre-eclampsia, in which case record every 30 minutes.
- **Temperature:** record every 4 hours.
- **Urine, ketones and volume:** ideally record every time urine is passed.

Maternal condition

Maternal vital sign observations are crucial in labour, in order to detect pre-eclampsia, haemorrhage (accompanied by a rise in heart rate, or, as it worsens, a fall in blood pressure) and sepsis (fever). A fall in blood pressure is usually a late and ominous sign. The pulse rate and respiratory rate are valuable early features of worsening maternal condition.

Fetal condition

The fetal heart rate should be measured every 15 to 30 minutes immediately after a contraction, for 1 minute, with the mother sitting or in the lateral tilt position.

The normal baseline fetal heart rate is 110–160 beats/minute. The fetus's baseline heart rate should remain stable throughout labour. Fetal heart rate accelerations are healthy features, whereas decelerations may suggest fetal compromise. This applies particularly if the decelerations do not recover immediately after the contraction (this is described as a late deceleration). A baseline rate of > 160 beats/minute (tachycardia) or < 110 beats/minute (bradycardia) may indicate fetal distress, as can a rising baseline.

Membranes and liquor

If the membranes are intact, write 'I'.

If the membranes are ruptured:
- if liquor is clear, write 'C'
- if liquor is meconium-stained, write 'M'
- if liquor is absent, write 'A'
- if liquor is bloodstained, write 'BS'.

If liquor is absent, or if there is meconium staining of liquor, draining, fetal distress should be considered and monitored for closely (meconium staining is present in 15–30% of all pregnancies, with a higher prevalence after 41 weeks' gestation).

Moulding of fetal skull bones (*see* Figure 2.3.11)

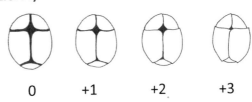

| 0 | +1 | +2 | +3 |

FIGURE 2.3.11 Degrees of moulding of the bones of the fetal skull.

Increasing moulding may be a sign of cephalo-pelvic disproportion, as the fetal skull bones overlap to aid passage through the maternal pelvis.

Key: 0 = bones are separated and sutures can be easily felt, + = bones are just touching each other, ++ = bones are overlapping but can be reduced, +++ = bones are severely overlapping and irreducible.

Stages of labour

Labour is divided into **latent** and **active** phases.
- The **latent phase** is cervical dilatation from 0 cm to 4 cm with gradual shortening of the cervix.
- The **active phase** is cervical dilatation from an effaced 4 cm cervix to full dilatation with good contractions. Progress should be at the rate of at least 1 cm/hour.

Latent stage of labour (0 cm to 4 cm cervical dilatation)

In the latent phase of labour, contractions usually start off as irregular, establishing into regular painful uterine contractions. In the primigravida, this can take up to a few days to occur, but usually takes less time in the multigravida.

The well-being of the mother and fetus in the latent phase should be assessed without unnecessary interventions, and mobilisation should be encouraged. Adequate hydration and nutrition are important, and the woman should be enabled to empty her bladder as required. During this time it is important to check the haemoglobin level and review the notes with regard to possible future problems with delivery.

Unnecessary vaginal examinations in the latent phase can lead to life-threatening infections in the mother and baby.

Active phase of labour
First stage

There should be regular painful contractions, and the cervix should efface and dilate at a rate of about 1 cm/hour from 4 cm to full dilatation (10 cm).

Vaginal examinations during labour must be recorded and only done by those caring for and monitoring the mother. They should not be undertaken more than 4-hourly unless there is a reason for doing so. During such examinations, the use of Hibitane cream or similar disinfectant cream can help to prevent infections. Care should be taken when diagnosing active labour as misdiagnosis can lead to unnecessary medical intervention and risk to the mother and fetus. The cervix should be 4 cm and effaced and there should be regular contractions. It should be noted that in multiparae the cervix is often soft and easily stretchable to 4 cm and even beyond. This can be the case in the latent phase and sometimes even before the onset of contractions.

The progress of labour
Measurement of cervical dilatation
Cervical dilatation is assessed by vaginal examination, which should be performed every 4 hours, unless there are indications to do so more frequently.

The cervical dilatation can be plotted on a partograph against time. When the patient is admitted in active labour, the dilatation is immediately plotted on the alert line, the first line drawn upwards on the graph illustrating a rate of 1 cm/hour from this first plot. If subsequent progress is satisfactory, the cervical dilatation will be on, or to the left of, this alert line in later vaginal examinations.

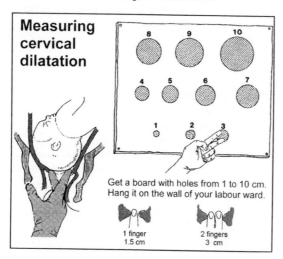

FIGURE 2.3.12 Measuring cervical dilatation. A cervical dilatation board shows the diameter of the cervix from 1 cm to 10 cm.

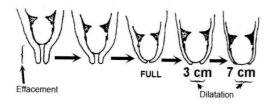

FIGURE 2.3.13 Effacement and dilatation.

Before the onset of labour, the cervix will usually be tubular. Effacement is the process whereby the cervix subsequently loses its length, to become flattened against the fetal presenting part.

In primigravid women, effacement occurs in early labour, followed by cervical dilatation. In multiparous women, the cervix commonly dilates before full effacement.

Diagnosis of the stages and phases of labour
Cervix not dilated = not in labour
Cervix dilated < 4 cm = first stage and latent phase

Cervix dilated 4–9 cm = first stage and active phase (usually 1 cm/hour) and onset of fetal descent
Cervix fully dilated (10 cm) = second stage (non-expulsive phase), no urge to push and fetus continues to descend
Cervix fully dilated (10 cm) = second stage (expulsive phase), urge to push and fetus reaches pelvic floor
Delivery of the baby = Onset of third stage
Delivery of the placenta = End of third stage

Bishop's Score: The early pre-labour/early labour changes that occur to the cervix can be quantified by using the Bishop's score which assigns a score of 0 to 2 for each of the following characteristics: dilatation, effacement, consistency, position of cervix and station of the head (see below). It is useful both for assessing progress in the latent phase of labour, and also for assessing the 'favourability' of the cervix for induction of labour. A patient with a favourable cervix has a Bishop score of 6 or more and is likely to be easier to induce. It should also be possible to rupture the membranes by the time the Bishop score is 6.

Characteristic	0	1	2	3
Dilatation	Closed	1–2 cm	3–4 cm	5 cm or more
Effacement	>4 cm	3–4 cm	1–2 cm	Effaced
Consistency	Hard	Medium	Soft	–
Station of head	–3 or above	–2	–1/0	+1/+2
Position of cervix	Posterior	Mid	Anterior	–

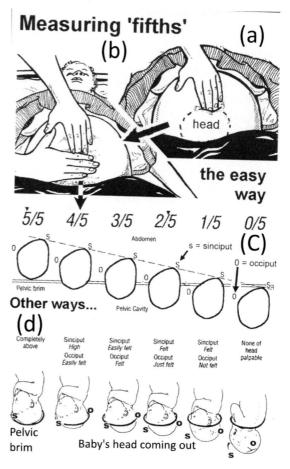

FIGURE 2.3.14 Measuring 'fifths'.

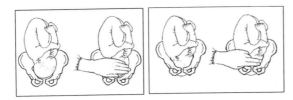

FIGURE 2.3.15 Fetal head descent palpated abdominally showing 4/5 and 2/5.

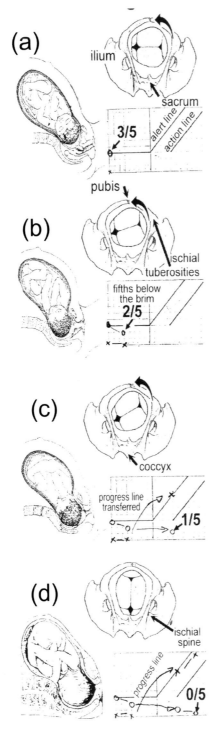

FIGURE 2.3.16 Descending fetal head showing vaginal appearance to palpation. Alongside each picture of the fetus is a view of the head from below and a partogram to show the stage of the mother's labour.

Descent of the fetal head

Dilatation of the cervix should be accompanied by descent of the head, although this may not occur until advanced labour. Sometimes descent does not occur until full dilatation, especially with the pelvis of African women.

The descent of the head is measured in fifths (20% increments) palpable above the pelvic brim.

Abdominal examination should always be performed immediately before vaginal examination, and plotted on the partogram with the cervical dilation.

Assessing fetal descent
By abdominal palpation

This method involves measuring by fifths of the head palpable above the symphysis pubis as described above.

- 5/5: head entirely above the inlet of the pelvis (head totally free)
- 0/5: head deep in the pelvis.

By vaginal examination

This method measures the descent of the head past the mother's ischial spines. When the presenting fetal head is at the level of the spines, this is designated '0'.

Figure 2.3.16a shows the occiput entering the brim of the pelvis on the left side, so the fetus is left occipito-lateral. Later drawings show the occiput moving round to the front so that in (d) it becomes anterior (OA). The mother was admitted soon after labour began. The baby's head is 3/5 palpable, it will soon engage in the pelvis and has started to flex. The membranes are intact, and the cervix is 2 cm long (uneffaced).

In Figure 2.3.16.b, the fetal head is now 2/5 palpable; it is more flexed and has just started to turn towards the front (anteriorly). The cervix is fully effaced but has not begun to dilate. The membranes are still intact.

In Figure 2.3.16.c, the fetal head is now 1/5 palpable; the neck is more flexed and has turned a little more. The cervix is now 7 cm dilated, so the progress line has been transferred to the alert line on the partogram. The membranes are still intact. Until now the mother has been allowed to move and walk about. She has chosen to lie down for delivery.

In Figure 2.3.16.d, the fetal head is 0/5 palpable, the occiput is anterior and the scalp is visible. The mother is almost fully dilated, so the first stage is almost over.

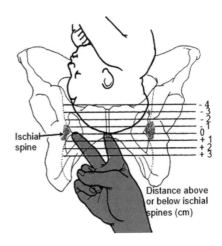

FIGURE 2.3.17 Measuring the descent of the vertex using the ischial spines.

Figure 2.3.17 shows the use of the ischial spines to measure descent of the head. Feel the vertex with your index finger and feel for an ischial spine with your third finger. Is the vertex higher or lower than the ischial spines? You may only be feeling caput. Measuring fifths abdominally is more reliable but can be difficult, especially in obesity.

Uterine contractions

For labour to progress satisfactorily there must be good contractions. They normally become more frequent and longer-lasting as labour progresses.

Uterine contractions are assessed by **palpation**, usually hourly in the latent phase, and every 30 minutes in the active phase. The frequency is measured by the number of contractions felt in a 10-minute period, and the duration is measured from the start of the contraction until it passes off (e.g. 3 in 10 minutes, each lasting for 45 seconds).

Management of the first stage of labour

1 **Place an IV cannula early on in all high-risk patients.**
2 If a fever develops give intravenous antibiotics (ampicillin 2 grams IV/IM 6-hourly plus gentamicin 80 mg IV/IM 8-hourly or 5 mg/kg IV/IM once every 24 hours).
3 If the first stage is prolonged, consider the following:
   - malpositions or malpresentations
   - pelvis too small or head too big
   - contractions too weak
   - membranes need rupturing (only if there are no malpresentations or malpositions)
   - dehydration, ketosis and/or exhaustion.

Pain control in labour

At present in low resource settings the only safe pharmacological treatment is nitrous oxide plus oxygen. Epidural anaesthesia is effective but requires careful monitoring (unlikely to be available), risks local infection, and can increase the need for Caesarean section. Opiate drugs, such as pethidine and morphine, have many potentially harmful effects on the woman and newborn infant.

Our recommendation is that, where possible, nitrous oxide plus oxygen should be made available for all women who need pain control, particularly the primigravida.

Nitrous oxide plus oxygen

It is recommended that a maximum concentration of 50% nitrous oxide and 50% oxygen should be used.

The labour ward must be adequately ventilated and the mask fit well to avoid contamination of others in the vicinity.

The drug is always self-administered to ensure its safety (if drowsiness occurs, the woman will drop the mask).

It should not be used for more than 24 hours, and can interfere with vitamin B_{12} metabolism if used continuously rather than intermittently (i.e. only during contractions).

The cylinder must not be mixed up with those containing 100% nitrogen. Nitrous oxide and oxygen mixture (Entonox) is supplied in a blue cylinder with white quadrants on the shoulder, whereas 100% nitrogen is supplied in a plain blue cylinder without white shoulders.

Treatment

The woman should inhale the gas only during painful contractions. After starting an inhalation, it takes 30 seconds to 1 minute for the nitrous oxide and oxygen mixture to act, and ideally the onset of the contraction should be anticipated, and inhaling started 30 seconds before it begins. Between contractions the mouthpiece or mask should be removed and the woman should breathe normally from room air.

Between patients the mouthpiece or mask must be cleaned and disinfected.

Side effects include drowsiness, dizziness, nausea and vomiting, and buzzing in the ears.

Nitrous oxide and oxygen is contraindicated in patients with impaired consciousness.

It does not modify uterine contractions or cause harm to the neonate.

Prolonged pregnancy

This is defined as a pregnancy that continues for more than 14 days after the expected date of delivery. This is a particularly difficult management issue in low-resource settings, where the dates of the last menstrual period may not be recalled by the time of antenatal presentation, and where early ultrasound scanning during pregnancy is unlikely to have been performed.

Prolonged pregnancy is associated with fetal distress, shoulder dystocia, poor progress in labour, and increased fetal, maternal and neonatal mortality.

If there is reasonable evidence that a patient is at or above 40 weeks' gestation, stretching and sweeping of the membranes in a suitably equipped healthcare facility can be helpful in starting off labour, and may thus avoid the need for formal induction of labour (see below).

Stretching the cervix and sweeping the membranes

First check the fetal position and ensure that the head is not high, and record the fetal heart rate. **If there has been any antepartum haemorrhage this procedure must not be undertaken because of the risk of placenta praevia.** The woman should empty her bladder.

A vaginal examination in the lateral tilt position using sterile gloves coated with an obstetric antiseptic cream (e.g. chlorhexidine) should be undertaken. **If there is any evidence of vaginal infection or spontaneous rupture of membranes, a membrane sweep must not be performed.**

The cervix should be assessed for effacement, whether it is soft or hard, and for dilatation. If there is no cervical dilatation or the head is not at a minimum of −3, then a sweep should not be undertaken.

If the cervix is closed but soft, it may be massaged until it allows the insertion of a finger. Once the cervical os is open (more likely post term), introduce a finger into the cervical os and pass it circumferentially around the cervix. This should separate the membranes and result in the release of local prostaglandins, increasing the likelihood of the onset of labour within 48 hours.

The whole procedure is uncomfortable but afterwards it should produce only slight pain or bleeding with irregular contractions. If pain or bleeding is marked, keep the woman under close observation in the healthcare facility.

The process can be repeated if labour does not start spontaneously after 36 hours.

Induction or enhancement of labour

This may be required if there is prolonged pregnancy, pre-labour prolonged rupture of membranes, placental abruption, or a hypertensive disorder. Ensure induction is indicated, as failed induction is usually followed by Caesarean section.

Artificial rupture of membranes (ARM)

This is undertaken to either induce or augment labour. Induction of labour usually also requires uterotonic drugs.

Slow progress in labour can often be corrected by ARM. However, in areas of high HIV prevalence, leaving the membranes intact for as long as possible may reduce the risk of perinatal transmission.

ARM risks infection and cord prolapse. It is contraindicated where placenta praevia is possible, in the first episode of active herpes infection, and in vasa praevia. It is more risky with a high fetal head or polyhydramnios.

Procedure for ARM

ARM is best delayed until the cervix is 'favourable' as this will reduce the length of time the membranes are ruptured (and hence risk of chorioamnionitis), and limit the duration of any oxytocin infusion used. It is also likely to result in a reduced risk of failed inductions and thus unnecessary caesarian sections. A favourable cervix is one where softening, dilatation and effacement has started to occur, and corresponds to a Bishop score of 6 or more.

It is therefore advised to 'ripen' the cervix with one of the following before ARM: misoprostol, a Foley catheter or an oxytocin infusion (all discussed below), whichever is considered the most appropriate.

- Listen to – and note – the fetal heart rate.
- Ensure that the woman has emptied her bladder.
- Palpate the abdomen. If the presenting part is well descended, cord prolapse is less likely.
- Ideally perform an ultrasound scan to identify the position of the placenta.
- Wearing sterile gloves and with chlorhexidine obstetric cream on your fingers, examine the cervix, and note the consistency, position, effacement and dilatation. Confirm the fetal presentation.
- With the other hand (again with obstetric cream) insert an amniotic hook or a Kocher clamp into the vagina.
- Guide the clamp or hook along the fingers of your first hand towards the membranes in the vagina.
- Place two fingers against the membranes and gently rupture them with the instrument in the other hand. Allow the amniotic fluid to drain slowly around your fingers.
- Check that no cord can be felt.
- Note the colour (clear, yellow, greenish or bloody) and smell of the fluid. If thick meconium is present, suspect fetal distress. Some light bleeding may occur.
- After ARM, listen to the fetal heart during and after a contraction. If the fetal heart rate is abnormal (less than 110 beats/minute or more than 160 beats/minute), suspect fetal distress.
- If delivery has not occurred within 18 hours, give prophylactic antibiotics (IV ampicillin 1 gram 6-hourly plus gentamicin 80 mg IV/IM 8-hourly or 5 mg/kg body weight IV/IM once every 24 hours) in order to help to prevent infection in the baby and the mother. If there are no signs of infection in the mother after delivery, discontinue antibiotics.

- If the liquor is foul smelling or there is a maternal fever or other indication of uterine infection/chorioamnionitis treat with the antibiotics as above but with the addition of metronidazole 500mg IV 8 hourly.
- Regularly monitor vital signs.

Oxytocin infusion
Indications

- If active labour is not established within 2–4 hours after ARM, and only if contractions are weak, begin oxytocin infusion. If there are strong contractions and no progress, look for a reason (e.g. obstructed labour).
- If labour is induced because of severe maternal disease (e.g. sepsis, eclampsia), begin oxytocin infusion at the same time as ARM.

Contraindications

- It is essential that obstructed labour is excluded before oxytocin is administered.
- Use oxytocin with great caution, as fetal distress can occur from hyperstimulation and, rarely, uterine rupture can occur. Multiparous women are at higher risk for uterine rupture (see below).
- Carefully observe all women receiving oxytocin. **They must never be left alone.**
- **Never use oxytocin in a woman or girl who has undergone two or more previous Caesarean sections, or who has a uterine scar for another reason, such as fibroid removal or traumatic uterine rupture.**
- If labour has been progressing and then stops in a multiparous woman there is likely to be a reason for this secondary arrest, such as cephalo-pelvic disproportion or malposition. The use of oxytocin (rather than Caesarean section) in this situation is dangerous, as uterine rupture may occur. However, in low-resource settings this concern has to be balanced against the risks associated with Caesarean section (assuming that this procedure is even available without transfer). We recommend that secondary arrest in a multiparous woman should result in urgent transfer to a facility where Caesarean section can be undertaken.
- Never use oxytocin where a previous classical Caesarean section has been performed. Provide a timed Caesarean section.

Concerns about oxytocin and the need for great care in its use

- If a woman has undergone one previous Caesarean section, the use of oxytocin is associated with a much increased risk of uterine rupture, and these patients must be delivered in a facility where immediate Caesarean section can be performed if required. Oxytocin may, in this latter setting, be used with great care and discontinued when adequate contractions are present.
- If more than four pregnancies after 24 weeks' gestation have been delivered, there is increased risk of uterine rupture. Oxytocin must be used with great care and discontinued when adequate contractions are present.
- Wait before starting oxytocin if misoprostol or another prostaglandin has been given within the previous 8 hours.

Administration of oxytocin

The individually needed effective dose of oxytocin varies greatly; so all patients must be monitored carefully.

Fluids can be calculated in drops per minute. Identify from the IV giving set what the 'drop factor' is (in standard giving sets it may be 10, 15 or 20 drops/1 mL). For micro-drop systems, (with burettes), 1 mL is 60 drops. Set the infusion rate with the flow controller below the chamber where the drops occur, and always count the rate over a full minute.

Cautiously administer oxytocin in IV fluids (Ringer-lactate or Hartmann's solution), gradually increasing the rate of infusion until active labour is established (three contractions in 10 minutes, each lasting more than 40 seconds). Maintain this rate until delivery. The uterus must relax between contractions.

A burette in-line IV giving set (see Figure 2.3.18) can help to prevent too much oxytocin being given.

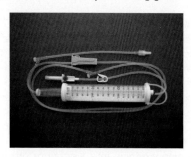

FIGURE 2.3.18 Burette for safer and more accurate administration of oxytocin.

When oxytocin infusion results in an active labour pattern, maintain the same rate until delivery.

Ensure that the woman is in the left lateral tilt or recovery position.

Record on a partogram every 30 minutes:
- rate of infusion of oxytocin (note that changes in the woman's arm position may alter the flow rate)
- duration and frequency of contractions
- fetal heart rate: listen every 30 minutes, always immediately after a contraction; if less than 100 beats/minute, stop the infusion.

Monitor pulse, blood pressure and contractions every 30 minutes. Keep a fluid balance chart. Regularly reassess for contraindications.

Details of oxytocin infusion

An ampoule of oxytocin usually contains 5 international units in 1 mL. Insert oxytocin 5 international units (5000 milliunits) in 500 mL of Ringer-lactate or Hartmann's solution. The concentration of this solution is 10 milliunits in 1 mL.

Start infusion at 2.5 milliunits/minute (i.e. at 5 drops/minute with a standard giving set with a drop factor of 20 drops/1 mL).

Increase infusion rate by 2.5 milliunits/minute (5 drops/minute using a standard giving set with a drop factor of 20 drops/1 mL) every 30 minutes until a good contraction pattern is established – that is, contractions lasting more than 40 seconds, and occurring 3 times in 10 minutes.

Maintain this rate until delivery is completed.

If there are not three contractions in 10 minutes, each lasting more than 40 seconds, with the infusion rate at 20 milliunits/minute (40 drops/minute if using a giving set with a drop factor of 20 drops/1 mL):
- In multigravida, further increases may risk uterine

rupture. The reason for this may be cephalo-pelvic disproportion or malposition. Therefore **consider Caesarean section**.
- In the **primigravida**, infuse oxytocin at a higher concentration (rapid escalation).
  - Change to a more concentrated solution with oxytocin 10 international units (10 000 milliunits) in 500 mL of Ringer-lactate or Hartmann's at a concentration of 20 milliunits/mL.
  - Give an initial infusion of 20 milliunits/minute (20 drops/minute if using a giving set with a drop factor of 20 drops/1 mL).
  - Increase the infusion rate by 5 milliunits/minute (additional 5 drops/minute if using a giving set with a drop factor of 20 drops/1 mL) every 30 minutes until good contractions are established.
  - **If good contractions are not established at 40 milliunits/minute** (40 drops/minute if using a giving set with a drop factor of 20 drops/1 mL), deliver by Caesarean section.

Do not use oxytocin 10 international units in 500 mL (i.e. 20 milliunits/mL) in multigravida.

If hyperstimulation occurs (i.e. any contractions lasting longer than 60 seconds or more than 4 contractions in 10 minutes), stop the infusion. The half-life of oxytocin is short (between 1 and 5 minutes), and therefore any hyperstimulation should stop with appropriate titration of the dose given. If hyperstimulation resolves, restart oxytocin infusion at half of the last dose given.

Consider terbutaline, 250 micrograms subcutaneously if the uterus does not relax.

Possible side effects of oxytocin infusion

These include the following:
- uterine hyperstimulation (see above).
- hyponatraemia due to water retention from vasopressin-like actions (unlikely if diluted with Ringer-lactate or Hartmann's and more likely with prolonged infusions). Monitor urine output carefully and, if possible, measure plasma sodium concentrations.
- hypotension, flushing and tachycardia if oxytocin is given as a bolus IV by mistake.

The use of oral misoprostol to induce labour

Because of its stability at high room temperatures and low cost, misoprostol is increasingly being used to induce labour, especially in low-resource settings. Close monitoring of uterine contractions is still essential, and misoprostol must not be used if there has been a previous Caesarean section.

Misoprostal is available as a vaginal or oral tablet or an oral solution. The latest Cochrane reviews suggest that oral misoprostol solution is the most appropriate.

Dose of oral misoprostol solution

A single misoprostol tablet is dissolved in drinking water (200-microgram tablet in 200 mL of water or 100-microgram tablet in 100 mL of water), and 20–25 mL of misoprostol solution (20–25 micrograms) are then given orally every 2 hours. It may be used in women with ruptured membranes, where the oral route has the additional benefit of avoiding vaginal installations with their increased risk of infection. Solutions are stable for up to 24 hours, but should then be discarded. For safety reasons it may be better to discard unused solutions and make up a 20- to 25-microgram dose every 2 hours. Review progress by a doctor after 100 micrograms have been given although the induction can be continued with further doses if necessary.

When induction of labour is urgent and delivery indicated within a short period of time (e.g. eclampsia) consider increasing the misoprostol dose to 50 micrograms orally every 2 hours. This may increase the speed of the induction but may also increase the risk of hyperstimulation. The recent Cochrane review recommends an oral dose of 20-25 micrograms and not more than 50 micrograms every 2 hours.

Oral misoprostol tablets
It is possible to cut 100-microgram misoprostol tablets into quarters that are 25 micrograms in size and administer them orally every 2 hours up to a maximum of six doses. However, this is not accurate, and there is a danger of giving an incorrect dosage. The oral misoprostol solution described above is safer.

The use of a Foley catheter to induce labour
An effective alternative to misoprostol is to use a Foley catheter to mechanically 'ripen' the cervix and induce labour. The Foley catheter tip is passed through the cervical os either during a sterile digital examination, or with the use of a sterile/high-level disinfected speculum and forceps. The inflatable bulb is introduced beyond the internal cervical os and then inflated with 10ml of sterile water. The catheter tip is then left in situ for up to 24 hours to allow cervical ripening and contractions to begin. It may fall out in the interim if the cervix dilates adequately. Once removed amniotomy and oxytocin can be commenced if needed.

This method is particularly useful in women at high risk of rupture as it does not risk hyperstimulation.

Delay in the first stage of labour
If progress is initially good, but then slows down or stops, there may be:
- malpositions or malpresentations
- obstructed labour
- an increased risk of shoulder dystocia.

Prolonged active phase (first stage) of labour
If cervical dilatation crosses the alert line, this warns that labour is slow and there may be problems. If possible, transfer the patient to an obstetric unit practicing comprehensive EmOC. If the action line (4 hours to the right according

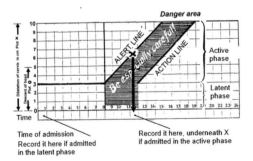

FIGURE 2.3.19 The partogram showing the portion relating to cervical dilatation. The numbers 1 to 24 represent the number of hours since the mother was admitted, but only if she was admitted in the latent phase.

A common mistake

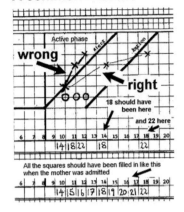

FIGURE 2.3.20 Correct placement of data on the partogram. A common mistake is to put the next record ('x' and 'o') in the next square, and not to allow for the time that elapses between one observation and the next.

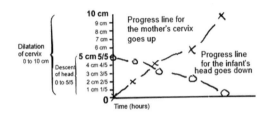

FIGURE 2.3.21 Lines on the partogram.

to the WHO, or 2 hours to the right according to recent evidence from South Africa) is reached, the mother must be reassessed to ascertain the reason for lack of progress and further management determined.

Other complications of the first stage of labour
Urgent help may be required to diagnose and manage cord prolapse (*see* Section 2.6.G), placental separation (*see* Section 2.5.D.iii) or ruptured uterus (*see* Section 2.5.F).

Second stage of labour
This begins when the cervix is fully dilated. Fetal descent occurs, but initially there may be no urge to push usually occurring only when the fetal head reaches the pelvic floor. It may be helpful for the mother to stand up or squat during this time to assist pushing. She must not lie flat on her back. (Note; some patients have an urge to push early in labour with a high head, generally with an occipito-posterior presentation)

Delivery of the baby may be allowed to take 2 hours from full cervical dilatation in the primagravida, and 1 hour in the multigravida, before there is cause for concern. The mother must not push if the cervix is not fully dilated.

During delivery, trauma to the perineum should be minimised. Routine episiotomy is not indicated, but should be performed if significant perineal trauma is anticipated, or to aid more rapid delivery if indicated. Anterior episiotomy/reversal of genital mutilation may be required in some women.

Episiotomy is recommended for the following:

- complicated vaginal delivery (breech, shoulder dystocia, forceps and some vacuum extractions)
- scarring from female genital mutilation (see above) or poorly healed third- or fourth-degree tears
- fetal distress.

Sometimes contractions become less strong when the cervix becomes fully dilated. After confirming the well-being of the mother and fetus, mobilise the mother, hydrate her orally, including sufficient calories to help to prevent ketosis, and then wait for up to 1 hour for the head to descend. If the mother is unable to tolerate oral fluids, administer IV glucose and fluids. However, be alert for the possibility of cephalo-pelvic disproportion. After 1 hour encourage pushing, provided that the cervix is fully dilated.

Ensure that delivery of the head is controlled so that there is not a sudden release of pressure on it as it delivers (this may damage the neonatal brain).

If there is fetal distress, or delivery has not occurred after 2 hours in a primigravida or 1 hour in a multigravida, assisted vaginal delivery should be considered. A ventouse or forceps may be considered so long as none of the head is palpable per abdomen. **The cervix must be fully dilated.**

Delivery of the baby

- Ask the mother to pant or give only small pushes with contractions.
- Control the birth of the head by placing the fingers of one hand against the baby's head to ensure that it does not deliver too quickly.
- Support the perineum with your other hand as it distends and the head is delivered.
- In low-resource countries, if meconium is present, suck it out of the baby's nose and mouth on the perineum as soon as the head is delivered.
- Call the paediatrician (if available) if you consider that the baby might need resuscitation.
- Once the head is delivered, ask the mother not to push.
- Feel around the baby's neck for the umbilical cord:
  - If it is round the neck but loose, slip it over the baby's head.
  - If it is so tight round the neck that it is preventing delivery of the baby's shoulders, double clamp it and cut it before unwinding it from the neck. Delivery can often be achieved with the cord left in place.
- Allow the baby's head to turn spontaneously.
- After the head has turned, place a hand on each side of the head and ask the mother to push gently without the need to wait for contractions.
- Avoid tears by delivering one shoulder at a time. Routine traction of the baby's head in an axial direction should be used and should result in delivery of the anterior shoulder.
- Lift the baby's head anteriorly to deliver the shoulder that is posterior.
- Support the baby's body as it slides out.
- After delivery of the baby, give the mother 10 units of oxytocin IM to reduce the risk of haemorrhage, **but only do this if the possibility of a second twin has been excluded by earlier ultrasound examination or by abdominal palpation.** Alternatively, 10 units of oxytocin plus 500 micrograms of ergometrine

(called Syntometrine) IM can be given, but never **give ergometrine if the mother has hypertension or pre-eclampsia,** as it can increase blood pressure and cause a cerebrovascular accident.

- Dry the baby, cover with a dry clean towel and assess the baby (see Section 3.1).
- If the baby does not need resuscitation, place on the mother's abdomen for 1 to 3 minutes to provide a transfusion of placental blood to the baby, but keep warm (for details, see Section 3.1).
- Then cut the umbilical cord and place the baby in skin-to-skin contact with the mother, ensuring that the body and head are covered to keep the baby warm. The baby may seek to suck on the breast which should be encouraged.
- If the baby needs resuscitation, cut and clamp the cord immediately, and proceed to open the airway and breathe for the baby (see Section 3.2).
- If the mother is not well, ask an assistant or relative to care for the baby.

Always prepare for the need to resuscitate the baby, especially if there is a history of eclampsia, prolonged or obstructed labour, bleeding, preterm birth or infection. Always have a bag-valve-mask of the right size available next to the mother, and ideally on a Resuscitaire®, in case assisted ventilation is required.

If the head retracts on to the perineum during delivery (the turtle sign), this suggests shoulder dystocia (see Section 2.5.F).

Active management of the third stage of labour

This is advised for preventing postpartum haemorrhage (PPH), and it consists of four possible interventions:

1. a prophylactic uterotonic drug after delivery of the shoulders of the baby and after ensuring that another fetus is not present in the uterus
2. early cord clamping and cutting
3. controlled cord traction
4. uterine massage after delivery of the placenta.

Of these, a uterotonic drug (see above), is the most important, with oxytocin the first choice because it causes uterine contraction to prevent atony rapidly with minimal adverse effects. Atony is the most common cause of PPH (around 80% of cases). If oxytocin is unavailable, or does not work, other uterotonic drugs should be used, including ergometrine or misoprostol.

All uterotonic drugs should be given within 1 minute of the complete birth of the fetus, to aid separation of the placenta by enhancing uterine contractions and reducing the risk of bleeding from an atonic (relaxed) uterus. **It is essential that you are certain there is not another fetus in the uterus before such drugs are given.**

Ensure that both oxytocin and ergometrine are protected from heat damage by close attention to the cold chain and their storage, otherwise they may not be effective. Ideally oxytocin should be stored in a fridge, but it can be kept at 15–30°C for 3 months. Oxytocin must never be frozen. Always store ergometrine in a fridge at 2–8°C. Misoprostol is not affected by ambient temperature.

Ergometrine is contraindicated in patients with heart

disease, hypertension, pre-eclampsia or eclampsia, as it raises the blood pressure by vasoconstriction, with the risk of cerebrovascular accidents.

Early cord clamping and cutting (the second intervention listed above) as part of the active management of the third stage of labour is no longer recommended unless the infant needs resuscitation (see above).

Controlled cord traction (the third intervention listed above) is optional where delivery is undertaken by a skilled birth attendant, but contraindicated if a skilled attendant is not available. It must not be undertaken if a uterotonic drug has not been given.

1 After the cord has been clamped, use cord clamp/ straight clamp to hold the cord close to the perineum.
2 Place the other hand just above the pubis, and counter the uterus during traction of the cord to prevent it from inverting (see Figure 2.3.22).
3 Keep slight tension on the cord and wait for a uterine contraction.
4 When the uterus becomes rounded or the cord lengthens, assume that the placenta has separated, and pull gently down on the cord to deliver the placenta. Do not wait for or expect a gush of blood before applying traction. Continue to apply counter traction on the uterus with your other hand.
5 If the placenta does not descend and deliver within 1 minute of cord traction the placenta is not separating. Therefore stop traction, wait for the next contraction and repeat the process.
6 As the placenta delivers, the membranes can tear off. To avoid this, hold the placenta in two hands and gently turn it until the membranes are twisted.
7 Gently pull to complete the delivery.
8 If the membranes do tear, wearing sterile gloves gently examine the upper vagina and cervix and use a sterile sponge forceps to remove any fragments of membrane that are present.
9 If the cord is pulled off the placenta, uterine contractions may still push it out, but if this does not happen a manual removal may be needed (see Section 2.13).
10 If the uterus is inverted, push it back immediately (see Section 2.6.H).

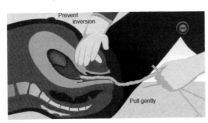

FIGURE 2.3.22 Controlled cord traction for active management of the third stage. Reproduced with the permission of Medical Aid Films, www.medicalaidfilms.org

In Figure 2.3.22 the operator's right hand is holding back the uterus while traction is applied to the cord.

Strong uterine massage (the fourth intervention listed above) should always be undertaken immediately after delivery of the placenta, until the uterus is contracted and remains so. Check the state of contraction of the uterus every 15 minutes for 2 hours, and repeat the massage if at any time the uterus becomes soft and relaxed.

All postpartum women and girls must be closely

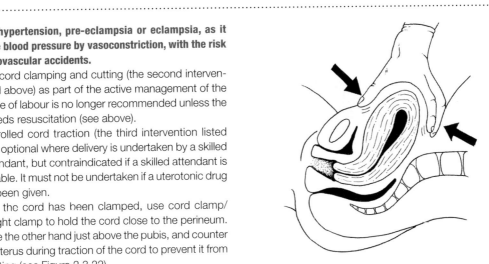

FIGURE 2.3.23 Strong massage applied to cause uterus to contract.

monitored to ensure that PPH does not occur. They should be examined every 15 minutes for the first hour after delivery, and then every 4 hours until 24 hours after delivery.

In order to prevent PPH during or after Caesarean section, oxytocin plus cord contraction is recommended in preference to manual removal of the placenta.

Expectant management of the third stage of labour if uterotonic drugs are not available

Unfortunately, it is not uncommon for hospitals to run out of uterotonic drugs. In this avoidable and dangerous situation, expectant/physiological management should be undertaken.

1 Place the baby on the mother's breast.
2 Leave the cord alone.
3 Observe for the following signs of placental separation:
   • the uterus becomes more rounded and contracted
   • there is lengthening of the cord at the introitus
   • the mother feels uncomfortable, feels a contraction and wants to 'bear down'.
4 Deliver the placenta.
   • Sit the mother upright
   • Encourage her to bear down with a contraction (only after separation of the placenta).
   • Catch the placenta. If membranes are dragging behind, gently twist a few turns and with slight traction and an up-and-down movement deliver the placenta plus the membranes.

Most placentas separate within 1 hour after birth. If this does not happen, seek help.

Controlled cord traction should not be undertaken prior to the separation of the placenta in the absence of uterotonic drugs.

Monitoring after the placenta has been delivered by active or expectant management

Monitor the patient's vital signs, blood pressure, pulse rate and volume, and the state of the uterus (is it contracted?) every 15 minutes for 2 hours after delivery of the placenta.

Examine the placenta for completeness.

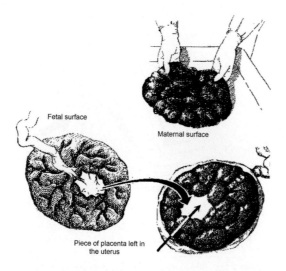

Fetal surface

Maternal surface

Piece of placenta left in the uterus

FIGURE 2.3.24 Examining the placenta in a sink. In this case the fetal and maternal surfaces show a piece missing, which has probably been left in the uterus.

Checking the placenta

Check that the placenta and membranes are intact. If they are not, there are retained products of conception which may pass spontaneously or that may need to be removed manually through the vagina.

Checking for tears

Examine the patient for tears in the cervix or vagina, and repair these as well as any episiotomy (*see* Section 2.13).

Skin-to-skin contact between mother and baby

If neither the mother nor the baby need resuscitation, ensure that the newborn baby is placed in skin-to-skin contact with the mother for at least 1 hour after birth, and encourage and support the baby to attach to and suck on the breast.

This approach recommended by the Baby Friendly Hospital Initiative (step 4) improves temperature control and respiratory function, increases milk production and helps to ensure weight gain for the baby.

Vitamin A for all recently delivered mothers

High-dose vitamin A should be avoided during pregnancy because of the risk of birth defects. A single dose of 200 000 units should be given to all postpartum mothers within 6 weeks of delivery, when the likelihood of pregnancy is very low, and when infants benefit most from its presence in breast milk.

Discharge of mothers and their babies from hospital after uncomplicated deliveries

In high resource settings there is evidence of lower economic costs associated with early discharge (e.g. at 6 hours after delivery compared with 48 hours). However, there is no conclusive evidence for or against the policy of early postnatal discharge in resource-limited healthcare facilities. Care should be taken when extrapolating the results of studies from countries with good socio-economic conditions to communities where resources are scarce. Consideration should also be given to different settings even within the same country (e.g. urban versus rural settings), and the cultural contexts in which the trials are conducted.

Postnatal care for mothers and their babies in resource-limited settings

In resource-limited African settings, 50% of postnatal maternal deaths occur in the first week after birth, with the majority occurring in the first 24 hours. The two most important causes of postnatal maternal death are PPH and puerperal sepsis. Mothers who are HIV positive are most at risk.

One in four deaths in childhood occurs during the neonatal period. Birth asphyxia is the most common cause, and occurs on day 1. Preterm babies most commonly die during the first week of life, and neonatal sepsis is most common after 7 days, especially in low-birth-weight/preterm babies. The origins and markers of many long-term childhood development problems occur or are seen in the first 6 weeks of life.

Despite a lack of research, mothers and their babies should remain in hospital for at least 24 hours after birth in low resource settings in order to ensure that breastfeeding is established and that any complications in the mother and baby are identified and treated. Those with high risk factors should remain in hospital for longer, and before going home all mothers should be trained to recognise danger signs in themselves and their babies.

The WHO has produced a landmark paper on postnatal care in Africa, and Tables 2.3.1 and 2.3.2 summarise their advice.

When and how many postnatal visits should occur?

The optimum number and timing of postnatal care (PNC) visits, especially in resource-limited settings, is a subject of debate. Although no large-scale systematic reviews have been conducted to determine this protocol, three or four postnatal visits have been suggested. Early visits are crucial because the majority of maternal and newborn deaths occur during the first week, most frequently on the first day, and this period is also the key time for promoting healthy behaviours. Each country should make decisions based on the local context and existing care provision, including who can deliver the PNC package and where it can be delivered.

The following information is offered as a guide.

First contact

If the mother is in a healthcare facility, she and her baby should be assessed within 1 hour of birth and again before discharge. Encouraging women to stay in the facility for 24 hours, especially after a complicated birth, should be considered. If birth occurs at home, the first visit should target the crucial first 24 hours after birth.

Follow-up contacts

These are recommended at least at 2–3 days, 6–7 days and 6 weeks after birth.

Extra contacts

Babies who need extra care (LBW babies or those whose mothers are HIV-positive) should have two or three visits in addition to the routine visits.

Where should postnatal care be provided and by whom?

The supervision and integration of postnatal care packages is essential.

TABLE 2.3.1 Routine postnatal care (PNC): What, when, where and who?

What should be routine postnatal care?

Preventive care practices and routine assessments to identify and manage or refer complications for both mother and baby, including the following:

Essential routine PNC for all mothers

1 Assess and check for bleeding; check temperature.

2 Support breastfeeding, checking the breasts and advising how to prevent mastitis.

3 Manage anaemia, promote nutrition and insecticide-treated bed nets, and give vitamin A supplementation.

4 Complete tetanus toxoid immunisation, if required.

5 Provide counselling and a range of options for family planning.

6 Refer for complications such as bleeding, infections or postnatal depression.

7 Counsel on danger signs and home care.

Essential routine PNC for all newborns

1 Assess for danger signs, measure and record weight, and check temperature and feeding.

2 Support optimal feeding practices, particularly exclusive breastfeeding.

3 Promote hygiene and good skin, eye and cord care.

4 If prophylactic eye care is local policy and has not been given, it is still effective up to 12 hours after birth.

5 Promote clean dry cord care.

6 Identify superficial skin infections, such as pus draining from the umbilicus, redness extending from the umbilicus to the skin, more than 10 skin pustules, and swelling, redness and hardness of the skin, and treat or refer if the baby also has danger signs.

7 Ensure warmth by delaying the baby's first bath until after the first 24 hours, practising skin-to-skin care, and putting a hat on the baby.

8 Encourage and facilitate birth registration.

9 Refer the baby for routine immunisations.

10 Counsel on danger signs and home care.

Extra care for low-birth-weight (LBW) or small babies and other vulnerable babies, such as those born to HIV-infected mothers (two or three extra visits)

The majority of newborn deaths occur in LBW babies, many of whom are preterm. Intensive care is not needed to save the majority of these babies. Around one-third could be saved with simple care, including the following:

1 Identify the small baby.

2 Assess for danger signs and manage or refer as appropriate.

3 Provide extra support for breastfeeding, including expressing milk and cup feeding, if needed.

4 Pay extra attention to warmth promotion, such as skin-to-skin care or kangaroo mother care.

5 Ensure early identification and rapid referral of babies who are unable to breastfeed or accept expressed breast milk.

6 Provide extra care for babies whose mothers are HIV-positive, particularly for feeding support (*see* Section 2.8.C).

TABLE 2.3.2 Early identification and referral or management of emergencies for mother and baby

Appropriate detection and management or referral is necessary to save the mother and the baby in the event of life-threatening complications.

Danger signs for the mother

1 Excessive bleeding.

2 Foul-smelling vaginal discharge.

3 Fever with or without chills.

4 Severe abdominal pain.

5 Excessive tiredness or breathlessness.

6 Swollen hands, face and legs with severe headaches or blurred vision.

7 Painful engorged breasts or sore cracked bleeding nipples.

Danger signs for the baby

1 Convulsions.

2 Movement only when stimulated, or no movement even when stimulated.

3 Not feeding well.

4 Fast breathing (more than 60 breaths/minute), grunting or severe chest in-drawing.

5 Fever (above 38°C).

6 Low body temperature (below 35.5°C).

7 Very small baby (less than 1500 grams or born more than 2 months early).

8 Bleeding.

At the hospital

This is more likely if the mother gives birth in hospital, but even then women and babies do not necessarily receive an effective PNC contact before discharge from the healthcare facility, and even if the mother comes to hospital for the birth, she may not return during the first few days after discharge. Where a waiting home is available, the mother and baby could remain there until it is considered safe for them to go home.

Through outreach services:

1 A skilled provider can visit the home to offer PNC to the mother and baby.

2 Home visits from a specially trained community health worker (CHW) linking to the hospital or other healthcare facilities for referral as required.

3 A combination of care in the healthcare facility and at home. PNC may be provided in the hospital following childbirth, and at home during the crucial first 2–3 days, with subsequent visits to a healthcare facility or clinic at 6–7 days and 6 weeks after the birth, when the mother is better able to leave her home.

Further reading

World Health Organization. Reproductive Health Library of videos on YouTube: www.youtube.com/user/WHOrhl

World Health Organization and UNICEF. *Baby Friendly Hospital Initiative*: www.unicef.org.uk/babyfriendly; www.unicef.org/newsline/tenstps.htm

World Health Organization (2006) *Opportunities for Africa's Newborns: Practical data, policy and programmatic support for newborn care in Africa*: www.who.int/pmnch/media/publications/oanfullreport.pdf

2.4 Pathways of care summarising the diagnosis of complications of pregnancy or delivery

(Please note that in all conditions included the presenting symptoms and clinical signs may be atypical and therefore diagnosis more difficult.)

2.4.A Abdominal pain in early pregnancy

TABLE 2.4.A.1 Abdominal pain due to obstetric or gynaecological causes

Presenting symptoms	Clinical signs on presentation	Investigations	Diagnosis	Treatment
Lower abdominal pain, intermittent and very sharp Vomiting	Mass in lower abdomen or on vaginal examination **Warning: when performing a vaginal examination in a patient with abdominal pain who may be pregnant, consider ectopic pregnancy**	Pregnancy test is helpful in early pregnancy	Ovarian cyst which may become twisted (consider torsion if there is severe pain and vomiting)	Consider surgery if this is safe and available
Lower abdominal pain Signs of early pregnancy: tiredness, nausea and/or vomiting (especially in the early morning), breast swelling, increased urinary frequency Light vaginal bleeding (takes > 5 minutes for clean pad to be soaked) Shoulder pain Fainting if ruptured Amenorrhoea with perhaps only one missed period Rectal pain	Shock if ruptured (pale, sweating, fast heart rate > 100 beats/minute), weak pulse volume, low blood pressure (systolic < 90 mmHg), drowsy, irritable, unconscious) **Caution must be exercised when performing a vaginal examination if an ectopic pregnancy is possible, because of the risk of rupture during and due to the examination** Vaginal examination may show signs of early pregnancy (soft uterus), closed cervix, light bleeding, tender mass in one fornix, tenderness with cervical movement	Pregnancy test positive Ultrasound	Ectopic pregnancy which may be ruptured	Prepare operating theatre for **immediate** salpingectomy Treat shock Group and cross-match 4–6 units of blood
Pelvic pain Pain on intercourse Vaginal discharge	Fever Tender lower abdomen Tender on vaginal examination but do not undertake this if ectopic pregnancy is a possibility	Raised white blood cell count Ultrasound High vaginal swab for microscopy, culture and sensitivity	Pelvic inflammatory disease	Antibiotics IV if severe: metronidazole plus: *either* a macrolide such as erythromycin or azithromycin *or* doxycycline or ofloxacin
Lower abdominal pain History of termination of pregnancy attempted (may not be given even if this has occurred) Vaginal bleeding	Fever Vaginal bleeding (moderate to heavy) Purulent vaginal discharge If very severe, peritonitis (see above)	White blood cell count Haemoglobin Blood culture	Septic abortion	Treat shock IV antibiotics May need an intervention such as manual vacuum aspiration to remove infected products of conception, or even hysterectomy (after stabilisation)

TABLE 2.4.A.2 Abdominal pain due to coincidental causes

Presenting symptoms	Clinical signs on presentation	Investigations	Diagnosis	Treatment
Lower abdominal pain Nausea and/or vomiting Anorexia Constipation may occur	Low-grade fever (> 37.5°C) Tenderness of the right iliac fossa, sometimes with rebound Tender in the right iliac fossa on rectal examination (care is needed if ectopic pregnancy is a possibility)	Pregnancy test Raised white blood cell count Ultrasound if skilled	Acute appendicitis	Appendicectomy
Severe abdominal pain Vomiting	High fever Abdominal distension Rigid abdomen Absent bowel sounds Shock (see above for signs)		Peritonitis	Treat shock IV antibiotics Nasogastric tube **Immediate laparotomy in operating theatre**
Pain on passing urine Increased frequency of passing urine Nocturia	Fever (unusual)	Microscope urine Stick tests for infection (if available) Urine culture and sensitivity (if available)	Cystitis	Antibiotics by mouth
Pain in the lower abdomen or loin Nausea and/or vomiting Increased frequency of passing urine with or without dysuria Rigors	High fever Tenderness of one of the loins over the kidney Normal bowel sounds	Microscope urine Stick tests for infection (if available) Urine culture and sensitivity (if available)	Pyelonephritis	IV antibiotics (IV gentamicin if patient has rigors or is shocked) In the case of shock, initiate immediate treatment

2.4.B Abdominal pain in late pregnancy

TABLE 2.4.B.1 Abdominal pain due to obstetric causes

Symptoms	Signs	Diagnosis	Investigations	Treatment
Intermittent lower abdominal pain Vaginal fluid loss before 37 weeks' gestation suggesting premature rupture of membranes Light vaginal bleeding*	Palpable uterine contractions Cervical dilatation Check for prolapsed cord if there is rupture of membranes	**Possible preterm labour**	Partogram	Give two 12 mg doses of betamethasone or dexamethasone IM 12 hours apart Tocolysis only to give time for the steroids to work. Nifedipine 20 mg orally, followed by 20 mg orally after 30 minutes. If contractions persist, therapy can be continued with 20 mg orally every 3–8 hours for 48–72 hours, with a maximum dose of 160 mg/24 hours
Intermittent lower abdominal pain Vaginal fluid loss after 37 weeks' gestation suggesting rupture of membranes Light vaginal bleeding	Palpable uterine contractions Cervical dilatation and effacement Check for prolapsed cord if there is rupture of membranes	**Term labour**	Partogram	*See* Section 2.3

(continued)

Symptoms	Signs	Diagnosis	Investigations	Treatment
Lower abdominal pain, intermittent and very sharp	Mass in lower abdomen or on vaginal examination. Difficult to feel in pregnancy per abdomen or per vagina as the uterus is enlarged	**Ovarian cyst** which may become twisted (this is very rare in late pregnancy)	Ultrasound	May need laparotomy
Severe constant abdominal pain Light or heavy vaginal bleeding* Fetal movements stop	Shock Tense and very tender uterus on abdominal examination Fetal distress or absent fetal heart	**Placental abruption**	Ultrasound	**Call for surgical and anaesthetic help** Left lateral tilt or recovery position IV fluid boluses for shock Cross-match 4 units of blood and freeze-dried plasma if available Deliver fetus as soon as possible if alive
There is a change (usually during labour) from intermittent labour contractions to a constant pain which may become less after rupture has occurred Sometimes there is an oxytocin drip in place Vaginal bleeding which may be light or heavy History of a previous Caesarean section or other operation on the uterus	Shock Abdominal distension Tender over the uterus, with more easily palpated fetal parts Absent fetal movements and heart sounds	**Ruptured uterus**	Ultrasound may help diagnosis, **but must not delay laparotomy**	**Call for surgical and anaesthetic help** Treat shock if present Cross-match 4 units of blood and freeze-dried plasma if available Prepare theatre for laparotomy after patient is stable
Foul-smelling watery vaginal discharge Lower abdominal pain Premature labour or premature rupture of membranes Light vaginal bleeding	Fever Tender over the lower abdomen and uterus Possible fetal distress	**Chorio-amnionitis**	White blood cell count Blood culture Discharge for microscopy, culture and sensitivity	IV antibiotics before urgent delivery, whatever the gestational age: Ampicillin 2 g IV every 6 hours *plus* gentamicin 80 mg IV/IM every 8 hours or 5 mg/kg body weight IV/IM once every 24 hours *plus* metronidazole 500 mg IV every 8 hours
Purulent, foul-smelling lochia Lower abdominal pain Light vaginal bleeding	Fever Tender uterus Shock	**Endometritis after birth (puerperal sepsis)**	Raised white blood cell count Blood culture Lochia for microscopy, culture and sensitivity	Treat shock IV antibiotics: Ampicillin 2 g IV every 6 hours *plus* gentamicin 80 mg IV/IM every 8 hours or 5 mg/kg body weight IV/IM once every 24 hours *plus* metronidazole 500 mg IV every 8 hours

(*continued*)

Symptoms	Signs	Diagnosis	Investigations	Treatment
Lower abdominal pain Rare in late pregnancy, but may present postnatally	Swinging fever Swelling in adnexa or pouch of Douglas Tender uterus Ultrasound	**Pelvic abscess**	Raised white blood cell count Blood culture Pus for microscopy, culture and sensitivity	IV antibiotics: Ampicillin 2 g IV every 6 hours *plus* gentamicin 80 mg IV/IM every 8 hours or 5 mg/kg body weight IV/IM once every 24 hours *plus* metronidazole 500 mg IV every 8 hours Surgical drainage
Upper abdominal pain	Headache Visual disturbance Oedema	**Severe pre-eclampsia with impending eclampsia**	Raised blood pressure Protein in urine > ++	Magnesium sulphate Urgent delivery of fetus

* Light bleeding is defined as taking longer than 5 minutes for a clean pad or cloth to become soaked. Heavy bleeding is defined as taking less than 5 minutes for a clean pad or cloth to become soaked.

TABLE 2.4.B.2 Abdominal pain due to coincidental causes

Symptoms	Signs	Diagnosis	Investigations	Treatment
Lower abdominal pain Nausea and/or vomiting Anorexia	Low-grade fever (> 37.5°C) Tenderness of the right iliac fossa, sometimes with rebound Tender in the right iliac fossa on rectal examination	**Appendicitis**	White blood cell count elevated Ultrasound if skilled	Appendicectomy
Severe abdominal pain Vomiting	High fever Abdominal distension Rigid abdomen Absent bowel sounds Shock (see above for signs)	**Peritonitis**		Treat shock Consider immediate laparotomy: call surgeon and anaesthetist and prepare operating theatre IV antibiotics: Ampicillin 2 g IV every 6 hours *plus* gentamicin 80 mg IV/IM every 8 hours or 5 mg/kg body weight IV/IM once every 24 hours *plus* metronidazole 500 mg IV every 8 hours Nasogastric tube on open drainage Immediate laparotomy in operating theatre
Pain on passing urine Increased frequency of passing urine Nocturia	Rarely fever	**Cystitis**	Microscope urine Stick tests for infection (if available) Urine culture and sensitivity if available	Oral antibiotics
Pain in the lower abdomen or loin Nausea and/or vomiting Increased frequency of passing urine	High fever Tenderness in one of the loins over the kidney Normal bowel sounds	**Pyelonephritis**	Microscope urine Stick tests for infection (if available) Urine culture and sensitivity if possible	Ampicillin 2 g IV every 6 hours *plus* gentamicin 80 mg IV/IM every 8 hours or 5 mg/kg body weight IV/IM once every 24 hours *plus* metronidazole 500 mg IV every 8 hours

2.4.C Vaginal bleeding in early pregnancy

In all cases a pregnancy test must be performed.

TABLE 2.4.C.1 Vaginal bleeding in early pregnancy

Symptoms	Signs	Diagnosis	Treatment
Light bleeding Cramping lower abdominal pain	Closed cervix	**Threatened miscarriage**	Wait and see
Light bleeding Abdominal pain, shoulder tip pain and/or rectal pain Feeling faint on standing up, or fainting	Shock Vaginal examination should be undertaken carefully (*see* Section 2.5.D.i)	Ectopic pregnancy	*See* Section 2.5.D.i
Heavy bleeding No history of products of conception passed Cramping lower abdominal pain	Dilated cervix Tender uterus that corresponds to dates Shock if bleeding is severe Severe anaemia if bleeding is prolonged	**Inevitable miscarriage**	Cross-match blood and freeze-dried plasma if available Treat shock if present Evacuate products of conception (ideally by manual vacuum aspiration) Give iron if the patient has anaemia
Light bleeding Mild cramping lower abdominal pain History of products of conception passed	Closed cervix Soft uterus that is smaller than expected for dates	**Complete miscarriage**	Check haemoglobin levels Give iron if the patient has anaemia
Heavy bleeding Nausea and/or vomiting Cramping lower abdominal pain Passage of some products of conception which look like grapes	Dilated cervix Soft uterus, larger than expected for dates	Molar pregnancy	Evacuate products of conception (ideally by manual vacuum aspiration). If symptoms persist and there is continued vaginal bleeding, repeat urine pregnancy test Measure HCG levels if possible Screen for pre-eclampsia (measure blood pressure, and urine for protein) Follow up for abnormal bleeding; if it occurs, perform a vaginal examination, ultrasound scan and measurement of HCG levels
A history of pregnancy and self-induced abortion may or may not be given Lower abdominal pain Prolonged light to heavy bleeding	Lower abdominal tenderness Foul-smelling vaginal discharge Pus coming from the cervix Fever Tender uterus with pain on moving the cervix Shock due to haemorrhage and/or sepsis	Induced abortion with infection	Treat shock if present IV antibiotics: Ampicillin 2 gram IV loading dose, then 1 gram IV every 6 hours *plus* gentamicin 80 mg IV/IM every 8 hours or 5 mg/kg body weight IV/IM once every 24 hours *plus* metronidazole 500 mg IV every 8 hours until the patient has been fever-free for 48 hours Manual vacuum aspiration (risk of uterine perforation): only when pulse and blood pressure are improving and after 24 hours of appropriate IV antibiotics and good urine output of > 30 mL/hour Correct DIC if there is a blood clotting disorder If the patient remains shocked after resuscitation and/or heavy vaginal bleeding continues, they will need earlier surgery After ensuring that there are no vaginal or cervical injuries, irrigate the vagina with sterile normal saline, Ringer-lactate or Hartmann's solution to remove any herbs or caustic substances that may have been used to induce the abortion

(continued)

Symptoms	Signs	Diagnosis	Treatment
A history of pregnancy and self-induced abortion may or may not be given Lower abdominal pain Prolonged light to heavy bleeding Severe abdominal pain Urinary or faecal incontinence. Faecal discharge from vagina	Severe abdominal tenderness with rigid abdomen and ileus if there is peritonitis Foul-smelling vaginal discharge Pus coming from the cervix Fever Tender uterus with pain on moving cervix Shock due to haemorrhage and/or sepsis	Induced abortion with injuries to genital tract and to bowel or bladder	Stabilise if shocked Laparotomy to repair injuries Manual vacuum aspiration (high risk of uterine perforation) after checking that there are no tears in the vagina or cervix which need repair Appropriate IV antibiotics as above

Light bleeding is defined as taking longer than 5 minutes for a clean pad or cloth to become soaked. Heavy bleeding is defined as taking less than 5 minutes for a clean pad or cloth to become soaked.

2.4.D Vaginal bleeding in late pregnancy

TABLE 2.4.D.1 Vaginal bleeding in late pregnancy

Symptoms	Clinical signs	Diagnosis	Treatment
Severe constant abdominal pain Light or heavy vaginal bleeding Reduced fetal movements	Shock Tense and tender uterus on abdominal examination Fetal distress or absent fetal heart rate	Placental abruption	**Call for surgical and anaesthetic help** Left lateral tilt or recovery position IV fluid boluses for shock Cross-match 4 units of blood and freeze-dried plasma if available Deliver fetus as soon as possible if viable, either by inducing labour or by Caesarean section
Vaginal bleeding which can be light or very heavy Bleeding can be precipitated by intercourse or artificial rupture of membranes No pain	Soft uterus Presenting part may be higher than expected Fetus may be distressed, non-viable or uncompromised with normal movements and normal fetal heart rate pattern Ultrasound will show placenta praevia **Do not undertake digital vaginal examination, as this may precipitate massive bleeding which can be fatal** Shock may be present, depending on the severity of bleeding and its duration	Placenta praevia	Call for surgical and anaesthetic help Treat shock if present If preterm and not bleeding too heavily, give steroids, admit for bed rest, and only perform a Caesarean section if there is a further bleed Cross-match ideally 4 units of blood
Usually a change from intermittent labour contractions to constant pain Oxytocin may be being used to augment contractions Vaginal bleeding which may be light or heavy History of a previous Caesarean section or other surgery on the uterus	Shock (especially an increasing heart rate detected ideally on partograph) Abdominal distension Tender over uterus, with more easily palpable fetal parts Absent fetal movements and heart sounds	Ruptured uterus	**Call for surgical and anaesthetic help** Treat shock if present Cross-match ideally 4 units of blood Prepare theatre for laparotomy while resuscitating the patient

(continued)

Symptoms	Clinical signs	Diagnosis	Treatment
Heavy vaginal and other bleeding	Bleeding from sites in addition to the vagina Signs of other conditions that may be responsible, such as: • placental abruption • pre-eclampsia or eclampsia (high blood pressure and proteinuria) • retained dead fetus • septicaemia, including intrauterine sepsis • incompatible blood transfusion • amniotic fluid embolism	Coagulation failure	Fresh blood transfusion Blood products such as platelets, fresh-frozen plasma and cryoprecipitate if available
Light vaginal bleeding Bleeding can be precipitated by intercourse or artificial rupture of membranes No pain	Fetal distress or death	Vasa praevia (placental blood vessels lying in the membranes and in front of the baby's head)	If diagnosed by ultrasound before labour, plan for Caesarean section

2.4.E Vaginal bleeding after delivery

TABLE 2.4.E.1 Vaginal bleeding after delivery

Symptoms	Signs	Possible diagnosis
Immediate heavy bleeding after birth	Uterus soft and not contracted	Atonic uterus
Immediate heavy bleeding after birth	Uterus contracted	Trauma to cervix, vagina or perineum
Bleeding which may be light if clot is blocking cervix	Placenta not delivered within 30 minutes of birth	Retained placenta
Bleeding which is usually light but continues for many hours	Portion of placenta missing Uterus contracted	Retained placental parts
Bleeding for > 24 hours	Portion of placenta missing Foul-smelling lochia may be present Fever may be present Severe anaemia	Retained placental parts with or without infection
Lower abdominal pain of varying intensity Immediate but usually light bleeding	Uterus not felt on abdominal palpation Inverted uterus may be seen at vulva Bradycardia may be present Shock	Inverted uterus
Usually during labour there has been a change from intermittent labour contractions to a constant pain which may become less severe after rupture has occurred Sometimes an oxytocin drip is in place Vaginal bleeding which may be light or heavy History of a previous Caesarean section or other surgery on the uterus	Shock Abdominal distension Tender over uterus	Ruptured uterus (more likely before delivery of the baby)

2.4.F The diagnosis of breathing difficulties in pregnancy

All of the symptoms and signs may not be present for all of the diagnoses listed in Table 2.4.F.1, and it is difficult to distinguish between some of them; some symptoms and signs will be a diagnosis of exclusion. It is therefore important to treat the treatable.

TABLE 2.4.F.1 Breathing difficulties in pregnancy

Symptoms that may be present	Clinical signs that may be present	Diagnosis
Weakness Tiredness	Pale conjunctiva, nail beds, palms of hands and soles of feet	Severe anaemia
Weakness Tiredness Dyspnoea	Signs of severe anaemia Oedema of legs Basal lung crepitations Tachycardia Gallop rhythm Enlarged liver Elevated jugular venous pressure (JVP)	Heart failure due to severe anaemia
Dyspnoea	Heart murmur Irregular heart rhythm Oedema of face and legs Basal lung crepitations Tachycardia Gallop rhythm Enlarged liver Elevated JVP	Heart failure due to heart disease
Dyspnoea Cough Pleuritic chest pain	Fever Tachypnoea Respiratory distress Reduced air entry Bronchial breathing Pleural rub Rhonchi Crepitations	Acute lower respiratory tract infection (pneumonia)
Dyspnoea Cough	Respiratory distress Tachypnoea Wheezing Rhonchi Reduced air entry	Asthma
Dyspnoea	Hypertension Proteinuria Oedema of face and legs Basal lung crepitations Tachycardia Gallop rhythm Enlarged liver Elevated JVP	Pulmonary oedema due to hypertension and severe pre-eclampsia
Dyspnoea Swelling of the leg Pleuritic chest pain	Tachypnoea Haemoptysis Leg pain/swelling Cyanosis Shock Central chest pain Elevated JVP Pleural rub	Pulmonary embolus

(continued)

Symptoms that may be present	Clinical signs that may be present	Diagnosis
Collapse Dyspnoea	Shock Apnoea Cardiac arrest Cyanosis Coagulopathy	Amniotic fluid embolus

2.5 Life-threatening complications of pregnancy and delivery

2.5.A The pregnant woman or girl with shock during pregnancy and the puerperium

Introduction

The pregnant patient who is shocked due to hypovolaemia (the most common cause of shock; see below) will be pale, cold and clammy, have a rapid weak pulse, and may have a reduced conscious level, be confused or be unconscious. If the shock is due to sepsis, the patient's skin may become warm from vasodilatation.

Shock results from an acute failure of circulatory function. Maintenance of adequate tissue perfusion depends on the following:

- a pump (the heart): failure leads to cardiogenic shock
- the correct type and volume of fluid (blood): failure leads to hypovolaemic shock
- controlled vessels (arteries, veins and capillaries): failure leads to distributive shock
- unobstructed flow: failure leads to obstructive shock
- red blood cells: failure leads to dissociative shock.

The most common causes of shock are hypovolaemia from any cause, septicaemia, the effects of trauma and very severe anaemia.

Classification of causes of shock

Common causes are shown in bold type (see Table 2.5.A.1), and all causes are described in more detail in the relevant sections of this book.

Diagnostic pointers

During assessment and resuscitation, a focused history of the previous 24 hours and previous illnesses should be obtained. This may point to the likeliest working diagnosis for emergency treatment.

- A history of vomiting and/or diarrhoea points to **fluid loss**, either externally (e.g. **gastroenteritis**) or into the abdomen (e.g. appendicitis and peritonitis, early stages of gastroenteritis).
- A history of bleeding. This may be vaginal bleeding, or 'silent' bleeding into the abdominal cavity (as in ectopic pregnancy, placental abruption or ruptured uterus).
- Fever or a rash points to **septicaemia**.
- Urticaria, angioneurotic oedema or a history of allergen exposure points to **anaphylaxis**.
- Heart failure points to **severe anaemia** (usually with severe pallor), valve disease or cardiomyopathy.
- A history of sickle-cell disease or diarrhoeal illness and low haemoglobin levels points to **acute haemolysis**.
- A history of major trauma points to blood loss, and, more rarely, tension pneumothorax, haemothorax, cardiac tamponade or spinal cord transection.

TABLE 2.5.A.1 Causes of shock

Cardiogenic	Arrhythmias Cardiomyopathy **Heart failure** Cardiac valvular disease Myocardial contusion
Hypovolaemic	**Haemorrhage** **Gastroenteritis** Volvulus **Burns** **Peritonitis**
Distributive (relative hypovolaemia)	**Septicaemia** Anaphylaxis Anaesthesia Spinal cord injury
Obstructive	Tension pneumothorax Haemopneumothorax Flail chest Cardiac tamponade Pulmonary embolism
Dissociative	**Very severe anaemia** Carbon monoxide poisoning

- Severe **tachycardia** or signs of heart failure point to an **arrhythmia** or a cardiomyopathy.
- A history of polyuria, sighing respiration and a very high blood glucose level points to diabetes (*see* Section 2.7.D on **diabetic ketoacidosis**).
- A history of drug ingestion points to **poisoning**.

Physiology of shock

Shock is defined as an acute failure of circulatory function, leading to impaired delivery of nutrients and oxygen to, and impaired removal of waste products from, the body tissues.

Shock is a progressive syndrome, but its effects can be divided into the following progression.

Phase 1 (compensated) shock

TABLE 2.5.A.2 Compensated shock

Physiology	Clinical effects
Sympathetic reflexes maintain cardiac output by: • increased systemic arterial resistance • decreased blood flow to non-essential organs • increased heart rate • constriction of the venous reservoir • angiotensin and renin release leading to renal preservation of salt and water and reabsorption of intestinal fluid	Normal systolic blood pressure (diastolic blood pressure may be increased due to vasoconstriction) Tachycardia Cool skin and increased capillary refill time Decreased urine output (< 0.5 mL/kg/hour, or < 30 mL/hour in the mother) Confusion/agitation

Phase 2 (uncompensated) shock

TABLE 2.5.A.3 Uncompensated shock

Physiology	Clinical effects
Failure of compensatory mechanisms with decreased tissue perfusion leading to: • increased anaerobic metabolism, leading to lactic acidosis • acidosis impairs cardiac function and cellular homeostasis, leading to a further decline in cellular metabolic functions • inflammatory mediators are released which further impair cell function and vital systems such as the coagulation cascade and platelet function	Hypotension Cold peripheries and markedly increased capillary refill time Acidotic breathing Absent urine output Impaired cerebral function

Phase 3 (irreversible) shock

The diagnosis of irreversible shock is a retrospective one.

Severe damage to vital organs leads to inevitable death due to diminished energy stores which cannot be replenished even if circulatory function is restored. Therefore early recognition and effective treatment of shock are vital.

Physiology of septic shock

Tissue perfusion is decreased through the action of bacterial toxins and host inflammatory mediators. This results in the following:

- abnormal distribution of blood in the microcirculation, sometimes with peripheral vasodilatation
- loss of intravascular fluid into the extravascular space due to capillary leakage
- depressed myocardial contractility due to toxins and acidosis
- although cardiac output may be normal or raised from baseline, it may still be too low to deliver sufficient oxygen and nutrients to the tissues, because in septic shock the cells do not use oxygen properly. There appears to be a block at the mitochondrial level in the mechanism of oxygen uptake. This progressive deterioration in cell oxygen consumption can lead to multiple organ failure.

Early (compensated) septic shock

This is characterised by the following:

- raised cardiac output with tachycardia

- (sometimes) decreased systemic resistance, warm extremities and a wide pulse pressure
- (sometimes) increased systemic resistance with cold extremities and a raised diastolic blood pressure
- hyperpyrexia and hyperventilation
- mental confusion.

All of these signs may be minimal. Mental confusion in particular needs to be looked for carefully, if septic shock is not to be overlooked at this stage. In the group with increased systemic resistance, decreased capillary return is a useful sign in these circumstances.

A pregnant patient may lose 1200–1500 mL of blood before showing obvious signs of shock (20% of circulating blood volume, 6–7 litres). Maternal signs of hypovolaemia are late.

Fetal distress may be the first sign of shock in pregnancy.

Graphs to indicate the progression of shock in relation to clinical signs
Stage 1

At first, with less than 1000 mL of blood loss, there are very few signs and symptoms. The patient may be slightly anxious, and the pulse and respiratory rate are slightly elevated but still within the normal range. Therefore, if this is the first recording taken, you may think it is normal for this particular patient, but it may in fact be abnormal for her (*see* Figure 2.5.A.1).

Note that in the anaemic mother the signs may be worse and the risks may be greater earlier than this.

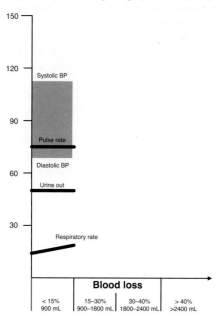

FIGURE 2.5.A.1 Stage 1 shock.

Stage 2

After further blood loss, the perfusion to organs is maintained by the body's stress response. This increases the diastolic pressure, with a resultant reduction in the pulse pressure, and the pulse rate continues to rise, reaching over 100 beats/minute (see Figure 2.5.A.2).

Meanwhile, urine is not being produced and the mother's respiratory rate starts to increase.

Note that in the anaemic mother the signs may be worse and the risks may be greater earlier than this.

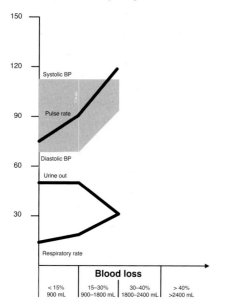

FIGURE 2.5.A.2 Stage 2 shock.

Stage 3

When 2000 mL of blood have been lost, a drop in blood pressure is observed, along with other signs and symptoms of hypovolaemia. It must be emphasised that

hypotension, which is commonly used as an indicator of the severity of blood loss, is in fact a very late sign.

Generally, the pulse rate should be lower than the systolic blood pressure. If the pulse rate is higher than the systolic pressure, the patient is in grave danger (see Figure 2.5.A.3).

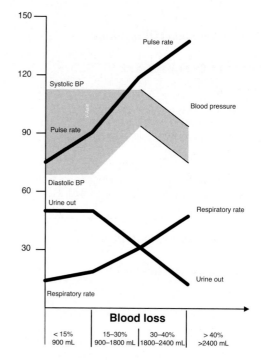

FIGURE 2.5.A.3 Stage 3 shock.

Note that in the anaemic mother the signs may be worse and the risks may be greater earlier than this.

Stage 4

If more than 2000 mL of blood are lost, this is an uncompensated very late stage of hypovolaemia, which could very rapidly result in death if emergency measures are not initiated immediately (see Figure 2.5.A.4).

Note that in the anaemic mother the signs may be worse and the risks may be greater earlier than this.

In late (uncompensated) septic shock:
- hypotension occurs as a result of decreased vascular resistance, and even with a normal or raised cardiac output, shock develops
- the cardiac output may fall gradually over several hours, or precipitously within minutes
- as tissue hypoxia develops, plasma lactic acid levels increase
- survival depends on the maintenance of a hyperdynamic state.

Choice of fluid for volume replacement

Crystalloid or colloid fluids are appropriate for volume replacement in shock (see Section 2.8.B).

However, dextrose/glucose infusions (particularly hypotonic ones such as 5% glucose or 0.18% saline in 5% glucose) do not constitute appropriate fluid resuscitation, and can be dangerous because they lower serum sodium levels, which can result in seizures and brain swelling.

Compared with colloids, crystalloid fluids:
- diffuse more readily into the interstitial space

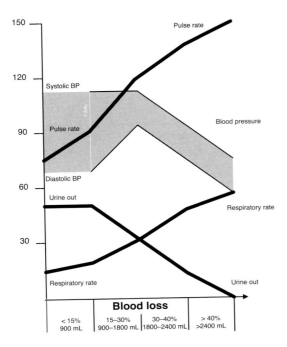

FIGURE 2.5.A.4 Stage 4 shock.

- may be associated with more peripheral oedema
- where capillary leak exists, allow more water to enter the interstitial space, because of the lower osmotic pressure
- need two to three times the volume of colloids to expand the vascular space
- have been reported to be associated with lower mortality.

Nevertheless, the use of both crystalloids and colloids is appropriate, although crystalloids (e.g. Ringer-lactate or Hartmann's solution or normal saline) are more likely to be available.

Choice of crystalloid

The fluid that was traditionally infused into the circulation for the management of shock was normal saline (0.9% sodium chloride). This fluid has increasingly been shown to be dangerous, especially in the sick patient. An infusion of normal saline causes a hyperchloraemic acidosis (a high chloride concentration leading to an acidosis) which, in the shocked patient, who is already acidotic, causes a deterioration in the health of cells in vital organs, even though perfusion of the cells has been improved by the increased circulating volume.

There are sodium-containing alternatives to normal saline that are safer as they approximate more closely to human serum/plasma in content (*see* Table 1.6.1), although they are slightly more expensive. We recommend the use of either of these alternatives – **Ringer-lactate and Hartmann's solution**, which are widely available – for all fluid replacement. Hospitals are advised to change their standard crystalloid from 0.9% ('normal') saline to Ringer-lactate or Hartmann's solutions as soon as possible.

As not all hospitals will have access to these solutions immediately, there may sometimes be no alternative but to start fluid replacement with normal saline. However, if more than 20 mL/kg needs to be given, then one of the safer alternatives should be used in very sick patients if at all possible.

Blood

If there is significant blood loss or pre-existing severe anaemia in the face of any blood loss, blood will be needed. Full cross-matching takes about 1 hour to perform. For urgent need, type-specific non-cross-matched blood (which is ABO- and rhesus-compatible, but has a higher incidence of transfusion reactions) takes about 15 minutes to prepare. In dire emergencies, O-negative blood must be given.

Fluids should be warmed, especially if they are needed in large volumes. In the absence of heaters, bags of fluid or blood can be warmed by placing them under the clothes next to the skin of a relative. Even this takes time, and another method is to pass the tubing of an IV set through a bowl containing warm water.

Primary assessment and resuscitation

Suspect or anticipate shock if at least one of the following is present:
- bleeding in early pregnancy (e.g. miscarriage, induced abortion, ectopic pregnancy or molar pregnancy)
- bleeding in late pregnancy or labour (e.g. placenta praevia, abruptio placentae, ruptured uterus)
- bleeding after childbirth (e.g. ruptured uterus, uterine atony, tears of genital tract, retained placenta or placental fragments)
- infection (e.g. induced or septic miscarriage/abortion, chorioamnionitis, endometritis, pyelonephritis)
- trauma (e.g. injury to the uterus or bowel during induced abortion, ruptured uterus, tears of the genital tract).

Primary assessment indicating shock

- Fast, weak pulse (≥ 100–110 beats/minute).
- Pallor (especially of the inner eyelids, palms or around the mouth).
- Sweatiness or cold clammy skin.
- Rapid breathing (> 30 breaths/minute).
- Anxiety, reduced conscious level, confusion or unconsciousness.
- Low blood pressure (systolic pressure less than 90 mmHg is a late sign).
- Reduced urine output (< 30 mL/hour).

Resuscitation

If heavy bleeding is the suspected cause of shock, take simultaneous steps to stop the bleeding. These consist of uterotonic drugs such as oxytocin or misoprostol, uterine massage, bimanual compression, aortic compression and condom catheter, and anti-shock garment in postpartum haemorrhage. Urgent surgical intervention may be required (e.g. for ruptured ectopic pregnancy).

Airway

Try at the same time to stop bleeding by surgical or specific medical treatments as urgently as possible.
- Use an opening manoeuvre if the airway is not open or is partially obstructed. Keep the airway open. If there is improvement but the airway closes without active opening support, consider airway adjuncts to maintain the airway if the patient is unconscious (P or U on the AVPU scale).
- **Suction** if necessary.
- The airway may need to be maintained and protected by **intubation**, using experienced senior help (if available).

Breathing

- Provide a high concentration of oxygen through a face mask with a reservoir bag if there is adequate spontaneous respiration.
- For patients with inadequate ventilation, respiration should be supported with oxygen via a **bag-mask**, and experienced senior help should be summoned (if available).

Circulation

- Gain IV access.
  - Use a short, wide-bore (16- to 18-gauge) IV cannula if possible for IV access.
  - Access via the internal or external jugular veins is a good option if peripheral access is impossible. Long saphenous vein cut-down may also be considered, and the new intraosseous drill can be used if all else fails (*see* Section 8.4.B).
  - **Applying pressure on the site of the bleeding can be valuable in many circumstances, including postpartum haemorrhage (*see* Section 2.5.D.iv) and external haemorrhage from major trauma.**
  - Try to obtain two vascular access sites to give large volumes quickly, and in case one line is lost.
  - A blood pressure cuff can be used to speed up infusions in emergency situations. Wrap the cuff around the blood/fluid bag and place it inside a non-compressible bag. (*see* Figure 2.5.A.5).
- Use the left lateral tilt position or recovery position to minimise aortic and vena caval compression, and to reduce the risk of aspiration in patients after 20 weeks' gestation.
- Elevate the legs by raising the foot of the bed.
- Consider using a non-pneumatic anti-shock garment (NASG).
- Give **an initial rapid bolus of 500 mL to 1 L of Ringer-lactate or Hartmann's solution or blood if the patient is haemorrhaging. A colloid at the same dose can also be given, if available.** It is essential that the bolus is given as rapidly as possible. In the absence of syringe pumps, it should be manually pushed in using a 20- to 50-mL syringe (using a three-way tap and link to an IV giving set).
- Further boluses of 500–1000 mL will usually be required in the first hour. Once more than 2 litres have been given IV, complications such as pulmonary or cerebral oedema may occur. Expert help, including CVP monitoring, is very valuable if it is available.

The concept of 'targeted crystalloid fluid-resuscitation' is important and requires urgent research into shock due to obstetric haemorrhage. Here the initial boluses of IV crystalloids required to treat shock would only be given to keep the vital organs (especially the brain, heart and kidneys) perfused before blood becomes available and, of most importance, surgery and specific medical treatments to stop the bleeding have started to take effect. The administration of too large a volume of IV crystalloids fluids may increase the blood pressure, damage clotting and disrupt early clot formation.

If this approach is used when giving boluses of crystalloid in shock due to bleeding (before blood is available and before procedures undertaken to stop haemorrhage are effective), only the amount necessary to keep the blood pressure at a level sufficient to perfuse the vital organs is given. There is no clear evidence to indicate the precise blood pressure that should be achieved in a woman in shock due to haemorrhage. However, **adequate perfusion of vital organs** may best be indicated by **a radial pulse which can be palpated and an alert conscious level.** During pregnancy, the adequacy of the fetal heart rate may also be helpful.

Our personal practice, especially in low resource settings, is to start with IV boluses of 500 mL of crystalloid and reassess after each bolus, always aiming to stop haemorrhage and obtain blood for transfusion as soon as possible. In situations where there is brisk active blood loss and delay in obtaining blood or effective intervention to halt the bleeding, several boluses of crystalloids may be required. The importance of undertaking measures to halt the bleeding and obtaining blood for transfusion rapidly cannot be overstated.

Tranexamic acid

If bleeding is the cause of shock, this inexpensive and safe drug can be helpful. The drug should be started as soon as possible after the onset of major haemorrhage, in order to be effective.

The loading dose is 1 gram over 10 minutes followed by an IV infusion of a further 1 gram over a period of 8 hours. The slow IV bolus dose is given by injecting 1 gram of tranexamic acid into a 100-mL bag of 0.9% saline and letting it run through over a period of about 10–20 minutes (the exact timing is not crucial). The 8-hour infusion is given by injecting 1 gram of tranexamic acid into a 500-mL bag of 0.9% saline and giving it over a period of 8 hours (approximately 60 mL/hour).

Keep the patient warm but do not overheat.

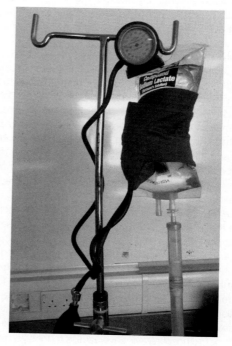

FIGURE 2.5.A.5 Pressure bag over the bag of Ringer-lactate or Hartmann's solution to increase infusion rate.

Transfuse blood as soon as possible to replace blood loss.

Determine the cause of bleeding

- If bleeding occurs **before the first 24–28 weeks of pregnancy,** suspect miscarriage, induced abortion, ectopic pregnancy or molar pregnancy.
- If bleeding occurs **after the first 24–28 weeks or during labour, but before delivery**, suspect placenta praevia, abruptio placentae or ruptured uterus.
- If bleeding occurs **soon after childbirth**, suspect atonic uterus, retained placental fragments, ruptured uterus, tears of the genital tract or occasionally an inverted uterus.
- In all cases consider the possibility of a primary or secondary blood clotting disorder.

Cases where infection is the suspected cause of shock

- Collect appropriate samples (blood cultures, urine, pus, swabs) for microbial culture before starting antibiotics, if facilities are available but do not delay giving antibiotics because of specimen collection.
- Give a combination of antibiotics to cover aerobic and anaerobic infections, and continue until the patient has been fever-free for 48 hours:
  - benzyl penicillin 2.4 grams initially, then 1.2 grams IV 6-hourly or ampicillin 2 grams initially, then 1 g IV/IM every 6 hours plus gentamicin 80 mg IV/IM 8-hourly or 5 mg/kg body weight IV/IM once every 24 hours plus metronidazole 500 mg IV every 8 hours
  - or ceftriaxone 2–4 grams IV once daily or cefotaxime 2 grams 12-hourly IV plus metronidazole 500 mg IV every 8 hours.
- **If the patient is in shock, do not give antibiotics by mouth or IM, as they will not be absorbed.**
- Reassess the patient's condition for signs of improvement.

Cases where haemorrhage due to trauma is the cause of shock

- Try and stop haemorrhage and if appropriate prepare for surgical intervention.
- Give 500 mL IV crystalloid fluid resuscitation boluses and reassess circulation after each bolus until blood is available (see above).

General issues

Avoid giving IV boluses of 5% dextrose or dextrose saline (4%/0.18%), as they cause hyponatraemia, and may result in cerebral oedema and death.

An antibiotic such as cefotaxime or ceftriaxone should always be given IV when a diagnosis of septicaemia is made obvious by the presence of a purpuric rash (suspect meningococcal infection).

BOX 2.5.A.1 Whole blood clotting time

If laboratory clotting tests are not available:

- ■ Transfer 2 mL of venous blood into a small dry clean plain glass test tube (approximately 10 mm × 75 mm).
- ■ Hold the tube in your closed fist to keep it warm (+ 37°C).
- ■ After 4 minutes, tip the tube slowly to see if a clot is forming. Then tip it again every minute until the blood clots and the tube can be turned upside down.
- ■ **Failure of a clot to form after 7 minutes, or formation of a soft clot that breaks down easily, suggests a blood clotting disorder.**

Take blood for the following investigations (if available): full blood count (FBC), renal and liver function tests, blood culture, cross-matching, blood clotting, glucose stick test and glucose laboratory test.

- Catheterise and monitor urine output.
- If peritonitis is possible, add metronidazole IV.

Cases where a blood clotting disorder is present and fractionated blood products are not available

- Use fresh whole blood (straight from the donor if possible). In general, in obstetric emergencies, volume overload is not a problem.
- If volume overload is a concern, allow the unit of fresh whole blood to stand for 30 minutes. The red blood cells will drop to the bottom, and the fluid/plasma above them containing clotting factors can be drawn off with a syringe and needle, and plasma alone can be given.

Central venous access

This can be valuable provided that the healthcare workers present have the skills needed to do this safely as it is potentially hazardous. The catheter should be inserted in the intra-thoracic inferior vena cava or superior vena cava via the femoral, internal jugular or subclavian vein routes. However, **it is essential that resuscitation is not delayed by trying to insert a central venous catheter. If there is a clotting disorder, never use the subclavian route**.

A normal central venous pressure (CVP) is 4–10 cmH$_2$O, and optimising the CVP can improve cardiac output with less risk of inducing heart failure. Take great care if the CVP is > 12 cmH$_2$O, as cardiac failure may be induced by excessive IV fluids, especially if severe anaemia, malnutrition or a primary cardiac disorder is present.

Reassess ABC **on a regular basis**.

Reassess the response to fluids to determine whether the woman's condition is improving. Signs of improvement include the following:

- decreasing pulse rate (a rate of ≤ 100–110 beats/minute)
- increasing blood pressure (systolic pressure ≥ 90–100 mmHg)
- improving mental status (less confusion or anxiety)
- increasing urine output (≥ 30 mL/hour).

Continue monitoring to ensure that the pulse rate and blood pressure do not deteriorate after improvement, indicating the return of shock.

If the mother's condition improves, adjust IV fluids to 1 litre over 6 hours, and continue management for the underlying cause of shock.

If more than 3 litres have been given IV in a mother, and if shock is still present, call for anaesthetic assistance.

Correct any hypoglycaemia.

Inotropes

An IV infusion of dobutamine and/or dopamine at 5–20 micrograms/kg/minute should be considered, especially if a third bolus of fluid is required. Sometimes adrenaline by IV infusion at 0.05–2 micrograms/kg/minute may be required.

These infusions can initially be given **carefully** through a peripheral vein until central venous access is obtained.

Patients who require ventilation and inotropic support should be cared for in a high-dependency or intensive-care unit with invasive monitoring (if available). Seek early advice.

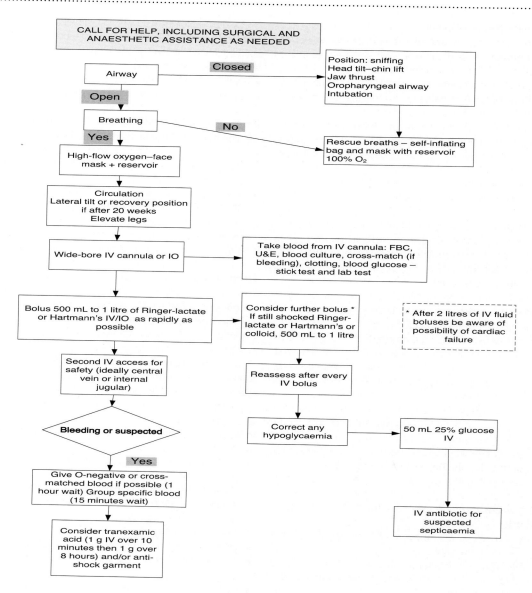

FIGURE 2.5.A.6 Shock in pregnancy or the puerperium: pathway of care. IV, intravenous; IO, intra-osseous; U&E, urea and electrolytes; PPH, postpartum haemorrhage.

2.5.B Severe anaemia, including sickle-cell disease

BOX 2.5.B.1 Minimum standards
- Oral and parenteral iron.
- Folic acid.
- Blood transfusion.
- Antimalarial drugs.
- Antihelmintic drugs.
- Haemoglobin measurements at healthcare facilities in the community.

Introduction

In normal pregnancy there is an increased total blood volume and a marked increase in plasma volume, so the haemoglobin concentration falls. Pathological anaemia is mainly due to iron deficiency, associated with depleted iron stores before pregnancy and poor diet. Malaria is another major cause of anaemia in pregnancy. Anaemic women cope poorly with blood loss at delivery. Where amoebiasis and other hookworms are endemic, these may worsen the anaemia.

Prevention of anaemia

Oral iron supplementation is advised during all pregnancies. It is particularly important in the mother who is anaemic before pregnancy or who has a poor diet. The WHO recommends an iron supplement of 60 mg/day for mothers with adequate iron stores, and 120 mg/day for those women without adequate iron stores. Give ferrous sulphate or ferrous fumarate 120 mg by mouth *plus* folic acid 400 micrograms by mouth once daily throughout pregnancy. Continue for 3 months postpartum. The mother may take the tablets after meals rather than in the morning if she prefers to do so.

In an endemic area, look for hookworm ova in the stools, and treat them if you find them. If a laboratory is not available to identify them, assume that they are present. Wait until around16 weeks of pregnancy and then treat with mebendazole ('Vermox') 500 mg as a single treatment.

If the mother has a large spleen and is anaemic, this is probably caused by malaria, which should be treated.

In areas where malaria is endemic, institute intermittent preventive treatment (IPT) with antimalarial drugs (*see* Section 2.8.D).

Severe anaemia is present if haemoglobin levels are less than 5.0 g/dL *or* if there are signs of heart failure and haemoglobin levels are less than 7.5 g/dL. This condition is very dangerous for both mother and baby.

Haemoglobin can be measured using either small drops of capillary blood or a venous sample. A portable battery-operated haemaccue (www.biomedcentral.com/content/pdf/1472-6890-11-5.pdf)) or a paper chart method can be used in rural areas where clinics are held.

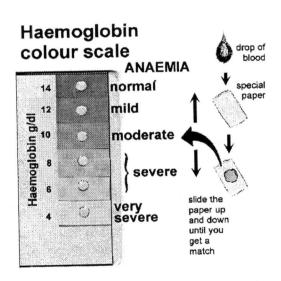

FIGURE 2.5.B.1 WHO test strip with colour scale for measuring haemoglobin in a rural area.

Presentation of severe anaemia

- The patient will be weak, with near white palms, soles and tongue, and **signs of heart failure** if the anaemia is severe (see below).
- In haemolysis, the urine may be **dark brown in colour** and there may be signs of jaundice.

Treatment of severe anaemia

If heart failure is not present, give ferrous sulphate 200 mg orally three times a day, vitamin C 1000 mg daily (this can increase haemoglobin levels by 1 gram/litre per week) and folic acid 5 mg once daily. If vitamin C is not available, iron tablets may be taken with orange juice to aid absorption.

Parenteral iron: parenteral administration produces a larger and more rapid rise in haemoglobin levels, and is more effective in replenishing ferritin levels, so might be

necessary for patients who cannot tolerate oral preparations or who are non-compliant, or if the anaemia is diagnosed late and rapid correction is required.

Parenteral iron is best given IV. Intramuscular injections are painful and may stain the skin. Do not give parenteral iron during the first trimester.

IV preparations: the side effects of intravenous iron preparations are less common with iron sucrose than with iron dextran. Side effects of iron dextran include arthralgia, myalgia, pyrexia, flushing and hypotension. Serious hypersensitivity is observed in approximately 1 in 200 patients with iron dextran (low-molecular-weight dextran) and 1 in 50 000 with iron sucrose.

Iron sucrose (Venofer®): 200 mg (elemental iron). For IV infusion, dilute 10 mL of iron sucrose (200 mg) in 100 mL of 0.9% saline and infuse immediately after dilution. The first 10 mL (20 mg) should be given slowly over 10 minutes and the remainder over 1 hour. No test dose is required for iron sucrose, as anaphylaxis is rare with this preparation. However, adrenaline must be available. A fall in blood pressure is possible if the iron infusion is given too quickly. IV infusions can be repeated weekly if the required rise in haemoglobin levels is not achieved, up to a maximum total dose of 1000 mg.

Do not overdose with iron, as this can affect the absorption of other essential elements from the diet and increase the oxidative stress of pregnancy.

Treat for malaria, give prophylaxis (*see* Section 2.8.D), and prevent future inoculations with impregnated bed nets.

Treat any chronic parasitaemia (e.g. hookworm, schistosomiasis).

Where hookworm is **endemic** (prevalence of 20% or more), give one of the following antihelmintic treatments:
- albendazole 400 mg by mouth once; **this must not be given in the first trimester** because it causes fetal anomalies
- *or* mebendazole 500 mg by mouth once or 100 mg twice a day for 3 days
- *or* levamisole 2.5 mg/kg body weight by mouth once daily for 3 days
- *or* pyrantel 10 mg/kg body weight by mouth once daily for 3 days.

Where hookworm is **highly endemic** (prevalence of 50% or more), repeat the antihelmintic treatment 12 weeks after the first dose.

Treatment of severe anaemia where there is heart failure

Give a high concentration of oxygen, bed rest and sit the patient upright (with lateral tilt as well if she is more than 20 weeks pregnant).
- Consider transfusion with packed cells if the haemoglobin concentration is less than 5.0 g/dL (with IV furosemide of 40 mg for each unit of packed cells). If blood cannot be centrifuged, let the bag hang until the cells have settled. Infuse the cells slowly and dispose of the remaining serum (*see* Section 1.7 on blood transfusion).
- Partial exchange transfusion may be helpful. Use a cannula in a large vein in the antecubital fossa, withdraw 20 mL of the patient's anaemic blood and infuse 40 mL of new blood (ideally packed red blood cells) over 5 minutes and repeat 5–10 times.

If labour occurs when the patient is severely anaemic:
- Deliver with the patient sitting up.
- Cross-match blood and have it available in case of postpartum haemorrhage (PPH).
- Avoid a prolonged second stage as this increases the risk of PPH.
- If there are signs of heart failure or maternal exhaustion shorten the second stage with a ventouse if possible.
- Manage the third stage actively (give oxytocin), and suture any tears without delay.
- **The mother is in great danger for at least 48 hours after delivery. Prescribe iron and folate during the puerperium.**

Sickle-cell anaemia in pregnancy

Sickle-cell anaemia is a disease in which the patient's red cells form sharp points when they lack sufficient oxygen. These pointed red cells are destroyed by the body, and as a result the patient becomes anaemic. Sickle-cell anaemia is harmful to pregnant mothers. It causes miscarriage and perinatal deaths. It also causes painful crises, which may be life-threatening. Infections, especially urinary and chest infections, are also more common.

BOX 2.5.B.2 Minimum standards
- A multidisciplinary team that includes an obstetrician, a midwife and a haematologist.
- Blood pressure and urinalysis monitoring.
- A facility for haemoglobin estimation and electrophoresis, and other laboratory tests.
- Analgesia, including paracetamol, NSAIDs and morphine.
- Blood transfusion.
- Oxygen.
- Penicillin prophylaxis.
- **Pneumococcal (PCV and Pneumovax), hepatitis B** and *Haemophilus influenzae* vaccines.
- Ultrasound scanning.

Before pregnancy

Ideally, women with sickle-cell disease (SCD) should be seen before pregnancy so that they can be told about how pregnancy and SCD can interact, and how to achieve the best outcomes. This is also an opportunity to screen for end-organ damage or manage existing problems, and perhaps to discuss contraception. These activities could be undertaken in the context of a regular specialist sickle-cell review.

Women should be encouraged to have their partner tested for haemoglobinopathy before becoming pregnant, so that the risk of having a child with SCD can be assessed. Prenatal diagnosis and possible termination of pregnancy may need to be discussed with the couple.

A history of previous Caesarean section and uterine curettage should be obtained because of the increased risk of placenta praevia.

An adequate nutritional assessment should be undertaken. The patient's pre-pregnant weight, height, and optimal weight gain in pregnancy should be recorded.

Women who are planning to conceive should be told about:
- the role of dehydration (from nausea and vomiting),

cold, hypoxia, overexertion and stress in the genesis of sickle-cell crises
- the increased risk of worsened anaemia, crises, acute chest syndrome (ACS) and infection (especially urinary tract infection) during pregnancy
- potential effects on the baby, such as prematurity, growth restriction and fetal distress. The rate of complications may depend on the type of SCD that is present
- the increased risk of induction of labour and Caesarean section
- the chance of their baby being affected by SCD
- the outcome of pregnancy in SCD is usually favourable. Smith *et al* (1996) reported that 99% (283 of 286) of pregnancies delivered after 28 weeks' gestation and resulted in live births, a rate that compares favourably with the rate of 99.29% for live births to African-American women in the same country (*see* Further reading at end of the section).

Tests for chronic disease complications and other relevant issues

These include:
- echocardiogram: used to screen for pulmonary hypertension that is associated with increased mortality. A tricuspid regurgitant jet velocity of more than 2.5 m/second is associated with a high risk of pulmonary hypertension
- blood pressure and urinalysis: identifies women with hypertension and/or proteinuria
- full blood count with a reticulocyte index
- haemoglobin electrophoresis
- serum iron, total iron binding capacity (TIBC) and ferritin levels
- renal and liver function tests: performed annually to identify sickle nephropathy and/or deranged hepatic function
- red cell antibodies: may detect an increased risk of haemolytic disease of the newborn
- measurement of antibodies to hepatitis A, B and C, and HIV
- rubella antibody titre
- tuberculin skin test
- pap smear, cervical smear, and gonococcus culture and screening for other sexually transmitted diseases; bacterial vaginosis testing should also be performed
- retinal screening (if an ophthalmologist is available); proliferative retinopathy is common in patients with SCD
- T2-star (T2*) cardiac magnetic resonance imaging: this screens for iron overload in the multiply transfused who have a high ferritin level; aggressive iron chelation before conception is advisable in iron-loaded women.

Medication and vaccination

- Penicillin (or erythromycin) prophylaxis: there is limited evidence of its effectiveness in pregnant women with SCD, although some authorities recommend it.
- Folic acid (5 mg daily) is useful both before and throughout pregnancy.
- Hydroxycarbamide (hydroxyurea) is helpful in severe SCD, but it is teratogenic in animals. Women on this medication should use contraception and stop hydroxycarbamide 3 months before attempting to conceive. If they become pregnant, the medication should be stopped and an ultrasound scan performed to look for structural abnormality. Termination is not indicated just

because of exposure to hydroxycarbamide, as it is still possible to deliver an unaffected baby.

- Angiotensin-converting enzyme inhibitors or angiotensin-receptor blockers are used in patients with SCD with significant proteinuria (a protein:creatinine ratio of more than 50 mg/mmol), but they are not safe in pregnancy and should be discontinued prior to conception.
- Chelation therapy (e.g. desferrioxamine) should be stopped prior to conception.
- Vaccination against the following is recommended before pregnancy (if not previously given): *Haemophilus influenzae* type b, conjugated meningococcal C, and pneumococcus, hepatitis B and influenza.

Antenatal care

Antenatal care should ideally be delivered by a multidisciplinary team that includes an obstetrician and a midwife with experience of high-risk antenatal care, and a haematologist with an interest in SCD.

Discussion about pregnancy, SCD and vaccination should cover the points listed under 'Before pregnancy' above. Providing information and education about SCD, improving the mother's nutritional status, malaria prevention and early detection of bacterial infection have a positive impact on SCD-related morbidity and mortality in Africa.

SCD may increase the risk of pre-eclampsia, so it is advisable to give low-dose aspirin (75 mg daily) from 12 weeks' gestation (unless there is an allergy). Because of the effects on fetal development, **non-steroidal anti-inflammatory drugs (NSAIDs) should only be given between 12 and 28 weeks' gestation**.

Iron supplements should only be given if there is laboratory evidence of deficiency (haemoglobin level less than 11 g/dL). Live attenuated vaccines should not be given until after delivery.

The woman's partner should be offered testing for haemoglobinopathy. If the partner is a sickle-carrier or has SCD, the risks of delivering an infant with SCD should be discussed. This should ideally occur within 10 weeks of conception, so that prenatal diagnosis and discussion about termination can be offered. Factors to be considered include coping skills for caring for a child with a serious illness, personal and cultural values with regard to childbearing, religious beliefs, the need and desire to have children, feelings and attitudes about abortion, and beliefs about self-determination versus fate as determinants of adverse events.

Pregnant women with SCD are likely to have an increased risk of venous thromboembolism, and their management should be tailored. Graduated **compression stockings** are an option. For hospital admissions, low-molecular-weight heparin is recommended (*see* Section 2.5.H).

Blood pressure and proteinuria assessment should occur at each visit because of the increased risk of pregnancy-induced hypertension in SCD. Any pre-existing proteinuria or renal impairment should be monitored more frequently. Women should be observed closely if their blood pressure rises above 125/75 mmHg, if their systolic blood pressure increases by 30 mmHg, or if their diastolic blood pressure increases by 15 mmHg, in association with oedema and proteinuria in the second trimester.

Urinalysis for protein should be performed at each antenatal visit, and midstream urine sent for culture and sensitivity if symptoms of urinary tract infection are present and routinely if resources allow microscopy.

Ultrasound scanning should ideally occur as follows:
- Women should be offered a viability scan at 7–9 weeks' gestation.
- They should be offered the routine first-trimester scan (at 11–14 weeks' gestation) and a detailed anomaly scan at 20 weeks' gestation. In addition, they should be offered serial fetal biometry scans (growth scans) every 4 weeks from 24 weeks' gestation.

Transfusion in women with SCD who are pregnant

- Routine transfusions are not required.
- Red cell units should ideally be matched for Rhesus (C, c, D, E, e) and Kell type.
- Ideally, cytomegalovirus seronegative units should be used.
- Decisions about transfusion should be made by an experienced haematologist (if available) and an obstetrician. One approach is to consider initiation of transfusions for women who have complications such as pre-eclampsia, severe anaemia, or increasing frequency of pain episodes.
- Each woman should have an individualised care plan that takes into account her previous sickle-cell and pregnancy history.
- Treatment of acute painful crisis is the same as that for non-pregnant patients, with hydration, oxygen and analgesics, although doses of the latter may be higher. Reassurance should be given that morphine use during pregnancy does not jeopardise the baby's health. However, if large doses of morphine are needed in late pregnancy, the newborn may require opioid weaning.

Intrapartum care

No randomised controlled trials are available to guide the timing of delivery. If there is a normally growing fetus, offer elective birth through induction of labour, or by elective Caesarean section if indicated for other reasons, between 38 and 40 weeks' gestation. In low resource settings the risks of induction and the uncertainty about due date must be balanced against the potential increased risk of late pregnancy complications such as abruption and pre-eclampsia in SCD. SCD is not a contraindication to attempting vaginal delivery, or vaginal birth after previous Caesarean section.

A 'group and save' for possible transfusion is acceptable for delivery unless there are atypical antibodies, when a cross-match should be requested (to reduce delays).

In women who have hip replacements it is important to discuss suitable positions for delivery.

During labour the following measures are recommended:
- Inform the multidisciplinary team (the senior midwife in charge, senior obstetrician, anaesthetist and haematologist) when labour is confirmed.
- Maintain warmth and hydration.
- Maintain continuous intrapartum electronic fetal heart rate monitoring if available, as there is an increased risk of fetal distress which may necessitate operative delivery. There is also an increased rate of stillbirth, placental abruption and compromised placental reserve.
- Intravenous fluids should be administered if oral hydration is inadequate. A fluid balance chart should be kept.

Changes during the intrapartum period:

- There is an increased frequency of sickle-cell crises and ACS.
- Cardiac function can be compromised because of chronic hypoxaemia and anaemia.
- There is an increased risk of painful crises with protracted labour (more than 12 hours). If the woman is well hydrated and labour is progressing, the labour should be carefully supervised. Caesarean section should be considered if labour is not progressing well and delivery is not imminent.
- There is an increased oxygen demand. Use of pulse oximetry to detect hypoxia is appropriate. If the oxygen saturation is 94% or less, oxygen should be given by nasal cannula.

Routine antibiotic prophylaxis in labour is not supported by evidence, but hourly observations of vital signs should be performed. A raised temperature (> 37.5°C) requires investigation. The clinician should have a low threshold for commencing broad-spectrum antibiotics.

Women should be offered anaesthetic assessment in the third trimester of pregnancy, as general anaesthesia should be avoided where possible. Regional (epidural) anaesthesia during labour where available may reduce the need for both general anaesthesia for delivery and high doses of morphine with lower body sickle pain. Regional analgesia (spinal) is recommended for Caesarean section.

Avoid pethidine because of the risk of seizures. Morphine is the most appropriate drug.

Postpartum care

- If the baby is at high risk of SCD (based on parental haemoglobinopathy results), early testing for SCD should be offered.
- Maintain maternal oxygen saturation above 94% and adequate hydration based on fluid balance until discharge.
- Low-molecular-weight heparin (or unfractionated heparin if former not available) should be administered while the woman is in hospital and for 7 days post-discharge following vaginal delivery, or for a period of 6 weeks following Caesarean section.
- Anti-thrombotic stockings are recommended in the puerperium.
- The risk of sickle-cell crisis is increased. Hydration and oxygenation should be maintained and early mobilisation encouraged. Crises should be managed as for non-pregnant women. NSAIDs can be given in the postpartum period and during breastfeeding. Breastfeeding should be encouraged.
- Postpartum contraceptive advice should be given. Progestogen-containing contraceptives, injectable contraceptives and the levonorgestrel intrauterine system are safe and effective in SCD. Oestrogen-containing contraceptives should be used as second-line agents.
- Barrier methods are as safe and effective in women with SCD as in the general population.

Further reading

Gladwin MT, Sachdev V, Jison ML *et al* (2004) Pulmonary hypertension as a risk factor for death in patients with sickle cell disease. *New England Journal of Medicine*, 350, 886–95.

Koshy M, Burd L, Wallace D *et al* (1988) Prophylactic red-cell transfusions in pregnant patients with sickle cell disease: a randomized cooperative study. *New England Journal of Medicine*, 319, 1447–52.

Oteng-Ntim E and Howard J (2011) *Management of Sickle Cell Disease in Pregnancy*. London: Royal College of Obstetricians and Gynaecologists.

Smith J, Espeland M, Bellevue R *et al* (1996) Pregnancy in sickle cell disease: experience of the Cooperative Study of Sickle Cell Disease. *Obstetrics and Gynecology*, 87, 199–204.

Sickle Cell Society (2008) *Standards for the Clinical Care of Adults with Sickle Cell Disease in the UK*. London: Sickle Cell Society.

National Institutes of Health (National Heart, Lung, and Blood Institute) (2002) *The Management of Sickle Cell Disease*, 4th edn. NIH Publication No. 02-2117. Bethesda, MD: National Institutes of Health (National Heart, Lung, and Blood Institute).

2.5.C Septic abortion or miscarriage

Introduction

Septic abortion is defined as abortion complicated by infection. Sepsis may result from infection if organisms rise from the lower genital tract following either spontaneous miscarriage or induced abortion. Sepsis is more likely to occur if there are retained products of conception and evacuation has been delayed. Sepsis is a frequent complication of unsafe abortion involving instrumentation.

Diagnosis

Consider the possibility of septic abortion in any woman or girl with a history of termination of pregnancy or attempted termination. Presentation is typically with some of the following symptoms and signs: lower abdominal pain, prolonged vaginal bleeding, tender uterus, foul-smelling vaginal discharge, purulent cervical discharge, fever and malaise.

Treatment

If septic shock is present, this will be shown by some of the following signs and symptoms:

- fast, weak pulse (≥ 100–110 beats/minute)
- pallor (especially of the inner eyelid, palms or around the mouth)
- sweatiness with cold or warm (vasodilated) skin
- rapid breathing (> 30 breaths/minute)
- anxiety, confusion or unconsciousness
- low blood pressure (systolic pressure < 90 mmHg is a late sign)
- reduced urine output (< 30 mL/hour).

Resuscitation then proceeds as described below.

Airway

- Use an opening manoeuvre if the airway is not open or is partially obstructed. Keep the airway open. If there is improvement but the airway closes without active opening support, consider airway adjuncts to maintain the airway if the patient is unconscious (P or U on the AVPU scale).
- Suction if necessary.
- The airway may need to be maintained and protected by intubation, using experienced senior help (if available).

Breathing

- Provide a high concentration of **oxygen** through a face mask with a reservoir bag if there is adequate spontaneous respiration.
- For patients with inadequate ventilation, respiration should be supported with oxygen via a **bag-mask**, and experienced senior help summoned (if available).

Circulation

- Gain IV access.
  - Use a short, wide-bore (16- to 18-gauge) IV cannula if possible for IV access.
  - The internal jugular and external jugular veins are good options for access if peripheral access is impossible. Long saphenous vein cut-down may also be considered.
  - Try to obtain two vascular access sites to give large volumes quickly, and in case one line is lost.
- Elevate the legs by raising the foot of the bed.
- Give an initial rapid IV/IO bolus of 500 mL to 1 litre of Ringer-lactate or Hartmann's solution. It is essential that the bolus is given as rapidly as possible.
- Further boluses of 500–1000 mL will usually be required during the first hour. Once more than 2 litres have been given IV, complications such as pulmonary or cerebral oedema may occur. If available, expert help, an anaesthetist, and the use of inotropes, sodium bicarbonate, and intermittent positive pressure ventilation (IPPV) with positive end-expiratory pressure (PEEP) are all potentially valuable.
- A fresh blood transfusion may also be important.

Antibiotics after taking specimens for culture if facilities are available (blood cultures, high vaginal swab and urine)

All patients, whether shocked or not, must be given the following antibiotics without delay:

- ampicillin 2 grams IV every 6 hours
- *plus* gentamicin 80 mg IV/IM 8-hourly or 5 mg/kg body weight IV/IM every 24 hours
- *plus* metronidazole 500 mg IV every 8 hours.

All of these should be continued until the woman has been fever-free for 48 hours.

Patients who do not appear to be shocked on first examination must still be frequently observed for the early signs of shock during the first 6–12 hours. The frequency of observations can then be reduced.

Start antibiotics as soon as possible and ideally before attempting manual vacuum aspiration (MVA).

The woman or girl may also need the following:

- MVA to remove infected products of conception. This is preferable to curettage, because perforation may already have occurred, or could easily do so because of the friable nature of the uterine wall
- hysterectomy after stabilisation if the infection cannot be controlled.

Further reading

Surviving Sepsis Campaign: www.survivingsepsis.org/GUIDELINES/Pages/default.aspx

---

2.5.D Obstetric haemorrhage

2.5.D.i Ruptured ectopic pregnancy

Introduction

An ectopic pregnancy is defined as the implantation of the fertilised ovum outside the uterus, usually within the Fallopian tube.

When it is a few weeks old it ruptures the tube, resulting in bleeding into the peritoneal cavity.

If the fetus is expelled ('tubal abortion') it leaves from the fimbrial end of the Fallopian tube with blood collecting as a haematoma, usually at about 8 week's gestation.

If the Fallopian tube ruptures, there is generally severe abdominal pain, with or without shock, depending on the amount of bleeding. Rupture usually occurs from 8 weeks' gestation onwards, but the timing can vary depending on the exact site of the pregnancy and the rate of growth of the pregnancy tissue. As a result rupture is possible before 8 weeks and beyond 12 weeks' gestation.

Cause of ectopic pregnancy

This is not known, but associated factors include the following:

- pelvic inflammatory disease leading to salpingitis (especially as a result of gonococcus, chlamydia or TB infection)
- if pregnancy occurs with an intrauterine contraceptive device in place (a rare occurrence)
- previous tubal surgery resulting in tubal ligation or tubal re-anastomosis
- previous ectopic pregnancy
- previous intra-abdominal infection (peritonitis).

Sites of implantation

Implantation in the Fallopian tube is most common (over 90% of cases), usually at the ampulla. Less common but more dangerous is implantation at the interstitial end. The fetus can also rarely implant on the bowel, pelvic peritoneum, cervix or ovary.

Clinical presentation: symptoms and signs

- Abdominal pain that is lower abdominal (which tends to be unilateral), cramping or stabbing, due to distension of the tube and peritoneal irritation from blood in the abdominal cavity. Rupture results in generalized abdominal pain, often associated with distention, guarding and rebound tenderness (peritonism).
- Shoulder tip pain, caused by blood irritating the diaphragm.
- Rectal pain or perineal discomfort caused by the presence of blood in the pouch of Douglas.
- Diarrhoea is an atypical symptom and can rarely be the main presenting complaint.
- Hypovolaemic shock occurs as soon as sufficient blood has been lost. Often there will be fainting or a feeling of faintness that requires the patient to lie down.
- A fast weak pulse (heart rate ≥ 100 beats/minute).
- Hypotension (a late sign after much blood has been lost: systolic pressure < 90 mmHg).
- Vaginal bleeding, which can mimic a normal menses (75%):
  - usually dark, and not heavy
  - may be irregular.
- Signs and symptoms of early pregnancy are unusual. They include tiredness, nausea and/or vomiting (especially in the early morning), breast swelling and urinary frequency.
- Anaemia if there is chronic slower bleeding.

In all women and girls of reproductive age with diarrhoea and/or dizziness or fainting, do a pregnancy test and consider the possibility of ectopic pregnancy.

Abdominal examination reveals muscle guarding and rebound tenderness and probably fever. The differential diagnosis is appendicitis. There may be abdominal distension with shifting dullness if there is free blood in the abdomen.

Pelvic examination: **caution must be exercised when performing a bimanual vaginal examination if an ectopic pregnancy is possible, because of the risk of rupture during and due to the examination.** Vaginal examination may show general pelvic tenderness, sometimes with a mass in the fornix, or increased tenderness on one side. There may be cervical excitation, bluish discoloration of the vagina and cervix and/or slight uterine enlargement.

Diagnosis

Consider this diagnosis in particular if any anaemia, shock or abdominal pain is greater than expected for the amount of vaginal bleeding. Check whether the woman or girl has any risk factors for an ectopic pregnancy.

Differential diagnosis: threatened miscarriage, acute or chronic pelvic inflammatory disease (PID), torsion or rupture of an ovarian cyst, acute appendicitis or peritonitis.

Tip test: Tilt the head down. If there is blood in the peritoneal cavity it will irritate the diaphragm; this is manifested

as shoulder tip pain. This test is useful if it gives a positive result, but a negative result does not exclude haemorrhage.

Do a pregnancy test in all potentially fertile women and girls with abdominal pain, fainting or shock. If they are unable to provide a urine specimen, consider using a urinary catheter to obtain one.

Ultrasound examination

If there is a positive pregnancy test but no intrauterine pregnancy is seen on the ultrasound scan, an ectopic pregnancy is likely. The likelihood of ectopic pregnancy increases if free fluid and/or an echogenic mass is seen.

Culdocentesis is not recommended, as it may delay surgery and introduce infection.

Primary assessment and resuscitation of shocked patients

Call for help. A surgeon and anaesthetist must be urgently requested, and the operating theatre must be prepared.

Airway

- Use an opening manoeuvre if the airway is not open or is partially obstructed. If there is an improvement, use airway adjuncts to support the airway or ask an assistant to hold it open.
- Suction if necessary.
- The airway may need to be maintained and protected by intubation using experienced senior help (if available).

Breathing

- Provide a high concentration of oxygen through a face mask with reservoir bag for patients with adequate spontaneous respiration.
- For patients with inadequate ventilation or depressed conscious level (P or U on the AVPU scale), respiration should be supported with oxygen by bag-valve-mask inflations and experienced senior help obtained, including an anaesthetist.

Circulation

- Elevate the legs and consider using a non-pneumatic anti-shock garment.
- Gain IV access.
- Use a short wide-bore IV cannula if possible (14- to 16-G).
- External jugular vein access is a good option if peripheral access is impossible. Long saphenous vein cut-down may also be considered, and, if the operator is adequately trained, central venous access ideally via the internal jugular vein can be extremely helpful, or the intraosseous route if this is not possible (see Section 8.4.B).
- Try to obtain two vascular access sites in order to give large volumes quickly, and in case one line is lost.
- Take blood for cross-matching of 4–6 units, full blood count, renal function tests (if available) and blood clotting.
- Give 500 mL to 1 litre of Ringer-lactate or Hartmann's solution by rapid bolus while awaiting blood for transfusion.
- Remember that young healthy women and girls can lose a lot of blood before they become shocked, especially if it is a slow leakage rather than a sudden large loss of blood.

The concept of **targeted crystalloid fluid resuscitation** is important in management. Here the initial boluses of IV crystalloids required to treat shock would only be given to keep the vital organs (especially the brain, heart and kidneys) perfused before blood and, most important of all, surgery have become available.

The administration of too large a volume of IV crystalloid fluids by increasing blood pressure and damaging the coagulation system could increase bleeding by disrupting early clot formation.

If this approach is adopted when giving boluses of crystalloid to patients who are in shock due to bleeding, before blood becomes available and here, of most importance, surgical intervention, only the amount needed to keep the blood pressure at a level sufficient to perfuse the vital organs would be given. There is no clear evidence to indicate the precise blood pressure that should be achieved in a woman in shock due to a ruptured and bleeding ectopic pregnancy. However, **adequate perfusion of vital organs may best be indicated by a radial pulse that can be palpated and an alert conscious level**.

Our personal practice is to start with IV boluses of 500 mL of crystalloid or ideally blood and reassess after each bolus always aiming for urgent surgical intervention and blood transfusion. Several boluses of crystalloids may be required before these actions are possible.

Disability

Conscious level on AVPU scale.

Central venous access

This is valuable if skilled staff are available to undertake it. Ideally it should be achieved using a multi-lumen catheter coated with heparin, if available, with the catheter placed in the intra-thoracic inferior vena cava (IVC) or superior vena cava (SVC).

A normal central venous pressure (CVP) (*see* Section 2.7.A for details of measurement) is +4 to +10 cmH$_2$O, and optimising the CVP can improve cardiac output with less risk of inducing heart failure. Take great care if the CVP is greater than 12 cmH$_2$O, as cardiac failure may be induced by excessive IV fluids, especially if severe anaemia, malnutrition or primary cardiac disorders are present.

Emergency treatment

If the diagnosis is ruptured ectopic pregnancy with shock, order blood for transfusion and immediately prepare the operating theatre. Obtain a surgeon urgently, and proceed to urgent laparotomy while resuscitation is under way. Do not wait for blood.

At laparotomy, perform salpingectomy. Repair of the tube carries a major risk of future ectopic pregnancy, and should not be undertaken in resource-limited settings.

Autotransfusion

If blood is unquestionably fresh and free from infection, it can be collected after the abdomen has been opened and transfused.

When the woman is on the operating table prior to surgery and the abdomen is distended with blood, it is sometimes possible to insert a needle through the abdominal wall and collect the blood in a donor set.

Alternatively, open the abdomen and proceed as follows:

- Scoop the blood into a basin and strain it through gauze to remove all clots.
- Clean the top portion of a blood donor bag (containing anticoagulant) with antiseptic solution and open it with a sterile blade.
- Pour the mother's blood into the bag and infuse it through a filtered set in the usual way.
- If a donor bag with anticoagulant is not available, add 10 mL of 0.3 molar sodium citrate to each 90 mL of blood.

Advice post salpingectomy for ruptured ectopic pregnancy

- If the other tube was macroscopically normal there is good chance of further successful pregnancy.
- The risk of a recurrent ectopic is 10% or more; that is 10 times the background risk therefore an early ultrasound scan is recommended (if available) as soon as a new pregnancy is suspected.
- Offer family planning advice.
- Consider treatment of pelvic inflammatory disease for the patient and her partner if there was intra-operative evidence of pelvic infection and no clear history of previous treatment.

2.5.D. ii Miscarriage

Types of miscarriage

Consider miscarriage or induced abortion in any woman or girl of reproductive age if more than 1 month has elapsed since her last menstrual period, and one or more of the following is present: bleeding, lower abdominal pain, partial expulsion of products of conception, dilated cervix, or smaller uterus than expected for gestation.

Spontaneous miscarriage

This is the loss of a pregnancy before fetal viability (28 weeks' gestation in low-resource settings). It occurs in at least 15% of pregnancies.

The stages of spontaneous miscarriage may include the following:

- **threatened miscarriage:** pregnancy may continue
- **inevitable miscarriage:** pregnancy will not continue and will proceed to incomplete or complete miscarriage
- **incomplete miscarriage:** products of conception are partially expelled.
- **complete miscarriage:** products of conception are completely expelled.
- **missed miscarriage:** is not associated with symptoms but found incidentally on routine ultrasound scan or when ultrasound is performed to investigate a pregnancy that is not growing as anticipated. The time from fetal demise to expulsion from the uterus varies widely and it is not uncommon for a miscarriage to remain *in situ* for many weeks.

Miscarriages can be complicated by infection (*see* Section 2.5.C).

Threatened miscarriage

Here there is light vaginal bleeding and sometimes cramping lower abdominal pain. On examination there is a soft uterus corresponding in size to the date of the last menstrual period, and the cervix is closed.

Ideally in the presence of bleeding the viability of the pregnancy should be assessed by sonicaid/Pinnard stethoscope (if gestation permits) or by ultrasound. However, if the bleeding is light and self-limiting and ultrasound is not easily available then a conservative approach can initially be followed. Advise the woman to avoid strenuous exercise and sexual intercourse but bed rest is not necessary. Follow her up in the antenatal clinic. If the bleeding continues, assess for fetal viability and if the equipment is available perform an ultrasound scan. There is no medication that can prevent progression to a complete miscarriage.

Inevitable miscarriage

This can be diagnosed clinically by the findings of an open internal cervical os and/or the passage of products of conception per vagina. If in doubt the diagnosis should be confirmed by ultrasound.

Incomplete miscarriage

Here there is a history of significant bleeding (greater than menstruation), often with passage of clots and fetal tissue and varying degrees of lower abdominal pain secondary to uterine contraction. Bleeding can vary in severity and the cervix may be open or closed. Often the bleeding has reduced and almost stopped in which case, a complete miscarriage is an important differential diagnosis.

Diagnose by visualisation or palpation of products of conception in or through the cervical os, or by visualisation of retained products of conception on ultrasound.

Management of miscarriage

There are three broad methods for managing miscarriage:

1 Expectant: No medical or surgical intervention is made but the patient is monitored for spontaneous resolution. This relies on ready access to emergency treatment and careful follow-up, and is therefore not commonly used in resource poor settings.
2 Medical: Medication is used to expedite or induce expulsion of the retained products of conception. In resource poor settings this is generally used only for later mid-trimester miscarriages (below).
3 Surgical: The uterus is surgically evacuated of the products of conception.

Surgical Management

If pregnancy is less than 16 weeks this is the preferred management method where access to care and follow-up are restricted.

If the pregnancy is 12 to 16 weeks gestation with an unfavourable cervix that is likely to be difficult to dilate, then consideration should be given to:

1 'ripening' the cervix with misoprostol 200 to 600 micrograms around 3 to 24 hours prior to the procedure
2 Using medical induction as for gestations of 16 weeks and over (below).
3 Expectant management – especially if the patient appears to be contracting and is otherwise stable
4 Performing the surgery under optimal conditions: in an operating theatre with local anaesthetic, the availability

of a general anaesthetic, and with an experienced practitioner available.

If the cervix is open and/or some products have already been expelled a sponge forceps can be used to remove products of conception if they are visibly protruding through the cervix. A manual evacuation of the uterus can then be performed to ensure evacuation is complete.

- Manual vacuum aspiration (MVA) (see Figures 2.5.D.ii.1, 2.5.D.ii.2 and 2.5.D.ii.3) is the preferred method of evacuation. **Evacuation by curettage should only be used if MVA is not available.**
- If evacuation is not immediately possible and there is significant bleeding, give ergometrine 200–500 micrograms IM *or* misoprostol 200 micrograms orally, sublingually or rectally.
- Proceed to evacuation as soon as possible.

If the pregnancy is more than 16 weeks; a late miscarriage:

A detailed account of how this can be managed is given on pages 182–3.

In summary management, as above, can be divided into Expectant, Medical and Surgical approaches.

Expectant management is most appropriate when the miscarriage is progressing on its own.

Medical management includes oxytocin, mifepristone and misoprostol.

Surgical management for retained placental tissue either by Manual Vacuum Aspiration/curettage or, after 24 weeks, manual removal of the placenta is sometimes required. It is very important that this complication, which can cause chronic vaginal bleeding, is recognised.

Safe evacuation of retained products

1 Explain the procedure and the reasons for undertaking it, and obtain consent.
2 This must be a surgically aseptic procedure, with the use of sterile gloves and gown. Apply antiseptic solution (such as 0.5% chlorhexidine) to the vagina and cervix (especially the os) by first inserting a high-level disinfected or sterile speculum into the vagina and then using a sterile or high-level disinfected sponge forceps with a cotton or gauze swab and giving three applications of antiseptic.
3 Where possible perform the procedure in the operating theatre. This is especially indicated if there is a risk of heavy bleeding (e.g. molar pregnancy, suspected coagulation disorder), if the procedure is poorly tolerated by the patient or if the cervical os is difficult to dilate or difficult to access.
4 Even when bleeding is not heavy, give oxytocin 10 units IM or ergometrine 200 micrograms IM before MVA to make the uterus firmer and reduce the risk of perforation.
5 Prepare the MVA syringe by closing the pinch valve and pulling back on the plunger until its arms lock. In the case of large amounts of retained products (e.g. molar pregnancy), prepare two or three syringes.
6 Bimanually examine the uterus to assess whether it is anteverted or retroverted prior to instrumentation and to access its size.
7 Provide an oral analgesic, paracetamol 1 gram, and if the cervix is not dilated sufficiently to pass the MVA

catheter, prepare 20 mL of 0.5% lignocaine **(without adrenaline)** with a 3.5 cm long 22- or 25-gauge needle to perform a paracervical nerve block.

8 Using a Cusco's or Sims' speculum or vaginal retractor, visualise the cervix. You will need an adequate light source.

9 Inject 1 mL of 0.5% lignocaine into the anterior or posterior lip of the cervix, whichever has been exposed, if a tenaculum is to be used.

10 Apply either a tenaculum or sponge (ring) forceps (the latter do not require administration of local anaesthetic, and are less likely to tear the cervix in incomplete miscarriage) to the lip of the cervix.

11 If the cervix is insufficiently dilated for the MVA catheter to be passed, perform a paracervical nerve block following slight traction applied to the cervical lip to identify the junction between the cervix and the vaginal wall where injections of lignocaine are to be made. Inject 2 mL of lignocaine just under the epithelium (no deeper than 3 mm) at 3, 5, 7 and 9 o'clock positions. **Ensure that the needle is not in a vein with each injection by drawing back the needle before injection, as IV injection of lignocaine is dangerous and can cause convulsions and cardiac arrest.** Wait 2 minutes and check that the cervix is anaesthetised by pinching it gently with forceps. If the pinch is felt, wait for another 2 minutes.

12 Grasp the lip of the cervix with the sponge forceps and apply gentle traction. Cervical dilatation with Hegar dilators is only needed where the cervical os is not dilated and is firm. Slowly introduce the dilators (the smallest one first) into the cavity, checking carefully whether the uterus is anteverted or retroverted, until the resistance felt on passage through the closed internal os is released and the dilator is felt to pass through it into the uterine cavity. Usually a dilatation of 10–12 mm is sufficient. Ensure that the cervix is not torn or a false passage created by the dilators.

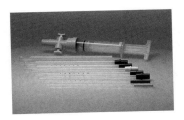

FIGURE 2.5.D.II.1 Manual vacuum aspiration kit including cannulae of different sizes.

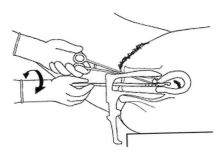

FIGURE 2.5.D.II.2 Inserting the MVA cannula.

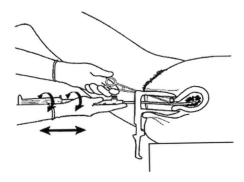

FIGURE 2.5.D.II.3 Evacuating the uterine contents.

13 Pass the MVA cannula gently with a rotating movement through the cervix into the uterine cavity just beyond the internal os.

Slowly push the cannula into the uterus until it touches the fundus. Measure the depth by dots visible on the cannula and then withdraw the cannula by about 0.5 cm. Note the depth of the cavity and do not pass instruments beyond this. The risk of uterine perforation is higher in cases complicated by sepsis, or in a postpartum uterus with retained products of conception (see Section 2.5.D.iv). Also be aware that as it is evacuated the uterus generally contracts and thus the cavity will be smaller by the end of the procedure. Attach the prepared MVA syringe to the cannula and release the pinch valves, allowing the vacuum to transfer to the cannula and the inside of the uterus.

Evacuate the uterine contents by gently rotating the syringe from 10 to 12 o'clock and moving the cannula back and forth within the uterus. Do not allow the cannula at this stage to be withdrawn past the cervical os into the vagina, as the vacuum will be lost. If the vacuum is lost or the syringe is more than half full, empty it and then re-establish the vacuum. Do not hold the syringe by the plunger arms while the vacuum is present, as they may become unlocked and the plunger will then slip back into the syringe, pushing materials back into the uterus.

14 To ensure that all products of conception have been removed, check that red or pink foam but no tissue is seen in the cannula. The uterus will have a 'gritty' feel when the cavity is empty, and haemostasis should be achieved. The uterus may contract around the cannula. Always examine the syringe contents after the procedure. An absence of products of conception in a patient with signs of pregnancy or a positive pregnancy test and continued bleeding suggests three possibilities. Either the miscarriage was complete before evacuation, or the products are still in the uterus (in which case evacuation needs to be repeated), or there is an ectopic pregnancy. Be very careful about the third possibility.

15 If MVA is not available and a curette is used, undertake the procedure up to Step 11 above. Apply the curette with firm but controlled movements in all four quadrants of the uterus (anterior wall, left lateral, posterior wall and right lateral). The uterus will have a 'gritty' feel when the cavity is empty, and haemostasis should be achieved. If there is ongoing bleeding ensure that the cavity is empty with additional gentle curettage.

16 IV antibiotics should be given as a single dose unless

there are signs of sepsis, in which case a full course of antibiotics should be given (*see* Section 2.5.C). All patients should be treated prophylactically for *Chlamydia trachomatis* with either azithromycin 1 g orally stat or doxycycline 100 mg orally twice daily for 7 days.

17 Anti-D immunoglobulin prophylaxis, if available and affordable, should be given to women with a Rhesus-negative blood group. In well-resourced countries, a dose of 250 IU of anti-D immunoglobulin is given before 20 weeks' gestation, and 500 IU after 20 weeks' gestation.

18 Give paracetamol, 500 mg to 1 gram orally, if needed for pain.

19 If an unsafe induced abortion is suspected, examine the woman for signs of infection and uterine, vaginal, bladder or bowel injury, and thoroughly irrigate the vagina with sterile Ringer-lactate or Hartmann's solution to remove any herbs, local medications or caustic substances before MVA is undertaken (*see* Section 2.5.C).

Follow-up and management after a miscarriage, especially where evacuation has occurred

Uncomplicated evacuations may not require follow-up. The patient should be encouraged to eat and drink and be mobile. She should be aware of the potential complications of miscarriage that include: retained tissue (sometimes requiring repeat evacuation), infection and haemorrhage. She should be advised to seek help if there are any symptoms suggestive of these complications, such as ongoing bleeding beyond 2 weeks, very heavy bleeding at any time, severe abdominal pain, offensive-smelling vaginal secretions, fever or malaise. Rigors or fainting potentially indicate severe complications, and the woman must return immediately to the hospital if these symptoms occur. Family planning must be discussed, and the woman advised to avoid pregnancy for at least 3 months.

In the case of mid-trimester miscarriages (>12 weeks' gestation), consideration should be given to the cause of the miscarriage as it is less common at this time and more likely to be secondary to a treatable factor. As a minimum, malaria (where endemic), syphilis and urinary tract infection should be excluded or treated.

Uterine perforation

Uterine perforation may occur following evacuation of the uterus in either a medical or non-clinical setting. The risk of complications, such as infection, perforation, and damage to visceral organs such as bladder and bowel, is high where procedures are performed in non-clinical settings, and in such cases a laparotomy will be required along with high-dose intravenous antibiotics (*see* Section 2.5.C).

In most perforations where only the uterus has been damaged, the hole will heal spontaneously. Keep the woman under close observation for at least 48 hours.

Symptoms and signs of perforation when it has occurred in a non-medical setting

These include severe abdominal pain, vaginal bleeding, weakness, and dizziness or fainting. On examination of the abdomen there will be guarding, rebound tenderness or a rigid abdominal wall. Frequently there will be signs of septic shock (*see* Section 2.5.A).

Complete miscarriage

Evacuation of the uterus is not needed. Observe closely for evidence of bleeding, and follow up the woman in the clinic.

Miscarriage beyond 16 weeks' gestation

Spontaneous miscarriage will generally result in expulsion of the complete fetus (this is also usually the case between 12 and 16 weeks' gestation) and placenta. These may be expelled together within the gestational sac or separately after rupture of the fetal membranes.

The patient may present with bleeding, pain, loss of liquor or a history of having already expelled the fetus before arrival. The examination may reveal an effacing and/or dilated cervix, bulging membranes, or fetal parts. The cervix may also be closed and the patient relatively asymptomatic despite a finding of fetal death on ultrasound. Ultrasound may reveal fetal cardiac activity despite evidence of an inevitable miscarriage.

Management of late miscarriage can be divided into Expectant and Medical management with Surgical management reserved for retained placental tissue after fetal expulsion and the rare cases where life-threatening haemorrhage occurs and delivery is not rapidly achievable by any other means.

If there are no signs of labour and especially if the cervix is unfavourable then the use of mifepristone is beneficial, but not essential if unavailable.

Expectant management

This is best reserved for patients where the delivery/miscarriage process is clearly ongoing and is likely to occur spontaneously without medical intervention. If the delivery is urgent due to the maternal condition, the patient must be monitored closely to ensure the labour is progressing so that it can be medically augmented promptly if required.

Medical management

If spontaneous delivery is not expected or delayed then delivery can be expedited medically. If chorioamnionitis is suspected then delivery is urgent and induction should be started without delay and the patient treated appropriately with antibiotics and other measures as indicated during the process.

The patient needs to be assessed for evidence of infection, bleeding or other associated disorders and treated accordingly.

The following investigations should be performed as a minimum: blood group and cross match, Hb, malaria RDT +/– malaria smear, urine analysis for possible infection.

If there are no signs of labour and especially if the cervix is unfavourable, then the use of mifepristone is beneficial if available but can be omitted. If the delivery is urgent then either the interval between mifepristone and misoprostol treatment can be reduced or they can be administered together.

1 Give mifepristone 200 micrograms orally.

2 Observe the patient in hospital for a period of 36 to 48 hours.

3 Obtain intravenous access and give misoprostol 100 micrograms vaginally or orally every 3 hours up to a total of 5 doses. Oral administration is advised following initial vaginal installation of the first dose of misoprostol and assessment, especially, in the presence of ruptured

membranes, to reduce the risk of ascending infection. A sterile technique must be followed whenever vaginal assessments are performed.

4 Review by a doctor if delivery has not occurred within 3 hours of the final dose.

Note: The dose of misoprostol should be reduced to 100 microgram beyond 27 weeks' gestation and to 50 microgram in women at higher risk of perforation e.g. grand-multiparae and after previous Caesarean section.

If mifepristone or misoprostol are not available, infuse oxytocin, 40 units in 1 litre of IV fluid (Ringer-lactate or Hartmann's solution) over 4 hours until expulsion of the products of conception occurs.

Following delivery, oxytocin 10 IU intramuscular should be given and the patient monitored for bleeding.

If the placenta is not expelled with or immediately following the fetus, retained tissue is likely even if the placenta is eventually expelled. Have a low threshold for exploration and evacuation.

Where gestation is around 24 weeks it may be safer to remove the placenta manually as after a term pregnancy. If not possible then MVA/curettage can be used.

Abortion

This is the deliberate termination of pregnancy before the fetus is viable.

- **Unsafe abortion** is a procedure performed by individuals who lack the necessary skills and/or in an environment that does not meet minimal medical standards. It may be attempted by 'medically' inducing the abortion or by 'surgically' expelling or removing products. The terms medical and surgical are used loosely here as 'medicines' used include highly toxic herbs as well as over-the counter medicines taken in overdose.

  Likewise 'surgical' is used to describe anything from unskilled use of routine surgical instruments to self-insertion of sticks or other objects into the uterus to disturb the pregnancy. Unsurprisingly, complications following unsafe abortion are common and unsafe abortion is a major contributor to maternal mortality.

- **Septic abortion** is abortion complicated by infection. Sepsis may result from ascending infection from the lower genital tract, and is more likely to occur if there are retained products of conception and evacuation has been delayed. It is a frequent complication of unsafe abortion involving instrumentation.

Molar pregnancy/gestational trophoblastic disease

This is relatively uncommon. Gestational trophoblastic disease refers to molar pregnancy (complete and partial moles), choriocarcinoma and placental site trophoblastic tumour.

Complete and partial molar pregnancies are distinguished by the presence of a fetus in the partial group. Complete moles usually result from duplication of a single sperm following fertilisation of an empty ovum. There is no evidence of fetal tissue. Partial moles usually result from dispermic fertilisation of an ovum. There is generally evidence of a fetus or fetal red cells. Only complete molar pregnancy is likely to progress to choriocarcinoma.

Signs of pregnancy are exaggerated. The uterus increases in size more rapidly than normal, vomiting is often but not always severe and constant, there may be pre-eclampsia in the early part of the second trimester, and βHCG levels are very high. The symptoms and signs that are typically present include heavy bleeding, a dilated cervix, uterus larger than dates and softer than normal, and partial expulsion of products of conception that resemble grapes. MVA is required to evacuate the uterus (with anti-D prophylaxis in Rhesus-negative women if available and affordable). Diagnosis in low-resource settings is very difficult, and requires good-quality ultrasound and ability to monitor blood βHCG levels before dilatation and curettage. The products of conception should be examined visually and ideally histologically.

Management of molar pregnancy

This is difficult and requires referral to hospital, ideally with expert facilities if these are available.

MVA will usually be required. There is a higher risk of bleeding, and therefore it is essential to cross-match blood prior to MVA.

Follow-up βHCG measurements, regular ultrasound and possibly chemotherapy will be needed (see below).

Chest X-ray and ideally liver function tests will also be required.

The woman should be strongly advised not to become pregnant within the next year, and family planning advice is particularly important.

Choriocarcinoma, a malignant condition, is the most serious form of mole. It may follow a normal pregnancy and be manifested as continuing vaginal bleeding. Metastasis may occur to the lungs and other organs, and specialist care will be required, including chemotherapy.

Further reading
World Health Organization (2012) *Safe Abortion: technical and policy guidance for health systems*, 2nd edn. http://apps.who.int/iris/bitstream/10665/70914/1/9789241548434_eng.pdf

2.5.D.iii Antepartum haemorrhage

Introduction

Antepartum haemorrhage (APH) is defined as bleeding from the uterus or vagina occurring after potential viability from 24–28 weeks' gestation. The main causes of APH are placenta praevia, placental abruption, and bleeding from cervical or vaginal lesions.

Bleeding from the cervix is common but is not usually heavy. It may be due to rapid cervical dilatation, cervical ectropion or polyps. Ectropions and polyps may become more vascular and friable in pregnancy, predisposing to bleeding. Endo-cervical and vaginal infections such as *Chlamydia*, *Neisseria*, *Trichomonas* and *Candida* can give rise to bleeding. Cervical carcinoma is another cause of APH.

Speculum examination should be performed in order to visualise the cervix and help to assess the likely cause

TABLE 2.5.D.III.1 Causes of major (> 500 mL) or massive (> 1500 mL) antepartum haemorrhage

Symptoms	Clinical signs	Diagnosis	Treatment
Severe constant abdominal pain Light or heavy vaginal bleeding (or non-visible bleeding in concealed abruption) Reduced or absent fetal movements Dizziness Shortness of breath Confusion	Shock Tense and tender uterus on abdominal examination Fetal distress or absent fetal heart rate	Placental abruption	Call for surgical and anaesthetic help Oxygen Left lateral tilt or recovery position IV fluid boluses for shock + blood Cross-match 4 units of blood and freeze-dried plasma if available; transfuse prior to delivery if possible, to try to correct any clotting abnormality Deliver the fetus as soon as possible if it is viable, either by inducing labour or by Caesarean section
Vaginal bleeding that may be light or very heavy Bleeding can be precipitated by intercourse or vaginal examination No pain	Soft uterus Presenting part may be higher than expected. Malpresentation is more common Fetus may be distressed, non-viable or uncompromised with normal movements and normal fetal heart rate pattern Ultrasound will show placenta praevia **Do not undertake digital vaginal examination, as this can puncture the placenta and precipitate massive bleeding which may be fatal** Shock may be present, depending on how heavy the bleeding is and for how long it has been occurring	Placenta praevia	Call for surgical and anaesthetic help Treat shock if present, including the lateral tilt or recovery position (see above) **Do not undertake digital vaginal examination, as this can puncture the placenta and precipitate massive bleeding which may be fatal** If preterm and not bleeding too heavily, give steroids, admit for bed rest and only go for Caesarean section if there is a further bleed Cross-match ideally 4 units of blood
Continuous abdominal pain Vaginal bleeding that may be light or heavy History of a previous Caesarean section or other surgery on the uterus	Shock (especially an increasing heart rate) Tense, distended and tender abdomen Easily palpable fetal parts Absent fetal movements and heart sounds Malpresentation – transverse lie Signs of cephalo-pelvic disproportion Scar from previous surgery Haematuria	Ruptured uterus	Call for surgical and anaesthetic help Treat shock if present Cross-match ideally 4 units of blood Prepare operating theatre for laparotomy while resuscitating patient Stop oxytocin infusion if *in situ*
Heavy vaginal and other bleeding	Bleeding from sites in addition to the vagina Signs of other conditions that may be responsible, such as: • placental abruption • pre-eclampsia or eclampsia (high blood pressure and proteinuria) • retained dead fetus • septicaemia, including intrauterine sepsis • incompatible blood transfusion • amniotic fluid embolism	Coagulation failure	Fresh blood transfusion Blood products such as platelets, fresh-frozen plasma and cryoprecipitate if available Antibiotics if appropriate
Vaginal bleeding that is light Bleeding can be precipitated by intercourse or artificial rupture of membranes No pain	Fetal distress or death	Vasa praevia (placental blood vessels lying in the membranes and in front of the baby's head)	If diagnosed by ultrasound before labour, plan for Caesarean section

of bleeding, as well as to aid evaluation of the severity of bleeding.

Bleeding from the vagina or vulva may result from local trauma or infection. Vulval bleeding may be due to vulval varices, and may be heavy.

Diagnosis

Important points in history taking include the following:

- Is the bleeding provoked or unprovoked?
  - Bleeding due to placenta praevia is likely to be unprovoked. However, bleeding may be precipitated by intercourse or vaginal examination.
  - Abruption is more likely after abdominal trauma.
  - Intercourse may cause bleeding from cervical or vaginal lesions.
- Is the bleeding painful or painless?
  - Bleeding due to placenta praevia is usually painless.
  - Bleeding due to placental abruption is initially painless, but as it continues contractions will occur and eventually become tonic with constant severe pain and a woody feel to the uterus.
- Is it fresh or old blood?
- Is the bleeding light or heavy?

Management of APH

This can be summarised as follows:

- ABC.
- Monitor vital signs.
- Gain IV access and give fluid resuscitation.
- Send blood for urgent haemoglobin, grouping and cross-matching, as well as Kleihauer test (if available).
- Catheterise the patient.
- Perform an abdominal examination: assess uterine tone, tenderness, presence of contractions, auscultation of the fetal heart.
- Do a speculum examination: assess for vaginal and cervical lesions, and severity of bleeding. If the placental site is unknown ideally an ultrasound scan should be performed first. If not possible, caution must be taken as bleeding from a placenta praevia may be exacerbated by vaginal assessment.
- Listen to the fetal heart.

Insert a venous cannula if any of the following are present: active bleeding, contractions, tenderness or increased tone of the uterus. If the patient is shocked, proceed to assessment and resuscitation (see below).

Investigations: haemoglobin, platelet count, clotting tests, urea and electrolytes, liver function tests. Cross-match 4 units if there is major (> 500 mL) or massive (> 1500 mL) haemorrhage or if the bleeding is rapid; group and save if there is loss of < 500 mL and the bleeding is not ongoing. Perform a Kleihauer test, if available, if the woman is Rhesus negative or if there is major abdominal trauma.

Management of the different causes of APH

Placenta praevia

Placenta praevia is an abnormally situated placenta in the lower uterine segment. It presents with painless bleeding,

often with no precipitating factor. Bleeding may be heavy and is bright red.

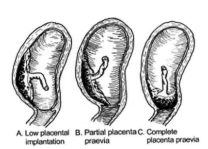

A. Low placental implantation   B. Partial placenta praevia   C. Complete placenta praevia

FIGURE 2.5.D.III.1 Increasing levels of low implanted placentas.

Prevention and protection

- Early detection of placenta praevia is very important to prevent serious bleeding.
- **Any bleeding during pregnancy must be investigated by an ultrasound scan.**
- Mothers with placenta praevia should have immediate access to an obstetric unit with facilities for Caesarean section.
- Mothers over 28 weeks pregnant with a placenta praevia and bleeding should stay in hospital until delivery by Caesarean section, or live very near to an obstetric unit that can perform Caesarean section.

Never allow a digital vaginal examination to be undertaken on a patient with known or suspected placenta praevia, as it can precipitate massive vaginal bleeding.

Careful speculum examination can help to exclude bleeding from the cervix or vagina but if placenta praevia is known to be present then undertake with extreme caution, ideally in the operating theatre.

Placental abruption

- Placental abruption refers to the premature separation of a normally situated placenta. The bleeding may be concealed or revealed, or mixed. It may be partial or complete (if complete, the fetus will be dead).
- The characteristic initial symptom is painless bleeding, which can be concealed or be associated with vaginal bleeding. As abruption becomes worse, contractions will occur and eventually become tonic with constant severe pain and a woody feel to the uterus. At this stage there will usually be shock, severe abdominal pain, and tenderness over the uterus. In early bleeding the uterus may still be soft to touch, but as the bleeding progresses it has a hard 'woody' feel due to uterine contraction. It may be difficult to palpate the fetal parts, the uterus may be large for dates and there may be signs of fetal distress or intrauterine fetal death. It is possible for large bleeds to be asymptomatic and even small bleeds can occasionally result in fetal death.
- Disseminated intravascular coagulation (DIC) is a common complication. A large placental abruption can occur without any visible vaginal blood loss (concealed haemorrhage).
- Remember that blood loss is invariably underestimated. Young healthy women will compensate and maintain their blood pressure until they lose around 20% of their circulating volume.

- The main risk factor for placental abruption is a previous abruption. Increased maternal age, maternal hypertension and trauma also increase the risk.

Ruptured uterus

Uterine rupture is full-thickness separation of the uterine muscle and the overlying visceral peritoneum, sometimes associated with extrusion of the fetus, placenta or both into the abdominal cavity.

- Bleeding from a ruptured uterus can occur either before (rare) or after the onset of labour, although the vast majority occur during labour itself.
- Risk factors for rupture include, obstructed labour due to cephalo-pelvic disproportion, multiparity (especially grand-multiparity), previous uterine surgery (including myomectomy and Caesarean section), and use of uterotonics (including misoprostol and oxytocin).
- A previous Caesarean section scar may rupture during labour. However, obstructed labour even without a uterine scar, particularly in a woman of high parity, may also cause uterine rupture.
- Excessive doses of oxytocin during labour can precipitate uterine rupture and oxytocin should be used with particular caution in multiparous women, especially if it is being used to augment rather than induce labour. Any mother who is receiving this drug during labour should be assessed closely for contraindications before its administration, and should not be left alone.
- **Extra careful consideration must be given to the administration of oxytocin in labour to a woman with a uterine scar, because of the increased risk of uterine rupture. This applies to women with previous myomectomy as well as to those with a previous Caesarean section.**
- **In any setting, including resource limited settings, women with uterine scars should only receive oxytocin before delivery when a high level of supervision is available.**
- Ideally, always use a burette in-line giving set to administer IV oxytocin, to avoid over-dosage.
- Rupture of the uterus can also occur following violence or major trauma.

Symptoms and signs

- Characteristically there is pain and tenderness over the uterus, with blood loss vaginally and cessation of contractions.
- Uterine rupture usually presents with shock, which is partly due to blood loss and partly due to increased vagal nerve stimulation (so there may be a slow pulse rather than a fast one). The baby is usually dead or has severe fetal distress.
- There may be a change in the nature of the pain in labour, from severe intermittent pain to a constant pain.
- Vaginal bleeding may or may not be present. Bleeding from a ruptured uterus can fail to drain vaginally due to an impacted fetal head, and usually the majority of bleeding is intra-abdominal in this situation.
- Maternal shock can be made worse by dehydration, exhaustion and acidosis if prolonged obstructed labour has preceded the rupture.
- The abdomen is tender to palpation, and the fetal parts can be too easily palpable.
- On vaginal examination, the presenting part may be

high or impacted; the fetal head may have retreated into the uterus.

- There may be a marked maternal bradycardia (< 60 beats/minute) due to increased vagal tone.
- The main differential diagnosis is placental abruption.

Management

1 Suspect uterine rupture in any patient with risk factors such as previous Caesarean section.
2 Primary assessment, resuscitation and emergency treatment for shock (see below).
3 Call the obstetrician and anaesthetist.
4 Obtain consent and prepare the operating theatre.
5 Perform urgent laparotomy.
6 Give prophylactic IV antibiotics (ampicillin, gentamicin and metronidazole).

For a discussion of the dangers of oxytocin during labour, and its management and contraindications, see above (and *see* Section 2.5.F).

Vasa praevia

- This is an uncommon but life-threatening condition for the fetus or neonate. In vasa praevia, fetal blood vessels run over or close to the cervix beneath the presenting part, unprotected by Wharton's jelly or placental tissue. These vessels are vulnerable to laceration and compression, most commonly at the time of delivery.
- Fetal or neonatal death can occur due to exsanguination or asphyxiation.
- Antenatal diagnosis can be made only by skilled ultrasound examination. Caesarean section is then needed to reduce the high mortality rate.

Failure of blood clotting

This may be due to a pre-existing coagulation problem, or to complications of the pregnancy causing excessive bleeding and disseminated intravascular coagulation (DIC) (consumption of the clotting factors).

Obstetric causes include the following:
- placental abruption
- pre-eclampsia or eclampsia
- retained dead fetus
- septicaemia, including intrauterine sepsis
- incompatible blood transfusion
- amniotic fluid embolism.

Primary assessment and resuscitation and secondary assessment and emergency treatment for bleeding in pregnancy

In any patient with vaginal bleeding and known or possible placenta praevia, a vaginal assessment should be avoided and performed with extreme caution if deemed to be essential. Ideally an ultrasound should be used to confirm the placental site.

The aims are as follows:
- to prevent shock and disseminated intravascular coagulation
- to achieve intact fetal survival if viability is possible in the circumstances.

Call for experienced obstetric and anaesthetic assistance (if available) and ensure that the operating theatre is ready

Airway

- Open the airway using chin lift or jaw thrust techniques if it is closed or partially obstructed. If there is an improvement, keep the airway open using either an assistant or an oropharyngeal airway if the patient is unconscious and this is tolerated without gagging.
- Suction if necessary.
- The airway may need to be secured by intubation using experienced senior help (if available).

Breathing

- Normal respiratory rates in a pregnant mother at rest are 15–20 breaths/minute. Tachypnoea can be due to acidosis.
- Provide high-flow oxygen by face mask with reservoir bag for adequate spontaneous respiration regardless of SaO_2. This increases fetal oxygen delivery as well as improving maternal tissue oxygenation.
- If ventilation is inadequate, especially when there is a depressed conscious level (P or U on the AVPU scale), airway and breathing should be supported by bag-valve-mask inflations with high-flow oxygen, and experienced senior help should be called, including an anaesthetist if available.

Circulation

- Normal heart rates in a pregnant mother at rest are 60–90 beats/minute.
- Normal blood pressure in a pregnant mother at rest is 95/60–135/85 mmHg.
- Remember to put the patient in the left lateral tilt position and elevate the legs.
- Monitor the heart rate and blood pressure, and reassess regularly. Aim to keep the heart rate at ≤ 110 beats/minute and the systolic blood pressure at ≥ 100 mmHg.

Recognise the signs of hypovolaemia. These include the following:

- tachycardia
- tachypnoea
- cold, pale, sweaty and possibly cyanosed skin
- alteration of mental state: confusion or unconsciousness
- fall in urine output to less than 30 mL/hour
- narrowed pulse pressure
- hypotension (this is a late sign).

Healthy women and girls who are pregnant can maintain a normal blood pressure when large volumes of blood are lost. Most, but not all, will demonstrate tachycardia if they are bleeding significantly, but bradycardia may also be observed.

Remember that young healthy women can lose a lot of blood before they become shocked, especially if it is a slow trickle rather than a sudden large loss.

Restore circulating volume

- Put the mother in the left lateral tilt or recovery position to minimise the effects of compression of the inferior vena cava or aorta. Lateral tilt can be achieved by using a pillow, blanket or rolled up towel. A wedge may be

used during obstetric procedures. Assistants can also manually displace the uterus.

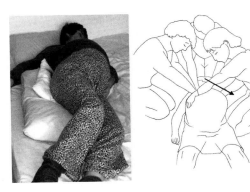

FIGURE 2.5.D.III.2 Manual displacement of uterus and left lateral tilt.

- Gain IV access and take blood for full blood count, cross-matching and blood clotting measurement. If IV access is not possible, consider intra-osseous needle insertion (*see* Section 8.4.B).
  - Use a short wide-bore IV cannula if possible, either 14G (usually orange) or 16G (usually grey).
  - External jugular vein access is a good option if peripheral access is impossible. Long saphenous vein cut-down may also be considered. If adequately trained personnel are available, central venous access, ideally via the internal jugular vein, can be extremely helpful. If access is not possible, consider intra-osseous needle insertion (*see* Section 8.4.B).
  - Try to obtain two vascular access sites to give large volumes quickly, and in case one line is lost. Do not waste time, and as soon as the first IV cannula is in place, give an IV fluid bolus.
  - Take blood for cross-matching (ideally 4–6 units), full blood count, renal function tests (if available), and blood clotting.
- Elevate the legs.
- Give an initial IV bolus of 500 mL to 1 litre of Ringer-lactate or Hartmann's solution as fast as possible using a three-way tap and 20- to 50-mL syringes to push in as rapidly as possible. If reassessment of the circulation shows little or no improvement, then a further 500 mL should be given and followed by blood transfusion as soon as this is available. (A normal adult has a circulatory blood volume of 5 litres, and during pregnancy this increases by 40% to 7 litres.)
- Apply an anti-shock garment (if available) to help maintain adequate central circulation.

Tranexamic acid can be of benefit in patients with continued bleeding. The loading dose is 1 gram over 10 minutes followed by an IV infusion of a further 1 gram over 8 hours. The slow IV bolus dose is given by injecting 1 gram of tranexamic acid into a 100-mL bag of 0.9% saline and letting it run through over about 10–20 minutes (the exact timing is not crucial). The 8-hour infusion is given by injecting 1 gram of tranexamic acid into a 500-mL bag of 0.9% saline and giving it over 8 hours (approximately 60 mL/hour).

- Ensure adequate transfusion; the best way to resuscitate the fetus is to resuscitate the mother. Inadequate transfusion is common, especially in cases of placental abruption.

- A central venous pressure (CVP) line can aid the decision as to whether more fluid is needed. However, insertion should not delay initial resuscitation, and must be undertaken by a competent person. If peripheral access is inadequate, this route may be used for volume replacement. If DIC is established, CVP insertion is more hazardous and the subclavian vein should be avoided, because it is not externally compressible.
- If shock is accompanied by a bradycardia of less than 60 beats/minute (e.g. in a patient with a ruptured uterus), give atropine 500–600 micrograms as an IV injection.

Blood products

- Fresh whole blood is preferable for managing obstetric haemorrhage.
- Use cross-matched blood where available except in an immediately life-threatening emergency, when group-specific blood should be used, as cross-matching may take up to an hour.
- The patient's blood group should be established during pregnancy, to facilitate the provision of blood when it is needed.
- All large-volume infusions should be warmed. In

particular, do not infuse cold fluid through a CVP line. The patient should also be kept warm, as hypothermia will exacerbate poor peripheral perfusion, acidosis and coagulation abnormalities. Any benefits of blood filters may be outweighed by their deleterious effect on the speed of transfusion. A good way of warming blood is to place the cold bag under the clothes of a relative next to their skin until the blood is warmed.

- Hand-inflated pressure bags are effective for giving blood and other fluids quickly (see Figure 2.5.A.5 on p. 170).

Identify and treat any blood clotting disorders.

- Assess bedside clotting: coagulopathy is defined as failure of a clot to form after 7 minutes, or formation of a soft clot that breaks easily (see Section 7.5 for details of whole blood clotting time measurement). Suspect and aggressively treat blood clotting disorders using warmed fresh blood, platelets (if the platelet count is $< 50\,000 \times 10^9$), fresh-frozen plasma (15 mL/kg) and cryoprecipitate as appropriate and if available.
- Freeze-dried plasma is being used in the military in adverse conditions, as it is shelf stable for 2 years and easily reconstituted with sterile water within minutes. It would be a very useful addition to the emergency stores

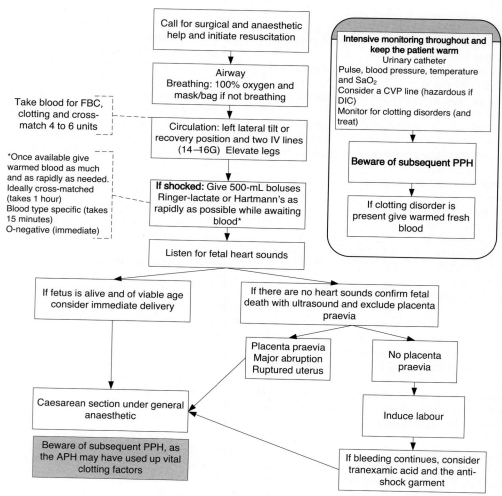

FIGURE 2.5.D.III.3 Pathway of care for massive antepartum haemorrhage (APH). FBC, full blood count; CVP, central venous pressure; DIC, disseminated intravascular coagulation; PPH, postpartum haemorrhage.

in resource-limited countries where the use of fresh or frozen plasma presents major storage problems.

- Urinary catheterisation is needed for measurement of hourly urine output. Aim for a rate of more than 30 mL/hour.

When the patient is stable, move her to a place where there is adequate space, light and equipment to continue resuscitation and treatment.

Fetal assessment
When the mother has been resuscitated:
- listen for fetal heart sounds
- if significant haemorrhage has occurred and the fetus is considered viable after birth in the prevailing circumstances, consider immediate delivery **only if this is safe for the mother**.

Anaesthetic issues
Cardiovascular instability is a relative contraindication to spinal anaesthesia.

- Rapid sequence induction agents with minimal peripheral vasodilator action, such as ketamine 1–2 mg/kg, should be considered.
- Adrenaline and atropine should be readily available in case cardiovascular collapse occurs on induction. Ventilation with high oxygen concentrations may be needed until the bleeding is controlled.
- Volatile agents have been associated with increased blood loss due to their relaxant effects on uterine muscle. Anaesthesia should be maintained with IV agents (usually ketamine) if uterine atony is a problem.
- If spinal anaesthesia is used, compensatory lower limb vasoconstriction is abolished, so profound hypotension may occur.

Delivery options
- Diagnose and treat the source of bleeding.
- Perform Caesarean section for major abruption or placenta praevia.
- Induce labour if the fetus is dead, there is no placenta praevia, the mother is stable and there is no significant ongoing blood loss.
  - Urine output should be monitored hourly and Caesarean section considered if labour does not become established fairly quickly. The longer the dead fetus remains *in utero*, the greater the likelihood of development of DIC.
  - **Expect and be prepared for massive postpartum haemorrhage, whether the baby is delivered vaginally or by Caesarean section.** In cases of severe APH that require surgery, discuss the possibility of hysterectomy.

It is often APH that weakens and PPH that kills, because APH uses up the clotting factors and platelets, leaving the woman in danger if PPH follows soon afterwards.

If no safe operating theatre facilities for Caesarean section are present, give oxygen, transfuse fresh blood and transfer the patient as soon as she is safe and stable. Ensure that IV fluids are in place, catheterise the patient, and ensure that she is nil by mouth.

Monitoring
Essential monitoring should include pulse rate and volume, blood pressure, respiratory rate, oxygenation (SaO_2 if available), temperature and fluid balance (with a urinary catheter). Regular checks of the haematocrit, clotting studies and blood gases will help to guide resuscitation.

Monitor blood glucose levels and treat any hypoglycaemia.

2.5.D.iv Postpartum haemorrhage

Introduction
The definition of a postpartum haemorrhage (PPH) is blood loss of more than 500 mL from a vaginal birth and more than 1 litre after a Caesarean section. It is common, occurring in 1–3% of all pregnancies. **Globally it causes 25–50% of maternal deaths, and is the leading cause of death in low-resource settings.**

Estimates of blood loss are inaccurate and tend to be low, often around half the actual loss. Blood is mixed with amniotic fluid and sometimes with urine. It is also dispersed on sponges, towels and linen, in buckets and on the floor.

The importance of any given volume of blood loss varies depending on the mother's haemoglobin level. A mother with a normal haemoglobin level will tolerate blood loss that would be fatal for an anaemic woman. This is why it is essential to ensure that every woman who reaches labour has an adequate haemoglobin level.

Even healthy non-anaemic women can have catastrophic blood loss.

Bleeding may occur at a slow rate over several hours, in which case the condition may not be recognised until the mother is shocked. Previously healthy women can compensate for substantial blood loss until a relatively late stage.

Risk assessment in the antenatal period does not necessarily predict women who will have PPH. However, identification and treatment of anaemia antenatally will allow women to better withstand life-threatening PPH.

Prevention of PPH
Active management of the third stage of labour
This is essential for prevention of PPH, and it consists of four possible interventions:
1. a prophylactic uterotonic drug after delivery, after checking that there is not a second twin present.
2. early cord clamping and cutting
3. controlled cord traction
4. uterine massage after delivery of the placenta.

Prophylactic uterotonic drug after delivery
This is the most important intervention. Oxytocin 10 IU IM or, especially if the mother is shocked, 5 IU by slow (over 1–2 minutes) IV injection is the first choice because it causes uterine contractions to prevent atony rapidly and with minimal adverse effects. Atony is the most common cause of PPH (around 80% of cases). Where oxytocin is

unavailable or does not work, other uterotonic drugs should be used, including:

- ergometrine 200 or 500 micrograms IM or misoprostol 600 micrograms sublingually or orally if the mother is fully conscious
- misoprostol 800 micrograms rectally if the mother is drowsy or unconscious.

All uterotonic drugs should be given within 1 minute of the complete birth of the fetus, to aid separation of the placenta by enhancing uterine contractions and reducing the risk of bleeding from an atonic (relaxed) uterus. **It is essential that, before giving such drugs, you are certain there is not another fetus in the uterus.**

Ensure that both oxytocin and ergometrine are protected from heat damage by paying close attention to the cold chain and their storage, otherwise they may not be effective. Ideally oxytocin should be stored in a fridge, but it can be kept at 15–30°C for 3 months. Oxytocin must never be frozen. Ergometrine should always be stored in a fridge at 2–8°C. Misoprostol can be stored at ambient temperature.

Remember that ergometrine is contraindicated in heart disease, hypertension, pre-eclampsia and eclampsia, as it raises the blood pressure by vasoconstriction, which increases the risk of cerebrovascular accidents.

Early cord clamping and cutting
This is not an essential part of the active management of the third stage of labour, and it is no longer recommended unless the infant needs resuscitation.

Controlled cord traction
This is optional where delivery is undertaken by a skilled birth attendant, but contraindicated if a skilled attendant is not available. Details are given in Section 2.3.

Strong uterine massage
This should always be undertaken immediately after delivery of the placenta until the uterus is contracted and remains so. Check the state of contraction of the uterus every 15 minutes for 2 hours, and repeat the massage if at any time the uterus becomes soft and relaxed.

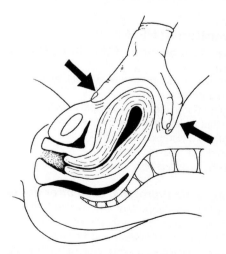

FIGURE 2.5.D.IV.1 Strong massage applied to cause uterus to contract.

The third stage

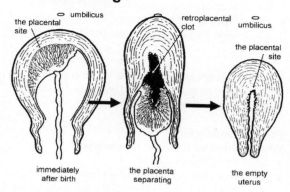

FIGURE 2.5.D.IV.2 The third stage.

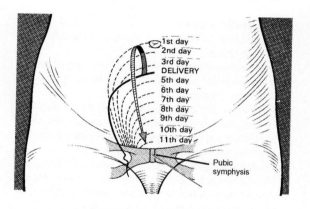

FIGURE 2.5.D.IV.3 The uterus during the puerperium.

In order to prevent PPH during or after Caesarean section, the use of oxytocin plus cord traction is recommended in preference to manual removal of the placenta.

How to manage the third stage of labour if uterotonic drugs are not available
Unfortunately it is not uncommon for hospitals to run out of uterotonic drugs. In this avoidable and dangerous situation, expectant and/or physiological management should be undertaken.
1. Place the baby on the mother's breast.
2. Leave the cord alone.
3. Observe for the following signs of placental separation:
   - a small gush of blood
   - a lengthening of the cord at the introitus
   - the mother feeling uncomfortable, feeling a contraction and wanting to 'bear down'.

Most placentas separate within 1 hour of birth. If this does not happen, seek help.
4. Deliver the placenta.
   - Sit the mother upright.
   - Encourage her to bear down with a contraction (only after placental separation).
   - Catch the placenta. If membranes are dragging behind it, gently twist a few turns and with slight traction and an up-and-down movement deliver the placenta plus membranes.

Controlled cord traction should not be undertaken prior to

TABLE 2.5.D.IV.1 Diagnosis of causes of PPH

Symptoms	Signs	Possible diagnosis
Immediate heavy bleeding after birth	Uterus soft and not contracted	Atonic uterus
Immediate heavy bleeding after birth	Uterus contracted	Trauma to cervix, vagina or perineum
Bleeding which may be light if clot is blocking cervix	Placenta not delivered within 30 minutes of birth	Retained placenta
Bleeding which is usually light but continues for many hours	Portion of placenta missing Uterus contracted	Retained placental parts
Bleeding for more than 24 hours	Portion of placenta missing Foul-smelling lochia may be present Fever may be present Severe anaemia	Retained placental parts with or without infection
Lower abdominal pain of varying intensity Immediate but usually light bleeding	Uterus not felt on abdominal palpation Inverted uterus may be seen at vulva Bradycardia may be present Shock	Inverted uterus
Usually during labour there has been a change from intermittent labour contractions to a constant pain which may become less after rupture has occurred Sometimes an oxytocin drip is in place Vaginal bleeding which may be light or heavy History of a previous Caesarean section or other operation on the uterus	Shock Abdominal distension Tenderness over uterus	Ruptured uterus (more likely before delivery of the baby)

the separation of the placenta in the absence of uterotonic drugs.

Monitoring after the placenta has been delivered by active or expectant management

1 Monitor the blood pressure, pulse and state of the uterus (i.e. whether it is contracted) every 15 minutes for 2 hours after delivery of the placenta.

2 Examine the placenta for completeness.

Causes of PPH

Primary PPH

This occurs within 24 hours of birth, and in around 80% of cases is due to uterine atony.

Remember the 4 T's: Tone, Tissue, Trauma, Thrombin.

- **Tone:** atonic uterus – failure to contract after birth.
- **Tissue:** retained placenta or placental fragments.
- **Trauma:** ruptured uterus, or trauma to the cervix, vagina or perineum.
- **Thrombin:** clotting defects, notably disseminated intravascular coagulation (DIC).

Remember also the following:

- **Haemorrhage may be concealed within the uterus or within the abdominal cavity.**
- **A ruptured uterus** can cause concealed bleeding, as can **bleeding following Caesarean section.**
- **An inverted uterus is associated with PPH.**
- **Any degree of PPH is dangerous if there has been severe anaemia before delivery.**

Secondary PPH

Secondary PPH (occurring from 24 hours or more after delivery up to 6 weeks after birth) is commonly associated with retained products of conception that undergo necrosis, become infected and prevent involution (sustained contraction) of the uterus. A **fever** suggests an infective component.

See p. 198 for details of the management of this problem.

Factors that predispose to PPH

These include the following:

- previous APH
- retained products of conception
- trauma to the uterus or birth canal (e.g. from instrumental delivery)
- uterine over-distension (e.g. due to multiple pregnancy or polyhydramnios)
- grand multiparity
- prolonged labour.

Management of PPH

First call for help (this must include a surgeon and an anaesthetist), palpate the uterus and massage it strongly and immediately, as it is most likely that an atonic uterus is the cause (see Figure 2.5.D.iv.1 and below).

Airway and breathing

- Ensure that the airway is open and remains so.
- Provide **high-flow oxygen** through a face mask with reservoir bag if there is adequate spontaneous respiration.

Give 100% oxygen (using a mask with reservoir and high flow rate).

- For patients with inadequate ventilation or depressed conscious level (P or U on the AVPU scale), respiration should be supported with oxygen via a **bag-valve-mask**, and experienced senior help should be summoned (if available).

Circulation
Primary assessment denoting shock
- Fast, weak pulse (≥ 100–110 beats/minute). Normal heart rates in a pregnant mother at rest are 60–90 beats/minute. Tachycardia is an early sign of shock.
- Low-volume (weak) pulse.
- Pallor (especially of the inner eyelid, palms or around the mouth).
- Sweatiness or cold clammy skin.
- Prolonged capillary refill time (> 3 seconds).
- Rapid breathing (> 30 breaths/minute). Normal respiratory rates at rest are 15–20 breaths/minute; tachypnoea can be due to acidosis.
- Low blood pressure (systolic pressure < 90 mmHg) is a **very late sign**. Healthy women and girls can maintain a normal or even high blood pressure while losing large volumes of blood.
- Nausea with or without vomiting.
- Anxiety, confusion or unconsciousness.
- Reduced urine output (< 30 mL/hour). Urinary catheterisation is needed for measurement of hourly urine output if the patient is shocked (normal output is > 30 mL/hour).

Procedures for stopping haemorrhage must be started immediately and then undertaken in parallel with IV fluid resuscitation.

Measures to stop further haemorrhage due to uterine atony
Rubbing up a contraction
Poor contraction of the uterus after delivery is the commonest cause of PPH. **Rub up a contraction of the uterus (do not just pinch the skin).**

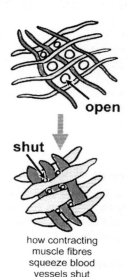

how contracting
muscle fibres
squeeze blood
vessels shut

FIGURE 2.5.D.IV.4 Contraction of uterine muscle fibres squeezes blood vessels shut.

As the muscle fibres are stimulated to contract, they compress the blood vessels running between the muscle fibres and help to stop bleeding.

Abdominal massage of the uterus
If the uterus is atonic, a contraction may be rubbed up by abdominal massage.
- Massage the fundus in a circular motion with the cupped palm of your hand until it is contracted.
- When it is well contracted, place your fingers behind the fundus and push down in one swift action to expel clots.

Uterotonic drugs
These drugs make the uterus contract.

Give 10 IU of oxytocin IM or 5 IU IV slowly, especially if the patient is already shocked, and repeat after 5 minutes if they are still bleeding and/or the uterus is not contracted. This is the drug of first choice.

Oxytocin starts to work 2–3 minutes after IV injection, but has a relatively short duration of action, and an infusion will be needed to maintain a contracted uterus. Following an oxytocin bolus, give an IV infusion of oxytocin 40 IU in 500 mL (60 drops/minute with a standard IV giving set where 20 drops = 1 mL) or 1 litre (120 drops/minute) of Ringer-lactate or Hartmann's solution over 4 hours.

Side effects include hypotension (due to vasodilatation when given as a rapid IV bolus) and fluid retention.

If the mother does not have eclampsia, pre-eclampsia or hypertension, **ergometrine** 200 to 500 micrograms IM in addition may help uterine contraction. If the first dose of oxytocin does not stop bleeding within a few minutes, give **misoprostol** (which, unlike oxytocin and ergometrine, does not need to be kept in a refrigerator). It is given rectally as 4 × 200 microgram tablets or pessaries (800 micrograms in total) or, if the patient is conscious, orally as 3 × 200 microgram tablets or 2 × 200 micrograms of powder sublingually.

Ergometrine, either as part of Syntometrine (oxytocin 5 IU and ergometrine 500 micrograms IM) or alone, is contraindicated in pre-eclampsia, as its hypertensive action increases the risk of convulsions and cerebrovascular accidents.

Urinary catheterisation
This may help the uterus to contract.

Bimanual uterine compression
If heavy PPH continues despite uterine massage, and with the placenta already delivered, this procedure can be very effective. If the placenta is still in place priority should be given to removing it as soon as possible.
- You must wear sterile or disinfected gloves (ideally long versions up to the elbow).
- Introduce your right hand into the vagina, clench your fist with the back of your hand positioned posteriorly and your knuckles in the anterior fornix.
- Place your other hand on the abdomen behind the uterus and squeeze the uterus firmly between both hands.
- Continue compression until the bleeding stops (i.e. there is no bleeding when compression is released), and the uterus is contracted.

Although this procedure is painful, it is highly effective and can significantly reduce or even successfully treat uterine haemorrhage. Therefore, if the bleeding is profuse, and the number of staff attending the patient allows, it is a good idea for one member of the team to commence bimanual compression while uterotonic drugs are prepared and given, and initial fluid resuscitation commenced.

Bimanual compression

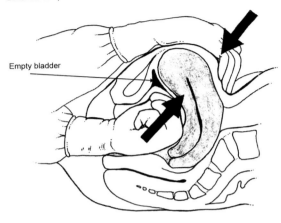

FIGURE 2.5.D.IV.5 Bimanual compression.

Aortic compression

If bleeding still persists, apply aortic compression.

- Apply downward pressure with a closed fist (with your thumb outside the fist) over the abdominal aorta directly through the abdominal wall.
- The point of compression is just above the umbilicus and slightly to the left.
- Aortic pulsations can be felt through the anterior abdominal wall in the immediate postpartum period. Press the aorta down on to the vertebral column.
- With your other hand, palpate the femoral pulse with four fingers parallel to and just below the inguinal ligament to check the adequacy of compression.
- **If the pulse is palpable during compression, the pressure exerted by the fist is inadequate.**
- **If the femoral pulse is not palpable, the pressure exerted is adequate.**

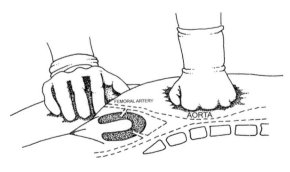

FIGURE 2.5.D.IV.6 Aortic compression.

Continue until the bleeding stops. If it does not stop, continue to exert pressure while transferring the mother to a facility where expert help is available.

Uterine tamponade

Uterine packing with a hydrostatic balloon such as a Rusch balloon or condom over a simple in–out urinary catheter can help to control haemorrhage from an atonic uterus that does not respond to the above measures. The uterus may also be packed with a sterile pack or gauze, although it is important to ensure any gauze used is tied together, counted carefully, and extended into the vagina to facilitate removal.

A condom catheter, which is inserted into the uterus as a sterile procedure and filled with 250–500 mL of sterile Ringer-lactate or Hartmann's solution or 0.9% saline to create a uterine wall tamponade, is an effective way of stopping uterine bleeding that is continuing despite the use of uterotonic drugs and procedures (see Figure 2.5.D.iv.7). **It is important to check that the balloon is fully inside the uterus as it is inflated, and to take measures to ensure that it does not become displaced into the vagina.** This can be done by packing the vagina with a pack or gauze swab.

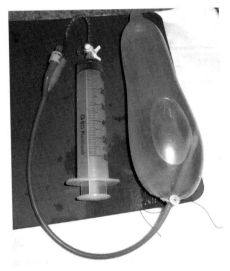

FIGURE 2.5.D.IV.7 Condom catheter inflated with sterile IV fluid.

Leave the balloon in position until the bleeding has stopped for up to 24 hours (the exact time needed is unclear). Before removing it, ensure that at least 1 unit of cross-matched blood for possible transfusion is available, with the possibility of making more available if required. Theatre staff and an anaesthetist should be warned in case bleeding occurs when the catheter is removed. One approach is to remove 50 mL every 30 minutes until it is fully emptied. Observe the patient closely for 4 hours after removal of the catheter, looking at vaginal blood loss and vital signs. IV antibiotics should be given when the catheter is put in place, and should be continued for 48 hours.

An alternative new approach (the EgAr device from The Gambia) useful in low resource settings involves inflating a condom with air rather than IV fluids (see Figure 2.5.D.iv.8). It includes the following components:

- a firm type of urinary catheter (used for temporary insertion and drainage of urine) rather than an indwelling Foley catheter, which is easily constricted
- a latex male condom from a sterile and unbroken pack
- the inflator (with its tube) of an aneroid blood pressure machine
- a surgical suture (preferably black silk) for tying the condom to the catheter
- a piece of sterile thread for tying the end of the condom after inflation to stop the escape of air

- sterile gauze to pack the vagina and maintain the inflated condom in the uterine cavity.

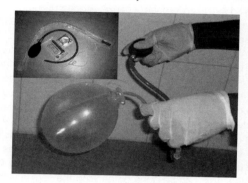

FIGURE 2.5.D.IV.8 Condom catheter inflated with air.

Using a sterile procedure throughout, the catheter is inserted into the condom, with the end part of the condom touching the tip of the catheter. The lower part of the condom is tied to the catheter using suture thread and inserted into the uterine cavity. The condom is then held in place inside the uterine cavity using the non-dominant hand, the lower end of the catheter is connected to the inflator of the blood pressure machine (with the valve closed), and the condom is then inflated with air until the bleeding is either arrested or greatly reduced. Pneumatic pressure is rapidly achieved after a few inflations. The uterus gradually increases in size (this can be seen abdominally) as the condom is being inflated, and the woman should experience no more than slight discomfort. Excessive inflation of the condom must be avoided, and pain indicates that too much air is being forced into the condom. If this happens, the volume of air can be easily reduced by loosening the valve of the inflator.

Compared with inflating the condom with fluid (assuming that IV fluid is available, which is not always the case), this technique is much faster and easier, and good control is achieved by using the valve on the inflator.

Fluid resuscitation

The aim of fluid resuscitation is to maintain perfusion of vital organs (the brain, heart and kidneys) during the manoeuvres described above.

1 **Elevate the patient's legs (raise the foot of the bed).**
2 Try to obtain two vascular access sites in order to give large volumes quickly, and in case one line is lost. Insert a wide-bore IV cannula (ideally two) (14- to 16G) and send blood for a full blood count, cross-matching (4–6 units) and clotting. If peripheral veins are difficult to access, the external jugular vein or long saphenous vein cut-down are good alternatives. If a skilled person is available, an internal jugular vein central line can be helpful, especially if the central venous pressure can be measured.
3 If venous access is not possible, consider inserting an intra-osseous line using the newly available drill system (*see* Section 8.4.B).
4 Give 500 mL of O-negative blood if it is immediately available. If not, standard practice is to give an initial **rapid** IV bolus of 1 litre of Ringer-lactate or Hartmann's solution (or of 0.9% saline if the former are not available) while waiting for blood for transfusion. It is essential that the IV bolus is given as rapidly as possible, with the aid of pressure bags or manual pressure. A blood

pressure cuff that is wrapped around the fluid bag and inflated can be used to speed up infusions (*see* Figure 2.5.D.iv.9). An alternative is to push the boluses in using a 20- to 50-mL syringe (with a three-way tap linked to the IV giving set).

5 **As soon as it is available give 1 unit of blood (500 mL) as rapidly as possible,** and repeat as required. Fresh blood is particularly useful for combating the coagulopathy that occurs in major blood loss if specific coagulation components such as platelets are unavailable. Remember that blood loss is usually underestimated.
6 Further 500- to 1000-mL boluses of IV crystalloid or blood, if available, will usually be required in the first hour. Once more than 2 litres have been given IV, complications such as pulmonary oedema may sometimes occur, so be alert for circulatory overload.

The concept of **targeted crystalloid fluid resuscitation** may be relevant here and requires urgent research. If this approach is adopted the initial boluses of IV crystalloids required to treat shock would only be given to keep the vital organs (especially the brain, heart and kidneys) perfused before blood becomes available and, most important of all, before specific treatments to stop the bleeding have started to take effect. Giving too much IV crystalloid fluid may theoretically increase bleeding by disrupting early clot formation and damaging the coagulation system. There is no clear evidence to indicate the precise blood pressure or clinical signs that should be achieved in a woman in shock due to PPH. **Adequate perfusion of vital organs may be indicated by a radial pulse that can be palpated and a fully alert conscious level.**

Until bleeding has been stopped and blood is available for transfusion, our personal practice, especially in low resource settings, is therefore to start with IV boluses of 500 mL of crystalloid and reassess after each bolus.

7 Keep the patient warm but do not overheat them, as this will cause peripheral vasodilatation and reduce the

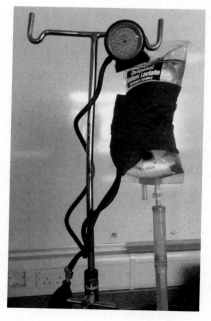

FIGURE 2.5.D.IV.9 Pressure bag over bag containing Ringer-lactate or Hartmann's solution.

blood supply to vital centres. Hypothermia will exacerbate poor peripheral perfusion, acidosis and coagulation abnormalities.

8 If there is evidence of a blood-clotting problem, give fresh-frozen plasma and/or other clotting factors (if available).

9 Further IV fluid administration should be guided by the response of the pulse rate, blood pressure and capillary refill time, and later by the hourly urine output. Aim for a pulse rate of ≤ 100–110 beats/minute and a systolic blood pressure that is ≥ 90–100 mmHg and stable.

Blood products

Fresh whole blood is the ideal choice if it is available. Full cross-matching of blood may take up to an hour and is often unavailable in resource poor settings. In an emergency, group-specific blood should be used. The patient's blood group should have been established during pregnancy, as this facilitates the provision of blood when it is needed. O-Rhesus-negative blood can be transfused in acute emergencies.

All large-volume infusions of blood should be warmed. A good way of warming blood is to place each bag of blood or fluid under a relative's clothes next to their skin. Do not infuse cold fluid directly through a central venous line.

New potentially valuable treatments for PPH
Tranexamic acid

If there is continuing bleeding, especially if it has been caused by genital tract trauma, this inexpensive and safe drug can be helpful. Recent evidence has shown that tranexamic acid can reduce mortality from major haemorrhage in major trauma in adults. The drug should be started as soon as possible, and within the first 3 hours after the onset of major haemorrhage, in order to be effective.

The loading dose is 1 gram over 10 minutes followed by an IV infusion of a further 1 gram over 8 hours.

The slow IV bolus dose is given by injecting 1 gram of tranexamic acid into a 100-mL bag of 0.9% saline and letting it run through over a period of about 10–20 minutes (the exact timing is not crucial).

The 8-hour infusion is given by injecting 1 gram of tranexamic acid into a 500-mL bag of 0.9% saline and giving it over a period of 8 hours (i.e. approximately 60 mL/hour). If there is a gap between the initial bolus and the subsequent infusion this probably does not matter too much, but ideally one should follow the other.

The non-pneumatic anti-shock garment (NASG)

This compression garment is made from neoprene, a stretchable material that recoils and applies pressure through the skin. It feels like a tight diving wet-suit to wear, and consists of five segments that compress the legs (segments 1, 2 and 3), the pelvis (segment 4) and the abdomen (segment 5) (see Figures 2.5.D.iv.10 and 2.5.D.iv.11). The abdominal segment includes a foam compression ball that presses on the area of the uterus. The segments are held in place by Velcro. It is a very promising, potentially life-saving technique for low-resource settings.

Preliminary pre- and post-intervention trials have shown that the NASG significantly reduces shock, blood loss, the need for emergency hysterectomy, and maternal mortality and severe morbidity associated with PPH and other

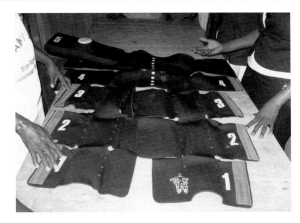

FIGURE 2.5.D.IV.10 NASG garment before it is placed on the patient. Reproduced with permission from Miller S, Martin HB, Morris JL. Anti-shock garment in postpartum haemorrhage. *Best Pract Res Clin Obstet Gynaecol.* 2008; **22**(6): 1057–74. © Elsevier

causes of obstetric haemorrhage. Randomised controlled trials by the World Health Organization and others are currently under way in Zambia and Zimbabwe.

The NASG is reported to reduce shock by compressing blood vessels in the lower parts of the body, thereby diverting up to 30% of total blood volume to the heart, lungs, brain and possibly the kidneys. There is evidence that, through the applied pressures of 25–50 mmHg, it decreases blood flow in the pelvis and, in PPH, blood loss from the atonic uterus.

It is particularly promising in settings where there can be delays in transfer to facilities where comprehensive emergency obstetric care is available, and where blood transfusion and surgery can be undertaken. In such settings, even in hospitals, blood transfusion is frequently delayed for between 1 and 3 hours, with O-negative blood rarely available and supplies of stored blood precarious. The NASG, by stabilising the patient, gives time for blood transfusion to become established and other treatments to be given, as well as very probably reducing the amount of blood that subsequently needs to be transfused.

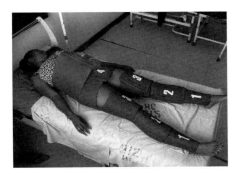

FIGURE 2.5.D.IV.11 NASG garment on a patient. Reproduced with permission from Miller S, Martin HB, Morris JL. Anti-shock garment in postpartum haemorrhage. *Best Pract Res Clin Obstet Gynaecol.* 2008; **22**(6): 1057–74. © Elsevier

As reported by the International Federation of Gynecology and Obstetrics (FIGO), 'The NASG is not a definitive treatment – the woman will still need to have the source of bleeding found and definitive therapy performed.' We would qualify this statement and substitute the word 'may' for 'will', as sometimes the bleeding, particularly in PPH, may be reduced during the application of the NASG, and advanced treatments such as surgery may not then be required.

The NASG is applied in sequence from the lower legs up to the abdominal compression segment (segment 5). With experience it can be applied by one person in 2 minutes, although it takes from 5 to 10 minutes if the healthcare worker is alone and unused to applying it. Help from others present, such as porters or relatives, can be valuable. In PPH due to uterine atony, it is particularly important that someone is massaging the uterus and giving the other treatments outlined above when the NASG is being applied. After the garment is in place the legs no longer need to be elevated and the uterus can still be externally massaged by placing one hand underneath the pelvic segment of the NASG. Vaginal examinations and repair of cervical or vaginal tears can be performed while the NASG is in place. The pelvic and abdominal segments can be opened for surgery such as emergency hysterectomy or B-Lynch sutures.

The NASG can be applied in addition to all the other measures for PPH described above when signs of shock first appear (*see* Section 2.5.A). The only contraindication to its use is known heart disease. The aim with all treatments is for a pulse rate of ≤ 100–110 beat/minute and a systolic blood pressure that is ≥ 90–100 mmHg and stable in a woman who is fully alert and has a urine output of ≥ 30 mL/hour.

The NASG is removed segment by segment when bleeding has been reduced to safe levels and the patient's cardiovascular stability has been maintained for at least 2 hours (systolic blood pressure ≥ 90–100 mmHg, heart rate ≤ 100–110 beats/minute and haemoglobin concentration of ≥ 7 g/dL). Removal begins at the ankles with 15-minute gaps between each segment that is opened, and clinical measurements being made before each segment is removed. If the systolic blood pressure drops by ≥ 20 mmHg and/or the heart rate increases by ≥ 20 beats/minute, reapply that segment of the NASG and consider additional treatments such as further blood transfusion.

Between patients, the NASG can be laundered in the same way as for bloodstained sheets. First soak the garment in 0.5% chloride solution for 15 minutes. Then wash and scrub it with a soft brush in soapy water. Finally rinse it in clean water and leave it to air-dry. Fold and store the garment when it is completely dry.

Each NASG can be used 50–100 times, and at present costs US$150–200.

Stopping bleeding due to trauma to the perineum, cervix or vagina

If the bleeding continues despite all of the measures described above, examine the perineum, vagina and cervix with a sterile speculum. Postpartum bleeding with a contracted uterus is usually due to a cervical or vaginal tear. Trauma to the lower genital tract is the second most frequent cause of PPH, and may coexist with an atonic uterus.

Examine the mother carefully and repair any tears. Bleeding from trauma can be substantial and may be fatal, especially if there is pre-existing severe anaemia. Suture packs, a torch, a Sims' speculum and sutures must always be immediately available on the PPH emergency trolley.

Initially stop the bleeding with sterile packing until a surgeon is able to repair the wounds.

It is essential to ensure that the uterus is contracted even when a traumatic cause is present.

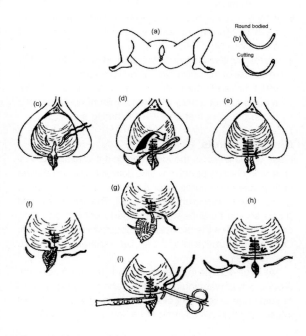

FIGURE 2.5.D.IV.12 Repairing a perineal tear.

Repairing a perineal tear

Get a good light, and start at the top of the tear. If difficult ask for help if available.

1 Anything except very minor tears should be repaired in the lithotomy or similar position as it provides a better view and is more comfortable for the surgeon/midwife.

2 Use a cutting needle on the skin and a round-bodied needle on other tissues.

3 Put the first stitch in above the highest point of the tear (apex). This is usually within the vagina.

4 When you get to the junction between the vaginal mucosa and the skin, put a needle through the loop and tie a knot.

5 Continue by applying stitches into the muscle and fascia to close any dead space (gaping of the vaginal skin) and again tie a knot once done.

6 Next close the skin by placing the needle in through the skin on one side, and then in through the sub-cutaneous tissues and out through the skin on the other side. If using interrupted sutures, the stitches are usually inserted ~ ½cm from the skin edges and ~1 cm apart from each other. Tie a knot after each stitch to oppose the skin.

Repairing a bleeding cervical tear

Place the patient in the lithotomy position and explain the procedure to the patient.

Get a good light and if at all possible an assistant.

Search all round the patient's cervix, if the cervix is not easily visible grasp it with a sponge holding forceps (or similar) and pull it into view. In order to visualise the entire cervix it is often necessary to follow the cervix round from anterior to posterior by pulling each segment down with the sponge holding forceps. Ideally two forceps are used and the next segment picked up with one set of forceps while traction is maintained with the other ('walking the cervix').

Once the cervical tear is identified start suturing it at its highest point (the apex).

If you cannot insert sutures, control the bleeding with a vaginal pack and transfer the patient.

Stopping bleeding due to retained placenta or retained products of conception
Examine the placenta and ensure that it is complete.

Retained placenta
A retained placenta is defined as occurring:
1 after active management of the third stage of labour (*see* Section 2.3), if the placenta is not delivered within 30 minutes of the birth
2 after expectant management of the third stage of labour, if the placenta is not delivered within 60 minutes of the birth.

Risk factors include a full bladder, a previous retained placenta, high parity, uterine fibroids, a history of previous uterine surgery and placenta praevia. The placenta may become trapped in the cervix or lower uterus. There may be no bleeding with a retained placenta, especially if there is abnormal adherence (placenta accreta).

A retained placenta occurs in around 2% of deliveries.

Management of retained placenta
If there is a clinically significant PPH, the placenta must be removed urgently. Call for help (including an anaesthetist and an obstetrician), insert a venous cannula, take blood for haemoglobin and cross-matching as for PPH, and ensure that the operating theatre is ready.

Massage the uterus, and if there is atony it should be managed as described for PPH above. However, although oxytocin should be used as necessary, **do not give ergometrine because it causes tonic uterine contraction, which may delay expulsion**.

Cause 1: The placenta is separated but trapped in the lower part of the uterus or cervix
If the **placenta is undelivered after 30 minutes of oxytocin stimulation**, and the **uterus is contracted and the placenta separated** (usually indicated by the gushing of blood and rising of the uterus into the abdomen as a firm, more movable structure as with a normal placental separation and delivery), attempt controlled cord traction. During this procedure, and at all times, keep one hand on the abdomen to support the uterus and prevent its inversion.

Avoid forceful cord traction and fundal pressure, as they may cause uterine inversion.

This situation usually responds to firm and persistent traction on the cord with the other hand countering this on the uterus to prevent inversion. Ensure that the bladder is empty. Ask the mother to empty her bladder, otherwise catheterise the bladder if necessary. If you can see the placenta, ask the mother to push it out; an upright position may help. Undertake a sterile vaginal examination and if you can feel the placenta in the vagina or cervix, remove it.

Cause 2: The placenta has failed to separate from the uterus
If controlled cord traction plus uterotonic drugs are

unsuccessful, manual removal of the placenta is likely to be required (see below).

If the cord has broken from the placenta, it is still possible for the placenta to be pushed out by contractions and by the mother.

Cause 3: The placenta is morbidly attached to the uterus
Very adherent tissue may be **placenta accreta**, a situation that is more likely to occur after a previous Caesarean section. Efforts to extract a placenta that does not separate easily may result in heavy bleeding or uterine perforation, which usually requires hysterectomy.

Therefore, if there is any suspicion of a morbidly adherent placenta the patient should ideally be referred to a hospital with operating facilities and a surgical team (if available). See pages below for more details on management.

Where there is significant haemorrhage, uterine and vaginal packing with gauze or balloon tamponade/condom catheter can halt the bleeding and eventually allow residual placenta to disintegrate and resorb/expel on its own. Hysterectomy will be needed if bleeding cannot be stopped by the measures described above.

If **bleeding continues**, assess clotting status using a bedside clotting test. Failure of a clot to form after 7 minutes, or formation of a soft clot that breaks down easily, suggests coagulopathy.

If there are **signs of infection** (fever with foul-smelling vaginal discharge), give antibiotics as for endometritis.

Manual removal of the placenta
This is a painful procedure associated with a high risk of infection unless it is undertaken using full sterile procedures. In many low-resource settings, manual removal of the placenta is undertaken without analgesia or anaesthesia, and often not even in the operating theatre.

Unless it is performed as an emergency for major PPH, we consider that manual removal of the placenta should be undertaken in an operating theatre with preceding morphine or ketamine in the presence of an anaesthetist. Elbow-length sterile gloves should be used. Provided that active PPH is not occurring, **the mother should first be adequately resuscitated with IV fluids/blood and oxygen**. The pulse rate, blood pressure, oxygen saturation and urine output should be closely monitored. Ideally, facilities for blood transfusion and, if necessary, emergency hysterectomy should be available.

After the placenta has been removed, massage the uterus to encourage tonic uterine contraction. An IV infusion of oxytocin 40 units in 500 mL or 1 litre of Ringer-lactate or

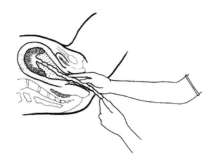

FIGURE 2.5.D.IV.13 Introducing one hand into the vagina along the cord.

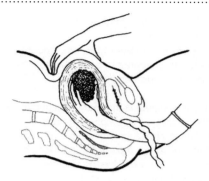

FIGURE 2.5.D.IV.14 Supporting the fundus while detaching the placenta. Reach the placenta from the implantation site by keeping the fingers tightly together and using the edge of the hand to gradually make a space between the placenta and the uterine wall

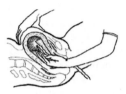

FIGURE 2.5.D.IV.15 Withdrawing the hand plus the placenta from the uterus.

Hartmann's solution should be administered over 4 hours to ensure continued uterine contraction.

A single dose of prophylactic antibiotics should be given just before all manual removals (2 grams of ampicillin IV or IM plus 80 mg of gentamicin IM/IV).

Treatment of PPH that continues despite all of the above interventions

Reassess the patient and determine whether bleeding is continuing and whether there is a clotting disorder. Assess the clotting status using a bedside clotting test. Failure of a clot to form after 7 minutes, or formation of a soft clot that breaks down easily, suggests coagulopathy.

If bleeding continues, re-examine the patient and ensure that the oxytocin IV infusion is running correctly (40 units of oxytocin in 500 mL of Ringer-lactate or Hartmann's solution over 4 hours).

Exclude the following:
- inverted uterus
- retained products of conception
- damage to the genital tract: check for bleeding from the cervix, vaginal walls and perineum.

If the above measures fail to control PPH, **do not wait too long.**

The following operative interventions are available:
- B-Lynch sutures
- hysterectomy, which may be life-saving, and should be considered early in order to reduce the risk of life-threatening coagulopathy.

Check the haemoglobin levels or haematocrit after resuscitation and when the patient is stable. Consider administering oral iron if the patient is anaemic.

Treatment of secondary PPH

This is particularly dangerous in low-resource settings. Severe and life-threatening anaemia can develop rapidly, and frequently the woman is admitted in shock and urgently requiring blood transfusion. Severe life-threatening septic shock can also develop.

Assess vital signs and temperature, and if the patient is shocked proceed as described above for massive PPH.

Assess the uterine size, and perform a speculum and vaginal examination and note the degree of bleeding, whether the blood is offensive, whether the cervix is still open, and whether there is cervical and uterine tenderness. Take a high vaginal swab for bacteriology (if available) before antibiotics are given.

Insert an IV line and take blood for haemoglobin, blood cultures, cross-matching and blood clotting (or clotting/bleeding time if unavailable) (as DIC may occur).

Urgently start 7 days of treatment with IV antibiotics, as the bleeding is often secondary to infection. This is especially likely if there is foul-smelling lochia, a fever, or there has been prolonged rupture of membranes prior to delivery.
- Give IV ampicillin 2 grams IV every 6 hours
  - *plus* gentamicin 80 mg IV or IM every 8 hours or 5 mg/kg body weight IV/IM once every 24 hours
  - *plus* metronidazole 500 mg IV every 8 hours.
- Alternatively, give ceftriaxone 2 grams IV or IM once daily *plus* metronidazole 500 mg IV every 8 hours.

Provide blood transfusion (ideally fresh blood) if the haemoglobin level is < 5 g/dL, or if it is < 7.5 g/dL with symptoms suggesting early cardiac failure or shock or if there is brisk ongoing blood loss.

Examine for suspected retained placental fragments, but beware of the high risk of uterine perforation. Feel inside the uterus using elbow-length sterile gloves, and try to remove any retained products manually or using ovum forceps. **Be very careful not to perforate the uterus.** Placental tissue that sticks to the uterus may be placenta accreta, which may result in heavy bleeding (see below for management). If the cervical os has already started to close, this approach might not be possible. If a curette is used, it should be blunt, and great care should be taken as the uterus will be soft and easy to perforate. A vacuum aspirator (as used for treating miscarriage) or digital curettage may be safer options. Laparotomy is occasionally needed to deal with the continued bleeding from an infected or ruptured uterine incision or infected placental bed.

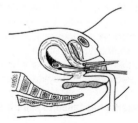

FIGURE 2.5.D.IV.16 Evacuating the uterus.

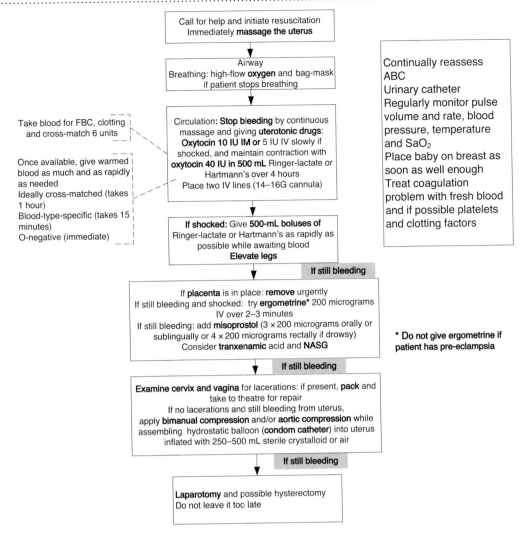

FIGURE 2.5.D.IV.17 Pathway of care for massive postpartum haemorrhage (PPH). Aim for a contracted and empty uterus. FBC, full blood count; NASG, non-pneumatic anti-shock garment; ABC, airway, breathing and circulation.

Management of placenta accreta

This serious complication is caused by the placenta being morbidly adherent to deeper layers in the uterine muscle or even external to the uterus. It is more common after a previous Caesarean section and in the presence of a placenta praevia. After Caesarean section an attempt should be made to assess the site of the placenta with ultrasound to determine whether it is likely to overlie the previous scar.

If the patient undergoes a new Caesarean section, or has a retained placenta, the procedure should be carried out by the most experienced practitioner possible and preparations made for major haemorrhage, i.e. experienced anaesthetic assistance, good intravenous access, cross matched blood and availability of the non-pneumatic anti-shock garment.

An option is to allow the placenta to be left *in situ* where it may separate and expel itself over time. This risks haemorrhage, infection and DIC and in these cases the mother must be made aware of these risks. She must be observed carefully for signs of infection, given prophylactic antibiotics (single dose of ampicillin 2 g IV/IM plus gentamicin 5 mg/kg body weight IV/IM) and warned about what to expect when the placenta is eventually expelled. She must have rapid access to emergency care and be monitored as an inpatient.

Alternatively, an attempt to remove the placenta can be made. Haemorrhage, as discussed, should be anticipated and the procedure performed in theatre with adequate intravenous access, monitoring, cross-matched blood available and the most experienced anaesthetic and surgical personnel possible.

An alternative option is an immediate hysterectomy in order to prevent later complications and the necessity for very close post-partum monitoring. The decision will need to be based on the patient's wishes, the resources available and the doctor's abilities. If there is no facility for emergency hysterectomy, the patient should be transferred to a facility where this is available.

Bleeding due to inverted uterus
See Section 2.6.H.

Anaesthetic issues when managing PPH
Cardiovascular instability is a relative contraindication to regional blockade.

Rapid sequence induction agents with minimal

peripheral vasodilator action, such as ketamine, should be considered (*see* Section 1.24). Adrenaline and atropine should be readily available in case cardiovascular collapse occurs on induction. Ventilation with high concentrations of oxygen may be needed until the bleeding is controlled.

Volatile agents have been associated with increased blood loss due to their relaxant effects on uterine muscle. Anaesthesia should be maintained with IV agents (ketamine or etomidate) if uterine atony is contributing to haemorrhage.

Disseminated intravascular coagulation (DIC)

Suspect and aggressively treat coagulopathy using warmed fresh blood, platelets, fresh-frozen plasma and cryoprecipitate as appropriate and available. DIC is more likely to occur if there has been a previous antepartum haemorrhage.

Sheehan's syndrome

Very rarely, massive PPH can cause pituitary infarction (also called Sheehan's syndrome). This presents initially as failure of breastfeeding, and later as no return of menstrual bleeding, as well as fatigue, low blood pressure and loss of pubic and axillary hair. Treatment is with replacement hormones, including oestrogen, progesterone, thyroid and adrenal hormones. Specialist endocrinological advice is necessary.

Monitoring

Once the bleeding has been controlled, frequent observations of respiratory rate, pulse rate, blood pressure, urinary output and oxygen saturation (if available) are vital both to detect problems and to monitor the response to treatment. At least 48 hours of close observations are required.

Further reading

A Textbook of Postpartum Hemorrhage: a comprehensive guide to evaluation, management and surgical intervention. www.sapienspublishing.com/pph_pdf/PPH.pdf

Videos on techniques used to treat PPH: www.glowm.com

FIGO Safe Motherhood and Newborn Health (SMNH) Committee (2012) *FIGO Guidelines: prevention and treatment of postpartum hemorrhage in low-resource settings*. www.figo.org/files/figo-corp/IJGO_2012%20PPH%20Guidelines.pdf

World Health Organization (2012) *WHO recommendations for the prevention and treatment of postpartum haemorrhage*. http://apps.who.int/iris/bitstream/10665/75411/1/9789241548502_eng.pdf

---

2.5.E Hypertension, pre-eclampsia and eclampsia

BOX 2.5.E.1 Minimum standards
- Blood pressure machine
- Urine protein testing sticks
- Magnesium sulphate
- Antihypertensive drugs (labetalol, hydralazine, methyldopa and nifedipine)
- Bag-valve-masks, oxygen and oropharyngeal airway
- Suction
- Patella hammer
- Pulse oximeter

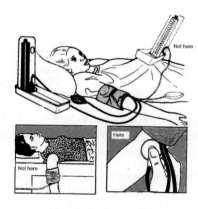

FIGURE 2.5.E.1 Measuring blood pressure.

Introduction

Hypertension in pregnancy occurs when the systolic blood pressure is ≥ 140 mmHg and/or the diastolic blood pressure is ≥ 90 mmHg. If the blood pressure is elevated, confirm this by making repeated measurements (see below).

Severe hypertension (systolic pressure ≥ 170 mmHg and/or diastolic blood pressure ≥ 110 mmHg) must be treated, because a systolic or diastolic blood pressure at or above these levels is associated with a risk of cerebral haemorrhage, hypertensive encephalopathy and placental abruption.

Measuring blood pressure and looking for hypertension

When you measure the blood pressure of a woman, she should be rested and seated at a 45-degree angle with the machine on the bed beside her. Do not prop it up on her abdomen. Also do not lie her down, as this causes compression of the central veins. Open the cuff out flat, and make sure that you place the centre of the inner bladder on the artery. A falsely high reading will be obtained if the cuff's bladder does not encircle at least 80% of the circumference of the arm.

If the blood pressure is consistently higher in one arm, this arm should be used for all subsequent measurements. Some automated blood pressure machines under-measure systolic blood pressure.

The systolic pressure is the onset of the first sound (Korotkov 1). The diastolic pressure is the complete disappearance of sounds (Korotkov 5). The normal systolic blood pressure in pregnancy is in the range 95–135 mmHg. The normal diastolic blood pressure is in the range 60–85 mmHg. Diastolic blood pressure measures peripheral resistance and does not vary with the woman's emotional state to the same degree that systolic pressure does. The blood pressure normally falls during the second trimester of pregnancy, reaching its lowest value by the end of the second trimester, and returning to pre-pregnancy levels at term.

If the systolic pressure is ≥ 140 mmHg and/or the diastolic blood pressure is ≥ 90 mmHg on two consecutive readings taken ≥ 4 hours apart, hypertension should be diagnosed.

In addition to a blood pressure of ≥ 140/90 mmHg, any increase in systolic pressure of ≥ 30 mmHg or in diastolic pressure of ≥ 15 mmHg over recent previous measurements requires close monitoring, even if the pressures do not reach 140 mmHg systolic or 90 mmHg diastolic.

The categories of hypertension in pregnancy

These can be classified as follows.

Pre-eclampsia

This is hypertension (blood pressure of ≥ 140/90 mmHg) that develops after 20 weeks' gestation, always in association with proteinuria (≥ 0.3 grams in a 24-hour specimen). This level correlates with ≥ 1+ on dipstick testing.

Pre-eclampsia is a multi-system disorder.

Other conditions cause proteinuria, and false-positive results are possible (e.g. due to contamination with normal vaginal discharge or amniotic fluid). Urinary infection may also produce proteinuria, but rarely ≥ 2+ on dipstick testing. Blood in the urine due to catheter trauma, schistosomiasis or contamination with vaginal blood may also give false-positive results.

Random urine sampling, such as the dipstick test for protein, is a useful screening tool. A change from negative to positive during pregnancy is a warning sign. If **dipsticks are not available**, a sample of urine can be heated to boiling point in a clean test tube. Add a drop of 2% acetic acid to check for persistent precipitates that can be quantified as a percentage of protein in the sample. Only clean-catch midstream specimens should be used. Catheterisation for this purpose is not justified, due to the risk of urinary tract infection.

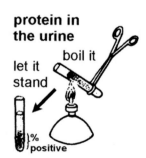

FIGURE 2.5.E.2 Testing for proteinuria without reagents/sticks.

Eclampsia is fitting associated with the syndrome of pre-eclampsia. Seizures can occur without any previous signs or symptoms.

The diagnosis of pre-eclampsia is made when there is hypertension after 20 weeks' gestation associated with significant proteinurea (≥ 0.3 grams/24 hours) (see above).

It is associated with a risk of developing one or more of the following:

- significant proteinuria (≥ 0.3 grams/24 hours) (see above)

- renal involvement (serum/plasma creatinine > 90 micro-mol/litre with or without oliguria)
- haematological involvement (low platelet count, haemolysis, DIC)
- liver involvement (raised transaminases, epigastric or right upper quadrant abdominal pain)
- neurological involvement (headache, persistent visual disturbances including photophobia, scotomata, blindness and retinal vasospasm, hyper-reflexia with sustained clonus, stroke)
- pulmonary oedema
- intrauterine growth retardation
- placental abruption.

HELLP is a syndrome that consists of **H**aemolysis, **E**levated **L**iver enzymes and **L**ow **P**latelets. It may complicate pre-eclampsia, sometimes with only mild or borderline hypertension and marginally abnormal proteinuria.

Pre-eclampsia and eclampsia are still one of the main causes of maternal mortality and morbidity in low-resource countries. In one study it was reported that 38% of eclamptic fits occur antenatally, 18% occur in the intrapartum period, and the remaining 44% occur postpartum, usually in the first 48 hours after delivery. Sometimes the first fit occurs postnatally.

Oedema occurs with the same frequency in women with and without pre-eclampsia. However, if oedema develops suddenly and is widespread, always screen for pre-eclampsia. Test for oedema by pressing with your finger for 1 minute over the bony part of the mother's tibia. If there is a dent when you take your finger away, oedema is present. If the mother has been lying down, look for oedema over the sacrum. Oedema can also make a finger ring tight. Oedema of the face is more likely to represent a sign accompanying pre-eclampsia.

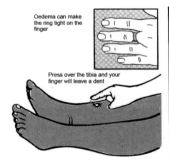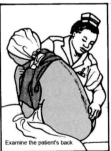

FIGURE 2.5.E.3 Testing for oedema of the ankles and lower back.

Gestational hypertension

This is hypertension that develops only after 20 weeks' gestation but with no other features of pre-eclampsia, and which resolves within 3 months after birth. Patients who present early in pregnancy (after 20 weeks) and with severe hypertension are more likely to develop pre-eclampsia.

Chronic hypertension

1 Essential hypertension (also called primary hypertension) occurs before 20 weeks' gestation, without cause (see below).
2 Hypertension may also be secondary to other medical conditions such as chronic renal disease, endocrine disorders or diabetes mellitus.

It is important to control the hypertension in these cases, keeping the blood pressure below 150/100 mmHg, but not permitting the diastolic pressure to go below 80 mmHg.

Pre-eclampsia in a woman with with chronic hypertension and gestational hypertension

Women with hypertension in pregnancy are at increased risk of developing superimposed pre-eclampsia and should be monitored more frequently for the presence of proteinurea and systemic features of pre-eclampsia from 20 weeks' gestation onwards but especially in the third trimester.

Pre-eclampsia
Risk factors

These include the following:

- first pregnancy
- multiple pregnancy
- family history of pre-eclampsia
- chronic hypertension (see above)
- renal disease
- hypertension/pre-eclampsia during a previous pregnancy
- diabetes mellitus
- molar pregnancy.

For those at high risk of recurrence, a systematic review of 59 trials involving 37 560 women found that low doses of aspirin reduced the risk of pre-eclampsia by about a sixth (17%), with a similar lowering of the risk of the baby dying (14%), and a small lowering of the risk of the baby being born too early (8%). Doses up to 75 mg appear to be safe and high risk women are advised to start taking it from 12 weeks' gestation and to continue until delivery of the baby.

Investigations

These include the following:

- urine dipstick test for protein and microscopy to exclude infection
- haemoglobin levels and platelet count
- urea and electrolytes, and creatinine
- liver function tests
- lactate dehydrogenase (LDH) and uric acid
- fetal growth assessment by ultrasound scan.

If there are signs of DIC, clotting studies should be undertaken (whole blood clotting time in low-resource settings; see below).

If there is severe hypertension in early pregnancy, investigations (if available) for the rarer causes such as molar pregnancy, autoimmune disorders, phaeochromocytoma, etc. may be indicated.

Management of pre-eclampsia and gestational hypertension

Pre-eclampsia progresses during pregnancy, and the only definitive treatment is delivery. If the patient is at term (i.e. after 36 weeks) then, after stabilisation of the mother, the baby should be delivered as soon as possible.

There is no evidence that bed rest improves the outcome for the mother or the fetus. Heavy physical labour is clearly inappropriate. However, women in low-income settings are commonly seen working in this way despite being in advanced pregnancy.

Mild cases can be cared for without hospital admission, but there need to be regular (at least weekly) checks on blood pressure and urine, and the family must be made aware of the warning signs of severe pre-eclampsia or eclampsia (see below).

If there is severe pre-eclampsia or eclampsia, if the blood pressure cannot be adequately controlled, or if there is pulmonary oedema, deteriorating renal or liver function, placental abruption or evidence of falling platelet counts or DIC, delivery is urgent but must always take place after stabilisation. In cases before 36 weeks' gestation, an injection of dexamethasone or betamethasone 12 mg IM, two doses 12 hours apart or 6 mg IM, four doses 12 hours apart, improves the likelihood of avoiding neonatal respiratory failure (see Section 3.1).

Stabilisation involves correction of severe hypertension, control of fluid intake and output, correction of blood-clotting disorders (in low-resource settings with fresh blood transfusion) and prevention or control of eclampsia (see below).

Antihypertensive drugs for pre-eclampsia

Mild pre-eclampsia does not require antihypertensive drugs.

If the systolic blood pressure is 150–160 mmHg and/or the diastolic blood pressure is 95–105 mmHg, treatment with oral antihypertensive drugs should be started.

Systolic pressure of ≥170 mmHg and/or diastolic pressure of ≥ 110 mmHg must be urgently treated with antihypertensive drugs. **However, it is essential that the blood pressure is not lowered too rapidly, as this can seriously affect the woman's cerebral circulation and the circulation to the placenta and fetus.** Aim for a systolic blood pressure of 150 mmHg.

Oral antihypertensive drug treatment
Methyldopa

This drug acts directly on the central nervous system and takes 24 hours to work. The dose is 250 mg three times a day initially, increasing every 2 days up to 750 mg three times a day. Side effects include dry mouth, postural hypotension, sedation and depression. Methyldopa is contraindicated in patients with depression or liver disease.

The simultaneous administration of oral iron and oral methyldopa can lead to a drug interaction that can result in clinically significant increases in blood pressure (> 15 mmHg increase in systolic pressure and > 10 mmHg increase in diastolic pressure).

Labetalol

This is a beta-blocker with mild alpha-blocking effects. The dose is 100–400 mg three times a day. Side effects include bradycardia, bronchospasm, weakness, scalp tingling (only for 24–48 hours), nausea and headache. Labetalol is contraindicated in patients with asthma.

Hydralazine

This is a vasodilator. The dose is initially 25 mg twice a day, increasing gradually to 50 mg three times a day. Side effects include uncontrolled hypotension, flushing, tachycardia, palpitations, headache and (uncommonly) a lupus syndrome.

Treatment of severe hypertension

It is vital that severe hypertension is controlled at any gestation, both before and after delivery.

Antihypertensive drugs should be given urgently to all patients with a systolic blood pressure of ≥ 170 mmHg and/or a diastolic blood pressure of ≥ 110 mmHg.

Without urgent treatment there is a risk of cerebral haemorrhage, eclampsia and pulmonary oedema.

The aim should be a gradual and sustained reduction in blood pressure with one or more of the drugs described below. Blood pressure should not be allowed to fall below 140/80 mmHg before delivery.

Hydralazine

This is the most widely available antihypertensive drug in low-resource settings. Give 5 mg IV slowly over a period of 5 minutes (it acts within 5 minutes). Repeat the BP after every 15 minutes and treat with further doses of 5 mg until the **diastolic** blood pressure is 90–100 mmHg and the systolic BP is 140–160. Repeat the hydralazine hourly as needed, or give hydralazine 12.5 mg IM every 2 hours as needed.

Alternatively, give hydralazine IV infusion, 20 mg in 200 mL of 5% dextrose at 0.5 mL (10 drops) per minute (20 drops = 1 mL for a standard giving set), and stop the drip when the diastolic blood pressure is ≤ 90 mmHg. Hydralazine may cause an increase in the maternal heart rate.

Side effects include uncontrolled hypotension, flushing, tachycardia, palpitations, headache and (uncommonly) a lupus syndrome.

Labetalol

Intravenous labetalol is preferable to hydralazine if the maternal pulse rate exceeds 120 beats/minute.

The labetalol dosage is 10 mg IV. If the response is inadequate (i.e. if diastolic blood pressure remains above 110 mmHg) after 10 minutes, give a further dose of labetalol 20 mg IV. Increase the dose to 40 mg and then 80 mg if a satisfactory response is not obtained after 10 minutes of each dose.

Alternatively, use an IV infusion of 200 mg in 200 mL of Ringer-lactate solution at 40 mg/hour, increasing the dose at 30-minute intervals as required to a maximum of 160 mg/hour.

Side effects include bradycardia, bronchospasm, weakness, scalp tingling (only for 24–48 hours), nausea and headache. **Labetalol is contraindicated in patients with asthma, as it may cause severe bronchospasm.**

Nifedipine

The slow release/modified action version of the tablets must always be used in this situation. Nifedipine is a calcium antagonist that can be administered as an initial 10 mg oral dose (onset of action within 10–20 minutes), with a repeat dose of 10 mg if there is an inadequate response after 30 minutes. Subsequent oral doses are 20 mg twice a day. Side effects include severe headaches associated with flushing and tachycardia. Oedema, weakness and constipation may also occur. Nifedipine is contraindicated in patients with aortic stenosis. It may inhibit labour.

Give prophylactic magnesium sulphate if hypertension is accompanied by proteinuria and/or if protein testing is not available by symptoms which suggest that eclampsia may occur (see below).

Eclampsia or severe pre-eclampsia

Although pre-eclampsia and eclampsia are most common in the primigravida, they can occur in multiparous patients.

Symptoms and signs of impending eclampsia

These include the following:

- headache, visual disturbances, epigastric pain and vomiting
- rapidly developing generalised (especially facial) oedema
- pulmonary oedema
- right upper quadrant tenderness
- recently developed hypertension ≥ 170/110 mmHg with proteinuria > 1 gram/24 hours or a rapid rise in blood pressure
- clonus and increased tendon reflexes
- HELLP syndrome.

Any headache or epigastric pain occurring in the second half of pregnancy should be investigated for pre-eclampsia (measure the blood pressure and test the urine for protein).

Differential diagnosis (*see* Table 2.5.E.1)

- A seizure:
  - in a patient with known epilepsy (*see* Section 5.16.E)
  - in severe malaria (*see* Section 2.8.D)
  - in head injury (*see* Section 2.7.E)
  - in meningitis/encephalitis (*see* Section 2.7.E).
- Intoxication (local anaesthetic overdose).
- Amniotic fluid embolus (*see* Section 2.5.I).

Maintain a high index of suspicion of pre-eclampsia or eclampsia even in those with malaria, migraine or epilepsy, as the conditions may coexist.

A small proportion of mothers with eclampsia have a normal blood pressure. Treat all convulsions as eclampsia until another diagnosis is confirmed.

Convulsions with signs of pre-eclampsia indicate eclampsia.

Convulsions due to eclampsia:

- can occur regardless of the severity of hypertension
- are difficult to predict, but rarely occur without increased tendon reflexes, headache or visual changes
- are tonic–clonic and resemble grand mal convulsions of epilepsy
- may recur frequently, as in status epilepticus, and may be fatal
- will not be observed if the woman is alone
- may be followed by coma that lasts for minutes or hours depending on the frequency of convulsions
- occur after childbirth in about 44% of cases, usually but not always within the first 24 hours after birth. The longer the gap between delivery and a fit, the more likely the diagnosis is to be **a condition other than eclampsia** (e.g. cerebral venous thrombosis).

The first eclamptic fit is usually self-limiting.

Control of blood pressure is essential in the management of severe pre-eclampsia or eclampsia where high blood pressure may cause a cerebrovascular accident (stroke). Magnesium sulphate is essential for preventing eclampsia and, if eclampsia occurs, for preventing further fits.

TABLE 2.5.E.1 Differential diagnosis of hypertension and convulsions in pregnancy

Symptoms	Signs	Results of investigations	Diagnosis	Treatment
None unless very severe	Blood pressure ≥ 140/90 mmHg before 20 weeks' gestation	Urine for protein negative Renal function tests normal	Essential hypertension	Consider antihypertensive drugs
None unless very severe	Blood pressure ≥ 140/90 mmHg before 20 weeks' gestation	Proteinuria ≤ 2+	Hypertension secondary to other disease such as renal impairment, or autoimmune disease	Treat hypertension with drugs if severe, and treat the underlying condition
None unless very severe	Blood pressure ≥ 140/90 mmHg after 20 weeks' gestation	No proteinuria	Pregnancy-induced hypertension	Treat hypertension with drugs if severe
None unless very severe	Blood pressure ≥ 140/90 mmHg before 20 weeks' gestation	Proteinuria ≤ 2+	Mild to moderate pre-eclampsia	Avoid work involving heavy labour
Headaches increasing in frequency and unrelieved by paracetamol Visual disturbance Upper abdominal pain Shortness of breath Passing small amounts of urine Oedema	Blood pressure ≥ 140/90 mmHg after 20 weeks' gestation Hyper-reflexia Passing less than 400 mL of urine in 24 hours Pulmonary oedema Facial and rapidly developing oedema	Proteinuria ≥ 2+	Severe pre-eclampsia	Urgent admission to hospital Magnesium sulphate
May be history of the above Generalised convulsions Unconscious	Generalised fitting Coma Blood pressure ≥ 140/90 mmHg after 20 weeks' gestation Facial and rapidly developing oedema	Proteinuria ≥ 2+	Eclampsia	ABC Magnesium sulphate
Difficulty opening mouth and swallowing	Spasms of the face, neck and trunk Arched back Board-like abdomen		Tetanus	ABC, Penicillin, anti-tetanus immunoglobulin Muscle relaxants (magnesium and/or diazepam) Nasogastric feeding
Past history of convulsions	Convulsions Coma Normal blood pressure	EEG abnormal	Epilepsy	ABC, blood glucose Anticonvulsant drugs
Chills/rigors Headache Muscle/joint pain	Fever Convulsions Coma Severe anaemia Jaundice	Blood smear for malarial parasites	Severe malaria	ABC, blood glucose Antimalarial drugs
Headache Stiff neck Photophobia Vomiting	Fever Stiff neck Reduced conscious level or coma Convulsions	Full blood count Blood culture Lumbar puncture (unless there is evidence of raised intracranial pressure)	Meningitis or encephalitis	ABC Antibacterial or antiviral drugs
Headache Blurred vision Photophobia History of migraine	Normal blood pressure	No proteinuria	Migraine	Paracetamol Bed rest in dark room
			Cerebral venous thrombosis	

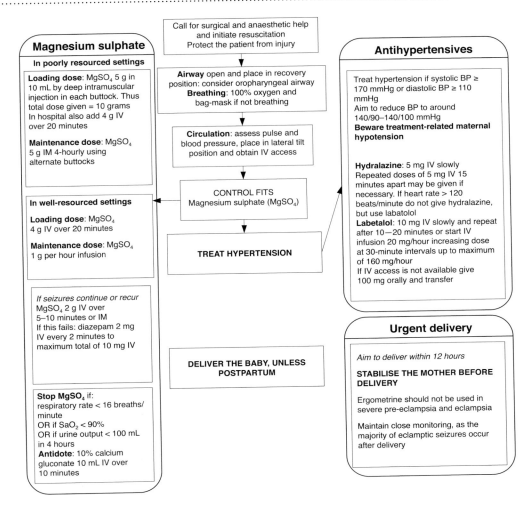

Magnesium sulphate

In poorly resourced settings

Loading dose: MgSO₄ 5 g in 10 mL by deep intramuscular injection in each buttock. Thus total dose given = 10 grams
In hospital also add 4 g IV over 20 minutes

Maintenance dose: MgSO₄ 5 g IM 4-hourly using alternate buttocks

In well-resourced settings

Loading dose: MgSO₄ 4 g IV over 20 minutes

Maintenance dose: MgSO₄ 1 g per hour infusion

If seizures continue or recur
MgSO₄ 2 g IV over 5–10 minutes or IM
If this fails: diazepam 2 mg IV every 2 minutes to maximum total of 10 mg IV

Stop MgSO₄ if:
respiratory rate < 16 breaths/minute
OR if SaO₂ < 90%
OR if urine output < 100 mL in 4 hours
Antidote: 10% calcium gluconate 10 mL IV over 10 minutes

Call for surgical and anaesthetic help and initiate resuscitation
Protect the patient from injury

↓

Airway open and place in recovery position: consider oropharyngeal airway
Breathing: 100% oxygen and bag-mask if not breathing

↓

Circulation: assess pulse and blood pressure, place in lateral tilt position and obtain IV access

↓

CONTROL FITS
Magnesium sulphate (MgSO₄)

↓

TREAT HYPERTENSION

DELIVER THE BABY, UNLESS POSTPARTUM

Antihypertensives

Treat hypertension if systolic BP ≥ 170 mmHg or diastolic BP ≥ 110 mmHg
Aim to reduce BP to around 140/90–140/100 mmHg
Beware treatment-related maternal hypotension

Hydralazine: 5 mg IV slowly
Repeated doses of 5 mg IV 15 minutes apart may be given if necessary. If heart rate > 120 beats/minute do not give hydralazine, but use labatolol
Labetalol: 10 mg IV slowly and repeat after 10–20 minutes or start IV infusion 20 mg/hour increasing dose at 30-minute intervals up to maximum of 160 mg/hour
If IV access is not available give 100 mg orally and transfer

Urgent delivery

Aim to deliver within 12 hours

STABILISE THE MOTHER BEFORE DELIVERY

Ergometrine should not be used in severe pre-eclampsia and eclampsia

Maintain close monitoring, as the majority of eclamptic seizures occur after delivery

FIGURE 2.5.E.4 Pathway of care for eclampsia when the mother is having convulsions.

Maternal complications of severe pre-eclampsia

These include the following:

- eclampsia
- cerebrovascular accident (stroke)
- renal failure
- HELLP syndrome, possible leading to rupture of the liver capsule
- pulmonary oedema
- placental abruption, possibly leading to DIC
- intrauterine growth restriction, fetal death.

Primary assessment, resuscitation and emergency treatment of convulsions in eclampsia

Call for help

- Never leave the patient alone.
- Prevent maternal injury during the convulsion.

Airway

- If the airway is not open, use an airway-opening manoeuvre and keep it open. Consider an airway adjunct such as an oropharyngeal airway or intubation. Do not attempt to insert an oropharyngeal airway while the patient is convulsing.

- The oropharynx may need gentle suctioning under direct vision, being careful to avoid inducing laryngospasm.
- The recovery position should be adopted to minimise the risk of aspiration of vomit.

Breathing

- If there is spontaneous breathing, give a high concentration of oxygen via a face mask plus reservoir. Give 100% oxygen (mask with reservoir and a flow rate of at least 5 litres/minute) regardless of the mother's oxygen saturation (this increases fetal oxygen delivery as well as improving maternal tissue oxygenation).

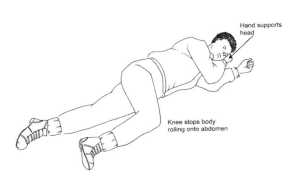

Hand supports head

Knee stops body rolling onto abdomen

FIGURE 2.5.E.5 The recovery position.

- If there is apnoea or hypoventilation, provide ventilation with bag-valve-mask-reservoir ventilation and 100% oxygen.

Circulation

- Look for signs of life (breathing, movement, gagging/coughing) or for a pulse at the carotid. If these are absent or you are not sure, initiate CPR (*see* Sections 1.12 and 1.13).
- If the mother is over 20 weeks' gestation, put her in the left lateral tilt position and/or manually displace the uterus to reduce vena caval compression, or put her in the recovery position.
- Secure IV or intra-osseous access.
- Monitor the blood pressure.
- Attach a pulse oximeter.
- Insert a urinary catheter with strict fluid input/output chart.

Insert a 14G or 16G IV cannula and take 20 mL of blood for full blood count, blood group, cross-matching (4 units = 2 litres) and clotting. Do a 20-minute whole blood clotting time (WBCT20) test if laboratory analyses are not available (*see* Section 7.5).

A central venous pressure (CVP) line may be a helpful monitor to avoid fluid overload, but the benefits must be weighed against the risks. If disseminated intravascular coagulation (DIC) is established, CVP insertion is more hazardous (you must avoid subclavian vein access).

Emergency drug treatment of eclampsia

Stopping the convulsion and preventing further convulsions

The majority of seizures are self-limiting.

Commence **magnesium sulphate** to prevent further fits.

Magnesium sulphate (MgSO₄) treatment

Magnesium sulphate is the anticonvulsant of choice.

If the mother is conscious, warn her that there will be a feeling of warmth passing through her body when magnesium sulphate is infused, and that this is not harmful. Failure to do so may result in the mother pulling out her IV cannula, and other potentially dangerous reactions.

Loading dose in well-resourced settings

Give 4 grams of MgSO₄ as 20 mL of a 20% solution of magnesium sulphate IV added to 80 mL of 5% dextrose solution given slowly over 20 minutes (total volume 100 mL). (To make 20 mL of a 20% solution, add 8 mL of 50% MgSO₄ solution to 12 mL of sterile water.)

If convulsions recur after completion of the loading regime, give 2 grams of MgSO₄ IV slowly over 10 minutes (10 mL of 20% solution is added to 90 mL of Ringer-lactate or Hartmann's solution).

Do not use the same IV line to inject other drugs if MgSO₄ is being given by IV infusion.

Loading dose in resource-limited settings

Give 5 grams of MgSO₄ (10 mL of 50% solution) by deep intramuscular injection in **each** buttock. Thus the total dose given is 10 grams. **(Sometimes 0.5 mL of 2% or 1 mL of**

1% lignocaine is given in the same syringe for each injection of 5 grams, to reduce the pain of the injections.) An aseptic technique is essential.

Maintenance dosage

- **Well-resourced countries:** Provided that there is close monitoring (ideally with a burette in giving set), give 1 gram of MgSO₄/hour IV for 24 hours (i.e. 25 mL/hour of the loading dose solution of 4 grams in 100 mL described above).
- **Resource-limited countries:** give 5 grams of MgSO₄ IM 4-hourly (plus 1 mL of 1% lignocaine, or 0.5 mL of 2%, in the same syringe) using alternate buttocks.

Alternative regime

This regime is recommended in Asia where pregnant women are smaller than those in Africa and there are more resources.

Loading dose: Give 4 grams of MgSO₄ as 20 mL of a 20% solution added to 80 mL of 5% dextrose solution slowly IV over 20 minutes (total 100 mL). (To make 20 mL of a 20% solution, add 8 mL of 50% MgSO₄ solution to 12 mL of sterile water).

Then immediately give 3 grams (6 mL of 50% solution) by deep intramuscular injection in **each** buttock. **(Sometimes 1 mL of 1% or 0.5 mL of 2% lignocaine is given in the same syringe, to reduce the pain of the injections.)**

Maintenance dose

Give 2.5 grams of MgSO₄ IM every 4 hours using alternate buttocks.

Treatment if seizures continue or recur

Give 2 grams of MgSO₄ if body weight is less than 70 kg, or 4 grams if body weight is over 70 kg, as an extra loading dose IV over 5–10 minutes or IM in low-resource settings.

Alternative regime

This regime is undertaken in some West African countries, and was recommended by the World Health Organization in 2003.

Loading dose: 4 grams IV of MgSO₄ over 20 minutes: add 8 mL 50% to 92 mL Ringer-lactate or Hartmann's solution. This is followed by 10 grams 50% MgSO₄ solution IM (5 grams in each buttock: deep IM injections with lidocaine as above in the same syringe). **Ensure that the needle is not in a vein.**

Maintenance dose: This is 5 grams MgSO₄ 50% solution with lidocaine every 4 hours into alternate buttocks.

If eclampsia recurs, and only after 15 minutes, give 2 grams of MgSO₄ over 5 minutes IV: add 4 mL of 50% to 16 mL of Ringer-lactate or Hartmann's solution.

Continued treatment with magnesium sulphate

Continue MgSO₄ for 24 hours after delivery or the last convulsion, provided that:

- respiratory rate is > 12–16 breaths/minute
- urine output is > 30 mL/hour (WHO figure is > 100 mL over 4 hours)
- tendon reflexes are present.

Discontinue magnesium sulphate when:

- blood pressure is stable and consistently below 150/100 mmHg
- diuresis has started
- there are no neurological symptoms.

Monitor the fetus by regular heart rate assessments.

A fluid balance chart must be kept (see below).

Remember to subtract the volume containing MgSO₄ infused from total maintenance infusion volume to avoid fluid overload.

When using magnesium sulphate, monitor hourly urine output, respiratory rate, SaO₂ and tendon reflexes every 15 minutes for the first 2 hours, and then every 30 minutes.

Progressive symptoms of magnesium toxicity

These include the following:

- double vision, confusion, slurred speech, nausea and weakness
- loss of tendon reflexes
- respiratory depression (< 12–15 breaths/minute) and/or SaO_2 < 94%
- respiratory arrest
- cardiac arrest.

If magnesium toxicity is suspected, stop the infusion and if severe signs such as very slow respiration, respiratory or cardiac arrest, administer antidote of 10 mL 10% calcium gluconate IV slowly over at least 1–2 minutes.

Stop the infusion of magnesium sulphate if:

- patellar reflexes are absent
- there is respiratory depression (respiratory rate < 12–15 breaths/minute) or a fall in oxygen saturation to ≤ 92% on a pulse oximeter. Give oxygen to keep oxygen saturation at 94–98%
- urine output is less than 30 mL/hour over the last 4 hours.

If respiratory depression develops, give 100% oxygen by face mask with reservoir, and give calcium gluconate 1 gram (= 10 mL of 10% solution) IV slowly over 1–2 minutes. Too rapid administration can result in loss of consciousness, cardiac arrhythmias and cardiac arrest.

If respiratory arrest occurs:

- give chest inflations with bag-valve-mask ventilation with 100% oxygen
- inject calcium gluconate 1 gram (10 mL of 10%) IV slowly over 5 minutes.

The magnesium sulphate infusion may be recommenced at a reduced dose, if this is considered necessary, once normal respiration and reflexes have returned.

Note for anaesthetists: there is an increased sensitivity to muscle relaxants (particularly non-depolarising agents) in patients on magnesium.

In patients with known renal disease or myasthenia gravis, magnesium sulphate is contraindicated and, if available, phenytoin should be used. The loading dose is 15 mg/kg (maximum dose 2 grams) over 20 minutes by slow IV injection. Subsequently a dose of 100 mg orally twice a day can be given. IV injection if given too rapidly can cause severe hypotension, cardiac arrhythmias or respiratory arrest.

Other anticonvulsant drugs

If repeated fits occur despite magnesium sulphate, give either rectal paraldehyde (10–20 mL as an enema mixed with 10 parts of Ringer-lactate solution; do not give if it is a brownish colour or smells of acetic acid; note that it crosses the placenta) or rectal diazepam (500 micrograms/kg or 10–20 mg; may cause neonatal hypothermia, hypotonia and respiratory depression).

Other causes of fitting should be considered if fits persist or recur despite magnesium sulphate. These include a cerebrovascular accident (stroke), malaria and meningitis.

If magnesium sulphate is not available, use diazepam (see below).

Diazepam

A bag-valve-mask must be immediately available in case the patient stops breathing.

Loading dose: diazepam 2 mg increments IV every 2 minutes up to 10 mg.

If convulsions recur, repeat the loading dose.

Maintenance dose: diazepam 40 mg in 500 mL of Ringer-lactate or Hartmann's solution, titrated to keep the mother sedated but able to be woken and without hypoventilation.

Maternal respiratory depression may occur when the dose exceeds 30 mg in 1 hour. Assist ventilation (e.g. bag-valve-mask, anaesthesia apparatus, intubation) if necessary, and do not give more than 100 mg in 24 hours.

Rectal administration: give diazepam rectally when IV access is not possible. The loading dose is 20 mg in a 10-mL syringe. Remove the needle, lubricate the barrel and insert the syringe into the rectum to half its length. Discharge the contents and leave the syringe in place, holding the buttocks together for 10 minutes to prevent expulsion of the drug. Alternatively, the drug may be instilled in the rectum through a catheter.

If **convulsions are not controlled within 10 minutes**, administer an additional 10 mg per hour or more, depending on the size of the woman and her clinical response.

Be prepared for neonatal resuscitation when diazepam has been administered, especially if it was used in large doses.

Severe pre-eclampsia

Stage 1: Prevention of fitting

If there are significantly increased tendon reflexes, often also with ankle clonus, before delivery or afterwards, and the patient shows other signs of impending eclampsia (e.g. confusion, jitteriness, severe headache), prophylactic 'anticonvulsant' therapy (magnesium sulphate where possible) should be commenced.

Other indications for magnesium sulphate treatment where eclampsia has not yet occurred include the following:

- persistent hypertension despite adequate antihypertensive drugs and good fluid management
- evidence of thrombocytopenia or liver dysfunction (if these can be measured).

The same regimen of magnesium sulphate (or diazepam if magnesium sulphate is not available) is used for prophylaxis as described above for the treatment of eclampsia. A loading dose alone may be sufficient.

Stage 2: Reduction of blood pressure and expansion of intravascular volume

Hypertension should be treated if the blood pressure is ≥ 170/110 mmHg as described above. Careful fetal monitoring during the commencement of treatment is vital, as a rapid fall in maternal blood pressure may cause fetal heart rate abnormalities, especially in a growth-restricted or compromised fetus.

If the gestation is less than 36 weeks, dexamethasone or betamethasone 12 mg IM in two doses 24 hours apart should be given to improve fetal lung maturity and decrease the risk of neonatal respiratory failure, if time allows.

Antihypertensive drugs

See pp. 202–3.

Volume expansion during antihypertensive treatment

Antihypertensive agents such as nifedipine and hydralazine act as vasodilators. In pre-eclampsia where intravascular volume is reduced, a small volume load should be given immediately prior to IV antihypertensive treatment (300 mL or Ringer-lactate or Hartmann's solution IV over 20 minutes). Colloid or starch, such as Haemaccel (500 mL), which remains for longer in the intravascular compartment, may be helpful. Clinical examination for signs of cardiac failure (see Section 2.7.A) should be sought before and after such treatment.

Stage 3: Anticipate and/or manage complications
Airway and breathing

- Keep the airway clear.
- The respiratory rate should be recorded regularly (ideally it should be 15–40 breaths/minute).
- **Beware of over-sedation, aspiration, pulmonary oedema and laryngeal oedema (which presents with stridor).**
- If the respiratory rate is less than 12–15 breaths/minute, particularly if the mother is receiving magnesium sulphate or opiates for pain control, action should be taken and other signs of toxicity sought (see above).
  - If an opiate is being used, naloxone may be required.
  - If magnesium sulphate is being given, stop this and give calcium gluconate (see above).
- Oxygen can be given using nasal cannulae (ideally with SaO_2 monitoring) if SaO_2 is less than 94%. Keep SaO_2 in the range 94–98%.
- Arrange for a chest X-ray if aspiration is suspected.
- An increased respiratory rate is an early sign of pulmonary oedema.

Circulation
Consider fluid balance/fluid overload (urinary catheterisation is important).

Usually there is net fluid overload in pre-eclampsia, but the fluid has leaked out of the intravascular compartment due to low oncotic pressure (partly due to hypoalbuminaemia) and increased capillary permeability.

Complications of excessive fluid in the wrong compartment include cerebral oedema, pulmonary oedema and laryngeal oedema (stridor).

Renal failure may develop secondary to the hypertension

or to intravascular hypovolaemia (or as a primary injury in severe pre-eclampsia).

Keep IV fluids at a rate of less than 100 mL/hour or less than 1 mL/kg per hour (the World Health Organization suggests a rate of less than 1 litre in 6–8 hours). Fluid restriction should be maintained until there is postpartum diuresis, which is easy to recognise as there is usually oliguria in severe pre-eclampsia. If there is APH or PPH, fluid restriction will probably not be appropriate.

- Insert an indwelling urinary catheter, and keep a strict intake–output chart with hourly running totals. The total maintenance fluid intake should not exceed 1.5–2 litres over 24 hours. If the average urine output is less than 30 mL/hour over a period of 4 hours this is usually due to the decreased intravascular volume, and will respond to a bolus of 200 mL of IV Ringer-lactate or Hartmann's solution, which can be repeated if necessary.
- In the presence of over-hydration, particularly with heart failure or renal impairment, furosemide 20–40 mg IV should be given. **Mannitol is not advisable because of the fluid load that results from its administration, and because of its rebound effects.**
- Beware of cardiac arrhythmias. Ideally monitor potassium levels regularly and ECG continuously.
- Magnesium sulphate is renally excreted, so careful observation for magnesium toxicity is required if there is oliguria.
- Fluid infusion equal to the same quantity as the urinary output in the preceding hour plus 30 mL is a useful guide to IV fluid administration.
- Central venous pressure (CVP) monitoring may be useful to guide management, especially if urine output is low. (Keep the CVP at up to + 6 cmH₂O in a spontaneously breathing patient.)

Additional organ involvement
Neurological complications

These include cerebrovascular accidents and cerebral oedema.

Undertake regular (2-hourly) neurological examination (including pupillary and tendon reflexes) and record the AVPU and/or Glasgow Coma Scale (GCS) scores. All patients should be able to open their eyes to stimulus, obey commands and respond to questions about their name and age. If not, they are over-sedated or may be developing cerebral complications.

The GCS Scale has three components, with a maximum possible score of 15:

E	Eye-opening response (E)	Spontaneous	4
		To speech	3
		To pain	2
		None	1
M	Best motor response (M)	Obeys command	6
		Localises to pain stimulus	5
		Withdraws	4
		Abnormal flexion/decorticate posture	3
		Extensor response/decerebrate posture	2
		No movement	1

V	Verbal response (V)	Oriented	5
		Confused	4
		Inappropriate words	3
		Incomprehensible sounds	2
		None	1

A GCS score of ≤ 8 indicates coma and an airway that is not protected by pharyngeal and/or laryngeal reflexes.

Cerebral oedema is usually localised to the occipital and parietal cortical areas, and is a result of cerebral vasospasm. Magnesium sulphate can help to prevent this. Mannitol is not indicated. Recurrent convulsions despite magnesium sulphate with or without other anticonvulsants may require intubation and controlled ventilation (if available).

Haematological complications
These include disseminated intravascular coagulation (DIC).
- Group and save and cross-match fresh blood.
- Check the full blood count, including a platelet count if possible.
- Do a whole blood clotting test as well as APTT (if available) (*see* Section 7.5). Failure of a clot to form after 7 minutes, or formation of a soft clot that breaks down easily, suggests coagulopathy.
- If the platelet count is > $100\,000 \times 10^9$, a major coagulation problem is unlikely. Spontaneous haemorrhage may occur with counts below $10\,000 \times 10^9$.
- In frank DIC, give whole fresh blood if there is bleeding.

Hepatic complications
These include jaundice, bleeding tendency, hepatic failure, hepatic sub-capsular oedema or hepatic rupture (the last two cause right upper quadrant or epigastric pain).

Delivery of the baby is urgent.

Fetal problems
These include intrauterine growth retardation, fetal distress in labour, preterm delivery as a result of obstetric intervention, fetal death due to placental abruption or fetal asphyxia in labour.

General nursing care
- Airway and breathing management should be undertaken as appropriate. This includes ensuring that SaO_2 remains normal at ≥ 94%.
- Maintain the patient in the lateral tilt or recovery position at all times before delivery.
- Indwelling aseptically placed urinary catheter and hourly urine output measurement.
- Care of eyes and oral hygiene.

The HELLP syndrome (Haemolysis, Elevated Liver enzymes, Low Platelet counts) syndrome is a dangerous form of severe pre-eclampsia.
- If the platelet count is < $50\,000 \times 10^9$ there is a high risk of bleeding, and if bleeding occurs in the absence of platelet transfusions, fresh blood may be helpful.
- Liver dysfunction may cause upper abdominal pain, and lowering of the blood pressure may be helpful.
- Delivery is urgent.

Stage 4: Delivery of the baby
The need for *in-utero* transfer should be considered, particularly if there are maternal complications that are likely to require a Caesarean section or high-dependency care. The need for delivery is dependent on the maternal and fetal conditions. Either Caesarean section or induction of labour may be appropriate, depending on the clinical findings. Although delivery will resolve the disease, it is inappropriate to deliver an unstable mother, even if there is fetal distress. Once eclamptic seizures have been controlled, severe hypertension has been treated and any hypoxaemia corrected, delivery can be expedited.

In severe pre-eclampsia, aim to deliver within 24 hours of the onset of symptoms. In eclampsia, aim to deliver within 12 hours of the onset of convulsions.

It is important to stabilise the mother's condition first. Then decide about the mode of delivery.

In selected patients, **labour may be induced** if the following conditions apply:
- the cervix is favourable
- the maternal condition is stable (i.e. eclampsia and blood pressure are controlled), there is no fetal distress and there is a cephalic presentation.

Assessment of the cervix
- If **the cervix is favourable** (i.e. soft, thin and partly dilated), rupture the membranes with an amniotic hook or a Kocher's forceps, and induce labour using an oxytocin infusion (*see* Section 2.3) or oral misoprostol (*see* Section 2.3 and below).
- If **vaginal delivery is not anticipated** within 12 hours (for eclampsia) or within 24 hours (for severe pre-eclampsia), deliver by Caesarean section.
- If there are **fetal heart rate abnormalities** (< 110 beats/minute or > 160 beats/minute), consider Caesarean section if this is safe for the mother.
- If **the cervix is unfavourable** (i.e. firm, thick and closed) and **the fetus is alive**, deliver by Caesarean section if the mother is adequately resuscitated.
- If **there are no facilities for Caesarean section** or if **the fetus is dead or too premature for survival**, deliver vaginally.

Aiming for vaginal delivery
If **the cervix is unfavourable** (i.e. firm, thick and closed) and the fetus is alive, Caesarean section should be performed. If the fetus is dead, consideration should be given to induction of labour using misoprostol (unless there has been a previous Caesarean section, in which case misoprostol is contraindicated).

There are many possible misoprostol regimens for induction of labour (vaginal misoprostol tablet, oral misoprostol solution or oral misoprostol tablet). Each has been widely used. The latest evidence is that oral misoprostol solution is the most appropriate treatment (Cochrane reviews).

Oral misoprostol solution: A single misoprostol tablet is dissolved in drinking water (a 200-microgram tablet in 200 mL of water or a 100-microgram tablet in 100 mL of water), and 20–25 mL of misoprostol solution (20–25 micrograms) are then given every 2 hours. The solution is stable for up to 24 hours at room temperature, but should then be discarded.

Oral misoprostol tablets: 100-microgram misoprostol tablets are cut to 25 micrograms size and administered orally every 2 hours up to a maximum of six doses. However, this may not be very accurate, so there is a danger of giving an incorrect dosage. The solution described above is much safer.

Caesarean section

If Caesarean section is performed, ensure that coagulopathy has been treated. Ensure that fresh blood for transfusion is available.

Spinal anaesthesia is usually safer than general anaesthesia for Caesarean section, unless there is a contraindication (e.g. maternal refusal, coagulopathy, thrombocytopenia, decreased conscious level, ongoing seizures). There does not appear to be an exaggerated decrease in blood pressure after spinal anaesthesia, and vasopressors (e.g. ephedrine) should be used cautiously in order to avoid a hypertensive response. An IV bolus of 500 mL of Ringer-lactate or Hartmann's solution may occasionally be required if the blood pressure does fall.

The use of general anaesthesia in severe pre-eclampsia or eclampsia is very hazardous. There may be laryngeal oedema, which makes airway management difficult, and increases in blood pressure during intubation and extubation, with an increased risk of intracranial haemorrhage. Drugs to weaken the vasopressor response to intubation should be used.

Local anaesthesia or ketamine in women with pre-eclampsia or eclampsia are contraindicated unless facilities and/or expertise dictate that these are the safest options in a given situation.

Stage 5: Management after delivery

- If the patient is post-eclampsia or at high risk of convulsions, continue to administer parenteral anticonvulsants (i.e. magnesium sulphate, or diazepam if magnesium sulphate is not available) for 24 hours after the birth. Continue for as long as the patient has increased tendon reflexes.
- **Do not give ergometrine to women with pre-eclampsia, eclampsia or high blood pressure, because it increases the risk of convulsions and cerebrovascular accidents.**
- Monitor the mother closely.
- Use antihypertensive agents if the diastolic blood pressure is > 105–110 mmHg or the systolic blood pressure is > 160 mmHg.
- Continue oxytocin infusion to keep the uterus contracted.
- **Syntometrine (which contains ergometrine, and can cause or worsen hypertension) is contraindicated.** Give oxytocin alone or with misoprostol, and avoid the possible hypertensive effects of ergometrine. If postpartum haemorrhage occurs, this should be managed as described in Section 2.5.D.iv.
- Keep the mother in the delivery unit or close observation area for at least 24 hours after the last fit.
- Review the need for further anticonvulsants and antihypertensive drugs.
- Regular monitoring is essential.
- It is not uncommon for the blood pressure to drop transiently following delivery only to rise again after 24 to 48 hours. Patients with severe pre-eclampsia and eclampsia should be monitored as in-patients for 72 hours after delivery so that dangerous post-partum rises in BP can be detected and treated.
- Plans for care should be communicated to the patient

BOX 2.5.E.2 Emergency box for eclampsia

Equipment	Quantity
Drugs	Magnesium sulphate 50%, 5 g in 10-mL ampoule × 10 ampoules
	Calcium gluconate 10%, 10-mL ampoule × 2 ampoules
	Hydralazine, 20 mg in 1-mL ampoule × 2 ampoules
	Labetalol, 200 mg in 20-mL ampoule × 1 ampoule
	0.9% Sodium chloride, 10-mL ampoule × 10 ampoules
	Diazepam, 5 mg/mL ampoules × 20
Intravenous fluids	500-mL bag of Ringer-lactate or Hartmann's solution × 1
	Giving set × 1
	IV blood giving set × 1
Venous access	20-gauge cannula (pink) × 2
	18-gauge cannula (green) × 2
	16-gauge cannula (grey) × 2
	Tourniquet × 1
	Fixation tape × 1 roll
Airway equipment	Guedel airways: sizes 4, 3 and 2
	Self-inflating bag-mask-valve
	Green oxygen tubing (2 metres) and high and medium concentration (MC) facemasks for oxygen delivery
	Yankauer sucker
Other equipment	50-mL syringe × 2
	20-ml syringe × 2
	10-mL syringe × 2
	Green needles × 2
	Patella hammer × 1
	Urinary catheter
	Charts for vital signs and fluid balance

and her attendants. The attendants should be educated about the use of the left lateral tilt position prior to delivery, the use of the recovery position after convulsions, the risk of aspiration of food, and care of the IV site.
- Before the mother goes home, the family and attendants should be warned about the risk of postnatal depression, especially if the outcome has been poor. The woman or girl should be followed up closely in the community.
- In women with severe pre-eclampsia/eclampsia a plan should be made to monitor the BP in the post-partum period, even in women who are not discharged on antihypertensive medication. This is because the BP is commonly labile during this period. One or ideally two checks (or more if the BP is poorly controlled) should be advised over the first 2 weeks following delivery. This may be done at a clinic local to the patient's residence, but may require that the patient stay in or near the hospital if no facilities exist close to her home.
- Women and their families should also be warned about

the symptoms of severe pre-eclampsia and advised that although delivery does usually resolve the disease, it can still worsen suddenly in the first 2 weeks following delivery (rarely up to 6 weeks).

- Antenatal care provided by the hospital during a future pregnancy is important. There is an increased risk of pre-eclampsia and hypertension if these problems have been present before.
- All patients are at risk of deep vein thrombosis (DVT), so close observation and appropriate treatment if DVT is identified are important (*see* Section 2.5.H). Anti-embolism stockings and low-molecular-weight heparin (or unfractionated heparin if the former is not available) prophylaxis should be considered early on.

Hypertension may take from many days to up to 3 months to resolve. Resolution will occur if the diagnosis is pre-eclampsia, unless there is an underlying medical cause.

Monitoring and preparation for emergencies

- Measure pulse rate and volume, blood pressure, respiratory rate and oxygen saturation regularly. A minimum of hourly if receiving $MgSO_4$ and more often if unstable.
- Monitor fluid intake and urinary output hourly.
- Monitor AVPU and GCS scores, reflexes and pupil responses hourly.
- Monitor the mother for confusion and visual disturbance.
- Monitor the fetus regularly.
- Record all drugs used.

Each maternity unit should have an emergency box to ensure that appropriate equipment and drugs are readily available.

2.5.F Prolonged and obstructed labour, uterine rupture and shoulder dystocia

Prolonged and obstructed labour

It helps to reduce prolongation of labour if mothers in labour are allowed to sit upright, or in a lateral or semi-upright position, **never flat on their backs**. They should be encouraged to stand, and be mobile in the first stage of labour for as long as is comfortably possible. The benefits of this include the assistance of gravity in the descent of the baby, the avoidance of pressure on the inferior vena cava (IVC), with all of the effects of compression on the circulatory dynamics, and possibly a reduction in the pain of contractions.

Recognition of prolonged or obstructed labour and early referral

Remember the three P's: Power (too little), Passenger (too big) and Passage (too small).

Prevention of prolonged labour

- Good antenatal care is essential, so that the presentation of the fetus is known (and ideally confirmed by ultrasound examination) before the onset of labour. **If the presentation is abnormal, the mother must be transferred to hospital as soon as she goes into labour.**
- Use of the modified WHO partograph.
- Optimal nutritional state in the mother.
- Absence of anaemia in the mother.
- Adequate fluids and glucose during labour.
- Ensuring adequate bladder emptying.
- Emotional support.

Risks associated with slow progress in labour

For the mother these include the following:

- infection
- uterine rupture
- fistulae
- death.

For the baby they include the following:

- infection
- insufficient oxygen supply to the brain and traumatic injury
- stillbirth
- neonatal death
- permanent brain damage.

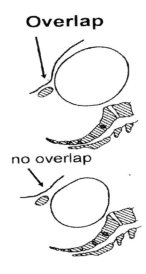

Overlap

no overlap

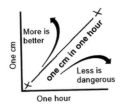

FIGURE 2.5.F.1 Cervical dilatation over time.

FIGURE 2.5.F.2 Obstruction of the fetal head's descent.

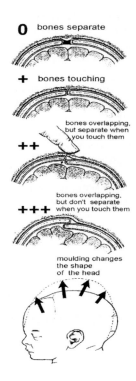

FIGURE 2.5.F.3 Development of increasing moulding of skull bones of fetus in labour. Increasing moulding is a sign of cephalo–pelvic disproportion.

Main causes of slow progress in labour
These include the following:
1 poor-quality uterine contractions
2 malpresentations and malpositions
3 disproportion between the size of the baby and the size of the pelvis; **it is important to exclude causes (1) and (2) before diagnosing this**.

All three of these causes require urgent transfer to hospital.
Bandl's ring
The presence of a Bandl's ring may be one sign that is seen in obstructed labour. It is often a late sign.

A Bandl's ring is a depression between the thickened upper segment and the thinned lower segment. A distended bladder sometimes forms a third swelling.

Moulding of the fetal head
Moulding refers to the overriding of the fetal skull bones that may occur during labour. Moulding should be assessed at the sagittal suture (not the lambdoid). During descent of the fetal head, the fetal skull bones move closer together. Moulding is described in three stages. The first stage (+) occurs when the bones touch, the second stage (2+) occurs when the bones overlap but are reducible, and the third stage (3+) is irreversible overlapping of the bones. Moulding, especially 3+, may suggest cephalo-pelvic disproportion, and should be looked at in conjunction with other clinical signs of obstructed labour.

Partogram in obstructed labour
Figure 2.5.F.4 shows the partogram for Mrs H, a mother who was admitted in active labour at 10 am.

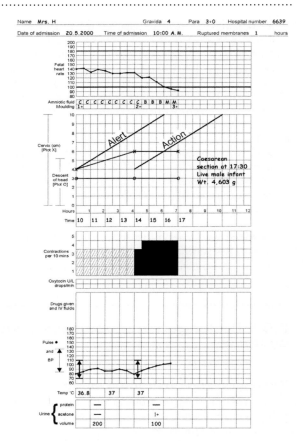

FIGURE 2.5.F.4 Partogram of obstructed labour.

- The fetal head is 3/5 palpable.
- The cervix is dilated to 4 cm.
- Three contractions occur in 10 minutes, each lasting for 20–40 seconds.
- Clear amniotic fluid is draining.
- There is fetal head moulding.

At 2 pm:
- The fetal head is still 3/5 palpable.
- The cervix is dilated to 6 cm and to the right of the alert line.
- There is a slight improvement in contractions (three in 10 minutes, each lasting for 40 seconds).
- There is second-degree moulding.

At 5 pm:
- The fetal head is still 3/5 palpable.
- The cervix is still dilated to 6 cm.
- There is third-degree moulding.
- The fetal heart rate 92 beats/minute.

Caesarean section was performed at 5.30 pm.

Note: The partogram for Mrs H is characteristic of obstructed labour. There is arrest of cervical dilatation in the active phase of labour, with no descent of the fetal head.

The presence of meconium and a falling fetal heart rate suggest fetal distress. All of these features, plus moulding of the fetal skull bones, point to cephalo-pelvic disproportion.

Oxytocin was rightly withheld, as Mrs H was multiparous, and this drug would therefore have increased the risk of uterine rupture in this patient.

Diagnostic issues in obstructed labour

The mother

- The patient may be dehydrated, tachycardic, ketotic (urine positive for ketone bodies, breath smells of ketones), febrile and exhausted, and there may be infected vaginal secretions.
- The bladder may be distended with retained urine, or it may be oedematous.
- Abdominal examination may reveal haemoperitoneum from a ruptured uterus. Blood may not appear vaginally, due to the impacted fetal head, which should be dislodged upwards to allow full assessment. If a ruptured uterus is suspected, a laparotomy should be performed (see below).
- Abdominal examination may reveal distended bowel from sepsis and ileus.

The fetus

- The lie and relationship of the fetus to the pelvis must be assessed.
- Despite visible caput at the introitus, 60% of the fetal head may still be palpable abdominally.

TABLE 2.5.F.1 Diagnosis of unsatisfactory progress of labour

Cervix not dilated	False labour
No palpable contractions/infrequent contractions	
Cervix not dilated beyond 4 cm after 8 hours of regular contractions	Prolonged latent phase
Cervical dilatation to the right of the alert line on the partogram	Prolonged active phase
Secondary arrest of cervical dilatation and descent of the presenting part in the presence of good contractions	Cephalo-pelvic disproportion
Secondary arrest of cervical dilatation and descent of the presenting part with large caput, third-degree moulding, cervix poorly applied to the presenting part, oedematous cervix, ballooning of the lower uterine segment, formation of a retraction band, and maternal and fetal distress	Obstruction
Less than 3–4 contractions in 10 minutes, each lasting from less than 40 seconds to 1 minute, with 1 minute of relaxation between contractions	Inadequate uterine activity
Presentation other than vertex with occipito-anterior	Malpresentation
Cervix fully dilated and the woman has the urge to push, but there is no descent	Prolonged expulsive (second stage) phase

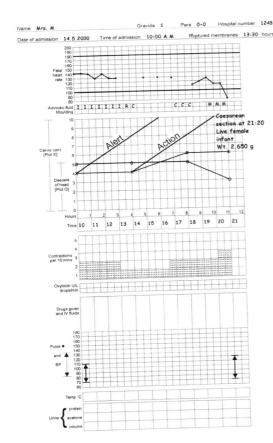

FIGURE 2.5.F.5 Partogram showing prolonged active phase of labour.

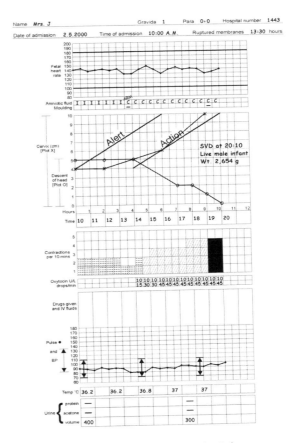

FIGURE 2.5.F.6 Partogram showing inadequate uterine contractions corrected with oxytocin.

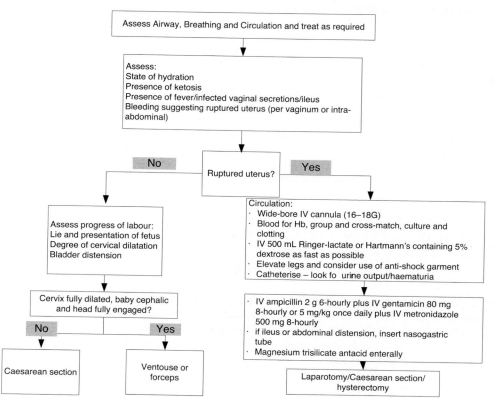

FIGURE 2.5.F.7 Pathway of care in obstructed labour.

The cervix in the primigravida whose partogram is shown in Figure 2.5.F.5 was 4 cm dilated on admission. Her contractions were ineffective at two in 10 minutes, decreasing to one contraction in 10 minutes. Her membranes ruptured 3.5 hours later, but her cervix dilated only a further 2 cm in 4 hours, with no further dilatation in the subsequent 3 hours. Fetal distress developed, with meconium and a falling fetal heart rate. Caesarean section was performed. It would have been advisable to start an oxytocin infusion at 13.30 hours, or at least by 15.30 hours.

The primigravida whose partogram is shown in Figure 2.5.F.6 started an oxytocin infusion at the time of membrane rupture, which increased the efficacy of contractions. She progressed to a spontaneous vaginal delivery. The fetal heart rate was satisfactory throughout.

Emergency treatment for obstructed labour

Assess ABC and resuscitate if required.
- Place a wide-bore IV cannula (14- to 16G).
- Place the mother in the left lateral tilt or recovery position.
- Send blood for haemoglobin, grouping and cross-matching, and electrolytes if possible.
- Give 1 litre IV of Ringer-lactate or Hartmann's solution containing 5% or 10% glucose over 1 hour as an infusion, or as rapidly as possible if the patient is shocked. Then reassess.
- Catheterise the patient to decompress the bladder, measure urine output and look for haematuria.
  - The presence of haematuria may suggest uterine rupture.
  - If there is concern about the viability of the vaginal

and bladder wall, the catheter may be kept *in situ* for up to 6 weeks to prevent or minimise the formation of a vesico-vaginal fistula.
- Give IV ampicillin (2 grams 6-hourly), gentamicin (80 mg IV/IM 8-hourly or 5 mg/kg body weight IV/IM once every 24 hours) and metronidazole (500 mg 8-hourly). Cefuroxime (1.5 grams 8-hourly, if available) can be given instead of ampicillin plus gentamicin.
- Measure the pulse rate, capillary refill time (CRT), blood pressure, temperature and urine output frequently.
- If uterine rupture has been excluded, shock may be due to hypovolaemia, sepsis or both.

If there has been recent food intake, or abdominal distension is present, the stomach should be emptied using a nasogastric tube, and then 10 mL of magnesium trisilicate oral suspension should be given to reduce the acidity of the gastric contents.

Overcoming slow progress in labour
- If the cervix is fully dilated and there is cephalic presentation and no signs of obstruction, instrumental delivery (ventouse or forceps) can avoid the need for Caesarean section. However, if the cervix is fully dilated and there is obstruction, instrumental delivery can make Caesarean section very difficult by causing further impaction of the fetal head.
- If the cervix is not fully dilated, in the primigravida with cephalic presentation, give an oxytocin infusion.
- If the cervix is not fully dilated, with abnormal presentation, perform a Caesarean section.
- If there is a ruptured uterus, a laparotomy and Caesarean hysterectomy must be performed.

Urgent referral is required if the above measures are not possible. Stabilise the mother's ABC before transfer if necessary.

Reasons for fetal death in obstructed labour

- Strong contractions with inadequate relaxation between contractions (sometimes made worse by inappropriate use of oxytocin) interfere with placental exchange.
- Excessive moulding of the head, in cephalic presentation, leads to intracranial haemorrhage. In breech presentation, the head may be trapped by an incompletely dilated cervix, or may not enter the pelvis because of disproportion.
- Ascending infection, amnionitis and severe intrauterine infection caused by prolonged ruptured membranes and labour, and/or unsterile vaginal examinations.
- Ruptured uterus.

Risks of Caesarean section in obstructed labour

These include the following:
- intra-operative haemorrhage
- post-operative shock
- generalised peritonitis
- the hazards of general or regional anaesthesia
- rupture of the uterine scar in subsequent pregnancies

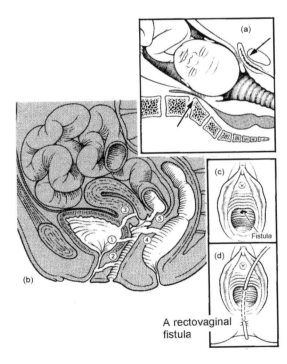

FIGURE 2.5.F.8 Mechanism and anatomy of vaginal fistulae. The arrows show where this mother's cervix, rectum and bladder are being pinched between the baby's head and the mother's spine and pubis. (a) The baby's head can press the mother's vagina and bladder against the symphysis pubis or the sacrum. This can make the tissues necrose (die) and cause a fistula. (b) The fistula can be in various places: 1, between the bladder and the vagina; 2, between the urethra and the vagina; 3, between the bladder and the cervix; 4, between the rectum and the vagina (rectovaginal fistula); 5, between the vagina and the small gut. (c) A vesico-vaginal fistula. (d) A catheter has been placed in a rectovaginal fistula.

- wound complications
- pelvic abscess
- visceral damage, especially to the bladder; it may be difficult to pass a catheter with a very impacted fetal head, and the bladder is often oedematous.

The management of uterine rupture in this setting depends on its site and extent. With a straightforward anterior rupture without extension, uterine repair (plus bilateral tubal ligation) may be most appropriate and safe.

If infection is present before a Caesarean section is performed, dangerous complications can follow. In one series of 107 Caesarean sections, performed in 156 patients with intrapartum infection, the following complications occurred:
- post-operative shock: 18 patients (17%)
- generalised peritonitis: 70 patients (65%)
- mortality: 13 patients (12%).

Rupture of the uterus

Complete rupture of the uterus is life-threatening to both mother and baby.

Causes

A previous Caesarean section scar may rupture during labour. However, obstructed labour, even without a uterine scar, particularly in a woman of high parity, may cause uterine rupture. It may be caused by inappropriate use of oxytocic drugs, especially in multiparous women, or in the presence of cephalo-pelvic disproportion. No woman who is receiving an oxytocin infusion should be left alone.

Ideally, always use a burette giving set to administer IV oxytocin to avoid dangerous over-dosage. **In the absence of a burette, refer to the progressive oxytocin dosage, and use as described in Section 2.3, making sure to slow or stop once labour is well established.**

Uterine rupture may be caused by violence or trauma during pregnancy, sometimes as a result of domestic violence (*see* Section 2.11).

Risk factors for uterine rupture

These include the following:
- malpresentation and malposition
- previous Caesarean section, especially if oxytocic agents

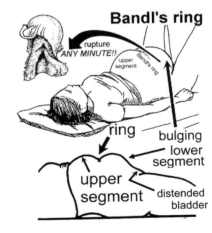

FIGURE 2.5.F.9 Bandl's ring in obstructed labour. Uterine rupture may be imminent.

are used, or if a classical Caesarean section scar is present

- previous uterine surgery (e.g. myomectomy), or uterine perforation at the time of dilatation and curettage (D&C) or manual removal of the placenta; this is often unrecognised
- the multiparous woman who has delivered normally before and has a significantly larger baby or a malposition in the current pregnancy, and is allowed a prolonged second stage.

Symptoms and signs

Uterine rupture usually presents with hypovolaemic shock, but vaginal bleeding can be concealed. The baby is usually dead.

Around 50% of ruptures occur at or near full dilatation.
- There is a change in the nature of the pain, from severe intermittent pain to a constant dull ache.
- Vaginal bleeding may or may not be present.
- There is maternal shock due to blood loss with or without vagal stimulation, as well as dehydration, exhaustion, and ketoacidosis in cases of prolonged obstructed labour.
- Abdominal distension occurs that is tender to palpation, the fetal parts may be very easily palpated, and there is absence of a fetal heart rate.
- On vaginal examination, the presenting part may be high or impacted.
- Uterine rupture may be preceded by the appearance of Bandl's ring (*see* Figure 2.5.F.9).

Suspect rupture in a patient with any of these risk factors.

Primary assessment and resuscitation

Call for help, especially for a surgeon and an anaesthetist, as urgent laparotomy will be required.

Airway

- If the airway is not open, use an airway-opening manoeuvre and keep it open. Consider an airway adjunct such as an oropharyngeal airway or intubation.
- The oropharynx may need gentle suctioning under direct vision, but be careful to avoid inducing laryngospasm.
- The recovery position should be adopted to minimise the risk of aspiration of vomit (*see* Figure 2.5.F.10).

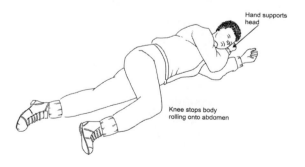

Hand supports head

Knee stops body rolling onto abdomen

FIGURE 2.5.F.10 The semi-prone or recovery position.

Breathing

- If there is spontaneous breathing, give a high concentration of oxygen via a face mask with reservoir. Give 100% oxygen (mask with reservoir and flow rate of at least 6 litres/minute) regardless of the mother's oxygen saturation. This increases fetal oxygen delivery as well as improving maternal tissue oxygenation.
- If the patient is apnoeic or hypoventilating, provide chest inflations with bag-valve-mask-reservoir ventilation and high-flow oxygen.

Circulation

Evaluate the pulse rate and volume, peripheral circulation (capillary refill time) and blood pressure.
- **If signs of life are absent, initiate CPR.**
- **Perform the left lateral tilt or manual displacement of the uterus.**
- **If the patient shows signs of shock, support the circulation as described below.**
    - Insert a 14- to 16G IV cannula and take 20 mL of blood for a full blood count, cross-matching (4 units = 2 litres) and clotting. Do a whole blood clotting time (WBCT) test if laboratory analyses are not available.
- Give 500 mL to 1 litre of Ringer-lactate or Hartmann's solution by rapid IV bolus.
- Reassess, and if shock is still present, give blood (if available) (500 mL as rapidly as possible after warming) or another 500 mL to 1 litre of Ringer-lactate or Hartmann's solution.
- If the patient is ketotic from prolonged obstructed labour, add 50 mL of 50% glucose to the second litre of Ringer-lactate or Hartmann's solution.
- Central venous access may be needed for volume replacement if peripheral access is not possible.

Emergency treatment

1. Obtain consent for laparotomy and hysterectomy.
2. Try to place a second IV cannula.
3. Perform urgent laparotomy under general anaesthesia.
4. The type of operation will depend upon the size and site of rupture, and the degree of haemorrhage.
5. Give IV prophylactic antibiotics (ampicillin 2 grams or cefuroxime 1.5 grams plus metronidazole 500 mg).

The rupture may extend anteriorly towards the back of the bladder, laterally towards the uterine arteries, or into the broad ligament plexus of veins, leading to massive haemorrhage.

Posterior rupture may occur, and is usually associated with intrauterine malformations, but has occurred in patients who have had a previous Caesarean section or uterine trauma, or after rotational forceps. Fundal rupture has been documented, and a detailed history usually elicits previous dilatation and curettage (D&C) or manual removal of the placenta.

Continuing haemorrhage is an indication for performing a total or subtotal hysterectomy. Subtotal hysterectomy is a simpler procedure than total hysterectomy, and has a reduced risk of ureteric or bladder damage.

The choice of uterine repair depends on the site of the injury. In one series of 23 cases of ruptured uterus, hysterectomy was undertaken in 15 cases (65%) and repair in the other 8 cases. Five successful further pregnancies were reported without repeat rupture (all delivered by Caesarean section). In another Middle Eastern series of 11 cases of uterine rupture, 8 cases had uterine repair, and all became pregnant again and were delivered by Caesarean section.

Shoulder dystocia (see video for download on www. mcai.org.uk)

Shoulder dystocia is caused by impaction of the shoulders against the bony pelvis. Special manoeuvres are required to deliver the shoulders. The reported incidence is between 0.15% and 2% of all vaginal deliveries. Shoulder dystocia carries a significant risk to the baby due to hypoxia, fractures of the clavicle and humerus, and injuries to the brachial plexus.

The problem lies at the **pelvic brim** where the anterior shoulder gets caught, while the posterior shoulder has usually entered the pelvis. Treatment therefore aims to encourage the anterior shoulder into the pelvis, or if this fails, either rotating the posterior shoulder round into the anterior position or delivering the posterior arm first. Traction on the head when the anterior shoulder is caught above the pelvic brim will not work and is dangerous.

Delivery should occur within 5 minutes of the delivery of the head. The longer the delay, the greater the risk of hypoxic injury to the baby.

Postpartum haemorrhage is common after shoulder dystocia, and there is a risk of serious vaginal and perineal lacerations.

Risk factors for shoulder dystocia

Antepartum risk factors include the following:

- fetal macrosomia
- maternal obesity
- diabetes
- prolonged pregnancy
- advanced maternal age
- male gender
- excessive weight gain
- previous shoulder dystocia
- previous big baby.

Intrapartum risk factors include the following:

- prolonged first stage
- prolonged second stage
- oxytocin augmentation of labour
- assisted delivery.

These risk factors often do not help in the prediction of individual cases of shoulder dystocia. Therefore the practice of emergency drills is essential for good management of the unexpected case.

Slow progress in labour, particularly in the multiparous patient or in the woman with a past history of a big baby or difficulty delivering the shoulders, should alert one to the possibility of shoulder dystocia.

During delivery, signs include the following:

- difficulty delivering the face and chin
- head retractions between contractions
- head bobbing
- the delivered head becomes tightly pulled back against the perineum (turtle sign).

As soon as the situation is suspected, a plan of action should be initiated.

Management of shoulder dystocia

If risk factors are present, try if possible to have an experienced obstetrician present in the second stage of labour. However, 50% of cases are unexpected.

Be prepared for the problem, including postpartum haemorrhage, which may follow.

Try each manoeuvre for 30–60 seconds only: if it does not work, move on. Try to recognise it early on and before applying any traction to the head, which can delay helpful procedures and cause Erb's paralysis.

The following acronym suggested by Advanced Life Support in Obstetrics (ALSO) is helpful (see www. also.org.uk):

HELPERR: **H** = Help
                E = Evaluate/Episiotomy
                L = Legs (McRoberts)
                P = Pressure (suprapubic)
                E = Enter (posterior arm and Wood's screw)
                R = Rotate (on to all fours)
                R = Repeat

1 **Call for help. This condition needs the most experienced team and extra helpers.**
2 **McRoberts manoeuvre (legs)** (see Figures 2.5.F.11 and 2.5.F.12). Both thighs are sharply flexed, abducted and rotated outwards, ideally by two assistants. Each assistant holds the leg in the region of the thigh and flexes the leg until the thigh lies parallel to the anterior abdominal wall. This will reduce the angle between the sacrum and the lumbar vertebrae to help to free the impacted shoulder. If two assistants are not available, the mother may be placed in the all fours position (see below).

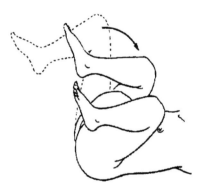

FIGURE 2.5.F.11 McRoberts manoeuvre, showing how important it is to fully flex both legs on to the mother's abdomen so that the thighs lie parallel to the anterior abdominal wall.

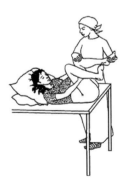

FIGURE 2.5.F.12 In McRoberts manoeuvre, with only one assistant the left leg is held flexed against the abdomen by a nurse, and the mother holds her right leg in this position.

3 **Suprapubic pressure with moderate traction (not fundal pressure).** Suprapubic pressure is applied to reduce the diameter between the shoulders and push the anterior shoulder underneath the symphysis pubis. It is important to know where the fetal back lies, so that pressure is applied in the right direction (i.e. from the fetal back forwards towards the fetal chest). If you are unsure of the position of the back, confirm it by vaginal examination. Pressure should be applied to the back of the shoulder with the heel of the hand, and sometimes a rocking movement may be helpful. Strong traction and fundal pressure should be avoided.

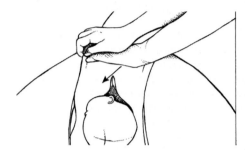

FIGURE 2.5.F.13 Suprapubic pressure.

4 **Apply moderate traction (harder pulling can make impaction worse and cause Erb's paralysis).** Once both McRoberts manoeuvre and suprapubic pressure are in place, moderate traction can be applied while discouraging maternal efforts (which can increase the impaction of the shoulders).

5 **Consider an episiotomy.** A medio-lateral episiotomy is recommended to allow more room for manoeuvres such as delivering the posterior shoulder, allowing the operator to use the sacral hollow, and reducing vaginal trauma.

6 **Deliver the posterior arm and shoulder.** Insert a hand up to the fetal axilla and hook the posterior shoulder down. Traction on the posterior axilla then brings the posterior arm within reach. Run your index finger or middle finger, or both, along the back of the fetal humerus, then flex the elbow at the antecubital fossa, which will disengage the arm, which can then be brought down (hold the hand and sweep it across the chest). Sometimes it comes out directly lying alongside the head, and sometimes it comes out with an element of rotation anteriorly.

7 **Internal rotational manoeuvres (Rubin's and Wood's screw manoeuvres).** These measures are rarely required.

Rubin's manoeuvre. The operator inserts the fingers of one hand vaginally, positioning the fingertips behind the anterior shoulder. The shoulder is then pushed towards the fetal chest.

Wood's screw manoeuvre. If Rubin's manoeuvre is unsuccessful, the fingers of the opposite hand may be inserted vaginally to approach the posterior shoulder from the front of the fetus. The combination of these two movements may allow rotation of the shoulders and aid delivery. If delivery of the posterior shoulder or arm is not successful, try to rotate the posterior shoulder 180-degrees in a corkscrew fashion (clockwise or anticlockwise) to bring it to an anterior position, from which the delivery can continue as normal (this rotation

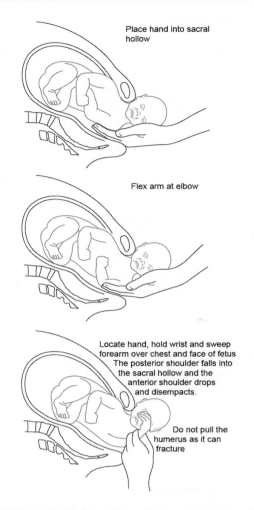

FIGURE 2.5.F.14 Delivery of the posterior arm. Reproduced with permission from Macdonald S, Magill-Cuerden J (ed.) *Mayes' Midwifery: a textbook for midwives.* Elsevier Health Sciences; 2010. © Elsevier

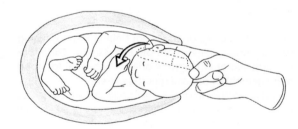

FIGURE 2.5.F.15 Rubin's manoeuvre.

releases the impacted anterior shoulder that ends up in the posterior pelvis). It is important not to twist the fetal head or neck during this manoeuvre.

8 **All fours position.** This is another procedure that can be useful if no help is available. The mother quickly positions herself evenly on hands and knees (Gaskin's manoeuvre). In many cases this alone relieves the dystocia. In addition, it can assist with the delivery of the posterior arm. The other manoeuvres described above can also be performed with the mother in this position. Early on try to deliver the posterior shoulder from this position. Sometimes pushing one leg forward into the

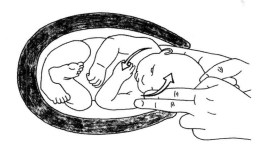

FIGURE 2.5.F.16 Wood's screw manoeuvre.

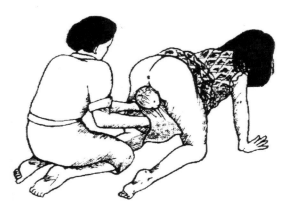

FIGURE 2.5.F.18 The all-fours position for shoulder dystocia (the method to use if you have no one to assist you). Guide the head downwards so that the posterior shoulder which has now become upwards with the adoption of the all-fours position is delivered.

'starting of a race' position can open up the pelvis from this position.

9 **Symphysiotomy.** If the baby is still undelivered, symphysiotomy should be considered.

10 Check the vagina and perineum for trauma, and repair accordingly.

11 Prepare for postpartum haemorrhage.

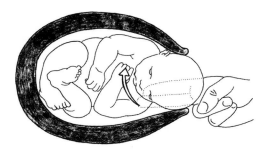

FIGURE 2.5.F.17 Reverse Wood's screw manoeuvre.

2.5.G Severe infection in the puerperal period

Diagnosis of infection after childbirth

TABLE 2.5.G.1 Symptoms and signs of infection, with diagnosis and treatment

Symptoms	Signs	Investigations	Diagnosis	Treatment
Rigors/chills Lower abdominal and/or pelvic pain Foul-smelling liquor Persistent light vaginal bleeding History of incomplete placenta delivered History of prolonged rupture of membranes, frequent unsterile vaginal examinations in labour	Fever (usually > 38°C) Tender uterus Shock Delayed rate of involution of uterus	Full blood count, including white blood cell count Blood culture Lochia for microscopy, culture and sensitivity	**Endometritis**	Treat shock urgently if present IV antibiotics Ampicillin 2 grams IV/IM every 6 hours *plus* gentamicin 80 mg IV/IM every 8 hours or 5 mg/kg body weight IV/IM once every 24 hours *plus* metronidazole 500 mg IV every 8 hours
Breast pain Rigors	Tender over breast Red wedge-shaped area of induration of one breast Fever > 38°C		**Mastitis**	If bacterial infection is suspected, give anti-staphylococcal antibiotics: flucloxacillin or cephalexin orally for 7 days
Breast pain Rigors, chills and/or malaise	Swinging fever Fluctuant swelling in the breast, possibly with pointing and draining of pus		**Breast abscess**	Surgical drainage If the patient is systemically very unwell, give anti-staphylococcal antibiotics IV: flucloxacillin or cefotaxime or ceftriaxone

(continued)

Symptoms	Signs	Investigations	Diagnosis	Treatment
History of Caesarean section Rigors, chills and/or malaise Severe abdominal pain Vomiting	High, swinging fever Swelling and redness around incision High fever Abdominal distension Rigid abdomen Absent bowel sounds Shock (see above for signs)		**Wound abscess** **Peritonitis**	Surgical drainage Treat shock Give IV antibiotics Nasogastric tube Immediate laparotomy in operating theatre
Lower abdominal pain Diarrhoea History of Caesarean section	Swinging fever Swelling in adnexae or pouch of Douglas Tender uterus Ultrasound	Full blood count, including white blood cell count Blood culture Pus for microscopy, culture and sensitivity	**Pelvic abscess**	Give IV antibiotics: Ampicillin 2 grams IV/IM every 6 hours *plus* gentamicin 80 mg IV/IM every 8 hours or 5 mg/kg body weight IV/IM once every 24 hours *plus* metronidazole 500 mg IV every 8 hours Surgical drainage
Pain in the lower abdomen or loin Nausea and/or vomiting Increased frequency of passing urine	High fever Tenderness of one of the loins over the kidney Normal bowel sounds	Microscopic examination of urine Stick tests for infection (if available) Urine culture and sensitivity if possible	**Pyelonephritis**	IV antibiotics (*see* Section 2.8.F) If the patient is in shock, initiate immediate treatment
Difficulty in breathing Cough, sometimes with expectoration Pleuritic chest pain	Fever Respiratory distress Signs of consolidation or effusion	Chest X-ray Ultrasound if there is effusion	**Pneumonia**	IV antibiotics (*see* Section 2.8.A)
Rigors Headache Muscle and/or joint pains	Fever Enlarged spleen Shock Reduced consciousness Jaundice Anaemia Fitting	Full blood count Thick film for parasites Blood glucose	**Malaria**	Antimalarial drugs (*see* Section 2.8.D)

Endometritis

This is the most serious and common cause of puerperal sepsis. It accounts for up to 15% of maternal deaths in resource-limited countries.

Infection of retained products of conception is the most common cause (suspect this if there is excessive vaginal bleeding or poor involution of the uterus). This can lead to long-term health problems, including infertility, chronic pelvic inflammatory disease and ectopic pregnancies.

Endometritis is defined as infection of the genital tract at any time between the onset of rupture of the membranes or labour and the 42nd day following delivery or abortion, in which two or more of the following are present:

- abdominal and/or pelvic pain
- fever of ≥ 37.5°C (can be masked by paracetamol or other antipyretic drugs)
- abnormal quantity of vaginal discharge
- foul-smelling discharge
- delay in the rate of involution of the uterus.

Puerperal sepsis can present with few symptoms (the woman feels unwell and usually has a fever). It can also progress rapidly to become life-threatening within hours.

Pathogens that cause sepsis

The pathogens most commonly responsible are group A beta-haemolytic streptococcus (often of community origin) and endotoxin-producing enterobacteria (e.g. *E. coli*). Less commonly involved are *Clostridium*, *Bacteroides*, *Chlamydia* and *Mycoplasma*. Bacterial infections are often mixed.

Risk factors

These include the following:

- prolonged rupture of membranes (> 48 hours before delivery)
- contact with others, especially children, with a bacterial throat infection (*Streptococcus*)
- frequent (particularly unsterile) vaginal examinations
- prolonged and obstructed labour
- instrumentation (e.g. forceps delivery)
- Caesarean section (especially in an emergency)

- retained products of conception
- lack of sanitary towels and hygienic materials to manage lochia during the postnatal period
- sickle-cell disease.

Pathogenesis
- Endotoxins are released from the cell wall of Gram-negative bacteria.
- Endotoxins can cause shock.
- Extensive tissue necrosis, even gangrene, may occur, especially in the uterus.

Prevention
- Antibiotic prophylaxis for prolonged rupture of membranes, manual removal of the placenta and Caesarean section.
- Antiseptic cream for vaginal examinations (e.g. Hibitane obstetric cream).
- Provision of sanitary towels and other hygienic items to all women and girls who have given birth, and where family poverty means that these items are not available.

Complications
These include the following:
- wound infection and wound dehiscence (burst abdomen)
- peritonitis
- ileus
- septicaemia, possibly accompanied by shock
- abscess formation in cul-de-sac and sub-diaphragmatic space
- adnexal infections
- ovarian abscess
- pelvic abscess
- breast infection or abscess
- deep vein thrombosis
- pulmonary embolus.

Investigations
These include the following:
- high vaginal swab if bacteriology facilities are available
- midstream samples of urine (MSSU) and microscopy of urine.

Treatment
Treat as an emergency, including IV fluid boluses if shock is present (see Section 2.5A), if there is persistent tachycardia (> 100 beats/minute), hypotension (systolic blood pressure < 90 mmHg), increased respiratory rate (> 25 breaths/minute), confusion or disorientation, oliguria (< 30 mL/hour), rash or bradycardia (< 50 beats/minute).

Give antibiotics until the patient has been fever-free for 48 hours or 7–10 days:
- ampicillin 2 grams IV every 6 hours
  - plus gentamicin 80 mg IV/IM every 8 hours or 5 mg/kg body weight IV/IM once every 24 hours
  - plus metronidazole 500 mg IV every 8 hours.

If fever is still present 72 hours after initiating antibiotics, re-evaluate the patient and consider revising the diagnosis.

Often a 1 to 2 week antibiotic course is completed orally once the patient has been fever free for 48 hours.

If retained placental fragments are suspected, perform a digital exploration of the uterus to remove clots and large pieces. Use ovum forceps or a large curette if necessary, but be very careful not to penetrate the uterine wall, which is very soft at this stage. Where general anaesthesia is not available, agents such as ketamine may be considered for this procedure.

If there is no improvement with conservative measures, and there are symptoms and signs of general peritonitis (abdominal pain, fever, and abdominal tenderness with rebound tenderness), perform a laparotomy to drain the pus, and if the uterus is the source do not leave it too late to perform a hysterectomy.

Wound infections

Wound infections may be superficial or deep. Superficial infections involve the skin and subcutaneous tissues, but not the rectus sheath (fascia). They may present with cellulitis or abscess formation. Cellulitis should be treated with antibiotics; this may prevent the development of a wound abscess.

Clear or purulent fluid exuding from the wound should raise concern that the infection is deep to the sheath. Where there is abscess formation, the wound should be opened by removing sutures to the skin and subcutaneous tissues, to allow drainage of pus. Antibiotics are not always required if an abscess is drained and the surrounding tissues appear healthy.

The wound may require debridement if tissue necrosis is suspected. If the sheath looks healthy and intact, the fascial sutures should be left in situ. The wound should be packed with a damp dressing, which must be changed every 24 hours.

If the sheath appears necrotic or infected, it should be opened and the peritoneal cavity inspected for collections of pus. If pus is present, it should be evacuated, and a broad corrugated drain left in situ in the peritoneal cavity to facilitate drainage post-operatively.

Necrotising fasciitis is a relatively uncommon but potentially life-threatening variant of wound infection, which presents with rapidly spreading cellulitis, with severe pain and tenderness. Urgent wide debridement of necrotic tissue is required, with antibiotics as for deep wound infection (see below). Secondary closure should be undertaken 2–4 weeks later, provided that the infection has resolved.

Antibiotic regimes for wound infections
Where possible, swabs should be taken for culture and sensitivity before starting antibiotics.

Superficial infections
Give ampicillin 500 mg by mouth, four times a day for 5 days, plus metronidazole 500 mg by mouth, three times a day for 5 days.

Deep infections
Give benzyl penicillin, 2 million units (1200 mg) IV every 6 hours, plus gentamicin 80 mg IV/IM every 8 hours or 5 mg/kg body weight IV/IM once every 24 hours, plus metronidazole 500 mg IV every 8 hours.

IV antibiotics should be continued until at least 48 hours after the pyrexia has settled.

The patient may then be switched to oral antibiotics, as described above.

Peritonitis

Treat shock, if present. Then:

- provide nasogastric suction
- infuse IV fluids for maintenance and replacement
- give antibiotics IV until the patient has been fever-free for 48 hours:
  - ampicillin/amoxicillin 2 grams IV/IM every 6 hours
  - *plus* gentamicin 80 mg IV/IM every 8 hours or 5 mg/kg body weight IV/IM once every 24 hours
  - *plus* metronidazole 500 mg IV every 8 hours.
- if necessary, perform a laparotomy to repair diseased or injured bowel.

Pelvic abscess

Give antibiotics before draining the abscess, and continue until the patient has been fever-free for 48 hours:

- ampicillin/amoxicillin 2 grams IV every 6 hours
- *plus* gentamicin 80 mg IV/IM every 8 hours or 5 mg/kg body weight IV/IM once every 24 hours
- *plus* metronidazole 500 mg IV every 8 hours.

If **the abscess is fluctuant in the cul-de-sac**, drain the pus through the cul-de-sac (culdocentesis) (see below). If **the spiking fever continues**, perform a laparotomy.

Bowel may be secondarily involved in the inflammatory process, and care must be taken to avoid bowel perforation.

Peritonitis may develop in association with a pelvic abscess. Prompt nasogastric suction and administration of intravenous fluids are important, as well as IV antibiotic therapy as described above.

Culdocentesis and colpotomy

Culdocentesis for the detection of pus

- Apply antiseptic solution to the vagina, especially the posterior fornix.
- Infiltrate with 1% lignocaine.
- Gently grasp the posterior lip of the cervix with a tenaculum and gently pull to elevate the cervix and expose the posterior vagina.
- Place a long needle (e.g. spinal needle) on a syringe and insert it through the posterior vagina, just below the posterior lip of the cervix (*see* Figure 2.5.G.1).
- Pull back on the syringe to aspirate the cul-de-sac (the space behind the uterus).
- If pus is obtained, keep the needle in place and proceed to colpotomy (see below).

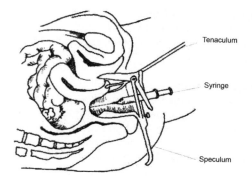

FIGURE 2.5.G.1 Culdocentesis: diagnostic needle aspiration of the cul-de-sac.

Colpotomy for a pelvic abscess

If **pus is obtained** on culdocentesis, keep the needle in place and make a stab incision at the site of the puncture.

Remove the needle and insert blunt forceps or a finger through the incision to break the loculi in the abscess cavity (*see* Figure 2.5.G.2).

- Allow the pus to drain.
- Insert a disinfected soft rubber corrugated drain through the incision. (If a surgical drain is not available, a makeshift drain can be prepared by cutting off the fingertips of a disinfected rubber glove.)
- If required, use a stitch through the drain to anchor it in the vagina.
- Remove the drain when there is no more drainage of pus.
- If **no pus is obtained**, the abscess may be higher than the pouch of Douglas. A laparotomy will be required for peritoneal lavage (wash-out).

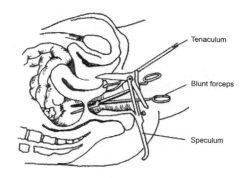

FIGURE 2.5.G.2 Colpotomy for pelvic abscess.

Mastitis

Mastitis may be infective or non-infective, ranging in severity from mild local erythema and tenderness through to abscess and septicaemia.

- Non-infective mastitis may be due to a blocked lactiferous duct, or to difficulties with breastfeeding technique. It may lead to infective mastitis.
- Infective mastitis is common in lactating women. It is usually caused by the bacterium *Staphylococcus*, which generally responds to a 7- to 10-day oral course of flucloxacillin or a cephalosporin, both of which are safe to take while breastfeeding.

Mastitis usually presents with a hot red swollen section of one breast. It may be associated with flu-like symptoms, namely pyrexia of 38°C or above, chills and myalgia.

Treatment

Continue breastfeeding. Although the symptoms of mastitis may discourage breastfeeding, it is important to try to continue. Regular breastfeeding will help to:

- remove any blocked breast milk from the breast
- resolve the symptoms of mastitis more quickly
- prevent mastitis from becoming more serious.

The milk from the affected breast may be a little saltier than normal, but is safe for the baby to drink. Any bacteria that are present in the milk will be harmlessly absorbed by the baby's digestive system and cause no problems.

Breastfeed frequently on the affected side, in order to empty the breast of retained milk. The baby can empty the breast more efficiently than a breast pump. However, if the baby is not feeding well, a **breast pump or hand expression** will be needed to get the milk out. It may be less painful if the affected breast is given to the baby second, after the let-down reflex has occurred.

Mastitis can usually be successfully treated by resting, drinking plenty of fluids and varying the baby's position at the breast. It is important to ensure that the baby is properly attached to the nipple, and that the breast is empty after the feed. It may be necessary to feed more frequently, and to express the remaining milk after a feed. Paracetamol is useful for pain control. Massaging the areas of tenderness may be beneficial.

Prevention of mastitis

The following advice should be given to any mother who has experienced mastitis:

- Relieve engorgement promptly. Milk that does not flow gets thicker and clogs the ducts.
- Breastfeed frequently. Do not restrict the length of feedings.
- If the mother feels her breasts getting full, she should encourage the baby to feed without waiting for the baby to initiate this.

Repeated mastitis

This is usually the result of irregular breastfeeding patterns, such as missing feeds and giving bottles in place of breastfeeding. Recurrent mastitis may also result from tiredness and stress.

With regard to antibiotic treatment, the bacterium involved in mastitis is usually *Staphylococcus*, and the two most effective antibiotics are cloxacillins and cephalosporins, which are safe to take while breastfeeding. A 10-day oral course is recommended.

2.5.H Pulmonary embolism

> **BOX 2.5.H.1 Minimum standards**
> - Oxygen.
> - IV unfractionated heparin.
> - Low molecular weight heparin.
> - Subcutaneous heparin.
> - Blood clotting measurements.
> - Anti-embolism stockings.

Introduction

If left untreated, as many as 24% of patients with deep vein thrombosis (DVT) will have a pulmonary embolism. However, when DVT is treated with anticoagulants (if that is possible), pulmonary embolism occurs in only 4.5% of cases, and the mortality rate is less than 1%.

Deaths are equally common antenatally and postnatally. Pregnancy is a thrombogenic state associated with a five- or sixfold increase in the risk of pulmonary embolism. The majority of DVTs in pregnancy are ileo-femoral, and these are more likely to embolise.

Anti-embolism stockings and early mobility after Caesarean section and after childbirth are the main ways of preventing this.

Additional risk factors

- **Operative delivery:** Caesarean section increases the risk of pulmonary embolism by two- to eightfold; the risk is greater after an emergency procedure than after an elective one.
- **Age:** The mortality from pulmonary embolism is 100 times higher in pregnant women over 40 years of age than in those aged 20–25 years.
- **Obesity.**
- **Congenital and acquired thrombophilia:** Patients with antithrombin III deficiency, protein C and S deficiency, activated protein C resistance, and lupus anticoagulant and antiphospholipid antibody are at increased risk of pulmonary embolism.

- Surgical procedures during pregnancy or the puerperium (especially Caesarean section).
- **Other risk factors:** Restricted activity, pre-eclampsia, dehydration, excessive blood loss and homocystinuria.

Clinical presentation

- Dyspnoea, tachypnoea, pleuritic chest pain, cough, haemoptysis and leg pain.
- Massive pulmonary embolism may be associated with cyanosis, circulatory collapse with hypotension, syncope or convulsions and central chest pain.
- Occasionally, patients present with unexplained tachycardia.

TABLE 2.5.H.1 Signs and symptoms of pulmonary embolism

Findings	Patients with proven pulmonary embolism (%)
Tachypnoea	89
Dyspnoea	81
Pleuritic pain	72
Apprehension	59
Cough	54
Tachycardia	43
Haemoptysis	34
Temperature > 37°C	34

Tachycardia and a few localised crepitations may be the only findings on physical examination.

Massive pulmonary embolism may produce right-sided heart failure with jugular venous distension, an enlarged liver, a left parasternal heave, and fixed splitting of the second heart sound.

Clinical evidence of DVT may not be found in patients with pulmonary embolism. Symptoms and physical findings must be interpreted with caution during pregnancy, because dyspnoea, tachypnoea and leg discomfort are common findings as pregnancy progresses.

Investigations

Request a full blood count, urine and electrolytes, oxygen saturation, and (when available) clotting studies and arterial blood gases.

Request an ECG and chest X-ray (if available). These investigations do not confirm or refute the diagnosis of pulmonary embolism.

- **ECG** is non-specific for the diagnosis of pulmonary embolism. The changes in electrical axis that occur in normal pregnancy make the ECG findings in pulmonary embolism even less specific. Sinus tachycardia is the most common abnormality. Right axis deviation and right ventricular strain pattern may be present with a large pulmonary embolism. The S1Q3T3 pattern is very rare.
- **Chest X-ray** helps to exclude pneumothorax and pneumonia. The non-specific radiological changes in pulmonary embolism include segmental collapse, a raised hemidiaphragm, consolidation and unilateral pleural effusion. A wedge-shaped infarction is a rare finding.

Primary assessment and resuscitation for possible pulmonary embolism (ABC approach)

Call for help.

Airway

- Use an opening manoeuvre if the airway is not open or is partially obstructed. If there is an improvement, use airway adjuncts to maintain the airway.
  - An oropharyngeal airway is usually appropriate only if the patient is unconscious.
- Suction if necessary.
- The airway may need to be maintained and protected by intubation using experienced senior help (if available).

Breathing

- Provide a high concentration of **oxygen** through a face mask with reservoir bag, if there is adequate spontaneous respiration.
- For patients with inadequate ventilation or depressed conscious level, respiration should be supported with oxygen via a bag-valve-mask and experienced senior help summoned (if available).

Give 100% oxygen (mask with reservoir and flow rate of at least 6 litres/minute) regardless of SaO_2, as it increases fetal oxygen delivery as well as improving maternal tissue oxygenation.

Circulation

- Place a wide-bore IV cannula (16- to 18G).
- Place the woman in a lateral tilt or recovery position if undelivered and more than 20 weeks' gestation.
- If possible, locally treat clinically suspected pulmonary embolism while awaiting confirmation from objective tests (if available) to prevent further thromboembolic complications and extension of the existing thrombus.
  - IV unfractionated heparin is the mainstay of treatment.
  - Initiate treatment with an IV bolus of 5000 IU of heparin given over 5 minutes.

- **Note:** there are serious potential risks of anticoagulation, in particular the risk of life-threatening haemorrhage in the 24 hours after delivery, especially after Caesarean section.
- Empirical anticoagulation should be undertaken only when the diagnosis is clear clinically.
- **Additional treatment options for shocked patients** (if available) include thrombolytic therapy using streptokinase, pulmonary embolectomy and transvenous catheter fragmentation of the clot (available only in well-resourced units). Expert advice should be sought (if available).

Secondary assessment and emergency treatment

Involve the senior obstetrician, the anaesthetist and the medical team (if available).

Transfer the patient to the **high-dependency area** (if available) and commence close monitoring of heart rate, blood pressure, central oxygenation (SaO_2 if possible), ECG (if available) and urine output.

Anticoagulation

Heparin is the anticoagulant of choice in pregnancy, as it does not cross the placenta. Rapid and prolonged anticoagulation prevents extension of the thrombus and its recurrence.

When available, acute therapy is with an IV bolus of unfractionated heparin, 5000 IU over 5 minutes, followed by an IV infusion of 1000–2000 IU/hour for 5–10 days. The dose is adjusted to maintain the activated partial thromboplastin time (APTT) at 1.5–2.5 times the control. Repeat the APTT every 6 hours during the first 24 hours of therapy, and thereafter monitor it daily.

Treatment may then be continued with subcutaneous heparin at a dose of 10 000 IU twice daily. Maintaining the APTT in the therapeutic range (1.5–2.5 times the control) following subcutaneous heparin may be problematic, and can lead to under- or over-anticoagulation. Low-molecular-weight heparin (LMWH) is ideal if available.

Before giving heparin, measure the platelet count (if available).

Rare complications of heparin treatment are allergy and thrombocytopenia. The platelet count should be monitored at the onset of treatment and monthly thereafter.

Warfarin crosses the placenta and is associated with characteristic damage to the fetus in the first trimester. Major fetal CNS abnormalities such as microcephaly and optic atrophy are also seen with warfarin use in the second and third trimesters. In addition, there is a higher risk of intracerebral bleeds from the trauma of delivery, and a higher risk of bleeding complications during labour and delivery. **For all these reasons, warfarin is not recommended in the antenatal period.** However, warfarin can be initiated in the postpartum period and overlapped with heparin until the INR is maintained at 2.0–3.0.

Can a patient be anticoagulated with heparin if APTT is not available?

This is difficult. You will need to weigh the risks of not treating against the risks of treating. The only good thing about this situation is that the half-life of heparin is short (a few hours).

- If the diagnosis is uncertain and/or the risk to the patient is low, do not give heparin.

- If the diagnosis is likely and the patient is unwell, give 5000 units IV as a bolus and then subcutaneous heparin in small doses of 5000 units 12-hourly. Increase to 10 000 units twice daily over a few days.
- If the diagnosis is certain and the patient is severely ill, give 5000 units IV as a bolus and start an infusion at 500 units/hour. Use your clinical judgement and increase slowly over 6 hours to 1000–2000 units/hour. Switch to subcutaneous heparin as soon as possible and be aware of bleeding complications.

LMWH as described above is a good alternative.

Anticoagulant treatment of deep vein thrombosis and/or pulmonary embolism

Following IV unfractionated heparin given as resuscitation (as described above), provide a heparin infusion of 1000–2000 IU/hour, and adjust the dose to maintain the APTT at 1.5–2.5 times the patient's control. Repeat the APTT every 6 hours during the first 24 hours of therapy. Thereafter monitor the APTT daily unless it falls outside the therapeutic range.

Another option is to treat with an LMWH such as enoxaparin given subcutaneously. The drug is available in syringes of 40, 60, 80 and 100 mg. The dose should be based on the patient's pre-pregnancy weight and should be given 12-hourly. The dose will vary depending on the drug used, but for enoxaparin is 1 mg/kg 12 hourly (note this is a greater total dose than the non-pregnancy dose of 1.5 mg/kg/24 hours). If coagulation tests are available, the aim is to achieve an APTT of 1.5–2.5 times the pre-treatment level. If these tests are not available, careful monitoring for signs of overdose, which can cause haemorrhage, should be undertaken and the mother should be warned of the symptoms to be alert for.

The mother can then be discharged home when she has been taught how to administer the injections and dispose safely of the needles.

Anticoagulation following pulmonary embolism or DVT should be continued throughout pregnancy and for at least 3 months postpartum.

LMWH should be continued for the duration of the pregnancy, and for at least 3 months after delivery. An expert should be consulted about the use of prophylactic heparin during any further pregnancy.

On entering labour, the mother should not be given any further doses of LMWH. If an elective Caesarean section is planned, the mother should have the usual dose of LMWH on the night before surgery, but the morning dose should be omitted. After delivery, as long as there are no concerns about bleeding, enoxaparin should be restarted 4 hours after a vaginal delivery and 8 hours after a Caesarean section. A once daily regimen may be used, especially after 3 days when concerns about haemorrhage are much reduced.

Shocked patients with a pulmonary embolus should ideally be managed on an intensive-care or high-dependency unit (if available). These patients will ideally have arterial blood pressure and central venous pressure (CVP) monitoring. They will also receive haemodynamic support with adequate fluid management and inotropes, in order to ensure maximal right heart filling.

All women at high risk of DVT or pulmonary embolism (e.g. those who have suffered these conditions before, in this or a previous pregnancy) should use anti-embolism stockings and receive subcutaneous heparin until they are fully mobile.

2.5.1 Amniotic fluid embolism

Introduction

Amniotic fluid embolism occurs when a bolus of amniotic fluid is released into the maternal circulation during uterine contractions. It becomes trapped in the maternal pulmonary circulation and causes cardiorespiratory collapse and clotting problems with disseminated intravascular coagulation (DIC). It is very rare, and extremely difficult if not impossible to treat without high-level resources.

Clinical presentation

Amniotic fluid embolism usually presents late in the first stage of labour. It has also been reported during first-trimester surgical termination of pregnancy, second-trimester termination, after abdominal trauma and after amniocentesis.

The diagnosis is essentially clinical and by exclusion and treatment of other possible causes. Amniotic fluid embolism may occur during labour (70%), during Caesarean section (19%) or immediately postpartum (11%).

The major signs include the following:
- acute hypotension or cardiac arrest

- acute hypoxaemia (dyspnoea, cyanosis or respiratory arrest)
- coagulopathy (laboratory evidence of DIC or fibrinolysis or severe clinical haemorrhage) if the patient survives long enough for DIC to become established (more than 30 minutes)
- the absence of other causes or symptoms.

Diagnosis
- This is based on the clinical presentation.
- Chest X-ray may show pulmonary oedema, adult respiratory distress syndrome (ARDS), or right atrial enlargement and prominent pulmonary arteries.
- The ECG may show a tachycardia and right ventricular strain pattern.
- Clotting studies may show thrombocytopenia and elevated fibrin degradation products or D-dimers. The clotting and bleeding times are very prolonged.

Differential diagnosis
- **Pulmonary embolus:** infrequent during labour, often

accompanied by chest pain, without development of coagulopathy.

- **Air embolism:** may follow ruptured uterus, pressurised IV infusion or Caesarean section. The distinguishing feature in air embolism is pre-cordial water-wheel murmur. There is no coagulopathy.
- **Septic shock:** unlikely in the absence of evidence of preceding infection and pyrexia.
- **Anaphylactic shock:** there is no coagulopathy.
- **Eclampsia:** usually preceded or accompanied by hypertension and proteinuria.
- **Toxic reaction to anaesthetic or local anaesthetic agents:** there is no coagulopathy.
- **Acute left heart failure:** usually more insidious onset. There is no coagulopathy.
- **Cerebral haemorrhage:** no cyanosis or hypotension. There is no coagulopathy.
- **Massive obstetric haemorrhage:** the history may help. Beware concealed abruption. Uterine atony may be a feature of both. Hypoxaemia in massive obstetric haemorrhage is less pronounced than in amniotic fluid embolism.
- **Aspiration of gastric contents:** usually occurs in an unconscious patient, or during induction of or emergence from general anaesthesia. There is no coagulopathy.

Management

Management is supportive, and aims to correct hypoxaemia, shock and coagulopathy and its consequences.

- Give 100% inspired oxygen by face mask and reservoir.
- If the patient is unconscious (P or U on the AVPU scale), intubation and assisted ventilation (if available) are needed.
- High positive end-expiratory pressure (PEEP) should be avoided.
- Two large-bore cannulae (16G) IV should be sited.
- Urgently cross-match blood, ideally at least 6 units of group-specific blood with retrospective cross-matching (if available) should be ordered. Check clotting factors (or clotting time) and platelets. Blood needs to be sent for a full blood count, clotting, fibrinogen and fibrinogen degradation product (FDP) levels (if available) immediately, and frequent repeated estimations of haematological parameters are required (if available).

- Cardiac arrest is managed according to protocols (*see* Section 1.13).
- If the woman is in labour, immediate delivery is required, by Caesarean section (under general anaesthetic) if vaginal delivery is not imminent. In cardiac arrest, if a cardiac output cannot be restored immediately, cardiac massage and ventilation should continue and Caesarean section should be performed.
- Circulatory support depends on the causes of decreased cardiac output. The available haemodynamic data indicate that high left heart filling pressures, reflecting a failing left ventricle, are a feature of the condition. In patients who survive the initial haemodynamic collapse, there is a high risk of secondary pulmonary oedema (70%). Inotropic support, ideally guided by monitoring of the central venous pressure (CVP), may be life-saving.
- If massive obstetric haemorrhage occurs, large volumes of fresh blood and blood products may be required.
- Monitoring of cardiac filling pressures may help to prevent fluid overload and pulmonary oedema.
- Place an arterial line if possible.
- Correct coagulopathy with fresh blood, platelets, fresh-frozen plasma and cryoprecipitate (rich in fibrinogen) if available.
- Massive haemorrhage may be due not only to coagulopathy, but also to coexisting uterine atony. Oxytocic drugs will be needed. Uterine tamponade may reduce blood loss while the coagulopathy is corrected.
- Patients who survive are at high risk for heart failure, ARDS and DIC. If the patient is sustaining a cardiac arrest, there is a high risk of neurological injury. As in other cardiac arrests associated with pregnancy, delivery may improve the success of resuscitation.

Outcome

The outcome is poor, even when optimum treatment and monitoring is available, so it is important to exclude other possible and treatable causes of collapse, including anaphylaxis, pulmonary embolism, haemorrhage, sepsis, myocardial infarction, eclampsia, intracranial haemorrhage, hypoglycaemia and drug toxicity (e.g. magnesium, local anaesthetics).

The outcome depends on the facilities for cardiorespiratory support and the ability to manage the DIC with blood and blood products.

2.6 Complications that require hospital care

2.6.A Ovarian cysts in pregnancy

Ovarian cysts in pregnancy may cause abdominal pain due to torsion or rupture. Laparotomy is required if torsion of an ovarian cyst is suspected. If the findings at laparotomy

are suggestive of malignancy (i.e. solid areas in the tumour, growth extending outside the cyst wall), the specimen should be sent for immediate histological examination if available and the woman should be referred to a tertiary care centre for evaluation and management.

Corpus luteum cysts are common and normal in the first trimester. They should **not** be removed surgically, as the corpus luteum will disappear as pregnancy progresses.

Asymptomatic ovarian cysts

If, on ultrasound, the cyst is found to be more than 10 cm in diameter, observe by regular ultrasound examinations for growth or complications. If there is torsion this will produce pain and the cyst will need to be surgically removed.

Surgery will pose a significant risk of miscarriage and premature delivery. In the case of a torted cyst, the resulting

necrosis and infection will themselves place the women and fetus at risk of acute complications and therefore prompt intervention is unavoidable.

Malignancy is difficult to diagnose even where access to advanced imaging such as MRI is available, and therefore a decision to operate on the basis of suspected malignancy is not advised in low resource settings, unless the index of suspicion is very high. If this is considered then it should take in to account the gestation of the pregnancy, the risk of pregnancy loss/prematurity, and the treatment available to the mother following delivery.

If the cyst is less than 10 cm in diameter and remains so on ultrasound examination, it will usually regress on its own and does not require treatment.

2.6.B Reduced fetal movements, intrauterine death and stillbirth

> **BOX 2.6.B.1 Minimum standards**
> - Pinard's stethoscope.
> - Doppler device for fetal heart rate monitoring.
> - Ultrasound scan.
> - Misoprostol and oxytocin or ergometrine.
> - Fresh blood for transfusion.

General management

Check for fetal heart sounds, and if they are present, measure the fetal heart rate.

If the fetal heart cannot be detected with a Pinard's stethoscope, Doppler device or ultrasound scan, refer to Table 2.6.B.1 below.

Diagnosis

TABLE 2.6.B.1 Diagnosis of reduced fetal movements

Symptoms	Signs	Investigation	Diagnosis	Treatment
Decreased or absent fetal movements Bleeding (but may not be external) Collapse Severe constant abdominal pain	Shock in the mother Tense and/or tender uterus Fetal distress or absent fetal heart sounds	Pinard's stethoscope, Doppler device or ultrasound scan	Placental abruption	Deliver the baby as soon as possible (see below) by Caesarean section if there are signs of fetal life
Decreased or absent fetal movements Bleeding (but may not be external) Collapse Severe constant abdominal pain	Shock in the mother Diffuse uterine tenderness with easily felt fetal parts Fetal distress or absent fetal heart sounds	Pinard's stethoscope, Doppler device or ultrasound scan	Ruptured uterus Major risk factors are prolonged labour, previous Caesarean section and use of oxytocin	Treat shock When the mother is stable perform laparotomy
Decreased or absent fetal movements If membranes are ruptured, meconium staining of liquor	Abnormal fetal heart rate (< 100 beats/minute or > 180 beats/minute)	Pinard's stethoscope, Doppler device or ultrasound scan Partogram should show alerts	Fetal asphyxia	Deliver the baby as soon as possible (see below) by Caesarean section if there are signs of fetal life
Absent fetal movements	Symphysis-fundal height decreases Absent fetal heart rate If membranes are ruptured, meconium staining may be present	Pinard's stethoscope, Doppler device or ultrasound scan Full blood count in mother Clotting screen, including measurement of platelet count in mother	Fetal death	Deliver baby as soon as possible (see below)

Fetal death in the absence of an abruption

Fetal death *in utero* (IUFD) may be the result of fetal asphyxia from placental failure, fetal infection, cord accident or congenital anomalies. Where syphilis is prevalent, a large proportion of fetal deaths are due to this disease.

Fetal death can be confirmed by abdominal ultrasound with confidence if there is a lack of fetal heart activity.

If fetal death *in utero* is diagnosed, inform the woman or girl and her family and discuss the options for management with them.

Common causes are infection (especially malaria and chorioamniominitis), abruption, and placental insufficiency. In the case of intrapartum IUFD, fetal hypoxeamia, often, but not always, associated with a prolonged obstructed labour or malposition, may be to blame. In the laboring patient uterine rupture must also be considered.

The following investigations should be performed as a minimum: blood group and cross match, Hb, malaria RDT +/− malaria smear and urine analysis to assess for urinary infection and pre-eclampsia. Syphilis is also common in some settings and may cause IUFD and premature labour.

If a clotting test shows failure of a clot to form after 7 minutes, or a soft clot that breaks down easily, suspect coagulopathy. Obtain fresh blood for transfusion and give broad-spectrum IV antibiotics, including metronidazole.

Expectant management

Explain to the mother that in 90% of cases the fetus is spontaneously expelled within 1 month of diagnosis. However, most mothers and their families will request delivery as soon as possible.

In addition, expectant management carries with it the risk of infection and DIC both of which complicate management and risk the mother's life. If this approach is used, it should be possible to monitor the patient for complications and there should be access to prompt and comprehensive treatment if they occur.

If IUFD is diagnosed in a laboring women, then once she has been assessed and treated for potential causes as above the labour can be allowed to continue with the usual monitoring. It is important to actively assess for life-threatening causes such as abruption and rupture.

Active management

If there is no evidence of active labour and no indication for urgent delivery by Caesarean section, induction of labour with misoprostol is an effective way of inducing labour. As is the case for mid-trimester miscarriage, mifepristone, where available, can be helpful in shortening the length of time it takes for misoprostol to work. This is especially the case where there is no evidence of labour, the cervix is unfavourable and the patient is primiparous.

The following drug regime is recommended for women with an IUFD of 26 weeks' gestation or more (see below for women with a previous Caesarean section and Section 2.5.D.ii for management of miscarriage before 26 weeks' gestation):

- Mifepristone 200 mg orally stat (omit if not available). Wait for 36 to 48 hours after giving this drug – shorten if any clinical concerns arise during this interval
- misoprostol 50 micrograms orally or vaginally every 4 hours to a total of 5 doses
- if delivery has not occurred by the fifth dose of

misoprostol, the patient should be reviewed by a doctor. Subsequent options for management include continued use of misoprostol (usually after a period of 'rest' for 12 to 24 hours), or use of oxytocin.

For women with an IUFD at term (37 weeks and over) an alternative is to use the same induction of labour protocol as described previously (Section 2.3 'Managing labour and delivery), for women with a live fetus, i.e. 25 micrograms of misoprostol every 2 hours.

Note: The evidence base for the optimum dose of misoprostol to be used in this scenario is poor, and it is recognised that higher doses of 100 micrograms or more every 4 to 6 hours, have historically been used. Recent evidence *suggests* that lower doses *may* be as efficacious, and it is with this in mind, as well as concerns about optimising safety, that the above dose has been recommended. Further research is needed into the optimal regimen, especially in resource poor settings.

Women who have undergone a previous caesarean section

In women with a previous Caesarean section, previous uterine surgery, or in grandmultiparae, there is a risk of dehiscence/rupture in labour that is likely to be increased with the use of misoprostol, and therefore its use should be avoided. Vaginal delivery is still the preferred mode of delivery if the fetus is dead, but care must be taken to minimise the risk as much as possible.

If the cervix is favourable (Bishop score 6 or more) and ARM possible, then especially in women who have delivered previously, ARM alone will often result in delivery over the following 24 hours. If labour does not become established following ARM, then oxytocin can be titrated, using the usual protocol to augment/induce the labour.

If the cervix is unfavourable, then the oxytocin infusion may be started with intact membranes, and continued until the cervix becomes favourable for ARM (usually < 8 hours). Oxytocin use is associated with a lower risk of dehiscence/rupture than induction with misoprostol, but still increases the risk as compared with spontaneous labour. Close monitoring of the infusion, to prevent hyperstimulation, and of the patient for signs of any complication, is therefore essential.

Alternatively, the cervix can be 'ripened' with a Foley balloon catheter as previously described. ARM may then be performed, and oxytocin used as above if necessary.

Whichever method is used, all women with risk factors for rupture/dehiscence must be identified and monitored carefully with this complication in mind. Early recognition is the key to preventing maternal morbidity and mortality.

The membranes should be kept intact for as long as possible to prevent infection. However, they may be ruptured if it is necessary to achieve delivery. Vaginal assessments should be performed in a sterile manner and as infrequently as possible. If the membranes have been ruptured for more than 18 hours, treat the patient with prophylactic antibiotics (ampicillin 2 grams IV stat followed by 1 gram every 6 hours). If there are **signs of infection** (fever and/or foul-smelling vaginal discharge), give antibiotics as described for endometritis (*see* Section 2.5.G).

Oxytocin

Although misoprostol is recommended as the first-line induction agent in the case of IUFD where there are no risk factors for dehiscence/rupture, Oxytocin may be used if misoprostol is not available or proves ineffective. It may also be used where the risk of rupture is high (as discussed above), and a titratable and short-acting agent is therefore preferred.

In practice oxytocin is more effective following rupture of the membranes, although of course it is preferable to keep these intact as long as possible to avoid infection. As a minimum, rupturing the membranes before the cervix becomes favourable (Bishop score > 6), should be avoided.

Try not to use oxytocin within 8 hours of using misoprostol.

Avoid Caesarean section if possible, except for unavoidable obstetric reasons such as transverse lie, suspected uterine rupture or major abruption.

Fetal death in the presence of an abruption
Adopt the active management approach described above.

Stillbirth
Introduction
Between 2.08 and 3.79 million stillbirths occur each year worldwide. Of these, 98% occur in low- and middle-income countries and 55% occur in rural families in sub-Saharan Africa or South Asia where facilities for giving birth are much poorer than in urban areas (less skilled birth attendants and comprehensive emergency obstetric care). Around 45% of stillbirths occur during birth (intra-partum). The global average rate is 19 in 1000 births, the rate in low-resource settings is ≥ 25 in 1000 births, and the rate in well-resourced settings is < 5 in 1000 births.

Most stillbirths are not registered and the body is disposed of without any recognition or rituals such as naming, funeral services, or even the mother holding or dressing her baby. In some cultural settings there is a belief that sinning by the mother or evil spirits are responsible for the stillbirth, and the dead baby may be seen as a taboo object. Families affected may be subjected to stigma and marginalisation. Some healthcare workers believe that few stillbirths are preventable, and that these babies were just 'not meant to live'. There is considerable suffering involved for the family, and mothers frequently become depressed or anxious after a stillbirth, with similar emotions to those experienced after the death of a child.

Definitions of stillbirth
An early stillbirth is defined by the International Classification of Diseases as a birth weight of ≥ 500 grams or, if this measurement is missing, ≥ 22 completed weeks of gestation or, if this is missing, a body length of ≥ 25 cm.

The World Health Organization defines stillbirth as a birth weight of ≥ 1000 grams or, if this measurement is missing, ≥ 28 completed weeks of gestation or, if this is missing, a body length of ≥ 35 cm.

Causes of stillbirth
The major causes, which are the same as the causes of maternal and neonatal mortality, are as follows:

- complications of childbirth
- maternal infections in pregnancy (e.g. syphilis)
- medical disorders of pregnancy (especially pre-eclampsia or hypertension)
- maternal under-nutrition and fetal intrauterine growth retardation
- congenital abnormalities.

Prevention
The most important issues in low-resource situations are to increase the number of skilled birth attendants who can manage antenatal and intra-partum care, to increase the number of healthcare facility-based births, and to prevent or treat syphilis and malaria during pregnancy.

Specifically, the following ten interventions have been subjected to systematic review and reported to reduce stillbirth rates:

1. taking folic acid before and soon after conception
2. insecticide-treated bed nets or intermittent drug treatment to prevent malaria
3. detection and treatment of syphilis
4. detection and management of hypertensive disorders in pregnancy
5. detection and management of diabetes
6. detection and management of fetal growth restriction
7. routine induction to prevent post-term pregnancy
8. skilled care at birth
9. basic emergency obstetric care
10. comprehensive emergency obstetric care.

The main aim is to strengthen the healthcare systems involved in antepartum and intra-partum care, which include in addition to the ten items listed above:

- prevention of malaria (see Section 2.8.D) and syphilis (see Section 2.8.H) in endemic areas
- the availability of emergency obstetric surgery, in particular Caesarean section, without delay and with attention to 'task shifting' to improve access, especially in rural areas
- improved antenatal care
- advocacy to address poverty and its consequences (stillbirth rates are inversely correlated with wealth and development)
- systems to manage and prevent domestic violence
- efforts to achieve sexual equality, improve reproductive health and improve the secondary education of boys and girls.

Ideally, bereaved families should form groups that advocate for change at all of the levels identified above.

Further reading
The Lancet Stillbirths series, launched in London, New York, Hobart, Geneva, New Delhi, Florence, and Cape Town on 14 April 2011. www.thelancet.com/series/stillbirth

2.6.C Fetal distress during labour

> **BOX 2.6.C.1 Minimum standards**
> Pinard's stethoscope
> Hand-held battery-operated ultrasonic fetal heart rate monitor

Introduction

In all clinical circumstances, the well-being of the pregnant woman takes precedence over that of the unborn baby, and there are often situations where resuscitation of the mother will automatically bring about benefits for the fetus.

Careful thought has to be given to the assessment and management of the fetal condition in labour. This is especially so in resource-limited countries, where severe shortages of both equipment and suitably trained personnel often mean that women do not receive the life-saving care which they require in labour.

In such situations, strict prioritisation of needs is required, and fetal well-being has to take second place to maternal survival.

When considering taking steps to monitor fetal well-being, the following factors must be taken into account:

1. the cost of monitoring equipment, including maintenance, and replacement of disposable items
2. the cost of training staff in the use of such equipment
3. the proportion of caregivers' time required to be allocated to assessment of fetal well-being
4. the availability of suitable interventions, should fetal distress be diagnosed
5. the potential risks to the mother of an intervention for the sake of fetal well-being
6. the availability of neonatal care facilities and expertise, following on from an intervention to deliver a distressed and possibly premature baby.

Methods of monitoring fetal well-being in labour range from the low-cost low-technology Pinard's stethoscope to the relatively expensive high-technology cardiotocograph.

Pinard's stethoscope

The Pinard's stethoscope is cheap, portable and resilient, and requires no electricity or battery. It is used to listen to the fetal heart through the maternal abdomen for 60 seconds immediately following a contraction. It should be recorded every 60 minutes in the latent phase of labour, every 15–30 minutes in the active phase of the first stage of labour, every 5 minutes in the second stage, and after every contraction when the woman is pushing in the second stage.

A healthy fetus will withstand the relative hypoxia brought about by the compression of the blood vessels in the placenta during a uterine contraction.

A simple ultrasound Doppler monitor (e.g. a Sonicaid) can be used instead of a Pinard's stethoscope, but it does require batteries.

Fetal heart rate monitoring by Pinard's/Sonicaid: normal ranges and abnormalities

It should be noted that evidence and guidance is lacking on the use of intermittent fetal monitoring in settings without access to continuous electronic fetal monitoring (CEFM).

Where CEFM is available any abnormality detected by intermittent monitoring results in the mother being transferred on to CEFM. Where this is not possible, it is even more difficult to determine whether fetal distress is present.

In addition, without the ability to perform fetal blood sampling (below), it is not possible to confirm whether the fetus is distressed before delivery, or to determine the degree of distress likely. It should be noted that approximately 50% of babies with pathological electronic fetal heart rate tracings are not in fact distressed.

The impact of intermittent fetal monitoring on Caesarean section rates and neonatal morbidity and mortality, in this context, is therefore unknown. Decisions on whether to pursue Caesarean section with its inherent risks for the current and future pregnancies, is extremely difficult in this context, where information on the fetal condition is so incomplete.

The normal fetal heart rate

Baseline: The baseline is the rate that is returned to after any episodes of variation such as an acceleration or a deceleration. In simple terms it is the most common heart rate for that baby.

When listening with a Pinard's this may be the rate over the first minute of listening. However, if part of the minute includes a period of more rapid heartbeat (an acceleration), or slower heart beat (deceleration) then it may be higher or lower than the baseline.

Therefore, if when listening, the fetal heart can be heard to be very slow or very fast for part or all of the period, auscultating this may not be the baseline and it will be necessary to continue listening over a longer period to gain more information.

The normal range for the baseline is between 120 and 160 bpm. A rate of 110 to 120 bpm is often also a normal finding, especially in babies at term or post term. A rate of 160 to 170 can also be a normal finding in a premature baby. A rate below 110 and above 170 is always considered to be abnormal.

Variability: It is normal for the fetal heart rate to vary with every beat. This variation occurs continually above and below the baseline and is usually by approximately 5 to 15 bpm from the lowest to the highest reading (although normal variation is up to 25 bpm). Variation is not easily detected by the Pinard's stethoscope as monitoring involves counting for 1 minute and it is therefore the average heart rate over that time that is obtained. With a Sonicaid, however, the fetal heart rate is often displayed and it can be seen to vary around a certain level (the baseline).

Variability is a positive sign, and generally suggests that the fetus is coping well with labour.

Accelerations: These are episodes where the fetal heart rate increases by 15 beats or more above the baseline and for more than 15 seconds. They can be heard on a Pinard's with practice, although they are easier to hear the higher and longer they are. They are easier to see on a Sonicaid, where the number displayed can be seen to increase over a period before falling back to its more usual level.

Accelerations are a positive sign as they represent fetal movement. If the fetus is distressed it will not move and the accelerations will stop. Although it is reassuring when they are present, accelerations are often not present during labour.

Abnormalities of the fetal heart rate

Tachycardia: This is a fetal heart rate above 160–170 bpm.

A tachycardia is often caused by a maternal pyrexia or tachycardia and in these instances it will often resolve once the maternal observations have normalised.

Decelerations: A deceleration is a reduction in the fetal heart rate 15 bpm or more below the base line for 15 seconds or more.

An early deceleration occurs at the onset of the contraction and recovers by the end of the contraction. It is a common feature during labour (especially the second stage) and is not usually associated with fetal distress, and therefore it is not routine to listen to the fetal heart rate during a contraction.

A late deceleration starts during or at the end of a contraction and persists beyond the end of the contraction. This is more commonly associated with fetal distress and if it occurs the fetal heart should be monitored following the next 2 contractions to see if it recurs. If it does, there is a significant chance that the fetus is distressed.

Bradycardia: A bradycardia is a deceleration that continues for over 3 minutes. It may occur during pregnancy or labour and may be associated with inferior veno-caval compression if the patient is lying supine, sudden drops in blood pressure from any cause or cord compression.

It may also represent the end stage of a prolonged period of fetal distress. If the cause of the bradycardia is self-limiting, then the fetal heart should recover, whereas if it has occurred due to period of prolonged distress or the insult is ongoing, it will not recover and will end in fetal death. Even if it resolves, a bradycardia of over 10 minutes may cause brain damage to the fetus and have implications for the neonate.

Cardiotocograph

The cardiotocograph is a relatively expensive, sophisticated but non-invasive item of equipment that requires expertise in its use and in its interpretation, as well as regular maintenance, and ongoing provision of disposables, such as print-out paper. It also requires a power supply (either mains electricity or batteries).

It has a high sensitivity for detecting possible evidence of fetal distress, but a relatively low specificity, such that an additional method of assessment of fetal well-being, usually scalp pH assessment, is required in order to avoid excessive intervention.

If a cardiotocograph is used in the absence of fetal blood sampling, there are certain fetal heart rate patterns which are very likely to be associated with serious fetal distress and that warrant urgent actions to protect the fetus, usually immediate delivery.

Fetal scalp pH assessment

This is achieved by fetal scalp blood sampling, which is carried out with the woman in the lithotomy position with a wedge to prevent aorto-caval compression or in the left lateral position.

A speculum is inserted in the vagina, the fetal scalp is visualised with the aid of a light source, and a blood sample is obtained using a lancet and a capillary tube.

A blood gas analyser (an extremely expensive item of equipment) is required for assessment of the sample.

Fetal blood gas analysis

This is used to detect fetal acidosis, which is a consequence of hypoxia.

A capillary sample is assessed for pH and base excess. Generally, a pH of ≥ 7.25 is considered to be normal, but it has to be borne in mind that acidosis may develop rapidly, and the sample therefore needs to be repeated if the CTG abnormality persists. A full guide to the interpretation and use of fetal blood gas analysis is not included here as it is not a technique available in the majority of resource poor settings.

Fetal blood sampling is contraindicated if the mother is infected with HIV or in high prevalence areas in the untested patient.

Clinical assessment of fetal well-being

A large amount of information may be gained by clinical assessment as follows.

History

- Gestational age is important, as an immature fetus withstands the stresses of labour less well than if it had reached term. Similarly, those with intrauterine growth retardation are at risk.
- A reduction in fetal movements should always give rise to concern, as it may reflect fetal distress (*see Section 2.6.B*).
- Pre-eclampsia, antepartum haemorrhage (APH), preterm pre-labour rupture of membranes (PPROM) or other obstetric or medical problems, prolonged pregnancy, multiple pregnancy, diabetes and previous Caesarean section all increase the risk of fetal distress.
- The use of oxytocin, a maternal fever, meconium- or bloodstained liquor, and prolonged first and second stage of labour also increase the risk.
- The duration of labour at the time of admission is crucial, as obstructed labour is a potent cause of severe maternal and fetal morbidity and mortality.

Examination of the maternal abdomen

- **Fetal size:** small or large for dates.
- **Amniotic fluid volume:** oligohydramnios (too little) or polyhydramnios (too much).
  - Oligohydramnios is often associated with poor fetal growth. Growth-restricted fetuses are more likely to become distressed in labour than are well-grown fetuses.
  - Polyhydramnios may be associated with fetal abnormalities or fetal infection *in utero*.
- **Abdominal tenderness with or without hardness feeling like wood:** consider placental abruption.
- **Colour of amniotic fluid after rupture of membranes:**
  - bloodstained: consider placental abruption

- meconium-stained: consider the possibility of a hypoxic episode causing fetal distress.
  (a) Passage of meconium is often a physiological (normal) phenomenon in a mature fetus.
  (b) In the presence of plentiful amniotic fluid, the meconium will be dilute. Where there is little fluid, it will be thick.
  (c) Meconium may signal fetal distress. It may also trigger neonatal respiratory problems through meconium aspiration, which occurs when a distressed fetus gasps *in utero* or during delivery.
  (d) During the final stages of a breech delivery, meconium may be passed because of the compression of the fetal abdomen. In this case, passage of meconium is not necessarily a sign of fetal distress.
- **Frank blood loss vaginally:** consider placental abruption, uterine rupture, placenta praevia and vasa praevia.
- **Haematuria in labour:** this may signal uterine rupture, usually in association with severe abdominal pain and tenderness, commonly in a woman with a previous Caesarean section scar or in a woman of high parity, particularly where labour is induced or augmented.

Management of fetal distress

- If fetal distress is suspected, attention should first be paid to detecting and treating maternal factors, including hypovolaemia, sepsis, obstructed labour and uterine rupture.

- The woman should be turned (tilted) on her left side or placed in the recovery position, to prevent aorto-caval compression.
- Facial oxygen should be administered at a high flow rate.
- Oxytocin should be discontinued if ongoing, and if still detected *in situ*, misoprostol tablets may be removed from the vagina.
- Antibiotic therapy will be indicated if infection (including chorio-amnionitis) is suspected.
- Vaginal examination should be performed to assess the feasibility of vaginal delivery, either spontaneously or by using forceps or ventouse.
- If suspected fetal distress continues despite the above measures and vaginal delivery is not rapidly achievable then a decision about whether to proceed to Caesarean section needs to be made. This is a difficult decision, which ideally takes into consideration a number of factors including: the obstetric history and wishes of the patient, the availability of neonatal care, the degree of fetal compromise suspected and the speed with which Caesarean section can be performed, the availability of hospital care and Caesarean section in subsequent deliveries, and the presence/absence of other relative indications for Caesarean section.
- If a decision is made to deliver by Caesarean section and a delay is anticipated (> 30 minutes), then a tocolytic such as terbutaline 250 microgram s/c may be beneficial if the contractions are felt to be contributing to the fetal distress.

2.6.D Multiple births

Introduction

Twins occur in around 1 in 80 pregnancies. Non-identical twin rates vary depending on age, parity and racial background; in Africa, rates are higher than the world average. The incidence of monozygous (identical) twins is relatively constant worldwide, at 3.5 in 1000 births.

Multiple pregnancies are associated with higher risks for both the mother and the fetus. Ultrasound scanning should be undertaken if the uterine size is larger than expected, or if abdominal examination of fetal parts leads to suspicion of multiple fetuses.

If ultrasound scanning facilities are not available, abdominal examination after delivery of any first baby should be performed to **exclude a second twin before oxytocin or Syntometrine is given to aid delivery of the placenta.**

Maternal risks associated with multiple pregnancy

These include the following:
- miscarriage
- anaemia
- preterm labour
- hypertension
- polyhydramnios
- operative delivery
- postpartum haemorrhage.

Fetal risks associated with multiple pregnancy

These include the following:
- stillbirth or neonatal death
- preterm delivery
- intrauterine growth restriction
- congenital abnormalities
- cord accident
- specific complications of twin pregnancies (e.g. twin-to-twin transfusion syndrome)
- difficulties with delivery.

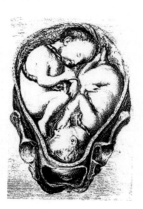

FIGURE 2.6.D.1 Twin pregnancy.

If a twin pregnancy is diagnosed, additional care should be provided. Iron and folate treatment must be ensured, due to the increased risk of anaemia. Preterm labour and delivery present the greatest risk of fetal illness and death. If the mother develops premature labour, a course of antenatal steroid injections should be given, betamethasone 12 mg IM, two doses 24 hours apart, *or* dexamethasone 6 mg IM four doses 12 hours apart.

Presentation of twins

- In 40% of cases both twins are cephalic.
- In 21% the second twin is a breech.
- In 14% the first twin is a breech.
- In 10% of cases both twins are breeches.
- In all remaining cases, one twin or the other, or occasionally both, are transverse.

In Figure 2.6.D.2, the first twin is the lower one.

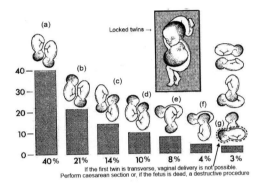

FIGURE 2.6.D.2 The range of different twin positions *in utero* at birth.

Antenatal monitoring in multiple pregnancy

- A 2-weekly check-up (urine for protein if blood pressure is elevated, ultrasound if possible) is recommended from 28 to 36 weeks; warn the woman about the risk of preterm delivery.
- Iron and folate treatment must be ensured as increased risk of anaemia is present.
- A weekly check-up is recommended from 37 weeks.
- Be alert for signs of pre-eclampsia and premature labour.

Twin delivery

Vaginal delivery is usually safe, but must be undertaken in a healthcare facility where comprehensive emergency obstetric care is available. If labour has not started by 39–40 weeks' gestation based on an accurate LMP or first trimester ultrasound, consider induction.

Summary of management during labour

Delivery of first twin

1. Insert an IV cannula. Maternal blood should be obtained for a full blood count and blood grouping. A blood sample should be kept for cross-matching.
2. Ensure that the lie of the first baby is longitudinal.
3. Augment contractions only when indicated.
4. Prepare two delivery packs with extra clamps. Remember that there are almost always two membranes to rupture with twins, so have an amniohook ready.

5. Make sure that the cervix is fully dilated.
6. Empty the mother's bladder.
7. Deliver the first baby as normal.
8. **Always clamp the maternal end of the cord of the first twin to prevent the second twin bleeding from it.**
9. As the first baby is delivered, stabilise the lie of the second twin to a longitudinal position by asking an assistant to place their palms firmly on either side of the uterus in a longitudinal direction. The baby's position should be stabilised in this way until the head or buttocks are fixed in the maternal pelvis. If the second twin is not longitudinal on assessment, undertake version (see below).
10. Tie a marker (e.g. gauze) to the clamp on the cord of the first baby to identify it.

Delivery of second twin

1. The second baby should preferably be born within 30 minutes.
2. Check the fetal heart rate of the second baby.
3. Stabilise the lie of the second twin, by external version if necessary (see above).
4. Provided the lie is longitudinal and contractions do not restart 5–10 minutes after delivery of the first baby, start an oxytocin infusion, increasing carefully to achieve adequate contractions. Note that contractions may not be felt by the mother, so it is important to keep your hand on the uterus to identify them.
5. When the presenting part is well into the pelvis, rupture of the membranes can be performed during a uterine contraction.
6. Delivery of the second baby should not be rushed, but assisted delivery should be considered if the second baby has not been delivered by 30 minutes after delivery of the first.
7. If the lie of the second twin is transverse, attempt external version.
8. If external version is successful, or the second twin is longitudinal, wait for the presenting part to enter the pelvis, then perform artificial rupture of membranes (ARM) and allow normal cephalic or breech delivery if there is no fetal distress.
9. If external cephalic version is unsuccessful, either carry out internal version with breech extraction or perform a Caesarean section.

    Internal podalic version: It is essential that as the baby descends, rotation of the fetus is encouraged to obtain a back-up (back anterior) position (as in breech delivery). Make sure that it is a foot, not a hand. Pull gently down into the birth canal so that the fetal back is encouraged to turn anteriorly. An attempt is made to pull the fetal foot as gently as possible in an attempt to pull it as low as the vulva before the membranes rupture. It may be that maternal effort will be sufficient once the baby's leg has been brought down into the vagina and the remainder of the delivery can then be managed as for an assisted breech delivery. Continued traction (avoiding soft tissues as for all breech deliveries) is permissible in this scenario, to facilitate descent of the buttocks, arm and head (breech extraction, *see* Figure 2.6.D.3).

10. If there is fetal distress or delay, perform an assisted vaginal delivery if cephalic. Note that cephalo-pelvic

disproportion is very uncommon in the case of the second twin.

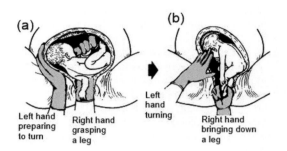

FIGURE 2.6.D.3 Internal version for transverse lie in a second twin.

Postpartum management of a twin birth

1 After the birth of the second baby, give 10 IU oxytocin IM after ensuring that there is no third baby in the uterus. Then give oxytocin 40 units IV in 500 mL of Ringer-lactate or Hartmann's solution over 4 hours, to reduce the risks of postpartum haemorrhage due to atonic uterus.

2 Deliver the placenta by controlled cord traction after giving oxytocin IM.

3 After the placenta and membranes have been delivered, examine and record on the chart the number of placentas, amnions, chorions and cord vessels. Check the placenta and membranes for completeness.

4 Check and repair any vaginal and perineal damage.

5 Monitor the mother carefully for postpartum bleeding over the next few hours.

6 Provide extra support to assist with the care of the babies.

7 At least a 24-hour stay in hospital is required.

8 Observe vaginal bleeding closely, because of the risk of postpartum haemorrhage.

Hooking or locking of heads

This is a rare complication during vaginal delivery.

Women may present with locked twins with the first trunk partially delivered. The head of the second twin will have entered the maternal pelvis, and needs to be pushed upwards to allow descent of the head of the first twin. If the first baby is already dead, it can be delivered by decapitation. After delivery of the body, the head is dis-impacted and the second twin is delivered. Finally, the first head is delivered with a vulsellum.

If the first baby is still alive (e.g. if the delivery is taking place in hospital), or if despite decapitation of the first baby the second one cannot be delivered, proceed immediately to Caesarean section if this is safe for the mother.

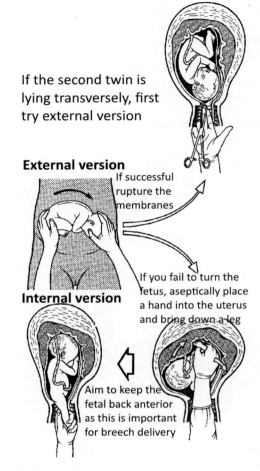

If the second twin is lying transversely, first try external version

External version

If successful rupture the membranes

Internal version

If you fail to turn the fetus, aseptically place a hand into the uterus and bring down a leg

Aim to keep the fetal back anterior as this is important for breech delivery

FIGURE 2.6.D.4 Transverse lie in a second twin, ensuring the correct foot is pulled so that the fetal back becomes anterior in the birth canal.

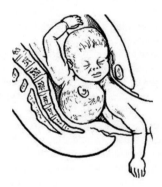

FIGURE 2.6.D.5 Locked twins.

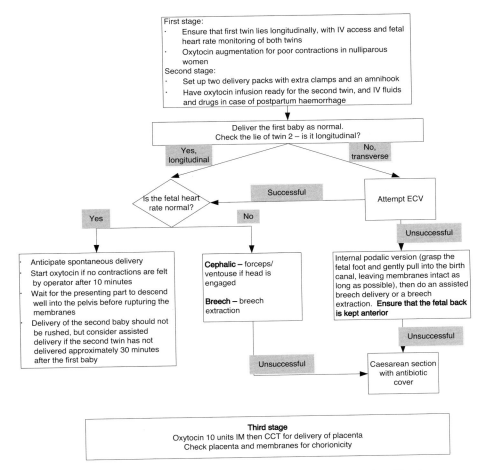

FIGURE 2.6.D.6 Pathway of care for delivery of twins. ECV, external cephalic version; CCT, controlled cord traction.

2.6.E Malpresentations and malpositions including breech delivery

Introduction

Malpresentations and malpositions can be due to maternal pathology (e.g. contracted pelvis, uterine fibroids) or fetal pathology (e.g. hydrocephalus), which ideally should be diagnosed antenatally. Most often there is no apparent cause.

Malpresentations are all presentations of the fetus other than a vertex presentation (e.g. face presentation, breech presentation).

Malpositions are abnormal positions of the vertex of the fetal head (with the occiput as the reference point) relative to the maternal pelvis.

A fetus in an abnormal position or presentation may result in prolonged or obstructed labour.

Management

Review the progress of labour using a partograph (*see* Section 2.2). Observe the mother closely. Malpresentations increase the risk of uterine rupture because of the potential for obstructed labour.

Note: Observe the mother closely. Malpresentations increase the risk of uterine rupture because of the potential for obstructed labour.

Assessment of the fetal position
Determining the presenting part

The most common presentation is the vertex of the fetal head.

If **the vertex is the presenting part**, use landmarks of the fetal skull to determine the position of the fetal head (*see* Figure 2.6.E.1). However, although the anterior fontanelle is larger than the posterior one and has four sutures leading from it, one of these is small and may be difficult to feel.

Determining the position of the fetal head

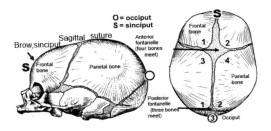

FIGURE 2.6.E.1 The fetal skull.

The fetal head normally engages in the maternal pelvis in an occiput transverse position.

With descent, the fetal head rotates so that the fetal occiput is anterior in the maternal pelvis (*see* Table 2.6.E.1). Failure of an occiput to rotate to an occiput anterior position results in a persistent transverse presentation. Rotation may also occur to an occiput posterior position.

An additional feature of a normal presentation is a well-flexed vertex (*see* Figure 2.6.E.2), with the fetal occiput lower in the vagina than the sinciput.

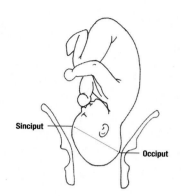

FIGURE 2.6.E.2 Well-flexed vertex presentation.

TABLE 2.6.E.1 Diagnostic features of malpositions and malpresentations

Position	Observations	Picture from introitus
Malpositions		
Occiput anterior	**On vaginal examination provided that the head is flexed** only the posterior fontanelle with three sutures entering it is felt	**Occiput anterior** **Left occiput anterior** **Right occiput anterior**
Occiput posterior	On **vaginal examination**, the posterior fontanelle is towards the sacrum and the anterior fontanelle may be easily felt if the head is deflexed On abdominal examination the lower part of the abdomen is flattened, and the fetal limbs are palpable anteriorly	**Occiput posterior** **Left occiput posterior**
Malpresentations		
Brow presentation is caused by partial extension of the fetal head so that the occiput is higher than the sinciput	On **abdominal examination**, more than half of the fetal head is above the symphysis pubis, and the occiput is palpable at a higher level than the sinciput On **vaginal examination**, the anterior fontanelle and the orbits are felt	

Position	Observations	Picture from introitus
Face presentation is caused by hyper-extension of the fetal head so that neither the occiput nor the sinciput are palpable on vaginal examination	On **abdominal examination**, a large amount of head is palpable on the same side as the back, without a cephalic prominence on the same side as the limbs On **vaginal examination**, the face is palpated, the examiner's finger enters the mouth easily and the bony jaws are felt	
Compound presentation occurs when an arm prolapses alongside the presenting part	Both the prolapsed arm and the fetal head present in the pelvis simultaneously	
Transverse lie and shoulder presentation	The fetus lies in the transverse position with usually the shoulder presenting On **abdominal examination**, neither the head nor the buttocks can be felt at the symphysis, and the head is usually in the flank On **vaginal examination**, a shoulder may sometimes be felt. An arm may prolapse and the elbow, arm or hand may be felt in the vagina	
Breech presentation occurs when the buttocks and/or the feet are the presenting parts	On **abdominal examination**, the head is felt in the upper abdomen and the breech in the pelvic brim. Auscultation locates the fetal heart higher than expected with a vertex presentation On **vaginal examination during labour**, the buttocks and/or feet are felt; thick, dark meconium is normal	**extended legs** **flexed legs** **footing** **a single footing presentation**

Malpositions of the fetal head

As the baby's head extends (deflexes), the diameter that has to pass through the mother's birth canal gets larger, until the baby becomes a brow presentation (14 cm). Then it gets smaller as the baby becomes a face presentation (see Figure 2.6.E.3).

Labour gets more difficult as the head extends, with brow and mento-posterior face presentations being impossible to deliver vaginally unless the baby is particularly small in relation to the mother's pelvis.

A face presentation is easier to deliver than a brow presentation. This is because the head has now become fully deflexed.

The vertex presentations in Figure 2.6.E.3 show the diameters of the skull. When the head is well flexed (a), the shortest diameter of the skull is entering the mother's pelvis.

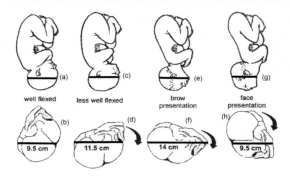

FIGURE 2.6.E.3 (a), (c), (e) and (g) are all vertex presentations. The only normal one is the well-flexed head (a). As (a) turns through to become (g), the baby's head becomes more and more extended (deflexed).

In a brow presentation (e), which is the most difficult type, the longest diameter is trying to enter it.

Management of malpositions
Occiput-posterior positions

Around 15–20% of term cephalic fetuses are in an occiput-posterior (OP) position before labour, and approximately 5% are OP at delivery. Most fetuses (around 90%) rotate to the occiput-anterior (OA) position, some maintain a persistent OP position, and others rotate from an OA to an OP position during labour and delivery.

Arrested labour may occur when the head does not rotate and/or descend. Delivery may be complicated by perineal tears or extension of an episiotomy because an instrumental delivery is performed or because a persistent OP presentation requires passage of a greater diameter. The newborn infant is more likely to need resuscitation.

Diagnosis of an OP position in the second stage is generally made by digital examination, but if there is uncertainty, ultrasound examination is both useful and accurate in the right hands.

Management
There is no effective method of facilitating rotation from OP to OA before labour begins.

First stage of labour
Manual rotation (see below) must not be attempted in the first stage of labour, as it can lead to a prolapsed cord or complex presentations (e.g. hand). It is also technically more difficult and may introduce infection.

1 If there are signs of obstruction or the fetal heart rate or pattern is abnormal (< 110 beats/minute or > 160 beats/minute, or abnormal dips) at any stage, deliver by Caesarean section if this can be safely undertaken.
2 If the membranes are intact, rupture them.
3 If there are no signs of obstruction, augment labour with oxytocin.

Second stage of labour
If the cervix is fully dilated:

● If the fetal head is more than 3/5 palpable above the symphysis pubis, or the leading bony edge of the head is above –2 station and there is fetal distress and/failure to descend, perform a Caesarean section.

● If the fetal head is less than 3/5 above the symphysis pubis, or the leading bony edge of the head is between 0 station and –2 station, try manual rotation (see below) if there is no clear progress in the second stage with an OP position after 30 minutes of pushing.

However, expectant management of the OP position is appropriate in the presence of a reassuring fetal heart rate, adequate space on clinical examination of the pelvis, and continued progress in the second stage. More than 50% of multiparous women and more than 25% of nulliparous women with persistently OP fetuses achieve spontaneous vaginal delivery.

Therefore it is not appropriate to routinely perform prophylactic rotation at the beginning of the second stage of labour.

Delivery from an OP position rather than rotation (see below) is more appropriate in women who, on clinical examination, are found to have ample room between the fetal occiput and the maternal sacrum/coccyx, and when the pelvis is too narrow to permit anterior rotation (women with an anthropoid pelvis with a narrow transverse diameter, and women with an android pelvis with a narrow arch).

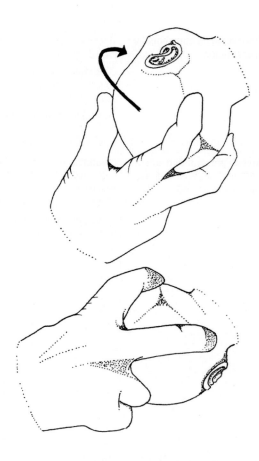

FIGURE 2.6.E.4 Finger rotation of occiput posterior to occiput anterior position. Reproduced with permission from Argani CH, Satin A. Management of the fetus in occiput posterior position. In: UpToDate, Post TW (ed.), UpToDate, Waltham, MA (accessed 5/8/14). © 2014 UpToDate, Inc. For more information visit www. uptodate.com.

Manual rotation

Successful rotation after the onset of the second stage of labour is more likely to be successful if it is performed before arrest occurs. Manual rotation can convert 90% of OP or transverse arrest situations to OA.

Manual rotation is more successful in multiparous women and young women.

Rotation is important if there is a need for a fast delivery and/or if there is minimal or slow descent after a trial of pushing.

First empty the bladder.

There are two methods for rotating the fetus.

1 A hand is inserted into the vagina with the palm upward. Digital rotation is performed by placing the tips of the index and middle fingers in the anterior segment of the lambdoid suture near the posterior fontanelle (see Figure 2.6.E.4).

The fingers are used to flex and slightly dislodge the vertex, rotating the fetal head to the OA position by rotation of the operator's hand and forearm. The thumb may also be used with gentle downward pressure more anteriorly on the parietal bone to aid this rotation. The fetal head should be held in place for a few contractions to prevent rotation back towards the posterior position.

2 The operator's four fingers are placed behind the posterior parietal bone with the palm up and the thumb over the anterior parietal bone. The right hand is used for the left OP position, and the left hand is used for the right OP position. The head is grasped with the tips of the fingers and thumb. During a contraction, the patient is encouraged to push and the operator attempts to flex and rotate the fetal head anteriorly. Occasional mild upward pressure may help to slightly displace the head and facilitate rotation (see Figure 2.6.E.5).

If rapid delivery is indicated, failed manual rotation may be followed by vacuum delivery from the OP position. Manual rotation performed prior to instrumental birth is associated with little or no increase in risk to the pregnant woman or to the fetus.

Ventouse or forceps delivery should never be attempted above 0 station or if the head is more than 1/5 above the symphysis pubis.

Delivery of a brow presentation (see Table 2.6.E.1)

In brow presentation, engagement is usually impossible, and arrested labour is common. Spontaneous conversion to either vertex presentation or face presentation can rarely occur, particularly when the fetus is small or when there is fetal death with maceration. It is unusual for spontaneous conversion to occur with an average-sized live fetus once the membranes have ruptured.

If the fetus is alive, deliver by Caesarean section if this can safely be undertaken.

If the fetus is dead and:

• the cervix is not fully dilated, deliver by Caesarean section

• the cervix is fully dilated, deliver after craniotomy.

If the operator is not proficient in craniotomy, deliver by Caesarean section.

Only if the fetus is small or very low in the vagina, a brow presentation might be delivered by vacuum extraction, forceps delivery or symphysiotomy.

Delivery of a face presentation (see Table 2.6.E.1)

Background

This presentation occurs in 1 in 500–1000 pregnancies. It is due to extension of the fetal neck, caused by either a fetal abnormality or progression from a deflexed occipito-posterior position in labour. Diagnosis is important, as a face presentation may be mistaken for breech presentation.

Diagnosis

Face presentation may be detected on ultrasound scan before labour, but the majority of cases are unpredictable because they arise in labour.

On abdominal examination, a large amount of head is palpable on the same side as the back, without a cephalic prominence on the same side as the limbs.

On vaginal examination, in early labour the presenting part is high. Landmarks are the mouth, jaws, nose, and malar and orbital ridges. The presence of bony gums (alveolar margins) distinguishes the mouth from the anus. The mouth and the zygoma ridges of the maxillae (upper jawbone) form the corners of a triangle, whereas the anus is on a straight line between the ischial tuberosities.

FIGURE 2.6.E.5 Manual rotation of occiput posterior to occiput anterior position. **Manual rotation of occiput posterior to occiput anterior position.** Reproduced with permission from Argani CH, Satin A. Management of the fetus in occiput posterior position. In: UpToDate, Post TW (ed.), UpToDate, Waltham, MA (accessed 5/8/14). © 2014 UpToDate, Inc. For more information visit www.uptodate.com.

Avoid damaging the eyes with trauma or use of antiseptics.

Ventouse must not be used.

In early labour, particularly with the occipito-posterior position and a multiparous patient, deflexion is common. In such cases, uterine contractions often cause increased flexion, and delivery will proceed as normal. However, if extension occurs, a brow presentation and finally the fully extended face will result. Most face presentations therefore only become obvious late in labour.

Descent is usually followed by internal rotation with the chin passing anteriorly. If the chin is towards the pubis (mento-anterior), the baby can often be delivered normally, although an episiotomy is usually necessary. If the chin lies towards the back, delivery will not occur and a Caesarean section will be required.

The widest biparietal diameter is 7 cm behind the advancing face, so even when the face is distending the vulva, the biparietal diameter has only just entered the pelvis. Descent is less advanced than vaginal examination suggests, even allowing for gross oedema. The head is always higher than you think.

Abdominal examination is vital.

The head is born by flexion, causing considerable perineal distension in the process and risking considerable perineal trauma, so **consider an episiotomy.** Anterior rotation having occurred, the neck comes to lie behind the symphysis pubis and the head is born by flexion. The shoulders and body are born in the usual way.

With satisfactory uterine action and the mento-anterior (MA) position, spontaneous delivery or easy 'lift-out' (forceps-only) assisted delivery will ensue in 60–90% of cases (*see* Figure 2.6.E.6).

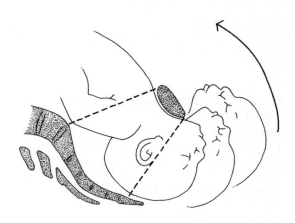

FIGURE 2.6.E.6 Mento-anterior position.

If spontaneous delivery of an MA face does not occur, a 'lift-out' forceps delivery can be performed (*see* Section 2.13 on forceps delivery).

In mento-posterior (MP) positions (*see* Figure 2.6.E.7), the neck is too short to span the 12 cm of the anterior aspect of the sacrum. In addition, the neck would have to be extended to pass under the symphysis, but it is already maximally extended. Delivery is impossible unless a very small fetus or one that is macerated allows the shoulders to enter the pelvis at the same time as the head.

Even with MP positions, anterior rotation will occur in the second stage in 45–65% of cases, so a persistent MP

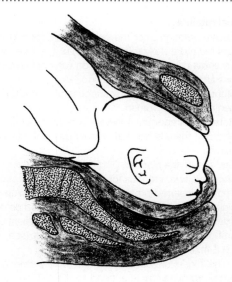

FIGURE 2.6.E.7 Mento-posterior position. Reproduced with permission from Macdonald S, Magill-Cuerden J (ed.) *Mayes' Midwifery: a textbook for midwives.* Elsevier Health Sciences; 2010. © Elsevier

position or mento-transverse arrest is encountered in only 10% of face presentations.

Persistent MP positions are usually delivered by Caesarean section (if this is possible and safe), in order to reduce fetal and maternal morbidity.

After birth, the oedema and bruising of the child's face may persist for some days, and may make feeding difficult.

Vaginal manipulation of persistent MP position has been successfully achieved with ultrasound guidance.

Management

- Make a diagnosis.
- Check for cord presentation or prolapse.
- Continuously monitor the fetal heart rate.
- Examine regularly to check that progress is adequate.
- Give oxytocin if progress is not satisfactory. (Caesarean section may be preferred to augmentation if facilities are available.)
- **Do not use scalp electrodes or perform fetal blood sampling.**
- If the position is MA, vaginal delivery should be possible.
- Perform an episiotomy.
- If the fetus is persistently presenting in an MP position, deliver by Caesarean section (if appropriate resources are available and it is safe to do so).

Delivery of compound presentations (*see* Table 2.6.E.1)

Here more than one part of the fetus is facing the cervix (e.g. an arm prolapsing alongside the presenting part). It is more common in prematurity.

Compound presentations, especially minor degrees involving just a hand can be managed expectantly in the early stages of labour, especially in the multiparous patient, and can sometimes be digitally encouraged back into the uterus. If they progress or persist and cause delay in the first or second stages of labour, then Caesarean section should be undertaken.

Transverse and oblique lies (*see* Table 2.6.E.1)

Background

These are associated with prematurity, uterine fibroids and placenta praevia, and consequently are associated with high maternal and fetal morbidity. Always try to identify the underlying pathology, if any.

If the membranes are intact in early labour, it is worth attempting external cephalic version (see below under breech).

The presentation of shoulder, limb or cord in the presence of ruptured membranes means that Caesarean section is the only option for delivering a viable infant. If the fetus is dead, unless it is very small and macerated, it is safer to perform a destructive procedure if an operator experienced in the procedure is available, and it is acceptable to the patient.

Practical points to remember

- Using ultrasound, try to identify the cause of the abnormal lie, if any.
- **Positively exclude placenta praevia with ultrasound before performing digital vaginal examinations. If there has been no vaginal bleeding, placenta praevia is still possible.**
- Caesarean section can be extremely difficult:
  - The lower segment will be poorly formed.
  - Fibroids, when present, can distort the anatomy and inhibit access.
  - Placenta praevia is associated with severe haemorrhage.
- A vertical uterine incision may sometimes be most appropriate for the above reasons.
- Keep the membranes intact while making and extending the uterine incision, as this aids manipulation of the fetus into a longitudinal plane for delivery.
- Delivery is usually best achieved by finding, grasping and bringing down a foot (recognisable by the heel) into the incision. If the foot is difficult to find, the back and buttocks should be identified and the legs followed until a foot is found.
- If delivery is still impossible, the uterine incision can be extended upwards in the midline, making an 'inverted T'. **If an extended uterine incision has been used, it is essential to undertake an elective Caesarean section in subsequent pregnancies, because of the risk of uterine rupture during labour.**

Breech delivery (*see* Table 2.6.E.1)

Background

At 28 weeks, 20% of babies are breech, but most fetuses will turn spontaneously so that only 3–4% will remain breech at term. There is a higher rate with prematurity. Vaginal delivery (although safer for the mother than Caesarean section) carries a higher risk of perinatal and neonatal mortality and morbidity due to birth asphyxia and trauma.

Hazards of vaginal breech delivery

Compared with the cephalic presentation at term, there is a greater risk of perinatal and neonatal mortality and morbidity, due principally to fetal congenital anomalies and birth trauma and asphyxia. In terms of maternal outcomes, vaginal birth is generally better for the mother than Caesarean

section, as the operative complications associated with major abdominal surgery and the resulting uterine scar are avoided. All of these factors are especially relevant in resource-limited countries.

Minimising problems

Options

- If there are no associated complications of pregnancy (e.g. previous Caesarean section, pre-eclampsia), explain the three options to the woman and her family:
  - external cephalic version (ECV)
  - trial of vaginal breech
  - elective Caesarean section (only if this is safe).
- On the basis of current evidence, all women with uncomplicated breech presentation at term should be offered ECV.
- If it is decided that an elective Caesarean section is the best option, wait until at least 39 weeks (babies may still turn spontaneously until then).
- A trial of vaginal breech delivery is appropriate if **both mother and baby** are of normal proportions.
  - The presentation should be either frank (hips flexed, knees extended) or complete (hips flexed, knees flexed, but feet not below the fetal buttocks).
  - There should be no evidence of feto–pelvic disproportion – that is, adequate pelvis (using clinical judgement) and estimated fetal weight < 4000 grams (clinical measurement).
  - In some smaller women it may be appropriate to exclude a vaginal breech option where the estimated fetal weight is < 4000 grams, provided that Caesarean section is safe.
  - There should be no evidence (on ultrasound) of hyperextension of the fetal head.

Fetal complications of breech presentation

These include the following:

- cord prolapse
- birth trauma as a result of extended arm or head, incomplete dilatation of the cervix, or cephalo–pelvic disproportion
- asphyxia due to cord prolapse, cord compression, placental detachment or arrested head
- damage to abdominal organs
- broken neck.

External cephalic version (ECV)

Background

Current recommendations in well-resourced countries are that ECV should be performed with the mother wide awake, but 'starved', having made her informed choice and having given consent for Caesarean section if necessary, close to theatre, after fetal monitoring has been carried out, and using ultrasound guidance, and tocolysis where necessary. These safety guidelines minimise the risks of maternal injury and fetal distress, allowing early detection and treatment if necessary. However, in resource-limited settings, the avoidance of breech delivery by ECV is highly beneficial, and the method described below is a reasonable compromise.

ECV may be performed between 37 and 42 weeks' gestation if there is a single uncomplicated breech pregnancy. There should be no previous uterine scars, previous antepartum bleeding, fibroids or a placenta praevia. On admission, the fetal heart should be listened to regularly. If available, ultrasound should be performed to demonstrate the fetal presentation, an adequate amount of liquor, a flexed fetal head and the position of the fetal legs. The mother should be awake and have given consent to the procedure.

The membranes must be intact, with adequate amniotic fluid and no complications of pregnancy.

Procedure

If possible, use ultrasound to demonstrate the fetal position, an adequate amount of liquor, a flexed fetal head, a free loop of cord, and the position of the fetal legs (extended or flexed).

- The mother lies on her side (usually her right), which will allow a forward somersault (from 'left sacro-anterior' position, which is the commonest breech position).
- The bed is tilted head down to allow gravity to assist in disengaging the breech.
- If the uterus is relaxed, an attempt is made to turn the baby, by disengaging the breech with one hand and flexing the head further with the other.
  - This should not hurt the mother, but it will be uncomfortable; the movement on her abdomen is made easier by using lubricant (e.g. sweet almond oil, talc, ultrasound gel).
  - The manoeuvres are illustrated in Figure 2.6.E.8.
- Ensure that the fetal heart rate is normal (110–160 beats/minute).
- In well-resourced settings only, and with relatively only slightly more success, and if the uterus is not relaxed, tocolysis may be helpful. Consider giving a dose of 250 micrograms terbutaline subcutaneously.
- The fetal heart rate should be listened to regularly during the procedure.
- Whether the ECV is successful or not, after the procedure listen carefully to the fetal heart every 5 minutes for 30–60 minutes. If this is normal, the mother is allowed home.
- If the first attempt is unsuccessful, consider bringing the mother back the next day for a repeat trial.
- If the fetal heart rate becomes abnormal, turn the woman on to her left side, and reassess every 5 minutes. If the

fetal heart rate does not become normal within 30 minutes, deliver by Caesarean section (if the facilities are available and it is safe to do so).
- In well-resourced settings where blood group including rhesus factor is universally collected, and where the mother is rhesus negative, 500 IU of anti-D immunoglobulin should be given after ECV. Unfortunately, anti-D immunoglobulin is expensive.

Figure 2.6.E.8 shows the steps involved in ECV. It illustrates how a right-handed person would turn a baby. If you are left-handed, turn the baby the other way.

(a) Place one hand below the breech, and your other hand above the head. Lift the breech out of the pelvis. Bring the head and breech closer together so as to flex the baby.

(b) and (c) Turn the baby by guiding the head forwards as you lift the buttocks up. In this way you make the baby do a forward somersault (i.e. turn head over heels).

(d) If you fail to turn the baby, try turning them with a backward somersault.

All mothers should be warned about the possible subsequent risks of reduced fetal movements, vaginal bleeding, rupture of the membranes and onset of labour. If ECV is successful, the pregnancy can be managed as a cephalic presentation. If it is unsuccessful, future management should be discussed and a decision made regarding whether to opt for elective Caesarean section or trial of vaginal breech delivery.

Trial of vaginal breech delivery

This is a difficult issue where there is limited availability of safe surgery, or surgery without delay. A trial may not be appropriate if:
- the mother is very small and/or the baby is large
- there is evidence of fetal–pelvic disproportion – that is, an inadequate pelvis (using clinical judgement) and an estimated fetal weight exceeding 4000 grams
- evidence (on ultrasound) of hyper-extension of the fetal head.

If there has been a previous Caesarean section or other scar in the uterus, a repeat Caesarean section may be preferable, although this will depend on the availability of safe surgery. Moving the woman to a waiting home next to a unit that provides comprehensive emergency obstetric care from 37 weeks' gestation (if available) may be a good option.

Procedure

- The mother should confirm her informed choice of vaginal delivery.
- If the mother is in hospital, an obstetrician, anaesthetist and operating theatre should be ready.
- Careful fetal monitoring and documentation of the partograph should be undertaken.
- The bladder must be emptied either naturally or with an in–out catheter.
- If spontaneous rupture of the membranes occurs, do a vaginal examination to check for cord prolapse. Meconium is common and not a sign of fetal distress.
- Amniotomy may be used to accelerate labour, where indicated, and careful use of oxytocin may be used to correct poor uterine activity if the mother is having her first baby. However, oxytocin should only be used in a well-resourced hospital. It should not be used for poor

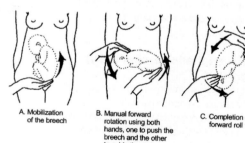

A. Mobilization of the breech

B. Manual forward rotation using both hands, one to push the breech and the other to guide the vertex

C. Completion of forward roll

D. Backward roll

FIGURE 2.6.E.8 External cephalic version.

progress due to poor uterine contractions in a mother who has previously given birth. Where available and safe, it is reasonable to perform a Caesarean section, rather than commencing oxytocin, even in primiparous women who are making inadequate spontaneous progress in labour.

- Caesarean section should be considered if there is poor progress or fetal distress.
- Ensure that a healthcare worker with adequate experience in delivering breech babies vaginally is present during the second stage.

The basic principle of delivering a breech is to avoid interfering.

- Active pushing should not be encouraged until the breech has descended to the pelvic floor and the cervix is fully dilated as confirmed by vaginal examination.
- Sitting the patient up at this stage may help to encourage descent of the breech. An **episiotomy** may well be required, but should not be performed until the anus is visible or until the baby's buttocks are distending the perineum.
- The breech will usually rotate spontaneously to lie with the sacrum anteriorly. **Rarely it will try to turn posteriorly, and this must be prevented by holding the baby by the bony pelvis and rotating the baby to the back-anterior position as it descends with maternal effort.**
- Extended legs are delivered by flexing the knee joint of the baby and then extending at the hips.
- The baby is **supported** only when the arms are delivered and the nape of the neck becomes visible. Avoid holding the baby's abdomen, as internal organs may be traumatised; the pelvis should be held gently to support the weight of the baby and prevent hyperextension of the fetal neck.
- As the mother pushes, the anterior shoulder tip will become visible. A finger is run over the shoulder and down to the elbow to deliver the arm, if this does not occur spontaneously. The other shoulder will rotate anteriorly spontaneously to allow similar delivery of the other arm. If the arms are not delivering spontaneously despite the shoulders being visible, the Løvset manoeuvre should be used (*see* Figure 2.6.E.9). Traction on

the baby combined with rotations as shown (multiple if necessary) will usually result in each arm dropping out of the cervix. Minimal assistance by the healthcare worker running a finger along the arm to disengage it may sometimes help.

- The baby lies supported as the head engages and the neck comes into view (*see* Figure 2.6.E.10).

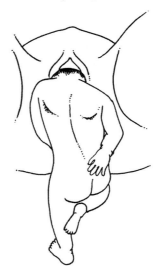

FIGURE 2.6.E.10 Breech delivery: the baby should hang until the hair line at the back of the neck is seen.

- Delivery of the head may then be performed by the Mauriceau–Smellie–Veit manoeuvre (*see* Figure 2.6.E.11). The right hand is placed in the vagina, the fetus is supported on the right forearm, the middle finger of the hand is passed into the baby's mouth, and the first and third fingers are placed **just below** the bony ridges of the lower part of the orbits (the maxilla). The eyes must not be compressed. Pressure is applied to flex and deliver the head. The left hand is used to press upwards and posteriorly on the back of the fetal head to encourage flexion.
- Alternatively, forceps may be used to achieve the controlled delivery of the head. An assistant should hold the baby's feet to elevate the body above the horizontal to

FIGURE 2.6.E.9 Breech delivery using Løvset method. Reproduced with permission from Macdonald S, Magill-Cuerden J (ed.) *Mayes' Midwifery: a textbook for midwives.* Elsevier Health Sciences; 2010. © Elsevier

An arm is extended alongside the head. Posterior shoulder is below sacral promontory and anterior shoulder above symphysis pubis

Clockwise

1) Fetus gently pulled down. MUST keep back uppermost to allow head to enter pelvis occipito-anterior.

2) Rotation 180 degrees brings posterior shoulder anterior to lie under symphysis and arm descends

Anticlockwise

3) Rotation in opposite direction brings down other arm

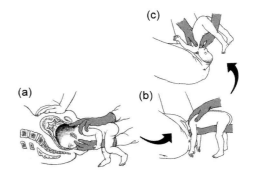

FIGURE 2.6.E.11 Breech delivery: delivering the head by the Mauriceau–Smellie–Veit manoeuvre. To help to deliver the head safely, lay the body on your forearm. Put the index and middle fingers of your left hand on the bony ridges below the eyes. Place your right index finger on the occiput, flex the head, and deliver the head slowly and in a controlled way.

allow the operator access to apply forceps. The nape of the neck must be in view before the baby's body is lifted upwards, or damage to the fetal neck may be caused. It is also essential that the baby is not lifted too high, as this will damage the neck.

If the head fails to descend into the pelvis (i.e. the nape of the neck does not appear), first check that the cervix is fully dilated. If it is not, it will need to be incised. If the cervix is fully dilated, if possible forceps (ideally Piper's) may be applied to the fetal head to facilitate delivery. Firm suprapubic pressure may be applied in the midline to encourage the unengaged head to flex and facili tate delivery. If this is unsuccessful, a symphysiotomy should be considered. All of these manoeuvres are potentially dangerous for the mother. If the fetus dies, a destructive procedure should be undertaken.

Elective Caesarean section for breech

This is advisable for the following:
- failed external cephalic version
- if vaginal birth is contraindicated, or the mother wishes
- double footling breech
- a very large fetus
- a small or malformed maternal pelvis
- a hyperextended or deflexed fetal head.

Before and at operation:
- Explain to the woman that she will have a scarred uterus, which may create problems in future pregnancies.
- Ensure that the presentation remains breech before anaesthetising the patient.
- Note that if the uterine incision is too small, there can be difficulty delivering the after-coming head.
- Remember to keep the fetal back upwards during delivery.

2.6.F Preterm pre-labour rupture of membranes (PPROM) and/or preterm labour

Introduction

PPROM is defined as spontaneous rupture of the membranes before the onset of labour and prior to 37 weeks' gestation. It occurs in 2–4% of single pregnancies and 7–20% of multiple pregnancies, and accompanies 60% or more of preterm births.

PPROM is associated with maternal mortality and morbidity with neonatal complications, which include cord prolapse, neonatal sepsis and respiratory failure, pulmonary hypoplasia and malpresentations.

Preterm labour is defined as labour that begins before 37 weeks' gestation. It has increasingly serious implications for the neonate the earlier it occurs.

Preterm labour may occur without PPROM. However, ruptured membranes are a common early consequence of premature labour. Likewise PPROM can occur before labour, but the risk of progression to labour following PPROM is high (see below).

There are multiple risk factors for preterm labour and PPROM. They include intrauterine infection, twin pregnancy, polyhydramnios, abruption, malaria, urinary tract infection/pyelonephritis and uterine anomalies (including large fibroids).

Clinical findings in the woman with PPROM and/or preterm labour

In PPROM the fluid may come out quickly as a sudden large flow, or it may trickle out over 1–2 hours, after which recognition is more difficult. Around 50% of women go into labour within 24–48 hours, and 70–90% within 1 week. The gap is longer the earlier in pregnancy the rupture occurs.

There may be no history or signs to suggest that PPROM has occurred, and therefore the woman may present with preterm labour. Preterm labour may also occur without PPROM.

It is important if possible to distinguish PPROM from urinary incontinence, bacterial/fungal vaginal infection or a 'show' of cervical mucus.

Premature labour is considered to be present if there are regular contractions (usually at least every 10 minutes) associated with cervical effacement and/or dilatation.

In its early stages it is very difficult to diagnose accurately, as the patient may present before cervical change has occurred, and it is then only with time that the cervical change becomes apparent.

Important differential diagnosis for premature labour, where cervical change has not yet occurred, include: Braxton Hicks contractions, urinary tract infection, musculoskeletal pain, constipation and diarrhoea.

Infection can itself result in premature labour and therefore patients presenting with threatened preterm labour should be assessed and treated for an underlying cause. Common examples of infections that precipitate premature labour include malaria and urinary tract infection/pyelonephritis.

Management of PPROM and/or preterm labour

Avoid doing a digital vaginal examination unless active labour is under way and/or birth is imminent, as it increases the risk of infection.

A sterile speculum examination should be undertaken to look for amniotic fluid passing through the cervix or in the posterior fornix. A swab should be taken of the fluid and sent to the laboratory for microscopy and culture (if bacteriological facilities are available), looking especially for group B streptococcus.

Monitor vital signs (temperature, heart rate and blood pressure), vaginal discharge (check sanitary towels regularly; do not use tampons), uterine activity and possible tenderness, and fetal heart rate, and where possible perform an ultrasound examination to assess the amniotic fluid index, presentation, gestation and placental site.

Also check a full blood count, maternal blood group, malaria RDT +/– smear and a midstream specimen of urine (MSSU). If available a CRP along with the white blood cell count may help to indicate an underlying infection.

Although there is no evidence that bed rest is appropriate, if it is undertaken apply anti-embolism stockings (if available) and encourage leg exercises to prevent deep vein thrombosis.

Inform the paediatrician (if available).

Sexual intercourse should not occur after PPROM.

When to consider antibiotics

1 Symptomatic ascending infection *in utero* in the mother (fever, maternal and/or fetal tachycardia, foul-smelling vaginal discharge, uterine tenderness and signs of systemic illness) needs **urgent treatment with IV antibiotics (ampicillin plus gentamicin plus metronidazole)**. If this is overlooked, the lives of both the mother and the baby will be in danger:

- ampicillin 2 grams IV/IM, then 1 gram IV 6-hourly
- *plus* gentamicin 80 mg IV/IM 8-hourly or 5 mg/kg body weight IV/IM once every 24 hours
- *plus* metronidazole (vial containing 500 mg in 100 mL) 500 mg or 100 mL IV infusion every 8 hours. Do not give metronidazole IM.

Usually there will be uterine contractions, but whether or not they are present the baby must be delivered as soon as possible.

2 Asymptomatic infection (no fever and no systemic signs of illness) is a more common problem which may progress to a life-threatening infection at any time. It is therefore essential that all women who have/or may have undergone rupture of membranes, are monitored regularly for the symptoms and signs of infection. These include: labour, generalised uterine pain, flushing and chills, body aches, fever (> 37.5°C), tachycardia, tachypnoea and fetal tachycardia.

3 If premature rupture of membranes is confirmed, the patient is stable, and a decision has been made to manage the patient expectantly (see below) then give prophylactic antibiotics as follows to help more safely to prolong the pregnancy:

a. Erythromycin 250 mg TDS plus amoxicillin 500 mg TDS both orally and for 7 days.

4 **All patients with confirmed premature labour should receive prophylactic antibiotics when in active labour as follows:**

a. IV ampicillin 2 grams IV/IM, then 1 gram IV 6-hourly. Discontinue antibiotics immediately after delivery if there are no signs of infection in the mother.

5 Maternal fever (> 38°C) or other indication of infection in labour (e.g. offensive liquor) requires that the mother be treated with IV penicillin/ampicillin, metronidazole and gentamicin as in 1. above. If this is the case, **the newborn infant should also be treated with IV antibiotics from birth without waiting for any signs of infection to appear (*see* Section 3.1).**

Minimising the risk of surfactant deficiency in the newborn with antenatal steroids

High-dose corticosteroids can improve surfactant production in the newborn, but steroids must not be given if there is evidence of tuberculosis or HIV infection. A transient increase in blood glucose levels can occur with the use of steroids in diabetes. Even one dose of steroids can be effective in improving lung maturity in the newborn.

Give betamethasone, 12 mg IM, two doses 24 hours apart *or* dexamethasone, 6 mg IM, four doses 12 hours apart. Maximum benefit is achieved 24 hours following the second dose and for 1 week thereafter. Although it is not evidence based, where delivery is urgent, it is common practice to accelerate the course of steroids by giving the two 12 mg doses of either betamethasone or dexamethasone 12 hours apart.

A second course of dexamethasone or betamethasone can be given if more than 2 weeks have elapsed since the first course of treatment was given, and delivery has not occurred but premature labour has restarted. No more than two courses should be given.

Stopping premature labour

There is evidence to demonstrate that labour can sometimes be delayed by treating the mother with tocolytic drugs. There is no evidence, however, that tocolysis alone is beneficial to the baby or mother. In fact their use is potentially dangerous, as delaying delivery may result in progression of the process which caused the premature labour in the first place, e.g. infection or abruption.

However, tocolysis may be useful to allow administration of antenatal corticosteroids (as above), thereby protecting the baby from lung surfactant deficiency. They may also allow transfer of the mother to a hospital where safer therapy can be provided for a preterm baby.

Tocolysis should not be given for more than 48 hours as this is the time taken for antenatal steroids to achieve their maximum therapeutic effects.

Premature labour is considered to be present if there are regular contractions at least every 10 minutes associated with cervical effacement and/or dilatation.

It is unsafe to try to stop labour if the membranes are ruptured.

Although tocolysis is not recommended after 34 weeks' gestation in well-resourced settings, it may possibly be helpful between 34 and 36 weeks' gestation in low-resource settings, as well as between 28 and 34 weeks.

If labour is well advanced and the cervix is more than 5 cm dilated, tocolysis will probably not be helpful.

Drugs used for tocolysis

There is always the option of not trying to stop uterine contractions, as the evidence of benefit is very limited. If antenatal corticosteroids are not going to be given and there is no need to transfer the patient, then tocolytics are not indicated.

Terbutaline

This is given in a dose of 250 micrograms subcutaneously every 6 hours.

Nifedipine

Nifedipine given orally is the most appropriate drug.

The side effects of nifedipine include facial flushing, headache, nausea, tachycardia, dizziness, a fall in blood pressure, heart failure and (rarely) increased liver enzymes.

Contraindications are situations where delivery is desired, such as antepartum haemorrhage, severe pre-eclampsia, infection, fetal distress and all cases of PPROM in low-resource settings. Nifedipine should not be given if the mother has heart disease.

Before starting nifedipine, measure urea and electrolytes and liver function tests (where available).

Regular and frequent measurements of the mother's vital signs, as well as the fetal heart rate, should be undertaken. Closely observe for signs of heart failure. If the blood pressure falls, give a bolus of 250–500 mL of Ringer-lactate or Hartmann's solution.

Doses of nifedipine:

- Initial dose: 20 mg of oral nifedipine.
- Up to three further doses can be given at 30-minute intervals if uterine contractions persist.
- If this stops labour, and the blood pressure is stable, give a maintenance dose of 20 mg three times a day for up to a total of 48 hours. The maximum daily dose is 120 mg of nifedipine.

How long to wait before inducing labour when there is PPROM

The decision on timing of delivery is difficult, and it depends on the stage of pregnancy, the availability of comprehensive emergency obstetric care, the quality of neonatal care available and the obstetric history and wishes of the patient.

If expectant management is undertaken women with PPROM should be resident in a healthcare facility where comprehensive emergency obstetric care is available. Induction of labour should be undertaken by 36 weeks as prolonging the pregnancy beyond this stage is of reduced benefit to the fetus.

In a resource poor setting it is reasonable to induce the pregnancy at a much earlier gestation, even if this will result in a neonatal death, in order to reduce maternal risk.

Patients should be monitored closely for any symptoms or signs of infection, and if any develop delivery should be achieved urgently (via induction or Caesarean section, whichever is indicated) regardless of gestation.

Suggested monitoring would include:

- Regular review for symptoms of infection, e.g. uterine pain, body aches, flushing, chills. The patient should be advised to report such symptoms as they occur.
- 2 to 4 times daily vital sign assessment – tachycardia (> 100 bpm), tachypnoea (> 20), and pyrexia (> 37.5° C) should raise suspicion of infection.
- At least twice weekly inflammatory marker assessment such as CRP (where available). Note: corticosteroid administration causes a transient increase in the maternal white blood cell count but does not affect CRP.

Clinical problems in the neonate associated with preterm birth

These include the following:

- Surfactant deficiency leads to increasing levels of respiratory difficulty with decreasing gestational age.
- There is an increased risk of infection and hypothermia.
- Nutritional problems: maturity is more important than weight with regard to the ability to feed and digest. Babies who are born before 36 weeks' gestation nearly always need some help with feeding. Breast milk is ideal, and everything possible should be done to help the mother to sustain her lactation until the baby is ready to feed reliably from the breast. A limited ability to suck and swallow usually appears from 32 weeks' gestation, but it remains unpredictable, unreliable and uncoordinated until 36 weeks' gestation. In the event that breastfeeding cannot be initiated immediately after birth, the mother should be encouraged to start expressing breast milk, to be given by nasogastric tube or cup and spoon. Partial breastfeeding can also help the mother to sustain her lactation, but in any event she should regularly express milk.

Further information on care of the prematurely born infant can be found in Section 3.

2.6.G Prolapsed umbilical cord

Incidence

Prolapse of the umbilical cord occurs in approximately 0.2% of all births, mostly in multiparous mothers. There is a significant risk of fetal death due to mechanical compression of the cord, and spasm of the cord vessels when they are exposed to cold air.

Risk factors for cord prolapse

The presenting part does not remain in the lower uterine segment due to any of the following causes.

Fetal causes

- Malpresentations (e.g. complete or footling breech, transverse and oblique lie).
- Prematurity or low birth weight.
- Polyhydramnios.
- Multiple pregnancy.
- Anencephaly.
- High head.

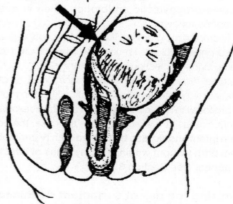

cord compressed

cord prolapsed

FIGURE 2.6.G.1 Sagittal view showing compressed cord.

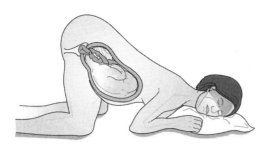

FIGURE 2.6.G.2 Prolapsed cord presenting. Reproduced with permission from Macdonald S, Magill-Cuerden J (ed.) *Mayes' Midwifery: a textbook for midwives.* Elsevier Health Sciences; 2010. © Elsevier

Maternal causes
- Contracted pelvis.
- Pelvic tumours.

Other predisposing factors
- Low-grade placenta praevia.
- Long cord.
- Sudden rupture of membranes in polyhydramnios.
- Artificial rupture of membranes (ARM).
- Manual rotation of the fetal head.

Management of cord prolapse

The longer the time between diagnosis of cord prolapse and delivery, the greater the risk of stillbirth and neonatal death. If the baby is dead, deliver in the safest way for the mother.

1 Assess fetal viability. If the baby is alive and of a viable gestation, and fetal heart sounds are heard with a Pinard's stethoscope or ideally a hand-held ultrasound fetal heart rate detector (e.g. Sonicaid), urgently relieve pressure on the cord by placing the woman in the knee–elbow or exaggerated Sims' position (Figure 2.6.G.3). Care should be taken not to stimulate the cord by handling it. Exposure to low temperatures should also be prevented if possible. This gives time for decision making.

2 Discontinue oxytocin if it is being used. You can buy time to allow the baby to be delivered by giving tocolysis with terbutaline 250 micrograms every 6 hours subcutaneously.

3 If the fetus is alive, prepare for either emergency vaginal delivery or emergency Caesarean section (if this can be undertaken safely).

4 If the cervix is fully dilated, and delivery is likely to be achievable within 5 minutes, encourage the patient to push and prepare to expedite the delivery by use of forceps or ventouse. The choice of instrument will depend on availability, operator experience and the position of the fetal head. If appropriate, forceps delivery is usually the most rapid method of achieving delivery, but must not be used by inexperienced staff. Rapid delivery is far more likely to be achieved in a multiparous woman.

5 If Caesarean section is safe and the only option (i.e. the cervix is not fully dilated, and the fetus is alive and viable), fill the bladder to raise the presenting part off the compressed cord for an extended period of time, so that the woman or girl can be transferred to the operating theatre. Insert 500 mL of sterile IV fluid into the bladder using an IV giving set attached to a Foley catheter. Inflate the balloon of the Foley catheter, clamp it and attach drainage tubing and a urine bag. The full bladder may also decrease or inhibit uterine contractions. The bladder must be emptied by unclamping the catheter before opening the peritoneal cavity for Caesarean section. **Mark the mother's abdomen to ensure that this is not forgotten. At skin incision, the bladder clamp must be released and the bladder emptied.**

6 Ensure that venous access is in place with a reliable IV cannula.

7 Transfer the woman or girl to the operating theatre in the exaggerated Sims' position on a trolley.

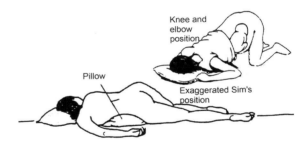

FIGURE 2.6.G.3 Maternal positions for immediately relieving pressure on prolapsed cord.

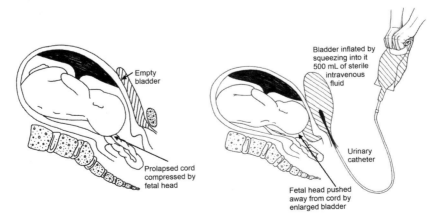

FIGURE 2.6.G.4 Treating prolapse of the cord by elevation of the fetal presenting part by inflating the bladder with sterile IV fluid.

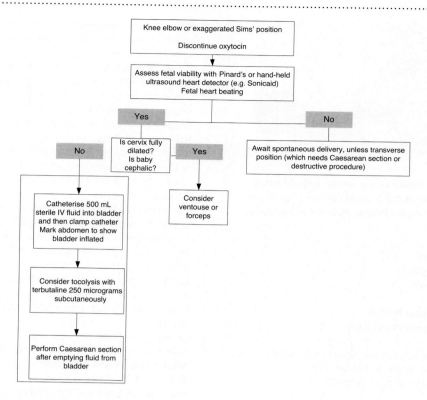

FIGURE 2.6.G.5 Pathway of care for prolapsed cord.

2.6.H Inverted uterus

Introduction
Definition
This occurs when the uterus, after or during delivery of the placenta, is inverted and may appear at the introitus. The inverted uterus has the endometrium and sometimes the placenta 'on the outside'.

Prevention
Prevent an inverted uterus by avoiding cord traction until the uterus is contracted and placental separation has occurred, and ensuring that the uterus is held back with one hand during cord traction.

Clinical signs
An inverted uterus most commonly presents as a pelvic mass, sometimes protruding from the vagina. If the inverted uterus does not protrude from the vagina, it may go undetected, resulting in a sub-acute or chronic inversion which is very dangerous and may even present as a sudden unexpected maternal death.

Symptoms and signs include severe lower abdominal pain in the third stage of labour, haemorrhage, shock out of proportion to blood loss, the uterus not being palpable on abdominal examination, and vaginal examination revealing a mass in the vagina.

Early recognition is vital, as **shock** is the most common complication. Shock out of proportion to blood loss may be due to increased vagal tone, which may also produce

a **bradycardia** (< 60 beats/minute), worsening the shock and confusing its diagnosis. Inversion is associated with haemorrhage in over 90% of cases. Alternatively, concealed bleeding may produce tachycardia and other signs of shock.

Incomplete inversion presents more subtly with continuing postpartum haemorrhage despite a contracted uterus. The fundus of the uterus may feel dimpled.

Suspect a diagnosis of inverted uterus if there is:
- shock with little obvious bleeding
- continuing postpartum haemorrhage despite an apparently well-contracted uterus
- associated lower abdominal pain
- a dimpled uterine fundus
- a fundus that is not palpable abdominally.

Management
The uterus must be replaced as soon as inversion is recognised, as a matter of urgency, as this becomes more difficult over time. Call for help and try to push it back while ABC resuscitation is being undertaken.

Primary assessment and resuscitation
Call for senior help, including a surgeon and an anaesthetist.

If shock is present, manage ABC as described below.

Manual replacement of the uterus
As soon as possible, and **wearing sterile gloves**, attempt manual replacement of the uterus by pushing the fundus

back through the cervix (the longer the delay, the more difficult it will be to achieve resolution).

It is important that the part of the uterus that came out last (the part closest to the cervix) goes in first.

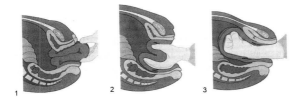

FIGURE 2.6.H.1 Bimanual replacement of inverted uterus. Reproduced with the permission of Medical Aid Films, www.medicalaidfilms.org

Do not attempt to separate the placenta until the inversion has been corrected.

However, if the inversion has been present for some time (e.g. if it occurred at home), and replacement is not possible without placental removal, then be prepared for possible severe bleeding if this is undertaken.

Hydrostatic correction

- If manual replacement is unsuccessful, hydrostatic correction should be attempted.
- Place the woman in the steep Trendelenburg position (lower her head about 0.5 metres below the level of the perineum).
- Prepare a high-level sterile douche system with a large nozzle, long tubing (2 metres) and a reservoir (1–2 litres of sterile Ringer-lactate or Hartmann's solution at room temperature, not from a refrigerator).
  - **Note:** This can also be done using Ringer-lactate or Hartmann's solution and an ordinary IV administration set.
- Identify the posterior fornix. This is easily done in partial inversion when the inverted uterus is still in the vagina. In other cases, the posterior fornix is recognised by the place where the ridged vagina becomes the smooth vagina.
- Place the nozzle of the douche in the posterior fornix.
- At the same time, with the other hand hold the labia sealed over the nozzle and use the forearm to support the nozzle.
- Ask an assistant to start the douche at full pressure (raise the water reservoir to at least 2 metres). Ringer-lactate or Hartmann's solution will distend the posterior fornix of

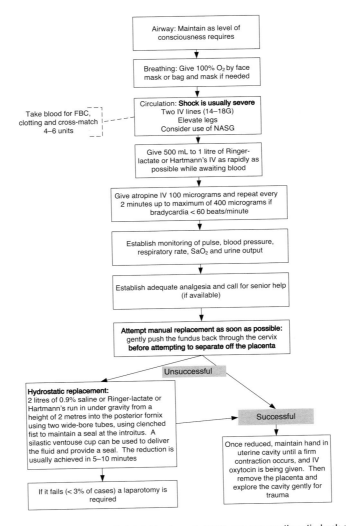

FIGURE 2.6.H.2 Pathway of care for inverted uterus. FBC, full blood count; NASG, non-pneumatic anti-shock garment.

the vagina gradually so that it stretches. This causes the circumference of the orifice to increase, relieves cervical constriction, and results in correction of the inversion.

- If a Silc Cup ventouse is available, this can be used to occlude the vagina and give a seal. Two IV infusion sets are inserted into the narrow end while the wide end lies against the inverted uterus vaginally.
- Terbutaline, 250 micrograms subcutaneously, may help to stop any uterine contractions that prevent correction of the inversion.

Manual correction under general anaesthesia

If hydrostatic correction is not successful, try manual repositioning under general anaesthesia, using halothane. Halothane is recommended because it relaxes the uterus, but be aware of the risk of possible atonic uterus and haemorrhage.

Airway

- Use an opening manoeuvre if the airway is not open or is partially obstructed. Keep the airway open. If there is an improvement but the airway closes without active opening support, consider using an airway adjunct to support the airway.
- Suction only under direct vision and only if necessary.
- The airway may need to be secured by intubation using experienced senior help (if available).

Breathing

Provide a high concentration of oxygen through a face mask with a reservoir bag if there is adequate spontaneous respiration. Give 100% oxygen (mask with reservoir and a flow rate of at least 6 litres/minute) regardless of SaO$_2$.

For inadequate ventilation or depressed conscious level (P or U on the AVPU scale), respiration should be supported with oxygen via a **bag-mask**, and experienced senior help should be summoned (if available).

Circulation

Primary assessment suggesting shock:

- **Fast, weak pulse** (≥ 100–110 beats/minute). Normal heart rates in a pregnant mother at rest are 60–90 beats/minute. Tachycardia is the first sign of shock.
- **Bradycardia** (< 60 beats/minute) may occur as a result of increased vagal tone due to the inversion.
- **Low-volume (weak) pulse.**
- Pallor (especially of the inner eyelid, palms or around the mouth).
- Sweatiness or cold clammy skin.
- **Prolonged capillary refill time** (> 3 seconds).
- **Rapid breathing** (> 30 breaths/minute). Normal respiratory rates in a pregnant mother at rest are 15–20 breaths/minute. Tachypnoea can be due to acidosis.

- **Low blood pressure** (systolic < 90–100 mmHg) **is a very late sign.** Healthy women and girls can maintain a normal or even high blood pressure while large volumes of blood are lost.
- Anxiety, reduced conscious level, confusion or unconsciousness.

If the woman or girl is shocked, obtain vascular access to give large volumes quickly. Insert two wide-bore IV cannulae (14- to 16G) and send blood for a full blood count, cross-matching (2 units) and clotting. If peripheral veins are difficult to access, the external jugular vein or long saphenous vein cut-down are good alternatives.

- Give an initial **rapid** bolus of 500 mL to 1 litre of Ringer-lactate or Hartmann's solution **or blood if available**. It is essential that the bolus is given as rapidly as possible. In the absence of syringe pumps, they should be pushed in manually using a 20- to 50-mL syringe (using a three-way tap and link to an IV giving set).
- Further 500- to 1000-mL boluses may be required in the first hour. Once more than 2 litres have been given IV, complications such as pulmonary or cerebral oedema may occur. If available, expert help, including CVP monitoring, is valuable.
- A blood pressure cuff can be used to speed up infusions in emergency situations. Wrap the cuff around the blood/fluid bag and place it inside a non-compressible bag.
- Keep the patient warm but do not overheat them, as this will cause peripheral vasodilatation and reduce the blood supply to vital centres. Hypothermia will exacerbate poor peripheral perfusion, acidosis and coagulation abnormalities.
- **Elevate the legs (raise the foot of the bed).**
- Give O-negative or group-specific blood if there is not time for full cross-matching. Have O-negative blood ready in the ward at all times if possible.
- Consider giving atropine 100 micrograms IV, and repeat every 2 minutes up to a maximum of 400 micrograms IV if bradycardia is < 60 beats/minute.
- Consider using the non-pneumatic anti-shock garment (NASG).

Post-procedure care

Once the inversion is corrected, infuse IV oxytocin, 40 units in 500 mL of Ringer-lactate or Hartmann's solution, over 4 hours. If **the uterus does not contract after oxytocin**, give misoprostol 3 tablets each of 200 micrograms orally or 600 micrograms of powder sublingually if the patient is conscious, or 4 × 200 micrograms rectally if she is drowsy.

The patient must be observed closely for haemorrhage.

Give a single dose of prophylactic antibiotics after correcting the inverted uterus. Use ampicillin 2 grams IV *plus* metronidazole 500 mg IV, and give appropriate analgesia.

2.6.1 Hyperemesis gravidarum

Introduction

Some nausea and vomiting is common in early pregnancy, with nausea affecting 70–85% of women. Around 50% of pregnant women experience vomiting. However, in a small proportion of patients severe vomiting (hyperemesis) can occur. This condition is more common if there is a larger than normal placental mass (e.g. in multiple pregnancy and molar pregnancy). Hyperemesis peaks at 11 weeks, with 90% of cases resolved at 16 weeks.

Associated conditions

Severe hyperemesis requiring hospital care is associated with the following:

- depression and severe stress
- multiple pregnancy
- molar pregnancy.

Consequences of hyperemesis

Consequences that are severe enough to require hospital care include the following:

- ketosis
- hypochloraemic alkalosis, hypokalaemia and hyponatraemia
- malnutrition with anaemia and hypoalbuminaemia
- ulcerative oesophagitis
- Wernicke's encephalopathy from thiamine deficiency
- worsened depression, may result in the patient seeking a termination of pregnancy
- hyperemesis is dangerous in type 1 diabetes and can result in ketoacidosis.

Investigations

- Ultrasound examination to exclude molar or multiple pregnancy.
- Urine for ketones and to exclude urinary tract infection.
- Blood for haemoglobin, urea and electrolytes.
- Special investigations as indicated to exclude serious medical problems affecting the gastrointestinal, genitourinary, neurological, metabolic or endocrine and psychological systems.

Treatment of severe hyperemesis

Intravenous 0.9% saline, 1 litre given over 4 hours initially and then repeated as required, is the most effective treatment for severe hyperemesis with dehydration.

Small volumes (100–200 mL every 2–3 hours) of WHO oral rehydration salts (ORS) powder dissolved in 1 litre of water giving Na^+ 75 mmol/litre, K^+ 20 mmol/litre and glucose 75 mmol/litre can be given in addition to IV fluids until vomiting settles and if tolerated.

After IV fluids have been started, anti-emetic drugs may not be required, but if vomiting continues try prochlorperazine 12.5 mg IM and then orally 5 to 10 mg three times daily. Alternatives include cyclizine, 50 mg IM, IV or orally TDS domperidone 10 mg orally or 30–60 mg rectally four times a day, and metoclopramide 10 mg IM, IV or orally three times

a day. If suppositories are available, rectal administration is ideal as it can be self administrated and avoids the oral route in the nauseous and vomiting patient. It is often necessary to use a combination of anti-emetics. If this is done it is often best to combine drugs with different mechanisms of action (e.g. cyclizine and metoclopramide) and to stagger their administration.

Supplements with thiamine should be given (IV if available) if there is evidence suggesting a severe deficiency may be present (Wernicke–Korsakoff syndrome). It should also be used prophylactically if the vomiting has been severe and/or protracted. See below for dosing.

If available, urea and electrolytes should be monitored (ideally daily) in women with severe hyperemesis. Women are at particular risk of hypokalaemia if the vomiting is severe and protracted. In a vomiting patient who is not tolerating any diet, potassium replacement should be considered even where blood measurement is not available. The daily requirement of potassium is approximately 60 mmol in a 60 kg woman, and will be higher in the vomiting patient.

Replacement should be undertaken with great care as too rapid replacement is dangerous.

A reasonable approach would be to add 20 mmol to 1 litre of 0.9% saline and to administer over 8 hours (42 dpm when using a standard giving set with a drop factor of 20). This provides a large margin of error as the infusion could be increased to >100 dpm before becoming hazardous.

Ringer's lactate does contain 5 mmol of potassium/litre and will provide some replacement if potassium is not available.

Hyperemesis is a risk factor for venous thromboembolism (DVT and PE). If a patient is admitted with severe hyperemesis she should be treated with anti-embolic stockings (if available).

Wernicke–Korsakoff syndrome

Symptoms of Wernicke's encephalopathy include the following:

- confusion
- loss of muscle coordination (ataxia)
- leg tremor
- vision changes
- abnormal eye movements (back-and-forth movements called nystagmus)
- double vision
- eyelid drooping.

Symptoms of Korsakoff syndrome include the following:

- inability to form new memories
- loss of memory, which can be severe
- making up stories (confabulation)
- seeing or hearing things that are not really there (hallucinations).

Treatment of severe hyperemesis where possible symptoms or signs of Wernicke–Korsakoff syndrome are present

Give an IV infusion of 10 mL of Pabrinex (Vials 1+2) in 100 mL of 0.9% saline over 1 hour (vials contain thiamine, ascorbic acid, nicotinamide, pyridoxine and riboflavin).

Subsequently, give oral thiamine 50 mg three times daily until vomiting has stopped.

Other management on discharge from hospital

Withhold iron tablets until vomiting has resolved, but ensure that they are taken subsequently, as iron-deficiency anaemia may have been an important consequence of the hyperemesis.

Try to help with any depression that is present and also, if resources to address intimate partner violence are available in the community, make sensitive inquiries of the woman or girl in case this is a contributing factor.

2.7 Medical disorders complicating pregnancy and delivery

2.7.A Heart failure during pregnancy, including rheumatic heart disease

---

BOX 2.7.A.1 Minimum standards
- Oxygen.
- Furosemide.
- Digoxin.
- Nitroglycerine sublingual tablets.
- Blood transfusion.
- Morphine.

Introduction

Serious cardiac pathology may present either as heart failure where respiratory distress is the most obvious finding, or as cardiogenic shock (see shock section later).

Causes of heart failure during pregnancy

There are five main causes of heart failure in pregnancy:
1. severe anaemia
2. structural heart disease
3. circulatory overload (e.g. excessive IV fluids)
4. hypertension in severe pre-eclampsia
5. hypertrophic cardiomyopathy (HCM) and peripartum cardiomyopathy.

Heart failure can result from:
- left ventricular volume overload (aortic and mitral valve incompetence) or excessive pulmonary blood flow (e.g. congenital heart defects)
- left heart obstruction (aortic stenosis, mitral stenosis, hypertension)
- primary pump failure (severe anaemia, myocarditis, cardiomyopathy or arrhythmia)
- over-transfusion (a particular risk in hospital with IV blood or fluid infusions, especially in the anaemic mother).

Clinical signs

These include the following:
- respiratory distress (raised rate and some chest wall recession)
- tachycardia out of proportion to respiratory difficulty

- raised jugular venous pressure
- gallop rhythm/murmur
- enlarged liver
- basal lung crepitations.

Jugular venous pressure

Normal levels of jugular venous pressure (JVP) are 4–5 cm above the sternal angle. In heart failure the JVP can be raised so that the external jugular vein is filled up to or above the angle of the jaw (see Figure 2.7.A.1).

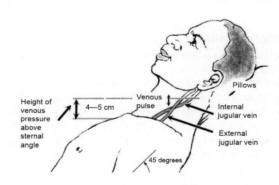

FIGURE 2.7.A.1 Clinical measurement of central venous pressure.

Treatment of severe decompensated heart failure

- Assess ABC.
- Sit the patient upright and **ensure bed rest**.
- Give a high concentration of **oxygen** via face mask with reservoir bag.
- If there are signs of shock (poor pulse volume or low blood pressure with extreme pallor and depressed conscious level), treat for **cardiogenic shock** with inotropes (if available).
- If there are signs of pulmonary oedema, give IV **furosemide 40 mg** (and repeat as required).

- Provided the patient is not hypotensive (systolic blood pressure > 90 mmHg) and has no serious obstructive valvular disease, give a **glyceryl trinitrate** tablet 500 micrograms sublingually and repeat up to a total of 3 tablets.
- Give **morphine** 3 mg over 5 minutes, and consider repeating after 15 minutes. Morphine is effective in reducing the afterload and, in addition, will reduce anxiety and pain both of which are likely to make heart failure worse.
- For patients with persisting heart failure load with **digoxin IV**, 250–500 micrograms over 10 minutes, then after 6 hours 125–250 micrograms over 10 minutes, then after a further 6 hours 125–250 micrograms over 10 minutes.

Or give an **oral digoxin** loading dose (instead of IV) of 375–750 micrograms, then after 6 hours 187.5–375 micrograms, then after a further 6 hours 187.5–375 micrograms.

- **Maintenance digoxin dose IV or oral:**
  - 125–750 micrograms once daily.
  - Reduce the dose in renal impairment. Be alert for low K^+ levels.
- Consider thromboprophylaxis. This treatment must take into account any bleeding risk and the timing of delivery.
- Check for severe anaemia (especially if the haemoglobin concentration is < 5.0 g/dL), for which partial exchange transfusion may be helpful. **Partial exchange transfusion can be achieved with a cannula in a large vein in the antecubital fossa. Withdraw 25 mL of anaemic blood and infuse 50 mL of new blood over 5 minutes, and repeat up to 10 times.** An alternative is careful transfusion of packed cells (hang the bag vertically for 15 minutes) to allow the red blood cells to separate from the plasma. Transfuse only the red blood cell component with 40 mg IV furosemide for each unit of 500 mL infused.

The following are useful investigations if available:
- full blood count (to exclude severe anaemia)
- serum urea and electrolytes
- infection screen, including blood cultures
- 12-lead electrocardiogram
- chest X-ray
- echocardiogram.

Subsequent treatment of heart failure
- Dietary sodium restriction.
- Loop diuretics (furosemide) for moderate/severe pulmonary oedema,
- Treatment with oral hydralazine or oral nifedipine (modified release version) as a vasodilator (instead of glyceryl trinitrate used in the acute scenario above).
- Treatment with a B-blocker (preferably a B1 cardioselective B-blocker such as atenolol) can be beneficial. They are NOT used in the acute presentation of a patient with severe decompensated heart failure. They are contraindicated in asthma and may be associated with intra-uterine growth restriction, but are not associated with congenital malformations.
- Continued treatment with digoxin (as above) should be considered if significant symptoms persist.

- Treatment of any underlying anaemia or poor nutritional status.
- Once the baby is delivered, treatment with hydralazine or nifedipine may be replaced with an ACE inhibitor such as enalapril or lisinopril. ACE inhibitors cause congenital abnormalities and therefore should not be used antenatally. They are contraindicated if the patient is hypovolaemic and in renal artery and aortic stenosis.

Management of heart failure during labour
- The mother must deliver sitting up.
- Give oxygen from a face mask throughout labour.
- Limit infusion of IV fluids to decrease the risk of circulatory overload, and maintain a strict fluid balance chart.
- Ensure adequate analgesia.
- **If an oxytocin IV infusion is required**, use a higher concentration at a slower rate while maintaining a fluid balance chart (e.g. the concentration may be doubled if the number of drops per minute is decreased by half).
  - Increase the rate of oxytocin infusion until regular strong contractions are established, and then maintain infusion at that rate.
- Avoid sustained, bearing-down efforts during the second stage if possible.
- If it is necessary to decrease the woman's workload during delivery, perform an episiotomy and assist delivery by vacuum extraction or forceps.
- Ensure active management of the third stage of labour. Oxytocin given on delivery of the baby must be given very slowly IV (5 units diluted in 20 mL of 0.9% saline over 5–10 minutes) to avoid hypotension.
- **Do not give ergometrine.**

Note: Heart failure is not an indication for Caesarean section.

Management of anaesthesia if Caesarean section is needed
It is assumed that epidural anaesthesia/analgesia is unlikely to be possible or appropriate in low-resource settings. Avoid spinal anaesthesia if there is a fixed cardiac output, such as aortic/mitral stenosis or heart failure associated with valvular disease. If you are giving a general anaesthetic, take precautions against aspiration and minimise the risk of an increase in blood pressure associated with intubation by premedication with either morphine (5 mg initially IV) or lignocaine (1 mg/kg IV). If the patient is considered to have insufficient cardiovascular stability for general anaesthetic, undertake Caesarean section under local infiltration anaesthesia.

In all of the above situations the surgeon should be ready to start operating **immediately** when anaesthesia is established, so that the operating time is as short as possible. As above, oxytocin given for active management of third stage must be given very slowly IV (5 units diluted in 20 mL of 0.9% saline over 5–10 minutes) to avoid hypotension.

Post-operative management must ensure adequate analgesia with morphine.

Cardiac consequences of rheumatic heart disease and their effects on pregnancy

Introduction

After an episode of acute rheumatic fever, there may be permanent valve damage. Rheumatic heart disease occurs when acute valve inflammation is followed by scarring and fibrosis, resulting in various degrees of shortening, thickening, rigidity, deformity, retraction and fusion of the valve cusps. The commonest valve lesions are mitral regurgitation, mitral stenosis and aortic regurgitation. Rheumatic heart disease is most severe and progressive in the following:

- patients who initially have severe carditis
- patients who have recurrent episodes of acute rheumatic fever. The prognosis is more favourable if recurrences are prevented. After single episodes, residual cardiac disease may disappear or improve, and valve damage only worsens in a few cases. It is therefore crucial to maintain continuous antibiotic prophylaxis to prevent further valve damage.
- Asymptomatic rheumatic valve disease often becomes clinically relevant during pregnancy. A history of rheumatic fever should be sought at booking and ideally the heart auscultated for murmers. It should be remembered as a differential diagnosis in a women presenting with shortness of breath, a cardiac arrhythmia or heart failure.

When a cardiology referral and/or surgical intervention is not available

- Medical management is supportive, aiming to maximise cardiac function. The most dangerous period is delivery and shortly afterwards. In general, the more normal the delivery the less stress there is on the heart.
- Regular follow-up and rational drug therapy can make a significant difference. Use routine medications (diuretics, B-blocker, digoxin and nitrates) to maximum effect.
- Bed rest and the avoidance of heavy work are essential.
- Treat anaemia and any other coexisting conditions.
- Advise hospital delivery.
- Venesection can be used to decrease venous load for the patient in life-threatening situations where preload is high.

Note that there is a risk of teratogenicity with ACE inhibitors during the first trimester, and problems with placental and renal function later in pregnancy. There is also diminished placental perfusion with diuretics although these should not be withheld if clinically indicated. ACE inhibitors may be used after delivery and during breastfeeding.

Effects of rheumatic heart disease
Mitral regurgitation

Mitral regurgitation is the commonest valve lesion.

Clinical features

These include the following:
- easy fatigue (caused by low cardiac output)
- shortness of breath on exertion (caused by pulmonary oedema and inability to increase cardiac output)
- orthopnoea, paroxysmal nocturnal dyspnoea and haemoptysis
- hyperdynamic apical impulse

- apical impulse displaced laterally and inferiorly
- a blowing apical pansystolic murmur radiating to the left axilla; there may be a third heart sound and a short low-frequency mid-diastolic murmur from increased trans-mitral flow
- there may be basal crepitations
- chest X-ray demonstrates cardiomegaly and left atrial enlargement (a double density on the right heart border and elevation of the left main bronchus)
- the ECG demonstrates left atrial enlargement (broad bifid P waves in lead II and a prominent negative component to the P in V1) and left ventricular hypertrophy
- signs of pulmonary hypertension.

Management

- Urgent referral for a cardiology opinion, as surgery is likely to be necessary (if available).
- Annual echocardiograph (if available), as progressive left heart dilation may result in irreversible left ventricular dysfunction if referral is delayed until symptoms develop.
- Medical treatment for heart failure, but patients who are unwell enough to require this may be more appropriately treated by mitral valve repair or mitral valve replacement with a mechanical valve or bioprosthesis, if possible locally.

Mitral stenosis
Features

- Mild stenosis does not cause symptoms, moderate stenosis causes shortness of breath on exertion, and severe stenosis causes easy fatigue, shortness of breath at rest, orthopnoea (shortness of breath on lying down), paroxysmal nocturnal dyspnoea and haemoptysis.
- There is a low-frequency mid-diastolic murmur that is maximal at the apex, accentuated by exercise.
- There is a loud first heart sound and diastolic opening snap.
- The murmur becomes longer as the severity of stenosis increases.
- In severe cases, there are signs of pulmonary hypertension.
- Chest X-ray and ECG show left atrial enlargement when there is moderate mitral stenosis, and chest X-ray shows pulmonary oedema when stenosis is severe.

Management

- Symptoms are treated with diuretics and a low-sodium diet. Digoxin is indicated only in rare cases where there is atrial fibrillation secondary to left atrial enlargement.
- Symptomatic patients and those with pulmonary hypertension should be referred for cardiology review (if available), as surgery is often necessary (open or closed mitral commissurotomy, mitral valve replacement and percutaneous catheter balloon mitral commissurotomy).

Aortic regurgitation

- This is less common than mitral regurgitation, and frequently occurs in combination with mitral valve disease.
- Symptoms occur when left ventricular dysfunction develops secondary to chronic left ventricular volume overload.
- Once the symptoms have appeared, deterioration is often rapid.
- Symptoms include exercise intolerance, shortness of

breath on exertion, orthopnoea (shortness of breath on lying down), paroxysmal nocturnal dyspnoea, haemoptysis and chest pain.

- Examination reveals a blowing decrescendo early diastolic murmur that is maximal at the mid to lower left sternal border. The murmur is loudest when sitting forward with the breath held in expiration.

Signs of moderate to severe aortic regurgitation

- The murmur lengthens and may be present throughout diastole.
- Hyperdynamic apex.
- Apical impulse displaced laterally and inferiorly.
- Wide pulse pressure.
- Collapsing pulses.
- Basal crepitations.
- Visible pulsations in the suprasternal notch and neck vessels.
- Systolic murmur at the upper right sternal border (from increased aortic valve flow).

Management

- Cardiology assessment, as surgery may be necessary (if available). Marked cardiomegaly on chest X-ray or multiple ventricular ectopics on the ECG should prompt referral.
- An echocardiogram is needed at least annually (if available), as it is important to assess left ventricular dilation and function to ensure that surgery is performed before irreversible left ventricular dysfunction develops.
- Exercise tolerance may be improved by medical treatment for heart failure.

- Surgical options include aortic valve reconstruction, aortic valve replacement with an aortic homograft or mechanical valve, and transferring the patient's own pulmonary valve to the aortic position (Ross procedure).

Aortic stenosis

The two commonest causes of aortic valve stenosis are progressive wear of a congenital bicuspid aortic valve and rheumatic fever (the most common cause in developing countries, and usually also with aortic regurgitation).

Clinical features

- Chest pain (angina from inadequate coronary artery perfusion).
- Fainting, usually with exertion or excitement.
- Shortness of breath due to heart failure.
- Sudden death.
- On examination, delayed upstroke and reduced magnitude of the carotid pulse and an ejection systolic heart murmur.
- The ECG shows left ventricular hypertrophy and sometimes ST changes of myocardial ischaemia.
- The chest X-ray shows a normal sized heart, dilated aortic root and pulmonary venous congestion. Sometimes there is calcification of the aortic valve.

Management

- Avoid strenuous exercise.
- Avoid endocarditis.
- Refer for a specialist opinion if possible.
- Diuretics can be helpful, but surgery is usually required.

2.7.B Asthma

BOX 2.7.B.1 Minimum standards
- ■ Oxygen.
- ■ Salbutamol by metered-dose inhaler and nebuliser.
- ■ Aminophylline.
- ■ Magnesium sulphate.
- ■ Adrenaline.
- ■ Prednisolone/hydrocortisone.

Assessment

Features of severe asthma
- Too breathless to feed or talk.
- Recession/use of accessory muscles.
- Respiratory rate > 40 breaths/minute.
- Pulse rate > 120 beats/minute.

Features of life-threatening asthma
- Conscious level depressed/agitated.
- Exhaustion.
- Poor respiratory effort.
- SaO_2 < 85% in air/cyanosis.
- Silent chest.

Asthma complicates 3–4% of pregnancies. Pregnancy is associated with worsening of the symptoms in one-third of affected mothers.

- A chest X-ray is indicated only if there is severe dyspnoea, uncertainty about the diagnosis, asymmetry of chest signs (possible pneumothorax) or signs of severe infection.
- Transcutaneous PCO_2, arterial or capillary blood gases (if available) can be helpful in very severe asthma.
- Continuous pulse oximetry is valuable (if available), as hypoxaemia is a major feature of all severe asthma attacks.
- **Do not give prostaglandins other than misoprostol (the latter is safe in pregnancy).** For the prevention and treatment of postpartum haemorrhage, give oxytocin 10 units IM or ergometrine 500 micrograms IM or both (Syntometrine IM).
- **Do not give labetalol for hypertension in patients with asthma.**
- The priority of treatment is to maintain good control of the patient's asthma. This will reduce the likelihood of acute exacerbations which can be life-threatening. In order that control is maintained the following are recommended:
  - It should be emphasised that inhaled salbutamol and steroids are not harmful to the fetus and should be continued in pregnancy.

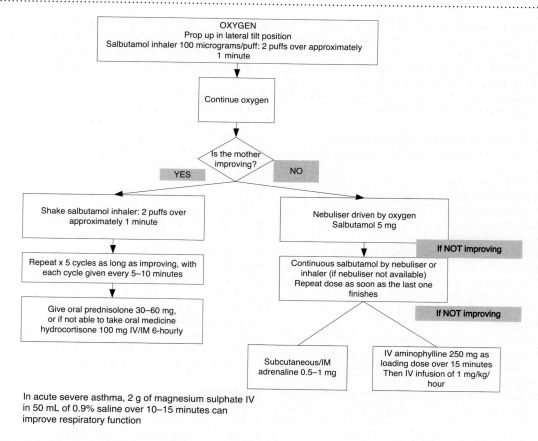

FIGURE 2.7.B.1 Pathway of care for pregnant mother with severe asthma.

— The aim should be for the patient to need her salbutamol inhaler no more than 1–2 times/day. If use in excess of this occurs, the patient should be commenced on inhaled steroids or have her current dose of inhaled steroids increased.

— If the maximum dose of inhaled steroids is reached, then long acting B₂-agonists and slow release theophylline should be considered if available.

— If not available, or ineffective, oral prednisolone can be added at the lowest dose required to maintain control. Oral prednisolone is associated with an increased risk of infection and gestational diabetes, and complicates control of established diabetes. Its long term use has other potential side-effects for the mother, such as osteoporosis, but it should not be withheld if required to maintain control of maternal disease.

Emergency treatment of severe asthma

- Assess ABC and resuscitate as needed.
- Give a high concentration of **oxygen** via a face mask with reservoir bag or nasal cannula. Attach a pulse oximeter and maintain SaO₂ in the range 94–98%.
- Sit the patient up.
- Give nebulised salbutamol 5 mg driven with oxygen half-hourly to 4-hourly via a nebuliser (or 10–20 puffs of a beta-2-agonist inhaler, such as salbutamol or terbutaline, giving one puff at a time through a spacer with a mouthpiece or face mask).
- Give oral prednisolone 30–60 mg, or if the patient is vomiting, IV/IM hydrocortisone 100 mg, followed by

100 mg 6-hourly. (**Note:** steroids will not show benefits for a number of hours.)

If the patient is not responding, or their condition is deteriorating:

- **Nebulised salbutamol** may be given continuously.
- In acute severe asthma, 2 g of **magnesium sulphate** IV in 50 mL of Ringer-lactate or Hartmann's solution over 10–15 minutes can produce significant bronchodilatation.
- As an alternative to magnesium sulphate, and if the patient is not already on oral theophylline or other methylxanthines, give a loading dose of IV **aminophylline** 250 mg over 15 minutes, monitoring the ECG for arrhythmias (if possible), followed by 1 mg/kg/hour by IV infusion.
- **IV salbutamol** 250 micrograms over 10 minutes **is an alternative** to magnesium sulphate or aminophylline, followed by IV infusion of 1–5 micrograms/kg/minute (but monitoring ECG and checking K⁺ levels regularly is necessary; extra potassium may be needed, and monitoring of plasma K⁺ levels is essential if this drug is given IV).
- In severe cases in the absence of other measures, **adrenaline** can be effective. It should be given subcutaneously or IM (dose = 500 micrograms to 1 mg), but may be given IV in life-threatening asthma as follows.

— Place 1 mg of adrenaline in 10 mL of 0.9% saline and give 1 mL of this solution. Wait for 1 minute and then keep on repeating 1 mL doses IV every minute until the patient improves or the whole 1 mg (10 mL) has

2.7.D Diabetes mellitus

> **BOX 2.7.D.1 Minimum standards**
> - Insulin.
> - Blood glucose measurements.
> - 0.9% saline or Plasma-Lyte 148.
> - Oral and IV potassium.
> - Mannitol.
> - Nasogastric tube.

Introduction

Diabetes mellitus is associated with increased maternal mortality and morbidity, as well as increased perinatal mortality and morbidity, including congenital malformations. Pregnancy causes changes in the maternal physiology to make it a diabetogenic state. Women who have pre-existing diabetes have an increased insulin requirement in pregnancy. Previously healthy women may develop gestational diabetes. Both type 2 diabetes and gestational diabetes are more common in certain ethnic groups, including South Asians, and are more common in those with a high body mass index (BMI).

Before the discovery of insulin, maternal mortality in diabetics and perinatal mortality in their infants were extremely high. Insulin has led to a dramatic improvement in maternal survival, but in comparison with non-diabetic pregnancy there is still a three- to fivefold increase in perinatal mortality, and an increase in congenital malformations. These risks can be reduced by strict attention to the control of the diabetes both before and during pregnancy.

Diabetes predisposes to pre-eclampsia.

Management

Before pregnancy

- Advise any diabetics of reproductive age about the importance of close monitoring and modified treatment in pregnancy.
- Obesity: give dietary advice.
- Tight control of diabetes: aim for blood glucose levels of less than 7.5 mmol/litre and HbA1c levels within normal limits.
- The mother should take folic acid 5 mg daily if planning pregnancy.

In early pregnancy

- Nausea and vomiting are common.
- Hypoglycaemia is common in insulin-treated diabetes. Provide glucagon at home if possible, and explain its use to other household members. Alternatively, counsel the patient to keep sugar-containing foods close by. Inform the patient and others about the signs of hypoglycaemia.
- It is not always necessary to convert mothers treated with oral hypoglycaemic agents to insulin. Metformin is commonly used in these circumstances (initially 500 mg with breakfast for 1 week, then 500 mg twice daily with breakfast and tea, and then 500 mg three times daily with breakfast, lunch and tea).
- As soon as possible, assess the gestational age. Early ultrasound scan can detect anencephaly, but 20 weeks'

gestation is usually the best time to look at the spine and heart if facilities are available.

During pregnancy
Type 1 diabetes (insulin dependent)

Close control of diabetes is needed. Expect insulin requirements to increase by up to 50% above pre-pregnant levels. There is an increased risk of congenital abnormalities, macrosomia, polyhydramnios, preterm labour and pre-eclampsia. Plan delivery with care. The risks of infection and development of diabetic ketoacidosis are high. Signs of hyperglycaemia include a gradual onset of drowsiness and polyuria, dehydration, hypotension, difficulty breathing, and a ketotic smell to the breath. Signs and symptoms of hypoglycaemia may be of rapid onset, leading to unconsciousness, particularly if the mother has taken insulin but has not taken her usual food. Awareness of impending hypoglycaemia in those with type 1 diabetes is often reduced in pregnancy. These patients must be advised about the possible effects on safety during driving.

The insulin requirement often escalates rapidly, especially in the late second and early third trimester, and in order to maintain control of the blood glucose, frequent medical review every 1 to 2 weeks coupled with frequent self-assessment of blood glucose levels, is likely to be required for women with type 1 diabetes.

Type 2 diabetes

Women who are diet-controlled before pregnancy require careful monitoring of blood sugar levels in pregnancy, and may need metformin and/or insulin.

Gestational diabetes

This is often undiagnosed, and should be suspected if any of the following are present:

- a family history of diabetes
- a past history of a large baby, stillbirth or gestational diabetes
- recurrent glycosuria
- a high BMI (overweight)
- a relevant ethnic background.

All women with diabetes should ideally be monitored more regularly in the antenatal clinic for complications such as

Diagnosis of diabetes with a glucose tolerance test

TABLE 2.7.D.1 Seventy-five-gram oral glucose loading dose results

	Fasting plasma glucose concentration (mmol/litre)	2-hour plasma glucose concentration (mmol/litre)
Diabetes	> 8	> 11
Gestational impaired glucose tolerance	6–8	9–11
Normal	< 6	< 9

pre-eclampsia, polyhydramnios and a large or small for gestational age infant.

Management of delivery in women with diabetes

For spontaneous labour, induction of labour and elective Caesarean section:

1 Measure glucose on admission and hourly during labour.
2 Site an IV line with 500 mL of 0.9% saline containing 10% dextrose and potassium chloride 10 mmol, and give at a rate of 60 mL/hour.

Avoid the routine use of insulin in labour in low resource settings because of lack of experience and lack of blood glucose stick tests. In mothers who were using insulin during pregnancy and those where blood glucose is > 7 mmol/litre on two successive occasions one hour apart in labour, the insulin requirements shown in Table 2.7.D.2 below can be used.

TABLE 2.7.D.2 Insulin requirements

Blood glucose concentration (mmol/litre)	Hourly subcutaneous injections of insulin
< 2.0	No insulin; dextrose only
2.0–4.0	1 unit
4.1–9.0	2 units
9.1–11.0	3 units
11.1–16.9	4 units

NOTE: for blood glucose, 1 mmol/litre = 18 mg/dL

- If the glucose level is > 17 mmol/litre, expert advice should be sought.
- Aim for a glucose level of 4–9 mmol/litre.
- Reduce insulin by half at delivery, and aim to resume the pre-pregnancy insulin dosage 24 hours after delivery. If the mother is breastfeeding, her insulin requirement may be lower.
- Women who have developed gestational diabetes usually have normal blood glucose levels soon after the delivery of the placenta. Their diabetic medication should be stopped postnatally, and their blood sugar levels should be monitored.
- Mothers who have had gestational diabetes should have a glucose tolerance test at 6 weeks postnatally. They are at risk of developing type 2 diabetes, and appropriate dietary and lifestyle advice should be provided. A fasting blood glucose test annually should also be recommended.

Diabetic ketoacidosis (DKA)

DKA is the commonest endocrine emergency, and should be suspected in patients with any of the following:
- dehydration
- abdominal pain
- ketone smell on the breath
- acidosis
- acidotic breathing
- unexplained coma.

Patients die from hypokalaemia and cerebral oedema.
Patients who are 5% dehydrated or less and are not clinically unwell usually tolerate oral rehydration and subcutaneous insulin.

Patients who are more than 5% dehydrated, or who are vomiting or drowsy or clinically acidotic, need emergency care as follows.

Primary assessment and resuscitation
Airway
- If the airway is not open, use an airway-opening manoeuvre, and consider an airway adjunct such as an oropharyngeal airway or intubation (if available and subsequently supported).
- The nares and oropharynx may need gentle suctioning under direct observation.
- If the patient is unconscious and the airway is unprotected, the recovery position should be adopted to minimise the risk of aspiration of vomit.

Breathing
Give a high concentration of oxygen through a face mask with a reservoir, if the airway is adequate.

If breathing is inadequate, ventilate with oxygen via a bag-valve-mask-reservoir device, and ask for experienced senior help to intubate (if this is available and sustainable).

Circulation
- Gain IV access using a short wide-bore cannula (14- to 16G).
- External or internal jugular vein access is an option if peripheral access is impossible. Long saphenous vein cut-down may also be considered.
- Take blood for a full blood count, urea and electrolytes, blood culture, cross-matching, glucose stick test and laboratory blood glucose (if available).
- Give a 500-mL rapid IV bolus of 0.9% saline or Plasma-Lyte 148.
- An antibiotic such as cefotaxime 1 gram IV 6-hourly, or the locally available equivalent, is an appropriate antibiotic for those in whom an infection is likely to have precipitated the DKA. Although, of course, antibiotic therapy must be tailored to the specific cause.

Diagnosis
- History:
  - polydipsia
  - polyuria
  - weight loss.
- Clinical:
  - acidotic respiration
  - dehydration
  - drowsiness
  - abdominal pain and/or vomiting.
- Biochemical:
  - high blood glucose on finger-prick test
  - ketones and glucose in urine.

Secondary assessment and emergency treatment
The following in particular need to be assessed.

Degree of dehydration
- 3%: dehydration is only just clinically detectable
- 3–5%: dry mucous membranes and reduced skin turgor

- 5–8%: as above, with sunken eyes and poor capillary return
- > 8% with shock: severely ill with poor perfusion, thready rapid pulse and reduced blood pressure.

Conscious level
- Assess AVPU.
- Institute hourly neurological observations.
- If the patient is less than **A**lert on admission, or their conscious level deteriorates, record the Glasgow Coma Scale score.
- Consider instituting cerebral oedema management (if available).

Cerebral oedema
Look for irritability, slow pulse, high blood pressure and papilloedema (a late sign).

Infection
DKA can cause a leucocytosis but not fever. If fever is present, look for and treat infection.

Ileus
- Insert a nasogastric tube.
- Ensure by clinical assessment, and by abdominal X-ray if appropriate, that there is no other cause of the acute abdomen, including intestinal obstruction.

Observations
- Strict fluid balance and urine testing of every sample.
- Hourly capillary blood glucose measurements.
- Twice daily weights.
- Initially hourly or more frequent neurological observations.
- Report immediately to medical staff (even at night) symptoms of headache or any change in either conscious level or behaviour.
- Report any changes in the ECG trace, especially T-wave changes (monitoring for hypokalaemia).

Investigations
- When it is safe to do so, weigh the patient. If this is not possible, use recent clinic weight or an estimated weight.
- Blood glucose.
- Urea and electrolytes (if available).
- Bicarbonate or arterial blood gases (if available).
- Haematocrit and full blood count.
- Blood culture.
- Urine microscopy, culture and sensitivity; check for ketones.
- Monitor the ECG to observe T waves (if available):
  - **hypokalaemia** causes flat T waves
  - **hyperkalaemia** causes peaked T waves.
- Other investigations if indicated (e.g. if fever is present).

Additional emergency treatment
General
- After resuscitation with fluid boluses, calculate the fluid requirement (see below).
- Avoid excessive fluid replacement, as this is a risk factor for cerebral oedema.
- **Do not give hypotonic IV solutions** (e.g. 0.18% saline with 4% glucose, or 5% glucose): they are risk factors for cerebral oedema.
- Continue to give IV fluids until the patient is drinking.

- After fluids are running, calculate the rate of insulin infusion (blood glucose levels will already be falling).
- Use a continuous low-dose IV infusion of insulin (there is no need for an initial bolus), or in resource-limited situations use regular subcutaneous injections of short-acting insulin based on a sliding scale according to blood glucose measurements. Details below.
- Continue to give IV fluids until the patient is tolerating enteral fluids.

Fluid and electrolyte management
- Calculate the patient's fluid requirement. This is equal to maintenance plus deficit (see Figure 2.7.D.1).
  - Maintenance
  - Deficit (litres) = percentage dehydration × body weight (kg)/100
  - Only plan to correct up to an 8% deficit, as any more risks over-infusion.
- Ignore the volume of fluids used to resuscitate/treat shock.
- Give the total fluid requirement over 24 hours:

Glucose > 12 mmol/litre: give 0.9% saline or Plasma-Lyte 148.

Glucose < 12 mmol/litre: give 0.9% saline or Plasma-Lyte 148 containing 5% dextrose (by adding 100 mL of 50% glucose to 900 mL of 0.9% saline or Plasma-Lyte 148).

Sodium 135–155 mmol/litre: correct by rehydration over 24 hours.

Sodium > 155 mmol/litre: correct by rehydration over 48 hours using 0.9% saline or Plasma-Lyte 148.

Expect the sodium level to rise initially as the glucose level falls and water is removed from the circulation.

If the plasma sodium level initially falls (as well as the glucose level), this may precipitate cerebral oedema.

Bicarbonate
- **Administration of bicarbonate is rarely, if ever, necessary.**
- Continuing acidosis usually indicates insufficient fluid resuscitation.
- Consider the use of bicarbonate in patients who are profoundly acidotic (pH < 7.0 if measurable) and shocked. Its only purpose is to improve cardiac contractility in severe shock.

The maximum volume of 8.4% sodium bicarbonate for half-correction of acidosis is calculated according to the following formula, and given over 60 minutes:

$$\text{Volume (mL 8.4\% NaHCO}_3) = \frac{{}^{1}/_{3} \times \text{weight (kg)} \times \text{base deficit (mmol/litre)}}{2}$$

If blood gas analysis cannot be undertaken:
- The kidneys will resolve the acidosis (if they are working) if the patient receives adequate fluid and insulin therapy.
- If you cannot measure pH, then do not give bicarbonate except in extremis.

Potassium
In diabetic ketoacidosis there is always massive depletion of total body potassium, although initial plasma levels may

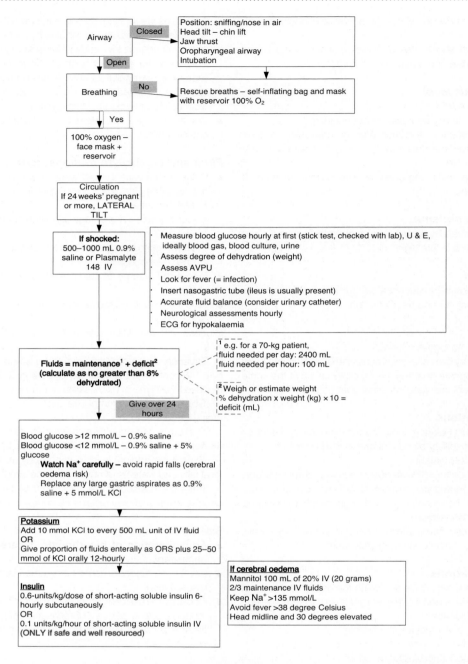

FIGURE 2.7.D.1 Pathway of care for severe diabetic ketoacidosis in pregnancy. AVPU scale: alert, responds to verbal stimulus, responds to pain, unresponsive; ORS, oral rehydration solution.

be low, normal or even high. Levels in the blood will fall once insulin is started.

Do not give potassium if any of the following are present:

- anuria
- peaked T waves on the ECG
- serum potassium level > 7.0 mmol/litre.

If biochemical assessment of the K+ is not possible, it should be assumed that K+ replacement is necessary as long as the urine output is adequate, and there are no peaked T-waves present on the ECG (where available).

- In resource-limited settings, hypokalaemia is most safely corrected enterally using ORS with or without

additional oral potassium supplements (aim for a total of 100 mmol/day).

- Potassium rich foods may also be given, e.g. coconut milk and bananas.
- If oral supplementation is not possible or the patient is severely ill: start IV potassium supplements with 20 mmol/litre of IV fluid given after the start of initiating therapy with insulin and fluids as long as sufficient urine is being passed at > 30 mL/hour.
- Run the IV infusion (20 mmol in 1 litre over 4 to 8 hours (42 to 84 drops per minute (dpm) if using a standard IV giving set with a drop factor of 20). It should not be given at a rate exceeding 20 mmol in 2 hours (126 dpm) as this is dangerous. Given the difficulty in accurately

monitoring transfusion rates without an electronic pump, a large margin of error should be used.
- Stop IV supplementation when the patient can take oral supplements.

Insulin

In **resource-limited settings**, give subcutaneous doses of short-acting soluble insulin 6-hourly at 0.6 units/kg/dose (i.e. 0.1 units/kg/hour). Give half the dose if the blood sugar level is falling too fast.

Always have an IV glucose solution (10% or 50%) available to treat any hypoglycaemia that develops.

In **well-resourced settings**, make up a solution of 1 unit/mL of human soluble insulin (e.g. Actrapid) by adding 50 units of insulin to 50 mL of 0.9% saline or Plasma-Lyte 148 in a syringe pump. Using a Y-connector, attach this to the IV fluids that are already running. Do not add insulin directly to the fluid bags. The solution should then run at 0.1 units/kg/hour (0.1 mL/kg/hour).

- If the blood glucose level falls by more than 5 mmol/litre/hour, reduce the infusion rate to 0.05 units/kg/hour.
- If the blood glucose level is less than 12 mmol/litre, and a dextrose-containing fluid has been started, consider reducing the insulin infusion rate.
- Do not stop the insulin infusion while dextrose is being infused, as insulin is required to switch off ketone production.
- If the blood glucose level falls below 7 mmol/litre, consider adding extra glucose to the infusion.
- If the blood glucose level rises out of control, re-evaluate the patient for sepsis or another condition.
- Discontinue the insulin infusion 30 minutes after the first subcutaneous injection, to avoid rebound hyperglycaemia.

Other management

Urine output
- Urinary catheterisation may be useful in patients with impaired consciousness.
- Document all fluid input and output.
- Test all urine samples for glucose and ketones.
- If a massive diuresis continues, the fluid input may need to be increased.

Gastric aspirate
- If large volumes of gastric aspirate occur, replace these volume for volume with 0.9% saline or Plasma-Lyte 148 plus 5 mmol/litre potassium chloride (KCl).

Biochemistry
- Check urea and electrolytes, blood pH/bicarbonate (if available), and laboratory blood glucose 2 hours after the start of resuscitation, and then at least 4-hourly.
- Do not expect ketones to have disappeared completely before changing to subcutaneous insulin.

Never give an IV insulin infusion without a syringe driver. This is not safe. It is better to use a sliding scale of subcutaneous rapid-acting insulin.

Cerebral oedema

Cerebral oedema in DKA:
- is unpredictable
- occurs more often in new diabetics
- has a mortality of around 80%.

Signs and symptoms
These include the following:
- headache
- confusion
- irritability
- reduced conscious level
- fits
- small pupils
- increasing blood pressure
- slowing pulse
- possible respiratory impairment.

Management
- Exclude hypoglycaemia.
- Give 20 grams of 20% mannitol over 15 minutes **as soon as cerebral oedema is suspected**. Repeat every 4–6 hours.
- Restrict IV fluids to two-thirds maintenance, and replace the deficit over 72 hours rather than 24 hours.
- Arrange for the patient to be intubated. Keep the $PaCO_2$ in the range 3.5–5.0 kPa (if this is possible and sustainable).
- Keep the sodium (Na^+) concentration higher than 135 mmol/litre.
- Keep the head in the midline and 30-degrees elevated.

If there is a fever, treat it actively with environmental measures, or with paracetamol, if more than 38.0°C.

2.7.E Reduced consciousness and coma

Introduction

In resource-limited countries, severe pre-eclampsia, eclampsia, malaria, meningitis (including TB), HIV infection, head injury and drug ingestion are the most common causes of reduced conscious level and coma in pregnancy.

Pathophysiology

Raised intracranial pressure (RICP) is an important component of the most severe cases. This can occur gradually or rapidly (e.g. due to intracranial bleeding or cerebral oedema). The initial physiological compensating mechanisms include a reduction in the volume of cerebrospinal fluid and in the volume of venous blood within the cranium. However, when these fail, the cerebral perfusion pressure (CPP) falls and arterial blood flow to the brain is reduced.

Cerebral perfusion pressure (CPP) = mean arterial pressure (MAP) – intracranial pressure (ICP).

A severely increased pressure within the skull will

cause pressure effects which are classically recognised in two main sites where brain tissue is pushed against the bone:

1 **Central syndrome:** cerebellar tonsils herniate through the foramen magnum. This is known as **coning**. The syndrome consists of slowing pulse, rising blood pressure and irregular respiration.

2 **Uncal syndrome:** the uncus (part of the hippocampal gyrus) is pushed through the tentorium. It may be unilateral. This leads to third cranial nerve compression and ipsilateral dilated pupil, followed by oculomotor palsy and failure of lateral gaze. Later effects include hemiplegia.

Raised intracranial pressure (RICP)

In a patient with impaired conscious level or with a Glasgow Coma Scale score of < 9, who was previously well and is not post-ictal, the following signs indicate raised ICP:

Absolute signs of raised ICP:
Papilloedema
Absence of pulsation of retinal vessels

Signs suggesting raised ICP:	
Abnormal oculo-cephalic reflexes **Do not test patients with neck injuries in this way**	(a) Rotation of the head to the left or right normally causes the eyes to move in the opposite direction; abnormal if there is no response or a random response
	(b) Flexure of neck usually causes eye gaze deviation upwards; abnormal if there is loss of this reflex
Abnormal posture May need to be elicited by a painful stimulus	(a) Decorticate: arms flexed, legs extended (b) Decerebrate: arms extended, legs extended (see Figure 5.16.A.3)
Abnormal pupillary responses	Unilateral or bilateral suggests raised ICP
Abnormal breathing patterns	Ranges from hyperventilation to Cheyne–Stokes breathing to apnoea
Cushing's triad	Slow pulse, raised blood pressure and abnormal pattern of breathing – a late sign of raised ICP

Primary assessment and resuscitation ABC

Call for help. Ideally an anaesthetist should be present to manage the airway and support breathing.

The first steps in the management of the patient with decreased conscious level are to assess and if necessary support airway, breathing and circulation.

Airway

The patient with a reduced level of consciousness is more likely to have a compromised airway as the tongue falls into the back of the mouth. There is also a risk of aspiration.

Look, listen and feel

Assess the airway, open it if closed and keep it open, either by assigning someone to continue airway-opening

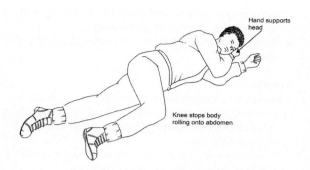

FIGURE 2.7.E.1 The semi-prone or recovery position.

manoeuvres or by using adjuncts such as an oropharyngeal airway (see Section 1.13). Never use such an airway if the patient is conscious enough to have a gag reflex, as it may worsen airway obstruction and cause vomiting. Give oxygen at a rate of 15 litre/minute or as high a flow rate as is available, via a tight-fitting face mask with a reservoir bag. If an anaesthetist is present, intubation can be performed to protect the airway; otherwise adopt the recovery position (see Figure 2.7.E.1). Careful suction of the nose and/or mouth may be helpful.

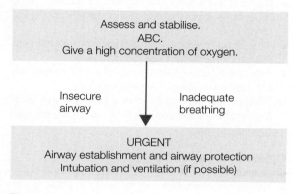

The patient will require support if:
- breathing is insufficient
- gag or cough reflex is absent
- GCS score is < 9, or AVPU score is P or U
- there is impending herniation due to raised ICP
- there is evidence of effects of inadequate breathing on other systems.

If the airway is adequate, give high concentration O_2 and support breathing if required.

Breathing

Assess the breathing for depth and frequency, and give high-flow oxygen via a face mask and reservoir bag. If breathing is absent or inadequate (gasping or agonal breaths only), provide assisted ventilation using a bag-valve-mask with a reservoir and oxygen.

Inadequate airway and breathing in coma can lead to a rise in arterial pCO_2 that can cause a dangerous rise in intracranial pressure.

Circulation

Inadequate perfusion of blood to the brain initially produces confusion and later causes coma. Measurement of the blood pressure in addition to other markers for shock is crucial in recognising hypovolaemia after haemorrhage, or unconsciousness after an eclamptic fit with hypertension.

If the intracranial pressure is high, cerebral perfusion will be compromised if hypotension occurs. However, excessive fluid administration should be avoided.

- Establish IV access quickly.
- Take blood samples and send them to the lab for a full blood count, blood smear for malarial parasites, electrolytes, liver function tests, blood glucose and blood culture.

Neurological failure

Assess neurological failure as follows:

- Use the AVPU scale.
- Check blood glucose levels: **If the blood sugar level is low or suspected to be low (< 2.5 mmol/litre or < 45 mg/dL)**, give 100 mL of 25% glucose IV over 15 minutes (dilute 50 mL of 50% glucose with 50 mL of Ringer-lactate or Hartmann's solution) and then give 10% dextrose in Ringer-lactate or Hartmann's solution over 4 hours (add 100 mL of 50% glucose to each 400 mL of Ringer-lactate or Hartmann's solution infused).
- Check the pupils for **signs suggesting raised intracranial pressure (RICP) or opiate overdose**.
- Check for **neck stiffness** which may suggest meningitis.
- Look for other signs of raised intracranial pressure, as outlined above.

Further assessment of conscious level can be aided by the Glasgow Coma Scale score and documentation of pupil function.

TABLE 2.7.E.1 Glasgow Coma Scale (GCS)

Response	Score
Eye opening	
Spontaneously	4
To verbal stimuli	3
To pain	2
No response to pain	1
Best motor response	
Obeys verbal command	6
Localises to pain	5
Withdraws from pain	4
Abnormal flexion to pain (decorticate)	3
Abnormal extension to pain (decerebrate)	2
No response to pain	1
Best verbal response	
Orientated and converses	5
Disorientated and converses	4
Inappropriate words	3
Incomprehensible sounds	2
No response to pain	1
Total	

A GCS score of < 9 is likely to need airway protection by intubation if skills are available to undertake this safely.

TABLE 2.7.E.2 Pupillary changes

Pupil size and reactivity	Causes
Small reactive pupils	Metabolic disorders
	Medullary lesion
Pinpoint pupil	Metabolic disorders
	Narcotic/organophosphate ingestion
Fixed mid-sized pupils	Midbrain lesion
Fixed dilated pupils	Hypothermia
	Severe hypoxaemic/ischaemic brain injury
	Barbiturate ingestion (late sign)
	During and post seizure
	Anticholinergic drugs
Unilateral dilated pupil	Rapidly expanding ipsilateral lesion
	Tentorial herniation
	Third cranial nerve lesion
	Epileptic seizures

Secondary assessment and emergency treatment

Secondary assessment occurs after stabilisation of ABCD. During secondary assessment, continue to monitor the patient, and if there is any change, reassess ABC and treat any residual problems.

Diagnostic pointers

As soon as possible during resuscitation, gain as much information about the history as possible:

- the possibility of eclampsia, which means that magnesium sulphate may be required
- recent trauma
- endemic area for infections such as malaria, sleeping sickness and encephalitis
- pre-existing neurological problem
- past history of epilepsy
- ingestion of poisons
- underlying chronic condition (renal, cardiac, diabetes).

Remember to treat the treatable components. The cause of coma may not be certain, so it is always important to address ABC. If the patient's condition is unstable or deteriorating, return to ABC.

Always consider the possibility of eclampsia and the need for magnesium sulphate.

If there is no other clear cause for the coma treat with antibiotics for presumed meningitis (usually a third-generation cephalosporin, or whatever is locally available and appropriate), and in endemic areas, also treat as for cerebral malaria (*see* Section 2.8.D).

Take the patient's temperature (core and peripheral).

- **Fever** may be associated with sepsis (but lack of fever does not exclude sepsis) or poisoning (ecstasy, cocaine or salicylates).
- **Hypothermia** is found in poisoning with ethanol or barbiturates.

Rash: **purpura** suggests meningococcal disease; **bruises** suggest trauma (consider domestic violence).

Evidence of **poisoning**, ingestion or drug use: smell, residue around nose/mouth, needle tracks.

Other issues in addition to ABC regarding the management of coma

The prognosis depends on the cause of coma and the state of the patient, in particular the level of consciousness on admission, and the initial response to appropriate interventions. The presumptive cause of coma guides the treatment. Consider the following interventions:

- Assess and **maintain electrolyte balance** (avoid **hyponatraemia**; use Ringer-lactate or Hartmann's solution plus added 5% glucose, **not 1/5 N dextrose saline**. Add 50 mL of 50% glucose to each 450 mL of Ringer-lactate or Hartmann's solution infused). If possible keep the serum sodium level in the normal range (135–145 mmol/litre).
- Treat seizures if present, and give prophylactic **anticonvulsants** if the patient has repeated seizures.
- Insert a **nasogastric tube** to aspirate the stomach contents. Perform gastric lavage in circumstances such as drug ingestion.
- Regulate the body temperature, and **avoid hyperthermia** (i.e. temperatures above 37.5°C).
- Undertake appropriate medical management of **RICP**, if noted:
  - Support ventilation (maintain a pCO$_2$ of 3.5–5.0 kPa, if measurable).
  - Give mannitol, 20 grams of 20% mannitol IV over 15 minutes, 2-hourly as required, provided that the serum osmolality is not greater than 325 mOsm/litre (if measurable).
  - Give dexamethasone (for oedema surrounding a space-occupying lesion) 10 mg initially IV, then 4 mg IV 6-hourly for 48 hours.
- **Catheterisation** is needed for bladder care and output monitoring, as well as for avoidance of retention, which can worsen RICP.
- Plan for continued **regular clinical assessment**, mainly nursing observations.
- **Prevent the patient from falling out of the bed.**
- **Provide nutritional support:** parenteral and/or oral feeding to prevent malnutrition during the period of unconsciousness.
- **Skin care:** prevent bed sores by turning the patient.
- **Eye padding:** to avoid xerophthalmia.
- Family **counselling, support and consent** in the case of invasive procedures.
- Appropriate surgical intervention if indicated.
- **Chest physiotherapy** to avoid hypostatic pneumonia.
- Restrict fluids to 60% of maintenance if evidence of water retention is seen.
- Prevent **deep vein thrombosis** by physiotherapy.
- Maintain **oral and dental hygiene**.
- Give appropriate care for central and peripheral venous access to **avoid infection** by maintaining sterility when handling the sites.
- Prevent hospital-acquired infection.

Reassessment

When the patient is stable, undertake a full examination of systems and neurological examination.

- Skin: rash, bruising, haemorrhage, neurocutaneous stigmata.

- Scalp: trauma.
- Ears/nose: discharge (blood, serous fluid, infection).
- Neck: tenderness, stiffness/rigidity.
- Odour: poisoning, ingestion, metabolic disorders.
- Abdomen: liver, spleen.
- Eyes: pupils, fundi (papilloedema, retinal haemorrhages, sub-conjunctival haemorrhages), movements.

Also assess the following:

- AVPU and Glasgow Coma Scale scores: re-evaluate regularly.
- Posture/tone: lateralisation.
- Deep tendon reflexes: lateralisation.
- If there are lateralising signs, and if the patient is stable enough, consider a CT scan (if available).

The CT scan may show cerebral oedema, haemorrhages, or hypoxic/ischaemic encephalopathy.

Specific topics in coma
Meningitis or encephalitis

The following organisms cause meningitis:

- *Neisseria meningitides*:
  - risk of mortality (> 5%) and permanent serious neurological sequelae.
- *Haemophilus pneumonia*:
  - less common where routine Hib vaccination is available.
- *Streptococcus pneumoniae*:
  - common in resource-limited countries
  - occurs with underlying immune compromise, especially HIV infection

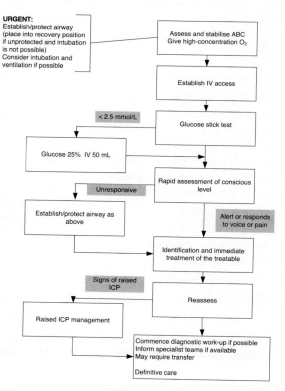

FIGURE 2.7.E.2 Pathway of care in coma. ABC, airway, breathing and circulation; ICP, intracranial pressure.

— may follow a head injury if there is damage to the dura and/or meninges.

There is a risk of coning and death if a diagnostic lumbar puncture is performed in a patient with significantly raised intracranial pressure.

Diagnosis of meningitis or encephalitis
Classic signs and symptoms include the following:
- headache

- vomiting
- neck stiffness
- opisthotonus
- photophobia
- rash
- altered consciousness.

Poisoning (*see* Section 7.4).
Malaria in pregnancy (*see* Section 2.8.D).
Eclamptic coma (*see* Section 2.5.E).

2.8 Infections complicating pregnancy, delivery and after birth

---

2.8.A Pneumonia

> **BOX 2.8.A.1 Minimum standards**
> - Oxygen.
> - Antibiotics (IV and oral).
> - Chest X-ray.

Clinical findings
A high fever is usually associated with pneumonia and bacterial tracheitis. In the absence of stridor and wheeze, breathing difficulties in association with a significant fever are likely to be due to **pneumonia**.

Examination of the chest may show reduced air entry, bronchial breathing and crepitations. Pleuritic chest pain, neck stiffness and abdominal pain may be present if there is pleural inflammation. Pleural effusions and empyema are complications.

Always consider HIV infection and TB.

Emergency treatment of pneumonia
- Assess ABC.
- Give oxygen through nasal cannulae or mask depending on flow rate required to maintain saturation (if available) as below.
- Attach a pulse oximeter (if available).
- Maintain SaO_2 in the range 94–98%, with nasal cannulae at a flow rate usually up to 5 litres/minute or if necessary by face mask with higher flow rates.

- Give antibiotics for 7 days:
  - ampicillin 2 grams IV/IM 6-hourly *plus* gentamicin 80 mg IV/IM 8-hourly or 5 mg/kg IV/IM every 24 hours for most cases of community-acquired pneumonia
  - cefuroxime 500 mg IV/IM 8-hourly or flucloxacillin 500 mg IM or IV slowly every 6 hours for suspected or bacteriologically diagnosed *Staphylococcus aureus*
  - erythromycin 500 mg every 6 hours orally for *Chlamydia* or *Mycoplasma pneumoniae*
  - *or* whatever is available locally and appropriate.
- Sit the patient upright.
- Maintain hydration.
  - Extra fluid may be needed to compensate for fluid loss from fever.
  - Fluid restriction may be needed because of inappropriate ADH secretion, revealed by oliguria < 30 mL per hour or rising blood urea levels.
- Chest X-ray is indicated.
- Large pleural effusions/empyemas should be diagnosed where possible by ultrasound, and pleural drainage undertaken under ultrasound cover (do not place a chest drain into the heart, liver or an undiagnosed tumour or hydatid cyst) (*see* Section 8.3). **Remember that in advanced pregnancy the diaphragm is elevated.**
  - Effusions/empyemas adjacent to the heart on the left side may cause pericarditis and cardiac arrhythmias. (Listen regularly for a pericardial rub, and ideally monitor an ECG if available until the patient is stable.)

2.8.B Severe dehydration and gastroenteritis

BOX 2.8.B.1 Minimum standards
- IV fluids containing appropriate amounts of sodium.
- Low-osmolarity oral rehydration solution (ORS).
- Nasogastric tubes.
- Urea and electrolyte measurements.
- Accurate weighing scales.

Introduction

Dehydration is loss of water, sodium and other essential electrolytes from the body. It causes death as a result of **shock** and **electrolyte emergencies** (*see* Section 2.5.A). Dehydration is a common cause of hospital admission, most commonly due to **acute gastroenteritis** and **diabetic ketoacidosis** (*see* Section 2.7.D).

A rapid clinical assessment (with support from biochemical tests, if **rapidly** available) in the very sick is the basis for treatment. The majority of patients can be treated with low-osmolarity oral rehydration solution (ORS) (by mouth or by nasogastric tube).

In patients with coincidental severe malnutrition, it is safer to use ORS with a lower sodium content, such as ReSoMal.

Classification of dehydration

Dehydration is classified according to clinical criteria. This may not apply in **severe malnutrition**, where caution is needed as signs may overlap and be misleading (*see* Section 5.10.B).

No dehydration (< 3% weight loss)

There are no clinical signs with this degree of dehydration, although there will be thirst in the fully conscious patient. The woman or girl who is not fully conscious will not feel thirsty.

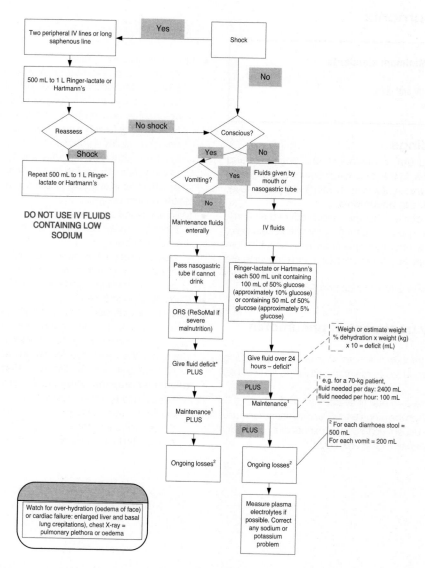

FIGURE 2.8.B.1 Pathway of care for gastroenteritis with severe dehydration (10% or more). ORS, oral rehydration solution.

Some dehydration (3–9% weight loss)

The following clinical signs are seen:

- increased thirst
- dry mucous membranes
- loss of skin turgor, tenting when pinched
- sunken eyes
- restless or irritable behaviour.

Severe dehydration (≥ 10% weight loss)

The following clinical signs are seen:

- more pronounced effects of the signs seen in moderate dehydration
- lack of urine output
- hypovolaemic shock, including:
  - rapid and feeble pulse (radial pulse may be undetectable)
  - low or undetectable blood pressure
  - cool and poorly perfused extremities
  - decreased capillary refill time (> 3 seconds): test this on the sternum of patients with light skins and on the thumbnail of those with dark skins
  - peripheral cyanosis
- rapid deep breathing (from acidosis)
- altered level of consciousness or coma.

Emergency treatment of severe dehydration

- Treat **shock** with an initial bolus of 1000 mL of Ringer-lactate or Hartmann's solution (*see* Section 2.5.A).
- Decide on the cause (e.g. acute gastroenteritis, diabetic ketoacidosis).
- Classify the extent of dehydration (see above).
- Calculate the **fluid deficit** (see below), add this to the maintenance and ongoing losses and give over 24 hours.
- The major danger in rehydration (once shock has been treated) is causing the plasma sodium level to fall rapidly. This may increase the transfer of water into the brain and result in **cerebral oedema**.
- Before the electrolyte results are known, or if such testing is not available, the safest fluid to give is Ringer-lactate or Hartmann's solution.

If the serum sodium level is higher than 155 mmol/litre, aim to lower it slowly over 48 hours or longer.

Calculating fluid requirements
Deficit

If an accurate recent pre-illness weight is available, subtract the current weight to estimate lost fluid (1 kg = 1 litre of fluid).

For example, a mother who weighed 70 kg is seen with diarrhoea and a weight of 65 kg.

In this case the estimated fluid loss is (70– 65) kg = 5 kg = 5000 mL deficit (i.e. 7% dehydrated).

If no recent weight is available, or the weight value given is considered to be unreliable:

- Decide the degree of dehydration.
- Weigh the patient.
- Use the formula: **percentage dehydration × weight (kg) × 10 = deficit (in mL)**.

For example, a mother whose weight is estimated to be 70 kg is 8% dehydrated.

In this case the estimated fluid loss is 8 × 70 × 10 = 5600 mL (233 mL/hour if replaced over 24 hours).

Maintenance

Estimated maintenance fluid requirements are **2400 mL/day** and **100 mL/hour**.

Ongoing losses

- **For each diarrhoeal stool:** 500 mL of ORS after each stool.
- **For each vomit:** 200 mL of ORS after each vomit. Give small frequent volumes (e.g. 20 mL every minute) with a spoon or syringe or cup.

Add deficit to maintenance and ongoing losses and aim to replace these over 24 hours.

For example, for a 70 kg mother who is 8% dehydrated, maintenance is 100 mL/hour, if there are no ongoing losses.

Total fluids needed per hour = 233 mL/hour (deficit) + 100 mL/hour (maintenance) = 333 mL/hour.

Severe acute gastroenteritis in pregnancy

Gastroenteritis is a common cause of dehydration and shock. Management starts with ABC, followed by assessment of the fluid deficit (extent of dehydration) and ongoing losses of fluid. Weigh the patient and keep an accurate fluid balance chart.

It is important to give fluids that:

- correct the deficit
- provide maintenance
- replace ongoing losses.

Differential diagnosis

Look for an abdominal mass or abdominal distension.

Consider the following:

- HIV infections
- surgical conditions, such as acute appendicitis, peritonitis or bowel obstruction (if suspected, resuscitate and call for surgical opinion)
- typhoid (high-grade fever, rash, hepatosplenomegaly and toxicity)
- antibiotic-associated colitis
- (rarely) inflammatory bowel disease.

Treatment if not shocked

- Start low-osmolarity oral rehydration solution (ORS) with 1–2 litres over 2–4 hours.
- The carer should give small amounts of ORS (e.g. using a small cup) frequently.
- Gradually increase the amount as tolerated, using a tablespoon, cup or glass.
- After 12–24 hours, review progress with regard to rehydration and progress to the maintenance phase or continue rehydration.

Severe dehydration (≥ 10% fluid deficit with or without clinical signs of shock)

- If the patient is shocked, assess and manage ABC, give oxygen if available, and start IV fluids immediately (use two intravenous lines if possible: use long saphenous vein cut-down or the external jugular vein if venous access is difficult).

- Give a 500 mL or 1-litre bolus of Ringer-lactate or Hartmann's solution IV as rapidly as possible.
- Reassess pulse, perfusion (capillary refill time) and mental status, and repeat the bolus if these are still abnormal.
- **Do not use low-sodium-containing IV fluids such as 0.18% saline with 4% glucose, which can be dangerous (they can cause hyponatraemia and cerebral oedema).** Instead use Ringer-lactate or Hartmann's solution, ideally also containing 10% glucose (obtained by adding 100 mL of 50% glucose to each 500 mL).
- **Hypokalaemia is a major complication which needs urgent attention.** Ideally measure serum K+ levels frequently. Provided that the patient is passing urine and IV potassium can safely be given, it should be added to the IV fluids given subsequent to the boluses given to treat shock. Ideally and if tolerated, potassium should be corrected by giving low osmolarity ORS enterally as soon as possible.

If it is necessary to add potassium to IV fluids given to correct dehydration, particularly if diarrhea is continuing and if measured serum K+ is < 2.0 mmol/litre or there are ECG signs of hypokalaemia, namely ST depression, T-wave reduction and prominent U waves, and only if safe to do so, great care must be taken.

In acute depletion, an infusion at the rate of 0.1 to 0.2 mmol/kg/hour (6 to 12 mmol/hour for a woman weighing 60 kg) of IV potassium can be used and the serum K+ level checked after 3 hours. The potassium for injection **must** be diluted before use and thoroughly mixed before being given. **The maximum concentration of potassium that can be given through a peripheral vein is 40 mmol/litre. The maximum infusion rate of potassium is 0.5 mmol/kg/hour.** Remember that Ringer-lactate or Hartmann's solution both already contain 5 mmol/litre of potassium.

Note: The injectable form of KCl usually contains 1.5 grams (i.e. 20 mmol of potassium in 10 mL), and can be given orally. The daily potassium requirement is 1–2.5 mmol/kg.

When shock has resolved, and the patient's level of consciousness has returned to normal, the remaining estimated deficit **must be taken by mouth or by gastric tube**, especially if **severe malnutrition** and/or **anaemia** is present (giving large fluid volumes IV can precipitate heart failure).

Assess the patient's hydration status frequently.

Oral fluids

Recommendations for oral replacement therapy in gastro-enteritis are as follows:

- Give low-osmolarity ORS (containing 75 mmol/litre of sodium) *or*, if the latter is unavailable, ORS containing 90 mmol/litre of sodium with an additional source of low-sodium fluid (e.g. water).
- The amount given should be in the range 300–500 mL/hour.
- Giving high-osmolarity fluids may contribute to hyper-natraemia, whereas giving water alone, or low-salt drinks, may cause hyponatraemia.
- Oral glucose within ORS enhances electrolyte and water uptake in the gut.
- 'Home-made' ORS can be prepared by adding a pinch of salt (1 mL) and a handful of sugar (5 mL) to a glass of clean potable water (250 mL).

Intravenous fluids

- Even in patients who are drinking poorly, try to give enteral fluids by mouth or by gastric tube until the IV infusion is running.
- Use Ringer-lactate or Hartmann's solution, which contains Na+ 131 mmol/litre, K+ 5 mmol/litre, HCO_3^- 29 mmol/litre and Ca^{2+} 2 mmol/litre.
- Hartmann's solution has no glucose to prevent hypo-glycaemia. This can be corrected by adding 100 mL of 50% glucose to 500 mL of Ringer-lactate or Hartmann's, giving approximately a 10% glucose solution (adding 50 mL to 450 mL of Ringer-lactate or Hartmann's gives a 5% solution).
- Ringer-lactate or Hartmann's solution with 5% dextrose added has the advantage of providing glucose to help to prevent hypoglycaemia.
- See above regarding potassium supplementation.
- **It is dangerous to use plain 5% glucose solutions, or 0.18% saline plus 4% glucose. They do not contain adequate electrolytes, do not correct the acidosis or hypovolaemia, and can cause dangerous hyponatraemia.**
- All patients should start to receive some ORS (at the rate of about 300 mL/hour) when they can drink without difficulty, which is usually within 1–2 hours. This provides additional base and potassium, which may not be adequately supplied by the IV fluid. Alternatively, give as soon as possible by gastric tube.

Over-hydration

Signs of over-hydration include the following:

- oedematous eyelids and generalised oedema, particularly ankle, facial and sacral oedema
- cardiac failure, especially in severe malnutrition or protein-losing enteropathy.
  - respiratory distress (raised rate and some chest wall recession)
  - tachycardia out of proportion to respiratory difficulty
  - raised jugular venous pressure
  - gallop rhythm/murmur
  - enlarged liver
  - basal lung crepitations.

A chest X-ray may be helpful for showing pulmonary plethora or oedema.

Management of over-hydration

- Stop giving ORS, but give plain water and food.
- Do not give a diuretic unless the patient is in cardiac failure.

When the oedema has resolved, resume giving ORS.

Reassess the following:
- ABC
- circulatory and hydration status
- plasma electrolytes if possible
- urine output and urine electrolytes
- give fluid according to plan; do not forget ongoing losses
- reassess regularly (including biochemistry if possible)
- do not forget glucose.

2.8.C HIV/AIDS

BOX 2.8.C.1 Minimum standards
- ■ Prevention of mother-to-child transmission (PMTCT).
- ■ Antiretroviral therapy (ART) for HIV-infected women.
- ■ Health education and community support.

Introduction

Prevention of mother-to-child transmission (PMTCT) of the human immunodeficiency virus (HIV) is possible, even in resource-limited settings, and the World Health Organization guidance (*Recommendations for a Public Health Approach*) published in 2010 on antiretroviral drugs for treating pregnant women and preventing HIV infection in infants suggests that elimination of mother-to-child transmission of HIV (MTCT) is a realistic public health goal.

Since the previous WHO guidance was published in 2006, new evidence has emerged on the use of antiretroviral prophylaxis to prevent MTCT, on the optimal time to initiate antiretroviral therapy (ART), and on safe feeding practices for HIV-exposed infants. This section draws heavily from the WHO 2010 and 2013 guidelines, which should be used and adapted within local settings. Once implemented, these recommendations could reduce the risk of MTCT to less than 5% in breastfeeding populations (from a background risk of 35%), and to less than 2% in non-breastfeeding populations (from a background risk of 25%), and will ensure increased maternal and child survival.

A woman will only know her HIV status if she has had an HIV test. HIV tests may be performed as a bedside point of care test (using capillary blood) or within a laboratory. An HIV-positive mother will pass her antibodies to her baby. These are harmless and are usually cleared by 18–24 months of age. It is transmission of the HIV virus that causes infection. An infant will have circulating maternal antibodies until 18–24 months of age, so the HIV antibody test is often not useful before this time, as it remains positive until the maternal antibodies have cleared.

When HIV infection is recent or the CD4 count is high, and a pregnant woman has no symptoms, HIV has little effect on pregnancy, and pregnancy has little effect on HIV. However, when HIV infection is advanced or the CD4 count is low, a woman is at risk of opportunistic infections, and HIV can directly affect the pregnancy, including increasing the risk of premature delivery, severe malaria and puerperal sepsis.

MTCT can occur when the baby is in the uterus, during delivery or during breastfeeding. Pregnant women should be encouraged to be tested for HIV because, if they are found to be HIV-positive, there are interventions at each of these stages that reduce the risk of MTCT, and there is also treatment to preserve the mother's own health. A negative HIV test provides an opportunity for health education, including promoting safer sex (e.g. use of condoms) to avoid the woman becoming HIV infected, particularly during pregnancy. Acquiring HIV during pregnancy carries a high risk of transmitting HIV to an unborn baby. HIV-negative women should be offered a repeat HIV test in the third trimester.

'Adult-to-child transmission' or 'vertical transmission' are other ways of describing MTCT, and are sometimes felt to imply less blame.

Prevention of mother-to-child transmission and ART in pregnancy

The WHO 2010 guidelines state that a woman with a CD4 count of ≤ 350 cells/mm³ (regardless of WHO clinical staging) or WHO clinical stage 3 or 4 (irrespective of CD4 count) (*WHO Case Definitions of HIV for Surveillance and Revised Clinical Staging and Immunological Classification of HIV-Related Disease in Adults and Children*, published in 2007) requires lifelong ART.

Updated consolidated ART guidelines published by the WHO in 2013 (www.who.int/hiv/pub/guidelines/arv2013/art/artadults/en/index1.html) now recommend that all pregnant and breastfeeding women should be commenced on ART (one simplified triple regimen), and that this should be maintained for at least the duration of MTCT risk (i.e. throughout breastfeeding). They suggest that, particularly in generalised epidemics, all pregnant and breastfeeding women with HIV should initiate ART as lifelong treatment. In pregnancy the focus is no longer on 'when or what to start' but on 'whether to stop' treatment after delivery. Ideally, a CD4 count should be obtained before deciding whether ART for PMTCT only (i.e. stopping after delivery) is an option.

As most women should continue ART following delivery, an effective link with HIV treatment programmes is essential.

The WHO 2013 guidelines are simplified, and they harmonise the approach to ART in adults and pregnancy. National programmes are encouraged to move from the previous Option 'A' to Option 'B' or 'B+'.

Option B+: all pregnant and breastfeeding women infected with HIV should be started on ART as lifelong treatment. This is particularly important in generalised epidemics where high fertility, long duration of breastfeeding, limited access to CD4 to determine ART eligibility, and high partner serodiscordance rates all increase the risks of transmission to the woman's partner and babies.

Option B: in some countries (e.g. where CD4 counts are available), in the case of women who are not eligible for ART for their own health, consideration can be given to stopping the ARV regimen after the period of risk of mother-to-child transmission has ended.

Single-dose nevirapine (sdNVP) for women in labour is no longer recommended (unless it is combined with other ART) because it causes the virus to develop high levels of drug resistance.

Option A (from the 2010 WHO guidelines) is no longer recommended, although some countries may not have the resources necessary to use options B or B+.

The treatment focus is shifting to consider ART for the mother's health, to utilise more effective ART drugs, and to extend coverage throughout the MTCT risk period. **All women should be started on ART in pregnancy.**

TABLE 2.8.C.1 WHO guidelines for ART in pregnancy for HIV-infected women who have not had previous ART

	For pregnant women for PMTCT only	For infants of mothers given a short course of ART for PMTCT
Option A (WHO 2010 guidelines)	AZT twice a day from 14 weeks sdNVP at onset of labour, and start AZT + 3TC for 7 days	Baby being breastfed: daily NVP from birth until at least 4–6 weeks of age *and* until 1 week after breastfeeding has stopped Baby being bottle-fed: daily NVP or sdNVP + AZT twice a day until 4–6 weeks
Option B	Preferred regimens: TDF + 3TC (or FTC) + EFV (as fixed-dose combination) Alternative regimens: AZT + 3TC + EFV or TDF + 3TC (or FTC) + EFV	Baby being breastfed: daily nevirapine (NVP) for 6 weeks Baby being bottle-fed: daily nevirapine (NVP) for 4–6 weeks or AZT twice a day for 4–6 weeks
	For pregnant women being given lifelong ART	**For infants of mothers on lifelong ART**
Option B+	Preferred regimens: TDF + 3TC (or FTC) + EFV (as fixed-dose combination) Alternative regimens: AZT + 3TC + EFV or AZT + 3TC + NVP or TDF + 3TC (or FTC) + NVP	Baby being breastfed: daily nevirapine (NVP) for 6 weeks Baby being bottle-fed: daily nevirapine (NVP) for 4–6 weeks or AZT twice a day for 4–6 weeks

Women diagnosed with HIV during labour or immediately postpartum

If a woman is diagnosed with HIV infection during labour or immediately postpartum, ART should be commenced immediately for PMTCT. This regimen can be modified later when the woman has been assessed (with CD4 count) with regard to whether she requires lifelong ART for herself.

Postpartum, women should be assessed and a CD4 count obtained. Ideally they should continue their triple-drug ART regimen lifelong unless their CD4 count is > 500 cells/mm³.

It will take weeks for the maternal viral load to be reduced, and therefore it is important to give the mother ART in labour which will cross the placenta (and enter the baby) in addition to starting ART prophylaxis in the infant.

TABLE 2.8.C.2 WHO guidance for ART for women diagnosed with HIV in labour/immediately postpartum

	For the mother	For the infant
Option A	sd-NVP in labour and AZT + 3TC twice a day for 1 week	Baby being breastfed: Daily NVP from birth for 6 weeks, consider extending to 12 weeks
Option B	Start (triple) ART immediately. Continue until 1 week after exposure to breast milk has ended	
Option B+	Start (triple) ART immediately. Continue lifelong	Baby being bottle-fed: Daily NVP from birth for 6 weeks

If a woman is diagnosed with HIV infection postpartum and plans replacement (formula or bottle) feeding, refer her for HIV care and evaluation for treatment.

HIV-exposed infants (children born to women with HIV) should be given co-trimoxazole prophylaxis from 4–6 weeks of age, and this should be continued until HIV infection has been excluded and the infant is no longer at risk of acquiring HIV through breastfeeding (World Health Organization, *Guidelines on Co-Trimoxazole Prophylaxis for HIV-Related Infections among Children, Adolescents and adults: recommendations for a public health approach*, published in 2006).

Delivery

Labour can be a worrying time for the HIV-positive woman, particularly because of possible underlying fears about her own HIV infection and the risk of infecting her baby. She will need reassurance and support, and it is important to ensure she knows that with all of the interventions that are given her baby is more likely to be HIV-negative than infected.

Get close to her, greet her and be seen to shake hands with her, to help to reduce the stigma around touching those infected with HIV. Support her relatives, and encourage her to tell her partner so that he can be tested for HIV. Promote safer sex and advise her to use condoms to prevent transmission of HIV.

Standard precautions should be used when caring for women in labour, whether or not they have HIV infection. Always wear gloves when touching body fluids, and dispose of single-use syringes and needles safely.

During delivery, to reduce MTCT:
- **avoid artificial rupture of membranes**
- **avoid prolonged rupture of membranes**
- **avoid unnecessary episiotomy, but also avoid a tear.**

Both blood and placenta will contain HIV, so wear gloves, an apron and eye protection. Avoid direct contact of blood on your skin. Blood on intact skin should be washed off immediately. HIV-positive blood on an open wound or splashed into the eye can transmit HIV and should be washed immediately (use soap and water for a wound, and water for an eye) and managed in the same way as a needlestick injury (with post-exposure prophylaxis with ART).

Other considerations for managing HIV infection in pregnancy

Anaemia

Screening for and treatment of anaemia should be routine in antenatal care for all pregnant women (World Health Organization, *Pregnancy, Childbirth, Postpartum and Newborn Care: a guide for essential practice*, 2nd edn, published in 2009). Iron supplements and folate supplements in areas with a high prevalence of iron deficiency are indicated for all pregnant women regardless of haemoglobin levels. Iron should be continued for 3 months after delivery. If possible, antenatal screening for anaemia should include laboratory measurement of haemoglobin levels, but anaemia can be assessed clinically if this is not available.

In women with severe anaemia, AZT should be avoided, and TDF or stavudine (d4T) should be used instead.

Malaria and worm infestations

The prevention and treatment of malaria and worm infestations is necessary in high-prevalence areas (*see* Sections 2.8.D and 6.3.C).

HIV-2 infection

HIV-2 is much less transmissible than HIV-1 (the MTCT risk is 0–4%).

Non-nucleoside reverse transcriptase inhibitors (NNRTIs) such as NVP and EFV are not effective against HIV-2, and a triple nucleoside reverse transcriptase inhibitor (NRTI) combination is recommended.

BOX 2.8.C.2 Treatment of HIV-2 infection

Mother requires treatment: AZT + abacavir (ABC) + 3TC

PMTCT only: AZT from 14 weeks and continued until delivery

Infant of mother with HIV-2: AZT twice a day until 4–6 weeks

Tuberculosis

The risk of active TB increases in pregnancy, and is around 10 times higher in HIV-infected women. It is associated with increased maternal mortality, premature labour, low birth weight and tuberculosis in the infant. HIV-infected women must be assessed for TB at each visit; any woman with a cough, fever, night sweats and weight loss should be evaluated for TB and started on TB treatment. ART is also required regardless of the CD4 count. Commence TB treatment first, followed by ART as soon as clinically possible (within 8 weeks of starting TB treatment).

Rifampicin interacts with many antiretroviral drugs, especially the boosted protease inhibitors. As is the case for all adults, EFV is the preferred NNRTI for HIV/TB co-infected pregnant women (starting after the first trimester).

For those women on TB therapy who are unable to tolerate EFV, give a NVP-based regime or a triple NRTI regimen such as AZT + 3TC + ABC or AZT + 3TC + TDF. In the presence of rifampicin, start full-dose NVP (a lead-in dose is not required).

Summary

Interventions during pregnancy, labour and delivery and postpartum can all significantly reduce the risk of MTCT of HIV. Therefore all pregnant women should be tested for HIV. The WHO 2007 guidelines (www.who.int/hiv/pub/mtct/pmtct_scaleup2007/en/index.html) summarise the essential services required for good-quality antenatal care, and these are listed below.

Package of routine quality antenatal and postpartum care for all women, regardless of HIV status

1 Health education, information on HIV and sexually transmitted infection (STI) prevention and care including safer sex practices, pregnancy including antenatal care, birth planning and delivery assistance, malaria prevention, optimal infant feeding; family planning counselling and related services.
2 Provider-initiated HIV testing and counselling, including HIV testing and counselling for women of unknown status at labour and delivery, or postpartum.
3 Couple and partner HIV testing and counselling, including support for disclosure.
4 Promotion and provision of condoms.
5 HIV-related gender-based violence screening.
6 Obstetric care, including history taking and physical examination.
7 Maternal nutritional support.
8 Infant feeding counselling.
9 Psychosocial support.
10 Birth planning, birth preparedness (including pregnancy/postpartum danger signs), including skilled birth attendants.
11 Tetanus vaccination.
12 Iron and folate supplementation.
13 Syphilis screening and management of STIs.
14 Harm reduction interventions for injecting drug users.

Additional package of services for HIV-positive women

1 Additional counselling and support to encourage partner testing, adoption of risk reduction and disclosure.
2 Clinical evaluation, including clinical staging of HIV disease.
3 Immunological assessment (CD4 cell count) where available.
4 ART when indicated.
5 Infant feeding counselling and support based on knowledge of HIV status.
6 ART prophylaxis for PMTCT provided during the antepartum, intrapartum and postpartum periods.
7 Co-trimoxazole prophylaxis where indicated.
8 Additional counselling and provision of services as appropriate to prevent unintended pregnancies.
9 Supportive care, including adherence support.
10 TB screening and treatment when indicated; preventive therapy (INH prophylaxis) when appropriate.

11 Advice and support on other prevention interventions, such as safe drinking water.

12 Supportive care, including adherence support, and palliative care and symptom management.

Essential postnatal care for HIV-exposed infants

1 Completion of ART prophylaxis regimen.

2 Routine newborn and infant care, including routine immunisation and growth monitoring.

3 Co-trimoxazole prophylaxis.

4 Early HIV diagnostic testing and diagnosis of HIV-related conditions.

5 Continued infant feeding counselling and support, especially after early HIV testing.

6 Nutritional support throughout the first year of life, including support for optimal infant feeding practices, and provision of nutritional supplements and replacement foods if indicated.

7 ART for HIV-infected children when indicated.

8 Treatment monitoring for all children receiving ART.

9 INH prophylaxis when indicated.

10 Adherence support counselling for caregivers.

11 Malaria prevention and treatment where indicated.

12 Diagnosis and management of common childhood infections and conditions, and integrated management of childhood illness (IMCI).

13 Diagnosis and management of TB and other opportunistic infections.

2.8.D Malaria

Introduction

Malaria, particularly falciparum malaria, is an important cause of maternal mortality and postpartum morbidity, severe anaemia, miscarriage, intrauterine growth retardation, intrauterine death, stillbirth, premature delivery, low birth weight (LBW), and perinatal and neonatal morbidity.

Plasmodium falciparum malaria is the most dangerous type. *P. vivax* malaria is less dangerous. Malaria destroys red blood cells and can harm the placenta. The main danger with falciparum malaria is cerebral malaria, which causes coma and death.

In most endemic areas of the world, pregnant women are the main adult risk group for malaria. The burden of malaria infection during pregnancy is chiefly caused by *Plasmodium falciparum*, the most common malaria species in Africa. The impact of the other three human malaria parasites (*P. vivax*, *P. malariae* and *P. ovale*) is less clear. Every year at least 30 million pregnancies occur among women in malarious areas of Africa, most of whom reside in areas of relatively stable malaria transmission.

In sub-Saharan Africa, poor nutrition, micronutrient imbalances (particularly vitamin A, zinc, iron and folate), HIV co-infection, poverty and limited access to effective primary healthcare and emergency obstetric services exacerbate the impact of pregnancy-associated malaria.

In Africa, perinatal mortality due to malaria is around 1500 deaths per day. In areas where malaria is endemic, 20–40% of all babies born may have a low birth weight, increasing the likelihood of infant mortality.

Malaria in pregnancy is a particular problem for women in their first and second pregnancies, and for women who are HIV-positive.

Studies have shown that in high transmission zones more than 50% of women have placental malaria infections at birth. This increases the risk of HIV viral transfer (especially if the parasite load is high), and prevents the transfer of maternal antibodies protecting against measles.

Malaria in pregnancy in low versus high transmission areas

The clinical presentation and severity of malaria in pregnancy differ in areas of high and low transmission due to differences in the level of immunity of the population. Although these settings are presented as two distinct epidemiologic conditions, in reality the intensity of transmission and immunity in pregnant women occurs on a continuum, with potentially diverse conditions occurring within a country.

In areas of epidemic or low (unstable) malaria transmission, adult women have not acquired any significant level of immunity and usually become ill when infected with *P. falciparum* malaria. Pregnant women resident in areas of low or unstable malaria transmission are at a two- or three-fold higher risk of developing severe disease as a result of malaria infection than are non-pregnant adults living in the same area. In these areas, maternal death may result either directly from severe malaria or indirectly from malaria-related severe anaemia. In addition, malaria infection of the mother may result in a range of adverse pregnancy outcomes, including spontaneous abortion, neonatal death, and low birth weight (LBW).

In areas of high and moderate (stable) transmission of malaria, most adult women have developed sufficient immunity that, even during pregnancy, *P. falciparum* infection does not usually result in fever or other clinical symptoms. In these areas, the principal impact of malaria infection is associated with malaria-related anaemia in the mother, and with the presence of parasites in the placenta. The resulting impairment of fetal nutrition contributing to low birth weight is a leading cause of poor infant survival and development. In areas of Africa with stable malaria transmission, *P. falciparum* infection during pregnancy is estimated to cause as many as 10 000 maternal deaths each year, 8–14% of all low-birth-weight babies, and 3–8% of all infant deaths.

The strategy for management of malaria in the pregnant population in **areas of high transmission** should include screening and treating of positive cases, intermittent presumptive treatment (IPTp) for rapid diagnostic test (RDT)-negative cases and use of insecticide-treated bed nets (ITNs).

In high transmission areas, in women who are known to be HIV-positive, or where the prevalence of HIV exceeds 10%, IPTp should be given monthly (and at least four times during pregnancy), see below.

In **areas of low transmission** the risk of malaria infection during pregnancy is greater, and can result in maternal death, and in spontaneous abortion in up to 60% of cases. Silent malaria is rare. The strategy in these areas involves ITNs, screening and treatment of positive cases, chemoprophylaxis if possible, and early diagnosis and prompt effective treatment of malaria.

TABLE 2.8.D.1 Comparison of occurrence of complications in areas of high and low transmission

Complication	Hyper-endemic areas	Low transmission
Hypoglycaemia	–	++
Severe anaemia	+++	+++
Pulmonary oedema	–	++
Acute renal failure	–	++
Hyperpyrexia	+	+++
Placental malaria	+++	+++
LBW babies	+++	+++
Abortions	–	+++
Congenital malaria	–	+++

A pregnant woman who has not lived in a malarious area has no immunity. Therefore if she goes to a malarious area she is at risk of developing severe malaria. She must take tablets to prevent malaria before she goes to that area and throughout her pregnancy, and sleep under a bed net when she gets there.

If a mother has had malaria before, she will have some immunity. Unfortunately, pregnancy reduces immunity. She is at risk from severe anaemia, but the other complications are unusual. Often her blood film will be negative, and she will have few symptoms. If she has fits they will probably be caused by eclampsia or meningitis, not malaria.

Partially immune primigravid mothers are at particular risk, especially during the last trimester. Early teenage primigravida are at greatest risk. This risk decreases with further pregnancies.

Screening and treating pregnant women during antenatal care

Since in most African countries over 70% of pregnant women make multiple antenatal clinic visits, these provide a major opportunity for prevention of malaria, along with other important diseases that affect pregnant women.

The rationale for screening and treating all pregnant women for malaria during routine antenatal care is that **even one attack at any time during pregnancy can have serious consequences** (i.e. low birth weight and maternal anaemia).

There is a four-pronged approach to malaria prevention and control during pregnancy:
1 intermittent preventive treatment (IPTp)
2 insecticide-treated bed nets (ITNs), or preferably long-lasting insecticide-treated bed nets (LLINs)
3 indoor residual spraying (IRS) with insecticides
4 case management of malaria illness.

Intermittent preventive treatment (IPTp)

This involves providing all pregnant women with preventive treatment doses of an effective antimalarial drug during routine antenatal clinic visits. This approach has been shown to be safe, inexpensive and effective. A study in Malawi evaluating IPT showed a decline in placental infection (from 32% to 23%) and in the number of low-birth-weight babies (from 23% to 10%). It also found that 75% of all pregnant women took advantage of IPTp when it was offered.

The drug recommended at present is sulphadoxine/pyrimethamine (SP, also called Fansidar). Starting as early as possible in the second trimester, IPTp-SP is recommended for all pregnant women in Africa at each scheduled antenatal care (ANC) visit (four visits are recommended by WHO during every pregnancy) until the time of delivery, provided that the doses are given at least one month apart. SP should not be given during the first trimester of pregnancy; however, the last dose of IPTp-SP can be administered up to the time of delivery without safety concerns.

IPTp-SP should ideally be administered as directly observed therapy (DOT) of three tablets sulfadoxine/pyrimethamine (each tablet containing 500 mg/25 mg SP) giving the total required dosage of 1500 mg/75 mg SP.

In areas where malaria is very common and antenatal clinic attendance is poor, all mothers, especially all primigravida, should be given a dose of SP when they first come to the antenatal clinic after quickening (when the mother first feels the fetus moving).

Although high levels of resistance to SP occur in many countries, it is not known at what level of SP resistance IPTp still gives a positive outcome in terms of improved haemoglobin levels in the mother and higher birth weights. A preventative effect provided by SP seems to exist even at relatively high levels of resistance.

For pregnant women who are HIV-positive, the dosage schedule for IPT should be augmented to at least four doses of SP, starting in the second trimester, the doses being given at least 1 month apart. This increased frequency is also recommended for all pregnant women with unknown HIV status living in areas of high HIV prevalence (over 10%).

Women who are HIV-positive experience increased vulnerability to malaria in all pregnancies, not just the first two pregnancies.

Note: HIV patients who are receiving co-trimoxazole preventive therapy should not take IPTp as adverse effects can occur.

Research to assess the safety, efficacy and programme feasibility of other antimalarial drugs for use in IPTp is ongoing.

Weekly chloroquine has in the past been shown to be effective in preventing malaria in pregnancy, especially in the case of *P. vivax* malaria. Adherence to this regime and loss of efficacy in the case of *P. falciparum* malaria make this regime less appropriate.

Insecticide-treated bed nets (ITNs) and long-lasting insecticide-treated bed nets (LLINs)

Nets decrease both the number of malaria cases and the malaria death rates in pregnant women. A study in an area of high malaria transmission in Kenya has shown that women who are protected by ITNs every night during their first four pregnancies produce 25% fewer underweight or premature babies. In addition, ITN use benefits the infant who sleeps under the net with the mother, by decreasing their exposure to malaria infection. ITNs should be provided to pregnant women as early in pregnancy as possible, and their use should be encouraged for women throughout pregnancy and during the postpartum period. Health education programmes, social marketing and lobbying to reduce the prices of ITNs and re-treatments are helping to encourage the use of ITNs by pregnant women.

Indoor residual spraying (IRS) with insecticides

IRS involves applying a long-lasting (residual) insecticide to the inside walls of houses and other structures where people sleep, to kill mosquitoes when they rest on the walls. It is a highly effective malaria prevention method in settings where it is epidemiologically and logistically appropriate. IRS must be applied prior to the transmission season (either annually, or twice a year if there are continuous or multiple seasons of transmission), and is carried out by a trained cadre of workers who move through a community spraying all appropriate structures. Its full potential is realised when at least 80% of houses in targeted areas are sprayed. Indoor spraying is effective for 3–6 months, depending on the insecticide used and the type of surface on which it is sprayed. DDT can be effective for 9–12 months in some cases. Longer-lasting forms of IRS insecticides are under development. The WHO approves the following pyrethroid class of pesticides; lambda-cyhalothrin, bifenthrin, alpha-cypermethrin, deltamethrin, cyfluthrin and etofenprox.

Case management of malarial illness

In areas of unstable (infrequent) *P. falciparum* malaria transmission, non-immune pregnant women exposed to malaria require prompt case management of febrile illness. Although at present there are no fully effective tools to prevent malaria among non-immune women, ITNs will decrease exposure to infective mosquito bites, and thus would be expected to be of benefit in decreasing symptomatic infections. Essential elements of the antenatal care package should therefore include malaria diagnosis, where available and needed, and treatment with antimalarial drugs that have an adequate safety and efficacy profile for use in pregnancy.

In view of the increasing evidence of the severe effects of malaria in pregnancy on both the woman and her unborn child, even when asymptomatic, all pregnant women presenting for antenatal care or delivery should be tested using an RDT. Since the sensitivities of both RDT and smear to detect low parasitaemias in pregnancy are not infallible, **both are recommended** where this is programmatically possible. Where this is not possible, RDTs are to be preferred.

All women who are found to be positive should receive an effective antimalarial drug, namely quinine in the first trimester and artemisinin-combination therapies (ACT) in the second and third trimesters. If they are found to be negative, they should receive a dose of SP as IPTp. Women should not be screened more often than monthly in the absence of signs or symptoms of malaria.

Patients with severe anaemia (haemoglobin < 7 g/dL) in a high transmission zone are in all probability infected, and should be treated with an effective antimalarial drug as well as iron/folic acid even if there are no other signs of malaria and negative smear or RDT, or if laboratory tests cannot be undertaken.

All patients with a positive biological test (RDT and/or microscopy) should be treated with an effective antimalarial drug. If you suspect malaria, but cannot examine a blood film or do an RDT, treat the mother anyway.

Asymptomatic (placental) malaria has the same implications in pregnant women as symptomatic malaria. Asymptomatic women should be routinely tested and treated.

In high transmission zones, many women suffer minor attacks of malaria for which they do not seek treatment. However, the placenta can still be infected. Women should be advised at each antenatal visit to come for treatment even if their symptoms are minor. **Both RDTs and smears may miss cases of placental malaria.** Because of the inability of biological tests to reliably detect placental malaria, patients with a negative biological test should receive SP as IPTp both to treat an undetected infection and to prevent further infection.

In low transmission zones, anaemia without a positive biological test and without symptoms or signs of malaria such as fever is probably due to other causes, and such patients should not automatically receive an antimalarial drug, but should be treated for the underlying cause (including treatment with iron and folate tablets).

RDTs versus microscopy in pregnancy

There is indirect evidence that only 30% of cases with placental malaria show peripheral parasitaemias. Although there is little evidence, it is more likely that RDTs will detect sequestered parasites because of accumulated antigenic product.

In Thailand and Assam, studies found that RDTs missed cases of parasitaemia found on slides (2.5% of patients in Assam). This is a much lower number of cases than the number missed by smears.

Ideally, use of both RDT and microscopy would detect most cases. However, this is usually impractical in the field setting. RDTs are preferable to microscopy in this setting for the detection of subclinical infections.

In cases of *P. vivax* malaria, placental malaria is difficult to detect. However, placental *P. vivax* malaria occurs infrequently because vivax malaria does not sequestrate. Detection of parasites in vivax is best done by microscopy.

Treatment of malaria
Drug safety in pregnancy

Guidelines on the treatment of malaria in pregnancy are made difficult by the lack of evidence about the safety of ACTs in pregnancy.

The recommendation is to ask the woman if she is

pregnant, and if she is not, to treat her with ACT. This is a pragmatic recommendation based on the fact that no serious adverse effects have yet been recorded in women who were inadvertently given ACT in the first trimester, and the fact that a 7-day course of quinine is rarely adhered to.

As a change from previous recommendations, the combination of artemether and lumefantrine (AL) is now considered as safe (or as unsafe) as the other combinations of AS + AQ, AS + SP and AS + MQ.

Drug resistance of *P. falciparum* to chloroquine and the antifolates has arisen throughout malaria-endemic areas.

Combination therapy (**artemisinin-combination therapies, or ACTs**) is considered best for malaria management (artemisinin-based compounds in combination with other classes of antimalarial drugs).

ACTs are highly effective and may help to delay development of resistance. It is important to ensure wide access to these drugs through effective delivery systems and affordable cost.

The risks of ACT in the **second and third trimester** are low. During these phases of pregnancy, ACTs should be used to treat both clinical and subclinical infections, due to the serious outcomes of these infections.

Quinine should always be used in the **first trimester**. However, if the life of the woman is threatened (i.e. when the risk to the mother outweighs the theoretical risk to the fetus), an ACT should be prescribed. Malaria is less often resistant to **quinine** than it is to other drugs, and this drug may be safely used throughout pregnancy if ACTs are not available.

ACTs in pregnancy: the use of ACTs in pregnancy has not been widely studied, but all of the current evidence points to their relative safety, even in the first trimester. Research into the safety and pharmacokinetics of antimalarial drugs in pregnancy is ongoing.

The following ACTs (arranged in alphabetical order) are currently recommended by the WHO for the treatment of uncomplicated *P. falciparum* malaria:

- artemether (ATM) + lumefantrine (LM): combined (fixed-dose combination, FDC) tablets ATM 20 mg/LM 120 mg in blister packs.
  - **Dose:** On day 1 give 4 tablets and then repeat 4 tablets between 8 and 12 hours later. Then give 4 tablets twice daily in the morning and evening on days 2 and 3.
  - Advise the patient to take doses with food, preferably fatty food. Consider supplying dried milk powder or Plumpy'Nut® to take with tablets.
- artesunate (AS) + amodiaquine (AQ): combined (fixed-dose combination, FDC) tablets AS 100 mg/AQ 270 mg in colour-coded blister packs.
  - **Dose:** 2 tablets per day for 3 successive days.
- artesunate (AS) + mefloquine (MQ): AS = 50 mg tablets, MQ = 250 mg tablets as base.
  - **Dose:** give 4 tablets of AS on days 1, 2 and 3, and 6 tablets of MQ on day 1 **and** 2 tablets of MQ on day 2 (or 8 tablets on day 1 only).
- artesunate (AS) + sulfadoxine + pyrimethamine (SP): AS = 50 mg tablets, SP = 25 mg (S) + 500 mg (P).
  - **Dose:** give 4 tablets of SP on days 1, 2, 3 and 4 **and** 3 tablets of SP on day 1.
- dihydroartemisinin (DHA) + piperaquine (PQP): combined (fixed-dose combination, FDC) tablets DHA 40 mg/PQP 320 mg.

- **Dose:** mother weighing 50–60 kg, 1 tablet three times a day for 1 day; mother weighing 60–70 kg, 1 tablet three times a day for 1 day plus additional ½ tablet at onset of day 1.
- quinine = usually 200 mg and 300 mg tablets.
  - **Dose:** give 600 mg 8-hourly over the first 24 hours or 30 mg/kg/day in three divided doses at 8-hourly intervals.
  - In South-East Asia where quinine sensitivity appears to be reduced, add clindamycin 7–13 mg/kg every 8 hours for 5 days.

Most pregnant women with malaria also lack folate, so give them folate tablets 5 mg daily.

If a pregnant woman is not immune, that is if she comes from an area without malaria transmission, she must have regular malaria tablets throughout pregnancy, especially in the last trimester.

Severe complicated malaria

This is usually *P. falciparum* malaria.

Severe malaria is a complex multi-system disease, and is a medical emergency.

Mortality approaches 100% without treatment, and death often occurs within the first few hours. Prompt initiation of antimalarial treatment in peripheral healthcare facilities and comprehensive management in hospital are necessary to prevent deaths.

Care should be provided within 15 minutes of arrival at a healthcare facility. **Triage systems** should be in place to pick up severely ill patients, referral should be rapid, and emergency facilities should be instituted in hospitals, with a high standard of medical and nursing care available 24 hours a day.

Any seriously ill or unconscious patient in a malaria endemic area must be tested for malaria by RDT (remember that parasites may not be present in the peripheral blood of a patient with cerebral malaria).

Even if a diagnostic test is not available, **the patient should be given an antimalarial drug (IV, IM or rectally, depending on the skill of the staff in the facility) before transfer to the hospital.** This can be repeated if transfer is impossible or is delayed for more than 12 hours. **A note of what has been given should be sent with the patient as soon as transfer can be arranged.**

Clinical features of severe malaria (WHO 2013)

- impaired consciousness (including unrousable coma)
- prostration, i.e. generalised weakness so that the patient is unable to sit, stand or walk without assistance
- multiple convulsions: more than two episodes within 24 hours
- deep breathing and respiratory distress (acidotic breathing)
- acute pulmonary oedema and acute respiratory distress syndrome
- circulatory collapse or shock, systolic blood pressure < 80 mmHg in adults and < 50 mmHg in children
- acute kidney injury
- clinical jaundice plus evidence of other vital organ dysfunction
- abnormal bleeding.

If any doubt exists about the diagnosis, it is safer to treat than not to treat before transfer.

Immediate measures (in hospital)

- Vital signs: temperature, pulse, blood pressure, and rate and depth of respiration.
- State of hydration.
- Estimation or measurement of body weight.
- Level of consciousness (AVPU or Glasgow Coma Scale scores).
    - **The depth of coma may be assessed rapidly by observing the response to standard vocal or painful stimuli (rub your knuckles on the woman's sternum; if there is no response, apply firm pressure on the thumbnail bed).**
- RDT and malaria smear (thick and thin film) for diagnosis and for continued monitoring of the progress of the disease. **Do not wait for a malaria smear result before initiating treatment, as it can take up to an hour.** If the RDT is positive, commence treatment immediately.
- Perform a lumbar puncture if the patient is unconscious, to eliminate meningitis.
- Measurement of glucose (finger prick test), haemoglobin, haematocrit and packed cell volume (PCV).
- Group and cross-match blood and **search for a suitable donor if there are no blood banking facilities.**
- Parenteral treatment (see below for details):
    - First choice: IV artesunate (2.4 mg/kg by slow IV injection at 0, 12 and 24 hours).
    - Second choice: IM artemether (loading dose of 3.2 mg/kg followed by 1.6 mg/kg every 24 hours).
    - If artemisinins are not available or the Ministry of Health has not authorised their use, commence with a loading dose of quinine 20 mg/kg (generally given in 10% dextrose to reduce the risk of hypoglycaemia) by slow infusion over 4 hours, followed by 10 mg/kg over 4 hours, every 8 hours for a minimum of 3 doses and continued until the patient is able to tolerate oral drugs. A full course of oral antimalarials must be completed once IV quinine has been discontinued. The loading dose of quinine may be omitted if the patient has definitely received a treatment dose of quinine within the previous 12 hours.

Every effort should be made to convince the Ministry of Health to allow the use of artemisinins to treat severe malaria in hospital, as mortality may be reduced by up to 30% over the use of quinine.

Additional measures where needed

- Insert a nasogastric tube to minimise the risk of aspiration pneumonia if the patient's level of consciousness is low. This can also be used to give food to prevent hypoglycaemia if the patient is unconscious for a long period and is unable to eat.
- Monitor for hypoglycaemia by laboratory or bedside testing if available (see below for more detailed advice).
- Insert an IV cannula and restore circulating volume.
    - Fluids should be given with caution and the need for them assessed on an individual basis after ascertaining the nutritional status and degree of dehydration present (see below for more details).
- In general, patients with metabolic acidosis who have not previously received parenteral fluids are dehydrated

and should be managed accordingly (see below for more details).

- Give oxygen, especially if metabolic acidosis is suspected or shock is present.
- Treat severe anaemia with a safe blood transfusion if the patient is showing signs of decompensation.
- Give anticonvulsants (diazepam is preferred initially, then phenytoin if convulsions persist) if the patient is fitting, to prevent long-term neurological damage (see below for more details).

Convulsions are common before or after the onset of coma. They are significantly associated with morbidity and sequelae. They may present in a very subtle way. Important signs include intermittent nystagmus, salivation, minor twitching of a single digit or a corner of the mouth, and an irregular breathing pattern.

- Prophylactic anticonvulsants have been recommended in the past, but recent evidence suggests that **phenobarbital is harmful.**
- IV broad-spectrum antibiotics should be given routinely in an unconscious patient.

The patient will need intensive nursing care at least until they regain consciousness. They may urgently need glucose or a blood transfusion if hypoglycaemia or haemolysis is severe.

Special issues with regard to severe malaria in pregnancy

Severe malaria is malaria with severe drowsiness, coma, vomiting, inability to walk, jaundice, fits or pulmonary oedema. These women are usually non-immune multigravida, or semi-immune primigravida, with *P. falciparum* malaria.

Severe malaria in pregnancy may be misdiagnosed as eclampsia. **If a pregnant woman living in a malarial area has fever, headaches or convulsions and malaria cannot be excluded, it is essential to treat the woman for both malaria and eclampsia.**

Pregnant women with severe malaria are particularly prone to hypoglycaemia, pulmonary oedema, anaemia and coma.

Malaria is especially dangerous during the last trimester.

Malaria drug treatment in pregnancy
Treat malaria in pregnancy urgently and early!

Calculate the dose in mg/kg. If you cannot weigh the patient, an average pregnant woman weighs about 60 kg, a small woman weighs around 50 kg and a large woman in resource limited settings around 80 kg.

Where available, artesunate IV/IM or artemether IM are the drugs of choice in the second and third trimesters. Their use in the first trimester must balance their advantages over quinine (better tolerability and less hypoglycaemia) against the limited documentation of pregnancy outcomes. **Artemesinin** and **artesunate** may be given rectally.

IV/IM artesunate

Artesunate IV/IM: 2.4 mg/kg by direct IV injection (over 5 minutes) or IM injection at 0, 12 and 24 hours, then once daily until oral therapy is possible.

A solution for parenteral use should be prepared for either IV (10 mg/mL) or IM (20 mg/mL) use, following the manufacturer's instructions, using the sodium bicarbonate and saline solution supplied to dilute the concentrated artesunate.

For a small pregnant woman (estimated body weight 50 kg), each dose would be 12 mL IV (10 mg/mL) or 6 mL IM (20 mg/mL).

Artesunate IM should be administered in the antero-lateral thigh, drawing back before injection to ensure that the needle is not in a vein.

IM artemether

Artemether IM: loading dose is 3.2 mg/kg on day 0, followed by 1.6 mg/kg daily for at least two more doses; then continue until oral therapy is possible. A full course of oral therapy should be taken once IM therapy is discontinued.

An 80 mg/mL presentation is preferred to reduce the volume of the injection.

For a small pregnant woman (estimated body weight 50 kg) each dose would be 2 mL IM (80 mg/mL).

Artemether IM should be administered in the antero-lateral thigh, drawing back before injection to ensure that the needle is not in a vein.

Artemether is not well absorbed in shock, and in this situation an alternative treatment (parenteral or rectal artesunate, or IV quinine) should be chosen.

Rectal artesunate

- It is recommended that this should be available in all rural settings, including those with trained village healthcare workers.
- It can be given at 12-hourly intervals.
- The minimum dose is 10 mg/kg. Larger doses are not harmful, but are not more effective.
- It can also be given to vomiting patients, or those unable to tolerate oral drugs.
- Rectal artesunate must always be followed by a full course of ACT when the patient is able to take oral drugs.

At present the WHO only recommends rectal artesunate as a pre-referral treatment. Where referral is not possible, ensure that a full course of ACT is given as soon as the patient is able to take oral treatment.

Artesunate is available as a rectal capsule: Rectocaps (Mepha), 50 mg and 200 mg.

A WHO-approved rectal capsule is to be available soon, as 100 mg and 400 mg presentation.

The dose is 10 mg/kg, and therefore an average-sized mother needs 600 mg per dose. Give three 200 mg rectal suppositories at 0, 12, 24, 36, 48 and 60 hours.

Follow-on treatment

When the patient has received at least three parenteral doses of artesunate or artemether, and is able to tolerate oral intake, give a full course (3 days) of **ACT** orally.

Quinine dihydrochloride
Always give quinine with glucose.

Do not confuse doses of salt and base. Quinine is usually prescribed as the salt (10 mg of quinine dihydrochloride = 8.3 mg of base).

Loading dose

Infuse quinine dihydrochloride 20 mg/kg body weight (usually 1.2 grams for the average 60 kg pregnant woman) in

500 mL of IV fluids (Ringer-lactate or Hartmann's solution plus 5% or 10% glucose) over 4 to 8 hours. Do not let it go in too quickly. Quinine is usually available in 2-mL ampoules of 150 mg/mL, where 1.2 g thus corresponds to 8 mL.

Do not give quinine in 5% dextrose solutions, as there is a danger of hyponatraemia. Add 50 mL of 50% glucose to 500 mL of Ringer-lactate or Hartmann's solution to produce Ringer-lactate or Hartmann's plus 5% glucose solutions. Add 100 mL of 50% glucose to 500 mL of Ringer-lactate or Hartmann's solution to give 10% glucose solutions.

Never give an IV bolus injection of quinine, as it is likely to cause cardiac arrest.

- If **it is definitely known that the mother has taken an adequate dose of quinine** (1.2 grams) within the preceding 12 hours, do **not** give the loading dose. Proceed with the maintenance dose (see below).
- If **the history of treatment is not known or is unclear**, give the loading dose of quinine.

Alternatively, omit the loading dose if the patient has received three or more doses of oral quinine in the last 48 hours, or mefloquine or halofantrine within the last 3 days.

- Wait 8 hours before giving the maintenance dose.

Maintenance dose

Infuse quinine dihydrochloride 10 mg/kg body weight (usually 600 mg for the average pregnant woman) in 500 mL of fluids (as above) IV over 4 hours. Repeat every 8 hours (i.e. quinine infusion for 4 hours, no quinine for 4 hours, quinine infusion for 4 hours, etc.) for 24 hours and then change to oral medication if the woman is conscious and able to swallow safely.

For follow-on oral treatment, give a **3-day course of ACT or 7 days of oral quinine**. If the combination AS + MQ is used, wait 12 hours after the last dose of quinine before giving MQ. Do not use AS + MQ if the patient developed neurological signs during the acute phase.

The dose of oral quinine dihydrochloride or quinine sulphate is 10 mg/kg body weight (usually 600 mg for the average size of pregnant woman) by mouth every 8 hours to complete 7 days of treatment. Ask the patient to swallow the tablets quickly with milk.

Monitor blood glucose levels for hypoglycaemia every hour while the patient is receiving quinine IV.

Quinine may increase the risk of hypoglycaemia, and it may cause haemolysis in patients with glucose-6-phosphate dehydrogenase (G6PD) deficiency, which may result in the passage of haemoglobin in the urine (this is called **blackwater fever**).

Make sure that plenty of fluids are given so that the urine output is adequate. Keep a strict fluid balance chart. Monitor the volume of fluid that you give, and the urine output. Do not overload with fluid.

If the haemoglobin level falls below 6 g/dL, try to give blood, but observe closely for fluid overload. When the patient is improving, give iron and folate tablets.

Intramuscular quinine

If you cannot place an IV line, you can give quinine IM, at a strength of not more than 60 mg/mL. Some ampoules are 60 mg/mL (usually 10-mL ampoules). Some ampoules are 300 mg/mL or 600 mg/mL. Dilute these in 0.9% saline or Ringer-lactate or Hartmann's solution to a concentration of

60 mg/mL (e.g. 600 mg of quinine in 10 mL of saline). If you do not dilute quinine, the mother may develop an injection abscess. Use the same dose as you would give IV. Give half the dose into each anterior thigh.

When giving quinine by IM injection, regularly draw back to ensure that the needle is not in a vein, as an IV injection of quinine is likely to cause cardiac arrest.

Fluid replacement

If the patient is unable to drink, maintain daily fluid requirements using the nasogastric (preferred) or IV (greater risk of fluid overload) route. Do not use 0.9% saline as it is an acid solution: use Ringer-lactate or Hartmann's solution. Measure urine output (a Foley catheter should be used in unconscious patients).

Weight	Daily fluid requirement	Hourly fluid requirement
In pregnancy	50 mL/kg	2.0 mL/kg

IV fluids

A Ringer-lactate or Hartmann's solution plus glucose mix is commonly recommended. Use a 10% glucose mix with Ringer-lactate or Hartmann's solution if hypoglycaemia is identified. Monitor carefully for fluid overload, especially when the IV route is used. Switch to the oral route as soon as possible. Fluids given should be included in the daily fluid requirement totals to avoid over-hydration.

Antibiotics

All patients who are in shock or who remain severely ill following resuscitation should receive a presumptive treatment with broad-spectrum IV antibiotics. Unconscious patients should have a lumbar puncture to exclude meningitis. Where this is not possible a presumptive treatment with a suitable antibiotic should be given.

Continuing hospital care of pregnant women with severe malaria

This should include the following:

- Nurse in the lateral position if the woman is more than 20 weeks' pregnant, to avoid inferior vena caval compression.
- If the patient is unconscious, nurse her in the recovery position, alternating sides frequently.
- Observe hourly pulse, blood pressure, respiratory rate and level of consciousness (using the AVPU scale: *see* Section 1.11).
- Frequently measure blood glucose levels (every hour if the patient has a reduced conscious level, especially when they are receiving quinine and/or where the level of consciousness does not improve).
- If the patient is conscious, regularly (4-hourly) determine blood glucose levels to exclude hypoglycaemia particularly if the patient is not eating well. This is especially important in pregnant women, particularly those receiving quinine therapy.
- A daily microscopic blood slide to determine the level of parasitaemia and to follow treatment efficacy.
- Regular haemoglobin measurement. The frequency will depend on the rate of red blood cell breakdown. This may be very rapid in cases of high parasite density.

- Blood transfusion where necessary with careful monitoring to prevent fluid overload. Packed cells should be used where possible. If overload is suspected, give a single dose of 20 mg IV.
- If the patient is unconscious or in shock, administer IV broad-spectrum antibiotics to manage septicaemia, pneumonia or meningitis, which are often associated with cerebral malaria.
- Oxygen is needed for patients in respiratory distress.
- Blood gases and urea and electrolytes should be measured where possible.
- Controlled IV fluids.
- Fluid balance charts: unconscious patients should be catheterised to measure urine output, facilitate correct fluid balance and detect possible renal failure.

Management of life-threatening complications of severe malaria

Severe anaemia (due to haemolysis)

Monitor haemoglobin levels daily.

Severe haemolytic anaemia: haemoglobin < 5 g/dL or haematocrit < 15%.

Severe anaemia may be the presenting feature in malaria. Patients with severe anaemia, especially pregnant women, should be tested for malaria.

- Establish safe transfusion as soon as possible.
- Transfuse with screened blood only if the patient is severely symptomatic. For patients with haemoglobin < 5 g/dL or haematocrit < 15%, recheck haemoglobin levels at least every 4 hours. Transfuse if haemoglobin levels start to fall or symptoms develop.
  - Packed cells are preferred for transfusion in pregnancy. Allow red blood cells to settle at the bottom of the bag, and stop the infusion when all of the cells have been used.
  - Perform microscopy following transfusion, and repeat or extend antimalarial treatment if parasitaemia is increasing.
- **Transfusion rates** may depend on the status of the patient. Exercise caution with malnourished patients.
- **Suggested rates:** two 500-mL units over 4–6 hours giving IV 20 mg of furosemide with each 500 mL.
- If the patient shows signs of fluid overload, give additional furosemide 20 mg IV, and repeat after 1–2 hours if indicated.

Give ferrous sulphate or ferrous fumarate 60 mg by mouth *plus* folic acid 5 mg by mouth once daily upon discharge.

Hypoglycaemia

This is defined as glucose levels of less than 2.5 mmol/litre (< 45 mg/dL).

Check for hypoglycaemia in patients who are unconscious, in shock or deteriorating, especially if they are malnourished, and in all patients receiving quinine. Often hypoglycaemia causes no symptoms until it results in coma and death. Watch for abnormal behaviour, sweating and sudden coma. Always give glucose with quinine. If the mother is drowsy, delirious or unconscious, do not assume that she has cerebral malaria; she is probably hypoglycaemic.

Treat with an IV glucose infusion over 15 minutes.

- If you give 50% glucose it irritates the veins, so dilute

50 mL of 50% glucose with 50 mL of Ringer-lactate or Hartmann's solution to make a 25% solution.

- Then give 500 mL of 5% dextrose in Ringer-lactate or Hartmann's solution over 8 hours (see above for details of how to prepare this).

If you do not have IV glucose, give sugar water by mouth or by nasogastric tube. Dissolve 4 level teaspoons (20 grams) in a 200 mL cup of clean water.

Retest 15 minutes after completion of infusion, and repeat the infusion if blood glucose levels remain low. Repeat until blood glucose levels recover, and then infuse with 5–10% glucose in Ringer-lactate or Hartmann's solution (according to hypoglycaemia risk) to prevent recurrence. Ensure regular feeding when oral intake can be sustained. Fluids used to treat hypoglycaemia must be included in the daily fluid requirements.

Hypoglycaemia is a major cause of death in patients with severe malaria, especially those who are pregnant. Remember that quinine will potentiate hypoglycaemia. Patients should receive regular feeding, including by nasogastric tube, when they are unable to take oral foods.

Fluid balance problems

Maintain a strict fluid balance chart and monitor the amount of fluids administered and urine output to ensure that there is no fluid overload. Assess the patient's clinical status regularly.

Note: Pregnant women with severe malaria are prone to fluid overload.

Acute renal failure (ARF)

This is defined as an abrupt decline in the renal regulation of water, electrolytes and acid–base balance, and continues to be an important factor contributing to the morbidity and mortality of malaria patients.

Oliguria or anuria is often associated with jaundice, anaemia and bleeding disorders.

Note: Dehydration is a common cause of low urine output.

- The basic principles of management are avoidance of life-threatening complications, maintenance of fluid and electrolyte balance, and nutritional support.
- The patient must be catheterised so that urine output can be accurately measured.
- Acute renal failure is suspected when the hourly urine output is < 30 mL/hour (over 4 hours). Blood concentrations of urea and creatinine are usually raised (> 2.9 mg/dL that is > 256 mmol/litre).
- Make sure that the patient is adequately hydrated, but avoid overload.
- If possible, monitor plasma electrolytes, especially serum potassium levels.

If urine output continues to be low despite adequate hydration, peripheral perfusion and normal blood pressure, give furosemide 40 mg IV.

If renal failure is established, restrict fluid to insensible loss (30 mL/hour) plus urine output. If possible, refer the mother to a tertiary care centre for management of renal failure. Consider peritoneal dialysis (if available).

Convulsions

If there are **convulsions**, consider whether the mother has eclampsia. Test the urine for protein and measure the blood pressure (*see* Section 2.5.E).

If the mother has eclampsia, treat this with magnesium sulphate. If she does not have eclampsia, prevent more convulsions with anticonvulsants.

Note: seizure activity in cerebral malaria needs to be looked for carefully, as it may just appear as a twitching of the thumb or mouth.

Give diazepam, 10 mg rectally or by slow IV injection over 2 minutes.

Do not exceed 10 mg per dose. Always have a bag-valve-mask of a suitable size available in case the mother stops breathing.

Alternatively, paraldehyde 0.1 mL/kg of body weight may be given by deep IM injection (usually 6 mL total dose) or 0.4 mL/kg of body weight (usually 24 mL) intra-rectally using a sterile glass syringe (a disposable plastic syringe may be used provided that the injection is given immediately after the paraldehyde is drawn up, and the syringe is never reused).

Consider preventing subsequent convulsions with phenytoin (see below).

Phenytoin
Loading dose

Infuse phenytoin 1 gram (approximately 18 mg/kg body weight) in 50–100 mL of 0.9% saline over 30 minutes (the final concentration should not exceed 10 mg/mL).

Note: Only 0.9% saline can be used to infuse phenytoin. All other IV fluids will cause crystallisation of phenytoin.

Flush the IV line with 0.9% saline before and after infusing phenytoin.

Do not infuse phenytoin at a rate exceeding 50 mg/minute, due to the risk of irregular heartbeat, hypotension and respiratory depression. Complete administration within 1 hour of preparation.

Maintenance dose

Give phenytoin 100 mg IV slowly over 2 minutes or by mouth every 8 hours beginning at least 12 hours after the loading dose.

Respiratory distress

Rapid laboured breathing: check for and treat secondary pneumonia (give antibiotics and oxygen) or anaemia (transfuse), or pulmonary oedema, which may occur with or without fluid overload. Check the fluid balance (reduce IV fluids), supply oxygen, nurse the patient in a semi-sitting position, and do a trial of furosemide, 40 mg IV, repeating this after 1–2 hours if indicated.

Slower laboured breathing (acidotic) (Kussmaul breathing): ensure appropriate fluid replacement (plus transfusion if indicated), and treat associated conditions and infections.

Metabolic acidosis

Deep breathing with a clear chest is a sensitive and specific sign for the presence of metabolic acidosis. It is the single most important determinant of survival, and can lead to respiratory distress syndrome. Metabolic (lactic) acidosis has been identified as an important cause of death in severe malaria.

Metabolic acidosis in severe malaria has been attributed to the combined effects of several factors that reduce oxygen delivery to tissues:

1 increased production of lactic acid by parasites (through direct stimulation by cytokines)
2 decreased clearance by the liver
3 a marked reduction in the deformability of uninfected red blood cells, which may compromise blood flow through tissues
4 dehydration and hypovolaemia, which can exacerbate microvascular obstruction by reducing perfusion pressure
5 destruction of red blood cells and anaemia, which further compromise oxygen delivery.

Management

- Maintain airway patency and oxygen delivery; intubate if the patient is unconscious, in severe shock, or otherwise unstable.
- Establish an IV line; replace an adequate intravascular fluid volume if the patient has tachycardia, hypotension or other signs of poor tissue perfusion, such as poor capillary refill time. **IV normal (0.9%) saline can be harmful in severe malaria, when there is frequently acidosis. Normal saline is a strongly acidotic solution and can make the acidosis much worse. Therefore use Ringer-lactate or Hartmann's solution for IV fluid replacement or in shock.**
- Monitor for cardiac arrhythmias.
- The use of sodium bicarbonate is controversial and generally should be avoided.

Pulmonary oedema is very dangerous. The mother may have it on admission, or it may develop after several days. Fast difficult breathing is the first sign. Frothy (bubbly) fluid may be coming from the mouth. Pulmonary oedema causes hypoxia, fits, coma and death. It can also be caused by too much fluid. Sometimes it is caused by malaria and too much IV fluid, so watch the jugular venous pressure regularly and ideally, if skilled, measure central venous pressure.

- Keep the patient upright; prop them up with pillows and lower the foot of the bed.
- Give high concentrations of oxygen using a face mask and reservoir.
- Give furosemide 40 mg IV. If there is no response (i.e. no increase in urine output), increase the dose progressively, every 4 hours, up to a maximum of 200 mg.
- If the woman might be receiving too much IV fluid, stop all drips.
- If the woman does not improve, withdraw 250 mL of blood into a transfusion bag. Give it back to her later.

Shock

Although severe malaria alone may cause shock (algid malaria), it is uncommon and bacterial sepsis often coexists, which must be treated.

Management includes initial assessment for severe anaemia, which can also be the cause of shock due to lack of oxygen-carrying capacity in severe anaemia. The management of severe anaemia, if this is responsible, is described above.

If the patient is not severely anaemic, and particularly if they are dehydrated, give rapid fluid replacement provided that there are no signs of pulmonary oedema:

- Ringer-lactate or Hartmann's solution IV, 500 mL over 30 minutes, then reassess. If there is no improvement

in capillary refill or tachycardia, repeat the infusion once or twice more, as required.

Give IV broad-spectrum antibiotics to treat septicaemia and any associated infections.

Abnormal bleeding

- Transfuse with fresh blood.
- Give vitamin K 10 mg IV or orally.
- Avoid IM injections and non-steroidal anti-inflammatory drugs (NSAIDs).

Coexisting infections

Treat any associated pneumonia, dysentery or endometritis (see Sections 2.8.A, 2.8.B and 2.5.G).

Congenital malaria

Congenital malaria is relatively rare; it occurs in up to 10% of affected pregnancies. This is because the placental barrier and maternal IgG antibodies that cross the placenta protect the fetus to some extent. All four species can cause congenital malaria, but P. malariae causes proportionally more than the other species.

Congenital malaria is much more common in non-immune populations, and the incidence increases during epidemics of malaria.

Fetal plasma quinine levels are about one-third of simultaneous maternal levels, and this sub-therapeutic drug level does not cure the infection in the fetus.

The newborn child can manifest with fever, irritability, feeding problems, hepatosplenomegaly, anaemia and jaundice. The diagnosis can be confirmed by a smear from cord blood or a heel prick, any time within 1 week after birth (HRP2 tests may not be relevant in the early days after birth, as the infant blood may include HRP2 from the mother). The risk of congenital malaria is higher in children born to mothers who have malaria during or shortly before delivery.

Prevention, diagnosis and treatment of non-falciparum malaria

Other forms of malaria are found all over the world and need to be prevented, diagnosed and treated.

P. vivax and P. ovale malaria

P. vivax and P. ovale malaria are recurrent due to the fact that the parasites can conceal themselves as the hypnozoite form in the liver. They can emerge and cause new attacks of malaria at regular intervals for up to 30 years. Most medications (except primaquine) only act on the erythrocyte stage of the parasite and therefore do not affect the hypnozoites.

Prevention

Long Lasting Impregnated Bednets (LLINs) with appropriate information should be supplied to prevent initial infection (and co-infection with other parasite species), but they will not prevent recurrent attacks once the infection is established. **Indoor residual spraying** should be used.

Diagnosis

The following methods can be used:

- microscopy
- RDTs: **HRP2 tests such as Paracheck will only detect P. falciparum**. pLDH tests such as CareStart will detect

other species. At present the sensitivity and specificity of pLDH in detecting *P. vivax* and other species of malaria are not clearly defined

- **Polymerase chain reaction (PCR)** can be used to distinguish between new and recurrent infections.

Treatment

At present, the treatment for *P. vivax* malaria (and the other non-falciparum species) is **chloroquine (CQ)**.

This should only be used for CQ-sensitive non-falciparum malaria.

It is available in the following formulations:

- 100 mg base tablets (chloroquine phosphate)
- 150 mg base tablets
- 50 mg base/5 mL syrup.

Chloroquine is sometimes found as a salt, but the WHO recommends use of the base product.

The regime described below is recommended by the WHO for use in settings where compliance may be difficult and dosing regimes need to be simplified.

Dose: 6 tablets 100 mg on days 1 and 2, then 3 tablets 100 mg on day 3 *or* 4 tablets 150 mg on days 1 and 2, then

2 tablets 150 mg on day 3. **Total dose** = 1500 mg base (= 2500 mg salt).

There is some evidence of resistance to chloroquine in India and Indonesia, but it is difficult to determine whether apparent failure of the treatment is due to recurrence from hypnozoites or to drug failure. There has been little evidence from efficacy studies.

Note: ACTs cure all types of malaria, but chloroquine is still effective (and cheaper) for treating most cases of *P. vivax*, *P. malariae* and *P. ovale*.

As mentioned above, chloroquine only kills the parasites in the red blood cells, and does not kill the pre-erythrocyte forms or the hypnozoites of the recurrent malarias *P. vivax* and *P. ovale* in the liver.

At present **primaquine** is the only drug available to tackle the hypnozoites and prevent recurrence.

Treatment with primaquine

Primaquine is the only drug at present available to prevent recurrent attacks of *P. vivax* and *P. ovale*. However, it is not recommended for pregnant women, so treatment with this drug should wait until the pregnancy has ended.

2.8.E Acute appendicitis

Introduction

Appendicitis should be suspected in any woman or girl with abdominal pain, whether she is pregnant or not. The diagnosis of appendicitis can be more difficult in pregnancy, due to the possibility of pregnancy-related conditions, including ectopic pregnancy, abruptio placentae, torsion of an ovarian cyst and pyelonephritis.

As pregnancy advances, the enlarging uterus displaces the appendix from its usual position, shifting the site of maximal tenderness towards the right upper quadrant (*see* Figure 2.8.E.1). In the third trimester, it may consequently mimic cholecystitis. The site of an incision for appendicectomy should be over the point of maximum tenderness.

Clinical management

If appendicitis is suspected clinically, give a combination of antibiotics before surgery, and continue until the woman is post-operative and fever-free for 48 hours:

- ampicillin 2 grams IV every 6 hours
- *plus* gentamicin 80 mg IV/IM every 8 hours or 5 mg/kg body weight IV/IM once every 24 hours
- *plus* metronidazole 500 mg IV every 8 hours.

Morphine 10 mg IV or IM may be administered as analgesia (*see* Section 1.16).

Immediate surgical exploration is required, regardless of the stage of gestation. Appendicectomy should be performed even if the appendix does not look infected.

Delaying diagnosis and treatment can result in rupture of the appendix, which may lead to generalised peritonitis. This has a high maternal mortality in pregnancy, as well as a significant risk of miscarriage or preterm labour.

If there are **signs of peritonitis** (fever, rebound tenderness and guarding), give antibiotics above as for peritonitis but continue until the infection has fully resolved (usually following surgery) and there has been no fever for 48 hours.

If **appendicitis occurs in late pregnancy**, the infection may be walled off by the gravid uterus. As the uterus rapidly decreases in size (involutes) after delivery, the infection may spill into the peritoneal cavity. In these cases, appendicitis then presents as generalised peritonitis.

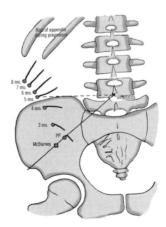

FIGURE 2.8.E.1 The changes in position of the appendix as pregnancy advances. Adapted from McGraw-Hill Companies, Inc. Reproduced with the permission of Chris Paschalidis.

2.8.F Cystitis and acute pyelonephritis

BOX 2.8.F Minimum requirements
- Microscopy and bacterial culture.
- Dipstick tests for leucocytes and nitrites.
- Antibiotics (e.g. ampicillin, gentamicin).
- Ultrasonography.

Acute cystitis

Cystitis is a common complication of pregnancy, and is characterised by dysuria, frequency, urgency and, if severe, by haematuria. Severe cystitis can progress to pyelonephritis if not treated. The presence of loin pain and tenderness, along with fever, suggests a diagnosis of pyelonephritis.

Asymptomatic cystitis is more common in pregnancy, carries a risk of progression to pyelonephritis, and is associated with an increased risk of premature delivery.

Diagnosis
- Use a dipstick leucocyte esterase test to detect white blood cells, and a nitrate reductase test to detect nitrites.
- Microscopy of a urine specimen (see Section 8.5) may show white blood cells in clumps, bacteria and sometimes red blood cells. Urine examination requires a clean-catch midstream specimen of urine to minimise the possibility of contamination. The results of bacterial culture, although not necessary before starting treatment, are helpful if there is treatment failure, and also for monitoring bacterial sensitivity in the population.

Treatment with antibiotics for uncomplicated cystitis
- Amoxicillin 500 mg by mouth three times a day for 5 days or cephalexin (or alternative available cephalosporin) 500 mg three times a day for 5 days.
- Trimethoprim/sulfamethoxazole 1 tablet 160/800 mg by mouth twice a day for 3 days. **This drug is best avoided in pregnancy** unless there is no alternative. It must be completely avoided in the first trimester. This antibiotic is a folate antagonist and therefore promotes congenital abnormalities, and in the third trimester it may cause haemolysis in the neonate.
- If treatment fails, check urine culture and sensitivity (if available), and treat with an antibiotic appropriate for the organism.

Acute pyelonephritis

Acute pyelonephritis is an acute infection of the upper urinary tract, mainly of the renal pelvis, which may also involve the renal parenchyma. It can precipitate premature labour.
- If shock is present or suspected, initiate immediate ABC treatment.
- Check urine culture and sensitivity (if available), and treat with an antibiotic appropriate for the organism.
- If urine culture is unavailable, treat with antibiotics until the woman has been fever-free for 48 hours:
  - ampicillin 2 grams IV every 6 hours
  - *plus* gentamicin 80 mg IM/IV every 8 hours or 5 mg/kg body weight IV/IM once every 24 hours.
- Once the woman has been fever-free for 48 hours, give amoxicillin/ampicillin 500 mg by mouth three times a day to complete 14 days of treatment.
- If there is no clinical response within 72 hours, review the results and antibiotic coverage.
  Alternative and/or second line treatment is with IV cephalosporins, e.g. cefuroxime 750 mg to 1.5 g 8-hourly.
- Perform a renal ultrasound scan. If any significant malformation of the kidneys or renal tract is noted, refer the patient for specialist advice.

2.8.G Tuberculosis in pregnancy

BOX 2.8.G Minimum standards
- Mantoux test/purified protein derivative.
- Sputum for acid-fast bacilli for stain and culture.
- Chest X-ray.
- Anti-tuberculosis therapy.

Introduction

Tuberculosis (TB) is generally becoming less common during pregnancy and in the fetus, even in high endemic countries, but remains a leading infectious cause of death during pregnancy and delivery, especially among women living with HIV. It is estimated that more than half a million women of child-bearing age die from TB (including HIV-related TB) each year, but the current epidemiology of TB in pregnancy is a reflection of the general incidence of disease. The infection has been associated with an increased risk of spontaneous abortion, perinatal mortality, small-for-gestational age and low birth weight in some studies. Poor outcome is attributable to delays in diagnosis or treatment, increasing the frequency of severe forms of extra-pulmonary disease.

Clinical findings

Signs and symptoms of TB are usually the same in both pregnant and non-pregnant woman. They include prolonged fever (especially at night), cough, weight loss, fatigue and breathing difficulty. Extra-pulmonary disease will present with organ-specific signs and symptoms such as lymphadenopathy, abdominal pain or mass, back pain, vaginal bleeding, pelvic inflammatory disease symptoms or infertility.

Diagnosis

Any woman who presents to an antenatal clinic with chronic respiratory symptoms, or has had close contact with a TB index case, or unexplained illness, should be screened for TB. This includes a tuberculin skin test, sputum for acid-fast bacilli (AFB) stain and culture for mycobacterium TB. A chest X-ray may have harmful effects on the fetus in the first trimester of pregnancy, but may be done with an abdominal lead shield. If clinically indicated a Chest X-ray is recommended as the risk to the fetus is very small and the mother's health a priority.

Additional newer tests, namely interferon gamma release assay (IGRA) or polymerase chain reaction (PCR) identification (if available), may complement diagnosis.

Extra-pulmonary TB is much more difficult to diagnose during pregnancy. After delivery, the placenta should be sent for histopathology, AFB stain and AFB culture to contribute to a diagnosis. The neonate should be evaluated thoroughly and treated accordingly.

Antituberculous treatment during pregnancy

During pregnancy, tuberculosis represents a greater hazard to the pregnant woman and her fetus than does its treatment. Therefore treatment should be commenced as soon as possible after a diagnosis has been made. Treatment for new patients with pulmonary TB is the same in pregnancy as it is for all other adults (see WHO guidelines 4th edition 2010 for full details: www.who.int/tb/publications/2010/9789241547833/en/).

In summary, new patients with pulmonary TB should be treated with a regime containing isoniazid (H) and rifampicin (R) for 6 months (see Table 2.8.G.1 for doses). There is an initial 2-month intensive phase of HRZE and then a 4-month continuation phase of just HR.

The optimal dosing frequency is daily throughout the 6-month course. However, provided directly observed treatment is practiced and the patient is not living with HIV infection or in a high risk setting for HIV the last 4 months of treatment can be given three times a week.

Isoniazid, ethambutol and rifampin are relatively safe for the fetus. In some countries, the routine use of pyrazinamide is discouraged because of inadequate teratogenicity data, but the WHO continues to recommend it as first-line therapy. The benefits of ethambutol and rifampin for therapy of tuberculosis disease in the mother outweigh the risk to the infant.

The use of these first-line antituberculous drugs in pregnancy is considered safe for the mother and the baby by the British Thoracic Society, International Union Against Tuberculosis and Lung Disease, and the World Health Organization.

The effects of other second-line drugs on the fetus are unknown, and their use during pregnancy must be undertaken only after a careful risk and benefit analysis.

Fixed-dose combinations (FDCs) are recommended in both children and adults, but drugs can be given separately as well. Tablets are the preferred formulation, even in children, as they prevent the emergence of resistance and improve compliance.

The WHO-recommended two-, three- and four-drug FDC schemes are simplified for clinical use according to body weight, and ensure that the doses remain within the therapeutic margins, and that underlying liver and renal impairment is considered (see Tables 2.8.G.1 and 2).

Drugs that are contraindicated during pregnancy

These include the following:

- streptomycin (which interferes with development of the ear and may cause congenital deafness)
- kanamycin, amikacin and capreomycin
- fluoroquinolones (ciprofloxacin, levofloxacin, ofloxacin and sparfloxacin)
- other second-line drugs (cycloserine, ethionamide and clofazimine).

TB treatment during pregnancy is the same for pregnant women as it is for non-pregnant women.

TABLE 2.8.G.1 Commonly used drugs for the treatment of TB in pregnancy

Drug	Daily dose (mg/kg/when given daily)	Daily dose when given three times weekly	Potential adverse reactions
Isoniazid (H) tablet, 100 mg, 300 mg	5 mg/kg (4–6 mg/kg) Maximum 300 mg	10 mg/kg (8–12 mg/kg) Maximum 900 mg	Mild hepatic enzyme elevation, hepatitis, peripheral neuritis, hypersensitivity
Rifampin (R) tablet, 150 mg, 300 mg, 450 mg	10 mg/kg (8–12 mg/kg) Maximum 600 mg	10 mg/kg (8–12 mg/kg) Maximum 600 mg	Orange discoloration of urine and other body fluids, vomiting, hepatitis
Pyrazinamide (Z) tablet, 500 mg	25 mg/kg (20–30 mg/kg)	35 mg/kg (30–40 mg/kg)	Hepatoxicity, hyperuricaemia
Ethambutol (E) tablet, 100 mg, 400 mg	15 mg/kg (15–20 mg/kg)	30 mg/kg (25–35 mg/kg)	Optic neuritis, decreased visual acuity, gastrointestinal disturbance, hypersensitivity
Four-drug FDC tablet, R 150 mg + H 75 mg + Z 400 mg + E 275 mg	Dosage recommendations are more straightforward, and adjustment of dosage is done according to patient weight category		
Three-drug FDC tablet, R 150 mg + H 75 mg + Z 400 mg			
Two-drug FDC tablet, R 300 mg + H 150 mg			
R 150 mg + H 75 mg			
Two-drug FDC tablet, H 150 mg + E 400 mg			

H = isoniazid, R = rifampicin, Z = pyrazinamide, E = ethambutol, S = streptomycin, FDC = fixed drug combination.

- A **three- to four-drug regimen** of isoniazid, rifampin and pyrazinamide with or without ethambutol is recommended for uncomplicated pulmonary TB (*see* Table 2.8.G.1).
- If pyrazinamide treatment is included in the initial drug regimen, after an **initial 2 months of three to four drugs**, therapy is continued with **two drugs** (isoniazid and rifampin) to complete **at least 6 months of therapy**.
- If pyrazinamide is not used, the two-drug period should be extended to at least 9 months.
- Prompt initiation of therapy is mandatory to protect the mother and the fetus.

Streptomycin should not be used in pregnancy, as it crosses the placenta and can cause auditory nerve impairment and nephrotoxicity in the fetus.

Vitamin K should be administered at birth to the infant of a mother taking rifampicin because of the risk of postnatal haemorrhage.

Pyridoxine (vitamin B$_6$) 10 mg daily is recommended for pregnant or breastfeeding women who are taking isoniazid-containing regimens.

Extra-pulmonary TB in pregnant women requires the same regimens as uncomplicated pulmonary TB. Some forms (e.g. meningitis, bone, joint) require a longer duration (9–12 months) of TB drugs.

If a woman has suspected resistant TB, attempts must be made to confirm drug resistance by appropriate cultures and therapy based on susceptibility results. Regimens are complicated and depend on susceptibilities, previous drug therapy, local susceptibility data, availability of second-line drugs and tolerability. **An expert in infectious disease must be consulted in such cases.** Pregnant women with resistant TB have a less favourable prognosis. They may sometimes require treatment with second-line drugs, including cycloserine, ofloxacin, amikacin, kanamycin, capreomycin and ethionamide. The safety of these drugs is not well established in pregnancy.

Breastfeeding and TB

The low concentrations of anti-TB drugs in breast milk do not produce toxicity in the nursing newborn. Therefore breast-feeding should not be discouraged for an HIV-seronegative woman who is planning to take or is taking anti-TB drugs. Anti-TB treatment is the best way to prevent transmission of tubercle bacilli to the baby. Mother and baby should stay together and the baby should continue to breastfeed. After active TB in the baby is ruled out, the baby should be given 6 months of isoniazid preventive therapy, followed by BCG vaccination (for advice on breastfeeding and HIV, *see* Section 6.2.D). Breastfed infants do not require pyridoxine supplementation unless they are receiving isoniazid.

Treatment of latent TB infection

In most pregnant women, treatment of latent TB infection (LTBI) – that is, treatment of asymptomatic pregnant women with a positive tuberculin test or IGRA result and normal chest X-ray – should be delayed until 2 or 3 months after delivery, even though no harmful effects of isoniazid (INH, the standard treatment regimen for LTBI) on the fetus have been documented.

However, in the following situations where there is a high risk of progressing to active disease, treatment for LTBI with isoniazid (INH), 300 mg daily should begin during pregnancy.

Treatment of LTBI should be started **during the first trimester** of pregnancy for:

- pregnant women who have HIV infection or behavioural risk factors for HIV infection, but who refuse HIV testing
- pregnant women who have been in recent close contact with an individual with smear-positive pulmonary TB.

Treatment of LTBI should be started **after the first trimester** of pregnancy for pregnant women who have had a documented tuberculin skin test conversion in the past 2 years.

Treatment of LTBI, if indicated, should be started 2 to 3 months after delivery for all other pregnant women, including those with radiographic evidence of old healed TB. The recommended duration of LTBI therapy is 9 months. If a woman who is taking isoniazid and/or rifampin for treatment of LTBI becomes pregnant, treatment should be interrupted and started again 2 or 3 months after delivery, unless one or more of the above risk factors are present.

Perinatal TB

Women who have only pulmonary TB are not likely to infect the fetus, but can infect their infant after delivery. Although protection of the infant from exposure and infection is of paramount importance, continuous close contact between infant and mother should be encouraged. Congenital TB is rare, but *in-utero* infections can occur after maternal bacteraemia. If a newborn infant has suspected congenital TB, a full evaluation should be done and treatment initiated based on individual circumstances and specific recommendations. Management of the newborn infant is based on categorisation of the maternal (or household contact) infection as follows:

- If the mother has completed TB chemotherapy during pregnancy, or has inactive disease, her infant should be given BCG at birth.
- If the mother has active disease or still requires treatment, the infant should be given isoniazid 10 mg/kg once daily for 3 to 6 months.
- Once the mother and infant are on appropriate treatment, the infant may breastfeed unless the mother has multidrug-resistant TB. A tuberculin test and chest X-ray are then performed on the neonate. If these are negative, BCG is given. If they are positive, full investigations for TB are undertaken. If no evidence of disease is detected, isoniazid is continued for another 3 to 4 months. If TB is suspected, full treatment is given at standard doses.

Monitoring

All pregnant women with TB must be carefully followed up monthly. At each visit, the patient needs to be checked for compliance, response to therapy, adverse effects and adjustment for any clinical event.

Directly observed treatment

Directly observed treatment: short-course (DOTS) remains an important WHO strategy for reducing the TB burden worldwide. In DOTS, healthcare workers observe patients as they take their medicine. DOTS is practised even for children, and parents can be asked to supervise treatment in the communities where DOTS is used. This is especially true for HIV-infected children, patients with multi-drug-resistant (MDR) TB or those with complicated TB, and has been shown to be successful.

The WHO has developed a new six-point **Stop TB Strategy**, which builds on the successes of DOTS. One of these is to 'pursue high-quality DOTS expansion and enhancement' through the following steps.

1 Secure political commitment, with adequate and sustained financing.

2 Ensure early case detection and diagnosis through quality-assured bacteriology.
3 Provide standardised treatment with supervision and patient support.
4 Ensure effective drug supply and management.
5 Monitor and evaluate performance and impact.

2.8.H Syphilis in pregnancy and the newborn infant

Introduction

Syphilis is a dangerous bacterial infection caused by *Treponema pallidum* which, when it occurs in pregnancy, can cause early fetal death, stillbirth, preterm birth, neonatal death or congenital infection. Mother-to-child transmission is a major problem, especially in resource-limited countries.

In a recent analysis, it was estimated that in 2008 worldwide there were between 1.2 and 1.6 million pregnant women with active syphilis, of whom 39% were living in Africa. In the absence of screening and treatment this would have resulted globally in 707 000 adverse pregnancy outcomes, including 286 000 stillbirths or early fetal deaths, 122 000 neonatal deaths, 82 000 preterm or low-birth-weight babies and 218 000 infected newborn infants. Additional mortality after the first month of life was estimated to be 10% by 1 year of age.

The cost of diagnosis and treatment per individual is US$2.

All countries must ensure that all pregnant women have access to antenatal care that includes diagnostic screening and treatment for syphilis.

Clinical features

Infection is either congenital (through *in-utero* transfer) or acquired (through sexual transmission or blood transfusion). The average time between acquired infection and the appearance of symptoms and signs is 21 days, but this period can range from 10 to 90 days.

Acquired syphilis has early and late phases. The early phase has primary, secondary, early latent (hidden and < 1 year), late latent (hidden > 1 year) and tertiary stages.

The early stages are more infectious and respond best to penicillin treatment.

The symptoms and signs can resemble those of many other diseases.

Primary stage

The chancre is firm, round, painless and usually single, but may be multiple at the location where syphilis entered the body. Chancres may not be visible in the vagina or anus. The chancre lasts for 3 to 6 weeks, and heals whether or not it is treated. If untreated, the infection progresses to the secondary stage.

Secondary stage

A non-itchy skin rash and/or mucous membrane lesions (sores in the mouth, vagina or anus) occur. This stage typically starts with the development of a rash on one or more areas of the body. The characteristic rash is rough red or reddish brown spots on the palms of the hands and the soles of the feet. However, rashes with a different appearance may occur on other parts of the body, sometimes resembling rashes caused by other diseases. Sometimes the rashes are barely visible. Large raised grey or white lesions, known as condylomata lata, may develop in warm moist areas such as the mouth, underarm or groin region. In addition, there may be fever, swollen lymph glands, sore throat, patchy hair loss, headaches, weight loss, muscle aches and fatigue. The symptoms will resolve with or without treatment, but if not treated the infection will progress to the latent and possibly late stages of disease.

Latent (hidden) and late stages

Without treatment, syphilis infection can persist without showing any signs or symptoms. **Early latent syphilis** is latent syphilis where infection occurred within the past 12 months. **Late latent syphilis** is latent syphilis where infection occurred more than 1 year ago.

Late stages (tertiary syphilis) develop in around 15% of people who have not been treated, and can appear 10–20 years after infection was first acquired. In the late stages of syphilis, the disease may damage the internal organs, including the brain, nerves, eyes, heart, blood vessels, liver, bones and joints. Symptoms of the late stages of syphilis include difficulty coordinating muscle movements, paralysis, numbness, gradual blindness and dementia.

When it invades the nervous system, at any stage of infection, syphilis causes headache, altered behaviour, and movement disorders that occur in Parkinson's and Huntington's disease.

HIV infection modifies the symptoms and signs described above, including hypopigmented skin rashes. There is also a greater likelihood of neurological involvement.

Where disease is prevalent, most cases are asymptomatic. At least 50% of women with acute syphilis have adverse pregnancy outcomes. The more recent the maternal infection, the more likely it is that the fetus and infant will be infected.

Congenital syphilis is divided into early (becoming apparent in the first 2 years of life) and late (becoming apparent after the first 2 years of life) types. At birth the following can be present: low birth weight, hepato-splenomegaly, pallor, jaundice and purpura, blisters or peeling of palms and soles. There can be difficulties in feeding and rhinorrhea. If not treated immediately, the newborn baby may remain asymptomatic but more commonly develops serious problems within a few weeks affecting many body systems. Untreated babies may become developmentally delayed, have seizures or die.

Late congenital syphilis can present with the following: blunted upper incisor teeth known as Hutchinson's teeth, inflammation of the cornea known as interstitial keratitis, deafness from auditory nerve disease, frontal bone bossing, a saddle nose (collapse of the bony part of nose), defects of the hard palate, swollen knees, saber like shins, short maxillae and protruding mandible. A frequently-found group of symptoms is Hutchinson's triad, which consists of Hutchinson's teeth (notched incisors), keratitis and deafness and occurs in 63% of cases.

Treatment (with penicillin) before the development of these late symptoms is essential.

Congenital syphilis may occur if the expectant mother has syphilis, but the risk is minimal if she has been given penicillin during pregnancy. Congenital syphilis does not cause congenital malformations as infection of the fetus in early pregnancy is lethal.

Treatment with penicillin is extremely effective (98% success rate) in preventing mother-to-child transmission.

Diagnosis

There are two types of blood tests available, namely non-treponemal tests and treponemal tests.

Non-treponemal tests (e.g. VDRL and RPR) are simple, inexpensive, and are often used for screening. Ideally, women with a reactive non-treponemal test should receive a treponemal test to confirm a syphilis diagnosis.

Their sensitivity increases from primary to secondary syphilis, and their specificity is high in the absence of another chronic condition.

The on-site RPR card test is quick and simple to use, allowing immediate treatment to be given. A simple strip of paper impregnated with treponemal antigen is used to test a finger-prick sample of blood.

Treponemal tests such as the *Treponema pallidum* haemagglutination assay (TPHA) and Rapid Syphilis Test have higher sensitivity and specificity and measure antibodies that are specific for syphilis. Treponemal antibodies appear earlier than non-treponemal antibodies and usually remain detectable for life, even after successful treatment, and therefore do not correlate with disease activity.

All pregnant women should be screened for syphilis at their first antenatal visit with an on-site RPR or other rapid test and to prevent congenital infection, preferably before 16 weeks' gestation and again in the third trimester.

All women who were not screened or tested during pregnancy should be screened at or immediately after delivery.

All infants born to mothers who have positive non-treponemal and treponemal test results should be evaluated for congenital syphilis.

Advise women who test positive that their partner(s) must also be investigated and treated if positive.

Test all women with a history of adverse pregnancy outcome (e.g. abortion, stillbirth, syphilitic infant) for syphilis.

Screen all women with syphilis for other sexually transmitted and HIV infections.

Treatment of pregnant women with syphilis

Early syphilis (primary, secondary or latent syphilis of not more than 2 years' duration)

Give benzathine benzylpenicillin, 2.4 million IU intramuscularly (check that it is not injected into a vein), in a single session. Because of the high volume, this is usually given as two injections at separate sites.

Alternatively, give procaine benzylpenicillin 1.2 million IU intramuscularly (check that it is not injected into a vein) daily for 10 consecutive days.

If the patient is allergic to penicillin, give ceftriaxone 500 mg IM/IV daily for 10 days. Erythromycin does not cross the placenta to treat the fetus.

Late latent syphilis (infection of more than 2 years' duration)

Give benzathine benzylpenicillin, 2.4 million IU intramuscularly (check that it is not injected into a vein), once weekly for 3 consecutive weeks.

Alternatively, give procaine benzylpenicillin, 1.2 million IU intramuscularly (check that it is not injected into a vein), once daily for 20 consecutive days.

If the patient is allergic to penicillin, give ceftriaxone 500 mg IM/IV daily for 14 days or (although this is less effective) erythromycin, 500 mg orally, four times a day for 30 days.

Treatment of congenital syphilis

All asymptomatic newborn infants born to seropositive mothers should be treated with a single IM dose of benzathine benzylpenicillin, 50 000 IU/kg, whether or not their mothers were treated during pregnancy. Routine CSF examination is not required.

Newborn infants with any signs of congenital syphilis should receive:

- aqueous benzylpenicillin, 100 000–150 000 IU/kg/day administered as 50 000 IU/kg/dose IV every 12 hours, during the first 7 days of life, and every 8 hours thereafter for a total of 10 days

or

- procaine benzylpenicillin, 50 000 IU/kg by IM injection, as a single daily dose for 10 days (ensure that it is not injected into a vein).

Early congenital syphilis generally responds well to penicillin. Recovery may be slow in seriously ill children with extensive skin, mucous membrane, bone or visceral involvement.

For older infants up to 2 years of age with confirmed congenital syphilis the treatment is the same as above.

If the patient is allergic to penicillin (this is unusual), give ceftriaxone 80 mg/kg IM/IV once daily for 10 days or give erythromycin, 7.5–12.5 mg/kg orally, four times a day for 14 days but erythromicin is less effective.

For infants older than 2 years, give aqueous benzylpenicillin, 200 000–300 000 IU/kg/day by IM/IV administered as 50 000 IU/kg/dose every 4–6 hours for 10–14 days.

An alternative regimen for penicillin-allergic patients after the first month of life is to give erythromycin, 7.5–12.5 mg/kg orally, four times a day for 30 days.

Jarisch–Herxheimer reaction

After starting penicillin treatment in some patients, the death of the bacteria results in the release of mediators that produce the adverse symptoms and signs such as myalgias, fever, headache and tachycardia, sometimes with exacerbation of whatever current syphilitic lesions are manifested (e.g. rash, chancre).

This reaction develops within several hours after

beginning antibiotic treatment, and usually clears within 24 hours after its onset. It is very rare in newborn infants.

Management consists of symptomatic treatment (e.g. antipyretics, analgesics) and observation. In pregnancy, treatment may induce early labour or cause fetal distress. Patients should be informed of the possibility of this reaction before undergoing antibiotic therapy. However, this risk should not preclude or delay therapy for syphilis. Women are advised to seek obstetric care after treatment if they notice any fever, uterine contractions, or a decrease in fetal movement.

2.8.1 Varicella zoster (chickenpox) in pregnancy

Introduction

Pregnant women and newborn infants are at risk of severe disease from varicella, involving serious effects on organs such as the lungs.

Varicella is transmitted from respiratory aerosols and skin lesions in chickenpox itself, and from the skin lesions but not aerosols in shingles (which is not infectious until the skin lesions appear).

In chickenpox, patients are infectious for 48 hours prior to emergence of the rash and until all of the skin lesions are crusted over.

The incubation period is 10–21 days.

Non-immune patients are those without a history of chickenpox or shingles or a completed vaccination profile. Immune status can be checked with blood varicella IgG measurement (if available).

Clinical features in pregnancy

Congenital varicella syndrome (CVS)

In the first or early second trimester infection may result in stillbirth, or the neonate may be born with a group of physical abnormalities known as congenital varicella syndrome (CVS). This is rare, occurring in 1–2.8% of women infected with chickenpox in the first 20 weeks of gestation (the period of maximum risk is between 12 and 20 weeks' gestation). There may be dermatomal scarring, limb hypoplasia, ocular abnormalities, low birth weight and early death. Survivors may have long-term developmental problems. An infant with CVS has a 30% risk of mortality in the first few months of life, and a 15% risk of developing herpes zoster between 2 months and 3 years of life.

Varicella pneumonia

Pregnant women with chickenpox may be more likely than non-pregnant women to develop severe pneumonitis. The risk is greatest in the third trimester, especially if lung disease is already present, or if the patient is a smoker or is immunocompromised (e.g. due to HIV infection).

Symptoms start as a non-productive cough, which can rapidly progress to respiratory failure within 36–48 hours. The cough becomes increasingly productive, with tachypnoea, dyspnoea, cyanosis and chest pain.

Perinatal infection

If a neonate is exposed (mother has a rash) around the time of birth (from 5 days before to 2 days after delivery), there is a 17–30% risk of dangerous perinatal infection. This is characterised by skin lesions, disseminated intravascular coagulation, pneumonitis and hepatitis, and it has a mortality of up to 30%.

Management

Maternal contact with varicella during pregnancy

If the patient is immune (see above for definition), no treatment or isolation is required.

If she is non-immune and an IgG test is not available and affordable, then if she has had a significant contact with chicken pox or shingles then give varicella zoster immunoglobulin (VZIG) (see below for details) within 4 days of contact if possible (maximum of 10 days after contact). Avoid contact with other pregnant women. The patient should be counselled regarding the signs of infection so that she can be treated early if it occurs.

Significant exposure to chicken pox occurs after very limited contact with an infected person (any face to face contact and as little as 15 minutes in the same room as an infectious patient). The risk of contracting chicken pox from exposure to shingles is very low if the infection is not in an exposed area.

Chickenpox during pregnancy

If this is **mild**, give oral aciclovir (see below for dose regimen) for 7 days, starting within 24 hours of the appearance of vesicles, and avoid contact with other pregnant women. In mild cases, aciclovir leads to little improvement. It is most important in women at risk of severe disease (immunocompromised, HIV infected, history of respiratory disease or smoking).

If it is **severe**, give IV aciclovir for 7 days. High-dependency care should be provided if available, as appropriate.

Prevention of neonatal chickenpox if the mother is infected from 7 days before to 7 days after birth

Give VZIG to the neonate as soon as possible after delivery. Isolate the mother and infant.

In addition, give IV aciclovir to the neonate if the onset of maternal symptoms was between 4 days before, and 2 days after the birth.

Infant in contact with chickenpox other than from mother, or from mother who develops chickenpox more than 7 days after the birth

If the mother is immune and the infant is full term at birth, no prophylaxis is needed. Mild illness may occur.

If the mother is not immune and the infant is less than 4 weeks of age, and full term at birth, give varicella zoster immunoglobulin (VZIG) (if available).

If the infant is preterm, and regardless of maternal immunity, give VZIG.

Regardless of whether VZIG is given, monitor the baby for signs of infection to enable early treatment should infection occur.

Shingles is very rare in infants and, if present, suspect HIV infection.

Doses of VZIG and aciclovir
In pregnancy
Aciclovir is of no benefit if commenced more than 24 hours after the appearance of chickenpox vesicles.

- Oral route: 800 mg five times daily for 7 days (mildly ill cases only).
- IV route: 10 mg/kg/dose every 8 hours for 7 days.

Side effects include nausea, vomiting, diarrhoea, headache and nephrotoxicity. Reduce the dose or dosage interval in patients with impaired renal function.

Varicella zoster immunoglobulin (VZIG): 1 gram IM. Anaphylaxis is rare, but ensure that adrenaline is available.

In the neonate
Aciclovir 10–20 mg/kg IV every 8 hours for at least 7 days. Side effects are as described above.

Varicella zoster immunoglobulin (VZIG): 250 mg by deep IM injection.

2.9 Mental health problems associated with pregnancy and the postnatal period

---

> **BOX 2.9.1 Minimum standards**
> - Screening tools for depression, such as the Edinburgh Postnatal Depression Scale (EPDS).
> - Selective serotonin reuptake inhibitor (SSRI) antidepressant drugs.
> - Ideally, an inpatient hospital facility for mothers and babies when the mother has puerperal psychosis.
> - Antipsychotic drugs.

> **BOX 2.9.2 Risk factors for development of maternal depression in low- and middle-income countries**
> - Poverty and high levels of economic stress
> - Low levels of social support
> - Domestic violence
> - Chronic maternal illness
> - Maternal anaemia
> - Lack of awareness among primary healthcare workers of depression as an illness
> - Social stigma associated with a family member being diagnosed with a mental illness
> - Families with four or more children, especially when the children are under 7 years of age
> - Having a preterm infant or an infant with a low birth weight
> - Having a child with a developmental disability
> - Having an unplanned or unwanted infant
> - Having a female child in a culture where there is a strong preference for male children
> - Lack of participation in family financial decisions, control of resources and reproductive health
>
> Adapted from Wachs, Black and Engle (2009).

Introduction

Childbirth poses a risk to a woman's mental health. This applies to all women and girls who become pregnant in all countries, irrespective of their social and cultural background. However, the background will influence how a mother presents and how quickly she receives appropriate care.

Much of the research about pregnancy-related mental illness and its effects on the new baby has been done in high-income countries where it has been possible to develop specialised services. However, there is evidence that mental health problems in mothers are as common in low- and middle-income countries. A number of risk factors that have been suggested as underlying maternal depression are listed in Box 2.9.2.

Perinatal psychiatric services have developed in many high-income countries, and involve liaison between psychiatric and obstetric services. The specialty covers women with pre-existing mental health problems who want to have a family, as well as mental illness that is first diagnosed antenatally and postnatally. Maintaining the mental health of a pregnant woman benefits the family, and in some cases can prevent problems from developing postnatally. The onset of depression and anxiety in pregnancy or postnatally can be especially worrying for a woman and her family because it is contrary to their expectations that this will be a happy time. The woman may not want to admit how she is feeling,

being ashamed both of her inability to feel joy about her newborn baby and of her perceived inability to cope, and fearing that she will be judged harshly for these feelings. This is especially important in countries and cultures where women and girls are not valued and their main role is perceived to be the production of healthy babies.

Mild antenatal and postnatal depression can be managed with minimal resources and does not require medication. Recognition of the condition and practical help from family and friends can be enough to prevent depression affecting the care of the baby. Reassurance from healthcare professionals can help the mother and her family to realise that she is not on her own in her feelings. To a depressed new mother it can feel as if every other mother is better than her, and to know that this is not the case can be extremely helpful. If antidepressants are available they may, in selected cases, speed up recovery (see below).

However, there are serious psychiatric conditions associated with childbirth that can necessitate prompt psychiatric treatment and admission of the mother to a psychiatric hospital, preferably with her baby. The most serious of these conditions, puerperal psychosis, has been described as the only true psychiatric emergency. Usually rare, this condition is more common in women who have had a manic episode and have been diagnosed with bipolar affective disorder. A history of a previous episode of puerperal psychosis considerably increases the risk of having another episode following subsequent pregnancies. Knowing that a woman is at risk provides an opportunity for prevention – either of the illness itself, or of the repercussions of the illness if it has not been possible to prevent it.

Antepartum psychiatric disorders

There is evidence that psychiatric symptoms occur as frequently antenatally as postnatally, with an estimated prevalence of 10–15%. The symptoms are often of mild depression and anxiety. Careful enquiry may reveal that the symptoms were present before conception. The development of a serious psychiatric condition in the antenatal period is no more common than at other times, but if a diagnosis is made during pregnancy, the decision to start medication has to balance the severity of the mother's illness against the adverse effects of medication on the fetus.

Women with mild symptoms usually present early in pregnancy, and may improve as the pregnancy progresses. Hyperemesis can make the first trimester miserable and lead women to express thoughts of rejecting the pregnancy. Sometimes this is mistaken for evidence of depression. The third trimester can be a time of anxiety about labour and the impending birth, especially for first-time mothers or those who have had previous complicated deliveries. The factors that make women and girls more vulnerable are listed in Box 2.9.3.

Supportive counselling is often sufficient to improve the mental health of most women, but if antidepressants are indicated, there needs to be a discussion about the risks and benefits before they are prescribed. The selective serotonin reuptake inhibitors (SSRIs) fluoxetine and sertraline seem to have the best safety profile, but new information is emerging as more women take antidepressants in pregnancy and clinicians continually evaluate the safety profile of this class of drugs. There is increasing evidence that the SSRI antidepressants, especially paroxetine, are associated with an increased risk of cardiac abnormalities in the baby if taken during embryogenesis. However, the risk is still relatively low (4%), and has to be balanced against the risks to the pregnancy if the depression is left untreated. If SSRIs are not available, tricyclic antidepressants can be effective, but prescribers must be wary of patients with suicidal ideation, as the tricyclic antidepressants are more dangerous than SSRIs when taken in overdose.

A woman with an established diagnosis of bipolar disorder may be taking a mood stabiliser such as **lithium, sodium valproate** or **carbamazepine**, and **these are associated with increased fetal malformations**, so consideration needs to be given to stopping them prior to conception. In women in whom relapse has occurred when stopping lithium, the balance between risks and benefits is probably in favour of continuing the drug. This is less likely to be the case for sodium valproate or carbamazepine.

BOX 2.9.3 Factors that increase the risk of antenatal depression and/or anxiety
- Previous obstetric loss
- Previous fertility problems
- Anxiety about the viability of the pregnancy
- Social and interpersonal adversity
- Feelings of ambivalence about the pregnancy
- Previous depression and/or anxiety associated with pregnancy

---

Postpartum psychiatric disorders

Psychiatric disorders that present postnatally are traditionally classified into three types as shown in Box 2.9.4. Other conditions can also present at this time, and it has been suggested that the term **postnatal common mental disorders** is more useful for distinguishing the milder depressive, anxiety and obsessional disorders from the more severe depressive disorders and puerperal psychosis.

BOX 2.9.4 Postpartum-onset psychiatric disorders
Maternity blues
Postnatal depression
- Mild
- Moderate
- Severe

Puerperal psychosis
Anxiety and obsessive-compulsive disorders

Maternity blues

This is generally a mild and self-limiting condition that affects over 50% of women, usually between day 3 and day 10 postnatally, but most commonly on day 5. A hormonal cause has been postulated for this transient condition, which is marked by variability of mood, feelings of confusion, irritability, insomnia and a feeling of not being able to cope. It is generally self-limiting, although if it is longer-lasting or more severe than usual, it can herald problems later in the postnatal period. Reassurance is usually sufficient to help the woman through this period, which usually last about 48 hours.

Postnatal depression

It is estimated that around 10% of woman develop symptoms of depression postnatally. The majority of these symptoms will be relatively mild and overlap with the process of adjusting to having a baby, particularly (although not exclusively) following the birth of a first child. In most cases a diagnosis will not be made until about 6 weeks after the onset of the depression.

Symptoms are not dissimilar to those that occur in non-puerperal depression, but sleep and appetite are often disrupted because of the baby's presence, so different questions may need to be asked in order to elicit a diagnosis. The mother may not recognise that she is depressed and so does not share how she is feeling. The commonly experienced anhedonia (inability to feel pleasure) is particularly difficult at this time, when the mother (and those around her) feels that she should be happy. This can lead her to conclude that she is a poor mother. Meanwhile others, particularly in western cultures, may state that there is a problem with bonding, which can exacerbate her guilt and low mood. Obsessional symptoms and irritability are also often reported.

The Edinburgh Postnatal Depression Scale (EPDS) is a screening tool (see Appendix) which has been translated into a number of languages and used across diverse cultural settings. It requires no psychiatric training to administer, and so can be used by healthcare workers to identify mothers who may be depressed.

Two recent studies in Ethiopia showed the EPDS to be less effective in rural areas than in urban ones. For rural Ethiopia the self-reporting questionnaire (SRQ) was considered to be superior. In urban areas the Kessler Psychological Distress Scale (which is used to assess psychological distress in various situations) and the EPDS were reported to be equally effective screening tools, but it was suggested that the Kessler Psychological Distress Scale may be more effective in detecting postnatal mental health disorders in this setting.

When the depression is mild, relatively simple interventions can be very effective, including listening to the mother's concerns, reassuring her that her feelings do not mean she is a bad mother, and giving practical help with the baby, allowing her to rest as much as possible. Antidepressants are not usually indicated in mild depression.

In cases of moderate depression with persistent low mood, reduced sleep and appetite, poor concentration, feelings of not being able to cope, and lack of improvement when practical help and support are given, antidepressants are likely to be needed. If available, sertraline or paroxetine are the SSRIs with the lowest relative infant dose (i.e. the amount passing to the infant through breast milk), so are the safest ones for breastfeeding mothers.

- **Sertraline:** starting dose is 50 mg, with a maximum dose of 200 mg daily.
- **Paroxetine:** starting dose is 20 mg, with a maximum dose of 60 mg daily.

The most commonly reported side effect for both of these drugs is nausea, which wears off after 2 to 3 weeks – the same time that it takes for the therapeutic effects to begin to appear – so the mother needs to be warned about this.

Imipramine and amitriptyline also appear to be safe in breastfeeding mothers.

- **Imipramine:** starting dose is 25 mg three times daily, increasing to a maximum total daily dose of 200 mg.
- **Amitriptyline:** starting dose is 25 to 100 mg total daily dose, given in three doses during the day or (usually more acceptably, because of its sedative effects) once at night. The maintenance dose is a total daily dose of 75 to 150 mg/day. Rarely a total daily dose of up to 300 mg may be used.

Side effects include sedation, postural hypotension, dry mouth, blurred vision, constipation, urinary retention and increased body temperature. In overdose imipramine and amitriptyline are cardiotoxic, and this has to be considered when prescribing for a mother who may be experiencing suicidal thoughts. However, if these are the only drugs available, this risk needs to be weighed against the ongoing suicide risk if the mother is not given antidepressants.

Severe postnatal depression affects about 3% of women and can merge with puerperal psychosis. It tends to occur early postnatally, and it is likely to be obvious that the mother is unwell. Sleep is evasive, even when the baby sleeps well through the night. Appetite will be markedly reduced, with marked weight loss. Most mothers, even when very depressed, will use all their energies on the baby and neglect themselves. Depressive delusions can develop, with the mother believing that the baby would be better off without her, and this leads to a significant suicide risk. The risk of the mother taking the baby with her in a suicide attempt, although rare, has to be considered, though again this should be managed by closely monitoring the mother while keeping her baby with her. Separating the mother from the baby can increase the woman's sense of desperation and feelings of failure as a mother.

Admission of the mother and baby to a suitable hospital setting (if available) is the ideal way to manage a woman with severe delusional postnatal depression. **Electroconvulsive treatment ECT), but only if given under general anaesthesia and safely**, is indicated, often fairly early after the onset of symptoms, as this can treat the mother quickly and reduce the amount of time she is unwell. Antidepressants should be given (see above for doses; the SSRI group is likely to be the best and safest option if available), and also antipsychotics if these are needed.

Once improved, the mother is likely to benefit from the supportive measures described for milder types of postnatal depression. It is not only possible but desirable to continue breastfeeding, whether or not the mother is being treated with antidepressants. If antipsychotics are also required, breastfeeding can continue. Adequate sleep for the mother can be achieved by her expressing breast milk and other family members giving this to the baby from a cup and spoon whenever the baby wakes during the night.

Puerperal psychosis

This is the most severe postpartum mood disorder, and symptoms can appear rapidly. The usual incidence is 1 in 500 deliveries. It is a great shock to the mother and her family when it develops with no prior warning. However, a previous diagnosis of bipolar disorder or puerperal psychosis increases the risk to as much as 1 in 2. This presents the clinician with an opportunity to identify women at risk antenatally, consider the options for prevention, and develop a plan of management for the puerperium should the mother become unwell.

Characteristically, the woman may have been mentally healthy during her pregnancy, which may have given her and her family hope that all would be well in the puerperium. Typically there is a sudden onset of symptoms, most commonly in the first 2 weeks following childbirth. Sometimes the symptoms appear to come on overnight. The symptoms vary, but tend to progress rapidly over the first few days, and characteristically include the following:

- perplexity and confusion
- overactivity

- insomnia
- marked behavioural changes.

These common presenting features are often accompanied by a fear that something will happen to the mother or the baby, or sometimes a belief that the baby is not her own. The woman is usually easily distracted, with grossly impaired concentration, and is unable to finish one task before trying to start another, in a markedly disorganised way. This significantly interferes with her ability to look after her baby. Pointing this out often causes her even more distress. This can reinforce delusional beliefs that the baby is not her own, or that others are going to take her baby away, especially if she is separated from the baby because of her illness. A strong affective component is often present, usually hypomania or labile emotions, although this can develop into a more typically depressive picture.

During the acute phase there is a risk of harm to the mother or child, mainly due to the mother's chaotic behaviour which may unintentionally lead to neglect of the infant, rather than to any deliberately harmful actions on her part. Rarely, a mother may describe delusional beliefs involving the baby that could lead to direct harm, but this is very unusual. Although these risks to the child obviously have to be borne in mind, it is important to note that most mothers do not want to harm their babies. This risk should be managed wherever possible by keeping the mother and baby together and supervising them very closely. Even when the mother is very unwell and unable to manage much of the baby's care herself, both mother and baby benefit from being in close proximity. The mother can then be encouraged to take over more of the baby's care as her mental state improves, re-establishing the mother–child bond.

Women or girls with puerperal psychosis will frequently need medication, and the type of drug will depend on the predominant symptoms. In settings where the choice of medication is limited, the older antipsychotics can be just as effective as more modern drugs, and, with monitoring, breastfeeding can be continued, although it should be remembered that the disorganised behaviour of the mother can make breastfeeding difficult. It is therefore very important to supervise this.

Chlorpromazine is an inexpensive and generally widely available 'typical' antipsychotic drug which is very effective but tends to have been superseded in well-resourced countries by the 'atypical' antipsychotics with their more acceptable side-effect profile. Nevertheless, chlorpromazine is efficacious and the dose can be titrated up quite rapidly from 50 mg four times daily to as high as 1000 mg daily. Side effects include sedation (which can be beneficial in the acute stages of illness), dry mouth, nausea and parkinsonism (mask-like face, slowing and stiffness of gait, and tremor), although the inherent anticholinergic properties of chlorpromazine mean that this is not so common as with some of the other typical antipsychotic drugs (e.g. haloperidol).

Haloperidol is given at a dose of 0.5–3 mg two to three times daily, with a maximum daily dose of 30 mg orally. It is also often used in emergency situations as an IM injection of 5 mg or 10 mg, with a maximum daily dose of 18 mg IM.

The atypical antipsychotic drugs include **risperidone**, for which the starting dose is 1 mg twice daily, with a maximum daily dose of 6 mg, and **olanzapine**, for which the starting dose is 10 mg, with a maximum daily dose

of 20 mg. Although these drugs have a low incidence of parkinsonism, they are associated with weight gain and an increased risk of type 2 diabetes.

If a woman on an atypical antipsychotic wishes to conceive, she may want to switch to a typical drug, as there is longer-term evidence for their safety. However, this introduces a risk of relapse, and she may not want to take that risk. Also if a woman has conceived while on an atypical antipsychotic, the balance is probably in favour of continuing it, although, if possible, the dose could be reduced.

In mothers who present with puerperal psychosis, the prognosis is generally good if treatment is available, but they may remain vulnerable for several months even when the psychotic symptoms remit. As the psychotic symptoms improve and insight develops, the mother may experience a period of depressed mood as she adjusts to what has happened. However, recovery is usually complete by 6 months, although there is a risk of relapse at other times, particularly in a subsequent pregnancy.

In a woman with a pre-existing diagnosis of bipolar disorder, the management of labour is important for reducing the risk of a puerperal psychosis. Where possible, sleep deprivation should be minimised in order to reduce the risk of the illness developing. The importance of letting the mother sleep when she can following childbirth should be emphasised to the family, and the father should be asked to undertake as much care as possible during the night.

The effectiveness of using prophylactic antipsychotic drugs has yet to be established. The trigger for puerperal psychosis appears to be biological, but so far the condition has proved difficult to prevent, even when treatment is continued through pregnancy. It is therefore essential to have a plan in place for what to do if the mother becomes unwell, and this can also reduce stress for the family.

Anxiety disorders and obsessive-compulsive disorders

Women and girls with a history of anxiety disorders and obsessive-compulsive disorders may relapse postnatally.

Anxiety can range from mild concerns about the health of the baby to extreme anxiety that the baby may be seriously unwell, with constant vigilance and fear of a sudden infant death. The mother may seek and receive much reassurance from family and healthcare workers, yet remain concerned.

Mothers may experience obsessional thoughts or images of their babies being harmed, and sometimes the thought is that they will be the person to harm the baby. This can cause great distress, as the mother may fear that she will act on these thoughts, and so will avoid caring for her baby and allow her family to do so instead, which will reinforce her belief that she is a bad mother. Careful diagnostic exploration to identify obsessional rather than psychotic symptoms is essential in such cases.

Non-delusional, non-psychotic obsessions have the following characteristics:

- They come into the mind fully formed.
- They are recognised as the mother's own thoughts and not placed there by someone else.
- They are not voices telling her to harm her child.
- They are repetitive and intrusive.
- They are difficult to push away.

This analysis should be followed by an explanation of the

nature of these thoughts. The mother will need encouragement to continue to care for her baby despite these abnormal thoughts, and to dispel the belief that she is a bad mother. These intrusive thoughts can lead to immense guilt and feelings of incompetence. Therefore allowing the mother to express her concerns and be reassured can be very therapeutic. Antidepressants may be indicated, even in the absence of other biological symptoms of depression.

Benzodiazepines such as diazepam must not be used regularly in pregnancy. When taken later in pregnancy they can cause withdrawal symptoms, hypotonia and agitation in the newborn.

Effect of maternal mental health disorders on the infant

For the majority of women experiencing symptoms of depression and anxiety during pregnancy or in the early postnatal period, their ability to care for their baby is not significantly compromised. However, there are many studies describing the adverse effects of maternal depression on early childhood development, and chronic depression does have deleterious effects on the whole family. This evidence needs to be taken seriously from a public health point of view to highlight the problem and aid development of services. However, it is also important to remember that for an individual mother the thought that she may be regarded as causing harm to her baby will reinforce the guilt that she is already feeling, and delay recovery. Several of the factors listed in Box 2.9.2, while predisposing to maternal depression, are also going to disadvantage the child, so addressing these where possible will benefit both mother and child.

Appendix

Edinburgh Postnatal Depression Scale (EPDS)

Name: _____

Address: _____

Your date of birth: _____

Baby's date of birth: _____ Phone number: _____

Instructions

As you have recently had a baby, we would like to know how you are feeling now. Please choose the answer that comes closest to how you have felt IN THE PAST WEEK, not just how you feel today.

Here is an example, already completed.

I have felt happy:

☐ Yes, all of the time

☐ Yes, most of the time (*This would mean: 'I have felt happy most of the time' during the past week*)

☐ No, not very often

☐ No, not at all

In the past 7 days:

Question 1

In the past week I have been able to laugh and see the funny side of things:

☐ As much as I always could

☐ Not quite so much now

☐ Definitely not so much now

☐ Not at all

Question 2

In the past week I have looked forward with enjoyment to things:

☐ As much as I ever did

☐ Rather less than I used to

☐ Definitely less than I used to

☐ Hardly at all

Question 3*

In the past week I have blamed myself unnecessarily when things went wrong:

☐ Yes, most of the time

☐ Yes, some of the time

☐ Not very often

☐ No, never

Question 4

In the past week I have been anxious or worried for no good reason:

☐ No, not at all

☐ Hardly ever

☐ Yes, sometimes

☐ Yes, very often

Question 5*

In the last week I have felt scared or panicky for no very good reason:

☐ Yes, quite a lot

☐ Yes, sometimes

☐ No, not much

☐ No, not at all

Question 6*

In the past week things have been getting on top of me:

☐ Yes, most of the time I haven't been able to cope at all

☐ Yes, sometimes I haven't been coping as well as usual

☐ No, most of the time I have coped quite well

☐ No, I have been coping as well as ever

Question 7*

In the past week I have been so unhappy that I have difficulty sleeping:

☐ Yes, most of the time

☐ Yes, sometimes

☐ Not very often

☐ No, not at all

Question 8*

In the past week I have felt sad or miserable:

☐ Yes, most of the time

☐ Yes, quite often

☐ Not very often

☐ No, not at all

Question 9*

In the past week I have been so unhappy that I have been crying:

☐ Yes, most of the time

☐ Yes, quite often

☐ Only occasionally

☐ No, never

Question 10*

In the past week the thought of harming myself has occurred to me:

☐ Yes, quite often

☐ Sometimes

☐ Hardly ever

☐ Never

Administered/reviewed by: _____ **Date:** _____

Source: Cox JL, Holden JM and Sagovsky R (1987) Detection of postnatal depression: development of the 10-item Edinburgh Postnatal Depression Scale. *British Journal of Psychiatry*, **150**, 782–6.

Instructions for using the Edinburgh Postnatal Depression Scale

1 The mother is asked to check the response that comes closest to how she has been feeling in the previous 7 days.
2 All of the items must be completed.
3 Care should be taken to avoid the possibility of the mother discussing her answers with others. Answers must come from the mother or pregnant woman.
4 The mother should complete the scale herself, unless she has limited English or has difficulty with reading.

Mothers who score above 13 are likely to be suffering from a depressive illness of varying severity. The EPDS score should not override clinical judgement. A careful clinical assessment should be undertaken to confirm the diagnosis.

The scale indicates how the mother has felt during the previous week. In doubtful cases it may be useful to repeat the tool after 2 weeks. The scale will not detect mothers with anxiety neuroses, phobias or personality disorders.

Scoring

Questions 1, 2 and 4 (without an asterisk) are scored 0, 1, 2 or 3, with the top box scored as 0 and the bottom box scored as 3.

Questions 3, 5, 6, 7, 8, 9 and 10 (marked with an asterisk) are reverse scored, with the top box scored as 3 and the bottom box scored as 0.

The maximum possible score is 30.

Possible depression is indicated by a score of ≥ 10.

Always look at item 10 (suicidal thoughts).

2.10 Female genital cutting

Introduction

What is female genital cutting?

Female genital cutting (FGC), also known as female circumcision or female genital mutilation, refers to all procedures involving partial or total removal of the external female genitalia, or other injury to the female organs for non-therapeutic reasons. It ranges from very simple to radical, and may be carried out between birth and puberty, or can be performed just before marriage or childbirth.

FGC varies across cultures, ethnic groups and tribal affiliations; there is also some variation in the types of cutting undertaken within cultures, ethnicity and tribes. The World Health Organization has estimated that 130 million women worldwide have undergone FGC. There are an estimated 2 million infants, girls and women at risk each year.

The European Parliamentary Committee on Women's Rights and Gender Equality states that around 500 000 women and girls living in Europe have been subjected to FGC.

A practice of performing a symbolic form of infibulation to accompany the usual ceremonies has been recently adopted in Somalia. The procedure consists of applying to the clitoris a small needle (sterile insulin needle) to obtain a drop of blood. The practice is called 'Sunna' and is not yet widespread in the country. It is performed only by enlightened women in that society, but hopefully it will attract others to adopt this approach while awaiting a time when all forms of this practice end.

Who performs FGC?

FGC is commonly performed by traditional medicine practitioners, including traditional birth attendants, local women or men, or female family members. Such individuals do not have formal medical training, and usually perform cutting without anaesthesia or asepsis with crude instruments such as kitchen knives or razor blades. It is not uncommon

for those who perform FGC to cut or damage more of the genital area than they intended to. Increasingly, doctors are also undertaking these procedures.

The health problems associated with FGC are life-threatening haemorrhage, sometimes death during or shortly after the procedure (from haemorrhage or infection), death during pregnancy, the need for assistance during childbirth due to interference with normal delivery, and the spread of HIV/AIDS and hepatitis due to the frequent use of unclean and unsterile instruments. There are also links to mental illness in the victims and to intimate partner violence.

Prevalence of FGC

FGC is practised in about 28 countries in Africa, Asia and the Middle East. A recent interview by Integrated Regional Information Networks (IRIN) in 2012 confirmed that FGC is still being practised in Pakistan. It is estimated that at least 50–60% of Bohra women undergo FGC; this is usually a symbolic snipping of the clitoris.

TABLE 2.10.1 Estimated prevalence of FGC by country

Country	Estimated prevalence of FGC in girls and women aged 15–49 years (%)	Year
Benin	16.8	2001
Cameroon	1.4	2004
Chad	44.9	2004
Central African Republic	25.7	2005
Djibouti	93.1	2006
Egypt	95.8	2005
Ethiopia	74.7	2005
Eritrea	95.0	1995

Country	Estimated prevalence of FGC in girls and women aged 15–49 years (%)	Year
Guinea Bissau	44.5	2005
Ghana	3.8	2005
Guinea	95.6	2005
Gambia	78.3	2005
Ivory Coast	41.7	2005
Liberia	45.0	
Mali	91.6	2001
Mauritania	71.3	2001
Nigeria	19.0	2003
Niger	2.2	2006
Sierra Leone	90.0	2003
Senegal	28.2	2005
Somalia	97.9	2005
Sudan, northern (approximately 80% of total population in survey)	90.0	2000
Kenya	32.2	2003
Togo	5.8	2005
United Republic of Tanzania	14.6	2004
Uganda	0.6	2006
Yemen	22.6	1997
Burkina-Faso	72.5	2005

Data taken from OHCHR, UNAIDS, UNDP, UNECA, UNESCO, UNFPA, UNHCR, UNICEF, UNIFEM and WHO (2008) *Eliminating Female Genital Cutting: an interagency statement.* www. un.org/womenwatch/daw/csw/csw52/statements_missions/ Interagency_Statement_on_Eliminating_FGM.pdf

Types of female genital cutting

The WHO has classified FGC into four types.

- **type 1:** excision of the prepuce, with or without excision of the clitoris, entirely or in part
- **type 2:** excision of the clitoris with partial or total excision of the labia minora
- **type 3:** excision of part or all of the external genitalia and stitching/narrowing of the vaginal opening (also known as infibulation). This type is most common in countries in the Horn of Africa, namely Sudan, Eritrea, Djibouti, Ethiopia and Somalia
- **type 4:** unclassified – includes pricking or incising of the clitoris or labia, cauterisation by burning of the clitoris, or introduction of corrosive substances or herbs into the vagina; sometimes the clitoris is buried rather than excised.

Around 90% of FGC is of types 1, 2 and 4, and 10% is of type 3 (infibulation). The type often varies depending on ethnicity.

The age at which FGC is undertaken varies between countries. In Ethiopia, Eritrea and Yemen most girls will have been mutilated in infancy. In Egypt, 90% are mutilated between 5 and 15 years of age.

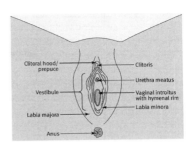

FIGURE 2.10.1 Normal female external genitalia.

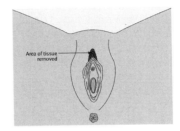

FIGURE 2.10.2 Area of tissue removed in type 1 female genital cutting.

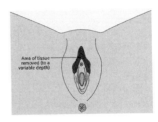

FIGURE 2.10.3 Area of tissue removed in type 2 female genital cutting.

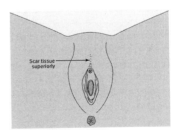

FIGURE 2.10.4 Appearance of genitalia after type 2 female genital cutting.

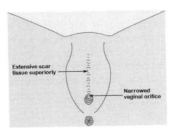

FIGURE 2.10.5 Appearance of genitalia after type 3 female genital cutting.

Implications and complications of FGC

FGC is dangerous to girls' and women's health and psychological well-being. It can cause urological, gynaecological and obstetric problems. Around 10% of girls and women are estimated to die from the short-term complications of FGC, such as haemorrhage, shock and infection. Another 25% die in the long term as a result of recurrent urinary and vaginal infections and complications during childbirth, such as severe bleeding and obstructed labour.

Short-term complications

These include the following:

- haemorrhage and anaemia
- severe pain (it is almost always the case that no local anaesthetic is given)
- shock (due to haemorrhage and/or pain)
- death from shock (due to haemorrhage and/or pain)
- difficulty passing urine or faeces
- urinary tract infection
- urethral meatus injuries, prolonged micturition, and dysuria
- injury to adjacent tissues
- damage to other organs
- fractures or dislocation due to restraint during the procedure
- infection due to tetanus, and bloodborne viruses such as HIV, and hepatitis B and C
- vulval abscess.

Long-term complications

These include the following:

- chronic pain
- chronic pelvic infection
- haematocolpos (obstruction to menstrual flow, leading to dangerous swelling of the vagina)
- keloid scarring
- decreased quality of sexual life, including pain on intercourse
- complications in pregnancy and childbirth, including obstructed labour (see below)
- psychological damage, including fear and anxiety during labour and delivery, as well as post-traumatic stress disorder and depression
- psychosexual effects; fear of and anxiety about sexual intercourse, difficulties with penetration, marital breakdown and divorce.

Complications during childbirth

Women who have undergone FGC are more likely to experience difficulties during childbirth, and their babies are more likely to die. A WHO study conducted in 2006 in six African countries showed an increased risk of possible obstetric complications in women who had been subjected to FGC compared with women who had not undergone this procedure. The same study showed an increased incidence of maternal death, Caesarean section, postpartum haemorrhage and neonatal resuscitation, as well as prolonged hospital stays, in women who had undergone FGC.

Management during pregnancy, labour and the postnatal period

Antenatal period

All women and girls who have been subjected to FGC should be identified at antenatal booking or the gynaecological clinic by asking questions such as 'Have you been closed?' or 'Did you have the cut or operation as a child?' Most women will then assume that you know about FGC, and further questions can be asked, such as 'Do you have any problems with passing urine or menstruation?' or 'How long does it take to pass urine?' Once the issue is raised, the woman may then feel comfortable discussing it further with the midwife or doctor.

Reversal of FGC (de-infibulation)

Reversal (de-infibulation) is best undertaken at 17–18 weeks' gestation (mid-trimester) by a specialist midwife or surgeon, to enable easy access to the vaginal orifice and urethra during labour. Performing reversal in the second trimester ensures complete healing prior to labour. Reversal is not recommended in the first trimester, as the procedure may be wrongly blamed for fetal loss.

Antenatal reversal is essential to assist in vaginal examinations using a speculum, and in urinary catheterisation. It may also prevent recurrent urinary tract infection. Local anaesthesia is encouraged for reversal, but general anaesthesia may be necessary if the woman suffers from flashbacks to childhood trauma.

Post-reversal care during the antenatal period should include adequate pain relief and promotion of personal hygiene. Some re-education may be necessary, as some women will have forgotten, or may never have known, what normal micturition or menstruation is like.

Labour

The aim is a normal delivery, with Caesarean section only for the usual obstetric indications. The woman should receive standard care in labour.

If the woman has not been seen antenatally, or if she has chosen not to have reversal undertaken, an individual assessment should be made on admission in labour, regarding the need for reversal and/or episiotomy to facilitate delivery.

If she has sustained FGC type 3 (infibulation), a midline incision should be made to expose the introitus and urethra, after infiltration with 1% lignocaine. Infibulated women should have a midline incision and medio-lateral episiotomy **only if necessary**.

Adequate **pain relief** is very important, especially as flashbacks may occur.

Bladder care is very important during labour, to avoid damage to the bladder and the urethra (catheterisation is not usually necessary; encourage frequent voiding).

Care following delivery

If suturing is needed, it should occur promptly. **Re-infibulation of FGC type 3 must not be carried out at this time.**

If a midline incision has been made to open a type 2 or 3 FGC to enable delivery, then each side of the incision is over sewn separately on either side. In this way the FGC is 'reversed' and haemostasis achieved.

Postnatal period

Immediate care following delivery should include the following:

- adequate pain relief.
- perineal care
- re-education. Some women will have forgotten or will

never have known what normal micturition or menstruation is like.

Following discharge from the healthcare facility, continued support for the woman should be provided. If reversal is performed in labour, there should be a post-reversal check 4 to 6 weeks later.

If the woman has delivered a baby girl, support and information should be given, encouraging her not to inflict or allow others to inflict the same procedure on her daughter.

Safeguarding children who are at risk of FGC
- The safety and welfare of the child is paramount.
- All agencies must act in the best interests of the rights of the child as stated in the UN Convention on the Rights of the Child (1989).
- In some countries, FGC is illegal.

Laws and FGC
The following countries in Africa have issued laws against FGC, although this does not mean that the prevalence of FGC has been significantly reduced:
- Benin (2003)
- Burkina Faso (1996)
- Central Africa Republic (1966)
- Chad (2003)
- Cote d'Ivoire (1998)
- Djibouti (1994)
- Egypt (Ministerial Decree) (1996)
- Ethiopia (2004)
- Ghana (1994)
- Guinea (1965)
- Kenya (2001)
- Niger (2003)
- Senegal (1999)
- Tanzania (1998)
- Togo (1998)
- Nigeria (multiple states) (1999–2002).

It is acknowledged that some families see FGC as an act of love rather than of cruelty. However, FGC causes significant harm in both the short and long term, and constitutes physical and emotional abuse of children.

All decisions or plans for the child(ren) should be based on good-quality assessments. They should be sensitive to issues of race, culture, gender, religion and sexuality, and should avoid stigmatising the child or the practising community as far as possible.

Accessible, acceptable and sensitive involvement with the health, education, police, children's social care and voluntary-sector services may be needed.

All agencies should work in partnership with members of local communities, to empower individuals and groups to develop support networks and education programmes.

Appropriate care for women and girls who have been subjected to FGC
- Provide access to information, support and services.
- Provide care pathways and guidelines for professionals.
- Ensure that information is accurate and up to date.
- Empower women and girls and encourage them to speak out and seek help.
- Engage and mobilise all concerned, and develop an understanding of cultural diversity.
- Be open and supporting, sensitive and non-judgemental.
- Encourage alternative rites to FGC. This is a strategy that retains all of the rites of passage or initiation that the girls would traditionally undergo, except for the genital cutting. The girls are still encouraged to learn essential domestic duties that would be useful when they get married.

Conclusion
FGC is a violation of human rights. It is essential to empower women and girls, to encourage women to have a voice, and to raise awareness of the dangers of FGC. Engagement with all concerned local communities is crucial, including community and religious leaders.

As has been expressed so beautifully by Uche Umeh, 'When culture kills, when culture silences, when culture is complicit then culture must be changed.'

It is essential to work with all professionals. We all have a duty and a responsibility to safeguard girls who are at risk of FGC, as the welfare of children is paramount.

2.11 Domestic/intimate partner violence and pregnancy

Introduction
Everyone has a fundamental right to be, and remain, safe from harm. **Domestic violence**, also described as **intimate partner violence**, is defined as 'any incident of threatening behaviour, violence or abuse (psychological, physical, sexual, financial or emotional) between adults who are, or have been, intimate partner or family members, regardless of gender or sexuality'. Family members are defined as mother, father, son, daughter, brother, sister and grandparents, whether directly related, in-laws or step-family.

The main characteristic of domestic violence is that the behaviour is intentional and is calculated to exercise power and control within a relationship.

Domestic violence is reported in up to one in five

pregnancies, often beginning or getting worse at this time. The risk of moderate to severe violence appears to be greatest in the postpartum period.

Injuries to the abdomen, genitals and breasts are most frequent in pregnancy, but can be multiple, affecting any part of the woman's body.

Women and girls who suffer domestic violence are at increased risk of miscarriage, premature labour, placental abruption, low-birth-weight infants, fetal injury and intrauterine fetal death. As a result of violence, women are five times more likely to attempt suicide.

The impact of domestic violence can be devastating, and creates long-term consequences for women and girls, such as anxiety and mistrust. The impact on children must also be considered, as domestic violence and child abuse are often linked to the same perpetrator.

Recognising domestic violence in pregnancy

Studies show that around 30% of women will suffer from domestic violence in their lifetime. The first incident of violence commonly occurs during pregnancy. For some of these women, the pregnancy might be unwanted, due to abuse, rape, or as a result of not having access to or not being able to negotiate contraceptive use.

Domestic violence in pregnancy may be suspected on the basis of the type of injury, as well as the mental health and emotional status of the woman.

Women who are being abused may book late, and be poor attendees at antenatal clinics. They may attend repeatedly with trivial symptoms, and appear reluctant to be discharged home. The partner may be constantly present, not allowing private discussion. The woman may seem reluctant to speak in front of her partner, or to appear to contradict him.

Abusive partners often seek to minimise the evidence of their violence (e.g. by targeting areas that are normally clothed). As with child abuse, the stated mechanism of injury often does not fit with the apparent injury. There may be untended injuries of different ages, or the late presentation of injuries.

Multiple injuries and bruising (especially to the face, arms, breasts and abdomen), loss of consciousness, and drunkenness are significant but non-specific markers of domestic violence.

A history of behavioural problems, or abuse of children in the family, may be suggestive of domestic violence.

Diagnosing domestic violence

Routinely ask mothers whether they have been subjected to violence. Questions such as the following may allow the woman to disclose that she is being subjected to violence:

- I have noticed you have a number of bruises. Did someone hit you?
- You seemed frightened by your partner. Has he ever hurt you?
- You mention that your partner loses his temper with the children. Does he ever do that with you?
- How does your partner act when he is drinking alcohol or on drugs?

Other strategies such as the use of questionnaires in the women's toilets/rest room may help those women whose partner is constantly by their side (*see* Appendix).

Community midwives and traditional birth attendants visiting women at home may have the privacy to discuss such sensitive issues.

The provision of interpreters is essential. **Family members should not act as interpreters in this situation, as free dialogue will probably not occur.**

A system for caring for and protecting mothers subject to violence should be advocated for by all healthcare professionals undertaking maternal and child healthcare. Multi-agency working is crucial, and should include liaison with police, social services and the judicial system.

All professionals must take any available steps to seek a safe haven and to protect and support women who are experiencing domestic violence. The impact of domestic violence on the unborn child should be acknowledged, as well as the potential impact on existing children. It is very important to perform a risk assessment on women. Access to information and support must be easily and readily available to pregnant women.

It is equally crucial to empower and counsel women to make their own choices. Underlying issues such as finance and housing should be addressed, and the woman should be directed to the appropriate agency or support group, or to a legal adviser.

Appendix

How do I know if I am experiencing abuse?

If you answer yes to one or more of the following questions, you may be in an abusive relationship.

- Has your partner tried to keep you from seeing your friends or family?
- Has your partner prevented you from continuing or starting a college course, or from going to work?
- Does your partner constantly check up on you or follow you?
- Does your partner accuse you unjustly of flirting or of having affairs?
- Does your partner constantly belittle or humiliate you, or regularly criticise or insult you in front of other people?
- Are you ever scared of your partner?
- Have you ever changed your behaviour because you're afraid of what your partner might do or say to you?
- Has your partner ever deliberately destroyed any of your possessions?
- Has your partner ever hurt or threatened you or your children?
- Has your partner ever kept you short of money so that you were unable to buy food and other necessary items for yourself and your children?
- Has your partner ever forced you to do something that you really didn't want to do, including sexually?

Further reading

Wellbeing Foundation Africa. *Eliminating Domestic Violence*. www.wbfafrica.org/resources/cat_view/1-resources/6-eliminating-domestic-violence.html

2.12 Post-operative care

Basic nursing issues

The patient should be discharged to the ward or recovery area with clear orders for the following:

- **Monitor ABC.**
- If the patient is unconscious (P or U on the AVPU scale) they should not be left alone until they are responding to voice. Put them in the recovery position and undertake airway opening as required.
- Check vital signs (temperature, pulse, respiratory rate, blood pressure and capillary refill time) every 15 minutes for the first hour, hourly for the next 4 hours, and then 2-hourly. Observations should be more frequent if there is a change in observation from a normal to abnormal value.
- Monitor SaO_2 (normal value is > 93%) after a general anaesthetic. Give **oxygen** as required until SaO_2 is > 93% in air or the patient's colour is normal. Remember that cyanosis may not be present if the patient is severely anaemic.
- Observe the mother closely until the effect of the anaesthetic has worn off.
- Control pain: if it is severe, the patient will need IV morphine.
- Record the rate and type of IV fluid (if the patient has ketosis, ensure that there is an adequate amount of glucose in the drip).
- Record urine output, surgical and nasogastric drainage, and vomiting.
- Record input versus output, and calculate the difference every 12 hours.
- Document other medications.
- Perform laboratory investigations.

The patient's progress should be monitored, and documentation should include at least the following:

- a comment on medical and nursing observations
- a specific comment on the wound or operation site
- any complications
- any changes made in treatment.

Prevention of complications

- Provide adequate pain control.
- Encourage early mobilisation:
  - deep breathing and coughing
  - active daily exercise
  - joint range of motion
  - muscular strengthening
  - availability of walking aids such as canes, crutches and walkers, as well as instructions for their use.
- Ensure adequate nutrition.
- Consider throboprophylaxis in those at high risk of thrombo-embolic disease (DVT/PE) (*see* Section 2.5.H: 'Pulmonary embolism').
- Prevent skin breakdown and pressure sores:
  - turn the patient frequently
  - keep urine and faeces off the skin.

Pain management (*see* Section 1.15)

Manage pain wherever the patient is seen (emergency department, operating theatre or on the ward), and anticipate their needs for pain management after surgery and discharge. Do not delay the treatment of pain unnecessarily.

In the first 12–24 hours after a major surgical procedure, such as Caesarean section, powerful opiate analgesia (usually morphine IV) will be needed (*see* Section 1.15 for details). Thereafter, the pain should be less severe, and regular codeine, non-steroidal anti-inflammatory drugs (NSAIDs), aspirin or paracetamol should be sufficient.

Wound care

Dressings protect the wound and absorb exudates. Usually the dressing applied in theatre can remain in place for 48 hours unless there is excessive or purulent exudate, when a new dressing should be applied as a sterile procedure after cleansing with sterile 0.9% saline. Swabbing a wound can be harmful as it damages the newly granulating tissue. It is also painful.

After 48 hours, provided that the wound is intact, it can be cleaned under a shower.

Removal of sutures should usually occur after 7 days. Use one hand to hold the knot with forceps, place the stitch cutter or scissors under the knot next to the skin, and cut the stitch where it emerges from the skin. Remove the suture by pulling on the knot, which prevents a potentially contaminated stitch being pulled through the wound. Observe the wound every 4–6 hours, without touching it, for evidence of dehiscence.

Monitoring

All patients should be assessed at a frequency that is determined by the severity of their condition. Even those who are not seriously ill must be regularly assessed.

Vital signs (temperature, pulse, respiratory rate, blood pressure, urine output and fluid inputs) should be recorded on a standard form or graph at least 4-hourly for 24 hours after the immediate post-operative recovery phase.

Do not forget anti-tetanus coverage when appropriate.

Progress notes need not be lengthy, but must comment on the patient's condition and note any changes in the management plan. They should always be signed by the person writing the note.

Notes can be organised in the 'SOAP' format as follows:

- **S**ubjective: how the patient feels.
- **O**bjective: findings on physical examination, vital signs and laboratory results.
- **A**ssessment: what the healthcare worker thinks.
- **P**lan: management plan (this may also include directives which can be written in a specific location as 'orders').

Specific post-operative issues
Post salpingectomy for ruptured ectopic pregnancy

- Counsel patient regarding operative findings and likely

future fertility (if the other tube is normal in appearance then fertility is around 70%).

- Counsel patient regarding risk of recurrence (1 in 10 or more) and the need for early ultrasound in any subsequent pregnancy If evidence of pelvic inflammatory disease intraoperatively, treat patient and partner unless clear history of recent treatment.
- Offer child spacing/family planning advice. The intrauterine contraceptive device (IUCD) is associated with ectopic pregnancy if the patient becomes pregnant while using it. If another contraceptive is available and acceptable/suitable then this should be used in preference.

Post Caesarean section
Monitoring

1 Regularly (at least 2- to 4-hourly initially) monitor vital signs, including temperature, heart rate, respiratory rate, blood pressure, urine output, AVPU and SaO_2.
2 Regularly palpate the uterine fundus to ensure that the uterus remains contracted.
3 Regularly check for excessive vaginal blood loss.

Fluids and nutrition

1 If uncomplicated, give liquids and solids after 4–8 hours.
2 Bowel function should be normal after 12 hours.
3 Remove the IV cannula when the patient is stable and eating and drinking.
4 If there is infection, obstructed labour or uterine rupture, wait until bowel sounds appear before giving oral fluids.

Urine output

1 Keep a fluid balance chart and ensure that adequate urine output is occurring.
2 Remove the urinary catheter after 8 hours if the urine is clear; if not wait, until it is.
3 Wait 48 hours before removing the urinary catheter if there is a history of severe pre-eclampsia, uterine rupture, prolonged or obstructed labour, massive perineal oedema, or puerperal sepsis with pelvic peritonitis.
4 If the bladder was damaged, leave the catheter in for 7 days and until the urine is clear. If the patient is not receiving antibiotics, give nitrofurantoin 100 mg or cefalexin 500 mg or amoxicillin 500 mg orally once daily until the catheter is removed.

Anaemia

1 If the mother is significantly anaemic (haemoglobin level < 6–7 g/dL), transfusion may aid recovery from the operation. If possible, consider giving 500 mL of fresh cross-matched blood from a relative or other donor. The need for blood transfusion is dependent on the starting Hb and how well the patient is tolerating the anaemia.

Wound care

1 Check the dressing without disturbing it every 6 hours for the first 48 hours. Look for bleeding or infection.
2 Change the dressing after 48 hours.
3 If blood is leaking, replace the dressing with a new one if it is more than half soaked.

Postpartum vaginal haemorrhage

1 Massage the uterus to expel blood and blood clots. The presence of blood clots will inhibit effective uterine contractions;

2 Give oxytocin 10 units IM and then infuse 40 units in 500 mL of IV fluids (Ringer-lactate or Hartmann's solution) over 4 hours. If bleeding is heavy, give misoprostol orally, 3 × 200 microgram tablets, or rectally, 4 × 200 microgram tablets (*see* Section 2.5.D.iv for further management of postpartum haemorrhage).

Infection

1 If there are signs of infection or the mother currently has fever, give ampicillin 2 grams IV every 6 hours, *plus* gentamicin 80 mg IV/IM every 8 hours or 5 mg/kg body weight IV/IM once every 24 hours, *plus* metronidazole 500 mg IV every 8 hours. If fever is still present 72 hours after initiating antibiotics, re-evaluate and revise the diagnosis.
2 Infection of the uterus is a major cause of maternal death. Delayed or inadequate treatment of endometritis may result in pelvic abscess, peritonitis, septic shock, deep vein thrombosis, pulmonary embolism, chronic pelvic infection with recurrent pelvic pain and dyspareunia, tubal blockage and infertility.
3 If retained placental fragments are suspected as a cause of infection, perform a digital exploration of the uterus to remove clots and large pieces. Use ovum forceps or a large curette if required.
4 If there is no improvement with conservative measures and there are signs of general peritonitis (fever, rebound tenderness and abdominal pain), perform a laparotomy to drain the pus.
5 If the uterus is necrotic and septic, perform a hysterectomy (subtotal is preferable, if the cervix is not necrotic).

General measures

1 Ensure that the mother cannot fall out of bed when recovering from a general anaesthetic or if she is very unwell with a reduced conscious level.
2 Ensure pain control.
3 Encourage early mobility and deep breathing exercises.
4 The patient should wear knee-length well-fitting anti-embolism stockings until she is fully ambulant.

At the time of discharge from hospital

1 Discuss the implications of Caesarean section for future pregnancy management.
2 Discuss the timing of future activities such as sexual intercourse and heavy lifting.
3 Provide details of warning signs as to when the mother should contact a trained healthcare worker for advice.

Wound abscess

- If there is **pus or fluid**, open and drain the wound. Remove infected skin or subcutaneous sutures and debride the wound. Do not remove fascial sutures unless deep infection is evident or suspected.
- If there is an **abscess without cellulitis**, antibiotics are not required.
- Place a damp sterile normal saline dressing in the wound and change the dressing every 24 hours.
- Advise the patient on good hygiene and the need to wear clean pads or cloths that are changed frequently.
- **If the infection is superficial and does not involve deep tissues, monitor for development of an abscess and give antibiotics for 5 days or until fever free for 48 hours:**

— Flucloxacillin/cloxacillin 250–500 mg by mouth four times a day for 5 days.

- **If the infection is deep, involves muscles and is causing necrosis (necrotising fasciitis), give antibiotics until the necrotic tissue has been removed and the patient has been fever-free for 48 hours:**
  - Flucloxacillin/cloxacillin 500 mg–1 gram IV 6 hourly plus penicillin G 2 million units IV every 6 hours, plus metronidazole 500 mg IV every 8 hours.

Necrotising fasciitis requires urgent wide surgical debridement. Perform secondary closure 2 to 4 weeks later, depending on the resolution of infection.

It is important to inform the mother on discharge that she is at risk of uterine rupture during her next pregnancy. Offer child spacing/family planning advice.

Other complications
Peritonitis
Signs and symptoms

These include severe generalised abdominal pain, nausea and vomiting, fever, absent bowel sounds, rigid abdominal wall and shock.

Treatment

1. Call a surgeon and an anaesthetist.
2. Provide nasogastric suction.
3. Treat shock if present, but always place a wide-bore IV line and infuse fluids.
4. Give antibiotics until the patient has been fever-free for 48 hours:
   - ampicillin 2 grams IV every 6 hours, *plus* gentamicin 80 mg IV/IM every 8 hours or 5 mg/kg body weight IV/IM once every 24 hours, *plus* metronidazole 500 mg IV every 8 hours.
5. If necessary, perform laparotomy for peritoneal washout.

Pelvic abscess

Give antibiotics before draining the abscess, and continue until the patient has been fever-free for 48 hours:

- ampicillin 2 grams IV every 6 hours, *plus* gentamicin 80 mg IV/IM every 8 hours or 5 mg/kg body weight IV/

IM once every 24 hours, *plus* metronidazole 500 mg IV every 8 hours.

If **the abscess is fluctuant in the pouch of Douglas (cul-de-sac)**, perform culdocentesis. If the **spiking fever continues**, perform a laparotomy.

Care of the patient after spinal anaesthesia
Observations
Standard post-anaesthetic observations

Sensation should return within 4 hours. If after 4 hours the patient remains numb and/or cannot move her legs, contact the anaesthetist urgently.

Analgesia

Severe pain may return suddenly when the effects of the spinal block have worn off. Give analgesia when the patient first experiences pain.

Fasting

Fasting is not needed unless it is a surgical requirement (e.g. after abdominal operations).

Posture

The patient does not have to lie flat. Allow them to sit up as soon as they are able to do so.

Mobilising

If not contraindicated by the surgery, the patient can get out of bed 2 hours after the return of normal sensation, but **only with assistance**. Before getting the patient out of bed, sit her up slowly. If she feels faint, dizzy or sick then lie her down, take her blood pressure and inform the anaesthetist.

Potential complications

- **Postural hypotension:** lie the patient on the bed, give or increase IV fluids and inform the anaesthetist.
- **Urinary retention:** encourage the patient to pass urine when sensation returns. If the patient has not passed urine and she has a palpable bladder, she may need a catheter.

2.13 Obstetric procedures

The importance of basic and comprehensive Emergency Obstetric and Neonatal Care in resource-limited settings

The availability of Emergency Obstetric and Neonatal Care (EmONC) indicates how well any healthcare system can respond to the obstetric and newborn complications that are the main causes of maternal and newborn deaths. The Averting Maternal Death and Disability Program (AMDD)

and the United Nations have defined nine essential EmONC services that directly treat these complications. These are termed signal functions.

The functional status of an EmONC facility depends on the 24-hour availability of these life-saving signal functions and whether they have been performed recently. To qualify as a basic EmONC (or BEmONC) facility, health centres and hospitals must have performed the following seven signal functions within the past 3 months:

1 administered IM or IV antibiotics
2 administered IM or IV anticonvulsants
3 administered IM or IV uterotonic drugs
4 performed manual removal of the placenta
5 performed removal of retained products of conception (manual vacuum aspiration)
6 performed assisted vaginal delivery (with vacuum extractor or forceps)
7 performed neonatal resuscitation with a bag and mask.

To qualify as a comprehensive EmONC (or CEmONC) facility, health centres and hospitals must have performed all seven basic services listed above plus the following two additional signal functions within the past 3 months:
1 blood transfusion
2 Caesarean section.

In order for these EmONC systems to work adequately, there must be effective coordination of the supplies of essential emergency drugs, medical and surgical supplies and equipment to every facility providing this care. Essential drugs must include oxytocin, magnesium sulphate, misoprostol, antibiotics and antihypertensive drugs. Essential supplies include sutures and urinary catheters. Essential equipment includes manual vacuum aspirators, vacuum delivery kits and self-inflating bag-and-mask ventilators for newborn resuscitation.

Urethral catheterisation
Method

Use an appropriate size of catheter, which is one that is smaller in diameter than the external urethral meatus (to minimise the risk of subsequent urethral stricture formation). Usually this will be size 10–14 French gauge.

Using sterile precautions (gloves, etc.), wash the area with gauze swabs soaked with antiseptic (although sterile water or 0.9% saline can be just as effective), and clean from anterior to posterior with downward movements (to avoid faecal contamination). Sterile lubricant should be used to aid passage of the catheter. Use a syringe of sterile water or 0.9% saline to inflate the balloon if it is a Foley catheter, with the woman lying on her back or in the left lateral tilt position if she is more than 20 weeks' pregnant. The catheter is inserted far enough (urethra length is around 4 cm) for urine to be seen in the tube. Attach a catheter bag (if

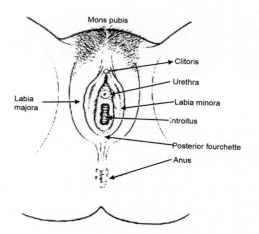

FIGURE 2.13.1 Normal female external genitalia showing urethra.

available). Secure the catheter to the thigh with tape to prevent traction damage to the bladder.

The balloon must be deflated before the catheter is removed.

Ventouse (vacuum) delivery
Introduction

The ventouse creates a vacuum in a cup attached to the fetal head to assist delivery. This technique is also called vacuum-assisted vaginal delivery or vacuum extraction (VE).

The advantages of the ventouse over forceps are that less training is needed, there is less risk of excessive traction, there are clear-cut rules on its use (e.g. the number of contractions during which traction is allowed), if the baby needs to rotate in order to be delivered this can occur spontaneously, and it can cause less injury to the mother.

The disadvantages are that it cannot be used for preterm delivery, face presentation, breech or after-coming head of breech, and if the mother is unable to provide expulsive efforts the ventouse is generally not effective. The equipment is more complex than forceps and more difficult to sterilise and maintain, and there can be more trauma to the baby (e.g. cephalhaematoma).

A number of different types of cups are available.

The original (Malmström) metal cup (see Figure 2.13.2) has the chain within a pipe leading to the cup. It may be difficult to sterilise the tube adequately.

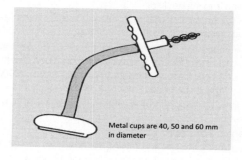

Metal cups are 40, 50 and 60 mm in diameter

FIGURE 2.13.2 The Malmström cup.

The Bird metal cup (see Figure 2.13.3) has two configurations:
1 The 5 cm **anterior metal cup** is used for occipito-anterior positions. The smaller 4 cm cup is reserved for the small fetus (e.g. a second twin, and particularly if the cervix is no longer fully dilated).
2 The **posterior metal cup** is used for occipito-posterior positions, particularly those with significant deflexion. This is often also the cup of choice for the deep transverse arrest, as the abnormal angle of the baby's head to the vertical, which is often marked, makes correct placement with the anterior cup highly unlikely.

The plastic cup (50 or 60 mm internal diameter) comes in two main forms:
- a silastic/silicon soft cup (see Figure 2.13.4) is the safest of all for the fetus, but has a slightly higher failure rate, especially with occipito-posterior positions
- the easy-to-use Kiwi OmniCup (see Figure 2.13.5), which is reusable but relatively expensive (www.youtube.com/watch?v=TgAcCi9rJhw).

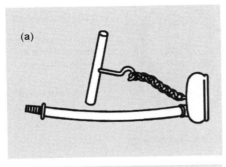

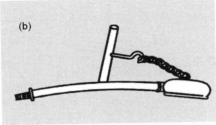

FIGURE 2.13.3 The two types of Bird metal cup. (a) Anterior cup. (b) Posterior cup.

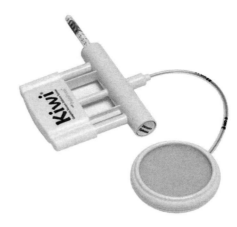

FIGURE 2.13.5 The Kiwi OmniCup.

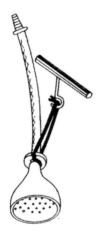

FIGURE 2.13.4 A soft plastic cup.

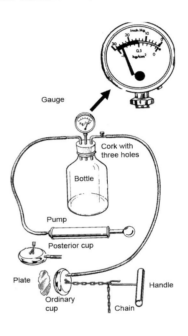

FIGURE 2.13.6 A simple vacuum extractor attached to a Bird anterior metal cup. This is Bird's modification of Malmström's extractor.

The application of negative pressure to the cup, including a vacuum gauge to show how much pressure is being applied, is shown in Figure 2.13.6.

Indications for an assisted delivery using the vacuum extractor

- Delay in the second stage of labour.
- Fetal distress in the second stage.
- Maternal conditions that require a short second stage (e.g. eclampsia, heart disease).
- Maternal exhaustion.

Contraindications

- Face presentation.
- Gestation less than 34 weeks.
- Breech presentation.
- Signs of obstructed labour.

Prerequisites

- Full dilatation of the cervix and engagement of the head (head at least at 0 station and no more than 1/5 above the symphysis pubis).
- The position of the fetal head in relation to the pelvis must be known.
- A fetus greater than 36 weeks' gestation, or with great care if between 34 and 36 weeks.
- Cooperation of the mother is helpful so that she can enhance contractions and traction by bearing down.
- Uterine contractions must be present.
- Ensure that a healthcare worker who is able to undertake neonatal resuscitation is present in case this is required.
- Ensure that the equipment is working, in particular that the vacuum reaches the correct value by testing the cup on the palm of the hand of the operator (covered by a sterile glove).

Basic rules

- If the patient is mobile, ask them to empty their bladder. If not, catheterise them. If the patient is catheterised, ensure that any within-catheter balloon is deflated.
- No additional anaesthetic is required (perineal infiltration with lidocaine will suffice if an episiotomy is planned).
- Lithotomy is the commonest position used, but delivery may be possible in a dorsal, lateral or squatting position. The mother should be in a 45-degree sitting position to aid expulsion.
- The delivery should be clearly achievable after three pulls, with evidence of descent with each pull.
- The head, not just the scalp, should descend with each pull.
- The cup should be reapplied no more than twice provided that it has been in the right position and the direction of pull is correct (and after one detachment an experienced operator, if available, should be summoned).
- If failure with the ventouse occurs despite good traction, do not try the forceps but proceed to Caesarean section (provided that it is safe, and available within a reasonable time).

Methods

First check your equipment. Attach the cup to the suction, and ensure the suction is working by testing it. This can be done by briefly holding the cup against your hand while suction is applied.

1 Examine the mother carefully using a sterile procedure and gloves and ideally an obstetric cream such as Hibitane. Estimate the size of the baby by abdominal examination, and ensure that the head is fully engaged (no more than 1/5 of the head should be palpable). The membranes should have ruptured.

2 Determine the position of the vertex and the amount of caput by vaginal examination. Identify the posterior fontanelle.

3 Describe the attitude of the presenting part as 'flexed' or 'deflexed'. In a flexed attitude only the posterior fontanelle can be felt, whereas any situation in which the anterior fontanelle can be felt or the posterior fontanelle cannot be found should be described as deflexed.

4 With two fingers press on the perineum posteriorly to widen the vaginal opening (see Figure 2.13.7).

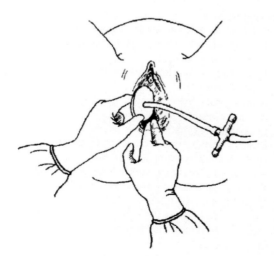

FIGURE 2.13.7 Inserting a Malmström cup.

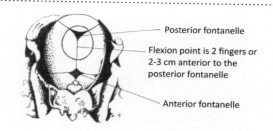

Posterior fontanelle

Flexion point is 2 fingers or 2-3 cm anterior to the posterior fontanelle

Anterior fontanelle

FIGURE 2.13.8 Placing the cup.

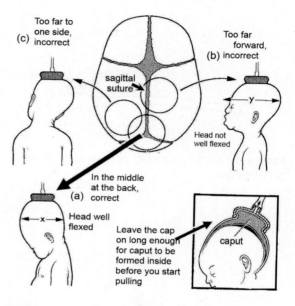

FIGURE 2.13.9 Correct and incorrect positions for the cup.

5 Insert the cup, avoiding the urethra. Apply the largest cup that will fit, with the centre of the cup over the flexion point, 2–3 cm anterior to the posterior fontanelle (see Figures 2.13.8 and 2.13.9). This placement will promote flexion, descent and autorotation with traction. Suction is applied to draw the fetal scalp into the cup.

6 Ensure that no maternal tissue is caught under the edge of the cup.

7 Place the middle of the cup 1–2 cm anterior to the baby's posterior fontanelle/posterior to the anterior fontanelle. This will flex the head during its passage through the pelvis.

- If you put it more towards the front it will tend to extend the head, so that it will be less easy to pull out. The distance 'Y' when the head is deflexed (bent backwards) is much longer than the distance 'X' when it is flexed (bent forward).
- If you put the cup to one side, the head will bend to one side.

8 Connect the cup to the pump (see Figure 2.13.6), and check for leaks prior to commencing the delivery.

- First increase the pressure to $0.2\,kg/cm^2$, and then, after checking again that there is no maternal tissue caught under the cup, increase the pressure to $0.8\,kg/cm^2$, but never any higher than this.
- Common problems include suction bottles not tightly screwed in or tubing loosely attached to the metal cup.
- The metal cup should have a meshed bottom plate, which functions to maintain a clear space between

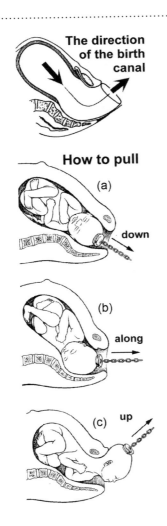

The direction of the birth canal

How to pull

(a) **down**

(b) **along**

(c) **up**

FIGURE 2.13.10 Delivery with the Bird anterior metal cup.

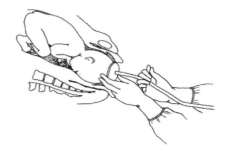

FIGURE 2.13.11 How to ensure that the vacuum cup is securely on the infant's head as you pull.

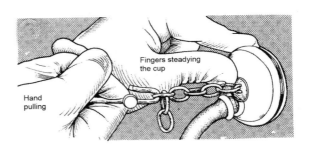

Fingers steadying the cup

Hand pulling

FIGURE 2.13.12 Guiding the cup with the fingers to detect any slippage while pulling.

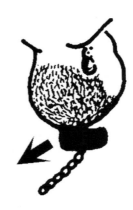

FIGURE 2.13.13 Cup slipping off with sideways traction.

the scalp and the cup so that an effective vacuum can be applied.

9 Only perform an episiotomy when the head stretches the perineum (to avoid blood loss), and only if the perineum is interfering with the delivery.

10 Check the application. Ensure that there is no maternal soft tissue (cervix or vagina) within the rim.

11 During a contraction, encourage the patient to push, and aid her expulsive efforts by applying traction to the cup/fetal head (method described below).

Delivery with the anterior metal or plastic cup

The metal or plastic cup is lightly lubricated with sterile delivery cream (e.g. chlorhexidine cream) and then inserted sideways into the vagina. To orientate the cup correctly, direct the chain towards the occiput, which will result in the vacuum pipe lying centrally. Take the pressure up to $0.2\,kg/cm^2$. Check that no maternal tissue is caught under the cup and then increase the pressure directly to $0.8\,kg/cm^2$, but never any higher than this. Begin traction with the next contraction after this pressure has been achieved.

Traction should be along the pelvic axis for the duration of the contraction (initially down, then progressively forwards, and finally upwards as the head delivers) and always perpendicular to the cup (see Figure 2.13.10).

Always pull in the direction of the birth canal.

1 Pull downwards towards the floor until the head is below the ischial spines.

2 Pull outwards until the head is stretching the perineum.

3 Finally pull upwards until the baby is delivered.

During traction keep one finger or thumb on the edge of the cup and another finger on the scalp so that the earliest sign of detachment or slippage is detected (see Figures 2.13.11 and 2.13.12).

With each contraction apply traction in a line perpendicular to the plane of the cup rim to help to prevent the cup slipping off (see Figure 2.13.13). Place a finger on the scalp next to the cup during traction to assess potential slippage and descent of the vertex (see Figure 2.13.12). **Slight** side-to-side movements may help to edge the head down the pelvic wall, but side-to-side movements must be small to keep the traction line perpendicular and prevent the cup from detaching.

As the head crowns, the angle of traction changes through an arc of over 90 degrees.

If the perineum is stretching as normal, it is simply supported with the hand that was on the cup. An episiotomy must only be undertaken if perineal resistance is preventing delivery.

Occasionally, an edge of the cup might lift off at the introitus (this is more likely to happen if there is caput present). If this occurs, one has to be careful not to catch maternal tissue under the cup as it reattaches. Therefore this should be rechecked before final delivery of the head.

Once the head has delivered, release the vacuum and take off the cup and complete the delivery normally.

Delivery with the posterior metal cup

For a deflexed head in an occipito-posterior position, the 'OP' cup or if this is not available a plastic cup, ideally a Kiwi OmniCup, should be used. It is applied as far back on the head as possible, again ideally in the midline over the occiput. To allow good placement of the cup, it sometimes helps to try to flex the head, with two fingers of the left hand pressing on the sinciput, while the right hand inserts the cup behind the head. Once correctly placed, the vacuum can be started and taken directly to the required level. (Because the cup lies parallel to the vagina it is unlikely to catch any maternal tissue.) The first pull will be in the direction required to flex the head. With flexion of the head, the presenting diameter immediately becomes less. Thereafter, traction will be along the pelvic axis. The delivery may be completed simply by a standard spontaneous rotation of the baby with maternal effort and gentle assistance. **It is essential not to try to twist the cup to rotate the baby. This will cause trauma, especially spiral tears of the scalp, with the rotational deliveries.**

Overall, occipito-posterior deliveries are the most likely to cause problems. The most difficult ones are those where the head is markedly deflexed or where there is excessive caput. Another difficulty sometimes encountered is that the suction pipe tends to kink once the head flexes, making the cup more likely to detach. If the cup detaches at this point (after flexion and rotation), put it back on again or perform a lift-out forceps.

Between contractions, check the **fetal heart rate** and **secure application of the cup**.

Note the following:

- Never use the cup to actively rotate the baby's head. Rotation of the baby's head will occur naturally with traction, if it is going to rotate.
- Do not continue to pull between contractions and expulsive efforts.
- With progress, and in the absence of fetal distress, continue the 'guiding' pulls to achieve delivery. Descent must be seen with each pull, and delivery should be clearly achievable following three pulls.

Causes and management of failure to deliver with the ventouse

Vacuum extraction has failed if:

- the head does not advance with each pull
- the fetus is not delivered or delivery is not imminent after three pulls
- the cup slips off the head twice at the proper direction of pull with a maximum negative pressure.

Every application should be considered a trial of vacuum extraction. Do not persist if there is no descent with every pull.

Generally delivery is achieved with three pulls. As a minimum, it should be clear after three pulls that the delivery is **definitely** going to be achieved imminently by the vaginal route.

Failures occur for the following reasons.

1 Inadequate initial assessment of the case:
    - The head being too high: a classic mistake is to assume that because caput can be felt below the ischial spines, the head must be engaged.
    - Misdiagnosis of the position and attitude of the head: attention to simple detail will minimise this.
2 Anterior or lateral placements will increase the failure rate.
    - If the cup placement is found to be incorrect, it may be appropriate to begin again with correct placement (i.e. midline over the flexion point).
3 Failures due to traction in the wrong direction.
    - Gentle sustained traction in the correct direction is what is needed, and sideways movements will be ineffective and increase scalp trauma and cup detachments.
4 Excessive caput.
    - Rarely, even with metal cups, adequate traction is not possible because of excessive caput.
    - In these cases, consideration must be given to delivery by Caesarean section unless the head is well down, in which case forceps can be used.
5 Poor maternal effort.
    - Maternal effort can contribute substantially to success.
    - Adequate encouragement and instruction should be given to the mother.
    - This may be a reason for preferring forceps to ventouse if the patient is under general anaesthetic.
6 The incidence of cephalo–pelvic disproportion (CPD) (true failure) is low. However, in settings where the majority of women deliver at home or in community clinics, it must be remembered that the patient is likely to have been fully dilated for some time before arrival in the hospital, if she has been referred for failure to progress in the second stage. CPD is likely to be relatively more common in this group.

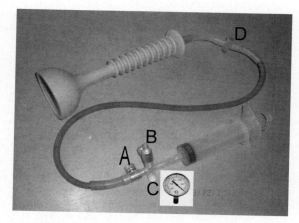

FIGURE 2.13.14 The EgAr device.

One of the main problems with using a ventouse in resource-limited settings is difficulty with the availability of reliable suction. Although this is integral to the Kiwi, these are expensive and usually disposable. A new technique to provide negative pressure for a plastic or metal cup (the EgAr device) has been developed in Gambia by a senior midwife and is described here.

The main components are two valves from out-of-use aneroid blood pressure machines, a 100-mL bladder syringe, a four-way open tap from a urine bag, a urine bag control valve, and a vacuum gauge (*see* Figure 2.13.14).

The blood pressure system valves are attached to the outflow control unit of a urine bag, which is then attached to the syringe. The valves are arranged in such a way that when the plunger of the syringe is pulled, air is withdrawn into the syringe through the first valve (i.e. valve A). When the plunger is pushed back, the air in the syringe is expelled through the second valve (i.e. valve B). Since the valves (when closed) allow air to flow in only one direction, the syringe can function both to create vacuum pressure by pulling the plunger, and also as an air pump when the plunger is pushed back.

A standard conventional vacuum delivery cup (either the metal or silicon type) is attached to the syringe through one of the blood pressure valves, using the tube from the blood pressure machine. Both valves are closed to ensure that air flows into the syringe only through the first valve (A) when the plunger is pulled, and is expelled only through the second valve (B) when the plunger is pushed back. The vacuum cup is attached to the fetal head and a few pulls (three or four) on the plunger create a negative pressure measured on the vacuum gauge attached to the fourth outlet of the four-way tap (D) sufficient to deliver the baby without the need for continuous pumping. Vacuum pressure is released when the baby is born through the valve (C) from the urine bag near to where the cup is attached.

If vacuum extraction fails, use vacuum extraction in combination with symphysiotomy (see below) or perform Caesarean section.

Vacuum extraction and symphysiotomy

Vacuum extraction may be used in combination with symphysiotomy in the following circumstances:

- the head is at least at −2 station or no more than 2/5 palpable above the symphysis pubis
- Caesarean section is not feasible or immediately available
- the provider is experienced and proficient in performing symphysiotomy
- vacuum extraction alone has failed or is expected to fail
- there is no major degree of disproportion.

Complications of vacuum extraction

Complications usually result from not observing the conditions of application, or from continuing efforts beyond the time limits stated above.

Fetal complications

- Localised scalp oedema (artificial caput or chignon) under the vacuum cup is harmless and disappears within a few hours.
- Cephalhaematoma (*see* Figure 2.13.15) requires observation, and will usually clear in 3 to 4 weeks.
- Scalp abrasions (common and harmless) and lacerations

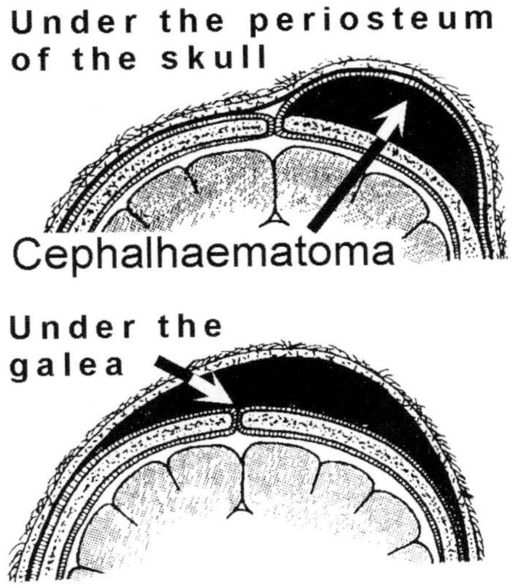

FIGURE 2.13.15 Fetal scalp bleeding complications of ventouse (vacuum extraction).

may occur. Clean and examine lacerations to determine whether sutures are necessary. Necrosis is extremely rare.

- Sub-galeal haemorrhage is more serious.

There have been reports of transmission of herpes viral infections from the mother to the fetal scalp following the use of a metal cup. It is theoretically possible that hepatitis or HIV infection may also be transmitted in this way. There is a lower risk of scalp injury using the flexible/plastic cups. Therefore for straightforward ventouse deliveries use the flexible cup when possible, bearing in mind that where rotation is needed as part of the delivery the metal cup is more successful. The metal cup can also deliver a stronger traction force.

Maternal complications

Tears of the genital tract may occur. Examine the woman carefully and repair any tears to the cervix or vagina, or undertake episiotomy repair.

Special indications for delivery with the ventouse

With the exception of second twin deliveries (where the cervix is in effect recently parous), vacuum extraction before full dilatation is generally only possible in multiparous women in which the cervix is soft and easily stretchable. This is definitely not always the case even with multiparous women, and great caution must be taken before proceeding to any vaginal delivery before full dilatation. Complications of such deliveries include cervical tears which can extend upward to involve the uterus, and therefore may require laparotomy for repair or even hysterectomy as for a ruptured uterus.

If the operator is uncertain about the degree of engagement, degree of cervical dilatation or the position of the head, a more experienced practitioner should assist (if available).

Forceps delivery after failure to deliver with the ventouse

There is no place for an attempt at forceps delivery if there has been no descent with the ventouse despite adequate traction. However, if traction has been inadequate (due to caput, leaking equipment or no maternal assistance), it may be justified to change to forceps. The most experienced operator should make this decision.

The ventouse is the instrument of first choice for operative vaginal delivery provided conditions for its use are safe and suitable.

Forceps delivery
Introduction
Forceps are particularly helpful in the delivery of the after-coming head of a breech, delivery of a mento-anterior face presentation, and delivery before 34 weeks (although this is controversial).

Conditions for possible use of forceps
These include the following:
- vertex presentation
- face presentation with chin anterior
- entrapped after-coming head in breech delivery; some operators will routinely control the delivery of the head here by using forceps, provided that the cervix is fully dilated.

At the very minimum, the sagittal suture should be in the midline and straight, guaranteeing an occiput-anterior or occiput-posterior position.

Outlet forceps
In resource-limited settings, forceps at the outlet can be helpful for delay in the second stage when the baby's head is near the outlet, but for all other situations the ventouse is preferred if suitable. The conditions for the use of outlet forceps are as follows:
- the fetal scalp is visible without separating the labia
- the fetal skull has reached the pelvic floor
- the sagittal suture is in the anterio-posterior diameter or right or left occiput-anterior or occiput-posterior position (rotation does not exceed 45 degrees)
- the fetal head is at or on the perineum.

The blade on the mother's left always goes in first, and the right blade fits on top of it.

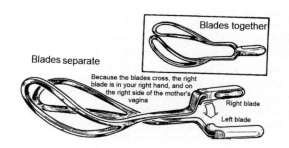

Blades together

Blades separate

Because the blades cross, the right blade is in your right hand, and on the right side of the mother's vagina

Right blade

Left blade

FIGURE 2.13.16 Outlet forceps.

Procedure
- Ensure that the head is engaged in the pelvis. Abdominal palpation must be undertaken, particularly in the case of face presentation.
- Urinary catheterisation is required.

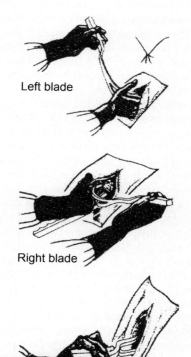

Left blade

Right blade

Blades locked

FIGURE 2.13.17 Applying outlet forceps.

- Pudendal block and perineal infiltration with 1% lignocaine is required.
- An episiotomy is usually required.
- Identify the position of the head. Occipito-transverse or occipito-posterior positions are indications for ventouse, and if the head is deflexed, for using the OP ventouse cup or Kiwi OmniCup.
- Ensure that the pair of forceps match. Assemble them and check. It may be useful to check the maximum diameter between the blades, which must be at least 9 cm.
- Lubricate the blades of the forceps with disinfectant cream (e.g. Hibitane).
- Wearing sterile gloves, insert two fingers of the right hand into the vagina on the side of the fetal head. Slide the left blade gently between the head and fingers to rest on the side of the head (see Figure 2.13.18).

A biparietal bimalar application is the only safe option.

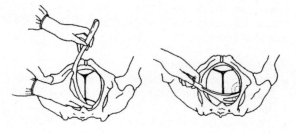

FIGURE 2.13.18 Applying the left blade of the forceps.

Repeat the same manoeuvre on the other side, using the left hand and the right blade of the forceps (*see* Figure 2.13.19).

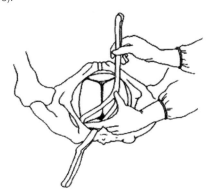

FIGURE 2.13.19 Applying the right blade of the forceps.

- Depress the handles and lock the forceps.
- Difficulty in locking usually indicates that the application is incorrect. In this case, remove the blades and recheck the position of the head. Reapply only if the head is in the appropriate position for the use of forceps.
- After locking check that the sagittal suture lies vertically in the midline between the shanks of the forceps. Also ensure that no more than two fingers can be placed laterally into the fenestrations of the blades. Note: these checks do not ensure correct placement but do help detect some instances of mal-placement.
- After locking, apply steady traction inferiorly and posteriorly with each contraction (*see* Figures 2.13.20 and 2.13.21). There should be both traction and pressure on top of the joined forceps.

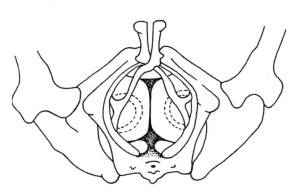

FIGURE 2.13.20 Locking the handles.

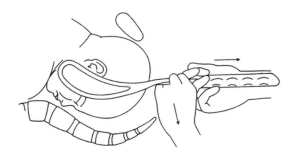

FIGURE 2.13.21 The correct way of applying traction with downward pressure.

Between contractions check the fetal heart rate and correct application of forceps.

- When the head crowns, make an adequate **episiotomy**.
- Lift the head slowly out of the vagina between contractions.
- The head should descend with each pull. Only two or three pulls should be necessary.
- Ensure that the head rather than the blades of the forceps are descending with each pull by feeling the fingers on the fetal head moving down. It is very harmful to the fetus if the blades slide down the side of the fetal head.

Failure of forceps
- The fetal head does not advance with each pull.
- The fetus is not delivered after three pulls.

Every application should be considered a trial of forceps. Do not persist if there is no descent with every pull.

If forceps delivery fails, consider a symphysiotomy or perform a Caesarean section.

- After repairing any episiotomy, ensure that swab and instrument counts are correct.
- Do a rectal examination to check the integrity of the rectal sphincter and the mucosa for tears.

Complications of forceps use
Fetal complications
- Injury to facial nerves requires observation. This injury is usually self-limiting.
- Lacerations of the face and scalp may occur. Clean and examine any lacerations to determine whether sutures are necessary.
- Fractures of the face and skull require close monitoring.

Maternal complications

Tears of the genital tract may occur. Examine the woman carefully and repair any cervical or vaginal tears and undertake episiotomy repair.

Caesarean section

The WHO suggests that systems should be in place to ensure that Caesarean section is performed in a minimum of 5% of all expected births.

Indications
- Obstructed labour.
- Obstetric haemorrhage (especially if ongoing or the mother or fetus is unstable).
- Severe maternal illness where urgent delivery is indicated and is not achievable rapidly by vaginal delivery (e.g. eclampsia where delivery is advised within 12 hours).
- Fetal distress.
- Malpresentation.
- Major placenta praevia.

Pre-operative considerations
- Check for fetal life by listening to the fetal heart rate.
- Examine for fetal presentation and to ensure vaginal delivery is not achievable.
- Avoid performing a Caesarean section if there is no maternal indication and the fetus is dead.
- Obtain informed consent from the mother.

Take a blood sample for haemoglobin or haematocrit, blood grouping and cross-matching if indicated. More than 2 × 500 mL units may be needed if antepartum bleeding or massive haemorrhage is anticipated.

- Transfer the patient to the operating theatre in the left lateral position with a wedge under the right buttock.
- Give antacid immediately prior to general anaesthetic (30 mL of 0.3% sodium citrate (preferable non-particulate) or 300 mg of magnesium trisilicate). This neutralises the stomach acid and minimises damage to the lungs if aspiration occurs.
- Start an IV infusion with a crystalloid such as Ringer-lactate or Hartmann's solution.
- Spinal or general anaesthesia with rapid sequence induction, or ketamine, or local infiltration may be used, depending on local circumstances.

(For choice of anaesthesia, *see* Section 1.24.)

In theatre, the operating table must be kept in the left lateral tilt position or a pillow placed under the woman's right lower back to reduce aorto-caval compression until after delivery.

Urinary catheterisation

The woman must be catheterised and her bladder emptied before starting the procedure, both to avoid injury to the bladder and to monitor urine output.

Remove the catheter after 8 hours if the urine is clear; if not, wait until it is.

Wait 48 hours before removing the catheter if there is:

- uterine rupture
- prolonged or obstructed labour
- gross perineal oedema
- puerperal sepsis with pelvic peritonitis.

If the bladder was damaged, leave the catheter in for 7 days. The urine should be clear of blood and remain so after 48 hours. If the woman is not receiving antibiotics, give nitrofurantoin 100 mg (or cefalexin 500 mg or amoxicillin 500 mg) orally once daily until the catheter has been removed.

Skin preparation

The presence of a large amount of pubic hair around the site of skin incision can interfere with healing. A suitable proportion of this should be shaved off **immediately before the skin is disinfected and the incision is made. There must not be a gap between shaving and operation.**

Tincture of chlorhexidine, iodophor and tincture of iodine are the recommended antiseptic products for preparing the patient's operative site. Apply three times to the incision site using disinfected ring forceps and a cotton or gauze swab. Do not contaminate the glove by touching unprepared skin. Begin at the proposed incision site and work outwards in a circular motion away from the incision site. At the edge of the sterile field discard the swab.

The use of alcohol or hexachlorophene as a single agent is not recommended unless the patient's skin is sensitive to the recommended antiseptic products. Impregnated adhesive film as skin preparation is not recommended.

All patients should be given a prophylactic antibiotic, ampicillin 2 grams IV, before the skin incision, and ideally thromboprophylaxis post-operatively (compression stockings, mobilisation, and 5000 units of heparin subcutaneously 12-hourly until the patient is discharged from hospital).

Prevention of exposure of staff to HIV and hepatitis

In many operations, micro-holes develop in gloves (not due to needlestick injuries). These micro-holes will of course be more prevalent if gloves are reused, as in some resource-limited settings. If there is a significant risk of HIV or hepatitis, double gloves or special thick gloves should be used. A clear plastic facial shield reduces exposure to blood.

Opening the abdomen

Abdominal and uterine scars are two separate issues. Classical section is a vertical uterine scar, usually but not always associated with a vertical abdominal scar. A vertical abdominal scar may be present with either a classical or lower segment uterine scar.

Skin incision

The choice of skin incision depends on the following:

- the gestational age of the fetus
- the indication for section
- the presence of previous scars
- the operator's surgical experience.

A low transverse incision is preferred to the vertical incision, as there is less likelihood of wound dehiscence and hernia. There are two possibilities, namely the Pfannenstiel incision and the Joel-Cohen incision.

The Joel-Cohen incision

The Joel-Cohen technique includes straight transverse incision through the skin only, 3 cm below the level of the anterior superior ileac spines (higher than the Pfannenstiel incision; see below). The subcutaneous tissues are opened only in the middle 3 cm. The fascia is incised transversely in the midline and then extended laterally with a blunt finger. Finger dissection is used to separate the rectus muscles vertically and laterally and open the peritoneum. All of the layers of the abdominal wall are stretched manually to the extent of the skin incision. The bladder is reflected inferiorly. The myometrium is incised transversely in the midline, but not to breach the amniotic sac, then opened and extended laterally with finger dissection. Interrupted sutures are used for the closure of the myometrium.

The Pfannenstiel incision

This consists of a curved skin incision, two finger-breadths above the symphysis pubis, transverse incision of the sheath, blunt separation of the rectus muscles, and incision of the parietal peritoneum in the midline.

The low vertical incision

The incision is made from the base of the umbilicus to the pubic hair line. This is preferred if better exposure is needed or local anaesthesia is used. It allows easier access to the upper abdomen, is indicated if the lower uterine segment is difficult to access due to adhesions from previous Caesarean sections, if the lie of the fetus is transverse with the back down, and if there are fetal malformations, large fibroids over the lower segment, a vascular lower segment due to placenta praevia, or carcinoma of the cervix.

Compared with Pfannenstiel-based Caesarean

section, Joel-Cohen-based Caesarean section has been shown to be associated with a reduction in blood loss, operating time, time to oral intake, fever, duration of post-operative pain, analgesic injections, and time from skin incision to birth of the baby.

The surgeon must ensure that the access to the uterus is adequate to deliver the fetus without difficulty, and in the presence of scarring a Pfannenstiel incision may give better exposure.

Length of incision

A minimum length of 15 cm is indicated (which accommodates an open Allis forceps).

Excision of the previous scar is not essential for better healing and cosmetic results unless there is keloid scarring.

General measures

- Handle tissue gently.
- Prevent bleeding.
- Eradicate dead space.
- Minimise the amount of desensitised tissue and foreign material in the wound.

Practical points

- Extend incision of the fascia, peritoneum and myometrium digitally or with scissors rather than with a scalpel.
- Transfer sharp instruments into a basin/tray.
- Retract tissue with instruments, reposition suture needles with forceps and remove the needle before the final tying of sutures.

Make the skin incision to the level of the fascia.

If the Caesarean section is performed under local anaesthesia, make a vertical incision that is about 4 cm longer than when general/spinal anaesthesia is used. A **Pfannenstiel incision** takes longer, retraction is poorer and it requires more local anaesthetic.

Make a 2–3 cm vertical incision in the fascia.

- Hold the fascial edge with forceps and lengthen the incision from side to side using scissors.
- Use fingers or scissors to separate the rectus muscles (abdominal wall muscles).
- Use scissors to make an opening in the peritoneum near the umbilicus. Use scissors to lengthen the incision up and down in order to see the entire uterus. Use scissors to separate the layers and open the lower part of the peritoneum, taking care to avoid bladder injury.
- Place a bladder retractor over the pubic bone.
- Use forceps to pick up the loose peritoneum covering the anterior surface of the lower uterine segment, and incise with scissors.
- Extend the incision by placing the scissors between the uterus and the loose serosa. Cut transversely about 3 cm on each side.
- Use two fingers to push the bladder downwards off the lower uterine segment. Replace the bladder retractor over the pubic bone and bladder.

Opening the uterus

- Use a scalpel to make a 3 cm transverse incision in the lower segment of the uterus. It should be about 1 cm below the level where the vesico-uterine peritoneal fold was incised to bring the bladder down.

- Widen the incision by placing a finger at each edge and gently pulling upwards and laterally at the same time.
- If the **lower uterine segment is thick and narrow**, extend the incision in a crescent shape, using scissors instead of fingers to avoid extension into the uterine vessels.
- **It is important to make the uterine incision large enough to deliver the head and body of the baby without tearing the incision.**

Uterine incision

A **high vertical uterine incision** is indicated if any of the following are present:

- an inaccessible lower segment due to dense adhesions from previous Caesarean section
- transverse lie (with the baby's back down) for which a lower uterine segment incision cannot be safely performed
- fetal malformations (e.g. conjoined twins)
- large fibroids over the lower segment
- a highly vascular lower segment due to placenta praevia
- carcinoma of the cervix.

A **lower transverse incision** is commonly used because:

- less dissection of the bladder is needed
- entry into the uterus is easier
- there is less blood loss
- there is a lower incidence of uterine rupture with subsequent pregnancies.

Lower vertical incision (De Lee's incision) can be useful if the lower uterine segment is poorly formed and thickened, in which case a transverse incision would be unwise.

If a lower transverse incision has been attempted and found to be inadequate, it can be extended upwards in a J-shaped incision to avoid blood vessels and enable adequate access.

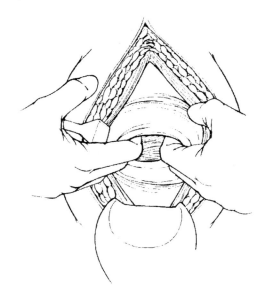

FIGURE 2.13.22 Enlarging the uterine incision.

Delivery of the baby and placenta

- To deliver the baby, place one hand inside the uterine cavity between the uterus and the baby's head.
- With the fingers, grasp and flex the head.

- Gently lift the baby's head through the incision (*see* Figure 2.13.23), taking care not to extend the incision down towards the cervix.

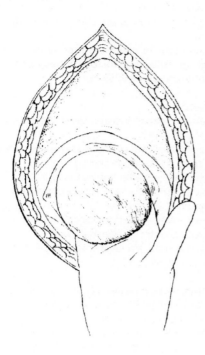

FIGURE 2.13.23 Delivering the baby's head.

- With the other hand, gently press on the abdomen over the top of the uterus to help to deliver the head.
- If the **baby's head is deep down in the pelvis or vagina**, ask an assistant (wearing sterile gloves) to reach into the vagina (which must be sterilised as described above) and push the baby's head up into the uterus. Then lift and deliver the head (*see* Figure 2.13.24).

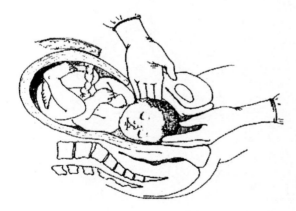

FIGURE 2.13.24 Delivering the deeply engaged head abdominally with assistance via the vagina.

Method of delivery of fetus

The head delivers into the wound in a transverse direction, so gentle rotation with lateral flexion of the neck is required. In the following circumstances this can be difficult or impossible:

- Caesarean section in the second stage of labour following failed forceps/ventouse, when the head is very low

- occipito-posterior position
- impacted breech
- transverse lie
- prematurity and oligohydramnios where the lower segment is poorly formed and thick.

Manoeuvres that may help include the following:

- an assistant can disengage and push the presenting part upwards from the vagina
- modified lithotomy position with a combined abdomino-vaginal approach
- application of forceps when the head is free
- grasping a foot and delivering by the breech in the presence of transverse lie
- uterine relaxation.

Other practical points

- If there is posterior placenta praevia, open the uterus and reach in below the placenta, separating it upwards until the membranes are reached, and then deliver the baby. If the placenta is anterior, as soon as you cut into it there will be haemorrhage from the fetus. **It is vital that the cord is clamped as quickly as possible.**
- **In all cases of fetal distress, quick delivery is required.**
- Suction the baby's mouth and nose when delivered, especially if there is meconium-stained liquor.
- Deliver the shoulders and body.
- Give oxytocin 5 units IV to aid delivery of the placenta, and then infuse 40 units in 500 mL of IV fluids (Ringer-lactate or Hartmann's solution) over 4 hours if there is a risk of haemorrhage.
- Clamp and cut the umbilical cord.
- Hand the baby to an assistant for initial care.
- Give a single dose of a prophylactic antibiotic after the cord has been clamped and cut, but only if not given prior to incision: ampicillin 2 grams IV *or* cefotaxime 1 gram IV.
- Keep gentle traction on the cord and massage the uterus through the abdomen.
- Deliver the placenta and membranes.

Delivery of the placenta

Spontaneous delivery after oxytocin has been given on delivery of the baby, and with controlled cord traction, is preferred to manual removal. Manual delivery of the placenta may be necessary, and routine checking of the cavity is essential to ensure that no retained placental fragments or membranes are present, as this cannot always be ensured by inspection of the placenta.

Closing the uterine incision
General principles

- Meticulous handling with re-approximation of tissues. Avoid strangulating tissue with tight knots.
- Haemostasis: isolate and ligate major bleeding vessels.
- Grasp minimal tissue while cauterising.

Exteriorisation of the uterus

This may be necessary in order to visualise the lower segment for suturing, and it may thereby reduce blood loss. It may cause vagal stimulation leading to bradycardia, and may be uncomfortable if performed under spinal or epidural anaesthesia. It is important to inform the anaesthetist of the need to exteriorise.

Suturing of the uterus

Sutures of polyglycolic acid suture are preferred to catgut. Use of thick suture causes more foreign body and tissue reaction, but if too thin it will cut through the myometrium. Usually the uterus is closed in two layers.

- Grasp the corners of the uterine incision with clamps.
- Grasp the bottom edge of the incision with clamps. Make sure that it is separate from the bladder.
- Look carefully for any extensions of the uterine incision.
- Repair the incision and any extensions with a continuous locking stitch using a robust absorbable suture such as No. 1 or 0 chromic catgut, polyglycolic acid or Vicryl (*see* Figure 2.13.25).
- A routine second layer of sutures is usually undertaken for the uterine incision, as it may help to reduce the risk of haemorrhage and subsequent uterine rupture through the scar.
- If there is any **persisting bleeding from the incision site**, close with figure-of-eight sutures.

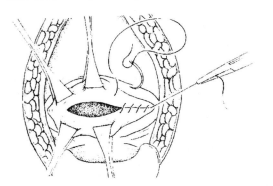

FIGURE 2.13.25 Closing the uterine incision.

Peritoneal closure of parietal and visceral peritoneum is safe. Healing and strength of the wounds are not affected. The duration of surgery is reduced and there is less tendency to form intra-abdominal adhesions.

Rectus sheath

Standard single-layer closure with a synthetic delayed absorbable suture is recommended. Place each suture 1 cm from the wound edge to allow healing. In vertical incisions, mass closure using synthetic permanent suture is appropriate, but the stitch should not be locking, as this increases post-operative pain and wound hernias.

Subcutaneous tissue and skin closure

Closure of Camper's fascia with continuous suture reduces the rate of wound disruption. The routine use of closed suction drainage in non-obese patients is not recommended.

Subcuticular or interrupted skin suturing may be undertaken. The type of suture material used for subcuticular suturing does not affect the outcome. Interrupted mattress sutures are recommended in obese patients and in cases where delayed healing is anticipated. Placement of clips has similar results.

If a Couvelaire uterus (swollen and discoloured by blood) is seen at Caesarean section, as a result of major placental abruption, close it in the normal manner and monitor closely for 48 hours after delivery.

- **Closing the abdomen.** Look carefully at the uterine incision before closing the abdomen. Make sure that there

is no bleeding and the uterus is firm. Use a sponge to remove any clots inside the abdomen.

- Examine carefully for any injuries to the bladder, and repair these.
- If there are **signs of infection**, pack the subcutaneous tissue with gauze and insert loose 0 catgut (or polyglycolic) sutures. Delay closure of the skin until the infection has cleared.
- If there are **no signs of infection**, close the skin with vertical mattress sutures of 3-0 nylon (or silk) and apply a sterile dressing.
- Gently push on the abdomen over the uterus to remove clots from the uterus and vagina. Swab out the vagina to remove any clots. Any bleeding subsequently noted will therefore be recognised as fresh loss.
- Ensure that there are no instruments or swabs left in the abdomen. One way of achieving this is to have a black or white board in the operating theatre on which is documented every swab or instrument used during the operation, and to ensure that these are available when the abdomen is closed.

Types of needle and suture material

In resource-limited settings it is often only possible to find two types of suture material for a Caesarean section, for example:

1 chromic catgut which can be used on a round-bodied needle for the uterus
2 polyglycolic acid which can be used on a round-bodied needle for the uterus and on a cutting/round-bodied needle for the rectus sheath and the skin.

Complications of Caesarean section

In cases of previous Caesarean section, other abdomino-pelvic operations or pelvic sepsis, bowel may be adherent to the undersurface of the peritoneum. Extra care must then be taken when opening the peritoneum, dividing it transversely under direct vision when possible.

In such cases, the peritoneum should be opened with a knife or scissors rather than with the fingers.

Bladder may be adherent to the lower segment, and care must be taken to push the bladder well down in order to avoid trauma to the bladder or ureters. Emptying the bladder pre-operatively reduces the likelihood of bladder damage.

Fibroids may obstruct access to the lower segment. A decision has to be made as to whether to make the uterine incision above, below or around the fibroids, or to cut through them. Alternatively, a classical (midline) uterine incision may be necessary, with its attendant greater risk of scar rupture in future pregnancies.

In cases of placenta praevia, the placenta is encountered on making the lower segment incision. This may lead to excessive bleeding.

The placenta may be morbidly adherent to a previous Caesarean section scar (placenta accreta). It is important not to traumatise the uterine wall by delivering the placenta piecemeal. It may be necessary to leave the adherent fragment *in situ*, and monitor carefully for bleeding and signs of infection. Postpartum hysterectomy may be required in this situation.

Caesarean section at full dilatation may be complicated by difficulty in dis-impacting the fetal head. An assistant should push firmly but gently from the vagina using sterile gloves and obstetric chlorhexidine cream on their fingers. Once the head is dis-impacted, fundal pressure is required.

Excessive bleeding at Caesarean section is most commonly due to uterine atony, lateral extension of the lower segment incision, or a combination of these two factors (*see* Section 2.5.D.iv on postpartum haemorrhage).

Where a trial of forceps has taken place prior to Caesarean section, care must be taken to identify and suture any vaginal tears, which may bleed heavily.

Uncontrolled bleeding
Primary haemorrhage
The cause of the haemorrhage, whether due to atony or trauma, should be determined. Help should be sought from senior colleagues (if available). The anaesthetist must be informed about the haemorrhage, and blood should already be cross-matched (at least 4 to 6 units). In cases of vertical extension into the vagina, suturing should be attempted from the lowest part of the tear before suturing the transverse incision. Massage the uterus to expel blood and blood clots. The presence of blood clots will inhibit effective uterine contractions.

Broad ligament haematomas
The leaves of the broad ligament need to be opened and the ureters should be identified before suturing the bleeding point.

Atonic uterus
If the uterus is atonic, massage it, continue to infuse oxytocin, and give:
- ergometrine 200–500 micrograms IM (must not be used if the patient has hypertension), if the mother is fully conscious
- *and/or* misoprostol 400–600 micrograms sublingually or orally or 800 micrograms rectally if the mother is drowsy or unconscious.

These drugs can be given together or sequentially.

Transfuse as necessary.

Have an assistant apply firm pressure with a fist over the aorta to reduce the bleeding until the source of bleeding can be found and stopped.

If bleeding is not controlled, *see* **Section 2.5.D.iv for details of the many methods of treatment that can be adopted. They include a hysterectomy.**

Breech delivery at Caesarean section
The fetal back should always be upwards during breech delivery. Gentle rotation of the fetal trunk may be required, being careful to grasp the bony pelvis and legs, thereby avoiding traumatising the fetal abdomen.

The baby is delivered as if performing a breech extraction vaginally. In summary, place the fingers of each hand into the groin of the baby and lift out the buttocks and legs.

Deliver the arms by the Løvset's manoeuvre; legs and the body up to the shoulders, then deliver the arms.

Flex the head and deliver using the Mauriceau–Smellie–Veit manoeuvre.

Complete the delivery as for a vaginal delivery.

Transverse lie delivery at Caesarean section
Assess the position of the fetus, including the position of the head, before opening the uterus. If the membranes are intact and there is liquor around the fetus, try to convert the transverse lie to a longitudinal lie.
- If **the back is up** (near the top of the uterus), reach into the uterus and find the baby's ankles.
- Grasp the ankles and pull gently through the incision to deliver the legs and complete the delivery as for a breech baby.
- If **the back is down**, a high vertical uterine incision may be preferred, but this is too late if only discovered once inside the uterus.
- Following the incision, reach into the uterus and find the feet. Pull them through the incision and complete the delivery as for a breech baby.
- To repair the vertical incision, three layers of suture will be needed.

Placenta praevia
If a low anterior placenta is encountered, find an edge of the placenta and move the placenta laterally or incise through it and deliver the fetus.
- An ultrasound scan prior to the operation will help the operator to judge whether it will be possible to manually displace the placenta in order to access the amniotic cavity.
- After delivery of the baby, **if the placenta cannot be detached manually**, the diagnosis is placenta accreta, occasionally seen at the site of a previous Caesarean scar.
- There are two approaches to this problem. The **placenta can be left** *in situ* **to degenerate spontaneously, or a hysterectomy may be performed**. If the former approach is followed, a careful watch will need to be kept for any signs of infection in the postnatal period, and prophylactic antibiotics will be required.
- Women with placenta praevia are at high risk of postpartum haemorrhage.
  - If there is bleeding at the placental site, under-run the bleeding sites with chromic catgut (or polyglycolic/Vicryl) sutures before closing the wound.
  - It may also be helpful to compress the lower segment vessels by packing the uterus or inserting a condom-catheter.
  - Watch for bleeding in the immediate postpartum period and take appropriate action.

Post-operative care
- Bowel function should be normal after 12 hours.
- If progress is uncomplicated, give liquids immediately and solids when the patient is passing gas per rectum.
- If there is infection, obstructed labour or uterine rupture, wait until bowel sounds reappear before giving oral fluids.
- Keep a dressing on the wound for 24 hours to ensure re-epithelialisation.
- If blood is leaking, reinforce the dressing or replace it with a new one if it is more than half soaked.

If bleeding occurs:
- Massage the uterus to expel blood and blood clots. The presence of blood clots will inhibit effective uterine contractions:
  - Give oxytocin 5 units IV slowly or 10 units IM and then infuse 40 units in 500 mL of IV fluids (Ringer-lactate or Hartmann's solution) over 4 hours

— *or* ergometrine 500 micrograms IM or misoprostol 400 micrograms sublingually or orally **provided that the mother is fully conscious**

— *or* misoprostol 800 micrograms rectally **if the mother is drowsy or unconscious.**

These drugs can be given together or sequentially.

- **If there are signs of infection or the mother has a fever**, give a combination of antibiotics until she has been fever-free for 48 hours:
  — Ampicillin 2 grams IV every 6 hours
  — *plus* gentamicin 80 mg IV/IM every 8 hours or 5 mg/kg body weight IV/IM once every 24 hours
  — *plus* metronidazole 500 mg IV every 8 hours.
- Give appropriate analgesic drugs.

Discharge the mother home when her temperature has been normal for at least 24 hours, and she is mobilising and able to eat and drink normally.

Symphysiotomy
Background
Symphysiotomy is performed for the management of cephalo–pelvic disproportion in selected situations in resource-limited countries or ill-equipped obstetric units. It may be required for the delivery of the trapped after-coming head with a breech delivery, or for shoulder dystocia. Symphysiotomy results in a temporary increase in pelvic diameter (up to 2 cm) by surgically dividing the cartilage of the symphysis under local anaesthesia. Symphysiotomy in combination with vacuum extraction is a life-saving procedure in areas where Caesarean section is not immediately available.

Symphysiotomy leaves no uterine scar, so the risk of ruptured uterus in subsequent pregnancies is not increased.

Caesarean section can have high morbidity and mortality rates in resource-limited healthcare facilities. Mortalities of up to 5% and uterine scar rupture in 7% of subsequent pregnancies have been reported. Symphysiotomy has a very low maternal mortality, with 3 deaths reported in a series of 1752 symphysiotomies. These deaths were unrelated to the procedure.

However, symphysiotomy has risks of complications, which include urethral and bladder injury, infection, pain and long-term difficulty in walking. Therefore it should only be performed when there is no safe alternative.

Symptoms following symphysiotomy include pain in the symphysis pubis and groin, hip or thigh pain, backache and stress incontinence.

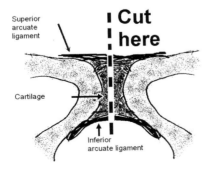

FIGURE 2.13.26 Site of the symphysiotomy incision.

The majority of mothers (73%) will have an uncomplicated vaginal delivery in a subsequent pregnancy.

Indications for symphysiotomy
- Trapped after-coming head in breech delivery, in the presence of full cervical dilatation.
- Shoulder dystocia, where all other methods have failed.
- A live fetus with vertex presentation **and** presumed cephalo–pelvic disproportion (i.e. prolonged second stage, no head descent after adequate augmentation, and failure or anticipated failure of vacuum extraction alone).
- At least one-third of the fetal head should have entered the pelvic brim.
- The cervix should be fully dilated, and the head should be at –2 station or no more than 3/5 above the symphysis pubis, with no overriding of the head above the symphysis.

Technique

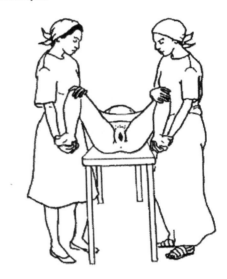

FIGURE 2.13.27 Legs abducted no more than 45 degrees from vertical.

Ask two assistants to support the woman's legs with her thighs and knees flexed. The thighs should be abducted no more than 45 degrees from the midline, **not** the lithotomy position.

Abduction of the thighs more than 45 degrees from the midline may cause tearing of the urethra and bladder.
- Infiltrate the anterior, superior and inferior aspects of the symphysis with 1% lignocaine solution.
  — Aspirate (pull back on the plunger) to make sure that no vessel has been penetrated. **If blood is returned in the syringe with aspiration**, remove the needle. Recheck the position carefully and try again. Never inject if blood is aspirated.
- **Infiltrate the local anaesthetic and wait for it to take effect.**
- Insert a firm sterile urinary catheter to identify the urethra.
- Apply antiseptic solution to the suprapubic skin.
- Wearing sterile gloves:
  — Place the index and middle fingers of the left hand into the vagina.

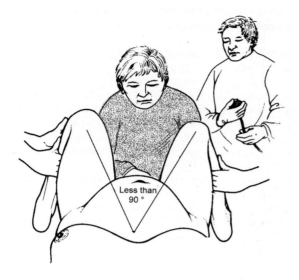

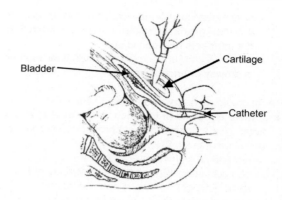

FIGURE 2.13.29 Sagittal view of symphysiotomy.

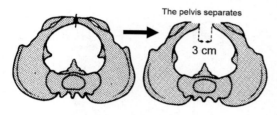

FIGURE 2.13.28 The position for holding the woman's legs for symphysiotomy.

— Using the index finger, push and hold the catheter, and with it the urethra, away from the midline to the patient's right side.
— The middle finger lies centrally under the symphysis to guide the incision.
● With the other hand, use a firm-bladed scalpel to make a vertical incision over the symphysis.
● Cut down through the cartilage joining the two pubic bones until the pressure of the scalpel blade is felt on the finger in the vagina.
— The symphysis pubis is incised in the midline at the junction of the upper and middle thirds. The point of the scalpel will be felt impinging on the vagina by the underlying finger of the left hand.
— The upper third of the uncut symphysis is used as a fulcrum against which the scalpel is levered to incise the lower two-thirds of the symphysis.
— The scalpel is then removed and rotated through 180 degrees, and the remaining upper third of the symphysis is cut.
● Once the symphysis has been divided, the pubic bones will separate.
1 The symphysis should open as wide as the operator's thumb. A large episiotomy is required to relieve tension on the anterior vaginal wall. Usually a vacuum extractor will be used to pull the fetus downward at this point.
2 Delivery of the head and trunk of the baby occurs in a downward direction, taking care to avoid the temptation to lift the baby up until it is completely delivered.
3 After delivery of the baby and placenta, the symphysis is compressed between the thumb above and the index

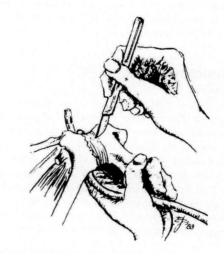

FIGURE 2.13.30 The symphysiotomy incision.

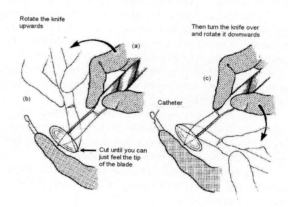

FIGURE 2.13.31 Cutting through the cartilage.

and middle fingers below for several minutes in order to express blood clots and promote haemostasis.
4 There is no need to close the incision unless there is bleeding.
5 Reinsert the urinary catheter.

Post-procedure care

● If there are signs of infection or the mother has a fever, give a combination of antibiotics until she has been fever-free for 48 hours:

— Ampicillin 2 grams IV every 6 hours
— *plus* gentamicin 80 mg IV/IM every 8 hours or 5 mg/kg body weight IV/IM once every 24 hours
— *plus* metronidazole 500 mg IV every 8 hours.

- Give appropriate analgesia.
- Apply a binder or sheet or elastic strapping across the front of the pelvis from one iliac crest to the other to hold the pelvis together to aid pelvic healing and reduce pain. Nurse the woman on her side to allow gravity to aid pelvic healing.
- Leave the urinary catheter in for at least 5 days.
- Encourage oral fluids to ensure a good urinary output.
- Encourage bed rest for 7 days after discharge from hospital.
- Encourage the mother to begin walking with assistance when she is ready to do so.
- If **long-term walking difficulties and pain** occur (2% of cases), treat them with physiotherapy.

Induction of labour for intrauterine death in the second or third trimester

See Section 2.6.B.

Destructive operations

Background

Destructive procedures are undertaken when a vaginal delivery must occur because:

- skilled staff are not available to carry out what may be a difficult or dangerous Caesarean section
- in neglected obstructed labour there is a risk of over-whelming infection following Caesarean section
- of the implications of a uterine scar for future pregnancies
- the patient does not give consent to Caesarean section.

Reasons for fetal death in obstructed labour

- Strong and continuous contractions (sometimes made worse by inappropriate use of oxytocic drugs or other non-prescription uterotonic drugs) interfere with placental exchange.
- Excessive moulding of the head, in cephalic presentation, can lead to intracranial haemorrhage. In breech presentation the head may be trapped by an incompletely dilated cervix, or may not enter the pelvis because of disproportion.
- Prolapsed cord.
- Ascending infection, amnionitis and intrauterine infection due to prolonged ruptured membranes and labour, and/or unsterile vaginal examinations.
- Ruptured uterus.

Destructive operations

Before a destructive procedure is undertaken the fetus must be dead.

Ensure that the mother is adequately resuscitated.
Ruptured uterus must be excluded.
Ensure adequate analgesia or anaesthesia.
The procedure can be performed under general or regional anaesthesia, or sedation and analgesia with morphine, midazolam and/or ketamine.

General issues relating to destructive procedures

- The operator must be competent at destructive deliveries.
- Destructive operations are most safely done at full dilatation, but may be performed when the cervix is 7 cm or more dilated. If there is hydrocephaly, it is best to drain the CSF at diagnosis without waiting for full dilatation, as the hydrocephalic head may cause uterine rupture.
- The bladder must be catheterised.
- Post-delivery care includes continuous catheterisation of the bladder, IV antibiotics and IV fluids.

Craniotomy

Craniotomy is used for the delivery of a dead fetus with cephalic presentation when labour is obstructed. Usually the head is impacted in the pelvic brim. If the head is mobile, craniotomy may be difficult and Caesarean section may be safer (if circumstances are suitable).

The head may need to be dis-impacted from the pelvis to facilitate urinary catheterisation.

A 3 cm incision is made on the posterior aspect of the skull using Mayo scissors. The index finger of the left hand is inserted into the incision and the suture and fontanelle are identified. The scissors are then pushed though the fontanelle into the cavity of the skull. Thereafter the brain is evacuated and Kocher's forceps are clamped on to the edges of the parietal bones. A weight is attached to the Kocher's forceps with a length of bandage. The mother's legs are taken out of the lithotomy stirrups and placed on two stools for support. Delivery will take place within a period ranging from a few minutes to several hours. This method can be used when the cervix is at least 8 cm dilated.

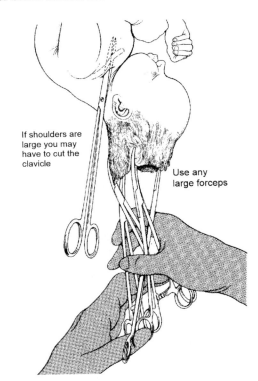

If shoulders are large you may have to cut the clavicle

Use any large forceps

FIGURE 2.13.32 Craniotomy. This baby's skull has been opened and the brain removed. These are not vulsellum forceps, but you can use such forceps.

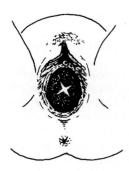

FIGURE 2.13.33 X-shaped fetal skull incision.

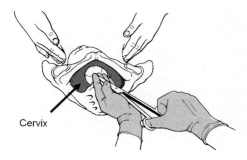

FIGURE 2.13.34 Perforating the skull: a life-saving operation. Your assistant is pushing the baby's head into the mother's pelvis. You have made an X-shaped incision in the skin of the baby's scalp. You have found a suture line, and are pressing a strong pair of scissors into it.

Breech presentation with an entrapped head and dead fetus

- Make an incision through the skin at the base of the neck.
- Insert a craniotome (or large pointed scissors or a heavy scalpel) through the incision and tunnel subcutaneously to reach the occiput.
- Perforate the occiput and open the gap as wide as possible.
- Apply traction on the trunk to collapse the skull as the head descends.

Craniocentesis (skull puncture) for hydrocephalus and obstructed labour and dead fetus

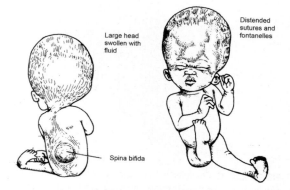

FIGURE 2.13.35 Hydrocephaly. A child with one abnormality often has several others as well.

Craniocentesis with a fully dilated cervix

- Pass a large-bore spinal needle through the dilated cervix and the sagittal suture line or fontanelles of the fetal skull (*see* Figure 2.13.36).
- Aspirate the cerebrospinal fluid until the fetal skull has collapsed. Then allow normal delivery to proceed.

Craniocentesis with a closed cervix

- Palpate for the location of the fetal head.
- Apply antiseptic solution to the suprapubic skin.
- Pass a large-bore spinal needle through the abdominal and uterine walls and through the hydrocephalic skull.

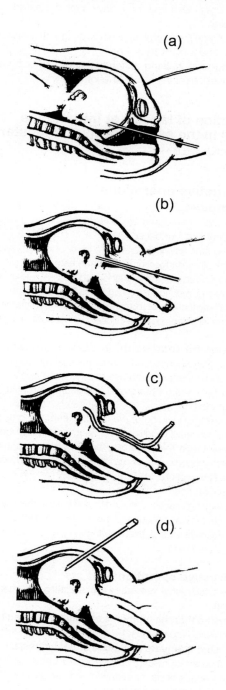

FIGURE 2.13.36 Draining a hydrocephalus. (a) Draining the vertex. (b) Draining the occiput. (c) Draining through a meningomyelocele. (d) Draining through the mother's abdomen.

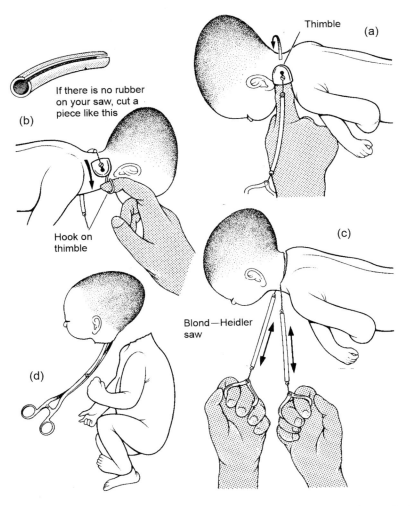

FIGURE 2.13.37 Decapitation of dead fetus. (a) Fix the saw to the thimble and push it over the neck. (b) Remove the thimble and fix the handles to each end of the saw. (c) Saw to and fro. (d) Grasp the stump of the neck.

- Aspirate the cerebrospinal fluid until the fetal skull has collapsed. Then allow vaginal delivery to proceed.

Craniocentesis in breech where the hydrocephalic head is stuck and the fetus is dead

- When the rest of the body has been delivered, insert a large-bore spinal needle through the dilated cervix and foramen magnum.
- Aspirate the cerebrospinal fluid and deliver the after-coming head as in breech delivery.

This can be managed similarly, by craniotomy with perforation of the head through the occiput. Where there is hydrocephalus and accompanying spina bifida, CSF can be withdrawn by exposing the spinal canal and passing a catheter into the canal and up into the cranium. Alternatively, the hydrocephalic head can be decompressed trans-abdominally using a spinal needle.

Decapitation

This procedure is summarised in Figure 2.13.37.

In cases of neglected obstructed labour with shoulder presentation and a dead fetus, decapitation is the treatment of choice. The lower uterine segment is very vulnerable. If the fetus is small, the neck can easily be severed with stout scissors. However, for the larger fetus, where the neck is not easily accessible, the Blond–Heidler decapitation tool is probably the safest instrument. If possible, an arm of the fetus is brought down in order to facilitate access and exposure of the neck. The saw is threaded around the fetal neck, and by keeping the handles at the ends of the saw close together, injury to the vagina is prevented and the neck can be severed with a few firm strokes. Delivery of the trunk is straightforward, and the after-coming head is delivered by grasping the stump with a heavy vulsellum.

Cleidotomy

Cleidotomy is indicated where the impacted shoulders prevent delivery of the dead fetus. The most accessible clavicle is divided first using stout scissors.

Evisceration

This is sometimes necessary for an abdominal tumour or very large fetus following craniotomy. An incision is made in the abdomen or thorax. The viscera are then extracted digitally. Once the bulk of the fetus has been reduced the fetus can be extracted easily.

TABLE 2.13.1 Possible situations of fetal death and the relevant procedures

Clinical situation	Procedure
Cephalic presentation:	
Head < 60% above the pelvic brim	Craniotomy
Head free or > 60% palpable	Caesarean section
Hydrocephalus	Perforation before full dilatation
Obstruction due to abdominal tumour	Embryotomy if the abdomen is accessible, otherwise Caesarean section
Impacted shoulders	Cleidotomy
Breech presentation:	
Obstruction due to after-coming head	Perforation of the head
Obstruction due to abdominal tumour	Embryotomy
Impacted shoulders	Cleidotomy
Transverse or oblique lie:	
Shoulder presentation or arm prolapse	Decapitation
Access to fetal neck difficult	Caesarean section
Ruptured uterus	Laparotomy – repair/ hysterectomy
Gross disproportion	Caesarean section

Complications of destructive operations

Instruments or sharp pieces of bone may cause a vesico-vaginal fistula. The vagina, cervix and perineum must therefore be carefully examined after the procedure.

Alternative to destructive operations

Symphysiotomy with episiotomy may avert the need for destructive operations if the fetus is still alive.

Caesarean section may be preferred, if available, especially if the operator is inexperienced in performing destructive procedures. However, caesarean section will create a risk for scar rupture during a subsequent pregnancy and in low resource settings this could result in maternal and fetal death.

Post-procedure care

- After delivery, examine and repair any tears to the cervix or vagina, or undertake episiotomy repair.
- Leave a self-retaining catheter in place until bladder injury has been excluded.
- Ensure adequate fluid intake and urinary output.

Episiotomy

Episiotomy should be considered in the case of:
- complicated vaginal delivery (e.g. breech, shoulder dystocia, forceps, vacuum delivery)
- scarring from female genital cutting
- fetal distress
- delay in the second stage
- previous third- or fourth-degree tears
- where significant perineal trauma is anticipated if it is not performed.

Procedure

- Apply antiseptic solution to the perineal area.
- Use local infiltration with 1% lignocaine. Make sure that there are no known allergies to lignocaine or related drugs.
- Infiltrate beneath the vaginal mucosa, beneath the skin of the perineum and deeply into the perineal muscle (*see* Figure 2.13.38) using 5–10 mL of 1% lignocaine solution.
- **Aspirate (pull back on the plunger) to be sure that no vessel has been penetrated. If blood is returned in the syringe with aspiration, remove the needle. Recheck the position carefully and try again. Never inject if blood is aspirated.**
- After local anaesthetic infiltration, wait for 2 minutes and then pinch the incision site with forceps. **If the mother feels the pinch**, wait a further 2 minutes and then retest.

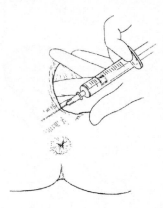

FIGURE 2.13.38 Infiltration of the perineum with local anaesthetic.

Do not perform an episiotomy until the perineum is thinned out **and** 3–4 cm of the baby's head are visible during a contraction.

Performing an episiotomy will cause bleeding, so it must not be done too early.

1 Wearing disinfected gloves, place two fingers between the baby's head and the perineum.
2 Use scissors to cut the perineum about 3–4 cm in the medio-lateral direction (*see* Figure 2.13.39). It is essential that the episiotomy cut is not made where, if it runs into a tear, it involves the anal sphincter. That is, it must be at an angle away from the anus, as shown in Figure 2.13.39.
3 Control the baby's head and shoulders as they deliver, ensuring that the shoulders have rotated to the midline to prevent an extension of the episiotomy.
4 Carefully examine for extensions and tears, and repair them (see below).

Repair of episiotomy

It is important that absorbable sutures or Vicryl are used for closure. Polyglycolic sutures are preferred to chromic catgut because of their tensile strength, non-allergenic properties and lower risk of infection and episiotomy breakdown. However, chromic catgut is an acceptable alternative.

Apply antiseptic solution to the area around the episiotomy.

- If the episiotomy is extended (torn) through the anal sphincter or rectal mucosa, which should not happen if the original cut has been away from the vertical

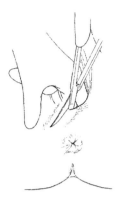

FIGURE 2.13.39 Using two fingers to protect the baby's head while making the incision.

(see above), manage as third- or fourth-degree tears, respectively.

- **Close the vaginal mucosa using continuous 2-0 suture.**
- Start the repair about 1 cm above the apex (top) of the episiotomy. Continue the suture to the level of the vaginal opening.
- At the opening of the vagina, bring together the cut edges of the vaginal opening.
- Bring the needle under the vaginal opening and out through the incision and tie.
- Close the perineal muscle using a continuous 2-0 suture.
- Close the skin using a subcuticular or interrupted 2-0 suture.

Complications of episiotomy

1 **Haematoma.** If this occurs, open and drain it. If there are **no signs of infection and bleeding has stopped,** reclose the episiotomy.
2 **If there are signs of infection,** open and drain the wound. Remove infected sutures and debride the wound:
   - If the **infection is mild,** antibiotics are not required.
   - If the **infection is severe but does not involve deep tissues,** give a combination of antibiotics:
     - Ampicillin 500 mg orally four times a day for 5 days
     - *plus* metronidazole 400 mg orally three times a day for 5 days.
   - If the **infection is deep and involves muscles,** give a combination of antibiotics until the necrotic tissue has been removed and the mother has been fever-free for 48 hours:
     - penicillin G, 2 million units IV every 6 hours
     - *plus* gentamicin 80 mg IV/IM every 8 hours or 5 mg/kg body weight IV/IM once every 24 hours
     - *plus* metronidazole 500 mg IV every 8 hours.
   - When **the mother has been fever-free for 48 hours,** give:
     - ampicillin 500 mg orally four times a day for 5 days
     - *plus* metronidazole 400 mg orally three times a day for 5 days.

Necrotic tissue requires wide surgical debridement. Perform secondary closure in 2 to 4 weeks (depending on resolution of the infection).

Repair of cervical tears

- If the mother is bleeding heavily it may be best to resuscitate and then pack the tear with sterile gauze. Bimanual compression may be required. Ensure that whoever repairs this is experienced. This might need referral to another hospital.
  - Repair only when the mother is stable and most of the bleeding has stopped, unless there is heavy ongoing blood loss despite compression in which case repair needs to be undertaken urgently while resuscitation continues
  - Apply antiseptic solution to the vagina and cervix.
- Anaesthesia is not required for most cervical tears.
  - For tears that are high and extensive, give morphine 10 mg IV slowly over 5 minutes (provided that shock is not present), or use ketamine.
- Ask an assistant to massage the uterus and provide fundal pressure.
- Gently grasp the cervix with ring or sponge forceps.
  - Apply the forceps on both sides of the tear and gently use the forceps to pull each part of the cervix down in turn so that the entire cervix is examined.
  - There may be several tears.
- One way of finding a high tear is to insert a suture as high as possible and then use it to provide traction to work up to the apex to obtain haemostasis, and then to work downward towards the introitus.
- Close the cervical tears with a continuous polyglycolic/Vicryl suture starting at the apex (upper edge of tear), which is often the source of bleeding (*see* Figure 2.13.40).
- **If a long section of the rim of the cervix is tattered and bleeding,** under-run it with a continuous polyglycolic/Vicryl suture. Often if the bleeding is persistent but mild, compressing the ragged edges with a sterile pack is the most effective way of halting the bleeding, if no specific delineated tear is identified.
- If **the apex is difficult to reach and ligate,** it may be possible to grasp it with artery or ring forceps. Leave the forceps in place for 4 hours.
  - Do not persist in attempts to ligate the bleeding points, as this may increase the bleeding.
  - After 4 hours, open the forceps partially but do not remove.
  - After another 4 hours, remove the forceps completely.
- A laparotomy may be required to repair a cervical tear that has extended beyond the vaginal vault.

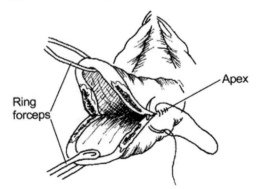

FIGURE 2.13.40 Repair of a cervical tear.

Manual removal of the placenta

If the placenta does not separate within 1 hour of delivery, or immediately if there is heavy bleeding:

- start an IV infusion
- ensure that the bladder is emptied either by the mother or by catheterisation
- give a slow IV injection of ketamine (1–2 mg/kg or 50–100 mg) or morphine (10 mg), ideally in the presence of an anaesthetist
- give a single dose of prophylactic antibiotics:
    - ampicillin 2 grams IV *plus* metronidazole 500 mg IV
    - *or* cefotaxime 1 gram IV *plus* metronidazole 500 mg IV.
- Ensure full aseptic drapes.
- Hold the umbilical cord with a clamp. Pull the cord gently until it is taut.
- Wearing sterile gloves (ideally covering the forearms) insert a hand into the vagina and follow the cord up into the uterus until you reach the edge of the placenta (*see* Figure 2.13.41). If the cervix is closed, gentle pressure with one or two fingers will usually relax it and make it open.
- Let go of the cord with the other hand and move the hand up over the abdomen in order to support the fundus of the uterus and to provide counter-traction during removal to prevent inversion of the uterus (*see* Figure 2.13.42).

If uterine inversion occurs, reposition the uterus immediately.

- Move the fingers of the hand laterally until the edge of the placenta is located.
- **If the cord has been detached previously,** insert a hand into the uterine cavity.
    - Explore the entire cavity until a line of cleavage is identified between the placenta and the uterine wall.

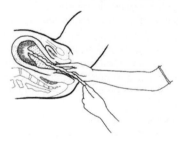

FIGURE 2.13.41 Entering the uterus along the cord.

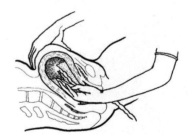

FIGURE 2.13.42 Supporting the fundus while detaching the placenta.

- Reach the placenta from the implantation site by keeping the fingers tightly together and using the edge of the hand to gradually make a space between the placenta and the uterine wall.
- Proceed slowly all around the placental bed until the whole placenta is detached from the uterine wall.
- If **the placenta does not separate from the uterine surface** by gentle lateral movement of the fingertips at the line of cleavage, suspect placenta accreta.
    - Consider laparotomy and possible subtotal hysterectomy.
    - Alternatively, the placenta can be left *in situ* to spontaneously degenerate.
    - The main risk is that of infection and delayed haemorrhage, and follow-up needs to be maintained to assess the woman for signs of sepsis.
- Hold the placenta and slowly withdraw the hand from the uterus, bringing the placenta with it (*see* Figure 2.14.43).
- With the other hand, continue to provide counter-traction to the fundus by pushing it in the opposite direction to the hand that is being withdrawn.

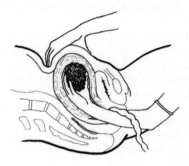

FIGURE 2.13.43 Withdrawing the hand plus the placenta from the uterus.

- Palpate the inside of the uterine cavity to ensure that all placental tissue has been removed.
- Give oxytocin 40 units in 500 mL of IV fluids (Ringer-lactate or Hartmann's solution) over 4 hours.
- Ask an assistant to massage the fundus of the uterus to encourage a tonic uterine contraction.
- If there is **continued heavy bleeding**, give 10 units of oxytocin IM. If this does not work, try ergometrine 200–500 micrograms (not if there is or has been hypertension) IM and, if that does not work, give misoprostol rectally as 4 × 200 microgram tablets or pessaries (800 micrograms total) or, **if the woman is conscious**, misoprostol orally 3 × 200 microgram tablets.
- Examine the uterine surface of the placenta to ensure that it is complete. If any **placental lobe or tissue is missing**, explore the uterine cavity under strict surgical asepsis to remove it.
- Examine the mother carefully and repair any tears to the cervix or vagina, or undertake episiotomy repair.

Problems

If the placenta is retained due to a constriction ring or if hours or days have passed since delivery, it may not be possible to get the entire hand into the uterus. Consider using a general anaesthetic to help to relax the cervix, and extract the placenta in fragments using two fingers or ovum forceps, but be very careful not to penetrate the soft uterine wall. If hours or days have passed and/or signs of sepsis are present, treat for puerperal sepsis with a full course of IV antibiotics (*see* Section 2.5.G).

Post-procedure care

Observe the mother closely until the effect of IV analgesia has worn off.

- Monitor the vital signs (pulse, blood pressure, respiration and temperature) every 15 minutes for the first hour and then every 30 minutes for the next 6 hours or until the patient is stable.
- Palpate the uterine fundus to ensure that the uterus remains contracted.
- Check for excessive lochia.
- Continue infusion of IV fluids.
- Transfuse as necessary, especially if the mother is severely anaemic before the procedure.
- Warn the mother of the increased risk of this occurring at the time of the next pregnancy, and therefore advise her to deliver in a well-equipped comprehensive EmOC facility.

Bilateral pudendal nerve block

Indications

This technique is indicated for some instrumental deliveries, for repair of larger tears, and for craniotomy or craniocentesis.

A pudendal nerve block targets the pudendal nerve as it enters the lesser sciatic foramen, about 1 cm inferior and medial to the attachment of the sacrospinous ligament to the ischial spine. The aim is to block the nerve proximal to its terminal branches. Here the nerve is medial to the internal pudendal vessels. The transvaginal approach is described here, as it is the most reliable.

Dilute 20 mL of 1% lidocaine to 40 mL with Ringer-lactate or Hartmann's solution, to make a solution of 0.5%. This is used starting with 15 mL on each side. The remaining 10 mL can be used to infiltrate the perineum during repairs if these are needed.

Adrenaline is not used with the lidocaine.

Ensure that IV access is in place.

The needle used should be around 15 cm in length and 20–22 gauge.

The procedure must be undertaken with surgical sterility after cleaning the vagina with chlorhexidine (Hibitane) obstetric cream, and always using sterile gloves.

Resuscitation equipment and medications should always be readily available in case an adverse reaction to the local anaesthetic occurs.

Procedure

Palpate the ischial spine through the vaginal wall.

A metal trumpet (see Figure 2.13.44) can facilitate the placement of the needle and limit the depth of submucosal penetration, but is not essential.

1. To perform a left-sided block, palpate the ischial spine with the index finger of the left hand, hold the syringe in the right hand, and guide the needle between the index finger and middle finger of the left hand toward the ischial spine (see Figure 2.13.45).
2. Place the end of the guide beneath the tip of the ischial spine.
3. Push the needle into the vaginal mucosa.
4. **Aspirate to ensure that the needle is not in one of the pudendal blood vessels, which could be very dangerous if lidocaine is injected.**
5. Inject 1 mL of local anaesthetic.

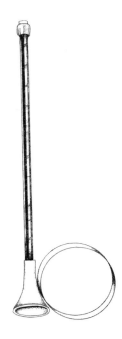

FIGURE 2.13.44 Metal trumpet to guide needle to site of pudendal nerve.

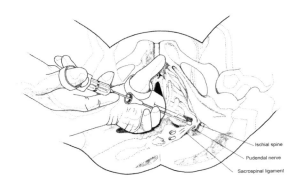

Ischial spine
Pudendal nerve
Sacrospinal ligament

FIGURE 2.13.45 Inserting the needle using a trumpet guide. © 2012 Christy Krames.

6. Advance the needle through the vaginal mucosa until it touches the sacrospinous ligament 1 cm medial and posterior to the ischial spine.
7. **Aspirate to ensure that the needle is not in one of the pudendal blood vessels, which could be very dangerous if lidocaine is injected, and infiltrate with 3 mL of local anaesthetic.**
8. Next, advance the needle further through the sacrospinous ligament for a distance of 1 cm until a loss of resistance is detected.
9. The tip now lies in the area of the pudendal nerve. At this point, the pudendal vessels lie just lateral to the pudendal nerve, so care must be taken to avoid intravascular administration. **Aspirate to confirm that the needle placement is not intravascular prior to injecting lidocaine.**
10. Inject another 3 mL of local anaesthetic solution into this region.

11 Subsequently, withdraw the needle into the guide and move the tip of the guide to just above the ischial spine.

12 At this new location, reinsert the needle though the mucosa and again inject 3 mL of local anaesthetic. **Aspirate to confirm that the needle placement is not intravascular prior to injecting lidocaine.**

To block the right side of the pelvis, repeat these steps using the right hand to hold the needle and needle guide.

The block usually takes at least 5 minutes to become effective, and lasts for between 20 and 60 minutes. Check bilaterally for pain before starting the procedure.

A smaller repeat dose (up to 5 mL of 0.5% lidocaine) on each side can be used if an adequate block is not seen.

A pudendal block does not provide adequate anaesthesia for deliveries that require uterine manipulation, postpartum examination and repair of the upper vagina and cervix, and manual exploration of the uterine cavity.

Under these circumstances, the addition of intravenous narcotics or ketamine may be required.

Vaginal examination in obstetrics

Vaginal examination should be performed only if it is essential, and the risk of infection must be minimised by hygienic hand washing and the use of a new set of examination gloves. At all times it is important to preserve the patient's dignity and privacy. In labour, a chlorhexidine obstetric cream can prevent ascending infection.

Always undertake abdominal palpation first.

Do not undertake vaginal examination if there is a possibility of placenta praevia, if there are ruptured membranes and the woman is not in labour, or if there is active herpes simplex infection in ruptured membranes unless the patient is in labour.

If you are using a speculum, offer to demonstrate it, explain how it is inserted and ensure that the correct size is used.

Document any blood loss, discharge and its characteristics, and any amniotic fluid and its characteristics. If female genital cutting is present, record this and describe the type.

Document the cervical length, position, dilatation, and application to the presenting part of the fetus. Determine if possible the presentation of the fetus and whether there is caput and/or moulding present. Evaluate pelvic size by examining the ischial spines and suprapubic arch.

At the end, provide a clean sanitary pad, auscultate the fetal heart, describe the results of the examination to the woman, and record the findings in the notes.

Section 3

Neonatal care

3.1 Preparation for and care of the baby at birth

BOX 3.1.1 **Minimum standards**
- Two clean dry towels.
- Firm work surface with padding.
- Stethoscope.
- Laryngoscope with straight blades size 0 and 1, spare bulbs and batteries.
- Set of ET tubes 2.5, 3.0, 3.5 and 4.0 with connectors to fit the inflation system.
- Umbilical catheter with fixating system.
- Adrenaline 1:10 000.
- Sodium bicarbonate 8.4%.
- Naloxone.
- Dextrose 10%.
- Ringer-lactate or Hartmann's solution.
- Soft suction device.
- Warming device.
- Food-grade plastic wrapping.

Introduction

Neonatal mortality in resource-limited countries runs at an unacceptably high level. The World Health Organization (WHO) estimates that worldwide there are 9000 neonatal deaths per day. Of these, approximately one-third are a result of neonatal infections, one-third are due to fetal hypoxia and a further one-third are due to prematurity and low birth weight.

If death and long-term or permanent disability are to be avoided, the management of neonatal emergencies must be both coordinated and effective. The care delivered in the first few minutes and hours of life is a major determinant of the outcome. Since in resource-limited countries almost half of the deliveries do not occur in hospitals, it is important that community-based skilled birth attendants (SBAs), traditional birth attendants (TBAs) and community health workers (CHWs) are encouraged to develop skills to recognise the vulnerable baby prior to delivery and provide effective intervention as required after birth.

Basic aspects of newborn care that apply to both community and hospital deliveries

In order to minimise the number of infants dying from birth-related problems (including perinatal asphyxia) or arriving at hospital with major complications which cannot be corrected, it is important for the hospital to work closely with the community.

The following approach has been shown to be helpful.
- All community-based healthcare professionals, including SBAs, TBAs and CHWs, should be able to undertake basic resuscitation of the newborn. Skills-based training involving manikins and the provision of a self-inflatable bag and mask to all these healthcare workers is essential, as delaying newborn resuscitation until the infant reaches the hospital will usually be too late, resulting in death or severe brain damage.

- Clean delivery kits should be available to all such health-care workers.
- There should be regular clinical audits and educational meetings with participation from all community-based healthcare workers.
- Community-based SBAs, TBAs and CHWs should ensure that mothers with pregnancy-related complications (e.g. preterm birth, breech presentation, twins) are identified and referred to the local hospital where there are good facilities for obstetric and newborn care.
- The local hospital must provide comprehensive emergency obstetric and neonatal care. Good management of labour and delivery is the key to intact neonatal survival.

Mothers who require referral to hospital for delivery include those with:
- peripartum bleeding
- malpresentation (breech, face, shoulder)
- preterm labour (< 35 weeks)
- twins
- abnormal fetal heart rate in labour.

The baby at risk of developing problems at birth
Preterm birth

Maturity matters more than birth weight. Prematurity is defined as gestation of less than 37 weeks (or less than 259 days from the first day of the mother's last menstrual period). In the absence of special facilities, mortality increases substantially in cases of gestation less than 32 weeks, and survival at less than 28 weeks is unlikely in resource-limited settings. When a preterm delivery is anticipated, realistic expectations should be discussed with the parents, and any limitations on resuscitative efforts should be agreed upon.

Preventative strategies

These may include **minimising the risk of surfactant deficiency** and **stopping premature uterine contractions**.

Minimising the risk of surfactant deficiency: this can be halved if the mother is given a short course of high-dose steroid treatment before delivery:
- dexamethasone, 12 mg IM, two doses 12 hours apart
- or dexamethasone, 6 mg IM, four doses 12 hours apart.

Stopping premature uterine contractions:
- Give 20 mg nifedipine orally. Up to three further doses can be given at 30-minute intervals if uterine contractions persist.
- If this stops labour, give 20 mg nifedipine orally three times a day for the next 3 days.

Other problems associated with preterm birth include the following:
- Even very small babies can survive preterm birth

successfully once the early problems associated with surfactant deficiency have been overcome, and as long as they are nursed in a clean environment and not allowed to get cold.

- Preterm babies are at increased risk of infection and hypothermia.

The main challenge is to give these babies enough nutrition for them to start growing again as soon as possible (*see* Section 3.3).

- Here, too, maturity is more important than weight. Babies born before 36 weeks' gestation nearly always need some help with feeding.
- Breast milk is ideal, and everything possible should be done to help the mother sustain her lactation until the baby is ready to feed reliably from the breast. A limited ability to suck and swallow usually appears from 32 weeks' gestation, but it remains unpredictable, unreliable and uncoordinated until 36 weeks' gestation. In the event that breastfeeding cannot be initiated immediately after birth, mothers should be encouraged to start expressing breast milk, to be given by nasogastric tube or cup and spoon.
- Partial breastfeeding can also help the mother to sustain her lactation, but in any event the mother should regularly express milk. Some mothers might find expressing breast milk difficult and may require help with this.

Infection

It is important to identify babies at risk of infection prior to delivery. If identified, the mother should be given antibiotics appropriately. Many of the babies who become infected during delivery develop respiratory signs very soon after birth, but in a few, the features are those of neonatal sepsis. In addition, there are a proportion of babies who are initially asymptomatic, and therefore prophylactic antibiotics should be commenced in the infant if there are risk factors for infection.

When to consider antibiotics for the mother and newborn

- **Symptomatic ascending infection** *in utero* needs urgent treatment. If this is overlooked, both the mother's and the baby's life will be in danger.
- **Asymptomatic infection is, however, a much commoner problem.** This occasionally progresses so rapidly once labour starts that, unless treatment is started at once, the baby will die even if the most appropriate antibiotic is given immediately after birth. Because such infection by definition is silent, it is important that treatment be considered in any mother going into active spontaneous labour before 35 weeks' gestation.
- **Membrane rupture can be both a sign of, and a risk factor for, ascending bacterial infection.** What most people mean by premature rupture of membranes (PROM) is really preterm pre-labour rupture of membranes (PPROM), where the membranes rupture before there is any overt sign of uterine activity or any detectable uterine contractions. When this happens in the preterm baby, it is often a sign of the start of some sort of ascending infectious process. This process has already weakened the amniotic membranes and may stimulate the onset of preterm labour. Antibiotics must be given to the mother.

- **Treatment with antibiotics should also be considered at any gestation if the mother's membranes rupture more than 18 hours before delivery.** If premature rupture of membranes occurs before the onset of premature labour contractions then infection is more likely.
- **Maternal fever (> 38°C) in labour** is a strong indication for initiating antibiotics for the mother. Similarly, foul-smelling or purulent liquor requires IV antibiotic treatment of the newborn from birth without waiting for any signs of infection.

- In mothers with PPROM who show signs of being clinically infected give IV antibiotics.
- In PPROM where there is no evidence of infection and no evidence of labour you can delay delivery by 1 week or more (on average) by giving the mother amoxicillin or, better still, erythromycin.
- In mothers who are in active labour 5 or more weeks before term and who give a clear history that the membranes had ruptured before they were able to detect any uterine contractions, the risk of the baby becoming infected during delivery can be reduced substantially by giving antibiotics IV (ideally probably both penicillin and gentamicin) during labour.

Antibiotic management of perinatal infection

Where facilities allow, a blood count, C-reactive proteins and blood cultures should be taken before starting antibiotics. Because a range of bacteria can be involved, treatment of the baby needs to protect against group B streptococcal, coliform and *Listeria* infection, making a **combination of ampicillin and gentamicin** the best strategy:

- Give ampicillin 50–100 mg/kg IV 12-hourly and gentamicin 5 mg/kg every 24 hours IV if more than 32 weeks' gestation, and 3 mg/kg if less than 32 weeks.

The WHO recommends that a neonate with risk factors for infection (i.e. membranes ruptured > 18 hours before delivery, maternal fever > 38°C before delivery or during labour, or foul-smelling or purulent amniotic discharge) should be treated with prophylactic antibiotics (IM or IV ampicillin and gentamicin) for at least 2 days. After this the neonate should be reassessed and treatment continued only if there are signs of sepsis (or a positive blood culture).

Hypothermia (*see Section 3.3*)

Hypothermia seriously increases the risk of surfactant deficiency and hypoglycaemia, and must be avoided.

Preparation for birth in the home and in hospital

For the majority of deliveries, only a minimum amount of resuscitation equipment is needed.

Equipment for basic resuscitation of the infant at home

The following equipment is needed:

- 2 clean dry towels
- a firm working surface (padded)
- a bulb suction device
- a well-fitting mask (size 0/1)

- a self-inflatable bag
- clean scissors or razor blade
- boiled string (two 6-inch lengths)
- woollen cap or head covering.

Management at delivery of a baby not needing resuscitation

Summary of management of the healthy baby at birth

- Deliver the baby on to the mother's abdomen or a warm surface, dry and cover.
- Clamp cord when pulsation stopped, usually between 2 and 3 minutes after birth and keep the baby between the mother's thighs level or below the placenta.
- Prevent hypothermia by nursing skin to skin with the mother.
- Initiate early breastfeeding.
- Minimise infection by hand washing, cord care and using clean materials.
- Give an injection of vitamin K.

Most babies do not need any resuscitation at birth but only require basic care to prevent infection and hypothermia. Extensive mouth suction, face mask oxygen, and vigorous stimulation in order to provoke a first gasp or cry are unnecessary rituals without clinical justification. As long as the baby becomes pink, and starts to breathe without distress, most babies should stay with their mothers and have a first feed at the breast within minutes of birth.

A simple approach would be to keep newborns without complications in **skin-to-skin contact** *with* their mothers during the first hour after birth to prevent hypothermia and **promote breastfeeding**. Colostrum, the initial milk with a clear, yellowish and thick appearance, is an extremely nutritious and concentrated feed rich in immunoglobulins (it is only present during the first 3 to 4 days). Mothers should be informed of its benefits and that it is ideal for their baby to feed on this as soon after birth as possible and as frequently as possible.

Preventing heat loss after birth

- Once any necessary resuscitation process has finished and as soon as the baby becomes pink, and starts to breathe without distress, they can be given to the mother for skin-to-skin contact and their first feed at the breast. This practice, among other benefits, not only prevents hypothermia but also helps in better uterine contraction following delivery.
- The practice of using water or oil to clean the skin within a few hours of birth before the body temperature has stabilised can make the baby dangerously hypothermic. A simple drying of the skin with a warm towel or sheet is all that is required.
- There is no more effective source of warmth than the mother's own body, so long as the baby is first well dried to minimise evaporative heat loss. A larger sheet or blanket can then be used to protect both mother and baby from the convective heat loss caused by draughts.
- Babies have relatively large heads. Covering the head with a shawl, blanket or woollen cap can significantly reduce heat loss.
- Heat and water loss through the skin can be a particular problem in babies born before 32 weeks' gestation.

This can be limited initially by wrapping all but the face in a clean plastic wrapping such as cling film or a food-grade plastic bag with a hole cut in the end of the bag for the baby's head to protrude, for a few hours after birth. **Remember that plastic over the face can cause death from suffocation.** If plastic bags or cling film are not available, the preterm baby must be wrapped well in a clean towel or blanket. However, plastic bags are very good for preventing heat loss, but only in conjunction with an overhead heat source or heated mattress. If the fluid in the bag gets cold it will cool the baby quicker than drying and wrapping.

- Heat supplementation can be provided by locally built and maintained incubators, overhead heating systems, and skin-to-skin (kangaroo) care.
- Ideally, the first bath should be delayed for at least 24 hours.

Managing the placenta, cord and umbilical stump

Babies often become relatively anaemic 4 to 6 months after birth because red cell production does not keep pace with body growth. This problem can be minimised by ensuring that blood intended for the baby is not left in the placenta at birth.

If the baby is held higher than the placenta (i.e. on the mother's abdomen) while the cord is still pulsating, blood will drain out of the baby and into the placenta, so hold the (covered) baby just below the placenta for 2 minutes if the cord is still pulsating. If the cord is clamped before it stops pulsating, this will also reduce the normal 'placental transfusion' at birth, especially if the uterus has not yet contracted.

If, however, blood is artificially 'milked' from the placenta into the baby, it is possible to leave the baby with so many red cells that the blood becomes thick and polycythaemic. Neonatal polycythaemia has many complications, including putting the circulation under strain, making the capillary circulation very sluggish, and increasing the risk of jaundice (see below).

It is recommended after a vaginal delivery to wait for 2 minutes before cutting the cord if it is still pulsating, to maximise the baby's haemoglobin, unless there is a need to start resuscitating the baby.

The cord must be cut cleanly, and the cut stump secured in a manner that minimises the risk of late haemorrhage. Remember that prevention rather than treatment is the key. A supply of fresh disposable razor blades is one widely adopted strategy in some communities where home birth is the norm.

The umbilical stump will shrink as it dries out. Plastic clamps that shut down further as the cord starts to shrink are very effective. They are relatively inexpensive, and they do make it possible to cut the stump about 2–4 cm from the skin. An elastic band, if carefully applied, is a cheap and well-tested alternative. A stump that is left too long provides a reservoir where bacteria can breed and multiply with great speed, and therefore should not be permitted. A length of 2–4 cm is ideal.

A short stump does not need to be covered except to keep it from snagging on clothes and blankets. Recent studies in resource-limited countries have shown that the application of 4% chlorhexidine solution immediately after birth can prevent omphalitis. Other possible antiseptics include surgical spirit or iodine.

Often the cord manifests a little 'stickiness', which may be of no concern. However, a local antiseptic should be applied if a red skin flare suggests early spreading staphylococcal cellulitis. Such babies must also be given an oral anti-staphylococcal antibiotic (cloxacillin or flucloxacillin). If the skin around the stump becomes oedematous with increasing redness, IV cloxacillin or oral flucloxacillin (25 mg/kg three times a day for 7 days) is usually the most logical choice. Babies who are systemically unwell always need urgent broad-spectrum antibiotic treatment, IV or IM, for septicaemia.

The risk of neonatal tetanus can be eliminated by ensuring that all mothers are immunised against tetanus with at least two injections of tetanus toxoid 1 month apart during pregnancy.

The risk of cross-infection during or after birth

Puerperal infection ('child-bed fever') is an illness that killed thousands of recently delivered women for more than two centuries. The fact that this could be eliminated if birth attendants washed their hands thoroughly **every time they moved from one woman to the next** was shown many years before it was ever realised that this lethal illness was caused by group A streptococcal infection. The arrival of antibiotic treatment has reduced the risk of death, but it has not lessened the need for meticulous hand washing before vaginal examination or delivery. Failure to observe this simple but important precaution also puts the baby at risk of cross-infection, especially if the baby is being cared for in a hospital setting.

The WHO estimates that infection is responsible for one-third of all neonatal deaths (over 3000 deaths a day). Kangaroo care has significantly reduced the number of neonatal deaths from infection by colonising babies with the mother's bacteria rather than those of the hospital.

Neonatal examination before discharge of a baby from the hospital

Before discharging the baby it is important that some basic checks are made. These include ensuring that the baby is feeding well, has passed meconium and urine and does not have any gross congenital abnormalities. Always check for jaundice. If there are qualified personnel available, a more detailed check could be undertaken. All examinations should be documented, including abnormalities, even if there is no other action which can be taken. It is also important to check local guidelines, if any.

Pre-Discharge Newborn Checklist

Name
Date of birth
Mode of delivery
Birth weight
Type of feed

Mother's name
Gestation
Need for resuscitation
Head circumference
Mother's blood group

	Tick if normal/Describe if abnormal	Common problems to look for
Head		Anencephaly, occipital encephalocele, microcephaly, large fontanelle, abnormal shape of head
Face		Abnormal looking facies
Ears		Low set ears, absent ears, ear tags
Eyes		White-coloured pupil, white cornea
Nose		Blocked nostrils with breathing difficulty
Lips		Cleft lip
Palate		Missing palate
Neck		Swelling on the neck, holding neck to one side
Clavicles		Lumps or bumps on the clavicle
Chest		Shape of chest
Abdomen		Scaphoid (empty) abdomen
Umbilicus		Omphalocoele, gastroschisis, hernia
Genitalia		Abnormal genitalia, undescended testis, hypospadias
Anus		Absent anus, abnormally placed anus
Spine		Spina bifida, meningomyelocele
Upper limbs		Absent limbs, contractures of limbs, not moving arm
Lower limbs		Not moving limbs, unequal limbs
Hands		Missing or extra digits
Feet		Abnormally shaped feet (talipes), missing or extra digits
Hips		Hip dysplasia (Barlow and Ortolani manoeuvres)
Jaundice		
Chest		Air entry (right and left)
CVS		Murmur, femoral pulse, cyanosis
Abdomen		Spleen, liver, kidney, palpable mass
Birth marks		

The following data should be recorded in the notes of every newborn baby.

Baby's name (if given at the time)

Mother's data

- Name, address, date of birth, and any identifying number
- Parity and previous obstetric history
- Blood group
- First day of last menstrual period
- **Results of any antenatal serology (e.g. rubella, syphilis, rhesus titres, HIV status)**
- Illness during the pregnancy
- Drugs taken during the pregnancy
- Family history of any illnesses

Father's data

- Full name, address and date of birth
- Family history of any illnesses

Labour and delivery data

- Time of onset: whether induction of labour or spontaneous
- Time membranes ruptured and any other known risk factors for infection (see below)
- Duration of first and second stage of labour
- Drugs given to the mother in labour
- Presentation and mode of delivery
- Full details of any resuscitation for baby or mother
- Time, dose, route of administration and full generic name of any drugs given to the mother

Baby data

- Temperature shortly after delivery, to document adequate thermoregulation
- Birth weight
- Head circumference (best measured after 24 hours when moulding has subsided)
- Length (ideally)
- Full physical examination, noting any abnormalities or evidence of birth trauma detected
- Details of dose, preparation and route of administration of any drugs given at delivery (e.g. vitamin K)
- **If not already given, ensure that vitamin K 1 mg IM is administered**

Follow-up home visits

Trials in South Asia have shown that three home visits in the first week of life (starting on the day of birth) by trained healthcare workers can reduce neonatal mortality by 30–60%. During their visits, the healthcare workers promote essential newborn care, examine babies for danger signs, and treat or refer when appropriate, counsel the families in how to recognise danger signs and emphasise the importance of prompt referral when they are identified.

The WHO and UNICEF recommend that skilled healthcare workers (nurses or midwives) should undertake these visits, but in many settings this is not possible. Volunteers have also been trained to do this, and recently the effectiveness of this has been shown in Ghana, where a fall in neonatal mortality followed two home visits during pregnancy and three visits in the first week of life.

Further reading

Van-Rheenen P (2011) Delayed cord clamping and improved infant outcomes. *British Medical Journal,* **343**, d7127.

WHO and UNICEF (2009) *WHO/UNICEF Joint Statement. Home visits for the newborn child: a strategy to improve survival.* www.unicef.org/health/files/WHO_FCH_CAH_09.02_eng.pdf

---

3.2 Resuscitation of the newly born

Introduction

Respiratory changes at birth in a healthy term infant

- During life *in utero*, the infant's lungs are full of lung tissue fluid. The fluid is removed during labour and at birth by the following mechanisms:
  - at the onset of labour, lung fluid production stops
  - as labour progresses, re-absorption of lung fluid occurs
  - about 35 mL of fluid are expelled from the lungs as a result of thoracic compression during vaginal delivery
  - the first breaths generate relatively high pressures to inflate the lungs, which has the effect of pushing this fluid into the circulation. These first breaths establish the infant's functional residual capacity.
- Surfactant is produced in the alveoli to prevent them collapsing completely during expiration.
  - Production starts slowly at 20 weeks' gestation, and increases rapidly from 30–34 weeks and thereafter.
  - Surfactant production is reduced by hypothermia, hypoxia and acidosis.

Caesarean section is associated with delayed clearance of pulmonary fluid, and reduces the initial functional residual capacity

Most infants breathe well and do not need active 'resuscitation' at birth. Simply drying the infant with a warm dry sheet/towel will in most cases stimulate a cry from the infant thus expanding the lungs (*see* Section 3.1). Attempts to clear the airway, to stimulate breathing, or to give facial oxygen are unnecessary. Therefore routine airway suctioning is not needed. Most infants make all the circulatory adjustments required at birth without external intervention as the lungs expand. All that the birth attendant has to do is to optimise the conditions needed for these changes to occur smoothly

Around 5% of infants do not breathe spontaneously after delivery. However, breathing can be started in almost all these infants by correctly applying bag-and-mask ventilation. With lung inflation there is an immediate and easily detectable rise in heart rate. It may be difficult to identify the infant's pulse rate by palpation at any site, so the best way to determine the heart rate is to listen over the chest with a stethoscope.

Far less commonly, infants are born cyanosed, shocked, limp and hypotonic. Around 1% do not respond to bag-and-mask ventilation, and need further help with advanced resuscitation.

Resuscitation at birth

Equipment needed for resuscitation

The following equipment is needed:

- Two clean dry towels.
- A firm working surface.
- Heat and light source.
- Sterile gloves.
- Sterile scissors.
- Sterile cord clamps.
- Food-grade plastic wrapping (cling film).
- Clock.
- Soft well-fitting face masks (size 0/1 and 00).
- A self-inflatable bag.
- A source of oxygen.
- A pressure-limiting device at 30 cmH$_2$0 if T-piece is used.
- A stethoscope.
- A laryngoscope, with straight blades size 0 and 1, and spare bulbs.
- A set of endotracheal tubes (2.5, 3.0, 3.5 and 4.0 mm) with adaptors to fit the inflation system.
- An endotracheal stylet.
- An umbilical venous catheter (or use a sterile feeding tube).
- A pulse oximeter (if available).
- A roll of zinc oxide tape for name-band.
- Syringes: 1 mL, 5 mL and 10 mL.
- Emergency drugs: 1 in 1000 adrenaline plus sterile water for dilution to make 1 in 10000.
- Ringer-lactate or Hartmann's solution.
- Glucose 10%.
- Nalorphine (naloxone) if opiates are used during labour.

Immediate preparation

Two clean dry towels are needed, one to dry the infant and one to keep them warm, a firm working surface in a warm well-lit area, a self-inflating bag with good soft well-fitting face mask (see below), and a suction device and a source of oxygen if possible is all that most infants who have not started breathing spontaneously need.

Self-inflating bag, valve and masks

A soft close-fitting face mask is essential. Access to a range of sizes of mask makes it possible to manage infants weighing as little as 500 g or as much as 5000 g at birth. It provides a near-airtight seal between mask and face in a way that mimics the effectiveness and efficiency of an endotracheal tube. Hence it is possible to use a mask as effectively as an endotracheal tube along with a self-inflating

bag to administer slow inflating pressures up to a maximum inspiratory pressure of 30 cmH$_2$O to the fluid-filled lung of an infant who is not breathing or who is making poor respiratory efforts at birth. The bag-valve-mask inflates the lungs, enabling the infant's respiratory centre to be oxygenated and initiate spontaneous respiration.

Suction devices

A range of simple suction devices, with a soft wide-bore tube (10 or 12) either mechanically or electrically operated, are available. Suction is rarely needed and should not be performed routinely. Mouth-to-mouth suction can be effective, but places the operator at risk of infections such as HIV or hepatitis. A double mucus trap may be used to help to prevent infected material being accidentally drawn into the mouth, but even this may be insufficient for user protection.

Circulatory access and drugs

An umbilical vein catheter may be used to administer drugs, but it is important to note that infants who require drugs during resuscitation have poorer outcomes and are at increased risk of death and long-term neurological sequelae. Ringer-lactate or Hartmann's solution, plasma expander or blood in the case of hypovolaemia due to fetal bleeding (see below) may occasionally be required and would use the umbilical vein route. The intra-osseous route is also now being used, either using a purpose-made needle and drill set or by using an venepuncture needle and the medial side of the tibial bone, below the growth plate (see Section 8.N). For a discussion of drugs, see below.

Timing

A clock will help you to document the duration of resuscitation and the timing of interventions.

Additional equipment

A heat and light source is needed plus food-grade plastic wrapping for infants under 32 weeks' gestation.

An oxygen source is helpful but not essential for infants who need advanced resuscitation.

A pulse oximeter can be of help in monitoring the improvement in oxygenation and detecting the occasional infant with sub-clinical cyanosis requiring further intervention or evaluation for cardiac or pulmonary disease. It is also useful to prevent hyperoxia when oxygen is used in resuscitation, especially in the preterm infant.

A roll of zinc oxide tape half an inch wide can be used to make a simple name band for infants not delivered in their own homes. Take six inches of this tape, write the date and the mother's name at one end, turn the last two inches of the other end back on itself (so the tape does not stick to the skin), and then turn this into a simple bracelet round the child's wrist. Ensure that the bracelet is loosely fitting to avoid a tourniquet effect.

Guidelines from the 2010 International Liaison Committee on Resuscitation (ILCOR)

The main changes that have been made to the Neonatal Life Support (NLS) guidelines relevant to resource-limited countries are as follows:

- The use of food-grade plastic wrapping (cling film) is recommended to maintain body temperature in very small preterm infants.
- Ventilatory resuscitation may be started with air. However,

where possible, additional oxygen should be available if there is no rapid improvement in the infant's condition.

- Adrenaline should be given by the IV route, as standard doses are likely to be ineffective if given via a tracheal tube.
- If there are no signs of life after 20 minutes of continuous and adequate resuscitation efforts, discontinuation of resuscitation may be justified.

Sequence of actions during resuscitation of the newborn

There are agreed guidelines from the 2010 International Liaison Committee on Resuscitation (ILCOR). The sequence below and that of 'Helping Infants Breathe' are both practical applications of these principles.

First call for help

Start the clock or note the time. Keep the infant dry and warm and assess their breathing and heart rate.

- Infants are born small and wet. They get cold very easily, especially if they remain wet and in a draught. Whatever the problem, **dry the infant well, including the head**. Remove the wet towel, and **wrap the infant in a dry towel**. It is helpful if the towels are warm.
- There is good evidence that for very preterm infants (30 weeks' gestation or earlier), placing the infant under a radiant heater after drying, and immediately covering the head and body, apart from the face, with clean plastic wrapping, is the most effective way of keeping these very small infants warm during resuscitation.
- **Drying the infant** immediately after delivery will provide significant stimulation during which **colour, tone, breathing and heart rate can continue to be observed**.
- It is important to **monitor the infant's breathing. Observing the colour, heart rate and tone helps to document the infant's condition and assess their response to resuscitation**.
- **Reassess** these observations regularly (particularly the heart rate), every 30 seconds or so, throughout the resuscitation process. The first sign of any improvement in the bradycardic infant will be an increase in heart rate.
- A healthy infant may be born blue but will have good tone, will cry within a few seconds of delivery, will have a good heart rate (the heart rate of a healthy newborn infant is about 120–150 beats/minute) and will rapidly become pink during the first 90 seconds or so. An ill infant will be born pale and floppy, not breathing, and with a slow or very slow heart rate.
- The heart rate of an infant is best judged by listening to the chest with a stethoscope. It can also sometimes be felt by palpating the base of the umbilical cord, but a slow rate at the cord is not always indicative of a truly slow heart rate, and, if the infant is not breathing, must not delay the immediate application of lung inflations. In addition, if the infant is not breathing, feeling for peripheral pulses is potentially harmful as it delays the onset of life-saving lung inflations. If a stethoscope is not available, you can listen to the heart by placing your ear on the infant's chest or using a Pinard's stethoscope.

Airway: Keep the airway open

- Before the infant can breathe effectively the airway must be open.

- The best way to achieve this in an infant who is not breathing well is to place the infant on their back with the head in the **neutral position** (i.e. with the neck neither flexed nor extended). Most newborn infants will have a relatively prominent occiput, which will tend to flex the neck if the infant is placed on their back on a flat surface. This can be avoided by placing some support using a folded nappy or cloth under the shoulders of the infant, but be careful not to overextend the neck.
- If the infant is floppy it may also be necessary to apply chin lift or jaw thrust.

The best way to stabilise an infant's condition at birth is to ensure that the upper airway remains unobstructed. The child will then have little difficulty in drawing air into its lungs for itself when it takes its first spontaneous gasp or cry. Unfortunately, books often talk of the need to keep the airway 'clear', giving the false impression that the infant is going to find it difficult to breathe unless all the fluid and mucus is first sucked out of the way. There is no evidence that this is ever necessary unless the infant is meconium stained or does not breathe well. **Moreover, blind deep suction of the nose or mouth can stimulate the vagus nerve, leading to bradycardia, apnoea and laryngospasm.**

However, the upper airway of any infant who is born limp and hypotonic certainly needs to be opened and maintained in just the same way as the airway of any other unconscious patient. In an unconscious patient, pharyngeal tone decreases even more than it does during sleep, causing the upper airway to narrow or close. When such a patient is laid on their back the tongue also falls back, further obstructing the airway. There are three key ways to counter this:

1. Hold the head in the neutral position *and*
2. Support the chin *or*
3. Push the jaw forward.

Because of moulding, most infants have quite a prominent occiput at birth. Lying supine (on their back) on a flat surface, the neck becomes flexed, and the airway becomes obstructed. Exactly the same thing can happen if the neck is over-extended. The aim is to ensure that the head is in a 'neutral' position – a posture most easily achieved by placing a small (2 cm high) pad under the infant's shoulders.

It is important that all healthcare workers who conduct deliveries are taught how to open the airway correctly.

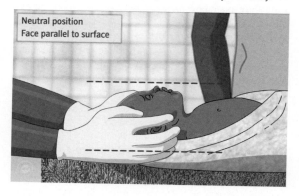

Neutral position
Face parallel to surface

FIGURE 3.2.1 Neutral position of the head and neck in a newborn. Reproduced with the permission of Medical Aid Films, www.medicalaidfilms.org

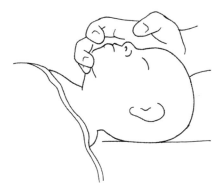

FIGURE 3.2.2 Chin lift in a newborn.

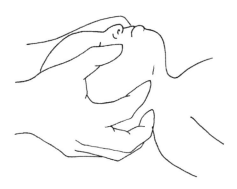

FIGURE 3.2.3 Jaw thrust in a newborn. Note that the operator's thumbs are in a position to hold a mask in place.

If tone is poor it may also be necessary to support the chin. It is important to support the bony part of the chin. Pressure anywhere else may merely push the base of the tongue backwards, making matters worse.

If tone is **very** poor it may be necessary to use one or two fingers under each side of the lower jaw, at its angle, in order to push the jaw forwards and outwards ('jaw thrust'), but this will require a second person to give the inflation and ventilation breaths with the bag-valve-mask.

Although it is rare for debris to completely block the trachea, this should be suspected if an infant tries to breathe but remains cyanosed and bradycardic, with laboured breathing and marked inter-costal and/or sternal recession. This is one of the few situations where tracheal intubation can be life-saving at birth.

Meconium

It is estimated that around 15% of infants have meconium-stained liquor at birth. Meconium aspiration syndrome (MAS) can occur in about 1 in 10 such infants. The development of MAS is not entirely dependent on suctioning at birth. It is possible for infants to aspirate meconium into the large airways *in utero* if there is hypoxia and gasping. However, some infants may aspirate meconium during delivery, and these are the ones in whom the risk of MAS can be reduced by suctioning when the infant's head is on the perineum.

Studies based on experience from Africa and India have shown that suctioning the mouth of infants with meconium-stained liquor during birth when the head is at the perineum has dramatically reduced the incidence of meconium aspiration syndrome (MAS) and death. There is subsequently no need for further suctioning after birth if the infant breathes well.

What to do if the trachea appears to be blocked

If the infant is born through meconium and is unresponsive (or 'not vigorous') at birth, the oropharynx should be inspected and cleared of meconium. If intubation skills are available, the larynx and trachea should also be cleared under direct vision. If meconium has entered the trachea, resuscitation here is only possible if the accumulated debris can be immediately removed. The easiest way to do this is to pass an endotracheal tube and then remove the debris by direct suction to the endotracheal tube. Sometimes the meconium debris is so large that it cannot be sucked through the tube. The tube can then be removed and replaced with a clean tube to clear the remaining obstructive material. Suction may also make it easier to see the larynx during intubation. Giving mask ventilation for the infant who is not breathing before the meconium has been cleared (as above) may force the meconium deeper into the lungs.

Breathing

- If the infant is not breathing adequately **give five inflation breaths as soon as possible** (unless the baby is very preterm, in which case such breaths may injure immature lungs: give ordinary ventilation breaths in this situation). Until now the infant's lungs will have been filled with fluid. Aeration of the lungs in these circumstances is best with slow inflations at pressures of about 30 cmH$_2$O with the bag and mask; these are called 'inflation breaths'. These initial ventilation breaths should last 2–3 seconds each. The aim is to mimic the initial breaths taken by a normal infant to open the airways, remove lung fluid and achieve its functional residual capacity.

- If the heart rate was below 100 beats/minute initially then it should rapidly increase as oxygenated blood reaches the heart. If the heart rate does increase then you can assume that you have successfully aerated the lungs and there is adequate tissue oxygenation. If the heart rate increases but the infant does not start breathing, then continue to provide regular ventilation breaths at a rate of about 30–40 breaths/minute until the infant starts to breathe.

- The chest may not move during the first one or two breaths as fluid is displaced. Adequate ventilation is usually indicated by either a rapidly increasing heart rate or a heart rate that is maintained at more than 100 beats/minute. Therefore reassess the heart rate after delivery of the first five breaths. It is safe to assume that the chest has been inflated successfully if the heart rate improves. Once the chest has been seen to move and the heart rate has increased, ventilation should be continued at a rate of 30–40 breaths/minute. Continue ventilatory support until regular breathing is established.

- If the heart rate does not increase following inflation breaths, then either you have not aerated the lungs or the infant needs more than lung aeration alone. By far the most likely possibility is that you have failed to aerate the lungs effectively. If the heart rate does not increase, and the chest does not passively move with each inflation breath, then you have not aerated the lungs.

Under these circumstances consider the following:
- — Are the infant's head and neck in the neutral position?
- — Do you need jaw thrust?
- — Do you need a second person's help with the airway or to squeeze the bag? A relative or ward orderly can be shown immediately how to effectively squeeze the self-inflating bag while you ensure that the mask is held firmly and in the best position on the face over the mouth and nose with the airway open.
- — Is there an obstruction in the oropharynx (laryngoscope and suction under direct vision)?

Bag-and-mask inflation of the lung

Having positioned the infant correctly it is then usually quite easy to use a self-inflating bag and mask to provide inflations.

Remember that the infant cannot breathe through the bag-valve-mask system, so do not leave the mask sealed to the face and expect the infant to breathe from the bag. The valve between the bag and the mask prevents this. When the infant is breathing, remove the mask and watch closely to ensure that adequate breathing continues.

Most infants will respond to bag-and-mask ventilation by gasping and then starting to breathe on their own without further support. If this does not happen, it is still easy to confirm that lung aeration has been achieved, because the heart rate will rise reliably and consistently above 100 beats/minute. If lung aeration has been achieved and the infant still has a slow heart rate, proceed to support the circulation (C). If oxygen is available, applying this through the bag and mask may also help.

It is essential that the skills of correct bag-and-mask ventilation are taught to all healthcare workers who conduct deliveries. This is best done on a mannequin. Correct bag-and-mask ventilation is the single most important skill needed to provide active resuscitation.

There is good evidence that most infants can be resuscitated using mask resuscitation without any need for tracheal intubation. However, in certain situations (e.g. infants less than 1000 g not responding to inflation, prolonged bag-and-mask ventilation with no spontaneous breathing, etc.) infants require early intubation, so the equipment and the skill to intubate should be available.

Deciding whether to use air or 100% oxygen for resuscitation of the newborn

Concern about the possible injurious effects of excess oxygen, particularly in preterm infants, and the apparent effectiveness of air in a number of randomised controlled human studies of resuscitation at birth, have resulted in a change in guidelines.

There is evidence to suggest that air is safer for initial resuscitation. However, where possible, it is recommended that additional oxygen should be available for use if there is not a rapid improvement in the infant's condition. Equally, hyperoxia should be avoided, especially in the preterm infant. If a pulse oximeter is available this can be done. Try to keep the SaO_2 between 88% and 95%.

When to cut and clamp the cord in an infant who needs resuscitation at birth

There are advantages to delaying clamping of the cord for 2 minutes after birth to allow placental transfer of blood to the infant (see above). However, it is important to ensure that by doing this there is no harm to the mother (e.g. if she needs resuscitation) or to the infant (e.g. if they require resuscitation). Usually the umbilical cord is clamped and cut immediately if the infant needs to be moved for active resuscitation.

Mouth-to-mouth resuscitation

Most current guidelines on neonatal care steer clear of discussing the role of mouth-to-mouth resuscitation. The risk of HIV infection or hepatitis has further fuelled that reluctance. However, there is no doubt that this can be a very effective way of reviving an apparently lifeless infant in the absence of equipment. Remember the following:
- Keep the upper airway open by optimising the position of the head and jaw as described above.
- Cover the infant's nose and mouth with your mouth (or cover the mouth of a big infant and just pinch the nose).
- Use the pressure you can generate with your cheeks, and try to aerate the lung by slow inflations for 2–3 seconds.
- Only use as much air for each breath as you can keep in your cheeks (i.e. do not 'blow' air into the infant, but just small puffs).
- Watch for chest movement, and allow time for lung recoil.
- Once the chest starts to move, sustain what has been achieved with 20–25 artificial breaths/minute.

Checking progress before moving on
- If the heart rate has **not** risen to over 100 beats/minute after the five initial breaths or within 30 seconds of adequate ventilation, something is wrong. The most likely problem is that you have not successfully ventilated the infant. **Never** move on to deal with the issues covered under letter C of the resuscitation alphabet until you are quite sure you have achieved objectives A and B. To do so is quite futile. Chest compression will never restore the circulation until the blood being massaged from the lung to the heart contains oxygen.
- Look to see whether the chest moves each time you apply mask pressure. Movement should not be difficult to see once the first few breaths have aerated the lungs. It is usually easier to judge success with your eyes than with a stethoscope. In a newborn, breath sounds can be heard when only the airway is being aerated, so are not a good way to judge ventilatory success.
- Check that the infant's head is well positioned. Check chin support and jaw thrust, and that the mask is correctly applied with no air leaks. Ask a second person to help you position the infant optimally and provide inflations by squeezing the bag while you hold the airway open and the mask in place.
- Few infants need support with their breathing once their lungs have been aerated. Most will gasp, cry or breathe just as soon as an attempt is made to get air into the lungs, and then continue breathing adequately.
  - However, a few may benefit from further support if they do not start to breathe regularly, or only gasp occasionally. Some may have suffered severe hypoxia *in utero*, and a few may be drowsy because of drugs given to the mother during labour. Check that the heart rate remains normal (above 100 beats/minute) and that there is no central cyanosis (best judged by looking at the colour of the tongue).
  - Try to assess whether there is hypoxemia (cyanosis

or SaO$_2$ less than 90% with a pulse oximeter), if the infant's breathing remains laboured and irregular or if the child's colour remains blue. Give oxygen then if it is available, preferably with SaO$_2$ monitoring. Hyaline membrane disease, meconium aspiration syndrome, pneumonia or transient tachypnoea of the newborn are most likely.

Other possibilities include:
— intra-partum pneumonia (common)
— diaphragmatic hernia
— pneumothorax
— pulmonary hypoplasia (possibly associated with a skeletal or renal abnormality)
— cyanotic congenital heart disease (although this usually takes a little time to appear)
— persistent fetal circulation.

- If breathing requires continuous support it is important to try and reduce mask inflation pressures to little more than half of what was needed to aerate the lung in the first place. It is easy to over-ventilate an infant with healthy lungs and to wash out so much of the carbon dioxide that normally provides the main stimulus to breathing that all such activity stops for a while. There is also increasing evidence that sustained over-ventilation can seriously reduce cerebral blood flow.

Endotracheal intubation

As discussed earlier, most infants who need resuscitation can be managed with bag-valve-mask intubation. However, occasionally endotracheal intubation is required, but this must be done by someone skilled and practised in the technique. It is most likely to be required for prolonged resuscitation, in meconium aspiration, and in preterm infants with surfactant deficiency. A straight-bladed laryngoscope is preferred, and tube sizes are around 3.5 mm for a term infant and 2.5 mm for a preterm infant. Sizes larger and smaller than these should be available.

Preterm infants

- Infants with surfactant deficiency may have difficulty in expanding their lungs, and in developing a normal functional residual capacity at birth.
- However, the preterm lung is quite a delicate structure with relatively little elastic support, and any use of undue pressure or excessive ventilation during resuscitation can damage the lungs.

While an inspiratory pressure of 30 cmH$_2$O may well be necessary to begin aerating the lungs at birth, the pressure should be reduced as rapidly as possible to a level that ensures that the chest is moving adequately. The key aim must be to conserve such surfactant as already exists by sustaining the lung's functional residual capacity (an objective best achieved by providing at least 5 cmH$_2$O of positive end-expiratory pressure (PEEP). Aim to achieve this consistently throughout transfer to the nursery. This can be achieved using nasal prongs (nasal PEEP), thus avoiding tracheal intubation altogether (see Section 8.2).

Circulation: chest compressions

- Most infants needing help at birth will respond to successful lung inflation with an increase in heart rate followed quickly by normal breathing. Chest compression should be started only when you are sure that the lungs are being aerated successfully.
- If the heart rate remains very slow (less than 60 beats/minute) or absent following 60 seconds of ventilation with good chest movements, start chest compressions.
- In infants, the most efficient method of delivering chest compressions is to grip the chest in both hands in such a way that the two thumbs can press on the lower third of the sternum, just below an imaginary line joining the nipples, with the fingers over the spine at the back. This can only be done if there is a second operator ventilating the lungs (see Figure 3.2.4).
- If you are alone, the two-thumb method is not possible, as ventilations also need to be provided. In this situation, use the first two fingers of one hand to depress the lower sternum, while the other hand holds the mask in place. Then move the hand from the sternum to squeeze the bag.
- Compress the chest quickly and firmly, reducing the antero-posterior diameter of the chest by about one-third.
- Because oxygenation is such an important part of neonatal resuscitation, **the recommended ratio of compressions to inflations in newborn resuscitation is 3:1**.
- Chest compressions move oxygenated blood from the lungs back to the heart and out into the ascending aorta. From there the two coronary arteries will then quickly deliver oxygen to the failing anoxic heart muscle. It is important to allow enough time during the relaxation phase of each compression cycle for the heart to refill with blood, at the same time ensuring that the chest is inflating with each breath.

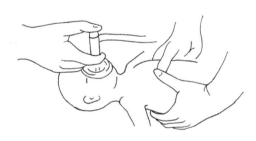

FIGURE 3.2.4 Two-thumb compression of the chest, with a second operator ventilating the lungs, here using a T-piece as an alternative to bag and mask.

- The rate of chest compressions is around 120/minute. However, with pauses for ventilation, the actual number of compressions is less than 120/minute.

Drugs

Rarely inflation of the lungs and effective chest compression will not be sufficient to produce adequate circulation and perfusion in infants. In these circumstances, drugs may be helpful. However, drugs are needed only if there is no significant cardiac output despite effective lung inflation and chest compression.

Very few drugs have proved to be of benefit in such circumstances. The drugs used are adrenaline (1:10 000) and dextrose (10%). Drugs are best delivered via an umbilical venous catheter. In those where IV access is not possible, the intra-osseous route may be used. Each injection of a drug should be followed with a bolus of 2–3 mL of Ringer-lactate or Hartmann's solution. Unfortunately, most of the infants in whom cardiac output only returns after such treatment require specialist neonatal care (often with mechanical ventilation) and do not survive to discharge. Most of those who do survive later develop profound disabling spastic quadriplegia.

Where the cause of the child's terminal apnoea is a sudden and much more abrupt hypoxic event (such as shoulder dystocia or an occasional case of late cord prolapse) these reservations may be less valid. Here there is at least anecdotal evidence that the outlook is much less bleak if the circulation can be restarted.

Acidosis not serious enough to precipitate circulatory standstill (asystole) will nearly always correct itself spontaneously within 90 minutes once the circulation has been restored and the infant starts to breathe for him- or herself. It does not therefore call for sodium bicarbonate, the use of which is controversial. Indeed, giving bicarbonate may increase carbon dioxide levels, worsening intracellular acidosis, and increases the amount of sodium that the potentially compromised kidney will need to excrete over the next few days.

- **Adrenaline:** The recommended dose of adrenaline is 10 micrograms/kg body weight (0.1 mL/kg body weight of 1:10000 solution). If this is not effective, a dose of up to 30 micrograms/kg (0.3 mL/kg body weight of 1:10000 solution) may be tried. Ideally, have ready-made and well-labelled 1:10000 adrenaline solutions available on all emergency trolleys. In situations where this is not available in a ready-made state it could be prepared by adding 1 mL of 1:1000 solution to 9 mL of normal saline or Ringer-lactate or Hartmann's solution. **It is potentially dangerous to leave inadequately labelled and made up doses of adrenaline around, as giving the same volume of 1:10000 as 1:1000 solution could cause cardiac arrest.** Do not use a higher dose by these routes (IV) as it is harmful.
- **Glucose:** The recommended dose of glucose is 200 mg/kg (2 mL/kg of 10% dextrose). Higher concentrations or larger doses can induce hyperglycaemia, which is associated with cerebral oedema and cerebral haemorrhage, and may lead to rebound hypoglycaemia. It is known that severe hypoglycaemia is rare immediately after birth, but tends to present after 1–2 hours. However, hypoglycaemia (**less than 2.5 mmol/litre (45 mg/dL)**) is a potential problem for stressed or hypoxic neonates, so 10% dextrose should be considered in cardiac arrest, as the heart will not recover in the presence of hypoglycaemia. This should be followed by an infusion of 5 mL/kg/hour of 10% glucose if there is confirmation of hypoglycaemia by a blood test. This should be continued until feeding is well established. **Never give any drug into the umbilical artery.**
- **Naloxone (nalorphine)** can be used to reverse profound opiate-induced respiratory depression, but has no real role in neonatal resuscitation. If it does prove necessary, it is best to give it intramuscularly and give a full 200-microgram 'depot' dose irrespective of body weight. If naloxone is given as a single dose IV it will be eliminated from the body faster than the opioid drug, causing a return of the respiratory depression, and therefore the infant will stop breathing again without a naloxone infusion. Naloxone

does not reverse the respiratory depressing effects of non-opiate drugs.

Acute blood loss as a cause of circulatory arrest (circulatory volume support)

- Sudden acute blood loss is a rare, but often unrecognised, cause of acute circulatory collapse. Bleeding from an aberrant placental blood vessel (vasa praevia) or snapped umbilical cord can rapidly lead to hypovolaemic death. The response to a rapid generous infusion of any IV fluid can be equally dramatic. Speed is of the essence. Circulatory collapse probably does not occur until the infant has lost 30–40 mL/kg of blood, but 20 mL/kg of Ringer-lactate or Hartmann's solution will usually reverse the immediate critical hypovolaemia rapidly. The initial intravenous fluid bolus should be **10 mL/kg** of Ringer-lactate or Hartmann's solution **or blood group O Rh-negative blood (if immediately available). This can be repeated *once* if there is no or only minimal response.** A similar response can be achieved with plasma, albumin or some artificial plasma-expanding agent (e.g. gelatin). A packed red cell transfusion using group-specific or group O Rh-negative duly cross-matched blood can be given later to correct the associated anaemia.
- Other less well-recognised causes of hypovolaemic collapse include acute feto–maternal blood loss, sudden twin-to-twin transfusion, and accidental incision of the placenta during Caesarean delivery and cord ligature that has come off and not been detected.

Apart from these specific indications, fluid should not be used during neonatal resuscitation. There is no evidence to suggest benefit from routine use, which only compounds the problem of fluid balance that can develop over the next 2 to 3 days if severe intrapartum stress causes secondary renal failure.

Environment

This is always at risk of being overlooked, but it should be the first issue to receive attention in all infants, before and at birth.

- A **clean, warm** and **well-lit** environment for resuscitation is the objective in all cases. It only takes a few seconds to dry the infant and provide a clean dry blanket for warmth. The room in which delivery takes place should also be clean, warm and free of draughts.
- Small infants in particular rapidly become cold, especially if left wet, which can be lethal. Enclosing the trunk and the limbs in a clear plastic drape or bag (plus a woollen cap if available) can greatly reduce evaporative heat loss. Indeed, infants born more than 10 weeks early have skin that is so thin that it is not really 'waterproof'. This will cause excessive evaporative heat loss to persist for several days after birth.

Family

- The mother's needs come first if you are on your own. Most infants are quite good at looking after themselves, once they are breathing and wrapped. If possible keep the infant with the mother.
- If you are not on your own, things become much easier. The 'ABC' summary really only comments on the care that should be given to the infant. Remember that

parents need to be told what is happening. They will fear the worst, more so if the infant was only taken away from them even for a few minutes at birth for stabilisation or resuscitation.

- If you tell the parents that their infant needed 'resuscitation' at delivery, they may well start to think that their child was in the process of dying. That might make you feel that you have done something useful, and it may make the parents very grateful. However, it will also make them feel that something must have gone 'wrong' during delivery, and it may lead them to worry that their child could be 'brain-damaged' as a result. The words that we use matter. Parents can easily read meanings into them that we never intended.

- Write down what you see and do, distinguishing fact from opinion and making no assumption as to the causation. Use adjectives with great care and do not make judgemental comments on the actions of others. Document everything.

Poor response to resuscitation

If the infant either fails to respond or shows a poor response to resuscitation, the most likely problem is inadequate oxygenation. The following steps should be considered:

- Check the airway and ventilation.

- Check for technical faults if using equipment.
  - Is the oxygen attached?
  - Is the airway blocked?
  - Is the endotracheal tube in the correct place?
- Re-examine the chest to see if a pneumothorax has developed. This is not common, but may cause a problem. Drain a tension pneumothorax with a small cannula over needle (21 gauge) in the second intercostal space in the mid-clavicular line. This should be followed by the insertion of a chest drain (see Section 8.3).
- Consider the possibility of a congenital heart lesion if the infant remains cyanosed despite breathing and having a good heart rate.
- Consider the possibility of maternal opiates or sedation, such as diazepam or phenobarbitone, if the infant is pink, well perfused, but requires assisted ventilation.
- Shock, caused by acute blood loss, should respond to a rapid bolus of 10–20 mL/kg of O-negative blood.
- Consider the possibility of hypoglycaemia.

Stopping resuscitation

Even with the most effective resuscitation, not all infants will survive.

If the infant has been without a cardiac output after 20 minutes of resuscitation and does not respond despite

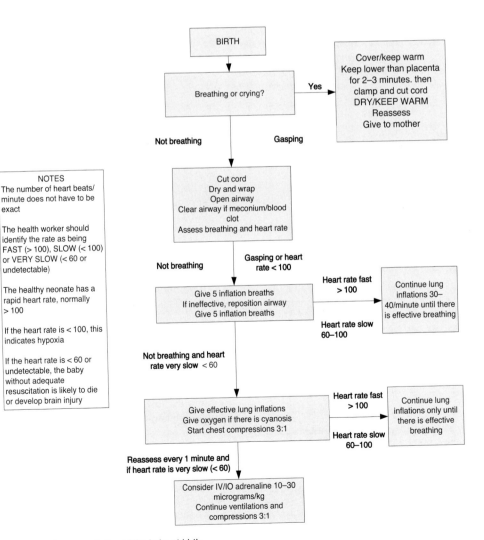

FIGURE 3.2.5 Algorithm for resuscitation of the baby at birth.

effective ventilations and chest compressions, the outcome is unlikely to be altered by the use of drugs, although these should be considered. The decision to stop resuscitation should be taken by the most senior healthcare worker present, and the reason for the decision should be clearly documented.

Explain sensitively to the parents that the infant has died. The infant should then be handled in accordance with cultural preference and practice.

Documentation

It is important to keep accurate records of the steps taken during resuscitation. The reason for any decision must be clearly documented, including the decision to start and end resuscitation. This is important irrespective of the immediate outcome of the resuscitation effort. As with any documentation, keep to the facts and make a complete record of all the steps taken, their timing, and the impact that they had on the infant's progress.

Remember to sign and date the record.

Vitamin K prophylaxis against haemorrhagic disease of the newborn

Following resuscitation/stabilisation, all newborn infants should receive vitamin K 1 mg IM. Vitamin K is given to prevent haemorrhagic disease of the newborn (HDN), which may cause significant bleeding and even death. The IM route is preferred as it provides a depot over many weeks.

Similarly, neonates requiring surgery, those with birth trauma, preterm infants and those exposed *in utero* to maternal medication that is known to interfere with vitamin K are at especially high risk of bleeding and must be given vitamin K 1 mg IM. This is often forgotten in the rush to get the infant to the nursery.

Resuscitation guidelines algorithm

As discussed earlier, all resuscitation guidelines are based on the international evidence-based science agreed in 2010 at the International Liaison Committee on Resuscitation. The algorithm shown in Figure 3.2.5 summarises the recommendations in the text.

Suggested reading

World Health Organization, London School of Hygiene and Tropical Medicine, Save the Children *et al.* (2011) Neonatal mortality levels for 193 countries in 2009 with trends since 1990: a systematic analysis of progress, projections and priorities. *PLoS Medicine*, **8**, e1001080.

Darmstadt GL, Lee ACC, Cousens S *et al.* (2009) 60 Million non-facility births: who can deliver in community settings to reduce intrapartum deaths? *International Journal of Gynaecology and Obstetrics*, **107**, S89–112.

Wall SN, Cousens S, Darmstadt GL *et al.* (2009) Neonatal resuscitation in low-resource settings: what, who and how to overcome challenges to scale up? *International Journal of Gynaecology and Obstetrics*, **107 (Suppl. 1)**, S47.

Lee ACC, Cousens S, Darmstadt GL *et al.* (2011) Care during labor and birth for the prevention of intrapartum-related neonatal deaths: a systematic review and Delphi estimation of mortality effect. *BMC Public Health,* **11 (Suppl. 3)**, S10.

Aschner JL *et al.* (2008) Sodium bicarbonate: basically useless therapy. *Pediatrics*, **122**, 831.

3.3   Clinical care of the infant in the early months of life

Prematurity and low birth weight

- A **low-birth-weight infant** is one weighing less than 2.5 kg at birth. Low birth weight may be attributable to preterm delivery or intrauterine growth restriction.
- A **preterm infant** is one born before 37 completed weeks have elapsed since the first day of the last menstrual period (259 days). Most preterm infants are born after 32 weeks' gestation.
- A **small-for-gestational age (SGA) infant** is one whose birth weight falls below the 10th percentile on a birth weight centile chart.

Probably at least 25% of SGA infants are just constitutionally small by virtue of maternal weight, and not secondary to poor placental perfusion. The mean birth weight of infants born to mothers 4 feet 10 inches (147 cm) tall is about 500 grams less than that of infants born to mothers 6 foot 0 inches (183 cm) tall. This discrepancy increases to about 1 kg if extremes of mid-pregnancy weight are also taken into account.

- **Intrauterine growth restriction (IUGR)** refers to a slowing of fetal growth velocity. Most but not all IUGR infants are SGA at birth. Some IUGR infants are just wasted.
- A **large-for-gestational age (LGA) infant** is one whose birth weight is greater than the 90th percentile on a birth weight centile chart.

For most clinical purposes it is sufficient to classify infants as 'low birth weight', 'preterm' or 'small-for-gestational age'.

Assessing gestational age

Sometimes a mother cannot recall the date of her last menstrual period. The infant's gestational age can then be assessed to within ± 2 weeks based on a combined physical and neurological score (*see* Table 3.3.1). Wasted infants underscore on physical criteria.

TABLE 3.3.1 Ballard's scoring system for gestational assessment

Sign	Physical criteria score							Sign score
	−1	0	1	2	3	4	5	
Skin	Sticky, friable, transparent	Gelatinous, red, translucent	Smooth, pink, visible veins	Superficial peeling and/or rash, few veins	Cracking, pale areas, rare veins	Parchment, deep cracking, no vessels	Leathery, cracked, wrinkled	
Lanugo	None	Sparse	Abundant	Thinning	Bald areas	Mostly bald		
Plantar surface	Heel–toe 40–50 mm: −1 < 40 mm: −2	> 50 mm no crease	Faint red marks	Anterior transverse crease only	Creases anterior two-thirds	Creases over entire sole		
Breast	Imperceptible	Barely perceptible	Flat areola, no bud	Stippled areola, 1–2 mm bud	Raised areola, 3–4 mm bud	Full areola, 5–10 mm bud		
Eye/ear	Lids fused loosely: −1 tightly: −2	Lids open, pinna flat, stays folded	Slightly curved pinna; soft; slow recoil	Well-curved pinna; soft but ready recoil	Formed and firm; instant recoil	Thick cartilage, ear stiff		
Genitals (male)	Scrotum flat, smooth	Scrotum empty, faint rugae	Testes in upper canal, rare rugae	Testes descending, few rugae	Testes down, good rugae	Testes pendulous, deep rugae		
Genitals (female)	Clitoris prominent and labia flat	Prominent clitoris and small labia minora	Prominent clitoris and enlarging labia minora	Labia majora and minora equally prominent	Labia majora large, labia minora small	Labia majora cover clitoris and labia minora		
Total physical maturity score								

Sign	Neurological criteria score							Sign score
	−1	0	1	2	3	4	5	
Posture								
Square window								
Arm recoil								
Popliteal angle								
Scarf sign								
Heel to ear								
Total neuromuscular score								

Notes on calculating the scores:

Posture: With the infant supine and quiet, score as follows:

- Arms and legs extended = 0
- Slight or moderate flexion of hips and knees = 1
- Moderate to strong flexion of hips and knees = 2
- Legs flexed and abducted, arms slightly flexed = 3
- Full flexion of arms and legs = 4.

Square window: Flex the hand at the wrist. Exert pressure sufficient to get as much flexion as possible. The angle between the thumb and the anterior aspect of the forearm is measured and scored:

- > 90° = −1
- 90° = 0
- 60° = 1
- 45° = 2
- 30° = 3
- 0° = 4.

Arm recoil: With the infant supine, fully flex the forearm for 5 seconds, then fully extend by pulling the hands and release. Score the reaction:

- Remains extended 180°, or random movements = 0
- Minimal flexion, 140–180° = 1
- Small amount of flexion, 110–140° = 2
- Moderate flexion, 90–100° = 3
- Brisk return to full flexion, < 90° = 4.

Popliteal angle: With the infant supine and the pelvis flat on the examining surface, the leg is flexed on the thigh and the thigh is fully flexed with the use of one hand. With the other hand the leg is then extended and the angled scored:

- 180° = −1
- 160° = 0
- 140° = 1
- 120° = 2
- 100° = 3
- 90° = 4
- < 90° = 5.

Scarf sign: With the infant supine, take the infant's hand and draw it across the neck and as far across the opposite shoulder as possible. Assistance to the elbow is permissible by lifting it across the body. Score according to the location of the elbow:

- Elbow reaches or nears level of opposite shoulder = −1
- Elbow crosses opposite anterior axillary line = 0
- Elbow reaches opposite anterior axillary line = 1
- Elbow reaches midline = 2
- Elbow does not reach midline = 3
- Elbow does not cross proximate axillary line = 4.

Heel to ear: With the infant supine, hold the infant's foot with one hand and move it as near to the head as possible without forcing it. Keep the pelvis flat on the examining surface. Score as shown in Table 3.3.1 above.

After assigning the score for the physical and neurological criteria, the sum of the two scores is then used to assess the gestation based on Table 3.3.2.

TABLE 3.3.2 Assessment of gestation from total score

Total score	Gestational age (weeks)
−10	20
−5	22
0	24
5	26
10	28
15	30
20	32
25	34
30	36
35	38
40	40
45	42
50	44

Low birth weight and/or preterm infants

Infants with birth weight in the range 2.25–2.5 kg

- These infants are normally strong enough to start feeding themselves. They need to be kept warm and closely observed for infection, but otherwise no special care is required.

Infants with birth weight in the range 1.75–2.25 kg

- These infants sometimes need extra care, but can normally stay with their mothers to receive feeding and warmth, especially if skin-to skin contact can be maintained. Close monitoring by a healthcare worker is required.
- Feeds can be started within 1 hour of delivery. Many of these infants will be able to suck and can be breast-fed. Those who cannot breastfeed should be given expressed breast milk with a cup. When the infant is sucking well from the breast and gaining weight on a daily basis, they can be weaned off cup feeds.
- These infants should be reviewed at least twice a day to assess their feeding ability, fluid intake and the presence of any **danger signs** (*see* Box 3.3.1 below), including signs of serious bacterial infection. Such problems will necessitate close monitoring in a neonatal nursery (if available) in a similar way to the very low birth weight. The risk of keeping the child in hospital (including hospital-acquired infections) should be considered.

Infants with birth weight below 1.75 kg

- These infants are at risk of hypothermia, apnoea, hypoxaemia, sepsis, feed intolerance and necrotising enterocolitis. The smaller the infant, the greater these risks. All infants with a birth weight below 1.75 kg should be admitted to a special care or neonatal intensive care unit (if available).

Other treatments for low-birth-weight and/or preterm infants
Oxygen

Oxygen should be administered via nasal cannulae, nasal prongs or a head box if there are signs of respiratory distress, such as moderate to severe recession (preterm infants may show mild recession with normal breathing), and definitely in the presence of cyanosis. **Pulse oximetry to measure oxygen saturation is a vital part of oxygen usage in the preterm infant.** Retinopathy of prematurity (ROP), previously known as retrolental fibroplasia, which leads to lifelong blindness in many cases, is caused by high blood levels of oxygen saturation in the preterm infant. There is no good evidence for the optimum oxygen saturation for preterm infants. On the one hand it is important to avoid hypoxia, which would lead to brain damage, as the infant is likely to have respiratory problems from surfactant deficiency, and on the other hand unrestricted oxygen may cause ROP, which would lead to blindness. Current advice is that the infant born at or before 32 weeks' gestation or weighing less than 1500 grams at birth should have a target oxygen saturation of 86–92%, which is higher than the oxygen saturation to which the fetus is exposed *in utero*.

Prevention of hypothermia

To prevent hypothermia, nurse the infant in skin-to-skin contact between the mother's breasts ('kangaroo care') or clothed in a warm room, or in an incubator. A hot water bottle wrapped in a towel can be useful for keeping the infant warm if no power for heating is available, but take care not to burn the infant. Aim for an axillary temperature of 36.0–36.5°C, with the feet warm and pink. When the mother is asleep or if she is ill, a clean incubator can be used. Incubators should be washed with disinfectant between infants, and should be of a basic design that can be used appropriately by the staff available.

Fluids

It is best to give fluids enterally. However, if the infant is not well enough (e.g. due to severe respiratory distress), give IV fluids (see Section 3.4). Initially, consider giving approximately 2–4 mL of expressed breast milk every 1 to 2 hours through a nasogastric tube. This can be adjusted depending on the weight and the amount of IV fluids that the infant is receiving. With increasing age and weight gradually increase the volume and timing of each feed (the maximum time interval between feeds should not exceed 4 hours). The total fluid intake of enteral feeds plus IV fluids per 24 hours should adhere to the following fluid management guidelines:

- 60 mL/kg on day 1
- 80–90 mL/kg on day 2
- 100–120 mL/kg on day 3
- 120–150 mL/kg on day 4
- 150–180 mL/kg thereafter.

Some infants can be fed with a cup. Use only expressed breast milk if possible. If 2–4 mL per feed is tolerated (i.e. there is no vomiting, abdominal distension, or gastric aspirates of more than half the feed) the volume can be increased by 1–2 mL per feed each day. Ideally, aim to have feeding established in the first 5 to 7 days so that the IV fluids can be tapered off. Reduce or withhold feeds if signs of poor tolerance occur. As the infant grows, recalculate the feed volume based on the higher weight. Feeds may be increased over the first 2 weeks of life to 150–180 mL/kg/day based on a 3- to 4-hourly feeding pattern.

How to give gastric feeds (see also Section 8.5 on gastric tube management)

Place the baby's lips on the breast even though he or she is unable to suck or attach before each feed. Place expressed breast milk (EBM) in the syringe. Only use fresh milk or milk that has been stored in a refrigerator, and that has not been out of the fridge for more than 1 hour in a hot climate. Check that the tube is in the stomach before every feed or administration of enterally given drugs. Also check that there is not more than 10% of the previous feed in the stomach by gentle aspiration using a 2- or 5-mL syringe. Connect the syringe containing EBM and remove the plunger, giving the milk by gravity over 10–15 minutes per feed. Only if the feed does not flow in should you gently push with the plunger for a few seconds only to get it started. Never push the whole feed in. Observe the infant closely during the feed for signs of respiratory distress that might be due to lung aspiration. Replace the tube every 7 days, or sooner if it is blocked.

Give enteral feeds only if there is no abdominal distension or tenderness, bowel sounds are present, meconium has been passed, and there is no apnoea, low aspirates, no vomiting and adequate stool output.

TABLE 3.3.3 Guide to volumes of each feed given every 3–4 hours at different infant weights

	Day 1	Day 2	Day 3	Day 4	Day 5	Day 6	Day 7	Day 8
Total (mL/kg/day)	60	80	100	120	140	150	160	170
1.25–1.4 kg	10	15	18	20	22	24	25	≥26
1.5–1.9 kg	15	17	19	21	23	25	27	≥27
2.0–2.4 kg	20	22	25	27	30	32	35	≥35
≥2.5 kg	25	28	30	35	35	≥40	≥45	≥50

Blood glucose levels

Check blood glucose levels every 6 hours until enteral feeds are established, and immediately if there are any danger signs of infection.

Infection or feed intolerance

Observe carefully and constantly for infection or feed intolerance.

Apnoea

Monitor for apnoea, ideally with a pulse oximeter (which are now affordable and available in many resource-limited countries), supplemented by close visual monitoring of the infant by the mother or a close relative.

Discharge and follow-up of low-birth-weight infants

Discharge when:

- there are **no danger signs** (see Box 3.3.1), including signs of serious infection
- the infant is gaining weight (at least 20 grams per day for 3 consecutive days) on breastfeeding alone

BOX 3.3.1 Danger signs associated with infection in the neonate

Common danger signs

- Infant feeding less well than before.
- Infant lying quietly and making few spontaneous movements.
- Hypothermia or fever > 38°C.
- Capillary refill time > 3 seconds.
- Respiratory rate ≥ 60 breaths/minute.
- Indrawing of the lower chest wall when breathing, *or* grunting.
- Cyanosis.
- History of a convulsion.

Less common but important signs

- Low respiratory rate (< 20 breaths/minute) or apnoea.
- Jaundice.
- Abdominal distension.

- the infant is able to maintain temperature in the normal range (36–36.5°C axillary) in an open cot or with skin-to-skin care
- the mother is confident and able to take care of the infant.

Low-birth-weight infants should be given all scheduled immunisations by the time of discharge from the health facility or soon after.

Counsel the parents before discharge on:
- exclusive breastfeeding
- keeping the infant warm
- the danger signs that necessitate seeking care (*see* Table 3.3.4), plus advice on when to return for healthcare
- basic life-saving manoeuvres to use in the event of an emergency, particularly mouth-to-mouth and nose ventilation if prolonged apnoea occurs.

Low-birth-weight infants should be followed up at regular intervals following discharge for weighing, assessment of feeding, and assessment of general health until they have reached 2.5 kg in weight.

TABLE 3.3.4 Danger signs for parents of discharged newborns

Seek advice immediately if any of the following occur:	Seek advice very quickly if any of the following occur:
Convulsion(s)	Infant refuses feeds
ANY bleeding	Minor diarrhoea or vomiting
Severe diarrhoea or vomiting	Minor breathing problems
Infant appears unresponsive	Infant is less active/interested
Severe breathing problems	Infant feels abnormally hot
Infant feels cold	Jaundice

Enteral feeding for the newborn infant in hospital

Type of milk

Breast milk will provide the nutrients required by almost all infants. However, for preterm infants the following supplements are needed:

Vitamin D supplementation

Term breastfed infants generally do not need extra vitamin D. However, this is only true if the mother has an adequate vitamin D status. Maternal vitamin D deficiency during pregnancy and lactation is common in resource-limited countries, contributing to the low vitamin D content of breast milk. Newborn infants of mothers who have dark skin or wear concealing clothes are also at greater risk of vitamin D deficiency at birth.

Large amounts of calcium and phosphorus are transferred from the mother to the infant during the last 3 months of pregnancy, helping the infant's bones to grow. Therefore a preterm infant may not receive sufficient amounts of calcium and phosphorus for this purpose. Vitamin D helps the body to absorb calcium from the intestines and kidneys. Very preterm infants require adequate vitamin D supplements. Liver problems such as cholestasis and prolonged use of diuretics or steroids may also cause problems with blood calcium levels.

Therefore, without further supplementation, preterm and also some full-term breastfed infants may be at risk of vitamin D deficiency. This risk may be minimised either by supplementing the mother with large amounts of vitamin D (4000 IU/day) during pregnancy and lactation, or by supplementing the infant directly (400 IU/day) during the period of lactation.

Phosphorus supplements

These may be needed in the case of very small infants, who can become hypophosphataemic (i.e. with plasma phosphorus levels of < 1.5 mmol/litre). If untreated, this may result in metabolic bone disease. The addition of a concentrated phosphorus salt (50 mg/kg/day of phosphorus) to feeds will prevent this. Adding 0.05 mL/kg of a 4 mmol/mL phosphorus solution to each of eight feeds per day will give 50 mg/kg/day of supplemental dietary phosphorus.

Vitamin A supplementation

In resource-limited countries, vitamin A supplementation of the newborn infant reduces mortality. Preterm infants are at high risk of vitamin A deficiency. This important subgroup of our infant population is not only born with inadequate body stores of vitamin A, but is also often unable to tolerate routine oral supplementation. Vitamin A supplementation programmes significantly reduce infant mortality as well as the incidence of xerophthalmia, respiratory infection, and morbidity from gastrointestinal disease. Oral supplementation of 4000 IU/kg/day has been recommended for very-low-birth-weight (VLBW) (< 1500 grams at birth) infants from establishment of full enteral feeding until discharge from the neonatal unit. Supplementing term newborn infants with vitamin A (100 000 IU as a single dose) within 48 hours of birth reduces infant mortality by almost 25%, with those of low birth weight deriving the greatest benefit. Alternatively, **a single dose of 200 000 units can be given to all postpartum mothers within 6 weeks of delivery, when the likelihood of pregnancy is very low, and when infants benefit most from the presence of vitamin A in breast milk.**

Vitamin K

All neonates should be given vitamin K 1 mg IM within 1 hour of birth. Those who require surgery, those with birth trauma, those who are preterm and those exposed before birth to maternal medication (that can interfere with vitamin K) are at high risk of bleeding and must be given vitamin K. If the need for surgery only becomes apparent some time after birth, we suggest that a repeat dose should be given before surgery.

Multivitamin preparation

A multivitamin preparation (preferably containing adequate vitamins A and D) for preterm infants may be commenced from 3 weeks of age. A supply of vitamin D (400 IU/day) is particularly important for bone mineralisation.

Iron supplements

Iron supplements for preterm infants are usually commenced from about 6 weeks of age. Preterm infants have reduced iron stores compared with term infants, especially if the umbilical cord is clamped early. The daily dietary iron supplementation is 2–4 mg/kg of elemental iron, up to a maximum of 16 mg/day.

Breast milk banking

The WHO recommends that low-birth-weight babies who cannot be fed their own mother's breast milk should receive donor milk. The high maternal mortality and morbidity in low-income countries mean that there are many infants who cannot be put to the breast within a few hours of birth, and donor milk is suitable for them. In addition, there is evidence that human donor milk reduces the incidence of severe infection and necrotising enterocolitis (NEC) in low-birth-weight babies, compared with formula milk.

It is possible to establish safe donor milk banks in resource-limited settings, provided that there is a microbiology laboratory able to process donor samples, and a power supply to keep the banked milk frozen. A nurse or other staff member must be trained in good hand hygiene, and the importance of labelling and storage. Only simple equipment is needed.

Milk can be collected from lactating mothers who are known to have tested negative to HIV and syphilis, and are non-smokers. Ideally they have also been screened for hepatitis infections. Milk is collected by hand expression under supervision (as 'drip milk' is lower in calories than expressed milk). A 1-mL aliquot from each donor's sample is sent to the microbiology lab. If colony-forming organisms are grown, the whole sample is discarded. Milk can be stored in a refrigerator while awaiting the microbiology results.

Milk is pasteurised by heating for 30 minutes at 62.5°C, and then cooled and frozen. Pasteurised frozen milk can be stored for up to 6 months from the date of collection. Supplementary formula feeding for the infants of mothers who cannot provide breast milk, or whose mothers have died, may be needed after discussion with the infant's carers.

Fluid and electrolyte management for the neonate in hospital

When giving fluid or blood intravenously, best practice is to use an in-line infusion chamber/burette to avoid fluid overload.

Fluid requirements

Body water content is high at birth and urine output is low for the first few days. Therefore giving large volumes of fluid in the first few days may make an infant oedematous and worsen any respiratory disease. **A simple general rule** is to start an ill newborn infant who cannot take enteral fluids (breast milk) on 60 mL/kg/day IV as 10% dextrose solution, increasing in daily steps of 20–30 mL/kg/day to a maximum of 140–180 mL/kg/day. However, in a small-for-gestational-age infant it may be necessary to begin with 70–90 mL/kg/day in order to meet the glucose requirements.

Ideally, use a 100-mL paediatric intravenous burette where 60 drops = 1 mL and therefore 1 drop/minute = 1 mL/hour.

So for an infant weighing 1.8 kg on day 1: 1.8 × 60 = 108 mL.

In each hour the fluid will be 108 ÷ 24 = 4.5 mL, which corresponds to 9 drops every 2 minutes.

The rate of insensible water loss (mainly through the skin) is high in some circumstances, particularly in infants under 29 weeks' gestation or when an overhead heater (radiant warmer) rather than an incubator is used. Helpful measures for reducing insensible water loss in such cases include the following:

- Place the infant from below the neck in a clean plastic bag to maintain humidity. Maintaining humidity helps to keep very premature infants warm by reducing evaporative heat loss.
- Clothe the infant, or wrap the body below the head with bubble wrap or aluminium kitchen foil (with the shiny side facing inward towards the infant).
- When an overhead heater is used, the infant should not be covered, and the heater output must be adjusted in direct response to the infant's skin temperature (typically achieved by a continuous temperature probe servo system). Alternatively, a plastic bag over the infant's body from the neck down can help to preserve heat.
- In the first week of life, high rates of insensible water loss will be reflected by high rates of weight loss (more than 10% of birth weight), and often an increase in the plasma sodium concentration to 150 mmol/litre or higher. If either occurs, the infant is dehydrated and fluid intake should be increased by 30 mL/kg/day. When nursing a low-birth-weight infant under an overhead heater, it is advisable to add an extra allowance of 30 mL/kg/day right from the start (i.e. start on day 1 at 90 mL/kg/day rather than 60 mL/kg/day).

Note, however, that even 30 mL/kg/day might not be enough to meet the insensible losses of a very preterm infant (29 weeks or less) under a radiant heater. Such infants are much better nursed in closed incubators.

In very-low-birth-weight infants, enteral feeds should be advanced slowly in 20–30 mL/kg/day increments. Infants who are being enterally fed but who are unable to breastfeed can be given expressed breast milk by orogastric tube or cup. A general plan for fluid enhancement is as follows:

- day 1: 60 mL/kg/day
- day 2: 85 (range 80–90) mL/kg/day
- day 3: 110 (range 100–120) mL/kg/day
- day 4: 135 (range 120–150) mL/kg/day
- day 5 and thereafter: 165 (range 150–180) mL/kg/day.

Monitor the fluid intake by weighing the infant daily and recording the frequency of urine output.

To weigh the baby, first place a blanket in the scales, set them to zero and then place the baby naked in the scales and cover the infant with the blanket to keep them warm. Fluid intake may need to be adjusted frequently to maintain fluid balance. Urine output can be monitored by measuring the difference between wet nappies (diapers) and a dry one using accurate scales. Generally expect at least eight wet nappies in a 24-hour period. Look out for signs of fluid overload (oedema) or dehydration. If possible measure the plasma electrolytes, but remember that these cannot be interpreted without information on body weight and urine output.

Electrolyte requirements when giving IV fluids
Sodium requirements

Infants over 48 hours of age need some sodium supplementation in a dose of 2–3 mmol/kg/day. This can most easily be given by adding 20 mL/kg of normal saline (0.9%) to the daily requirement of 10% glucose to make up the total daily fluid volume needed. This gives approximately 3 mmol of sodium per kg.

Adding sodium is open to many errors. Ready-made neonatal fluids are available in some countries, and may be used to avoid this problem in some situations. The sodium requirements of very preterm infants may be much higher, as urinary sodium losses may approximate 10 mmol/kg/day in those of 29 weeks' gestation or less.

Sodium can be commenced on the third day of life (after 48 hours) in infants receiving intravenous fluids, but if there is respiratory distress it is wise to wait until the diuresis associated with recovery begins (this is often delayed until the third or fourth day of life).

Potassium requirements

Potassium supplementation in a dose of 1–2 mmol/kg/day will meet requirements and can be provided by adding mathematically correct and smal amounts of potassium chloride to a 10% glucose fluid. If IV potassium is given, the plasma potassium concentration must be monitored daily. Potassium can be added to fluids but this should be done very carefully. **Remember that too much IV potassium can be fatal.** The concentration of KCl in peripheral IV solutions should never exceed 40 mmol/litre. **Do not add KCl until the urine output is well established.**

Remember that it is best to give potassium and calcium supplements orally, unless very low serum values are identified.

Glucose requirements

Infusing glucose at the following rates will match the normal hepatic glucose output and therefore maintain the blood glucose concentration at an acceptable level:

- term infant: 3–5 mg/kg/minute
- preterm, appropriate weight for gestation: 4–6 mg/kg/minute
- small for gestational age: 6–8 mg/kg/minute.

A solution of 10% glucose at 60 mL/kg/day will give 4 mg (0.22 mmol) glucose/kg/minute.

These infusion rates provide minimal glucose requirements to maintain a normal blood glucose level, but higher rates will be required for growth. Consider hyperinsulinism as a cause of the problem if an infant requires higher rates of infusion to maintain normoglycaemia. Always use 5% or ideally 10% glucose/dextrose for peripheral IV infusions; an umbilical venous catheter will be needed if high glucose requirements or limits on fluid volume necessitate a more concentrated solution which will be damaging to thin peripheral veins.

Composite maintenance fluid

An alternative way to make a simple composite maintenance fluid is by adding the following to give a total volume of 100 mL:

- 1/5 dextrose saline (0.18% normal saline with 5% dextrose) = 71 mL
- 7.4% KCl = 2 mL
- 10% calcium gluconate = 2 mL
- 25% dextrose = 25 mL
- **Total volume = 100 mL.**

Each 100 mL of the above solution would contain dextrose 10%, KCl 2 mEq, Ca 2 mEq and sodium 2.5–3 mmol. **Any such mixture must be prepared under sterile conditions.**

Remember that KCl should not be added until urine output is well established.

Drug use in the newborn infant

Relatively few drugs are needed to deal with most common neonatal emergencies.

The IV route should be used if the infant is already being given IV fluids, as this will reduce the amount of pain to which the child is subjected. There are dangers associated with rapid administration or breaking into an existing IV line, leading to an increased risk of sepsis. Erecting an IV line merely to administer drugs also risks exposing the child to dangerous fluid overload, unless a syringe pump can be used to control the rate at which fluid is infused.

Common emergency problems that require hospital care in the first month of life

Many emergencies can be prevented by attention to good feeding practices, providing adequate warmth and preventing infection. The more preterm or low birth weight the infant, the more likely it is that the following complications will occur:

- feeding difficulties
- poor temperature control, especially hypothermia
- infection – prevention and early recognition and safe management are essential
- polycythaemia
- respiratory distress and apnoeic attacks
- bleeding
- jaundice and neonatal anaemia
- reduced conscious level and seizures, including hypoglycaemia
- surgical problems.

Feeding difficulties

Infants born after 34 weeks are generally mature enough to suck and swallow well, but may be less demanding of feeds than term infants. Attention to the following can help all newborn infants, especially those born preterm, to establish breastfeeding:

- Encourage early and prolonged skin contact.
- Encourage small frequent feeds by waking the infant every 2 to 3 hours and putting them to the breast.
- If the infant will not latch on and suck, the mother can be encouraged to express breast milk and offer it to the infant by cup and/or spoon or if not accepted by orogastric or nasogastric tube.
- If an otherwise well infant on breast milk feeds is experiencing inadequate growth, an inadequate milk supply may be the problem. There are several possible causes for this, which can usually be identified by listening to the mother and then watching the infant feed. A relaxed mother will have a good 'let-down' reflex which gives the infant the more calorie-rich hind milk as well as the fore milk. The mother can tell when she has 'let down' by a tingling feeling in her breasts, and the infant starts to swallow rapidly. The infant must latch on properly for feeding to be successful, and this may need some assistance from the midwife. The best way to increase the milk supply for a hungry infant who is not thriving is to increase the feed frequency. Breast milk works on

a demand-and-supply system, so the more the infant demands, the more the breast supplies. If the infant is not feeding vigorously enough to increase the milk supply, the mother should express milk after feeding and give it to the infant as described above.

- Avoid giving formula or breast milk by bottle. A small feeding cup (about the size of a medicine measuring cup, with a smooth rim) or a spoon can be used to feed the infant.
- Give expressed breast milk via orogastric or nasogastric tube if the infant is too unwell to suck or drink from a cup.
- As the infant becomes stronger, encourage a transition to demand breastfeeding.

Feeding problems

- **Ingested meconium/blood.** Infants who have swallowed a lot of meconium or blood before birth may retch and appear distressed after birth. Such problems almost always settle within a few hours without any intervention.
- **Uncoordinated feeding.** Infants born before 32 weeks' gestation often have difficulty sucking and swallowing in a coordinated way. Most will initially need some tube feeds. They are not likely to start gaining weight until they are taking at least 120 mL/kg of milk a day. Infants need to be fed regularly at least once every 4 hours, day and night. Breast milk can be supplemented with formula milk at this time if donor milk is not available. However, every effort needs to be made to sustain the mother's lactation by expression and by keeping the mother in hospital to be near her infant.
- **Regurgitation.** Hurried frequent feeding may cause regurgitation. A poorly developed cough reflex can cause the infant to inhale milk into the lung, resulting in possible pneumonitis and even pneumonia. Newborn infants benefit from frequent small feeds every 2 to 3 hours. Feeds should be increased gradually over the first 3 to 5 days of life. Patience is required. Dehydration (and the risk of hypoglycaemia) need to be monitored, and can be prevented during this period by giving supplemental gastric or IV fluids so that total fluid intake (i.e. taking the gastric/IV and the oral intake together) does not fall below 120 mL/kg per day.
- **Feeding tubes.** Tube feeding is the best option for infants who have not yet developed a coordinated suck and swallow reflex. Nasogastric tubes are popular, easier to secure and less easily pushed out by the infant's tongue, but they can almost completely block one nostril, significantly increasing the work of breathing. Therefore orogastric tubes are preferred if respiratory distress is present. Alternatively, a fine-bore nasogastric tube can be left in place and changed as required (up to a maximum of 7 days). Small frail infants should be handled as little and as gently as possible, and can be left lying undisturbed in their cots during a tube feed so long as the head end of the cot is elevated 25 cm.

Temperature control and hypothermia prevention and treatment

Hypothermia can be due to a cold environment, but remember that **starvation** or **serious infection** can present as hypothermia.

Normal temperatures for newborn infants are **36.5–37.5°C (axillary)** if measured over 3 minutes, and lower (around **36.0–36.5°C**) if measured over at least 1 minute. Rectal thermometers are difficult to use and can be dangerous. If the trunk is cold, the infant is almost certainly hypothermic.

Use a **low-reading digital thermometer**, not a mercury thermometer. If the axillary temperature is less than 32°C, hypothermia is severe; if it is in the range 32–35.9°C the infant has moderate hypothermia. If the infant's temperature does not register on the normal thermometer, assume that they have hypothermia.

Hypothermia can be prevented by the following measures:

- Dry the infant well immediately after birth and place them in skin-to-skin contact with the mother. This is especially important for low-birth-weight infants who do not have other complications. For those with medical problems, warm the infant by skin-to-skin care. If there are adequate resources and staff, an overhead radiant heater **or** an air-heated incubator (set at 35–36°C) can be used.
- 'Kangaroo care' (skin-to-skin contact with the mother between her breasts and covered with a blanket) is the most effective method for all infants, especially for those of low-birth-weight. Randomised trials in both well-resourced and resource-limited countries have shown significant advantages to this technique for the infant and the mother, including an increased prevalence of breastfeeding, a reduced incidence of apnoea and a reduced risk of infection. Take care when examining the infant not to allow the temperature to fall (ideally room temperature in the hospital ward should be higher than 25°C).
- A cot heated **with a hot-water bottle with the top screwed in tightly and wrapped in a clean towel** can be just as effective if the above are not available. Ordinary domestic radiant heaters or electrical blower type heaters can also be effective.
- Cover the infant's head with a warm woollen hat and dress them in **warm, dry clothes**. Keeping the nappy dry is also very helpful.
- Avoid overheating by monitoring the axillary temperature 4- to 6-hourly.
- Feed the infant 2-to 3-hourly, and continue with 4-hourly feeds during the night.
- Avoid washing the infant before they are 24 hours of age.
- Do not leave the infant where there are any draughts.
- The infant should sleep either with or next to the mother during the night.

The development of incubators earlier in the twentieth century significantly reduced the mortality of preterm infants, but they are expensive, and require regular maintenance, thorough cleaning and sufficient numbers of trained staff. The nursing of infants in incubators is covered by standard texts, but Table 3.3.5 gives the settings from which to start, adjusting the incubator temperature up or down to maintain the infant's axillary temperature at 36.0–36.5°C.

TABLE 3.3.5 Incubator temperature guidelines

Weight of baby (grams)	Day 1	Day 2	Day 3	Day 4 and subsequently
< 1200	35.0°C	34.0°C	34.0°C	33.5°C
1200–1500	34.0°C	34.0°C	33.5°C	33.5°C
1500–2500	33.5°C	33.0°C	32.0°C	32.0°C
> 2500	33.0°C	32.5°C	31.0°C	30.5°C

Do not use antipyretic drugs to control fever in a newborn infant. Instead control the environment (e.g. remove some clothes, adjust incubator temperature) and always consider the possibility of serious infection.

Prevention of neonatal infection

A newborn infant with risk factors for infection (membranes ruptured more than 18 hours before delivery, mother with fever > 38°C before delivery or during labour, or foul-smelling/purulent amniotic fluid) should be treated with prophylactic antibiotics (ampicillin and gentamicin IM or IV) for at least 2 days. After 2 days the infant should be reassessed and treatment continued if there are signs of sepsis (or a positive blood culture).

Simple measures that can prevent infection in the newborn include the following:

- Ensure a **clean delivery environment** for the mother and infant, including disinfectant cream for all maternal vaginal examinations (e.g. Hibitane cream).
- **Good cord care:** the WHO recommends that the cord be kept clean and dry. It should not be covered. Local applications of creams, ointments, etc. are generally not required except in high-risk settings, where application of an antiseptic is recommended. An antiseptic solution or cream such as 4% chlorhexidine has recently been shown to reduce omphalitis and resulting neonatal mortality. It should be applied immediately after birth and for several days thereafter if possible, preferably after every nappy change. Similarly, there is extensive successful experience with the application of surgical spirit or iodine solution to the cord.
- **Exclusive breastfeeding.**
- Strict procedures for **hand washing** or the use of hand sprays or hand rubs for all staff and for families before and after handling infants.
- **Not using water for humidification** in incubators (where *Pseudomonas* can easily colonise).
- **Cleaning incubators with an antiseptic before use** (if skin-to-skin mother care is not possible).
- **Strict sterility for all invasive procedures.**
- **Sterile injection practices.**
- **Remove intravenous drips** when they are no longer necessary.
- **Keep invasive procedures (e.g. blood sampling, unnecessary IV cannulation) to a minimum**, only undertaking them when they are essential.

Early-onset sepsis (first 72 hours)

Early-onset sepsis usually occurs as a result of bacteria acquired by vertical transmission from mother to infant during labour and delivery. The most frequently observed organisms vary from one part of the world to another. Gram-negative enteric bacteria (especially *Escherichia coli and Klebsiella* species) predominate in many regions. Gram-positive cocci are also common, and include group B beta-haemolytic streptococcus, other streptococcal species, *Staphylococcus* and *Enterococcus*. Rarely *Listeria monocytogenes* is isolated from newborn infants with sepsis, especially when there are foodborne epidemics.

Maternal risk factors for early-onset sepsis

These include the following:
- maternal fever (especially 38°C or higher) before delivery or during labour
- pre-labour rupture of membranes
- prolonged rupture of membranes (18 hours or longer)
- preterm labour
- maternal bacteriuria during pregnancy (including *E. coli* and group B beta-haemolytic streptococcus)
- prior infected infant (group B beta-haemolytic streptococcus).

Early-onset sepsis in the newborn usually results from bacteria acquired from the mother at or shortly before delivery. These infants mostly present with respiratory distress, and have bacteraemia or pneumonia. However, vaginal cultures cannot be used to determine the choice of antibiotics when treating the symptomatic newborn.

Late-onset sepsis

Organisms are less likely to reflect those of the maternal genital tract, although the same pathogens may be identified in infants presenting from home. The most common infections are focal ones such as conjunctivitis, omphalitis, skin infections and meningitis. A circumcision wound can also be the site of serious infection.

In the hospital setting, infection is more commonly due to nosocomial pathogens, including coagulase-negative staphylococci, Gram-negative enteric bacteria (e.g. *Klebsiella oxytoca, Klebsiella pneumoniae, Enterobacter cloacae*), *Staphylococcus aureus*, *Pseudomonas* species, streptococcal species and *Enterococcus*. Fungal sepsis must also be considered. Investigate as for early-onset sepsis, with the inclusion of a lumbar puncture and suprapubic urine for analysis and culture if indicated, and treat empirically with parenteral broad-spectrum antibiotic therapy directed towards the most commonly encountered pathogens for the particular nursery. Once cultures are positive, therapy can be directed accordingly. (For details of treatment of sepsis, see Section 3.4.)

Laboratory evaluation of the unwell infant

In an infant who is generally unwell with no clinically obvious infective focus, the following investigations should be performed:
- **Blood culture (about 1 mL of venous blood):** This should be obtained from a peripheral vein after preparing

the skin with an antibacterial wash such as povidone-iodine and/or 70% ethanol or isopropyl alcohol. Blood culture is the gold standard for neonatal sepsis, but it is not 100% sensitive. The sensitivity may be further reduced if intrapartum antibiotics were administered to the mother antenatally. The results can be assessed at 48 hours.

- **White blood cell and differential cell count are not helpful in most situations.**
- **Chest X-ray:** This may be helpful if there are any respiratory signs, but not if it means taking the infant to another department in the hospital. A portable chest X-ray is ideal.
- **Lumbar puncture if indicated:** cytology, chemistry, Gram stain and culture. Not routinely done on all infants with suspected infection unless there are neurological signs.
- **C-reactive protein (CRP):** This is an inexpensive and useful test which may take 12 hours to become positive after the onset of an infection if this is present.
- **Blood glucose concentration.**
- **Serum bilirubin concentration:** if the infant appears jaundiced.
- **Surface cultures (ear canal, umbilical stump) and gastric aspirate cultures:** these do not correlate with either the likelihood of sepsis or the causative agent in septic infants. **These cultures should not be obtained.**
- **Midstream or suprapubic aspirate of urine for culture:** This procedure is of little value in the infant with suspected sepsis shortly after birth, but may be positive in infants with new-onset symptoms later in the first week (≥ 3 days). A urinary tract infection should always be considered in neonates with late-onset sepsis.

In seriously sick infants with suspected sepsis, priority should be given to the structured ABC approach, while simultaneously obtaining a blood culture followed by prompt administration of antibiotics. Other tests, such as a lumbar puncture if needed (see above), can be performed once the infant is stable and antibiotics have been started. (For details of treatment of sepsis, *see* Section 3.4.)

Infants who are vulnerable to maternal factors

The infant of a diabetic mother

If a diabetic mother is poorly controlled, her infant may be large for gestational age, putting him or her at risk of slow progress in labour and perhaps shoulder dystocia. At birth, the infant, although large, behaves in a similar manner to a preterm infant. There is a major risk of hypoglycaemia, caused by the intrauterine over-stimulation of the infant pancreas to produce abnormally high levels of insulin. The infant must be monitored at least hourly for hypoglycaemia in the first 6 hours, and should then be monitored 4-hourly for hypoglycaemia, which should be treated as described above with an infusion of 10% dextrose. The infant of a diabetic mother has immature lung maturation and is liable to surfactant deficiency (*see* Section 3.4), poor feeding and jaundice. Polycythaemia is also more likely.

The infant of a mother who is dependent on alcohol or drugs of addiction

These infants have been exposed to significant levels of narcotic drugs or alcohol *in utero*, causing an increased risk of congenital abnormalities and of abnormal neurological development and behaviour during childhood. Soon after birth they may show hyper-irritability and convulsions, requiring treatment and gradually reducing sedation as they are 'weaned off' the addictive drugs to which they have been exposed. These infants are also at risk of having been exposed to bloodborne viruses such as HIV and hepatitis B and C.

Birth injuries
Swellings around the head

- The commonest is a **caput succedaneum**, which is oedematous tissue over the occiput present after a vaginal delivery. This usually resolves within a few days and is of no consequence, requiring no intervention.
- A **cephalhaematoma** is a lateral (sometimes bilateral) fluctuant swelling, well circumscribed by the sutures. It does not cross the midline and anatomically represents a sub-periosteal haemorrhage. There may be an associated skull fracture, but neither this nor the swelling itself usually needs treatment. The only important complication can be worsening of jaundice as the blood is degraded and reabsorbed. **Never aspirate blood from a cephalhaematoma, as this can cause a serious infection.**
- A **subaponeurotic haemorrhage** (bleeding between the skull periosteum and the scalp aponeurosis) is the least common but most dangerous scalp swelling. It represents haemorrhage beneath the aponeurosis of the scalp. Onset and progression is often insidious, with progressive pallor due to significant haemorrhage. The boggy swelling of the head, extending from above the eyes to the occiput, may only be noticed after the infant has developed hypovolaemic shock. The infant may develop bruising behind the ears and around the eyes. This must be recognised early, as these infants often need urgent transfusion. Injection of vitamin K should be given.

Nerve palsies

- **Facial nerve palsies** are sometimes associated with forceps delivery. They usually resolve within a few days, requiring little intervention.
- **Brachial plexus trauma** may follow shoulder dystocia or a difficult breech delivery, and reflects traction injury to the upper roots of the brachial plexus. The arm is flaccid and the wrist flexed. This can most clearly be demonstrated by eliciting an asymmetric Moro reflex. Look for signs of respiratory distress, as the phrenic nerve on the same side is sometimes affected. An X-ray should be obtained to exclude a pseudoparesis associated with clavicular fracture or syphilitic osteitis. The humerus should also be included in the X-ray to rule out **humeral fractures**, which may occasionally be present. Most brachial plexus palsies resolve within 3 to 4 weeks of delivery, but rarely they can be permanent. Once fractures have been ruled out, the mother can be shown how to perform passive movements to reduce the possibility of joint contractures developing. Refer

the infant for a surgical opinion if they are not better by 4 weeks.

Fractures

The most common types are **skull and clavicular fractures**. These usually require no specific treatment. However, significant skull fractures must be evaluated for intracranial bleeding. There should also be consideration of whether the injury is a birth-associated one or a subsequent inflicted injury perpetrated by a caregiver.

Common external congenital abnormalities

Talipes equinovarus

Talipes equinovarus is a fixed inversion and flexion deformity of the foot at the ankle, in which the foot cannot easily be put in a normal position. It is helpful to note that this form of fixed talipes is usually associated with the presence of a groove on the medial aspect of the foot. Treatment is required. The foot should be splinted and strapped in the position closest to normal, and an orthopaedic surgeon's advice must be sought (*see* Section 5.17). Whenever talipes is present, be sure to examine the hips carefully for evidence of developmental dysplasia (also known as 'congenital dislocation of the hip'). It is also important to examine the back for a spinal defect and evidence of neurological deficit.

The common variation (positional talipes) where the foot can easily be brought into the normal position does not require treatment.

Extra digits

These are very common. It is important to distinguish a simple skin tag from a true extra digit containing bone or cartilage. The latter may be associated with other congenital anomalies, particularly of the heart, spine, kidney or gut. Skin tags are inherited and are of cosmetic significance only. Skin tags are often held by only a thin pedicle of tissue, which can be ligated at the base, usually causing the tag to fall off a few days later.

Supernumerary nipples and pre-auricular skin tags

These are often found and are of cosmetic concern only. No intervention is required.

Further reading

World Health Organization (2012) *Born Too Soon: The Global Action Report on Preterm Birth*. www.who.int/pmnch/media/news/2012/preterm_birth_report/en/index.html

---

3.4 Neonatal illnesses and emergencies

Sepsis in the neonate

Recognising and treating neonatal infection

Bacterial sepsis (septicaemia) in the newborn infant may present with any number of subtle non-specific changes in activity or physical findings. A change in feeding pattern, vomiting, irritability, pallor, diminished tone and/or decreased skin perfusion is suggestive of neonatal infection. Other presenting physical findings may include lethargy, apnoea, tachypnoea, cyanosis, petechiae or early jaundice. There may be fever, but this is not common, especially with bacterial infections occurring in the first week. However, temperature instability with hypothermia may be seen. Abnormal glucose homeostasis (hypoglycaemia or hyperglycaemia) and/or metabolic acidosis are commonly associated findings. Infants, especially preterm infants, are very prone to infection and can become ill very rapidly once infection takes hold. Antibiotic treatment is only likely to work if started early, but the recognition of early infection is not easy. A WHO study showed that more than a third of all deaths in the first month of life in most resource-limited countries were caused by infection. It also found that more than 80% of these infants, when first seen, had **one or more of the following eight danger signs associated with infection in the neonate**:

- infant feeding less than well than before
- infant lying quiet and making few spontaneous movements
- hypothermia or fever > 38°C
- capillary refill time > 3 seconds
- respiratory rate ≥ 60 breaths/minute
- indrawing of the lower chest wall when breathing, *or* grunting
- cyanosis
- history of a convulsion.

Less common but important signs include the following:
- low respiratory rate (< 20 breaths/minute) or apnoea
- jaundice
- abdominal distension
- skin infections.

All neonates with signs of sepsis need immediate hospital admission if they are not already there, and must be treated with IV antibiotics for at least 10 days after blood and other appropriate cultures have been taken.

Ampicillin (or penicillin) plus gentamicin are the first-line drugs to be used. Consider adding cloxacillin or flucloxacillin if there are signs suggesting that *Staphylococcus aureus* is a cause (e.g. skin pustules, abscess, omphalitis). Blood cultures are ideal although not always possible before starting antibiotics. If the infant does not respond within 48 hours, consider changing the antibiotic. If there is a possibility of meningitis, risk of resistance or Gram-negative organisms, a third-generation cephalosporin such as cefotaxime or ceftriaxone should also be added.

Causes of early-onset sepsis (first 72 hours)

Early-onset sepsis usually occurs as a result of bacteria acquired by vertical transmission from mother to infant during late pregnancy, labour and delivery. The most frequently observed organisms vary from one part of the world to another. Gram-negative enterics (especially *Escherichia coli* and *Klebsiella* species) predominate in many regions. Gram-positive cocci are also common, and include group B beta-haemolytic streptococcus, other streptococcal species, *Staphylococcus* and *Enterococcus*. Less commonly, *Listeria monocytogenes* is isolated from newborn infants with sepsis, especially when there are foodborne epidemics.

These infants mostly present with respiratory distress. However, vaginal cultures cannot be used to determine the choice of antibiotics when treating the symptomatic newborn.

Late-onset sepsis

Organisms are less likely to reflect those of the maternal genital tract, although the same pathogens may be identified in infants presenting from home. The most common infections are focal infections such as conjunctivitis, omphalitis, skin infections and meningitis. A circumcision wound can also be the site of serious infection.

In the hospital setting, infection is more commonly caused by nosocomial pathogens, including coagulase-negative staphylococci, Gram-negative enteric bacteria (e.g. *Klebsiella oxytoca*, *Klebsiella pneumoniae*, *Enterobacter cloacae*), *Staphylococcus aureus*, *Pseudomonas* species, streptococcal species and *Enterococcus*. Fungal sepsis must also be considered. Investigate as for early-onset sepsis (see below), with the inclusion of a lumbar puncture and suprapubic urine for analysis and culture if indicated, and treat empirically with parenteral broad-spectrum antibiotic therapy directed towards the most commonly encountered pathogens for the particular nursery. Once cultures are positive, therapy must be directed accordingly.

Laboratory evaluation of the unwell infant

In the case of an infant who is generally unwell with no clinically obvious infective focus, the following investigations should be performed if laboratory facilities are available:

- **Blood culture (about 1 mL of venous blood):** This should be obtained from a peripheral vein after preparing the skin with an antibacterial wash such as povidone-iodine and/or 70% ethanol or isopropyl alcohol. Blood culture is the gold standard for neonatal sepsis, but it is not 100% sensitive. The sensitivity may be further reduced if intrapartum antibiotics were administered to the mother antenatally.
- **White blood cell count (WBC) with differential cell count is generally unhelpful in this setting.**
- **Chest X ray:** This may be helpful if there are any respiratory signs, but not if it means taking the infant to another department in the hospital. A portable chest X-ray is ideal (if available).
- **Lumbar puncture if indicated:** cytology, chemistry, Gram stain and culture. Not routinely done on all infants with suspected infection unless there are neurological signs.
- **C-reactive protein (CRP):** This is an inexpensive and useful test which may take 12 hours to become positive if an infection is present. A negative test at 48 hours in a well infant suggests that antibiotics can be stopped.

- Blood glucose concentration.
- **Serum bilirubin concentration** if the infant appears jaundiced.
- **Surface cultures** (ear canal, umbilical stump) and gastric aspirate cultures do not correlate with either the likelihood of sepsis or the causative agent in septic infants. **These cultures should not be obtained.**
- **A midstream or suprapubic aspirate of urine for microscopy and culture:** This procedure is of little value in the infant suspected of having sepsis shortly after birth, but it may have a greater yield in infants with new-onset symptoms later in the first week (≥ 3 days). A urinary tract infection should always be considered in neonates with late-onset sepsis, and the same antibiotics should be used as for other serious infections unless cultures dictate otherwise.

In seriously ill infants with suspected sepsis, priority should be given to the structured ABC approach, while simultaneously obtaining a blood culture followed by prompt administration of antibiotics. Other tests, such as a lumbar puncture, can be performed once the infant is stable and antibiotics have been started.

Specific neonatal infections
Meningitis and/or septicaemia

Meningitis may occur at any time in the neonatal period, and is frequently fatal, with some survivors experiencing long-term sequelae. Survival and later prognosis depend on early diagnosis and rapid treatment. Confirmatory diagnosis from a lumbar puncture may take several hours. Therefore it is urgent and appropriate to start antibiotic treatment empirically as soon as the diagnosis is suspected.

Presenting features of meningitis: These include lethargy, reduced or complete lack of willingness to take feeds, irritability, a high-pitched cry, apnoeic episodes, lowered conscious level or even coma, hypotonia, convulsions, generalised signs of accompanying sepsis, and a bulging or tense anterior fontanelle. **Always measure and record the head circumference.**

However, once signs such as the above are present, treatment may be unsuccessful and survivors may be handicapped. **Therefore any infant with the following danger signs should be started on antibiotics IV and the relevant investigations undertaken:**

- infant feeding less well than before
- infant lying quiet and making few spontaneous movements
- hypothermia or fever > 38°C
- capillary refill time > 3 seconds
- respiratory rate ≥ 60 breaths/minute
- indrawing of the lower chest wall when breathing, *or* grunting
- cyanosis
- history of a convulsion.

Less common but important signs include the following:

- low respiratory rate (< 20 breaths/minute) or apnoea
- jaundice
- abdominal distension
- skin infections.

Treatment of suspected bacterial septicaemia with or without early meningitis

- Ensure that the **airway** is open and keep it open.
- Ensure that the infant is **breathing** adequately, and if they are apnoeic, gasping or have a very low respiratory rate, consider **ventilation** using a bag and mask until they are breathing adequately.
- If the infant is cyanosed, give them **oxygen** until they are pink or show normal oxygen saturation in air (> 92%).
- Insert an **IV cannula**, using full sterile precautions. Umbilical vein catheterisation may be the most effective way to gain vascular access quickly in a shocked infant less than 1 week old (*see* Section 8.4.B). Otherwise it might be necessary to site an **intra-osseous** line or cannulate a **scalp vein**.
- Take samples for full blood count, CRP, blood culture, lumbar puncture, blood glucose and other tests (urine microscopy and culture, chest X-ray, biochemical tests) if needed (and available). Failure to sterilise the skin rigorously can render blood culture results uninterpretable. Chlorhexidine, 0.5% aqueous solution, is a very effective antiseptic. Use two different swabs, applying each for 10 seconds, and then leave the skin to dry for 30 seconds. A keyhole drape and no-touch technique will reduce the risk of recontamination, especially when performing lumbar puncture or suprapubic aspiration.
- If possible, check **blood glucose levels**, but if facilities do not allow this, give 2 mL/kg of 10% glucose IV over 2–3 minutes as an initial bolus, followed by 5 mL/kg of 10% glucose per hour for the next few days while enteral feeds are established. An infant who becomes alert and active immediately following the initial bolus is suggestive of hypoglycaemia (i.e. a blood glucose concentration of < 2.5 mmol/litre, or < 36 mg/dL), and this may be part of the problem. If an IV line cannot be inserted and hypoglycaemia is suspected, give expressed breast milk or 10% glucose by nasogastric tube or sublingual sucrose. Further intermittent monitoring of the blood glucose level should be undertaken and the infusion continued until it is clear that the infant is well enough to be fed orally.
- Give the first dose of **ampicillin and gentamicin** (or **cefotaxime** *or* **ceftriaxone**) intravenously using the dose regimen outlined at the end of this section. Remember to use the high meningitic dose if meningitis is suspected, and continue it for the duration of therapy if meningitis is confirmed. If IV access is not immediately possible, give the initial antibiotic dose IM. Never wait for the results of cultures before starting antibiotics. Any delay can reduce the infant's chances of survival as well as leading to permanent damage if meningitis is present.
- Start an IV infusion of 60 mL/kg/24 hours of 10% dextrose (or 1/5 normal saline with 5% dextrose) if at all possible.
- If the infant is shocked, give an IV bolus of 10 mL/kg of Ringer-lactate or Hartmann's solution. This can be repeated twice (giving a total of 30 mL/kg) if the infant remains shocked. The use of inotropes (dopamine and dobutamine) (if available) can be considered in such situations, although the outlook is bleak if they are needed.
- If the child has any respiratory symptoms, take a portable chest X-ray (if facilities are available). Do not take a sick infant to an X-ray department for this, as the resulting information is not worth the risks of moving them. Look regularly to see whether cyanosis is developing, or use

a pulse oximeter (if available) and give supplemental oxygen, preferably using nasal cannulae rather than a head box. Infants who become infected during delivery develop respiratory symptoms with progressive signs of septic shock within a few hours of birth. Do not give anything by mouth to an infant who is breathless, especially if there is additional evidence of oxygen dependency.

Points to consider

- Undertake the **ABC approach**. Oxygen may be needed. If the conscious level is impaired, the airway may be at risk.
- Be alert for the presence of seizures, and treat them as appropriate. **Always consider meningitis as a possible cause.** If there are any features suggestive of meningitis, perform a lumbar puncture at the same time as blood cultures or within 2 hours of starting antibiotic treatment, because the blood culture is sterile in 15% of infants with early meningitis. **Do not delay antibiotic therapy pending the undertaking of a lumbar puncture.** Treat seizures with phenobarbitone 20 mg/kg IM or by slow IV injection. If needed, continue with phenobarbitone at a maintenance dose of 3–5 mg/kg/day. Diazepam or midazolam can also sometimes be used to control seizures. However, always have a bag and mask available if diazepam or midazolam are given to stop fitting, as these drugs cause temporary apnoea in some patients, which can easily be managed with bag-and-mask ventilation until the infant is breathing adequately.
- Microscopic examination of the CSF (in meningitis the white blood cell count is ≥ 25 cells/mm^3), low glucose levels and high protein levels with or without Gram stain can provide early confirmation of meningitis. **Remember that a differential white blood cell count or a differential count in the CSF do not help with the decision to initiate or continue antibiotic treatment.**
- Surface swabs and gastric aspirate cultures have no diagnostic significance. However, urinary tract infection can occasionally be the primary focus of a Gram-negative septicaemic illness. Simple microscopy on a clean catch or suprapubic urine specimen may be used to rule out a urinary tract infection. Identification of a urinary tract infection may suggest the need for ultrasound imaging of the renal tract and long-term prophylactic antibiotics.
- Watch for, prevent and correct any sign of hypothermia (skin-to-skin mother care).
- Antibiotics can be stopped after 48 hours if the blood cultures are negative **and** the infant is clinically well. If available, a normal CRP at 48 hours can help to exclude sepsis. If blood cultures are not available, continue the antibiotics for the full course appropriate for the site of infection (meningitis 14–21 days).
- Think also of herpes infection, congenital TORCH infection (newborn intrauterine-acquired infections, including toxoplasmosis, parvovirus B19, syphilis, HIV, varicella, coxsackie, rubella and cytomegalovirus) or neonatal malaria (rare) in a malaria-endemic region.

Antibiotic treatment

- **Beta-lactam antibiotics plus aminoglycosides** act synergistically in treating some of the most frequently encountered neonatal pathogens. Commonly used agents are ampicillin and gentamicin, but alternative broad-spectrum coverage may be used. Penicillin may be used if ampicillin is not available, but it has a narrower spectrum, limited to Gram-positive bacteria. Ampicillin may also provide better coverage for certain Gram-positive pathogens, including *Listeria*.

- **Third-generation cephalosporins** such as cefotaxime and ceftriaxone may be used, but some Gram-positive bacteria may not be covered (e.g. *Enterococcus*, *Listeria*) if a penicillin derivative is not included. Infants with suspected Gram-negative meningitis and accompanying early-onset sepsis may benefit from inclusion of a third-generation cephalosporin which offers a theoretically greater penetration and killing power for enteric bacteria in the cerebrospinal fluid. These antibiotics may be given intramuscularly if IV access cannot be obtained. **Frequent use of these drugs may contribute to the development of multi-drug-resistant strains of bacteria in nurseries.** Ceftriaxone has a longer half-life and can be dosed once daily.

- **Cloxacillin** (IV or oral) is preferable if septic spots are present, as these are usually caused by coagulase-positive staphylococci.

- **Second-line antibiotics** (e.g. ciprofloxacin, vancomycin, meropenem, piperacillin-tazobactam, linezolid) may be helpful for treating nosocomial infections and resistant organisms. However, their use should be limited to proven multi-drug-resistant organisms. Advice can always be sought on these from nearby referral centres. Inappropriate use of these expensive antibiotics may lead to even more multi-drug-resistant organisms (the so-called 'superbugs'). It is recommended that these agents should only be used in specified clinical settings.

Empirical antibiotic therapy includes antibiotics used for neonatal sepsis (i.e. a beta-lactam antibiotic plus an aminoglycoside) and a third-generation cephalosporin (e.g. cefotaxime or ceftriaxone) with excellent CSF penetration and bactericidal effect on sensitive Gram-negative bacteria. Therapy can be adjusted once the bacteria have been identified and antibiotic sensitivities determined. The duration of treatment is at least 14 days for uncomplicated Gram-positive bacteria and 21 days for Gram-negative bacteria.

The most frequently used initial combination is ampicillin and gentamicin (see the neonatal formulary at the end of this section). Benzyl penicillin may be preferable for known or suspected group B streptococcal infection. Cefotaxime or ceftriaxone is the drug of choice for most Gram-negative organisms, and ceftazidime is used for *Pseudomonas* infection.

Investigations for meningitis

- Lumbar puncture is potentially helpful if meningitis is suspected, and should be considered in all newborn infants with neurological signs. It is important to only attempt lumbar puncture once the infant has been stabilised, and ideally within 2 hours of initiating antibiotic treatment. Lumbar puncture is more likely than blood culture to identify the organism responsible, and within a shorter period of time.

- Cerebrospinal fluid (CSF) cell counts, chemistry and Gram stain would often point towards meningitis. An elevated CSF leucocyte count (≥ 25 white blood cells/mm^3) with pleocytosis is characteristic of neonatal meningitis. The CSF protein level in meningitis may be high (> 2.0 g/litre in a term infant), and the CSF glucose level is typically low ($< 30\%$ of blood glucose value). Gram staining may reveal bacteria, but antibiotic therapy should not be directed on the basis of this result, as rapidly growing bacilli may be mistaken for cocci, or the state of the organism may result in variable staining.

- Sometimes the CSF picture in preterm infants who have sustained an intra-ventricular haemorrhage can show a mild reactive pleocytosis in the first few weeks of life, which can be quite misleading. If there is clinical suspicion this should be treated as bacterial meningitis until cultures are known to be negative.

- If a 'bloody tap' is obtained it is best to treat the infant as having meningitis, and repeat the lumbar puncture after 24–48 hours. The finding of many white cells or bacteria is significant even if the CSF is bloodstained.

Diarrhoea in the newborn
Special points to remember

- Encourage frequent breastfeeding, as it helps in both preventing and treating diarrhoea in the newborn.

- If the infant is dehydrated, give low-osmolarity oral rehydration solution (ORS) in addition to breast milk.

- In the case of sick infants or those infants who are unable to feed orally, consider IV fluids.

- If bloody diarrhoea occurs, it is best to assume that the infant has dysentery, and initiate antibiotic therapy. Avoid the use of co-trimoxazole in the light of much better and more effective antibiotics with better side-effect profiles.

- In the case of the septic and unwell infant, give IV antibiotics as outlined in Table 3.4.1 (p. 358).

Sometimes what is described as diarrhoea by the mother is in fact the normal loose breastfed stools of some infants in the first few days of life. Usually the number of stools passed per day declines quickly, and in some breastfed infants may be as infrequent as once daily.

Congenital syphilis (*see* Section 2.8.H)

Congenital syphilis may be acquired from an infected mother via trans-placental transmission of *Treponema pallidum* at any time during pregnancy.

Clinical signs in infants may include any of the following:

- low birth weight with a heavy placenta
- palms and soles showing a red rash, grey patches, blisters or skin peeling
- abdominal distension due to large liver and spleen
- jaundice
- anaemia
- some low-birth-weight infants with syphilis show signs of severe sepsis, with lethargy, respiratory distress, skin petechiae or other signs of bleeding.

Investigation

No newborn infant should be discharged from hospital without determination of the mother's serologic status for syphilis at least once during pregnancy, and also at delivery in communities and populations in which the risk of infection with congenital syphilis is high.

If you suspect syphilis, perform a venereal disease research laboratory (VDRL), rapid plasmin reagent (RPR) or rapid syphilis test.

Treatment
All newborns of mothers with syphilis should be investigated and treated.

Infants should be treated for congenital syphilis if they have proven or probable disease demonstrated by one or more of the following:

1 physical, laboratory or radiographic evidence of active disease
2 a reactive result on maternal or infant VDRL testing where the mother has not had 3 weekly doses of benzathine penicillin.

Parenteral penicillin G remains the preferred drug for treatment of an infant with any signs of congenital syphilis.

Asymptomatic neonates born to VDRL-positive or RPR-positive women should receive 37.5 mg/kg (50 000 units/kg) of benzathine benzyl penicillin as a single IM dose into the anterolateral thigh. Ensure that the needle is not in a vein when this drug is given, by drawing back and ensuring that no blood is in the needle, as it can cause cardiac arrest and severe CNS damage if given IV.

Symptomatic infants require treatment with:

- procaine penicillin 50 000 units/kg or 50 mg/kg as a single dose by deep IM injection daily for 10 days.

Caution: Accidental intravascular administration may result in cardiac arrest and/or neurological damage

- *or* benzyl penicillin (aqueous crystalline penicillin G) 30 mg/kg or 50 000 units/kg IV, 12-hourly for 7 days and then 8-hourly for 3 days.

Treat the **mother and partner** for syphilis, and check for other sexually transmitted infections.

The infant of a mother with tuberculosis (*see* Section 2.8.G)

- If the mother has active lung tuberculosis and was treated for less than 2 months before birth, or was diagnosed with tuberculosis soon after birth, the infant should be evaluated for congenital tuberculosis.
- Women with tuberculosis who have been treated appropriately for 2 or more weeks and who are not considered contagious can breastfeed. Reassure the mother that it is safe for her to breastfeed her infant.
- Do not give the tuberculosis vaccine (BCG) at birth. Instead give prophylactic isoniazid 5 mg/kg body weight orally once daily. Separation is not necessary unless the mother (or household contact) has possible multi-drug-resistant tuberculosis.
- At the age of 6 weeks, re-evaluate the infant, noting weight gain and taking an X-ray of the chest if possible. Congenital TB is most often intra-abdominal, so look for signs suggesting this. If there are any signs or findings suggestive of active disease, start full anti-tuberculosis treatment according to national guidelines. If at the age of 6 weeks the infant is doing well and tests are negative, continue prophylactic isoniazid to complete 6 months of treatment.
- Delay BCG vaccination until 2 weeks after treatment is completed. If BCG vaccine has already been given, repeat it 2 weeks after the end of the isoniazid treatment.
- If the mother is suspected of having multi-drug-resistant tuberculosis, an expert in tuberculosis disease treatment should be consulted.

Infant of a mother with HIV infection
See Section 2.8.C.

Skin, eye and mucous membrane infections
Conjunctivitis

Most conjunctivitis presents as 'sticky eyes', but this may not always be of bacterial origin, especially if it occurs in the first few days. However, a bacterial process must be considered in all cases. Infants with a serous discharge without significant conjunctival inflammation may simply have blocked naso-lacrimal tear ducts. This usually responds to gentle pressure/massage applied in a downward motion along the nose immediately adjacent to the eyes. The discharge may be cleaned from the eye with sterile 0.9% saline drops. Show the parent how to clean the infant's eyes with sterile normal saline or boiled and cooled clean water. The eyes should be wiped from the inside to the outside edge using a clean cotton wool swab for each eye. The hands should always be washed before and after the procedure.

If the condition worsens or if there is conjunctival inflammation or a purulent discharge, use of topical therapy should be considered. Erythromycin, tetracycline, neomycin or chloramphenicol ophthalmic ointments or drops may be considered. Sometimes this condition is due to chlamydia. Apply the ointment 2 to 4 times a day for 5 days after washing away any pus with sterile normal saline as described above. Treat this level of infection as an outpatient, but review every 48 hours.

Gonococcal conjunctivitis
A severe rapidly progressive purulent conjunctivitis occurring within the first few days must always be assumed to be due to *Neisseria gonorrhoeae*, which must be promptly identified and aggressively treated in hospital with parenteral antibiotics and irrigation. Most strains are now resistant to penicillin. Swab the eye for microscopy (Gram-negative intracellular diplococci) and culture (special medium is required, such as Thayer–Martin agar with incubation under increased carbon dioxide). Treatment should be initiated immediately before culture confirmation. Treatment with IV penicillin for 7 days has been used successfully, but because of increased worldwide resistance (penicillinase-producing gonococcus), a third-generation cephalosporin is often selected as the first-line therapy:

- ceftriaxone 125 mg IM, as a single dose
- *or* cefotaxime 25 mg/kg (maximum 125 mg) IM, as a single dose
- *or* cefixime 20 mg/kg orally, as a single dose.

It is important to repeatedly clean the eye, or irrigate with saline until pus formation stops. It is vital to prevent corneal rupture and subsequent blindness.

In the case of a presumed or diagnosed gonococcal or chlamydial infection, the mother and partner should also be treated.

In countries with a low rate of sexually transmitted diseases, staphylococcal and Gram-negative organisms are more likely to be responsible. Staphylococcal infections can be treated with cloxacillin or flucloxacillin 30 mg/kg orally or IV every 6–8 hours for 5 days.

Chlamydial conjunctivitis

Chlamydia trachomatis is a common cause of infectious conjunctivitis in the newborn infant. It typically presents between 5 and 14 days. The presentation can vary from mild to moderate conjunctival erythema, and from scant mucoid discharge to copious purulent discharge. Eyelid oedema, chemosis or pseudomembrane formation may also be present. Corneal involvement is unusual initially, although untreated chlamydia conjunctivitis can result in varying degrees of conjunctival scarring and corneal infiltrates.

Chlamydia can be confirmed by culture or rapid antigen detection, but these are highly specialised procedures that may not be readily available. Without a positive laboratory diagnosis, treatment is based on clinical severity. If the condition is mild, clean the eye only. If it is moderate, use a topical antibiotic and consider giving erythromycin 10 mg/kg orally, 6-hourly for 14 days. This effectively treats this infection and may also eradicate upper respiratory tract colonisation. Drug interactions with erythromycin include increased serum levels of digoxin, theophylline and potentially caffeine.

If the condition is severe, beware gonococcal infection, irrigate and use IV or IM cefotaxime or ceftriaxone.

Ensure that the mother is appropriately referred for treatment.

Skin pustules

Skin pustules are most commonly caused by *Staphylococcus aureus*. Most often these occur in small clusters in an otherwise healthy asymptomatic infant. Topical therapy with chlorhexidine 0.5% may be all that is needed in most of these cases. Oral therapy with a penicillinase-resistant penicillin (e.g. flucloxacillin 25 mg/kg 6-hourly) or first-generation cephalosporin (e.g. cephalexin 25 mg/kg 6–12-hourly for 7 days) may also be used if extensive pustules are found. If septicaemia is suspected, septic investigations and IV antibiotics after hospitalisation may be needed. Sometimes staphylococcal pustules can be difficult to distinguish from **erythema toxicum** (a benign, non-infectious newborn rash).

Umbilical infection

A clinically relevant infection of the umbilical stump (omphalitis) presents as redness and oedema of the skin extending from the umbilicus. This should be distinguished from the ooze resulting from an umbilical granuloma, which may develop after a few weeks. If there is skin redness plus oedema extending from the umbilicus, appropriate antibiotics, usually anti-staphylococcal, should be used. Clean the area with soap and warm water and remove or drain pus and crusts. Dry and paint the area with antiseptic such as gentian violet, or use a simple alcohol swab to clean the area at the time of every nappy change. If there is only a 'sticky cord', manage it with local treatment only. Pus can be easily removed with a swab, whereas normal cord degeneration cannot be removed.

Cellulitis

This is most commonly caused by streptococci, but *Staphylococcus aureus*, Gram-negative enterococcus and anaerobes should also be considered when infection occurs at sites where there have been breaks in the skin. Treatment with **parenteral antibiotics** (e.g. Flucloxacillin, a penicillinase-resistant penicillin, and gentamicin, an aminoglycoside) should be directed against both Gram-negative

and Gram-positive bacteria. Omphalitis may become rapidly progressive and spread to deeper tissues. Infection with *Clostridium* is common in the setting of poor maternal immunity or poor umbilical cord care, and can cause neonatal tetanus.

Scalded skin syndrome

This is a rare infection caused by toxin-producing staphylococcal organisms which leads to a toxic reaction producing the effect of both serious infection and burns. Treat it with IV cloxacillin or flucloxacillin.

Superficial candidiasis ('thrush' and 'monilial' rash)

Superficial candidiasis of the oral mucosa ('thrush') commonly manifests as white patches which are not easily scraped with a spatula. The nappy area may also be affected ('monilial' rash). Unlike irritant dermatitis, the erythema extends into skin folds and there may be small raised erythematous lesions. Treat with oral nystatin suspension, 1 mL after feeds (divide it between each cheek with a small syringe). Topical nystatin ointment may be used to treat the skin rash, but only in combination with oral nystatin. Keep the nappy area dry. Apply local treatment to the mother's nipples if they are also infected.

Warning: Excess and inappropriate antibiotic usage, besides being costly and generating a lot of nursing work, also leads to multi-drug resistance. Excess use can cause overt *Candida* infection (thrush), and also risks the eventual emergence of multi-drug-resistant organisms, especially in a hospital setting. The widespread use of ampicillin has caused many coliform organisms to become increasingly resistant to this antibiotic, while units that use cefotaxime extensively are starting to encounter serious *Enterobacter* and other multi-drug-resistant Gram-negative sepsis.

Drugs used to treat severe infection in the neonate

Ampicillin (or amoxicillin)

Give 100 mg/kg per dose IM or IV where meningitis is a possibility, and 50 mg/kg per dose in other situations. Give one dose every 12 hours in the first week of life, every 8 hours in an infant aged 1–3 weeks, and every 6 hours in an infant older than this. Oral dosing can sometimes be used to complete a course of treatment.

Benzyl penicillin

Give 60 mg/kg (100 000 units/kg) IV if meningitis or tetanus is a possibility. Give 30 mg/kg (50 000 units/kg) per dose in all other situations, including syphilis. Time the interval between each dose as for ampicillin. Oral dosing (with phenoxymethylpenicillin) can sometimes be used to complete a course of treatment.

Cefotaxime

Give 50 mg/kg per dose IV or IM. Time the interval between each dose as for ampicillin, except in meningitis, where doses are given 6-hourly.

Chloramphenicol

This remains a useful antibiotic, although there is a serious risk of death from liver failure if the dose suggested here is exceeded. **Warning: The problem is not the dose** but incorrect mixing, as the bottle contains 1000 mg, so it is easy to overdose. Give a 25 mg/kg loading dose IM followed by 12.5 mg/kg once every 12 hours to infants less than 1 week old. Give this dose every 8 hours to infants aged 1–4 weeks, unless there is evidence of liver damage or renal failure. Infants older than this can be given 12.5 mg/kg once every 6 hours from the outset. Oral dosing can be used to complete any course of treatment. (The dose can be doubled in those over 1 month of age with severe infection.) Be very careful if the IV dose has to be diluted to obtain the correct dosage.

Cloxacillin (or flucloxacillin)

Give 100 mg/kg per dose IM or IV if serious infection is present, and 50 mg/kg per dose in other situations. Time the interval between each dose as for ampicillin. Oral treatment can often be given to complete a course of treatment (25 mg/kg standard, 50 mg/kg severe, 100 mg/kg in infections such as osteomyelitis).

Erythromycin

Give 12.5 mg/kg per dose orally once every 6 hours. There is no satisfactory IM preparation.

Eye drops (and ointments)

Prophylactic chloramphenicol 0.5% eye drops or 1% eye ointment can be used to minimise the risk of gonococcal infection (IM/IV ceftriaxone is being used for overt infection). Tetracycline ointment 1% should be used (with oral erythromycin) to treat chlamydia conjunctivitis (this condition is not prevented by silver nitrate use). *Pseudomonas* infection requires treatment with systemic antibiotics and topical gentamicin 0.3% eye drops.

Gentamicin

Give 5 mg/kg IM or IV once every 24 hours. If the infant weighs less than 2 kg, give 4 mg/kg per dose. Leave 36–48 hours between each dose if there is renal failure.
- If the infant is less than 32 weeks' gestation, give 4–5 mg/kg 36-hourly.
- If the infant is more than 32 weeks' gestation, give 4–5 mg/kg 24-hourly.

Hepatitis B vaccine

Give 0.5 mL IM into the thigh as soon as possible after or within 12 hours of birth. Remind the mother that the infant will require booster injections at 6 weeks and 14 weeks after birth. Infants born to mothers infected during pregnancy or who are known high-risk carriers with a positive

hepatitis B e-antigen should also be given 200 units of hepatitis B immunoglobulin (HBIG) IM into the other thigh within 24 hours of birth. Breastfeeding can safely continue.

Isoniazid

See Section 6.1.N for the latest advice on the treatment of children with TB or suspected TB.

Metronidazole

Give a 15 mg/kg loading dose and 7.5 mg/kg per dose once every 12 hours in infants less than 4 weeks old, and every 8 hours in children older than this. Treatment can be given IV or orally, but solubility makes IM use unsatisfactory. If the IV route is used, start the maintenance dose 24 hours after loading. If the oral route is used, give the first dose 12 hours after loading.

Miconazole

This controls infection with candida ('thrush') more effectively than topical nystatin. Use the oral gel at least four times a day and the skin cream twice a day for at least 7 days. Topical treatment with 0.5% aqueous gentian violet for not more than 4 days may be equally effective. Oral nystatin drops (1 mL four times a day) can be used to reduce heavy intestinal tract carriage.

Nevirapine

See Section 2.8.C and national protocols for the latest advice on the use of Nevirapine in the prevention of mother-to-child transmission of HIV infection.

Procaine and benzathine penicillin

Give asymptomatic infants born to mothers with evidence of untreated syphilis a single 37.5 mg (50 000 units/kg) dose of benzathine penicillin **IM** injection. **Never give this drug IV.** Infants thought to be infected at birth are often given procaine penicillin 50 mg/kg (50 000 units/kg) IM once a day for 10 days, but repeated IM injections can cause a sterile abscess with subsequent muscle fibrosis and atrophy. IV benzylpenicillin for 10 days (as specified above) is just as effective. Infants born to mothers who have been fully treated for syphilis (1.8 grams, or 2.4 mega-units, of benzathine benzylpenicillin) at least 4 weeks before birth need no further treatment after birth.

Zidovudine

See Section 2.8.C and national protocols for the latest advice on the use of Zidovudine in the prevention of mother-to-child transmission of HIV infection.

TABLE 3.4.1 Antibiotics and other drugs for use in the neonatal period

Drug	Route	Single dose	Frequency	Postnatal age	Gestation
Ampicillin	IV, IM	50–100 mg/kg	12 hourly	< 7 days	Any
		50–100 mg/kg	8 hourly	7–21 days	Any
		50–100 mg/kg	6 hourly	> 21 days	Any
	Reduce dose frequency in severe renal impairment and birth asphyxia				
	Use higher doses in case of suspected Group B strep infection or meningitis				

Drug	Route	Single dose	Frequency	Postnatal age	Gestation
Benzyl Penicillin	IV, IM	25–50 mg/kg	12 hourly	< 7 days	Any
		25–50 mg/kg	8 hourly	7–21 days	Any
		25–50 mg/kg	6 hourly	> 21 days	Any
	Reduce dose frequency in severe renal impairment and birth asphyxia				
Cefotaxime	IV, IM	50 mg/kg	12 hourly	< 7 days	Any
		50 mg/kg	8 hourly	> 7 days	Any
	Reduce dose by 50% in severe renal impairment				
Ceftazidime	IV, IM	50 mg/kg	12 hourly	< 7 days	Any
		50 mg/kg	8 hourly	> 7 days	Any
	Reduce dose interval to 24 hours in severe renal impairment				
Ceftriaxone	IV, IM	50 mg/kg	24 hourly	Any	Any
	Avoid in infants < 36 weeks' gestation or if jaundiced. Follow special IM preparation instructions				
Chloramphenicol	IV, IM	12.5 mg/kg	12 hourly	< 7 days	
		12.5 mg/kg	8 hourly	> 7 days	
	There is a serious risk of death from liver failure if the dose suggested is exceeded				
	Oral dosing can be used to complete any course of treatment				
Clonazepam	IV infusion	100 micrograms/kg	(***loading dose***)		
		10–30 micrograms/kg/ hour	**Not for > 3 days**	Not for > 3 days	
	Up to 200 micrograms/kg/24 hours may be required in first 48 hours				
	Use slow IV over 20 minutes				
	Caution: respiratory depression and increased pulmonary secretions particularly if accumulation occurs				
	If not ventilated use lower does because of respiratory depression				
Cloxacillin	IV, IM	50 mg/kg	12 hourly	< 7 days	Any
		50 mg/kg	8 hourly	> 7 days	Any
	Double the dose in severe infection and if CNS is involved				
	Increase dose interval to 24 hours in severe renal impairment				
Erythromycin	PO	12.5 mg/kg	6 hourly		
	There is no satisfactory IM preparation				
Gentamicin	IV	5 mg/kg	48 hourly	< 7 days	< 29 weeks
		4 mg/kg	36 hourly	> 7 days	< 29 weeks
		4 mg/kg	36 hourly	< 7 days	30–33 weeks
		4 mg/kg	24 hourly	> 7 days	30–33 weeks
		4 mg/kg	24 hourly	< 7 days	> 34 weeks
		4 mg/kg	24 hourly	> 7 days	> 34 weeks
	Trough and peak levels are not needed				
Isoniazid	*See Section 6.1.N for details on its use.*				
Metronidazole	IV, PO	5 mg/kg	(***loading dose***)		
		7.5 mg/kg	12 hourly	< 28 days	
		7.5 mg/kg	8 hourly	> 28 days	
	Infuse over 30 minutes				
	Injection solutions can be given rectally				

(continued)

Drug	Route	Single dose	Frequency	Postnatal age	Gestation
Miconazole	Oral gel		6 hourly		
	Skin ointment		6 hourly		
	This controls infection with Candida ('thrush') better than topical nystatin *Use for at least 7–10 days*				
0.5% Aqueous Gentian violet	Apply		Once daily for 4 days		
Oral nystatin drops	PO	1 mL	6 hourly		
	Can be used to reduce heavy intestinal tract carriage				
Nevirapine	*See* Section 2.8.C for details on its use.				
Paraldehyde	Rectal	0.2 to 4 mL/kg	(***loading dose***)		
		Can repeat once 4–5 hours later			
	Use injection rectally or ready-diluted rectal solution *Dilution with an equal volume of olive oil or any edible oil* *If using a plastic syringe administer immediately* *IM injections may cause sterile abscessed (maximum 1 mL at one site)*				
Phenobarbitone	IV, IM, PO	20 mg/kg	(***loading dose***)	*followed by maintenance 12–24 hours later*	
	Slow IV over 5 minutes. Loading dose may be repeated by at 10 mg/kg if clinically indicated				
		3–5 mg/kg/24 hours	Once daily	*Once daily generally but with time may need to be give 12 hourly*	
	Monitor plasma levels *Therapeutic range: 15–30 mg/L although increasing up to 40 mg/L should be considered in resistant seizures*				
Phenytoin	IV, PO	15–20 mg/kg	(***loading dose***)		
	Give IV infusion over 20–30 minutes diluted in 10 mL of normal saline				
		1.5–3 mg/kg	12 hourly		
	Slow IV over 20–30 minutes *Usual maximum dose 7.5 mg/kg 12 hourly* *Therapeutic range 5–17 mg/L*				
	Oral dose is poorly absorbed particularly in premature infants *Wide variation in levels, so monitor and adjust dose and interval accordingly* *Measure trough level. May not reach steady state for up to 14 days*				
Procaine penicillin	IM	10 mg/kg	Single dose		
	Give to asymptomatic babies born to mothers with evidence of untreated syphilis				
		100 mg/kg	Once daily		
	Babies thought to be infected at birth are often give once daily for 10 days ***Never give this drug IV*** *Rarely repeated IM injections can cause a sterile abscess with subsequent muscle fibrosis and atrophy* *Alternatively* *IM or IV benzylpenicillin for 10 day (as specified above) is just as effective* *Babies born to mother fully treated for syphilis need not further treatment after birth* *(Maternal treatment = 1.8 grams or 2.4 mega units of benzathine benzylpenicillin at least 4 weeks before birth*				
Zidovidine	*See* Section 2.8.C for details on its use.				

Polycythaemia

This potentially harmful condition occurs in up to 4% of births and risk factors are: being both small or large for gestational age or wasted, born to mothers with diabetes and being one of a multiple birth. Milking of the umbilical cord at birth, by increasing the amount of blood transferred into the baby, can also produce this condition.

Polycythaemia is defined as a venous haematocrit > 65% or Hb > 22 g/dL. Capillary samples can have higher haematocrit and if > 65% should be confirmed by venous sample.

Screen high risk babies at 2, 12 and 24 hours by capillary blood measurement of PCV and then if > 65% confirm by venous sample.

Above a PVC of 65%, the viscosity of blood increases exponentially and can produce dangerously reduced capillary perfusion in many organs which, when most severe, can produce cerebral, renal or mesenteric vein thrombosis.

Clinical presentation

The baby can be hypotonic, drowsy, have poor sucking, be irritable, jittery and, when severe, have convulsions. These are important danger signs.

There may also be jaundice, hypoglycaemia, and hypocalcaemia. With a high PCV the blood glucose reading may be falsely low with a normal serum glucose.

Management

First exclude dehydration and if present treat by supervised feeding and if necessary increased enteral or even IV fluids. The best way to check for dehydration is to weigh the baby and compare weight with that at birth. Normally babies lose 5–7% of their body weight in the first 3–4 days and regain their birth weight level by 10–14 days. If the baby's weight at 24 hours of age has dropped by 5% or more from the birth weight then dehydration is present.

Check blood glucose and bilirubin levels and treat appropriately (see below).

If venous PCV is 65–70% and no signs, bilirubin is below phototherapy levels, and no hypoglycaemia is present treat conservatively by regular examination for the signs described above, ensure adequate fluid intake by direct observation of feeding and regular accurate weighing before and after feeds.

If venous PCV is 70–75% and there are no danger signs, treat polycythaemia by giving additional fluid of 20 mL/kg per day enterally or IV. Also treat jaundice with phototherapy and hypoglycaemia with glucose, if necessary IV.

If PCV is > 75% or there are any danger signs as described above then partial exchange transfusion (PET) should be undertaken urgently.

PET involves the exchange of 20 mL/kg by repeatedly taking off aliquots of blood of up to 5 mL at a time and replacing IV with equal volumes of Ringer-Lactate or 0.9% saline. Ideally blood will be taken from a peripheral vein but, if this is not possible, either use an umbilical venous catheter placed aseptically or a peripheral arterial cannula. At the end of the procedure, re-check the PCV, Hb, bilirubin and blood glucose levels (ideally also blood calcium value).

Continue to monitor the clinical state of the baby and the PCV until it is shown to fall below 60%. Re-check blood glucose and bilirubin levels as appropriate.

Respiratory disorders

Features of respiratory distress in the newborn

These include the following:

- tachypnoea (respiratory rate > 60 breaths/minute)
- recession of the chest wall and sternum
- expiratory grunting
- nasal flaring
- prolonged apnoea (lasting for more than 20 seconds) or intermittent shorter apnoea with cyanosis or severe falls in oxygen concentration (< 90%)
- gasping
- tachycardia
- SaO$_2$ < 92% in air

- cyanosis is a relatively late presentation of a respiratory or cardiac cause.

These signs are relatively non-specific, arising from conditions that affect the respiratory system, as well as from cardiac, neurological and metabolic abnormalities.

Cardinal signs that characterise distress due to respiratory disorders

- **Central cyanosis in room air.**
- **Tachypnoea:** respiratory rate > 60 breaths/minute (always measure over at least 1 minute, as the infant's breathing may be irregular).
- **Retractions (recessions):** tugging of the soft tissues between the ribs or at the edges of the rib cage.
- **Grunting:** a prolonged expiratory effort, usually with an audible noise.

Two of these signs are sufficient to make the diagnosis. Cyanosis may not be present, especially if the infant is receiving oxygen.

If pulse oximetry is available, the SaO$_2$ in infants with respiratory impairment will usually be less than 92% in air (often less than 90% in more severe cases).

Causes of early respiratory distress

'Early' respiratory distress (presenting in the first 12 hours of life) may result from a number of causes, including the following:

- **'transient tachypnoea of the newborn'** associated with a delay in clearing of fetal lung fluid
- **congenital pneumonia or sepsis** (e.g. group B streptococcus sepsis)
- **surfactant deficiency** (hyaline membrane disease or respiratory distress syndrome)
- **pneumothorax**
- **meconium aspiration**
- **congenital abnormalities** of the lung or airways (including diaphragmatic hernia)
- **hypothermia.**

Maternal fever during labour and prolonged rupture of the membranes (more than 18 hours) particularly point to **pneumonia** or **sepsis**. Pneumonia may also be due to congenital syphilis. **Pneumothorax** should be considered if the infant has been resuscitated using positive-pressure ventilation (although it has also been described as occurring spontaneously in about 1% of normal term infants). **Transient tachypnoea** is more common among infants delivered by elective Caesarean section (in the absence of spontaneous labour). **Surfactant deficiency** and **infection** are the most likely causes in preterm infants.

Congenital heart disease does not usually cause early respiratory distress. Cyanosis/severe hypoxaemia is the more likely presentation (see Section 5.4.A).

Respiratory distress associated with heart failure normally occurs after the first week of life, in association with tachycardia, pallor, sweating, hepatomegaly and excessive weight gain.

Causes of respiratory distress in the newborn
Common causes
- Lack of surfactant causing respiratory distress syndrome in the preterm infant.
- Infection acquired before or during delivery.
- Transient tachypnoea of the newborn (wet lung).

Less common causes
- Meconium aspiration.
- Persistent pulmonary hypertension of the newborn.
- Pneumothorax.

Rare causes
- Pulmonary hypoplasia.
- Congenital abnormalities (e.g. diaphragmatic hernia, choanal atresia, tracheo-oesophageal fistula).
- Pulmonary haemorrhage.
- Metabolic causes (inborn error of metabolism).

Non-respiratory causes
- Congenital heart disease.
- Hypothermia.
- Severe anaemia.

Principles of treatment of respiratory diseases of the newborn
- Ensure that the **airway** is open and that it remains so. Thick secretions from the throat may be cleared by intermittent suction using direct observation
- Ensure that the infant is **breathing**. If the infant is apnoeic, gasping or has a very slow respiratory rate, use chest inflations with a bag valve mask to re-establish breathing.
- The infant should be offered enough supplemental oxygen to treat any degree of central cyanosis and ideally to keep SaO_2 in the normal range (86–92% in preterm and 92–96% in term infants). It should never be in the hyperoxic range (above 96%), especially in a preterm infant who is receiving additional inspired oxygen.
  - Oxygen should be given either with an oxygen concentrator or from cylinders. An oxygen supply must be available at all times in areas where newborn infants are treated.
  - Pulse oximetry should be employed (if available) to assess initial disease severity, to monitor subsequent progress, and to ensure that such supplies of oxygen as are available are optimally used. Wind-up versions of pulse oximeters are available (www.PET.org.za).
  - Tents and incubators are not an efficient way of giving oxygen. Giving oxygen into a clear plastic hood (head box) placed over the head stops the oxygen supply from dropping every time a tent or incubator door is opened. **Oxygen is an expensive resource and must not be wasted by giving it into incubators.**
  - **Nasal cannulae optimise the efficient use of the available oxygen supply.** They prevent wasting of oxygen, and also make it very much easier to move and handle the infant without disrupting the supply. However, they make it rather more difficult to quantify how much oxygen is needed to control cyanosis.

- Infants should ideally have their actual oxygen needs monitored and adjusted at regular intervals.
  - Measuring the inspired oxygen concentration needed is one way of assessing the infant's changing condition. This can be done using a combination of a pulse oximeter with an inspired oxygen monitor placed in a head box next to the infant's face.
  - A simpler alternative for achieving this objective involves titrating the oxygen flow to maintain saturation on the pulse oximeter in the range 92–96% for term infants and lower, at 86–92%, for preterm infants, as described earlier.
- Keeping the infant fully clothed with a pulse oximeter attached makes it possible to dispense with any other monitoring of pulse and respiration, thus keeping the infant warm with minimal handling.
- If assisted ventilation is available and there is very severe respiratory failure, an arterial or capillary blood gas measurement can be helpful for determining the severity of respiratory acidosis and the need for ventilator support such as nasal continuous positive airway pressure (nCPAP) or intubation and ventilation.
- Infants with serious respiratory distress should not be offered feeds until their condition has stabilised. Support expression of milk by the mother so that she is ready to provide breast milk when her infant has recovered. In such situations, IV infusion of 10% glucose (60 mL/kg/day) is safest. If there are no facilities for IV infusion, breast milk or 10% glucose may be given in limited quantities (up to 60 mL/kg/day) by orogastric tube. **Nasogastric tubes may contribute to upper airway resistance, so an orogastric tube is preferred in infants with respiratory distress, although it is more difficult to keep in place, so compromise may sometimes be necessary.**
- Infants less than 2 days old should be started on an IV infusion of 10% dextrose at 60–90 mL/kg/24 hours. For infants more than 3 days old sodium chloride should be added to 10% dextrose to provide 2–3 mmol/kg/day and used at the age-appropriate giving rates (see fluid management section on p. 347). It is recommended that in neonates it is best to use a paediatric burette (chamber) where 1 mL = 60 micro-drops (1 drop/minute = 1 mL/hour). **Caution: A standard infusion set gives 20 drops/mL and can lead to dangerous fluid overload if it is not carefully controlled.**
- Give antibiotics IV or IM (the IV route is preferable) at least for the first 48 hours in all infants with respiratory distress, as bacterial infection is a likely reason for the infant's respiratory problems. Take blood for culture first wherever possible. Antibiotics can be stopped if the blood culture results are negative and the infant is well after 72 hours.
- In order to gain further insight into the probable cause of the problem, a portable chest X-ray machine (if available) can be useful.
- Take stringent steps to prevent nosocomial cross-infection within the unit. This can be a particular problem not only with some bacterial infections (e.g. *E. coli*, *Klebsiella*), but also with some troublesome viral infections (e.g. respiratory syncytial virus, RSV) that are more commonly seen later in the first month of life.

Management issues in specific respiratory conditions

Primary surfactant deficiency (respiratory distress syndrome (RDS), or hyaline membrane disease)

The principles of treating IRDS are as follows:

1 Minimal handling of the infant.
2 Supplementary oxygen.
3 IV fluids.
4 No oral feeding.
5 Continuous positive airways pressure (CPAP).
6 Avoidance of hypothermia.

- Surfactant deficiency is by far the commonest cause of respiratory distress in a preterm infant in the first 3 days of life. It is a self-limiting condition, because birth always triggers a gradual increase in surfactant production. The challenge therefore is to support the infant for the first 2–3 days (72 hours) of life without doing further damage to the lung, until such time as the deficiency resolves itself.

- The key features of RDS (cyanosis, an expiratory 'grunt', tachypnoea, and intercostal and/or subcostal recession) become clinically obvious within 4 hours of birth. Supplemental oxygen, minimal handling and IV fluid, keeping the infant 'nil by mouth', have been the standard ingredients of care for the last 50 years. Elective surfactant administration (which is expensive) and ventilation (which is complex) have become the standard approach to management in the last 20 years. However, it is now becoming clear that the very small infant can pay a high price for chronic tracheal intubation, which by interrupting ciliary flow can interfere with the way that necrotic material is normally cleared from the lung.

- Most infants will manage well for themselves as long as they are offered help in preventing the lung from closing down and becoming airless for the 72-hour period it takes for the surfactant production to 'switch on'. The expiratory grunt that is a characteristic feature of this condition is the infant's own method of sustaining

positive end-expiratory pressure (PEEP) and holding the alveoli open. Making the infant breathe against a constant positive airway pressure gradient achieves the same result. By applying this pressure at the nose (nasal CPAP), the complications associated with tracheal intubation can often be avoided.

- To be maximally effective, we now know that CPAP should be applied as soon as there is any evidence of respiratory distress in a preterm infant. CPAP given via paired short cannulae or a specially made nasal mask is probably best, as it minimises airway resistance.

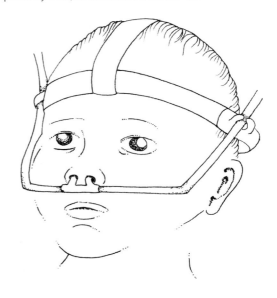

FIGURE 3.4.2 Nasal continuous positive airway pressure (CPAP) equipment in place.

Even though the 3-mm nasal cannulae that are normally used to provide supplemental oxygen can provide some CPAP, especially when higher flow rates are applied (6–8 litres/minute), there is a need for an air–oxygen blender to ensure that excessive and harmfully high concentrations of oxygen are not given. Humidification of the air–oxygen mixture is also required. Purpose-built CPAP systems with special nasal cannulae are better able to provide pressures of 5–8 cmH$_2$O (a system specially designed for resource-limited settings based on an oxygen concentrator has recently become available: www.diamedica.co.uk). In general, all that is then required is a controlled flow of blended humidified air and oxygen with a simple device for producing controlled adjustable CPAP. Regular nursing attention is necessary to make sure that the nasal cannulae remain correctly positioned and do not cause necrotic pressure damage to the nose. This is a skill that does not take long to acquire.

Transient tachypnoea of the newborn

This is almost indistinguishable from RDS. However, unlike RDS, the signs do not progress with time in the hours after birth. Most of these infants are born at or near term. All are tachypnoeic, and a few are obviously cyanosed for 6–12 hours after birth. The condition seems to be caused by a delay in clearing lung fluid after birth. All of these infants will recover on their own so long as handling is kept to a minimum and they are not fed until their respiratory signs

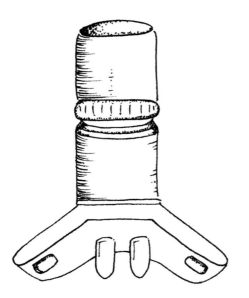

FIGURE 3.4.1 Nasal continuous positive airway pressure (CPAP) nasal prongs.

have subsided. Some need supplemental oxygen, but few need it for more than 72 hours. The condition appears to be more common after Caesarean section.

Aspiration pneumonia

Aspiration of particulate matter can occasionally almost completely block the trachea. More commonly it can also cause a chemical pneumonitis. Meconium can be particularly irritant in this regard, making the term infant very oxygen dependent for the best part of a week. Aspiration of particulate matter may also trigger **persistent fetal circulation** (see below).

Contrary to the findings of some studies originating from well-resourced centres in the developed world, suctioning meconium-stained infants during deliveries as soon as the head is on the perineum has made a dramatic difference to the risk of meconium aspiration syndrome in India and South Africa.

Nevertheless, with minimal handling, IV fluid and supplemental oxygen, most of these infants can be expected to make a complete recovery provided that there has been no associated hypoxic cerebral damage. Providing unnecessary respiratory support may actually make matters worse by increasing the risk of pneumothorax. Antibiotics should probably be given until it is clear that there is no associated bacterial infection.

Aspiration after birth can cause a similar picture. Milk can block the trachea, but it seldom causes much of an inflammatory reaction. However, gastric acid can be much more damaging. Recurrent minor unrecognised reflux and aspiration is probably more common than a single massive episode of aspiration, and it can certainly over time render the infant quite oxygen dependent. Infants who are hypotonic and have a poor cough reflex or repeated apnoea are probably at particular risk in this regard. **Aspiration is common after an apnoeic event.**

Bacterial pneumonia

This should be managed as outlined in the section on suspected infection, remembering that there may be septicaemia as well as pneumonia.

Persistent fetal circulation

- This is relatively common in resource-limited countries, and is a potentially life-threatening condition leading to poor lung perfusion after birth. It may complicate fetal hypoxia, meconium aspiration, early bacterial pneumonia, diaphragmatic hernia, respiratory distress syndrome or (very occasionally) be a primary disorder.
- After birth the pressure in the pulmonary vessels remains high, so that the normal fall in pressure in the right atrium, right ventricle and pulmonary arteries does not occur. As a result of this, the blood flows via the fetal circulation (i.e. the foramen ovale and ductus arteriosus) from the right side of the heart to the left. This blood has not been oxygenated, so the infant soon becomes cyanosed. It is difficult to differentiate this from a congenital cardiac malformation. Serious cyanosis in an infant with a well-aerated lung on chest X-ray and progressive acidosis can cause rapid self-perpetuating cyclical deterioration.
- The treatment in the first instance is oxygenation, minimal handling, IV fluids and avoidance of oral feeds. Metabolic acidosis should be vigorously and rapidly corrected or even over-corrected. Drugs that cause

pulmonary vasodilation, such as sildenafil or magnesium sulphate, have been used to some effect. However, they can lead to serious hypotension and should be used very selectively in a controlled environment in specialised centres.

- Survival is more likely in a unit that is capable of providing sustained respiratory support, and early transfer should be considered when possible.

Pneumothorax

This is present more frequently than expected, and may occur spontaneously in up to 1–2% of infants. It is often asymptomatic, and may be associated with meconium aspiration, too high inflation pressures used during mechanical ventilation or resuscitation, and respiratory distress syndrome. It does not automatically need to be treated, unless there is progressive respiratory distress. Confirmation by chest X-ray (if available) is often too time-consuming, especially in the case of a rapidly developing tension pneumothorax. It may be possible to diagnose a pneumothorax clinically by simple observations. The abdomen is often distended by downward displacement of the liver and spleen. The breath sounds may be reduced on the affected side. **A hyper-resonant chest with mediastinal shift (trachea deviated away from the side of the suspected pneumothorax) and rapidly deteriorating clinical condition with severe hypoxaemia and/or cardiovascular compromise (bradycardia, hypotension) strongly suggests a tension pneumothorax. This requires an immediate needle thoracocentesis followed (if this results in an immediate improvement in respiratory and cardiovascular function) by the insertion of a chest drain into the fourth or fifth intercostal space in the mid to anterior axillary line (see Section 8.3). In an emergency situation with a rapidly deteriorating cardiac and respiratory function, this must be done without prior X-ray confirmation.** Transillumination can be useful if a 'cold light' (fibre-optic light source) is available (the affected side may glow brightly).

A pneumothorax that does not result in severe respiratory distress, and is not under tension, may spontaneously resolve without mechanical removal of the pleural air, but oxygen and careful monitoring are required.

Lung hypoplasia due to oligohydramnios

Chronic loss of liquor for many days before birth can occasionally impede lung growth enough to threaten survival, but what looks like a serious problem at delivery can occasionally resolve quite rapidly after 1–2 days. However, where the oligohydramnios is due to bilateral renal agenesis or dysplasia, the prognosis for survival is very poor. The stiffness of the small malformed lungs in these cases causes marked intercostal and subcostal recession with unrelievable cyanosis. Chest X-ray will often reveal an untreatable pre-terminal pneumothorax. The infant's face may appear flattened and there may be limited extension of the elbows and knees due to oligohydramnios.

Congenital malformations

The most common congenital defect causing respiratory distress soon after birth is **diaphragmatic hernia**. This occurs in 1 in 4000 births, and more commonly affects the left side. Clinical examination reveals respiratory distress, and reduced air entry on the affected side with a displaced apex beat and scaphoid abdomen. The chest X-ray is diagnostic. It used to be thought that early surgery improved the likelihood of survival, but it is now known that this is not the case. Therefore immediate transfer does not have to be considered until the child's initial respiratory problems have stabilised. During the interim period, an IV line and open nasogastric tube should be in place to keep the gut empty of gas, and feeding should be withheld. Restricted lung growth means that only about 50% of these infants have any chance of survival. Use a headbox rather than nasal cannula oxygen, and place an open nasogastric tube to prevent bowel distension, which makes the condition worse.

Management of diaphragmatic hernia

This includes the following:
- oxygen supplements
- minimal handling
- IV fluids and withholding of oral feeds
- a nasogastric tube to keep the stomach empty
- stabilisation of respiration with mechanical ventilation following intubation or continuous negative extra-thoracic pressure (CNEP) can be helpful if available
- transfer to surgical care if the infant responds to treatment.

A number of rare generalised skeletal abnormalities that affect rib growth also cause severe untreatable lung hypoplasia.

Congenital heart disease can occasionally cause overt cyanosis from birth, but there are seldom any associated signs of respiratory distress (*see* Section 5.4.A).

Apnoeic/hypoxaemic episodes

Apnoea is the cessation of respiration or a hypoxaemic event associated with signs of cardiorespiratory decompensation (bradycardia, cyanosis and pallor). Apnoeic episodes are common in preterm infants under 32 weeks' gestation ('apnoea of prematurity'). In term infants, apnoea usually signifies an underlying pathological condition.

Apnoea of prematurity

This is often characterised by a brief cessation of respiration that responds to gentle tactile stimulation, and may vary significantly in duration and severity, especially in very-low-birth-weight infants. Sometimes, isolated bradycardia with brief oxygen desaturation events is identified without a clinically apparent apnoea. The aetiology of apnoea of prematurity is often a mixture of impaired central nervous system respiratory control ('central apnoea'), intrapulmonary shunting and upper airway obstruction. Sometimes recurrent apnoea is associated with gastro-oesophageal reflux, particularly in neurologically compromised infants with poor airway-protective reflexes. Oral theophylline or caffeine, by its effect on the respiratory centre, may reduce or even eliminate the severity and frequency of apnoeic events. Caffeine has become the preferred methylxanthine by some neonatologists, because it has a long half-life (allowing once daily dosing), fewer side effects and serum levels do not have to be monitored. Continuous positive airway pressure (CPAP) or rarely mechanical ventilation may become necessary to control recurrent apnoea.

The diagnosis of 'apnoea of prematurity' is one of exclusion, as various other processes may cause or exacerbate apnoea. In the case of a preterm infant, these include the following:
- respiratory distress (surfactant deficiency, pneumonia, pulmonary oedema due to a persistent ductus arteriosus)
- intraventricular haemorrhage
- hypoglycaemia
- over-heating or hypothermia
- sepsis
- severe anaemia may also contribute to apnoea.

Pulmonary parenchymal disease

Any condition that causes decreased lung compliance or impaired gas exchange can contribute to apnoea. Appropriate pulmonary support should be provided for adequate gas exchange, and the underlying pulmonary condition should be treated.

Airway obstruction

This may result from simple malpositioning of the head (e.g. hyper-flexion or hyper-extension of the neck), especially in preterm infants. Congenital airway anomalies such as tracheo-oesophageal fistula or an aberrant thoracic blood vessel compressing the trachea (vascular sling) may also present as apnoea. Maintaining proper head positioning or surgical correction of the underlying anomaly should be provided.

Infection

Infection must always be excluded and antibiotics administered until infection has been ruled out by subsequent clinical findings and laboratory results (complete blood counts, chest X-ray, blood cultures, etc.).

Convulsions (see below)

Convulsions may present primarily as apnoea. This possibility should be considered especially in term or near-term infants with no other identifiable cause of apnoea. In such cases there may be a poor response to positive pressure ventilation. Convulsions in the first 1 to 3 postnatal days are usually due to intrapartum hypoxia. If there is a history of an operative vaginal delivery (e.g. forceps) or other birth trauma, this may indicate the possibility of an intracranial haemorrhage.

Maternal medication

A common cause of apnoea in the newborn can be intrapartum morphine or pethidine administration for maternal pain or sedation during the last 4 hours before delivery. The effects can be reversed by administering naloxone hydrochloride (100 micrograms/kg, usually given IM). Naloxone should not be given if there is a history of drug abuse with narcotics in pregnancy, as acute neonatal narcotic withdrawal may be precipitated (*see* Section 3.3).

Exposure to high levels of magnesium sulphate has also been associated with apnoea in the immediate postnatal period. This is usually a self-limiting process that very rarely requires mechanical ventilation.

Continuous monitoring, preferably with a pulse oximeter, is needed especially if the infant becomes bradycardic or cyanosed with the apnoea.

Treatment

- Gentle stimulation is usually all that is required to start the infant breathing again.
- Bag-and-mask resuscitation may occasionally be called for, and there should always be equipment immediately available and ready to use (not locked away in a cupboard) should this be necessary.
- If available, oral caffeine may reduce the number of episodes in a preterm infant. Caffeine seldom causes the tachycardia and other side effects associated with

theophylline. It is advisable to continue caffeine for 4–5 days after cessation of apnoea. Recurrent apnoea that does not respond to caffeine occasionally requires a period of nasal CPAP or mechanical ventilation.

- If an apnoea monitor is available it can be used, but a pulse oximeter with the alarm turned on for hypoxaemia is much safer, as apnoea (absent ventilation) can occur despite continued breathing movements. This will also identify any baseline low oxygen saturation which, when treated, may help to prevent apnoea.

TABLE 3.4.2 Caffeine doses for apnoea of prematurity given intravenously or orally

Preparations	Each dose	Dose frequency	Notes on administration
Caffeine citrate	20 mg/kg	Loading dose	If oral dose is too large, divide into two and give 1 hour apart
	5–8 mg/kg maintenance	Once daily	
Caffeine base	10 mg/kg	Loading dose	Give IV loading dose over 30–60 minutes diluted as much as possible
	2.5–4 mg/kg maintenance	Once daily	

Haemorrhage in the neonate

Causes of haemorrhage

An infant's blood volume approximates 80 mL/kg of body weight. Peripartum haemorrhage of relatively small amounts of blood can therefore result in hypovolaemic shock in the newborn. Common causes may include a slipped ligature on the umbilical cord, intrauterine feto–maternal haemorrhage (diagnosed by the Kleihauer–Betke test), or subgaleal haemorrhage. Vasa praevia or an accidental incision of the placenta during Caesarean section are other causes.

The Kleihauer–Betke test is a blood test used to measure the amount of fetal haemoglobin transferred from the fetus to the mother's bloodstream. It is usually performed on Rhesus-negative mothers to determine the dose of Rho(D) immune globulin needed to inhibit the formation of Rh antibodies in the mother and prevent Rh disease in future Rh-positive children. It is also the standard method of quantitating feto–maternal haemorrhage.

The test exploits the differential resistance of fetal haemoglobin to acid. A standard blood smear prepared from the mother's blood is exposed to an acid bath. This removes adult haemoglobin, but not fetal haemoglobin, from the red blood cells. Subsequent staining makes fetal cells (containing fetal haemoglobin) appear rose-pink in colour, whereas adult red blood cells are only seen as 'ghosts'. The percentage of fetal to maternal cells is calculated under a microscope.

Bleeding in the first week of life is uncommon, but may signify haemorrhagic disease of the newborn or clotting factor deficiency.

Presenting features

The infant will appear pale with weak peripheral pulses, tachypnoea and a tachycardia that may exceed 200 beats/minute. Blood pressure may be low or undetectable even in a term infant but is very difficult to measure in neonates. **The haematocrit and haemoglobin concentration may be normal in an infant with acute hypovolaemic shock, and are an unreliable early indicator of the amount of blood lost in the first few hours after the bleed.** Obvious blood loss rarely results in hypovolaemic shock. Common sites of blood loss include the umbilical stump and the gastrointestinal tract. In the latter case, there may be doubt as

to whether blood is of maternal origin (blood swallowed at delivery or from a bleeding nipple) or infant origin. In some cases this can be resolved by the Apt test.

Apt test

Mix 1 part of the blood-containing fluid (vomitus, gastric aspirate or liquid stool) with 5 parts of distilled water. Centrifuge it, and then mix 1 mL of the supernatant with 0.25 mL of 0.25% sodium hydroxide (NaOH). A yellow-brown colour signifies maternal blood, whereas fetal haemoglobin remains pink. The solution must be pink to start with.

Treatment

- In an emergency in a shocked infant take a blood sample for blood grouping and cross-matching. Give O Rh-negative or cross-matched blood (20 mL/kg) at a rate depending on the degree of shock (usually the first 10 mL/kg can be safely given over 5 minutes), monitoring the response and reducing the rate of infusion as improvement occurs. Sometimes a further 10–20 mL/kg of cross-matched blood may be necessary.
- If O-negative or cross-matched blood is not available, use 10–20 mL/kg of 4.5% albumin or Ringer-lactate or Hartmann's solution.
- If there is overt bleeding, take a blood sample for blood grouping and cross-matching, haemoglobin, platelet count, film and clotting studies. Then give 1 mg of vitamin K (phytomenadione or phytonadione) IV. If bleeding continues, give 20 mL/kg of fresh-frozen plasma (if available). Administer platelets if the count is < 60 000/mm³. Bleeding due to haemorrhagic disease of the newborn usually stops within 30 minutes of vitamin K administration.

The neonate with jaundice

Many infants become jaundiced for a few days after birth. This is because bilirubin released from the breakdown of red blood cells has to be excreted by the infant after birth. *In utero*, bilirubin would cross the placenta to reach the maternal liver, from where it would be processed and eliminated. The neonatal liver takes time to develop normal functioning. The serum bilirubin level usually rises after the first 24 hours of life and peaks at 100–300 µmol/litre by 3 to 5 days after birth.

Causes of physiological jaundice in the neonatal period include the following:

- increased breakdown of red blood cells in the first few days of life
- reduced lifespan of red blood cells (70 days, compared with 120 days in the adult)
- less efficient metabolism of bilirubin by the immature liver enterohepatic circulation of bilirubin.

'Physiological jaundice' is common, affecting at least one-third of normal term infants. Jaundice can be considered physiological and does not require treatment or investigation if the following criteria are met:

- Jaundice is not present in the first 24 hours of life.
- The infant is well, and free from signs of infection, without enlargement of the liver or spleen.
- The bilirubin concentration does not exceed 300 µmol/litre (approximately 17 mg/dL) at any stage (term infants only). A much lower acceptable level is set for preterm infants.
- The bilirubin concentration reaches a peak on the fourth or fifth day of life.
- The jaundice has fully resolved by the end of the second week of life.

The risk of jaundice can be reduced by encouraging early unrestricted demand breastfeeding.

There is no evidence whatsoever to support the widely held belief that giving extra water for the infant to drink either reduces the risk of jaundice or is helpful in treatment. In fact the opposite has been shown. Giving water is likely to reduce the frequency of breastfeeds and increase the risk of jaundice. Dehydration should be avoided by encouraging frequent breast feeds.

Assessing the degree of jaundice

Various means of estimating the degree of jaundice make it easier to determine which infants really need any intervention. Healthcare professionals can sometimes make a rough estimate of the degree of jaundice by looking at the skin colour (this is best undertaken in natural daylight), but it can only be divided into simple categories such as 'slight', 'moderate' or 'severe'. The face is often the first part of the body to show signs of jaundice. The trunk usually only becomes yellow as jaundice deepens. Finally, the palms of the hands and soles of the feet become jaundiced. These observations are just estimates, and sometimes have to be confirmed by other means. Jaundice in the newborn infant can be missed in infants with dark skin, but can be more easily judged once the skin is blanched free of blood by finger pressure.

Bilirubin encephalopathy (kernicterus) in the absence of overt haemolysis is excessively uncommon in the **term** infant, unless the serum bilirubin level exceeds 425 µmol/litre.

Note:
- µmol/litre divided by 17.1 = mg/dL
- mg/dL multiplied by 17.1 = µmol/litre.

Several electronic devices have been developed for assessing skin colour, but none have yet been shown to work significantly better than the simple 'icterometer' devised in 1960 and still in use. Jaundice is assessed by pressing the clear plastic of this simple device against the tip of the nose (or against the gums or tongue in a dark-skinned infant, where it has been shown to be accurate in a South African study), and then matching the colour of the skin against the icterometer's colour scale. Levels in excess of 350 µmol/litre are unlikely to be missed if a blood sample is taken once the icterometer reads ≥ 3.5. This too little known device, which costs only US$39, is still made by Cascade Health Care Products of Salem, Oregon, in the USA. Measuring the degree of jaundice by this method is of no value once phototherapy has been started.

The bilirubin concentration can be most simply and accurately measured by simple spectrophotometry of serum obtained by centrifuging blood in a capillary tube. Several easily operated machines are available. Ward-based devices for assessing the bilirubin content of a spun micro-haematocrit tube optically are accurate until the level exceeds 350 µmol/litre, and are adequate for most clinical purposes. If these devices are used, staff should be trained in this technique, and the machine should be calibrated daily and checked with control specimens of known bilirubin content. Using dirty tubes (or cuvettes), haemolysed or lipaemic samples can produce significant errors. Use plastic tubes, not glass ones, to avoid HIV infection if the tubes break.

The accurate measurement of values in excess of 350 µmol/litre is only possible in a biochemistry laboratory. A laboratory spectrophotometer reading is needed before initiating an exchange transfusion.

Direct or conjugated bilirubin presents no threat to the brain. It only accounts for a small fraction of the total serum bilirubin level in the first week of life. Decisions about treatment should therefore be based on the total serum bilirubin level, remembering that even laboratory estimates have limited precision.

Collecting blood

- Only a small amount of blood is needed to check the bilirubin level. Although described as a heel prick, sticking a needle into the heel runs a high risk of entering the underlying bone, and can lead to osteomyelitis, so should be avoided.
- It is safe to take blood from any part of the back third of the foot.

Try to use a disposable 2.4-mm blood lance, but never use the same lance for more than one infant, because of the risk of transmitting hepatitis or HIV infection. It is not necessary or appropriate to try to sterilise the skin first, so long as it is clean. A spring-loaded lance does seem to render the procedure less painful. The infant will also show fewer signs of distress if held or given something to suck during the procedure.

Grip the foot firmly enough to make it go red but not white. Stab the back of the foot just once and then squeeze gently and intermittently to stimulate blood flow. The use of a standard lance should optimise blood collection because it helps to ensure that the skin is punctured to a standard depth. A shallower prick is unlikely to reduce the pain inflicted because it will almost certainly prolong the procedure. A double puncture may help if a lot of blood is needed. Slight finger pressure exerted through a cotton ball on the site for about a minute is usually enough to stop any further bleeding after the procedure is over. The healthcare worker should be careful not to prick their own finger.

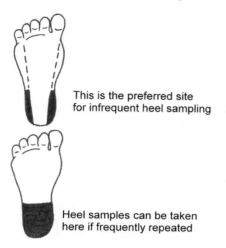

This is the preferred site for infrequent heel sampling

Heel samples can be taken here if frequently repeated

FIGURE 3.4.3 Unsuitable (top) and suitable (bottom) positions from which to obtain capillary blood from the foot of a neonate.

Biliary atresia

In prolonged jaundice (jaundice persisting beyond 14 days of age), it is important to determine not only the total bilirubin concentration but also **the proportion of conjugated bilirubin**. Conjugated bilirubin is not neurotoxic, but its presence signifies the presence of biliary obstruction attributable to potentially serious conditions such as neonatal hepatitis or biliary atresia.

The history can be informative if laboratory investigations are not available. The presence of pale unpigmented stools or dark urine would be suggestive of biliary obstruction. Urine can also be tested with a reagent strip for bilirubin (if positive for bilirubin, the diagnosis of biliary obstruction is supported, provided that the infant is not receiving phototherapy when unconjugated bilirubin appears in the urine).

It is important to identify biliary atresia promptly, as operative intervention is more likely to be successful if undertaken within 8 weeks of birth. Even mild jaundice merits review if the stool becomes grey or putty coloured rather than yellow or green. Similarly, in the absence of a neonatal screening programme (a situation that is prevalent in the majority of resource-limited countries), it is important that congenital hypothyroidism and glucose-6-phosphate dehydrogenase (G6PD) deficiency are identified. This can be done by tests including T_4, TSH, G6PD assay, bilirubin (total and direct), complete blood picture and reticulocyte count.

Breast milk jaundice

Around 10% of breastfed infants are still slightly jaundiced 1 month after birth. Laboratory investigations seldom reveal anything that needs treatment, and the infant is otherwise well. This scenario may be suggestive of breast milk jaundice. However, it is important that other common causes, including congenital biliary atresia, hypothyroidism and G6PD deficiency, are ruled out. Remember that breast milk jaundice is a diagnosis of exclusion.

Ill infants with continuing jaundice should be given a prophylactic 1 mg IM injection of vitamin K if it is not clear that they received such an injection at birth, to minimise the risk of potentially fatal late vitamin K deficiency bleeding.

Pathological jaundice

There is an increasing risk that high levels of unconjugated serum bilirubin will breach the blood–brain barrier, causing critical damage to many cells in the brain. This becomes more likely if, in the presence of haemolysis, the unconjugated serum bilirubin level is allowed to rise above 350 µmol/litre. Indeed, in a small preterm infant who is also ill, the safe limit may be nearer to 250 µmol/litre, or sometimes even less.

Once this happens there is nothing that can usefully be done to reverse the resultant brain damage. Infants may manifest this by seizures, or by becoming stiff with arching of the back and neck signifying a severe encephalopathy. Many of these infants will die after becoming severely ill. The survivors will almost all become severely deaf, and the majority may develop athetoid cerebral palsy.

Causes of abnormally raised bilirubin levels

These include the following:
- haemolytic disease
- neonatal sepsis
- polycythaemia
- severe malnutrition
- hypothyroidism
- congenital infection (usually obstructive jaundice):
  - syphilis
  - toxoplasmosis
  - cytomegalovirus
  - rubella
  - hepatitis.

In the first week of life, the following factors may lead to jaundice that is sufficiently severe to require treatment:
- **Preterm delivery:** Even moderate prematurity significantly increases the risk of early or severe jaundice and associated sequelae. Consequently, the bilirubin treatment charts give lower treatment thresholds for infants born at 31–34 weeks' gestation. At less than 31 weeks, treatment is started at even lower bilirubin levels.
- **Haemolytic disease:** This may be isoimmune (e.g. Rh or ABO incompatibility) or due to red blood cell disorders (e.g. hereditary spherocytosis, G6PD deficiency).
- **Infection:** Haemolysis and impaired elimination of bilirubin may be associated with septicaemia. Congenital infection (e.g. syphilis) may also be associated with jaundice, but other features such as rash, hepatosplenomegaly and thrombocytopenia will be present, and there is usually a significant conjugated bilirubin level.
- **Polycythaemia**.
- **Rarer causes:** These include inborn errors of metabolism (e.g. galactosaemia), congenital hypothyroidism, other intrauterine infections and neonatal malaria.
- **Obstructive jaundice:** This rarely presents in the first week of life, but is important in the differential diagnosis of prolonged jaundice.

Haemolysis

Clinically noticeable jaundice within 24 hours of birth, especially if the mother is blood group O and the infant is blood group A or group B, or the mother is Rhesus negative and the infant is Rhesus positive, should suggest the possibility of a haemolytic disease.

Term infants with physiological jaundice seldom need treatment with phototherapy unless there is an unusually high rate of red cell breakdown. However, phototherapy should be started as soon as jaundice becomes apparent if there is evidence of haemolytic disease. The trend in the bilirubin level should then be checked twice a day (the level cannot be assessed from skin colour once phototherapy has commenced).

Investigation

A good principle to remember is to measure bilirubin levels and investigate if:

- jaundice appears on day 1 in any infant
- jaundice appears on day 2 in any preterm infant
- the palms of the hands or soles of the feet are yellow in any sick neonate and in any infant of any age.

Jaundice should never last for more than 3 weeks.

In an infant who develops jaundice in the first 24 hours, the most likely causes are infections, haemolytic disease and polycythaemia. The history and examination may be helpful. It is important to determine whether the mother has previously had affected infants, or if she is known to have a hereditary haemolytic disorder, or if risk factors for infection or clinical signs of sepsis exist. Hepatosplenomegaly could be suggestive of congenital infection.

The following should suggest a high risk for haemolysis:

- red cell antibodies in the mother's blood
- a positive Coombs' or direct antiglobulin test on blood samples from the umbilical cord
- a packed cell volume > 65%, Hb > 220 g/litre
- a family history of G6PD deficiency or congenital spherocytosis
- a history of previous children being seriously jaundiced in the first week of life
- otherwise unexplained neonatal anaemia at birth (haemoglobin level < 140 g/litre or haematocrit < 40%).

Useful laboratory tests include the following:

- the mother's and infant's ABO and Rhesus blood groups.

Save serum to cross-match if exchange transfusion is needed

- direct Coombs' test (if positive this indicates an isoimmune haemolytic anaemia)
- complete blood count and reticulocyte count (anaemia and reticulocytosis indicate haemolysis, high PCV suggests polycythaemia and/or abnormal white blood cells indicate possible infection)
- peripheral blood smear (abnormal red cell morphology and/or fragmented red cell forms suggest a specific red cell disorder and/or haemolysis)
- G6PD screen
- syphilis serology
- thyroid function tests (T_4, TSH)
- urine test for non-glucose-reducing substance (for possible galactosaemia)
- ultrasound scan of liver.

Treatment

The bilirubin treatment charts (*see* Table 3.4.3) show intervention levels for the two principal treatments (i.e. phototherapy and exchange transfusion). In general, the smaller the infant and the sicker the infant, the more urgent the need to intervene. Bilirubin in plasma is normally bound to albumin, but in a sick acidotic infant less binding occurs, and more 'free' bilirubin will be available to enter the central nervous system. Therefore consider intervening about 40 µmol/litres below the indicated line in such circumstances.

The specific bilirubin levels for which phototherapy and exchange transfusions need to be considered in infants born before 31 weeks' gestation are less certain. A frequently used guideline is to **initiate phototherapy when the bilirubin level approaches 85 µmol/litre/kg birth weight (which equals approximately 5 mg/dL/kg birth weight), and to consider an exchange transfusion for levels above 170 µmol/litre/kg birth weight (which equals approximately 10 mg/dL/kg birth weight).**

TABLE 3.4.3 WHO recommendations (2012) for phototherapy and exchange transfusion levels of unconjugated bilirubin

	Phototherapy		Exchange transfusion	
Age	Healthy newborns ≥ 35 weeks' gestation	Newborns < 35 weeks' gestation or any risk factors	Healthy newborns ≥ 35 weeks' gestation	Newborns < 35 weeks' gestation or any risk factors
Day 1	Any visible jaundice		260 mmol/litre (15 mg/dL)	220 mmol/litre (10 mg/dL)
Day 2	260 mmol/litre (15 mg/dL)	170 mmol/litre (10 mg/dL)	425 mmol/litre (25 mg/dL)	260 mmol/litre (15 mg/dL)
Day 3+	310 mmol/litre (18 mg/dL)	250 mmol/litre (15 mgd/L)	425 mmol/litre (25 mg/dL)	340 mmol/litre (20 mg/dL)

Phototherapy

This uses light in the blue-green region of the spectrum (**not ultraviolet**) to convert bilirubin to its water-soluble isomer **lumirubin**, which can be excreted in urine and stools.

In infants who are very yellow, it is best to use light from a bank of at least six 60-cm 20-watt fluorescent strip lights suspended not more than 30 cm above the unclothed infant (lights placed 60 cm from the infant are only about half as effective). Placing a white sheet under and round the infant will increase the effectiveness of any treatment. While under phototherapy, it is important to monitor body temperature

and to protect the infant from draughts. It is also standard practice to mask the eyes to protect them from the bright light. The infant should be nursed naked in an incubator, under a radiant heater or in a cot, allowing maximum skin exposure. Feeding, especially breastfeeding, should continue without interruption, as more frequent breastfeeding is helpful not only in eliminating meconium from the bowel but also in enhancing bilirubin clearance via the stools and urine. During phototherapy, the infant can be removed for breastfeeds as necessary (intermittent treatment has been shown to be as effective as continuous treatment). Fluid other than breast milk (e.g. breast milk substitute, water, sugar water) should not be given. However, the total daily fluid intake may need to be increased by about 10%, especially in preterm infants, in order to minimise additional water losses from evaporation and convection.

Troublesome side effects of phototherapy include rashes and profuse watery stools, but these are rare and do not require treatment. Phototherapy can be stopped when the serum bilirubin level is 50 mmol/litre (3 mg/dL) below the phototherapy threshold.

Exchange transfusion

Bilirubin levels that rise above certain threshold values place the infant at risk of developing bilirubin encephalopathy (kernicterus). In such cases, the bilirubin level needs to be immediately lowered with a double-volume exchange transfusion. A volume of the infant's blood equal to the body weight in kg × 2 × 80 mL is exchanged in small aliquots with O Rhesus-negative blood, or blood cross-matched against maternal antibodies.

Double-volume exchange transfusion is recommended in **term infants** if:

- they are haemolysing or are ill and have a bilirubin level higher than 300 µmol/litre
- they are well and not haemolysing but their bilirubin level is higher than 425 µmol/litre.

The **functions of exchange transfusion** include the following:

- removal of maternal antibodies
- removal of antibody-coated red blood cells before they haemolyse
- correction of anaemia
- lowering of total bilirubin levels, if there is sufficient time for equilibration between intravascular and extravascular levels.

Exchange transfusion is generally only undertaken if the rate of red blood cell breakdown is likely to exceed the ability of phototherapy to control bilirubin levels. This is very likely to occur in infants with a positive Coombs' test who are already anaemic (because of fetal haemolysis) at birth. A cord blood haemoglobin level of less than 140 grams/litre serves to identify most of these infants.

Human immunoglobulin 500 mg/kg, given as an IV infusion over 2 hours, reduces the number of infants who require an exchange (especially if due to Coombs' positive Rhesus or ABO incompatibility). It also decreases the number who require a 'top-up' transfusion for late neonatal anaemia.

Exchange transfusion

1 Calculate the infant's circulating volume (= 80 mL/kg). Twice this amount of blood will be required. Do not exceed this (usually 1 bag of whole blood = 450 mL). Do not use blood that is more than 4 days old.
2 Check that the blood has either the same ABO group as the infant or is blood group O Rhesus-negative and in addition is compatible with the mother's serum.
3 Ensure that the infant is closely monitored throughout the procedure.
4 This is a sterile procedure, so gloves and gowns must be worn and universal precautions applied.
5 Secure umbilical vein access. Pass the umbilical venous

catheter (UVC) as described in Section 8.4.B, and check its position with an X-ray (if available). Ideally it should be positioned in the vena cava just outside the right atrium, but a position below the liver is also acceptable if the line will sample and flush easily. A line positioned in the liver should not be used.

6 Ideally, use a blood warmer (especially for low-birth-weight infants). Otherwise warm the blood bag by placing it under the mother's clothing next to the skin.
7 Set up a closed circuit with either a four-way tap, or two three-way taps. The four links are:
   - the infant
   - the syringe for removing and replacing blood
   - the blood to be transfused
   - the route for discarding the infant's blood.
8 Make sure that the total blood in and out is recorded. Plan to spend 1.5–2 hours on the procedure.
9 Decide on the size of aliquot you will be exchanging with each draw and infusion. This is roughly as follows:
   - baby weighing < 1500 grams: 5 mL
   - baby weighing 1500–2500 grams: 5–0 mL
   - baby weighing 2500 grams: 10–15 mL.

If you use small aliquots, remember to add an allowance for the 'dead space' in the tubing between the syringe and the baby. You should draw out each aliquot over 2–3 minutes to avoid abrupt changes in blood pressure, and replace over 3–4 minutes with the observer keeping a running total.

10 Send the first aliquot for measurement of bilirubin, electrolyte and calcium concentrations.
11 Halfway through the procedure check the blood glucose, calcium and potassium concentrations.
12 Measure them again, together with the bilirubin concentration, at the end of the procedure.
13 Sometimes it is necessary to exchange more than once in quick succession. Symptomatic hypocalcaemia may occur as the citrate in donor blood binds calcium. This responds best to halting the procedure for 15 minutes. Giving calcium gluconate is of little benefit and may be hazardous, so is best avoided.

Although the potassium concentration of the blood is often 8–10 mmol/litre, this does not usually cause significant hyperkalaemia.

Exchange transfusion should only be undertaken once all of the attendant risks have been considered. Even in experienced hands, 1% of infants may suffer a sudden cardiac arrest during or shortly after the procedure. This should respond to prompt intervention using the approach adopted when dealing with cardiac arrest at birth, but the infant needs to be monitored closely, and staff need to be prepared for such a possibility if this is not to prove fatal. Air embolism can kill within minutes, and faulty technique can cause sudden hypo- or hypervolaemia, or introduce later sepsis. The use of donor blood more than 5 days old can cause serious hyperkalaemia and an arrhythmia. Blood used straight from the fridge at 4°C can impose a major cold stress. Cytomegalovirus (CMV) infection may occur if the blood does not come from a CMV-negative donor. It is also critical to avoid causing HIV or hepatitis B or C infection. In addition, there is a definite but poorly understood risk that the procedure will trigger serious necrotising enterocolitis. If possible it is best to avoid the use of heparinised blood.

Because of all these risks, if at all possible exchange transfusion should only be undertaken in a neonatal unit where the staff are experienced in the use of this procedure.

The neonate with anaemia
Causes of anaemia
These include the following:

- haemorrhage
- twin-to-twin transfusion
- feto–maternal transfusion
- placental abruption
- haemolysis due to
  - Rhesus incompatibility
  - ABO incompatibility.

Treatment of anaemia
Haemolysis may continue for several weeks after birth even if it is not severe enough to require intervention in the first week of life. An attempt should therefore be made to check all infants with a positive Coombs' test for late anaemia when they are about 6 weeks old. Infants with a capillary haemoglobin level of less than 80 grams/litre or a haematocrit (PCV) of less than 25% should then receive a 'top-up' transfusion of 20 mL/kg of cross-matched or group O Rhesus-negative blood given over 2 hours. Red cell concentrate or packed cells are preferable. Daily folic acid (1 mg/day) for at least 1 week can help to reduce anaemia.

The neonate with seizures, spasms or reduced conscious level

Seizures (also called fits or convulsions) have been reported to affect about 0.1% of term infants and 10% of those weighing less than 1500 grams at birth.

Presenting features
Seizures may be subtle (apnoea, staring, lip smacking/grimacing, deviation of the eyes, cycling movements of the limbs) or more obvious (tonic extensor posturing or clonic movements). Involvement of a limb or one side of the body does not necessarily imply a focal cause in the neonate. A bulging anterior fontanelle may suggest intracranial haemorrhage or infection. It is important to **always measure and note the head circumference**. Sometimes involuntary movements (e.g. extreme jitteriness) or benign myoclonic jerks can be difficult to distinguish from seizures. The presence of associated autonomic instability and/or lateral eye deviations may signal seizure activity, whereas the absence of these findings or elimination of these movements when the limbs are restrained indicate a non-seizure event.

Causes of seizures
These include the following:

- hypoxia
- hypoglycaemia
- meningitis
- drug-related seizures
- sepsis
- polycythaemia
- tetanus
- hypocalcaemia
- hyper- or hyponatraemia
- metabolic abnormalities
- **hypoxic ischaemic encephalopathy:** this is the most common cause of seizures in a term infant. Onset is usually within the first 24 hours, and it almost never starts after the third day
- **intracranial haemorrhage, subarachnoid haemorrhage or cerebral infarctions:** these are also common causes of neonatal seizures. With subarachnoid haemorrhage, seizures may or may not be focal. However, unilateral tonic–clonic seizures are often observed with cerebral infarction. Although **intraventricular haemorrhage** occurs most frequently in low-birth-weight infants or at gestational ages under 32 weeks, very rarely it may manifest in term or near-term infants with neonatal seizures. Always give 1 mg IV vitamin K
- **infection:** although meningitis is not the commonest cause of neonatal convulsion, it must always be excluded by lumbar puncture and antibiotics commenced urgently pending the results of culture
- **metabolic causes** of seizures may include:
  - **hypoglycaemia:** always check blood glucose levels
  - **hypocalcaemia:** check plasma calcium and magnesium levels
  - **hyponatraemia and hypernatraemia:** seizures are uncommon unless the plasma sodium level is < 120 mmol/litre or > 160 mmol/litre. Seizures in infants with hypernatraemia may result from associated cavernous sinus thrombosis. A rapid fall or rise in serum sodium level, as may occur with too rapid therapeutic correction, may be more injurious than the absolute value of serum sodium level. A slow correction is desirable in such situations
- **bilirubin encephalopathy** (see above section on jaundice)
- rare **inborn errors of metabolism** (e.g. urea cycle defects, non-ketotic hyperglycaemia) require measurement of serum amino acids, urine fatty acids, serum lactate, serum pyruvate and blood ammonia levels. Measuring the anion gap can also be quite helpful. A high value may be suggestive of an inborn error of metabolism.
  Note: anion gap = (Na + K) − (Cl + HCO₃). Normal anion gap = 5–17 mEq/litre in neonates
- **maternal substance abuse**, particularly opiate withdrawal
- **tetanus** remains a problem in many low-resource countries.

TABLE 3.4.4 Differentiating between seizures and jitteriness

Well but jittery infant	Infant with clonic seizures
No abnormal eye movements	Abnormal eye movements
No apnoea	Apnoea
No colour changes	Pallor or cyanosis
No heart rate changes	Tachycardia
Easily triggered by handling and stopped by gentle passive flexion of the affected limb	Independent of handling
Rhythmical movements	Jerky with fast and slow components that are not equal

When managing neonatal seizures it is best to focus on the limited number of conditions where immediate treatment can have a major impact on long-term outcome. There are many situations where seizures are simply the outward sign of damage that cannot be reversed, even though it may be possible to stop continuing seizure activity from making matters worse.

Focal seizures can sometimes be the sign of what was otherwise a silent haemorrhagic infarction of part of the brain. While investigation would explain what was going on, it would not alter management.

If the infant is alert and well between episodes of seizure activity, appears normal on examination, and is feeding normally, sometimes it may be perfectly appropriate to do nothing.

Investigations

These should include the following:
- lumbar puncture and blood culture
- full blood count, PCV, CRP
- blood glucose, calcium, urea and electrolytes, and blood ammonia (if available)
- arterial blood gas analysis to help further assess acid–base status
- cranial ultrasound (if available)
- intracranial imaging (head computed tomography if available)
- baseline and follow-up electroencephalograms (if available) may aid diagnosis and treatment
- save urine, plasma and CSF for metabolic studies (if available) if seizures are protracted.

Treatment

Management of a neonate with seizures is as follows:
- Airway.
- Breathing.
- Circulatory access.
- Give glucose, IV or intra-osseous (2 mL/kg of 10% glucose).
- Give antibiotics, IV or IM, as there is a strong possibility of meningitis or sepsis.
- Stop the seizures with an anticonvulsant:
  - phenobarbitone, 20 mg/kg over 5 minutes IV or IM
  - paraldehyde, 0.2 mL/kg IM or 0.4 mL/kg rectally
  - diazepam 300 microgram/kg IV slowly or 500 microgram/kg rectally.
- Treat hypoglycaemia if present.
- Monitor the heart rate and respiratory rate, and oxygenation (ideally with pulse oximetry). Treat low SaO_2 or cyanosis with oxygen.
- Consider anticonvulsant therapy: the earlier the fits appear, the more frequent they are (more than two or three per hour) and the longer they last (more than 3 minutes), the more likely it is that anticonvulsants will be needed. Fits that interfere with respiration need to be treated and may require respiratory support.

Emergency treatment of hypoglycaemia

Hypoglycaemia is a common cause of seizures in infants. Ideally, do a rapid bedside test for low blood glucose levels and act accordingly, but if this test is not available then a test dose of 2 mL/kg of 10% glucose should be given IV or, if venous access is not available, intra-osseously.

Anticonvulsant treatment

Phenobarbital is the first-line drug for neonatal seizures. Give a 20 mg/kg IV loading dose slowly followed by 3–5 mg/kg once every 24 hours. Seizure control may be achieved more quickly if the first dose is given IV, but this loading dose must be given slowly, over at least 5 minutes, to minimise the risk of shock, hypotension or laryngospasm. Some texts recommend the use of a higher dose if the standard dose fails, but this can cause respiratory depression. **Always have a bag-valve-mask available to support ventilation.** With hypoxic encephalopathy usually only a loading dose is needed. Seizures have been reported to respond to this dose 40% of the time. An additional 10 mg/kg may be required if seizures persist or recur (70% response rate).

Phenytoin is the second-line drug for neonatal seizures. Initial seizure control with this drug requires the presence of a saline-filled IV line (because the drug crystallises out in dextrose solutions). The same problem also renders the IM route unavailable. Give a 20 mg/kg loading dose (diluted in 10–15 mL of normal saline) IV slowly over 10–20 minutes (monitor for hypotension and cardiac arrhythmia, making sure that the drug does not leak into the tissues), and then 2 mg/kg IV or by mouth once every 8 hours. Infants more than 2 to 3 weeks old may need a considerably larger maintenance dose. Oral absorption of phenytoin may be quite unpredictable, so this would need to be monitored. Phenytoin is dangerous in infants with hypoxic ischaemic encephalopathy who may also have ischaemic hypoxic heart injury.

Paraldehyde is the third-line drug for neonatal seizures. Give a single 0.4 mL/kg dose mixed with an equal volume of mineral oil by the rectal route. This route offers excellent bioavailability of the drug. The same dose can be repeated once if seizures persist. Give within 10 minutes after preparation when using a plastic syringe (because paraldehyde interacts with many plastics). Paraldehyde can also be given by the IM route. However, problems with muscle necrosis make this a less desirable route.

Diazepam is an alternative to phenobarbital as first line treatment for neonatal seizures. However, it is vital that hypoglycaemia has been excluded and treated before giving this drug. A working bag-valve-mask of suitable size must be ready next to the infant before this drug is given. It can be given IV at a dose of 300 microgram/kg over 5 minutes or rectally in a dose of 500 microgram/kg. The rectal dose can be repeated once after 10 minutes if the infant is still fitting.

Clonazepam: The loading dose is given as 100 micrograms/kg by slow IV infusion. It should not be administered for more than 3 days.

Midazolam: This has an immediate effect but a short duration of action. It can be given into the buccal cavity or IV. Like diazepam it can cause respiratory depression, so a bag and mask must be available when it is used, and the infant must be monitored closely.

Anticonvulsants may precipitate a need for respiratory support. Therefore always have a bag-valve-mask available.

Once seizures are controlled, maintenance therapy (which is rarely needed) with a single agent (usually phenobarbitone) is often possible. Discontinuation of treatment depends on the underlying aetiology, but aim to withdraw anticonvulsants as soon as possible.

It is essential to consider the four main treatable causes of fitting, namely **hypoglycaemia, hypocalcaemia,**

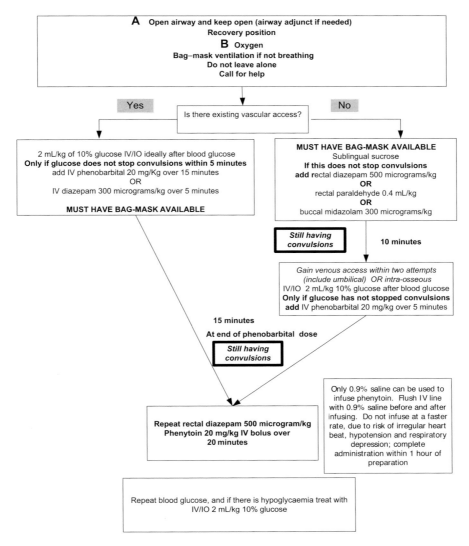

A Open airway and keep open (airway adjunct if needed)
Recovery position
B Oxygen
Bag–mask ventilation if not breathing
Do not leave alone
Call for help

Yes   Is there existing vascular access?   No

2 mL/kg of 10% glucose IV/IO ideally after blood glucose
Only if glucose does not stop convulsions within 5 minutes
add IV phenobarbital 20 mg/Kg over 15 minutes
OR
IV diazepam 300 micrograms/kg over 5 minutes

MUST HAVE BAG-MASK AVAILABLE

MUST HAVE BAG-MASK AVAILABLE
Sublingual sucrose
If this does not stop convulsions
add rectal diazepam 500 micrograms/kg
OR
rectal paraldehyde 0.4 mL/kg
OR
buccal midazolam 300 micrograms/kg

Still having convulsions   10 minutes

*Gain venous access within two attempts
(include umbilical) OR intra-osseous*
IV/IO 2 mL/kg 10% glucose after blood glucose
Only if glucose has not stopped convulsions
add IV phenobarbital 20 mg/kg over 5 minutes

15 minutes
At end of phenobarbital dose

Still having convulsions

Only 0.9% saline can be used to infuse phenytoin. Flush IV line with 0.9% saline before and after infusing. Do not infuse at a faster rate, due to risk of irregular heart beat, hypotension and respiratory depression; complete administration within 1 hour of preparation

Repeat rectal diazepam 500 microgram/kg
Phenytoin 20 mg/kg IV bolus over
20 minutes

Repeat blood glucose, and if there is hypoglycaemia treat with
IV/IO 2 mL/kg 10% glucose

FIGURE 3.4.4 Pathway of care for a neonate who is having convulsions.

meningitis and **tetanus**, as any delay in diagnosis could have serious consequences.

Hypoglycaemia (glucose < 2.5 mmol/litre or < 45 mg/dL)

Hypoglycaemia is a common problem in the nursery; it can occur in infants who appear well, as well as in those who are sick. It is important to identify any infant at risk and implement preventative and curative measures as early as possible. **Untreated symptomatic hypoglycaemia can result in brain damage.**

Infants at risk of developing hypoglycaemia include the following:

- infant of diabetic mother
- preterm infant
- small-for-gestational-age or wasted infant
- large-for-gestational-age infant
- post-term infant
- sick infant with infections and respiratory failure
- infant who is not receiving adequate breast milk.

The definition of hypoglycaemia is controversial, and no studies have determined an absolute value at which organ dysfunction will occur. However, it is known that a prolonged low level of symptomatic hypoglycaemia is associated with brain injury. At the time of writing, most neonatologists prefer to maintain blood glucose levels above 2.5 mmol/litre (45 mg/dL).

Causes of neonatal hypoglycaemia
Increased utilisation of glucose (hyperinsulinism)

- Infants of diabetic mothers.
- Respiratory distress.
- Abrupt interruption of high glucose infusion.
- Polycythaemia.
- Hypothermia.

Rare causes of hyperinsulinism include:

- erythroblastosis fetalis
- islet-cell hyperplasia
- Beckwith–Wiedemann syndrome
- insulin-producing tumours
- maternal beta-agonist tocolytic therapy
- rarely malpositioned umbilical arterial catheter infusing a high concentration of glucose into coeliac and mesenteric arteries (T11–T12), stimulating insulin release.

Decreased production/stores of carbohydrate
- Prematurity.
- Small-for-gestational-age or wasted infant.
- Inadequate caloric intake.

Mixed increased utilisation and/or decreased production from other causes
- Perinatal stress (e.g. due to hypoxia, sepsis, shock, hypothermia).

Rare causes
- Defects in carbohydrate metabolism (galactosaemia, fructose intolerance, glycogen storage disease).
- Endocrine deficiency (adrenal insufficiency, hypothalamic insufficiency, glucagon deficiency).
- Defects in amino acid metabolism (maple syrup urine disease, propionic acidaemia, methylmalonic acidaemia, tyrosinaemia).

Diagnosis of hypoglycaemia
- There are few data on normal blood glucose levels in the first week of life, particularly for healthy breastfed term infants. **Moreover, there is little evidence that a transient low blood glucose concentration in term infants who show no physical signs is harmful. However, asymptomatic hypoglycaemia may rapidly progress to symptomatic hypoglycaemia.** Fits due to hypoglycaemia typically start in a previously well infant on or after the second day of life.
- Indications for measuring the blood glucose concentration of a term infant include lethargy, poor feeding, temperature instability, respiratory distress, new-onset apnoea/bradycardia, jitteriness, pronounced hypotonia, diminished consciousness and seizures. The association between such signs and low blood glucose levels is described as 'symptomatic hypoglycaemia'.
- Beware of blaming 'hypoglycaemia' alone for these signs. **Remember that an infant who seems drowsy may be infected, and low blood glucose concentration may merely be an associated finding**. It is important to try to establish the underlying cause of the problem.
  - Although laboratory estimates of blood glucose concentration are ideal for diagnosing and managing this condition, reagent strips can be helpful.
  - The blood glucose concentration in the first 6 hours of life is very often low (1.5–2.0 mmol/litre). There is no evidence that this is harmful for otherwise healthy term infants, who adapt by mobilising other fuels. Consequently, early testing (under 6 hours of age) is pointless, unless neurological signs are present or there are other conditions that necessitate testing.
  - In newborn infants the serum glucose concentration is about 0.5 mmol/litre lower than that of whole blood.

When to test
- **Symptomatic infants** (lethargy, poor feeding, temperature instability, respiratory distress, new-onset apnoea/bradycardia, jitteriness and seizures) should be tested immediately.
- **Infants at risk** should be tested within 1 hour after birth (as such infants rapidly become hypoglycaemic after delivery) and then 3-hourly until blood glucose levels are stable at 2.5 mmol/litre (45 mg/dL) or higher. Continue to monitor until feeds are well established.
- In infants with **hypoglycaemia**, check the blood glucose concentration every 20–30 minutes from the beginning of treatment, then hourly until it is stable at 2.5 mmol/litre (45 mg/dL) or higher. Continue to monitor frequently (every 4–8 hours) during treatment, and while decreasing supplemental IV glucose infusions.

Laboratory diagnosis
- **Reagent strips** are useful and rapid, but in general are less reliable than laboratory plasma glucose measurements. Reagent strips may show a glucose level as much as 15% lower than plasma glucose levels. Whenever possible, it is preferable to use a calibrated glucometer.
- **Laboratory plasma glucose determinations** (if available) are useful for confirming hypoglycaemia detected by reagent strips, but blood samples must be processed promptly for accurate values, as glycolysis occurs in standing whole blood samples. **Do not wait for laboratory confirmation before initiating therapy.**

Management of hypoglycaemia
Infants at risk of hypoglycaemia but appearing to be well
- Initiate early feeding within 1 hour after birth with breast milk or formula (only if breast milk is not available) and repeat every 2–3 hours.
- Feeding with 5% glucose is not recommended in infants, because milk provides more energy.
- Infants of diabetic mothers are unlikely to develop hypoglycaemia on the second day of life if tests in the first 24 hours are satisfactory.

Infants with symptomatic hypoglycaemia who are unable to feed or who failed correction of glucose levels with enteral feeding
- Establish an IV line using sterile precautions, and take a sample for blood culture and other biochemical tests (if available).
  - Give an IV glucose bolus 200 mg/kg over 5 minutes (2 mL/kg of 10% glucose in water). If the infant almost immediately becomes more alert and active 'on the end of your needle' you have made the diagnosis, even before the laboratory report comes back.
  - In such situations it is then important to keep the blood glucose level stable by starting a sustained infusion of 10% dextrose at 5 mL/kg/hour (or 5–8 mg/kg/minute) for the next 2 to 4 days while gradually building up oral feeds.
- If further episodes of symptomatic hypoglycaemia occur, the bolus should be repeated and the infusion rate increased by 10–15%.
- An infant who seems drowsy may be infected, and a low blood glucose concentration may be an associated finding rather than the main cause of the problem. It is important to exclude infection and initiate antibiotics if indicated.
- When administering boluses, never use higher concentrations of glucose (> 10%) because of the risk of intra-ventricular haemorrhage and/or cerebral oedema.
- The concentration of glucose in the maintenance fluids

can be adjusted in accordance with the total daily fluid requirements.

- If using concentrations higher than 12.5%, a central venous line or umbilical venous catheter needs to be inserted because of the risk of tissue damage in the event of fluid extravasation.
- Most infants will correct hypoglycaemia with infusion of 5–8 mg/kg/minute; not infrequently, however, infants with severe intrauterine growth restriction or wasting and those with hyperinsulinism may require infusion rates of up to 12–15 mg/kg/minute.
- When normal blood glucose levels have been stable for 12–24 hours and the infant is tolerating enteral feeding, decrease the IV glucose infusion by 10–20% each time levels are higher than 2.5 mmol/litre (45 mg/dL).
- Always decrease the IV infusion gradually because of the risk of precipitating hypoglycaemia.
- If you are unable to gain IV access, a feed of breast milk should be started if the infant is conscious. Hypostop Gel, an oral glucose mixture containing 500 micrograms of glucose/mL, can be helpful (if available). Apply 1–2 mL to the oral mucosa.
- If hypoglycaemia persists beyond the first 48 hours of life and requires large infusions of glucose (greater than 8 mg/kg/minute), evaluation for endocrine or metabolic disorders should be considered.

Meningitis
See p. 353.

Tetanus

Do not forget tetanus. Neonatal tetanus has to be considered if a previously well and still conscious infant starts to develop increasingly frequent muscle spasms 3–14 days after birth. This becomes more relevant if there is any doubt about the way the umbilical cord was managed at birth, or if there is no proof that the mother was ever immunised with tetanus toxoid vaccine. Involuntary muscle contractions are typically triggered by quite light touch or sound, and the hands and jaw are often held firmly clenched.

- **Airway** and **breathing** are frequently compromised. Secure and maintain the airway, and ensure adequacy of ventilation. **Oxygen** may help if the spasms are causing cyanosis, but in severe cases survival may be dependent on the availability of **respiratory support**, sometimes with **tracheostomy** to protect the airway. Intubation may trigger very dangerous spasm of the airway and must be undertaken by a skilled professional.
- Insert an IV line for drug and antibiotic administration.
- Give high-dose **benzyl penicillin** 60 mg/kg IV one dose every 12 hours in the first week of life, every 8 hours in an infant aged 1–3 weeks, and every 6 hours in an infant over 3 weeks of age. Oral dosing (with **phenoxymethylpenicillin**) can sometimes be used to complete a course of treatment.
- Give an 150 unit/kg dose of IM human tetanus immunoglobulin. **Other IM injections must be avoided altogether, as they will provoke spasms.**
- If the infant/child is in **acute spasm**, this should be terminated by giving **diazepam by bolus IV infusion over 15 minutes (dose 200 micrograms/kg) or rectally (400 micrograms/kg)**. Ensure that for IV infusion, diazepam is diluted to 100 micrograms/mL, and that extravasation (very irritant) does not occur. Slow and

incomplete absorption means that IM diazepam is not effective. **Always ensure that a bag and mask are immediately available when giving diazepam, in case apnoea occurs.**

- Also give an IV loading dose of 25–40 mg/kg of magnesium sulphate over 20–30 minutes.
- Subsequently give 10–20 mg/kg of magnesium sulphate IV 2- to 4-hourly to control spasms. If this is not available or does not control spasms, give IV diazepam 200 micrograms/kg every 4–6 hours.
- Stop diazepam if magnesium sulphate alone controls the spasms.
- Reduce the dose of diazepam if apnoeic episodes occur.
- **Always have a bag and mask available in case the patient stops breathing as a result of the diazepam plus magnesium.**
- When stable, a nasogastric tube, ideally passed by an anaesthetist, will allow fluids, food and drugs to be given with minimal disturbance. Feeds need to be given frequently (ideally hourly) and in small amounts due to reduced gut motility. **Regular breast milk feeds via a nasogastric tube are essential.**
- Excision of the umbilical stump is not indicated.
- The disease itself does not induce immunity, so after recovery tetanus vaccine must be given for future prevention.
- **Treat any obvious umbilical infection** with an additional broad-spectrum antibiotic.
- **Minimise handling, provide care in a quiet dark room** and **give frequent small tube feeds**.
- **Immunising the mother** (give two 0.5-mL doses 1 month apart) will prevent a similar tragedy in any future pregnancy.
- **Severe cases may need muscle paralysis and ventilation in a specialist unit (if available).**

Treatment of neonatal tetanus
- Airway and Breathing: Oxygen as needed and tracheostomy may be required.
- Benzyl penicillin.
- Human tetanus immunoglobulin.
- Consider giving diazepam IV or by the rectal route to control spasms (with bag and mask available).
- Magnesium sulphate has been recently shown to help prevent spasms in tetanus.
- Minimise handling.
- Give frequent small tube feeds of breast milk.

Other causes of neonatal seizures
Rule out any other cause, including biochemical causes other than hypoglycaemia.

Remember that biochemical disturbance may not be the main underlying problem. In many infants, the evidence of hypoglycaemia or any other biochemical disturbance is only a sign of another more serious underlying illness. Of these, by far the most important treatable condition is meningitis. Unless the infant is otherwise entirely well it is important not to miss this possibility.

- Other important diagnostic possibilities include hypocalcaemia, hyponatraemia and hypernatraemia. Often a history and clinical features will aid the recognition of these biochemical abnormalities, and a serum level will clinch the diagnosis. Any existing problem will be made worse if hypernatraemia is corrected too rapidly.

- Fits due to hypocalcaemia (a serum total calcium level of < 1.7 mmol/litre), with or without hypomagnesaemia, are generally benign and occur unexpectedly in an otherwise well but hyper-reflexic child more than 2 to 3 days old. As with hypoglycaemia, signs may settle 'on the end of the needle' if the infant is given 1–2 mL/kg of 10% calcium gluconate in equal dilution as a **slow** IV infusion. Such seizures usually respond extremely well to oral supplementation. It is appropriate to investigate the mother for an unrecognised endocrine abnormality (if facilities allow this). **Do not allow IV calcium to go outside the vein as it will cause severe tissue damage.**
- Toxic substances provided by a traditional healer create important causes of seizures and reduced conscious level in neonates in some countries.

Bilirubin encephalopathy

Infants with brain damage due to jaundice are stiff and semi-conscious, but seldom have fits. Signs usually appear quite abruptly 3 to 6 days after birth, but by the time they appear it is too late to initiate treatment.

Inborn errors of metabolism

Other more complex biochemical disturbances are usually associated with metabolic acidosis and progressively deepening coma in a child who was initially well for 1 to 2 days after birth. They are generally too complex to treat without substantial biochemical support, but it may be appropriate to take specimens for later diagnostic evaluation, because many of these conditions are familial and genetically determined. **Pyridoxine deficiency** is one of the few rare treatable conditions.

Hypoxic-ischaemic encephalopathy

This is an abnormal neurological state of infants who have suffered significant lack of oxygen and/or circulation to vital organs before, during or immediately after birth. It is characterised by the following:

- signs of fetal distress in labour, cord blood pH < 7.0, and low Apgar score (≤ 3 at 5 minutes) despite appropriate resuscitation measures
- neonatal neurological abnormalities soon after delivery
- evidence of multi-organ dysfunction such as oliguria (signifying acute tubular necrosis), increased transaminase levels (hepatic necrosis), necrotising enterocolitis or myocardial dysfunction.

Hypoxic-ischaemic encephalopathy-related problems in the days after birth

- **Reduced consciousness and/or convulsions:** treat with phenobarbital and check glucose levels to rule out hypoglycaemia.
- **Apnoea:** this is common after severe perinatal asphyxia, and is sometimes associated with convulsions. Manage with oxygen administered by nasal cannulae and resuscitation with bag and mask.
- **Inability to suck:** feed with expressed breast milk via a nasogastric tube. Beware of delayed emptying of the stomach, which may lead to regurgitation of feeds.
- **Poor motor tone:** the infant may be floppy or have limb stiffening (spasticity).

Sarnat's clinical grading system (see Table 3.4.5) may be used to help to guide treatment and give some indication of the prognosis.

Treatment

- Treatment is generally supportive, with close attention to monitoring of good respiratory function, glucose levels and fluid balance. Avoid hyponatraemia, which may result from inappropriate antidiuretic hormone secretion and excessive IV hypotonic solutions. Acute renal failure is often present; if so, restrict fluids to measured urine output and gut losses plus 15 mL/kg/24 hours for full term and 24 mL/kg/24 hours for preterm infants (to reflect insensible losses), and avoid giving potassium supplements.
- Seizures are treated as described above. Note, however, that increasing doses of anticonvulsants may precipitate a need for mechanical ventilation and confound the clinical staging criteria below, which apply only to non-sedated infants.
- Keep the axillary temperature at 35.5–36.0°C. Avoid overheating.

Cooling infants for 72 hours under carefully controlled conditions has shown improved neurological outcomes. This should only be undertaken by experienced teams.

Prognosis

The prognosis is good in stage 1, guarded in stage 2 and very poor in stage 3.

About 50% of stage 2 infants will recover without sequelae. Infants in stage 3 will either die or be left severely disabled. A decision must therefore be made with the family about the implementation or continuation of intensive care in such cases.

TABLE 3.4.5 Sarnat's grading of hypoxemic-ischaemic encephalopathy

	Mild (stage 1)	Moderate (stage 2)	Severe (stage 3)
Conscious level	Hyper-alert	Lethargic	Stuporose
Muscle tone	Normal	Hypotonic	Flaccid
Seizures	Rare	Common	Severe
Feeding	Sucks weakly	Needs tube feeds	Needs tube feeds or IV fluids
Respiration	Spontaneous	Spontaneous	Absent

Management

Once bacterial meningitis has been excluded, intrapartum hypoxia or birth trauma will turn out to be the underlying problem in most infants presenting with fits in the first 2 to 3 days of life. Most of these infants already look stressed and unwell within a few hours of birth. The onset may be a little more sudden and abrupt in the preterm infant who suffers a sudden intra-ventricular haemorrhage. These infants usually become progressively more stuporose and unresponsive over time, and there is relatively little that can be done to improve the long-term outlook. An attempt should be made to minimise hypoxia, and anticonvulsant treatment is sometimes initiated in the hope that it will reduce the number of apnoeic episodes. Many of these infants are too ill to accept even tube feeds, and, where this is the case, it may be appropriate to minimise the risk of hypoglycaemia by giving IV glucose. Unfortunately, an infusion of more than 3 mL/kg of 10% dextrose per hour may result in water retention if there is accompanying renal failure. The outlook is fairly bleak for infants who have not recovered and started to feed normally within 1 week of birth.

Other less common causes

Drug-related seizures: Accidental infiltration of the fetal scalp during the injection of lidocaine into the maternal perineum prior to episiotomy can cause fits simulating intrapartum hypoxia. With supportive treatment there is every prospect of complete recovery.

Some infants born to **drug-dependent mothers** show signs of drug withdrawal, starting 1 to 2 days after delivery. A small minority may have seizures. Minimal handling in a quiet dark room with small frequent feeds and a more gradual withdrawal from the drug to which they have been exposed is the only treatment usually necessary.

Congenital brain abnormalities: It is said that up to 10% of otherwise unexplained neonatal seizures are associated with the existence of some underlying cerebral problem (often cortical dysgenesis). Some of these infants will benefit from continuing anticonvulsant treatment.

Other miscellaneous neonatal problems

Gastrointestinal problems

- **Oesophageal atresia** should always be considered in the infant with a history of polyhydramnios or excessive frothy salivation following delivery. Surgery is much more likely to be successful if it can be performed before aspiration pneumonia develops. Pass a large-bore catheter as far down the oesophagus as possible and aspirate frequently. If an X-ray shows that the tube has stopped at the level of the heart and has not entered the stomach, the diagnosis is made. Such an infant needs urgent referral for surgery, with steps taken to suck the blind upper oesophageal pouch clear of all accumulating secretions at least every 15 minutes before and during transfer. Site an IV line and ensure that the infant does not become hypoglycaemic.
- **Severe vomiting**, often associated with abdominal distension, in the first few days of life suggests the existence of a problem that requires referral for surgical review. This is particularly true if the vomit is green (bile stained), as this is suggestive of **duodenal atresia** or bowel obstruction requiring urgent surgical intervention. If severe vomiting develops in a infant who has passed changing stool, the diagnosis of **volvulus, pyloric stenosis** or **intussusception** must be considered. Duodenal atresia is more common in infants with Down's syndrome. A paediatric surgical opinion should be sought if available.

Necrotising enterocolitis (NEC)

This is a very serious condition with a mortality of approximately 20–40%. Preterm or small-for-dates infants are at increased risk of developing this condition. Prevalence is inversely related to birth weight and gestation. NEC is more common in ill infants. Although it is more common in infants who have received feeds, about 15–20% of affected infants may never have been fed. It is much less common in infants fed exclusively on human milk. NEC may occur in epidemics due to cross-infection in the nursery.

Presenting features

The condition should be suspected in an infant who had started to accept oral feeds and then develops an ileus or becomes lethargic and starts passing a bloody stool. The problem is caused by the sudden focal invasion of bacteria into an area of ischaemic gut, and an abdominal X-ray will often show gas accumulating within the gut wall.

Common signs of NEC include the following:

- abdominal distension or tenderness
- intolerance of feeding
- bile-stained vomit or bile-stained fluid up the nasogastric tube
- blood in the stools.

Features of multisystem failure, such as coagulopathy, petechial haemorrhage, oliguria and haematuria, may be associated with NEC.

Investigations

A plain abdominal X-ray may show an abnormal gas pattern in the form of:

- **free intra-peritoneal air**, best seen with a left side down (lateral decubitus) X-ray, where free air may be easily seen overlying the dense hepatic tissue
- **intramural gas (pneumatosis intestinalis)** or **gas in the portal tracts of the liver**.

A complete blood count with differential cell count, blood culture and serum electrolytes should be obtained. Regular weighing, frequent blood pressure measurements, and continuous heart and respiratory rate monitoring are required.

Treatment

- Stop all enteral feeds for at least 5 days and provide IV fluids, typically 120 mL/kg/day of 10% glucose with added electrolytes. Adjust fluids as indicated based on weight change, urine output and serum electrolyte values.
- If available, place an orogastric tube on low-pressure continuous suction or leave the tube open with intermittent gastric aspiration (every 4 hours). The goal here is to keep the intestines decompressed. The volume of gastric fluid aspirated is usually relatively small, so replacement fluid is seldom required.
- Start parenteral broad-spectrum antibiotics (usually ampicillin and gentamicin). Because of the probable association of Gram-negative anaerobes, also give metronidazole, especially if there is pneumatosis, perforation or evidence of peritonitis. Broader-spectrum antibiotics may be considered in the presence of extensive disease or poor response, or based on culture results.
- Treat any accompanying shock with Ringer-lactate or Hartmann's solution or colloid, such as 4.5% albumin, 10 mL/kg over 15 minutes. Repeat if necessary.
- Measure the haemoglobin concentration daily and transfuse if it falls below 10 g/dL. If the infant is bleeding, give 1 mg vitamin K IV and fresh-frozen plasma 10 mL/kg (if available).
- The principal goal of therapy is to rest the bowel and treat any contributing or evolving bacterial infection with antibiotics. The duration of this therapy is usually

10–21 days, depending on the severity of the process. Serial abdominal X-ray studies (if available) are indicated early in this disease to monitor for pneumatosis intestinalis or perforation. Ideally, parenteral nutrition should be given at this time in place of simple 10% glucose and electrolytes. Enteral feeds (breast milk) are reintroduced slowly at the end of antibiotic therapy (initially 20–30 mL/kg/day), with careful monitoring for abdominal distension or other signs of obstruction.

In seriously ill infants or infants who do not improve after 48 hours a surgical opinion should be sought.

Even in hospitals with good surgical support, perforation of the bowel is not necessarily an indication for a laparotomy. The conventional surgical approach has been laparotomy with resection of the perforated and adjacent necrotic bowel. A stoma and mucus fistula may be created with later anastomosis. An alternative surgical approach is to place a peritoneal drain, with laparotomy reserved for later complications, if they develop (e.g. bowel obstruction from adhesions or bowel wall strictures). Although there is some controversy about which approach is best, studies suggest that the overall mortality may be similar with either approach.

Immediate mortality is quite high, but many cases resolve without surgical intervention (although a stricture may occasionally develop about a month later in the affected area of gut), where it is usually possible to reintroduce feeds after about 5 days. An infant who is sucking and showing interest in feeding is usually ready for feeding. Intestinal perforation is generally the main indication for surgical intervention, but the prognosis really depends on whether there is generalised peritonitis and whether some part of the gut has become totally dead and gangrenous.

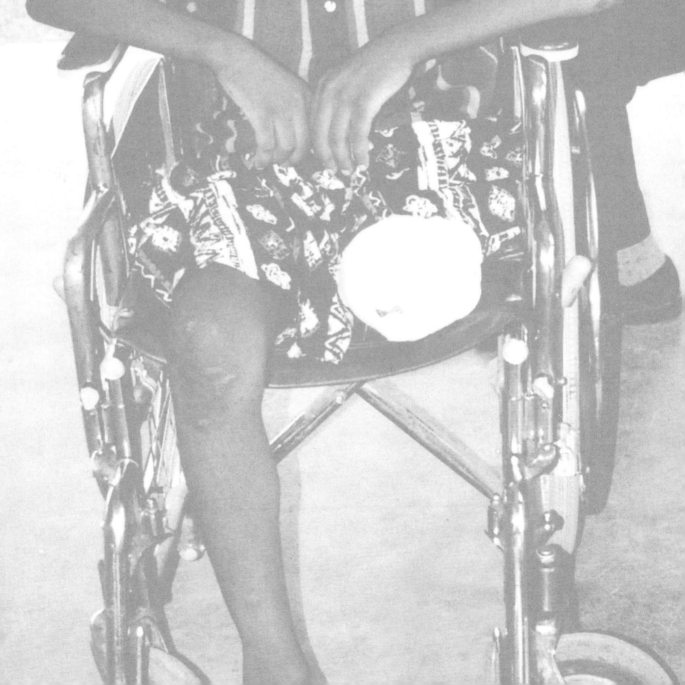

Section 4

Children in hospital

4.1 The differential diagnosis of common or serious presenting symptoms and signs in children

4.1.A The child with diarrhoea

There are several groups of causes of diarrhoea. For the management of acute and chronic diarrhoea, *see* Sections 5.12.A and 5.12.B.

Causes of diarrhoea

Infective
- Acute (< 14 days).
- Persistent (> 14 days).

Viruses, bacteria and parasites are the agents of infection.

Secondary diarrhoea
- Malnutrition.
- HIV.
- Disaccharide intolerance.
- Malaria.

Chronic (non-infectious)
- Food intolerance:
  - Milk protein, soy protein
  - Coeliac disease (gluten sensitivity)
  - Multiple food intolerances.
- Inflammation:
  - Crohn's disease
  - Ulcerative colitis.
- Pancreatic disease:
  - Cystic fibrosis
  - Shwachman syndrome (cyclic neutropenia).

Miscellaneous
- Non-specific 'toddler's diarrhoea'.
- Irritable bowel syndrome.
- Excessive intake of squash/fruit drinks.

History
- Duration of symptoms.
- Nature of stool (e.g. fatty, floating, watery, with blood).
- Number per day.
- Dietary intake.
- Other accompanying symptoms.
- History of foreign travel.

- Possible food poisoning exposure.

Examination
- Chart growth/nutritional status.
- Document degree of dehydration.
- Look for fever, anaemia, lymphadenopathy, hepatosplenomegaly and finger clubbing.
- Look for signs of vitamin or mineral deficiency, oral ulcers and anal fissures.
- Look for candidiasis.

Investigations

TABLE 4.1.A.1 Investigations in the child with diarrhoea

Investigation	Looking for:
Stool Microscopy (warm stool for *Entamoeba histolytica*), white blood cell count (WBC), red blood cell count (RBC), ova, parasites Culture	Infection
Stool pH (< 5.5) Clinitest tablets or Benedict's solution	Lactose intolerance
Stool Fat globules	Pancreatic disease
Hydrogen breath test	Lactose intolerance
Blood culture (high temperature, rigors)	Septicaemia (e.g. *Salmonella*)
Urea, creatinine, electrolytes (if oliguria)	Haemolytic uraemic syndrome Hyponatraemia/ hypernatraemia
Full blood count	Hidden bleeding
Albumin	Chronic diarrhoea
X-ray of abdomen, ultrasound scan	Ileus, bowel perforation
Urine microscopy	Haemolytic uraemic syndrome

4.1.B The child with jaundice

Causes of jaundice
- Neonatal jaundice (*see* Section 3.4).
- Excess haemolysis (pre-hepatic):
  - sickle-cell disease (*see* Section 5.11.B)
  - thalassaemia (*see* Section 5.11.C)
  - hereditary spherocytosis (*see* Section 5.11.C)

— malaria (*see* Section 6.3.A.d).
- Liver disease (*see* Sections 5.7.A and 5.7.B):
  — hepatocellular
  — obstruction to bile secretion
  — infective hepatitis
  — acute liver failure
  — chronic liver disease.

History
- Family history of hereditary haemoglobinopathy or liver disorder.
- Blood transfusion.
- Anorexia.
- Abdominal pain.
- Pruritus.
- Colour, nature and contents of stools and urine.

Examination
- Assess growth/nutritional state.
- Look for skin signs of chronic liver disease (e.g. spider naevi, clubbing, leuconychia, liver palms, scratches from pruritus).
- Assess liver and spleen (for enlargement and tenderness).
- Check for anaemia.

- Check for ascites.
- Look for frontal bossing or maxillary overgrowth (sickle-cell disease or thalassaemia).
- Observe colour of stool and urine.

Investigations

TABLE 4.1.B.1 Investigations in the child with jaundice

Investigation	Looking for:
Full blood count and film	Anaemia
Reticulocytes	Haemolysis
Haemoglobin electrophoresis	Sickle-cell disease and thalassaemia
Urine	Bilirubin and urobilinogen
Liver function tests: Liver transaminases	Bilirubin conjugated (liver disease or biliary obstruction) or unconjugated (haemolysis) Hepatitis
Serology	Identification of viral causes
Coagulation	Liver failure
Auto-antibodies	Chronic active hepatitis

4.1.C The child with lymphadenopathy

Common causes of generalised lymphadenopathy
- HIV infection.
- Infectious mononucleosis.
- Tuberculosis (TB).
- Leukaemia.
- Hodgkin's and non-Hodgkin's lymphoma.
- Cytomegalovirus (CMV), toxoplasmosis.
- African trypanosomiasis.

Infective causes of local lymphadenopathy
- Local skin (especially scalp) infections.
- Tuberculosis (TB), *see* Section 6.1.N.
- Environmental mycobacteria.
- Cat scratch disease.

History
- Known epidemiology of HIV and trypanosomiasis in the area.
- Contact with TB.
- Chronic ill health (e.g. malignancy, HIV, TB).
- Determine whether nodes are static or increasing in size.

Examination
- Chart growth and nutritional status.
- Check for fever.
- Check for liver or spleen enlargement.
- Check for purpura or anaemia.
- Check for *Candida* infection.
- Conjunctivitis, red cracked lips and persistent high fever, if present, suggest possible Kawasaki's disease.

TABLE 4.1.C.1 Investigations in the child with lymphadenopathy

Investigations	Looking for:
Full blood count	Atypical lymphocytes, leukaemic picture
Thick blood film	Trypanosomiasis
Bone marrow	Malignancy
HIV tests	HIV
Paul-Bunnell test	Infectious mononucleosis (positive 60%)
Erythrocyte sedimentation rate (ESR) and C-reactive protein (CRP)	Infection, TB
Mantoux test	TB, environmental mycobacteria
Serology	Epstein–Barr virus, CMV, toxoplasmosis
Chest X-ray	TB, malignancy
Lymph node biopsy	Diagnostic (lymphomas, etc.)

4.1.D The child with abdominal pain

Note that this group includes adolescent girls who may be pregnant.

Causes of acute and chronic abdominal pain

- Idiopathic:
  - Irritable bowel syndrome (intermittent stool variability).
  - Migraine (headaches with photophobia).
- Psychogenic.
- Gastrointestinal:
  - Appendicitis (central pain moving to right lower abdomen).
  - Peptic ulcer (upper abdominal pain, vomiting, blood in vomit/melaena stool).
  - Gastroenteritis (contact history, watery and/or bloody diarrhoea).
  - Intussusception (redcurrant-jelly stool, spasms of pain, mass in left lower abdomen).
  - Oesophagitis (retrosternal pain).
  - Inflammatory bowel disease (loose bloody, mucousy stool, weight loss, systemically unwell).
  - Constipation (hard, painful infrequent stool).
  - Bowel obstruction (bile-stained vomiting, abdominal swelling).

TABLE 4.1.D.1 Investigations in the child with abdominal pain

Investigation	Looking for:
Full blood count	Anaemia, eosinophilia, infection
Erythrocyte sedimentation rate (ESR)/C-reactive protein (CRP)	Inflammation
Urea, electrolytes	Renal disease
Amylase	Pancreatitis
Liver function tests	Liver dysfunction, hepatitis
Urine stick test: blood, protein, glucose	Glomerulonephritis, nephritic syndrome, diabetes, urinary system calculi
Urine microscopy for organisms, casts, culture	Infection, glomerulonephritis
Stool, ova, cysts, parasites, white blood cell count (WBC) and red blood cell count (RBC)	Infestation, dysentery, inflammatory bowel disease
Pregnancy test	*See* Section 2
Ultrasound scan (abdomen and pelvis), X-ray (straight abdominal film)	Bowel obstruction, constipation, lead poisoning, ovarian cyst, pregnancy, calculi
Barium studies and endoscopy	Peptic ulcer, inflammatory bowel disease
Barium studies and endoscopy	Peptic ulcer, inflammatory bowel disease

Differentiating between organic and non-organic (psychological) abdominal pain

	Organic	*Non-organic*
Nature of pain	Day and night	Periodic, often peri-umbilical
History	Weight loss/reduced appetite Lack of energy Fever Change in bowel habit Urinary symptoms Intestinal symptoms Vomiting: • bile stained • continuous • blood Rectal bleeding	Migraine School and family problems Isolated vomiting, not bile stained
Examination	Appears ill Weight loss Distension Absent or accentuated bowel sounds Shock Abdominal mass: • constipation • other	Normal, thriving

- Food intolerance (e.g. milk protein, gluten) (dietary history).
- Meckel's diverticulum.
- Henoch–Schönlein purpura (purpuric rash and/or arthropathy).
- Sickle-cell disease (history, anaemia).
- Urinary tract:
  - Infection.
  - Calculi.
  - Hydronephrosis.
- Liver:
  - Hepatitis.
- Pancreas:
  - Inflammation (pancreatitis).

- Malignancy:
  - Lymphoma.
- Gynaecological:
  - Dysmenorrhoea.
  - Pelvic inflammatory disease.
  - Ovarian cyst.
- Pregnancy related (see Section 2).
- Respiratory:
  - Pneumonia/pleurisy.
- Trauma.
- Poisoning:
  - Lead.

4.1.E The child with anaemia

Anaemia, especially that due to iron deficiency, is very common in resource-limited communities. Anaemia can be caused by a combination of inadequate nutrition and recurrent infections, such as malaria. Intestinal parasites such as hookworm are important causes. Genetic disorders such as sickle-cell disease and thalassaemia should always be considered in relevant ethnic groups. Acute worsening of anaemia may present as heart failure in young children.

For children aged < 6 years, normal haemoglobin concentration is > 11.0 g/dL (haematocrit is > 33%), see Section 5.11.A.

- Moderate anaemia: haemoglobin concentration is 6–9.3 g/dL.
- Severe anaemia: haemoglobin concentration is ≤ 6 g/dL, severe pallor (palmar/conjunctival), may have heart failure; gallop rhythm, enlarged liver and pulmonary oedema (fine basal crepitations in the lungs).

Causes of anaemia
Decreased production
- Prematurity: at 6–8 weeks postpartum.
- Hypochromic: iron deficiency (diet, blood loss, chronic inflammation).
- Normochromic: chronic infection or inflammation:
  - nutritional: malnutrition, scurvy
  - infiltration: leukaemia, malignancy
  - metabolic: renal and liver disease.
- Megaloblastic:
  - folic acid deficiency: infection, coeliac disease, anticonvulsants, haemolysis
  - vitamin B_{12} deficiency: intestinal resections, Crohn's disease, vegan diet.
- Hypoplastic: sickle-cell crises, drugs (e.g. chloramphenicol), malignancy.

Increased haemolysis
- Haemoglobinopathies: sickle-cell disease, thalassaemia major.
- Non-immune: drugs, infection, hypersplenism, burns, haemolytic uraemic syndrome, disseminated intravascular coagulation, porphyria, snake venoms.
- Enzyme deficiency: drug-induced and spontaneous glucose-6-phosphate dehydrogenase (G6PD) deficiency, glutathione synthetase deficiency, pyruvate kinase deficiency.
- Immune: Rhesus and ABO incompatibility, autoimmune (e.g. reticuloses), Mycoplasma infection, systemic lupus erythematosus, drugs.
- Membrane defects: spherocytosis, elliptocytosis, stomatocytosis, erythropoietic porphyria, abetalipoproteinaemia.

Blood loss
- Perinatal:
  - placental and cord accidents
  - feto–maternal, twin-to-twin transfusions
  - birth injury (e.g. cephalhaematoma, sub-aponeurotic haemorrhage, severe bruising)
  - haemorrhagic disease of the newborn.
- Epistaxis.
- Trauma.
- Alimentary tract: haematemesis, rectal bleeding, hookworm.
- Blood clotting disorder (e.g. haemophilia, thrombocytopenia).
- Renal tract: haematuria.

History
- Symptoms of anaemia: lethargy, tiredness, shortness of breath on exertion, poor growth.
- Obvious blood loss: epistaxis, haematemesis, haematuria, blood in stools.
- Assess the diet (e.g. inadequate weaning diet).
- Steatorrhoea.
- Chronic infection, inflammation.
- Drugs: especially antibiotics, antimalarial drugs, anticonvulsants, analgesics, cytotoxic agents.

Examination
- Chart growth/nutritional state.
- Conjunctivae, nails and palms for pallor.
- Stomatitis.
- Jaundice.
- Bruising, lymphadenopathy or petechiae.
- Hepatosplenomegaly.
- Tachycardia, flow murmur, cardiac failure.

Investigations

TABLE 4.1.E.1 Investigations in the child with anaemia

Investigation	Looking for:
Full blood count	Haemoglobin concentration, white blood cell count, platelet count
Blood film	Red blood cell morphology, malaria, target cells, haemolysis
Haemoglobin electrophoresis	Sickle-cell disease, thalassaemia
Mean corpuscular volume (MCV), reticulocytes	Iron deficiency, haemolysis
Coombs' test	Haemolysis
Bone marrow	Leukaemia, malignant infiltration, aplasia
Bilirubin, liver function tests	Direct/indirect bilirubin
Urinalysis	Red blood cells, casts, bacteria, white blood cells, protein, culture
Serum ferritin	Iron stores
Barium meal/endoscopy	Inflammatory bowel disease
Platelets and clotting	Coagulation disorder
Stool microscopy, culture and occult blood	Hookworm (egg count), gastrointestinal blood loss

4.1.F The child who is vomiting

The history of the acute, recurrent or chronic nature of this symptom indicates the approach to the diagnosis.

Common causes (depending on age)
Infants
- Gastroenteritis.
- Gastro-oesophageal reflux (distinguish from possetting).
- Overfeeding.
- Bowel obstruction:
  - pyloric stenosis
  - intussusception
  - congenital bowel anomalies.
- Infection:
  - urinary tract in particular
  - meningitis
  - otitis media
  - pertussis.
- Poisoning:

Children
- Gastroenteritis.
- Appendicitis (with pain).
- Infection:
  - especially urinary tract
  - meningitis (including TB)
  - malaria.
- Bowel obstruction.
- Ingestion of drugs or poisons.
- Migraine.
- Pregnancy.
- Bulimia (but rarely does a child admit this).
- Raised intracranial pressure (RICP).
- Hypertension.
- Diabetic ketoacidosis.

History
- Accidental drug ingestion.
- Check whether it is vomiting, regurgitation or possetting (especially in an infant).
- Is it associated with coughing or a whoop?
- Is it projectile?
- Does it contain blood or bile?
- Is there any diarrhoea or constipation?
- Is there abdominal pain?
- Are there urinary or ear symptoms?
- Is there a family history of migraine?
- Are there difficulties in coordination during physical activity? Consider the possibility of a middle ear or brainstem problem.

Examination
- Does the child look ill?
- Is the child febrile? Is there neck stiffness, a full fontanelle and/or a rash?
- Measure the head circumference, especially in infants, and check fontanelles and sutures.
- Is the child dehydrated? Is there an odour?
- Assess growth and nutritional status.
- Examine vomit:
  - bile-stained vomit suggests bowel obstruction
  - blood (coffee grounds).
- Full examination (include blood pressure, fundoscopy and anorectal examination as indicated).
- Abdomen:
  - test feed for pyloric stenosis: swelling or visible peristalsis
  - tenderness or mass
  - check whether bowel sounds are present and, if so, what they are like.

Investigations

TABLE 4.1.F Investigations in the child who is vomiting

Investigation	Looking for:
Urine microscopy	Urinary tract infection
Full blood count	Infection
Thick film	Malaria
Urea and electrolytes	Pre-renal or renal failure, pyloric stenosis
Blood culture	Infection
Lumbar puncture	Meningitis
Stool microscopy and culture	Ova, cysts, parasites, bacteria and viruses
Liver function tests	Hepatitis
Abdominal ultrasound	Masses, obstruction, free fluid
Straight abdominal X-ray/chest X-ray	Bowel obstruction, free air
Barium studies and/or endoscopy	Specific diagnosis
Pregnancy test	Pregnancy
Mantoux test	TB, meningitis
Brain imaging	Raised intracranial pressure

4.1.G The child with a rash

Causes of a rash

Macular rash
- Viral infections such as measles, sometimes meningococcal infection.
- Juvenile rheumatoid arthritis.
- Erythema marginatum: rheumatic fever.

Papular (vesicles, pustules) or bullae (blisters of various sizes)
- Chickenpox.
- Herpes simplex.
- Impetigo.
- Scabies.

Purpuric, petechial, ecchymosis
- Meningococcal disease.
- Henoch–Schönlein purpura.
- Dengue fever.
- Thrombocytopenia.

Desquamation with or without mucosal involvement
- Scalded skin syndrome.
- Toxic epidermal necrolysis.
- Kawasaki disease.
- Post-scarlet fever.
- Post-toxic shock syndrome.
- Stevens–Johnson syndrome.
- Epidermolysis bullosa.

Erythema multiforme
- Allergic reaction to drug or infection.
- Stevens–Johnson syndrome if very severe (then with bullae and mucous membrane redness).

TABLE 4.1.G.1 Investigations in the child with a rash

Investigation	Looking for:
Full blood count, erythrocyte sedimentation rate (ESR), C-reactive protein (CRP)	Systemic bacterial infection (e.g. meningococcal disease)
	Kawasaki disease
	Thrombocytopenia
Blood culture	Bacterial infection
Skin swab	Bacterial infection
Skin scraping	Scabies
Throat swab and antistreptolysin O titre (ASOT)	Streptococcal infection
Urinalysis (red blood cell count, casts, protein)	Nephritis (e.g. Henoch–Schönlein purpura)
	or connective tissue disorders
Skin biopsy	Epidermolysis bullosa
Auto-antibodies	Connective tissue disorders

Erythema nodosum

Lesions begin as flat, firm, hot, red, painful lumps approximately 2.5 cm across. Within a few days they may become purplish, then over several weeks fade to a brownish, flat patch. Erythema nodosum is most common on the shins, but it may also occur on other areas of the body (buttocks, calves, ankles, thighs, and arms).

- Streptococcal disease.
- TB.
- Connective tissue disorders.
- Sarcoidosis.
- Drugs.

4.1.H The child with failure to thrive

Approach to failure to thrive

- Failure to thrive is due to inadequate delivery of nutrients to developing tissues.
- It is usually manifested by failure to gain weight as expected.
- In extreme circumstances, height (length) and head circumference may be affected. Plot the mid-parental height.
- The majority of cases are related to gastrointestinal disorders: poor intake/malabsorption.
- Observe feeding, mother's interaction, child's behaviour, vomiting, diarrhoea and weight gain before embarking on investigations.
- Investigations should take place when a likely system and/or disorder has been identified.
- Always remember the possibility of child abuse.
- See relevant sections on gastroenterology, chronic infections, organ failure, hyperimmune disorder.

Failure to thrive: gastrointestinal disorders

- Oropharynx: cleft palate.
- Oesophagus: incoordination of swallowing (e.g. cerebral palsy).
- Stomach:
  - Gastro-oesophageal reflux
  - Pyloric stenosis.
- Digestion:
  - Pancreas: cystic fibrosis
  - Liver: cirrhosis.
- Small gut disorders:
  - Milk protein intolerance
  - Coeliac disease
  - Carbohydrate malabsorption
  - Protein-losing enteropathy
  - Short gut syndrome
  - Crohn's disease.
- Large gut disorders:
  - Ulcerative colitis
  - Crohn's disease
  - Hirschsprung's disease.

Causes of failure to thrive

TABLE 4.1.H.1 Mechanisms of failure to thrive

Mechanism	Systems involved:
Inadequate intake	Anorexia
	Breastfeeding failure
	Feeding mismanagement
	Swallowing disorders
Loss	Vomiting
	Diarrhoea
	Malabsorption
Structural dysfunction of organs	Brain (cerebral palsy, learning difficulties)
	Respiratory
	Cardiac
	Urinary tract
	Gastrointestinal tract
Increased requirement for nutrients or metabolites	Infection
	Connective tissue disorders
	Immune disorders
Failure of end-organ response	Metabolic (e.g. amino acid disorders, organic acid disorders)
	Endocrine (e.g. thyroid disorder)
	Malignancy
	Chromosomal abnormalities
Emotional and/or psychological	Parental problem: • Neglect • Abuse • Family dysfunction Child problem: • Feeding/behaviour disorders • Anorexia nervosa • Bulimia

4.1.I The child with fits, faints and apparent life-threatening events (ALTEs)

Common causes of fits, faints and ALTEs

- Febrile convulsions.
- Epileptic seizures.
- Hypoglycaemia.
- Infantile apnoea/hypoxaemic events.
- Premature birth.
- Respiratory infection (e.g. bronchiolitis, pertussis).
- Sleep-related upper airway obstruction (see Section 5.1.D).
- Vaso-vagal episodes (simple faints).
- Cardiac arrhythmias.
- Cyanotic breath-holding.
- White breath-holding (reflex anoxic seizures).

History

- Cyanosed:
  - Occurs with infant apnoea
  - Some febrile convulsions/epileptic seizures.
- Extreme pallor:
  - Vasovagal
  - Cardiac arrhythmia.
- Trauma/illness related (especially to head): white breath-holding.
- Emotional upset: cyanotic breath-holding.
- Snoring/inspiratory stridor during sleep, often with chest recession and restlessness: sleep-related upper airway obstruction (see Section 5.1.D).
- Exercise related: cardiac arrhythmia (see Section 5.4.C).
- Drug abuse.
- Fabricated or induced illness (see Section 7.6).
- Convulsions (see Sections 5.16.D and 5.16.E).
- Preterm infant in first few weeks (see Section 3.4).
- Respiratory illness.
- Diabetes/starvation (see Section 5.8.A).

Examination

- Growth and nutritional status.
- Signs of respiratory infection.
- Signs of anaemia (associated with cyanotic breath-holding and infant apnoea).
- Signs of fever.
- Neurological examination (to exclude or identify neurological abnormalities).
- History of breath-holding (see Section 5.16.I).
- Signs of cardiac disorder.
- Blood pressure lying and standing, for vasovagal episodes.
- Mouth and throat for enlarged tonsils or retrograde/small mandible for predisposition to sleep-related airway obstruction (the latter is also common in sickle-cell disease and Down's syndrome).

Investigations

TABLE 4.1.I.1 Investigations in the child with fits, faints and ALTEs

Investigation	Looking for:
Full blood count	Anaemia, infection
Blood glucose concentration	Hypoglycaemia
Haemoglobin electrophoresis	Sickle-cell disease
ECG	Wolf–Parkinson–White syndrome and long QT syndrome
	Structural lesion of heart
Oxygen saturation during sleep	Low baseline SaO_2 predisposes to infant apnoea/hypoxaemic events
	Should be > 94% (at sea level) (see Section 9, Appendix)
	Especially common in preterm infants and infants aged < 6 months with respiratory infection
Video (if available) during sleep (parents can do this with a mobile phone)	Sleep-related upper airway obstruction
EEG and video during episode	Epileptic cause
Chest X-ray	Lung disease in infantile apnoea/hypoxaemic events

4.1.J The child with generalised oedema

The major differential diagnosis relates to the presence or absence of hypoalbuminaemia.

Common pathophysiology

- Heart failure:
  - Jugular vein pressure increased, liver enlarged, triple rhythm, murmurs, basal lung crepitations.
  - Cardiovascular disorders.
  - Severe anaemia.
- Acute glomerulonephritis.
- Low serum albumin:
  - Nephrotic syndrome.
  - Liver disorders.
  - Protein-losing enteropathy (e.g. malabsorption, intestinal lymphangiectasia).
  - Malnutrition.
- Increased vascular permeability:
  - Anaphylaxis (history).
  - Shock.
- Over-hydration (particularly excessive IV solutions such as 5% dextrose).

History

- Shortness of breath, chest pain (pericarditis).
- Blood in urine (nephritis).
- Facial swelling (nephrotic syndrome or acute glomerulonephritis, anaphylaxis).
- Nutritional history (malnutrition).
- Gastrointestinal symptoms (protein-losing enteropathy).
- Exposure to allergen or sting (anaphylaxis).
- Excess and/or inappropriate IV fluids.

Examination

- Chart growth and nutritional status, and look for features of kwashiorkor and vitamin deficiencies.
- Cardiovascular system, including blood pressure.
- Rash with or without wheeze/stridor (anaphylaxis).
- Widespread purpuric rash/very ill patient (meningococcal septicaemia).
- Jaundice or other signs of liver disease.
- Anaemia and lymphadenopathy.
- Enlarged liver and/or spleen.
- Ascites (especially nephrotic syndrome). Ascites may be transudate (e.g. nephrotic syndrome) or inflammatory (e.g. TB, peritonitis). Abdominal malignancy may cause ascites and obstructive oedema of the lower limbs.

Investigations

TABLE 4.1.J.1 Investigations in the child with generalised oedema

Investigation	Looking for:
Full blood count	Anaemia
Urinalysis: • Dipstix: protein, blood Bilirubin Microscopy: red blood cell count, casts	Nephrotic syndrome, nephritis Liver disease Nephritis
Stool	Hookworm
Serum albumin	Low albumin levels
Imaging: abdominal ultrasound	Hepatosplenomegaly Malignancy Ascites (transudate/inflammation)
Echocardiogram	Cardiac disorders
Ascitic fluid Colour: clear, cloudy, bloody, chylous Cells: white blood cell count, malignant cells Protein: < 25 grams/litre transudate 　　　　 > 25 grams/litre exudate	Inflammation (e.g. from TB) Infection, malignancy
Ziehl–Neelsen stain Culture:	TB TB/general

4.1.K The child with headaches

- Headaches are common in children.
- They should be taken seriously if they persist.
- Their prevalence increases with age.

Acute headache

Common causes of acute headache include the following:
- Febrile illness.
- Meningitis/encephalitis.
- Acute sinusitis: pain and tenderness (elicited by gentle percussion) over the maxilla; there is usually a history of preceding upper respiratory tract infection and a postnasal discharge may be present.
- Head injury.
- Raised intracranial pressure.
- Intracranial haemorrhage (severe sudden headache, with rapid loss of consciousness).
- Migraine.

A careful history and physical examination will usually reveal the cause.

Raised intracranial pressure (RICP)

- Headache may be sudden or gradual in onset, often occipital in location and becomes progressively more severe.
- Made worse by lying down (in contrast to migraine and tension headache, which are relieved by lying down), by coughing, stooping and straining, and may wake the child from sleep.
- Worse in the morning and often associated with nausea and vomiting.
- Other signs of raised intracranial pressure may be present, such as impaired consciousness, bilateral abducens sixth nerve palsies (false localising sign) and, when severe, bradycardia and hypertension.
- Papilloedema is a late sign.
- Localising neurological signs may be present, depending on the site of the lesion. Ataxia suggests a posterior fossa tumour; cranial nerve palsies suggest a brainstem lesion; visual field defect suggests a craniopharyngioma; unequal pupils suggest a supratentorial lesion such as subdural haematoma.
- In endemic areas, cerebral malaria and neuro-cysticercosis are important causes.

Benign intracranial hypertension

- Raised intracranial hypertension without any space-occupying lesion or obstruction of the CSF.
- Can be caused by drugs (corticosteroids, especially during withdrawal, ampicillin, nalidixic acid) and sagittal sinus thrombosis.
- Most without cause, especially in young adolescent girls.

Recurrent or chronic headaches

Two common causes are anxiety (tension) and migraine.

Tension headache

- This affects around 10% of schoolchildren.
- Typically the headache is symmetrical and described as hurting or aching over the cranial vault.
- The headache develops gradually and is not associated with other symptoms.
- It is induced by stress (e.g. due to school examinations, assignments, etc.) and can coexist with migraine in the same child.
- It may be caused by isometric contraction of the head and neck muscles in anxious children.

Migraine

See Section 5.16.J.

Conversion (hysterical) headache

- Headache can be a conversion symptom used by the child to gain attention.
- The initial headache may have been due to an organic cause (e.g. febrile illness), but its persistence and recurrence are due to psychological factors.

Management of headaches

See also Section 5.16.A relating to an acute onset of headache.
- A detailed history and a careful full examination should be undertaken in order to rule out serious underlying causes.
- Investigations are rarely needed.
- X-ray of the sinuses will confirm sinusitis and CSF examination will confirm meningitis/encephalitis.
- A CT scan of the brain is essential if raised intracranial pressure is suspected or if there are localising neurological signs.
- Treatment is directed at the underlying cause and at pain relief.
- Benign intracranial hypertension can be alleviated with corticosteroids (dexamethasone 0.6 mg/kg/day in two divided doses) and/or acetazolamide (8 mg/kg 8-hourly, increasing to a maximum of 32 mg/kg/day) and repeated lumbar puncture.
- For tension and conversion headaches, counselling and stress management are important.

Relief of pain

For most headaches, simple analgesics alone or combined with non-steroidal anti-inflammatory drugs (NSAIDs) will suffice (e.g. paracetamol with or without ibuprofen). Remember that frequent or recurrent use of analgesics can **cause** headaches.

4.1.L The child with respiratory distress

Presenting features

- Tachypnoea.
- Increased effort of breathing: tracheal tug, inter/sub-costal recession.
- Poor feeding, sleep disturbance.
- Grunting.

- Unable to speak in sentences.
- Positioning: sitting up/forward, neck extension, splinting chest.
- Tachycardia.
- Altered mental state: agitation (hypoxaemia)/drowsiness (hypercapnia).
- Pallor/cyanosis (late sign).

Causes

TABLE 4.1.L Causes of respiratory distress

Common cause	Findings on examination
Upper airway obstruction	Stridor, hoarse voice, drooling, sitting up, head held forward
Inhaled foreign body	Suggestive history, tracheal deviation, unilateral hyper-expansion on chest X-ray
Asthma	Hyper-expansion, wheeze, reduced air entry, reduced peak flow, hypoxaemic ($SaO_2 < 94\%$ at sea level)
Bronchiolitis	Inspiratory crackles, wheeze, hypoxaemic ($SaO_2 < 94\%$ at sea level)
Pneumonia	Fever, grunting, pleuritic or abdominal pain, signs of consolidation or effusion. Clubbing indicates chronic disease (e.g. bronchiectasis)
Tuberculosis	Contact history, lymphadenopathy, fever, weight loss
Pneumothorax	Unilateral hyper-resonance on percussion, tracheal deviation, apex displacement
Cystic fibrosis	Recurrent respiratory infections, failure to thrive, fat malabsorption, family history
Heart failure/pulmonary oedema	Sweaty, gallop rhythm, hepatomegaly, heart murmurs, basal lung crepitations, raised jugular venous pressure (JVP)
Sickle-cell disease/acute chest syndrome	Hypoxaemia ($SaO_2 < 94\%$ at sea level), chest pain

Investigations

TABLE 4.1.L.2 Investigations in the child with respiratory distress

Investigation	Looking for:
Oxygen saturation (pulse oximeter)	Hypoxaemia < 94% at sea level
Chest X-ray	Lung disorder
ECG, echocardiogram	Heart disorder
Mantoux	TB
Erythrocyte sedimentation rate (ESR), C-reactive protein (CRP)	Inflammation
Full blood count	Infection
Haemoglobin electrophoresis	Sickle-cell disease
Bronchoscopy	Foreign body
Sweat test or DNA analysis	Cystic fibrosis

4.1.M The child with pyrexia (fever) of unknown origin (PUO)

Definition

Pyrexia of unknown origin (PUO) is defined as a minimum temperature of at least 38.3°C for 1–3 weeks with at least 1 week of hospital investigation. It is very important to determine whether fever is continuous or recurrent by plotting it on a chart (*see* Section 9, Appendix).

Baseline investigations
- Full blood count and film.
- Erythrocyte sedimentation rate (ESR)/C-reactive protein (CRP).
- Blood cultures.
- Thick film and/or rapid diagnostic test (RDT) for malaria (endemic areas/recent foreign travel).
- Mantoux test.
- Epstein–Barr and other viral serology.
- Urine microscopy/culture.
- Chest X-ray.
- Lumbar puncture (if meningeal signs are present).

TABLE 4.1.M.1 Relatively common causes of pyrexia of unknown origin in children

	Cause	Specific investigation
Bacterial infection	Tuberculosis	Chest X-ray, tuberculin skin test, lumbar puncture
	Campylobacter	Stool culture
	Typhoid	Blood and stool culture; serology, but unreliable. Clinical signs
	Brucellosis	Serology
	Cat scratch disease	Lymph node biopsy
	Rheumatic fever	Throat swab, anti-streptolysin O titre (ASOT)
Localised infection	Hidden abscess	Abdominal ultrasound scan
	Bacterial endocarditis	Blood cultures, echocardiogram
	Osteomyelitis	X-ray, bone scan
	Pyelonephritis	Urine microscopy and culture
	Cholangitis	Abdominal ultrasound scan
Spirochaete infection	*Borrelia*	Serology
	Syphilis	Serology
	Leptospirosis	Serology blood and urine culture
Viral infection	HIV	Serology
	Epstein–Barr virus	Serology, Paul-Bunnell test, blood film; atypical lymphocytes
Chlamydia infection	*Psittacosis*	Serology
Rickettsial infection	Q fever	Serology
Fungal infection	Histoplasmosis	Serology and culture
Parasitic infection	Giardiasis	Fresh stool microscopy
	Malaria	Blood film, rapid diagnostic test
	Trypanosomiasis	Thick blood film
	Toxoplasmosis	Serology
	Toxocariasis	Serology, blood eosinophil count
	Leishmaniasis	Serology, bone marrow
Connective tissue disorder	Juvenile idiopathic arthritis	Auto-antibodies
	Systemic lupus erythematosus	Auto-antibodies
Neoplasia	Lymphoma	Node biopsy
	Leukaemia	Blood film/bone marrow
	Neuroblastoma	Urinary VMA
	Wilms' tumour	Ultrasound or CT scan
Miscellaneous	Kawasaki disease	Erythrocyte sedimentation rate (ESR), platelets, clinical findings
	Inflammatory bowel disease	Barium studies/endoscopy
	Fabricated illness	Surveillance

4.2 Caring for children and young people in hospital

4.2.A Nursing sick children

BOX 4.2.A.1 Key points
- Children are not 'small adults'.
- Good basic care is essential and may reduce the need for further intervention.
- Have a system for allocation of nurses to patients. Any system is better than no system.
- Keep the sickest children in the place where they can be seen most easily.
- Provide information for children and their families and involve them in decision making. This reduces anxiety, improves their compliance and will make your care more effective.
- Empower the parents to provide care. This is better for the child and will help you.

Introduction

The spectrum of professional nursing care is vast, and ranges from the challenges of meeting basic human needs, key assessment and monitoring roles, to complex case management. Irrespective of the particular arena of nursing, the priority is to ensure that healthcare retains a focus on humane actions that increase the quality and effectiveness of care.

Much can be achieved by a skilled 'child-friendly' approach that leads to minimal intervention and trauma and includes the family as caregivers and, where appropriate, the child in decision making.

Children are unique, both as individuals and as a group, with rights enshrined by the UN Convention on the Rights of the Child (UNCRC) 1989. They are not 'small adults' – they have physical, psychosocial and physiological needs and responses that are different from those of adults. Effective nursing requires knowledge of these differences (recording vital signs means little without an understanding of the normal range).

Role and education of nurses

The role and status of nurses, together with the education that they receive, varies widely, although there are steps to increase standardisation. Many countries provide no specific training in the nursing of sick children. Good care is often delivered despite many challenges, but optimum care can only be consistently achieved by education and professional accreditation that relates specifically to the holistic physiological, physical and psychosocial care of the child and their family.

The increasing demands of healthcare sometimes result in an overlap of roles undertaken by nursing and medical staff. In many situations, the nurse may be the most experienced or skilled healthcare professional present.

The value of involving families in care

Hospitalisation is often a frightening experience in an unfamiliar environment, where the family no longer have their usual control over everyday life. Nurses should aim to return much of that control back to the child and family, and work to ensure that they receive the best care possible, given the environment and resources at their disposal.

The potential benefit and contribution of the parents cannot be overestimated. If the child's family is available, they should be encouraged and supported to participate in the child's care. Parents provide valuable information about what is normal for their child and how this may have changed. Since they know their child best they are often the first to notice small changes in his or her condition that may later prove significant. However, this critical knowledge can only be utilised for the benefit of the child if the contribution of families is recognised and valued.

Nurses as communicators and advocates

Nurses are central to communication between the multidisciplinary team and the family. They have a key role as an active advocate for the child, although this is often easier to say than to do. The hierarchical cultures in some healthcare systems can conspire against this, often to the detriment of the child. It is the responsibility of all healthcare professionals to promote an environment in which the views of all involved in the child's care, but especially the views of the child and their parents, are heard.

Inappropriate and unnecessary painful interventions and investigations, long hospitalisations without good reason and unnecessary separations from the family cannot be justified and are an abuse of children's rights under the UNCRC. Hospitals and other healthcare settings present numerous potential risks to children. It is the responsibility of every healthcare facility to be a place of safety, and of every healthcare worker to protect the best interests of children.

Basic nursing care
Organising care

In many places a small number of nurses have to look after many children. This makes it very difficult to provide good care, and this is a major (and sometimes overwhelming) challenge for nurses.

It is important to organise nursing care well and efficiently, particularly when resources and the number of nurses are low. Even when there are good resources, poor organisation will result in suboptimal and inequitable care.

A system of allocating certain numbers of patients to nurses, or grouping children by the acuteness of their needs, can help to make the best use of available resources and ensure some continuity of care. However, any system of care is likely to be better than no system at all.

In busy settings is it also important to place the sicker children (particularly children without a parent present) in beds where they can be easily and most frequently seen – for example, near to the nurses' station.

The importance of basic care

Although patients may sometimes require complex treatment, there are basic needs that will always have to be met. Unfortunately, these are sometimes viewed as being of secondary importance, but providing good basic care often reduces the need for further intervention, and can enhance other therapies (e.g. the beneficial effect of improved nutrition on wound healing), whereas poor basic care has the opposite effect (e.g. the adverse effects of stress on respiratory and cardiac function). Where therapeutic options are limited due to lack of availability, limited financial resources, etc., or perhaps where no further curative treatment is possible, the provision of good basic personal care is particularly relevant. It is invariably viewed as part of the nursing role, but in fact the underlying approach required is common to all healthcare professionals, and it should be understood that the provision of such care is rarely a simple task. It requires understanding, skill and patience, and is a subject that justifies a separate or expanded publication. Only the bare essentials are covered in this manual.

Information, participation and comfort

Hospitalisation often represents a traumatic change in the life of a patient. Much that was previously familiar and predictable in their life has now been replaced by an unfamiliar environment and fears about an uncertain immediate (and maybe long-term) future over which they have little control. Our words and facial expressions convey a stream of messages, but we often have little understanding of how we are perceived. Effective communication plays a vital role in the care of patients, and has a dramatic impact on their experience of and response to treatment.

Both the patient and their family have a need to trust those who are caring for them, to be told what is wrong and also to know what is going to happen to them. This is a major factor in helping them to adjust to the situation, develop coping strategies and make decisions about their own care.

The 'information needs' of children are often neglected, sometimes because it is assumed that their understanding is limited. However, even young children have a need to be given information in a language that is understandable to them. In the absence of reliable information, a child's fantasy may well be far more distressing than the reality.

These issues are also very important in preparing the patient (and their family) for a procedure. They need to be told truthfully and sensitively what will happen, particularly if it might be painful. If the patient is not warned, their trust in those around them can be destroyed, future procedures will be feared, their anxiety will be increased and the nursing task will be made more difficult.

Communication is a two-way process. It involves both conveying the message effectively and having an understanding of the thoughts and feelings of the other person. Children and their families should be allowed and encouraged to participate in decisions that affect them. This requires a willingness and ability to engage with them and

actively listen to them, and to interpret non-verbal signs that often tell a different story to the words that are actually spoken. Patients need to express their worries and anxieties. Young children do not always have sufficient vocabulary to convey how they feel, so the use of play and other activities, such as drawing, is a useful way to enable them to express themselves and to give them control.

Factors that may appear trivial to an adult may be important to a child. There may be issues causing distress that can be easily resolved, and in cases where there is not a solution, the feeling of isolation that is often experienced by these children can be helped by having someone to share their anxieties with.

Where the situation is grave, families sometimes struggle to discuss distressing subjects with their child. Although these are difficult and emotional situations, even very young children are extremely sensitive to the distress and anxiety of their family. They often have a much greater level of awareness than is generally realised, and failing to acknowledge the reality of their position may intensify their feelings of isolation by denying them the opportunity to express how they feel or to ask questions.

This all takes time, which may well be in short supply (another reason for encouraging family involvement), so it is important to make the most effective use possible of the little time you may have with a patient. The way you approach, talk to and touch the patient can make a big difference to the way they feel. It helps to build trust and it influences their compliance. Touch is a powerful tool and can convey more than words in terms of comfort and reassurance. Having their personal needs attended to may unfortunately be one of the few times during the day that a patient has the opportunity for human touch, so it is important to be kind, gentle and thoughtful in your approach.

Personal hygiene and protection of privacy and dignity

Personal care can contribute significantly to the way a sick or dying patient feels, and can prevent further problems such as sores at pressure areas. Attention to personal hygiene needs should always be given in a manner that protects the dignity of the patient. Even very small children often feel shy or uncomfortable when being attended to by an unfamiliar person, and this is particularly the case with older children and teenagers. It is another very good reason for encouraging the family to be involved in the patient's care, as well as helping to fulfil the natural wish of many parents to participate in this way.

When washing the patient, extra attention should be paid to skin folds, the neck, the back, the ears and the genitals, and the child should be encouraged to do as much as they are able. Patients who are malnourished, who have been sick for a long time or who have malignancies can have fragile skin that easily breaks down and requires special attention. An effective method that can be used by both professional and family carers is to gently change the patient's position at frequent intervals. This relieves the pressure on any given part of the body, and prevents reddening and breakdown of the skin. Pain relief should be given to prevent discomfort (see Section 1.15) and, when possible, pressure-relieving measures are also helpful.

Good mouth care is very important, and the patient should be encouraged to maintain this when in hospital. For children who have not brushed their teeth before, this is a good opportunity to start, and help needs to be given to those who are unable to do this. In patients who are very sick or who are dying, mouth care can help to prevent many problems, including bad breath, bleeding, infection, ulceration and pain, that can significantly add to their suffering. For these patients the following measures can be helpful:

- using a soft toothbrush or mouth sponge to clean the patient's mouth regularly
- using wet mouth swabs if the patient's oral intake is low
- using lip balm for dry lips.

Hydration and feeding

Children can quickly become dehydrated, particularly if they suffer from diarrhoea, vomiting and/or fever, or when they are too tired and lethargic to drink. Any caregiver should be able to recognise the observable signs of dehydration (for signs and symptoms, see below and Section 5.12.A).

Severe dehydration: two or more of the following signs are present:

- Lethargy/unconsciousness
- Sunken eyes
- Unable to drink or drinks poorly
- Skin pinch goes back very slowly (2 seconds or more).

Some dehydration: two or more of the following signs are present:

- Restlessness/irritability
- Sunken eyes
- Thirsty/drinks eagerly
- Skin pinch goes back slowly.

Other signs include the following:

- Reduced urine output/concentrated urine
- Increased pulse rate
- Increased respiratory rate
- Dry mouth
- Sunken fontanelle, where relevant.

A swift response to a patient who either is, or is likely to become, dehydrated can prevent a further deterioration and the need for IV fluids. Oral rehydration solution (ORS) powder to be mixed with boiled and cooled water (and also daily zinc supplementation) should be available in all hospitals, but in its absence the following will be suitable:

- To 1 litre of boiled water that has been allowed to cool add 6 level teaspoons of sugar and half a level teaspoon of salt (the solution should taste no saltier than tears).
- Dhal water, rice water, bean broth, fruit juices and thin porridge cereal are also effective.
- Breastfeeding mothers should be advised to breastfeed their child more often during episodes of diarrhoea.

Trying to persuade a patient, particularly a sick young child, to drink is not always easy:

- Encourage the patient to drink small amounts and often.
- Give them an age-appropriate explanation of why this is important.
- Involve the patient and decide together with them how much they will try to drink each hour.
- A child under 2 years of age needs to drink between a half and a quarter of a 250-mL cup for every watery stool.
- A child over 2 years of age needs to drink between a half and one full 250-mL cup for every watery stool.

For small children or those who are too tired to drink by themselves, the following measures can be helpful:

- Use a small cup, spoon or syringe.
- Encourage the child to play, or to participate by using the syringe him- or herself.
- Give small rewards for drinking.
- Give praise when fluid is taken.

Patients often lose their appetite when they are ill. In short acute episodes, the main priority is fluid intake and the replacement of salts. However, in longer periods of illness it is essential to ensure an adequate nutritional intake.

Anxiety caused by separation from their family can cause children to lose their appetite, and when they find themselves in an unfamiliar environment such as a hospital, a choice over whether or not to accept food or drink may represent the only control that the child still possesses.

Feeding difficulties often cause distress to families. The parents of a child who is dying may feel that a lack of nutrition will contribute to or hasten their child's death. These anxieties should be understood. It should also be explained to the parents that loss of appetite is sometimes part of the deterioration process, and the patient should be encouraged to eat what they want.

It is important to recognise and manage other factors that have an effect on oral intake, such as sore mouth, nausea, vomiting and constipation.

Try the following:

- Provide familiar food for the patient, and let them choose the food if possible.
- Encourage children to feed themselves if they are able to do so, and encourage the parents to help.
- Avoid performing invasive procedures immediately before or during a meal.
- Try giving small amounts of food often, rather than two or three large meals a day.
- Avoid giving the child highly spiced or strong-smelling foods unless such foods are the cultural norm for them.
- Give food at familiar times for the child, and try to make mealtimes fun.
- Praise the child when they eat, but do not criticise or punish them when they cannot.

Where possible, keep an accurate written record of all the patient's fluid and dietary intake, and also their output (urine, stool and vomit) (for an example of a chart, *see* Section 9, Appendix). Compare the total intake and total output over a given time period (usually 24 hours), and add an amount for insensible losses through perspiration and breathing (approximately 15 mL/kg/day, or more if the child has fever or is in a hot environment). Alongside clinical observations, this will give an indication of the patient's hydration level, and will also give warning of a patient who is becoming dehydrated. In reality, written records are often inaccurate and frequent weighing (e.g. once each day at the same time, wearing clothes of similar weight) can provide a valuable guide to fluid balance.

Elimination

For the management of constipation and diarrhoea, *see* Sections 5.12.A and 5.12.C.

The elimination habits of children vary with the individual, but often change when they are sick or in hospital. There are many possible causes of this, including the disease process, surgery, injury, and medication. Anticipating problems can do much to help. However, awareness of basic issues is always important.

- Maintain an adequate level of hydration.
- Obtain information about the child's normal elimination pattern.
- Children may be too frightened to go to the toilet in a strange place.
- Pain (e.g. from a urinary tract infection, anal fissure or post delivery in pregnant adolescent girls) may cause a patient to retain and deny the need to go to the toilet. Analgesia and simple measures such as sitting the patient in warm salty water can help to ease the pain and encourage urination or defecation.
- A patient who is passing bloodstained stools may be frightened and need reassurance.
- Praise and encouragement are important and effective.

Further reading and resources

Huband S, Hamilton-Brown P and Barber G (2006) *Nursing and Midwifery: A Practical Approach*. Oxford: Macmillan Education.

Maternal and Child Healthcare Initiative (MCHI): http://media.wix.com/ugd/dd2ba4_ef4f40edd7a8993a8621a-2caea7e4338.pdf

Nicholson S and Clarke A (2007) *Child Friendly Healthcare: a manual for health workers*. www.cfhiuk.org/publications/cfhi_manual.htm

WHO and UNICEF (2010) *Facts for Life*, 4th edition. New York: UNICEF. www.who.int/maternal_child_adolescent/documents/9789280644661/en/

World Health Organization (2014) *Pocket Book of Hospital Care for Children: guidelines for the management of common illnesses with limited resources*, 2nd edition. Geneva: World Health Organization. www.who.int/maternal_child_adolescent/documents/child_hospital_care/en/

4.2.B Nursing care for adolescents

Introduction

Adolescents are not small adults. Between the ages of 10 and 19 years their needs are complex as they make the difficult transition from dependency to responsible and independent adulthood. They are feeling their way towards this independence but at the same time may not feel confident, even if they are reluctant to admit this. When they are ill enough to require hospital care, frequently because of pregnancy and delivery, these pressures are even more marked.

Changes in adolescence that are relevant to hospital care

Sexual risk in adolescence

Adolescents, particularly girls, are vulnerable to sexual exploitation, especially if they are living in poverty. They may not know how to negotiate whether to have sex or not, or how to protect themselves from sexually transmitted infections (STIs) and pregnancy. They may have no caring adult to turn to. There are many stories of adolescent girls being coerced into unwanted sexual activity by those in positions of responsibility. They may be promised high school marks, or clothing, or money they need to help their families. They may fear reporting this, feeling that they will be shamed or not believed. They may be raped by men whom they know or to whom they are related, or by strangers, particularly in times of conflict and displacement. They may be endangered when rape is seen as bringing shame on the family. It may be difficult or impossible to prevent pregnancy, or they may not know how to do so. They may fail to report a pregnancy until it is too late for much of the antenatal care that is available. They may attempt to abort the fetus with extreme risk to their own life because they do not know what else to do. At the very least, these young women are vulnerable to STIs, including HIV and human papilloma virus (HPV) (the latter being a cause of cervical cancer). Such diseases (*see* Section 6.1.J) may be silent, or these young women may not know what to do or who to tell about symptoms that they experience. There is a high risk that pelvic inflammatory disease will result in infertility.

Pregnancy and childbirth

For an adolescent girl, pregnancy itself brings additional threats. She may not yet have completed her own growth and physical development. Her pelvis may not be fully developed, and the risk of obstructed labour and its consequences, namely fetal damage or death, maternal death or fistulae, is greater than for older women. She needs good nutrition for her own growth but has to provide for the fetus, and then for lactation, at the same time. The potential for malnutrition is high unless she has access to all the nutrients she requires. For this reason it is important that her nutrition status is monitored during pregnancy. She should also be given advice, help and micronutrient supplementation.

Other health dangers await pregnant adolescent girls. They are at greater risk of developing anaemia and pregnancy-induced hypertension, including pre-eclampsia and eclampsia. Stillbirth and neonatal mortality rates are higher in this age group, and babies are often of low birth weight. These girls may also have undergone female genital cutting (FGC) (*see* Section 2.10), with the many and lifelong health problems this may cause, and even social exclusion because of resulting fistulae or death from obstructed labour. Overall, complications of pregnancy and childbirth are the leading cause of death among female adolescents according to the World Health Organization (WHO).

Despite the dangers, many girls achieve a successful pregnancy outcome and become competent mothers. They may have to do this without the support of the baby's father or even their parents, and will have their education disrupted or even ended. They will often have to bring up the child in poverty, perhaps also being excluded socially. Others are married at a very young age, not necessarily willingly. Any adolescent mother (and father) will need help with parenting and the development of life skills to prevent their circumstances from spiralling downward. Family planning advice will be very important to enable these young women to avoid further pregnancies too soon, which would add to the downward spiral.

Mental health problems

Mental health problems are not confined to adults. Apart from having psychiatric disorders such as schizophrenia, young people may be depressed and confused, bullied, abused emotionally and psychologically as well as physically, and have to take part in activities that cause great stress. They may be forced to become child soldiers, they may have to take responsibility for other children in their family and even care for adult relatives such as parents with AIDS, and they may experience personal loss. An unhappy home life may lead to self-harming, to life-threatening eating disorders and to attempted suicide, any of which may result in hospital admission.

Malnutrition

It is not just in pregnancy that young people become malnourished. Malnutrition may occur because of poverty, or lack of access to healthy foods, or because of peer pressure and habit. This has substantial implications for their growth and development, their general health in the future, and their ability to recover from adolescent illness.

Implications for hospital care

Hospital care for adolescents is particularly difficult. Providers need to be sensitive to the needs and fears of these young people, and avoid being judgemental. A bad experience or poor-quality services may lead to adolescents failing to return, and possibly spreading the word to their friends. For a girl to have to attend an antenatal clinic alongside older and obviously married women is hard. To have to sit in a family planning clinic alongside women from her own community, and to have to tell a nurse (who may be a relative or who may know her parents) that she is sexually active is even harder. Young men will find it equally difficult to attend for contraceptive advice, and for adolescents of both sexes, attending an STI clinic could be an ordeal that they do not wish to repeat. At the same time, the pressures on young people are often so great that bad experiences are not effective deterrents to risky behaviours.

Dignity, privacy and confidentiality

Hospital care can be an experience of dignity and acceptance, or of rejection and embarrassment. Adolescents are unlikely to have special areas or wards except in the most well-resourced units. However, some kind of arrangement is needed to ensure that they are not nursed in the same space as very much older people, or with young children, and certainly not in mixed-sex areas. Facilities for privacy are needed, such as curtains around beds and interview spaces, and some arrangement should be made to ensure that interviews and conversations cannot be easily overheard.

Preservation of dignity, privacy and confidentiality is as important for adolescents as it is for adults. Going through puberty can make adolescents particularly self-conscious and even traumatised when examinations, such as those of their genitals, are performed insensitively or roughly. This may be especially difficult for young women (or men) who have experienced violence or sexual assault. Adolescent males may also feel great shame that an assault has happened and that they have been unable to prevent it. Therefore every effort needs to be made by care providers, from healthcare professionals to cleaners and porters, to maintain the privacy, dignity and confidentiality of these young people.

Confidentiality can be a particular issue when patients are minors, under the age of consent for the country in which they live. Parents or guardians may need to be given information that young people would prefer was not shared. There is no clear answer about how much those responsible should be told if the adolescent indicates that information should be withheld. Carers will need to be guided by their ethical codes and make decisions according to the best interests of each individual young person, as well as to the prevailing laws.

Parents or guardians may have legal powers to decide what treatment adolescents should receive, such as giving consent for surgery, but every effort needs to be made to take the young person's wishes and views into account. In some countries, even a court of law will take a child's wishes into account as they near the age at which they have the right to make decisions.

Services for young people with a disability

Care providers need to be particularly vigilant in providing services for young people living with disabilities, especially mental or learning disabilities. These people are vulnerable to abuse, to finding services inaccessible or inappropriate, and to misunderstanding of their needs. When they are away from their normal environment, as when in hospital, they may become withdrawn, confused and possibly uncooperative. Ensuring that young people with a disability feel secure and well treated is the responsibility of all grades of staff.

Emergency services

Emergency services for young people should not be neglected. Young women may need gynaecological assistance, for example, for the consequences of female genital cutting or sexual assault. They may need access to post-exposure prophylaxis for HIV, or to emergency contraception where this is acceptable, or to post-abortion care. Mental health problems may be acute and arise as emergencies, especially following major emotional stresses, when illnesses such as schizophrenia first arise, or when young people self-abuse or attempt suicide.

Building relationships

Trust is of primary importance for young people. Services that take into account the need to build trusting relationships are likely to be more acceptable, and therefore more effective and better used. Continuity is important, so that adolescents do not see a new face every time they attend for healthcare or counselling, but instead have the opportunity to develop a relationship of trust. This is a significant management issue, but it is important in terms of service uptake, effective use of human and other resources, and overall effectiveness of treatment programmes.

Advocacy

Healthcare providers have a strong advocacy role for adolescents, particularly in the context of working together, as for example in professional associations. This may involve campaigning for better services, talking to colleagues about their behaviours, or providing professional development opportunities. It may involve listening to young people, working with them, or campaigning against harmful local practices such as female genital cutting, early and/or forced marriage, ritual sexual initiation by older men, and erroneous and damaging beliefs (e.g. that having sex with young girls will cure HIV).

Hospital care summarised

The WHO suggests that services need to be accessible, acceptable, equitable, appropriate and effective. This means that young people need:

- appropriate, acceptable, accessible and gender-sensitive hospital and community services
- carers who have approachable, accepting and non-judgemental attitudes
- confidentiality, preservation of dignity and privacy
- accurate and honest information
- choice and some control over what happens to them
- avoidance of inappropriate hospital inpatient facilities where possible
- targeted health promotion
- targeted services, for example:
  - for young people with long-term physical disability or illness
  - for young people with learning and developmental disability
  - for family planning
  - for STIs and HIV
  - for pregnant adolescents, including post-abortion care, emergency contraception (if permitted), antenatal, labour and postnatal services, and nutrition services

  - for young mothers, whether supported or not, and young fathers
  - for displaced adolescents (e.g. refugees, internally displaced persons, the homeless)
- emergency health and counselling services for support in crisis
- advocates who understand their needs and can support them both as a group and individually (e.g. with families).

Finally, nurses, midwives and doctors may be the only people whom adolescents feel able to talk to, especially as others, such as parents, teachers and religious leaders, may be seen as authority figures. This vital role goes way beyond simply providing medical, surgical or obstetric care.

Further reading and resources

Huband S, Hamilton-Brown P and Barber G (2006) *Nursing and Midwifery: a practical approach*. Basingstoke: Macmillan Education.

Sawyer S, Afifi R, Bearinger L *et al.* (2012) Adolescence: a foundation for future health. *The Lancet*, **379**, 1630–40. (Special issue on adolescence.)

World Health Organization (2002) *Adolescent Friendly Health Services: an agenda for change*. www.who.int/maternal_child_adolescent/documents/fch_cah_02_14/en/

World Health Organization (2011) *Young People: health risks and solutions*. www.who.int/mediacentre/factsheets/fs345/en/index.html

World Health Organization (2012) *Adolescent Pregnancy*. www.who.int/mediacentre/factsheets/fs364/en/index.html

World Health Organization (undated) *Adolescent Friendly Health Services*. www.who.int/maternal_child_adolescent/topics/adolescence/health_services/en/index.html

WHO (undated) *Adolescent Health Web Page*. www.who.int/topics/adolescent_health/en/index.html

4.2.C The child with a disability in hospital

> ### BOX 4.2.C.1 Minimum standards
> *Prevention of avoidable disability*
> - Good antenatal care, including folic acid, iodinisation of salt, iron, antimalarial drugs and anti-tetanus immunisation.
> - Good care during delivery, including access to obstetric surgery and blood transfusion.
> - Effective neonatal resuscitation and care of the newborn.
> - Injury prevention.
> - Effective immunisation programme.
> - Good management of acute illness and injury.
>
> *Management of existing disability*
> - Access to diagnostics.
> - Multidisciplinary care.
> - Aids for disabled children.
> - Promoting equality of opportunity for children with a disability.

Introduction

Around 10% of children in most developing countries are disabled in some way. All children who are hospitalised for

illness or injury are at risk of becoming disabled due to their condition and/or their management.

Disabled children: definitions

- Disorder is a medically definable condition or disease.
- Impairment is the loss or abnormality of physiological, anatomical or psychological structure or function.
- Disability is any restriction, due to an impairment, in the child's ability to perform an activity in the normal way for a child of that age.
- Handicap is the impact of the impairment or disability on the person's pursuits or achievement of goals that are desired by him or her or expected of him or her by society
- Special needs refers to children who have needs greater than the normal needs of children of their age.

In 2001, the WHO introduced a new system of classification, The International Classification of Functioning, Disability and Health (commonly known as ICF) (www.who.int/classifications/en/) which uses two lists, a list of body functions and structure, and a list of domains of activity and participation. Since an individual's functioning and disability occur in a context, the ICF also includes a list of environmental factors. The ICF replaces the previous classification based on 'impairment', 'disability' and 'handicap', and shifts the emphasis to functioning. The ICF puts the notions of 'health' and 'disability' in a new light. It acknowledges that every human being, through illness or injury, may develop a disability. It 'mainstreams' the experience of disability and recognises it as a universal human experience. Furthermore, the ICF takes into account the social aspects of disability, and does not see disability only as a 'medical' or 'biological' dysfunction, but includes contextual factors, such as environmental factors. The ICF encourages assessment of the impact of the environment on the person's functioning. For example, hospital staff should be vigilant about preventing the development of contractures in a comatose child because they are concerned to ensure the best functioning of the child when he or she recovers.

Children's rights

Article 23 of the UN Convention on the Rights of the Child (www.ohchr.org/en/professionalinterest/pages/crc.aspx) defines the right of disabled children to special care, education and training designed to help them to achieve the greatest possible self-reliance and to lead a full and active life in society. It also encourages states to develop free and accessible services where possible, and to share information with other countries regarding the latest findings of research into the management of disabling conditions.

The main care of children takes place in the community. Children with special needs and chronic illness and their parents are entitled to receive the same standard of care as any other family when their child is in need of acute care for any other condition described in this book. The attitude of healthcare professionals should reflect this important principle. Many cultures in resource-limited countries have a greater degree of acceptance of disabled people than is found in more well-resourced countries. However, some cultures regard disability as a punishment or as a cause of shame. Accepting, encouraging and supportive behaviour of healthcare providers towards children with disabilities will go some way towards dispelling these attitudes.

Planning of services

Ministries of health and hospitals should consider establishing a register of disabled children, but only after careful consideration of the aims of registration, the likely benefits and costs, and the resources available.

The aims of a service for disabled children

These are as follows:
- to provide health services which ensure that children reach their maximum potential, optimising their independence and ability to lead a high-quality life
- to ensure that disabilities are promptly identified and treated where possible
- to promote active involvement of disabled children and their families in all aspects of healthcare, working in partnership with healthcare professionals
- to promote access to the healthcare facility for families with disabled children
- to provide comprehensive, integrated and coordinated services both in the healthcare facility and in the community, utilising outreach and community-based services, including community-based healthcare workers

- to enable health services to work with other key agencies, such as social services and education and training services.

The prevention of impairment and disability in children

This is the main issue in resource-limited countries, where facilities to support such children are very limited. Of most importance are the quality of antenatal care, the quality of neonatal resuscitation (see Section 3.2), the prevention of cerebral oedema due to inappropriate fluid management (see Section 5.12.A), the prevention of hypoxic-ischaemic cerebral injury (see Section 3.2), provision of adequate nutrition, the avoidance of accidents and protection from abuse (see Section 7.6). Adequate immunisation to combat poliomyelitis, measles, malaria, TB and meningitis, which are major causes of disability, is also mandatory.

Antenatal, peripartum, infant and child care

- Doctors and nurses working in hospital maternity services should work closely with local leaders, women's groups, and the Ministry of Health to improve pregnancy outcomes. This will involve promotion of early attendance at antenatal clinics. Detection and treatment of diseases such as syphilis and malaria, which can cause intrauterine growth retardation (IUGR) and prematurity, management of HIV and prevention of mother-to-child transmission, and the detection and management of intestinal worms and nutritional deficiencies are all essential.
- Every attempt should be made to provide good nutrition for women who may become pregnant. Folic acid supplements at the time of conception are vital for preventing spina bifida and other congenital abnormalities.
- Iodinisation of salt is inexpensive and should be universal.
- Iron-deficiency anaemia during pregnancy is associated with low-birth-weight babies and should be screened for and prevented. Malaria in pregnant women is another cause of low birth weight and prematurity, and should be prevented or, if contracted, be treated vigorously (see Section 2.8.D). Ministers of Health should be persuaded of the value of providing malaria prophylaxis or intermittent preventive treatment (IPT) for all pregnant women in endemic areas.
- Immunisation against tetanus (see Section 1.17) is essential.
- Obstetric care within hospitals should aim to prevent impairments due to complications of labour and delivery. Crucial to this is the availability of oxygen, obstetric surgery and anaesthesia, and a blood transfusion service.
- Effective neonatal resuscitation should be available 24 hours a day in every maternity unit and for all home deliveries. Staff must be trained and should have the basic equipment (see Section 3.2) necessary to prevent those causes of birth asphyxia which arise after the delivery of the baby.
- Simple interventions such as not bathing immediately after birth, prevention of hypothermia, and 'kangaroo care' for low-birth-weight babies should be taught to village health workers and traditional birth attendants in regions where they play an important role in home deliveries.
- Recognition of danger signs and the setting up of

community-based referral systems to deal with emergencies should be implemented at village level.

- Breastfeeding must be encouraged (see Section 3.3), and special support must be given to help mothers provide breast milk for babies with developmental impairments that make sucking or attachment difficult.
- Adequate training and facilities for the correct management of dehydration in gastroenteritis (see Section 5.12.A), hypoxic-ischaemic injury (e.g. in injuries) (see Section 7.3.C) and severe anaemia from malaria (see Section 6.3.A.d) all reduce the frequency of preventable brain damage.
- Paediatricians in hospitals should advocate for programmes of injury prevention and the prevention of injuries to children resulting from conflict, displacement or other social factors.

Management of disabled children: identification and primary diagnosis

All babies should be systematically examined at birth and, if possible, at 6 weeks of age to detect preventable disabilities such as dislocated hips and congenital cataracts. In regions where most babies continue to be born at home, community health workers (CHWs) should be trained to detect these problems or to encourage mothers to attend for postnatal checks at a clinic where these can be undertaken.

Postnatal services should be established in all healthcare facilities that provide antenatal care and delivery services.

Protocols for postnatal care should be developed based on WHO guidelines.

Signs or symptoms of an emerging disability should be actively sought. Findings which suggest that the child may be disabled should be communicated to the parents in a culturally sensitive manner in accordance with locally developed guidelines. This communication must include information about the local availability of services and social support.

Comprehensive interdisciplinary assessment

- This should always include the child's strengths as well as their weaknesses, and an assessment of their home circumstances and educational needs.
- It should result in decisions about management, including any immediate surgical or medical treatments available to alleviate the condition.
- It should include an assessment of sensory, motor, behavioural and intellectual capabilities as outlined below.

Convening a team to plan long-term management

- The team will include those people whose skills and training are relevant to the needs of the child. The team is often led by a named paediatrician.
- Representatives from outside agencies such as education and social services must be included if they are available.
- A care manager or key worker should be appointed, who will act as a liaison between professionals and the parents to ensure that the child fully benefits from the available resources.

Development of local guidelines for clinicians

- Hospital staff should aim for an early diagnosis and identification of treatable causes of disability.
- Resources to support the child and their family should be sought.
- In the absence of social support, hospitals must develop sensitive policies to inform parents of the diagnosis and expected prognosis in a way that is compatible with the best outcome for the child.
- Such policies should be decided by each hospital, and all personnel should be informed of the policy.
- Culturally sensitive disclosure of information about the diagnosis and expected prognosis should be given by a senior clinician who has experience in this area and is aware of local attitudes and beliefs regarding disability and the services available to the child and their family.
- Services should be developed as resources allow.
- Policies with regard to the intensity of resuscitative treatment given to children with various impairments should be developed by doctors, other healthcare professionals, representatives of the local community, including disabled people, and politicians. These policies must take into account ethnic and cultural issues and local support available for the care of severely disabled children. Such policies must be reviewed frequently. A hospital ethics committee can be valuable in this respect (see Section 1.20).
- Development of services for and the rights of disabled people should be promoted wherever possible. Front-line staff should feel confident that they know and can work within the framework of the policy.

Diagnosis

All newborn babies should be examined before leaving hospital by a member of staff (usually a nurse or midwife, or a paediatrician if one is available), who has been trained to perform a competent neonatal examination. Any possible impairment must be reviewed by an experienced paediatrician.

The neonatal examination

- **General:** Signs of dysmorphism should be looked for. The baby should be examined for tone and observed to have normal limb movements. Disordered tone, feeding difficulties, irritability and seizures should be noted.
- **Hips:** The hips should be checked for dislocation, remembering the three major risk factors, namely family history, female gender and breech presentation. Dislocated or dislocatable hips should be referred to an orthopaedic specialist.
- **Jaundice:** Any jaundice in the first 24 hours should be taken seriously and monitored appropriately. Causes of jaundice, such as blood group incompatibilities, glucose-6-phosphate dehydrogenase deficiency and sepsis, should be diagnosed and treated. Severe jaundice can lead to deafness and cerebral damage (see Section 3.4).
- **Cardiovascular system:** This should be examined looking in particular for cyanosis and equality of pulse volumes, and listening to heart sounds. If abnormalities are detected, the baby should be referred to a paediatrician (see Section 5.4.A).

- **Hearing:** Behaviour should be observed, although hearing defects are difficult to detect in the neonatal period without special equipment.
- **Vision:** The child's eyes should be examined for infection, which must be treated with suitable medication. The absence of cataracts should be ascertained by the presence of a good red reflex in each eye (*see* Section 5.15).

Comprehensive assessment of disabled children

Most children in resource-limited countries are born at home, and therefore children with disabilities are more likely to present at the hospital in later life.

History

A complete paediatric history, including antenatal, perinatal, postnatal and family history, should always be taken. Many countries have found that the 'Ten Questions' are helpful for establishing the prevalence and distribution of various disabilities:

1. Compared with other children, did he/she have any serious delay in sitting, standing or walking?
2. Compared with other children, does he/she have difficulty seeing, either in the daytime or at night?
3. Does he/she appear to have difficulty hearing?
4. When you tell him/her to do something, does he/she seem to understand what you are saying?
5. Does he/she have difficulty in walking or moving his/her arms, or does he/she have any weakness and/or stiffness in the arms or legs?
6. Does he/she sometimes have fits, become rigid or lose consciousness?
7. Does he/she learn things like other children of his/her age?
8. Does he/she speak at all? Can he/she make himself/herself understood in words. Can he/she say any recognisable words?
9. For 2-year-olds: 'Can he/she name at least one object (for example, an animal, a toy, a cup, a spoon)?' and 'Compared with other children of his/her age, does he/she appear in any way to have difficulties in learning?'
10. For 3- to 9-year-olds: 'Is his/her speech in any way different from normal (not clear enough to be understood by people other than his/her immediate family)?'

Examination

A full clinical examination of all physical, sensory and psychological systems should be undertaken.

Additional issues

- Determine how the child and their family have adapted their lives in response to the child's difficulties.
- Determine the extent to which the available treatment, training and management will improve the situation.
- Evaluate the emotional adjustment of the child and their family to the disability.
- Investigate the educational facilities available to the child and how they may be adapted to his/her needs.
- Determine the child's and family's strengths, abilities and positive personality traits which can be encouraged to help them to cope with the disability.

Protocols for particular conditions

These should be developed to ensure that the child is thoroughly investigated initially and reviewed at regular intervals to ensure that they can reach their maximum potential.

For example, a protocol for a child with Down's syndrome could include the following:

- full medical examination
- chromosome studies (if facilities are available)
- ECG and chest X-ray with echocardiography (if available)
- development of a care plan with the parents/carers as partners
- audiological assessment
- visual assessment
- assessment by a speech therapist (if available) to promote communication skills
- assessment by an occupational therapist (if available) to determine any aids or equipment which may be of help
- thyroid function test at appropriate intervals.

Sensory impairments

Liaison between health services and local education facilities is particularly important for the support and understanding of children with sensory impairments.

Visual impairment
Evaluation (*see* Section 5.15)

Most newborn babies can focus on and follow the mother's face and large brightly coloured objects. Impaired vision can therefore be detected soon after birth. It is normally the mother who will suspect this because the baby is not looking at her when she is breastfeeding. There may be roving eye movements.

- Use appropriate objects to confirm visual impairment – for example, human face for neonates, toys for older infants, and pictures (whose dimensions correspond to Snellen letters) for older children.
- Determine whether visual impairment is an isolated problem or associated with other developmental defects (e.g. cerebral palsy) by undertaking a detailed history and physical examination.
- Check for the red reflex as follows. Shine a light on the pupil from arm's length. Normally it will appear red because of light reflected from the retina. If it appears white, consider the possibility of dense cataract, severe retinopathy of prematurity, or retinoblastoma. If the red reflex is normal, check the pupillary response to light. If the latter is normal, a local cause (i.e. optic nerve or retinal degeneration) is unlikely, and impaired vision is then most probably due to occipital lobe damage.
- Check the retina and optic nerve by fundoscopy to exclude optic atrophy and retinal degeneration. If in doubt, refer the child to an ophthalmologist.

Causes of visual impairment

Common causes of blindness in children include optic atrophy, congenital cataracts and retinal degeneration, and in resource-limited countries they include vitamin A deficiency, measles, onchocerciasis and meningitis.

Trachoma remains a major cause of blindness in many developing countries. Early detection and treatment can prevent blindness. Prevention activities should include hygiene. Mass drug administration in affected areas can be considered.

Close liaison between paediatricians and

ophthalmologists is required to develop policies to detect and treat visual defects as early as possible.

Management of impaired vision

- **Treatable causes:**
  - **Cataract:** Children with congenital cataract should be referred to an ophthalmologist as soon as possible for early treatment. If no treatment is available, the parents should be shown ways of stimulating residual vision by playing with bright lights and presenting visual stimuli to the child as much as possible.
  - **Xerophthalmia:** Treat with vitamin A (*see* Section 5.10.A).
  - **Eye infections** (*see* Section 5.15).

Community healthcare workers should have training sessions on eye care emphasising simple hygiene measures and sources of food rich in vitamin A to be found in local diets.

- **Non-treatable causes:**
  - Perform a visual assessment and provide suitable visual aids.
  - Surgical correction of squints should be undertaken (when possible).
  - Mobility training should be provided for blind children and their carers.

The family will need support and advice about appropriate schooling, changes to the home, and mobility training.

Hearing impairment

Hearing loss is a hidden defect and may easily be missed if healthcare workers are not vigilant. Because hearing defects often lead to lack of development of speech and language, the child is sometimes assumed to have learning difficulties and may be further isolated from their family and society because of this. All children who present with failure to develop language should have a good-quality hearing assessment.

Hearing is essential for language development, so early detection of hearing impairment is essential. A newborn responds to sudden noise with the startle response. A normal baby will listen to the mother's voice. Formal hearing assessments in the newborn are possible using the acoustic cradle. The distraction test is used at 4 to 8 months of age, and audiometry is used in older children.

There are two types of hearing loss:

- **Conductive hearing loss:** The commonest cause is recurrent/chronic infective otitis media (*see* Section 5.1.C).
- **Sensorineural hearing loss:** The commonest causes are meningitis, cerebral malaria, genetic defects, drugs (e.g. excessive doses of aminoglycosides) and intrauterine infections. A hearing aid is required, and the child may need to learn a sign language.

Children with the following are at risk of hearing impairment:

- family history of sensorineural hearing loss
- dysmorphic features
- abnormalities of the pinnae
- severe birth asphyxia
- severe neonatal jaundice
- other neurological abnormalities
- postnatal infections (e.g. meningitis, measles)

- treatment with ototoxic drugs (e.g. gentamicin, streptomycin).

It is most important to identify and treat causes of conductive deafness, such as chronic otitis media (*see* Section 5.1.C).

- Treatable causes of sensorineural hearing loss are very rare.
- Hospitals in association with community health services and education authorities should seek to develop services for early identification and prompt treatment of children with irreparable hearing problems. These should include simple audiological assessment and the provision of hearing aids.

Neurological problems
General advice

- Parents and carers should be given information and training so that they can modify daily activities to promote the development of the child and enhance functioning (e.g. information on prevention of contractures). Lifting, carrying, seating, playing and bathing will all need to be discussed and demonstrated.
- Physiotherapy should be commenced as early as possible to prevent the development of contractures in hypertonic children.
- Good positioning and movement are helped by appropriate aids and appliances (*see* Section 4.2.D).
- Local people are often resourceful in developing appropriate equipment for their own children out of locally available materials (*see Disabled Village Children* referenced on p. 405). Advice from occupational therapists and physiotherapists is very useful (if available).
- Communication aids may also be required, and the advice of speech and language therapists is very useful.
- Children with motor difficulties often have feeding difficulties, and may not have the same access to food sources as children without impairments. Hospital staff, community health workers and family members should receive training on safe feeding techniques in order to improve the nutritional state of these children.
- Feeding may require the placement and management of a nasogastric tube, and parents or carers should be shown how to undertake this.
- A care plan should be developed and a key worker appointed to monitor long-term plans to support the parents and keep them informed and involved in the long-term planning of services for their child.
- Aids to enable the child to have mobility, an effective means of communication and access to education should be developed in the community.
- All hospitals should seek to develop specialist therapy services to help such children.

Neural tube defects

(See also section on paraparesis and incontinence below.)

- Where possible, neural tube defects should be prevented by adequate maternal nutrition, including folic acid and vitamins at the time of conception.
- Children born with neural tube defects should be treated urgently to prevent worsening of their condition (*see* Section 5.16.K).
- Parental wishes in terms of surgical treatment are very important.
- Later complications involve the urinary tract and bowel

function. Poor blood flow to the lower limbs associated with a lack of sensation and mobility may result in pressure sores.

- Many children with spina bifida require alternative means of mobility.
- Spina bifida occulta may result in clumsiness and continence problems. Some of the associated problems may be improved by surgical intervention.

Delayed development (see Tables 4.2.C.1 and 4.2.C.2)

Delayed development presupposes knowledge of normal development. Development proceeds in an orderly fashion, but there is considerable variation in the age at which milestones are achieved.

TABLE 4.2.C.1 Normal milestones in development

Age	Milestone
Birth	Focuses with eyes and responds to sound
4–6 weeks	Social smile
6–7 months	Sits without support, transfers objects from one hand to the other
9–10 months	Pulls to stand, pincer grasp, waves bye-bye
12 months	Stands, walks with one hand held, two or three words, stranger anxiety
15 months	Walks, drinks from cup
18 months	Says ten words, feeds with spoon
2 years	Runs, draws straight line, says two-word sentences
3 years	Draws circle, draws cross, says three-word sentences, dresses in simple clothes without assistance
4 years	Stands on one leg, fluent speech **Note:** in societies where access to pens and paper is very limited, even adults find drawing a line or a circle difficult as such an action is outside their experience

Developmental assessment

The purpose of developmental assessment is threefold:
1 to confirm normal or delayed development
2 to identify possible causes of delayed development
3 to plan a strategy for intervention.

To achieve these aims, a detailed history and physical examination are essential. Particular emphasis is placed on perinatal and developmental history. As well as looking for signs and symptoms of severe malnutrition or micronutrient deficiencies, allowance must be made for prematurity. Evidence of microcephaly, dysmorphic features and signs of neglect must be looked for, and a detailed neurological examination, including primitive reflexes, undertaken. The following questions must be addressed:

- Does the child have global delay (i.e. delay in all areas of development)?
- Is the delay confined to one area of development? If it is confined to the motor area, this suggests a possible neuromuscular disorder. Delayed speech development with normal motor and social skills could suggest a hearing disorder.
- Has the child lost previously acquired skills, and if so,

TABLE 4.2.C.2 Warning signs in development

Age	Sign
10 weeks	Not smiling
3 months	Not responding to noises or voice, not focusing on face, not vocalising, not lifting up head when lying on stomach
6 months	Not interested in people, noises or toys, does not laugh or smile, has squint, hand preference, primitive reflexes still present
9–12 months	Not sitting, not saying 'baba' or 'mama', not imitating speech sounds, no pincer grasp
18 months	Not walking, no words, no eye contact, not naming familiar objects, not interested in animals, cars or other objects Passive – not moving about exploring, excessive periods of rocking and head banging
3 years	Unaware of surroundings, not imitating adult activities, little or no speech, long periods of repetitive behaviour, unable to follow simple commands
4 years	Unintelligible speech
At any age	Parental concern, regression of acquired skills

has the loss been progressive? This suggests a neuro-degenerative disorder.

Delayed walking (not walking by 18 months)

- Family history of late walking and otherwise normal: give reassurance.
- Global delay (especially in language and social skills): the child probably has mental impairment.
- Child failing to thrive, and showing signs of malnutrition and poor nurture: this suggests neglect.
- Cerebral palsy with upper motor neuron signs (spasticity, clonus, brisk reflexes) or dystonia, ataxia and involuntary movements.
- Neuromuscular disorders (see Sections 5.16.F, 5.16.G and 5.16.H) with flaccid weakness, wasting or fasciculation of muscle, absent or diminished reflexes.
- Congenital dislocation of the hips or rickets can cause delayed walking.

Delayed language development

For meaningful speech to develop, the infant must be able to hear, and have intact language pathways and normal oropharyngeal structures. The child must also receive verbal communication.

The following approach to evaluating a child with language delay is useful:
- Is there a hearing defect?
- What is the problem in language delay? Is it in understanding or in expressing thoughts, or both?
- Is the delay confined to language or is it part of global delay (consider severe learning difficulty)?
- Is there any dysfunction or defect of the mouth and pharynx (obvious on physical examination)?

If the child cannot communicate and has normal intelligence, they will try to compensate by using gestures and/or signs. They are also likely to be frustrated and angry. The child whose language delay is part of a general learning difficulty is likely to be more passive and less frustrated.

Does the child have a problem with social interaction? Consider autism, signs of which include loss of social interaction, little or no non-verbal communication, no eye contact, and repetitive ritualistic behaviour.

Cerebral palsy (see Table 4.2.C.3)

Cerebral palsy refers to the disturbance of movement and/or posture that results from a non-progressive lesion of the developing brain. The commonest causes are hypoxic-ischaemic insult to the brain occurring prenatally or perinatally, or occasionally postnatally (e.g. meningitis, head injury). There are several different types of cerebral palsy, including the following:

- spastic diplegia (common with prematurity)
- spastic quadriplegia and spastic hemiplegia
- dyskinetic type (abnormal non-purposeful writhing movements induced by voluntary activity).
- ataxic type (involves mainly the cerebellum and is rare).

Diagnosis

The child normally presents with delayed development and is found to have abnormalities of tone, delay in motor development, abnormal posture or movements, and persistence of primitive reflexes. The diagnosis is made on clinical grounds and investigations are not required.

Evaluation

Assess the functional status of the child with regard to the motor system (this is best performed by a physiotherapist), and identify associated problems.

Management

The child with cerebral palsy has multiple problems and invariably will require care from a multidisciplinary team. The doctor and the physiotherapist play a prominent role. Physiotherapy advice enables the parents to move and handle the child in their daily activities to improve mobility and aim to prevent contractures. Parents need support in ensuring both that the educational needs of the child are met and that the child is integrated as fully as possible into society.

Deterioration in children with cerebral palsy

Children with cerebral palsy usually remain stable. If a child shows apparent deterioration consider the following possible causes:

- pain from dislocation of the hips
- dyspepsia from gastro-oesophageal reflux
- non-convulsive status epilepticus
- deterioration in mobility during growth spurt
- wrong diagnosis – the child may have a progressive neurodegenerative disease.

Paraparesis and incontinence

Paraparesis (paralysis of both legs) is usually due to a spinal cord problem. This may be congenital, as in spina bifida, or acquired (e.g. following trauma, infection or malignancy). Some causes are treatable if diagnosed early (e.g. TB of the spine). Burkitt's lymphoma with paraparesis is a sign of advanced disease and is often associated with a poor prognosis. Both thorough clinical assessment to establish the level of the lesion, and reassessment to look for

TABLE 4.2.C.3 Problems in children with cerebral palsy

Problem	Action
Visual and hearing impairment	Refer to appropriate specialist
Epilepsy	Anti-epileptic drugs
Contractures	Physiotherapy and (rarely) surgery
Dislocation of hips	Surgery to relieve pain
Feeding difficulties, failure to thrive	Monitor intake
	Correct positioning for feeding
	Increase energy content of food
	Consider gastro-oesophageal reflux
Recurrent aspiration	Close attention to feeding position, pacing of feeds, and positioning
Respiratory infections	Antibiotics
Gastro-oesophageal reflux	Feed thickener (starch), H_2-receptor antagonist (e.g. ranitidine) or proton-pump inhibitor (e.g. omeprazole)
	Exclude oesophageal stricture and/or aspiration
Constipation	Diet and stool softeners
Learning difficulties	Additional help with education

changes, are essential. Any suspected space-occupying lesion needs surgical advice.

Many children with paraparesis **will** suffer preventable complications **unless** carers and staff are aware of the risks of the following:

- **Poor nutrition:** many children with paraparesis find it difficult to eat and drink. They need good food to enable them to withstand infection, keep their muscles from wasting, prevent constipation and maintain good skin.
- **Contractures:** all joints need to be moved through their full range of movement to prevent contractures developing. If the child has presented late and contractures are already established, a programme of gradual passive stretching may help to improve the range of movement.
- **Pressure sores:** these are prevented by ensuring that the child is moved regularly. The child can often learn to do this by using their arms and upper body strength to pull on a suspended strap or ring to move their own position. The child can use a mirror to inspect their own skin to look for sore patches. Established pressure sores take a long time to heal. They must therefore be kept clean and free from pressure.

Rehabilitation should start immediately, but will depend on whether the child's spine is stable. A creative approach to mobility, using locally available materials (see *Disabled Village Children* by David Werner), is more likely to succeed than waiting for sophisticated rehabilitation equipment to be purchased.

Incontinence is usually associated with paraparesis, and can be both socially and medically disastrous. Some children have neuropathic bladders which are usually full, empty incompletely and may lead to reflux nephropathy, hydronephrosis and renal damage. These children need intermittent clean catheterisation to prevent back pressure and infection. Clean catheterisation may be required up to every 3 or 4 hours. This technique can be easily learned by a carer or by the older child. Other children have bladders that are not full and which empty themselves frequently. These children are at less medical risk of kidney problems, but it is much more difficult to enable them to be socially dry without complex surgery to enhance the size of the bladder.

Most children with bowel continence problems associated with paraparesis will be constipated due to their relative immobility. A healthy diet and plenty of fluids will prevent constipation. Bowel evacuation in young children is often managed by abdominal massage. Older children can learn to use a Shandling catheter, which is a plastic tube that is passed up the rectum for a washout of the bowel contents with saline.

Learning difficulties and developmental delay

- Children who do not meet their expected developmental milestones should be assessed for possible causes.
- Some children have specific learning difficulties and may be assumed to have general learning difficulties unless they are carefully assessed. Full psychological assessment is helpful (if available).
- Treatable causes (e.g. hypothyroidism, abuse/neglect, malnutrition, anaemia, etc.) should be ascertained. Problems such as autism and attention deficit disorder, with or without hyperactivity, should be documented.
- In planning services for these children, social and educational involvement is essential.

Severe learning difficulties

Severe learning difficulties (formerly referred to as mental retardation) are suspected when there is global developmental delay especially in language, social and fine motor skills. Gross motor milestones may be normal. Causes include fetal alcohol syndrome, hypoxic-ischaemic injury to the brain, Down's syndrome, fragile X syndrome and neurocutaneous syndromes, among others. **Treatable causes should be excluded** (e.g. hypothyroidism, phenylketonuria).

The parents will need considerable support in coming to terms with the diagnosis and its implications. They should be encouraged to stimulate the child's cognitive, language and motor development. Provide advice on appropriate play activities, suitable toys and reading material. Some children will be able to attend mainstream schooling but will need additional help; others will be better supported in special schools (if available). Their progress must be continuously monitored and associated problems dealt with. They deserve the same care as normal children.

Autism and communication disorders

- Autism usually presents in the second or third year of life.
- It is primarily a communication disorder associated with an absence of or disordered speech and language development.
- It is often associated with obsessional behaviours or interests.
- It may or may not be associated with mental retardation.
- It is often associated with learning difficulties because of inability to understand social situations.

The following should arouse the suspicion of autism: no babbling by the age of 1 year, no pointing by the age of 1 year, no single-word utterances by 16 months, no spontaneous two-word utterances by 24 months, and any regression in social skills and language.

Developmental coordination disorder

About 5% of children have difficulties with coordination which may affect their ability to perform motor tasks such as writing or sport. It is important to exclude a serious neurological cause and identify that the child cannot do these activities well, so that teachers and others do not conclude that the child is 'lazy'.

Attention deficit disorder

This is a major problem associated with the following:

- difficulty with concentration
- impulsivity
- difficulty in predicting the outcome of actions, so the child does not learn from their mistakes
- a strong association with hyperkinesis/hyperactivity
- poor listening skills.

Attention deficit disorder improves with maturity.

Treatment is difficult. The most important points are to recognise the disorder, explain it to the parents and provide them with family and/or other support to cope with it. **Stimulants, such as methylphenidate, used by an experienced health worker, may be very helpful.**

Behaviour disorders

- Exclude attention deficit disorder and other developmental impairments.
- Try to exclude abuse, although a behaviour disorder may coexist with abuse (*see* Section 5.9).

Psychiatric disorders (see Section 5.9)

- These are rare in young children.
- Severe malnutrition, deprivation and abuse can lead to depression and the signs of frozen awareness/watchfulness (*see* Section 7.6 on child abuse).

Surgically treated disabilities such as hare lip and cleft palate are addressed in the section on surgical problems (*see* Section 5.19).

Transition to adulthood for children with disabilities: a human rights perspective

The transition from childhood to adulthood takes time, and the process of adolescence is experienced and managed in very different ways in different cultures. This transition is much more challenging for disabled children whose abilities to achieve independence may be constrained by their condition. Disabled children are at higher risk of abuse and exploitation, and are likely to be more vulnerable as they pass through adolescence into adulthood. It is best to view this transition from a **human rights perspective**. Thus the disabled child has rights as stated within the UN Declaration of the Rights of the Child, and the same perspective informs any consideration of the transition to adulthood.

Conditions, cultures and economies

Different cultures and economies make it relatively easy or difficult for young people with different types of conditions to integrate and find a role. For example, a young person with a severe physical disability, such as spastic quadriplegia, but of normal intelligence may find it relatively easy to find a fulfilling role as an adult in a technologically advanced urban environment where there are relatively few physical barriers for wheelchair access. However, a young person with learning difficulties and good mobility may find it difficult to find a fulfilling role in such a society. By contrast, a less technologically advanced society can be much more accepting of the young person with learning difficulties, for whom there are many welcome roles in the rural economy, and the intellectually competent but physically impaired young person may find it much more difficult to find fulfilment in such an environment.

There may be very different cultural expectations of young men and young women, and deep-seated prejudices and cultural taboos that cause further disablement and devaluing of young disabled people unless the human rights perspective is paramount.

Child-friendly and child-safe environments

- All buildings that are used as healthcare facilities and playgrounds for children should be surveyed with the needs of their disabled users in mind.
- When new buildings are planned, it should be remembered that wheelchairs need wider doors and that where steps are needed ramps should also be provided.
- If the building has several floors, lifts should (when possible) be in place. If this is not possible, clinics serving disabled people should be located on the ground floor.
- Areas used by visually impaired people should be well lit, with steps and drops highlighted. Written notices should be as large and clear as possible.
- Special facilities may need to be provided for deaf and blind children to access information.

The challenges of transition
Independence

Good practice includes involving children in decision making about their own lives well before they enter adolescence. Learning from failures as well as successes is part of normal development. Many children in resource-limited communities are expected to work on the land or in industry, to look after livestock or to take responsibility for the care of their younger siblings at an age when they are not developmentally equipped to do so. Many children who have been involved in civil war and other armed conflict have been deprived of an ordinary childhood and may have had 'independence' forced upon them at an early age (see Section 1.23). Disabled children may have similar experiences or worse (e.g. being used as beggars), which deprive them of their human right to a childhood. If 'independence' means the insecurity of street children progressing to prostitution or a life of petty crime, this is not the sort of independence that young people need.

At the other extreme, disabled children worldwide are often overprotected by their families, who may feel ashamed, or there may be cultural taboos and beliefs about the origins of particular conditions. The parents may wish to do everything for their disabled child, but this can result in the child not learning from experience. The end result may be that the disabled young person does not get the opportunities for education and training that would enhance their self-esteem and ability to at least make some contribution to society, rather than be seen merely as an object of pity and charity.

Enabling the disabled child to become an integrated member of adult society is a challenge that requires the following:

- imagination, resources and flexibility on the part of the health, education and social services
- active engagement with the young person, their family and their community
- a real commitment to working with the strengths of the young person and minimising their weaknesses by reducing the barriers to their participation in society
- anticipating difficulties in advance and balancing the risk of failure against the benefits of increasing independence.

Information

Disabled young people often do not have access to information about their own condition, necessary health education to prevent secondary problems developing, training and employment opportunities, self-help groups and their rights.

Sexuality

The challenge of emerging sexuality is often more difficult for the disabled young person. Young people commonly have inaccurate information about the basic facts of sexual development, and disabled young people often miss out on the opportunity to learn these facts in a straightforward way. Many young people may be unaware of any genetic implications of their own condition, although it is more common to assume that there are genetic risks to their offspring when this is **not** the case.

Families, and indeed some healthcare professionals, may make inaccurate assumptions about the ability of disabled young people to have normal sexual experiences. These young people may have their own inaccurate beliefs which may cause much unnecessary suffering unless they have the opportunity to understand the facts about their own bodies. Even when there are some physical problems that will affect sexual experience (e.g. lack of genital sensation for some young people with paraplegia), this does not preclude an active and fulfilling sexual relationship.

Services for the transition to adulthood

Healthcare facilities that provide services for children with disabilities should develop expertise in enabling children to make the transition to adulthood. This expertise is likely to be achieved by developing shared knowledge among a group of relevant professionals working in partnership with young people. The service should be able to offer the following:

- information that is relevant and up to date
- individual counselling
- opportunities to meet other young people with similar difficulties
- careers advice
- a service to loan out equipment to increase independence
- close links with education facilities and any social and housing services.

Further reading

- Werner D (1987) *Disabled Village Children: a guide for community health workers, rehabilitation workers and families*. Palo Alto, CA: Hesperian Foundation.

4.2.D Care of children and young people with a spinal cord injury

> **BOX 4.2.D.1 Minimum standards**
> - Cervical collars.
> - Dexamethasone.
> - Physiotherapy.
> - Jewett brace.
> - Urinary catheters (in–out and Foley).
> - Glyceryl trinitrate.
> - Laxatives.
> - Suppositories.
> - Parent training.

Introduction

The acute and immediate management of children and adolescents with a traumatically injured spine in the context of major injury is described in Sections 7.3.A and 7.3.G. Much of the important advice given in this section is adapted from the following excellent book, which is essential reading for all healthcare workers in resource-limited settings:

- Werner D (1987) *Disabled Village Children: a guide for community health workers, rehabilitation workers and families*. Palo Alto, CA: Hesperian Foundation.

Mechanisms

- The following conditions predispose to spinal injuries: achondroplasia, Klippel–Feil syndrome, Down's syndrome and juvenile rheumatoid arthritis.
- Injuries can occur during birth and from abuse.
- Most of the injuries occur in road traffic accidents, sports, falls from trees or donkeys, bullet wounds and diving accidents.
- Non-traumatic causes include transverse myelitis (e.g. epidural abscess, tuberculosis of the spine, neuroblastoma, astrocytoma, eosinophilic granulomata, lipoma, teratoma and aneurysmal bone cysts).

Diagnosis

- In the conscious patient, localised tenderness in the spine, and impairment or loss of sensation, voluntary motor power and reflexes can help to determine the level of vertebral involvement.
- In the semiconscious or unconscious patient, hypotension associated with bradycardia, dilated peripheral veins in the lower limbs, paradoxical respiration, lack of spontaneous movement of limbs, lack of response to painful stimuli applied by pressure over bony prominences at various levels, and urinary retention are all signs suggestive of a spinal cord injury.
- Around 10–20% of injuries are in more than one site. Therefore an X-ray of the whole spine is necessary.
- Other associated injuries are common, and loss of sensation may delay their diagnosis.

Level of the injury

The magnitude of the area of the body that is affected will depend on the level of the injury. The higher the injury is, the greater the area of the body that is affected.

In paraplegia:

- there is loss of controlled movement and feeling in the legs

- the hips and part of the trunk may be affected (the higher the injury, the greater the area of the body that is affected)
- there may be partial or complete loss of urinary and bowel control
- there may be spasticity (muscle spasms) or hypotonia in the legs.

Complete and incomplete injuries

When the spinal cord is damaged so completely that no nerve messages get through, the injury is said to be 'complete'. Feeling and controlled movement below the level of the injury are completely and permanently lost. If the injury is 'incomplete', some feeling and movement may remain. Alternatively, feeling and controlled movement may return (partly or entirely) little by little over a period of several months. In incomplete injuries, one side may have less feeling and movement than the other.

X-rays often do not show how complete a spinal cord injury is. Sometimes the backbone (spinal column) may be badly broken, yet the spinal cord damage may be minor. And sometimes (especially in children) the X-ray may show no damage to the backbone, yet the spinal cord injury may be severe or complete. Often only time will tell how complete the injury is.

Neurological deterioration

This may be caused by:

- further mechanical damage and/or further non-mechanical damage to neural tissue during treatment
- hypoxia, hypotension and sepsis that develop due to poor management of the multisystem malfunction.

Acute management of spinal cord injuries: overall approach

For acute ABC management in the context of major traumatic injury, *see* Sections 7.3.A and 7.3.G.

- Aim to prevent complications related to multisystem dysfunction by good ABC resuscitation.
- Aim to contain the 'biomechanical instability' of the spinal column by preventing movement at the site of the fracture.
- Dexamethasone should not be given routinely to children with spinal injuries, as there is no evidence that steroids improve the neurological outcome, and the risk of complications is high.
- Dexamethasone should only be considered if there are signs of neurological deterioration following acute spinal injuries. The recommended dose is 500 micrograms/kg immediately, followed by 50 micrograms/kg every 6 hours for 48 hours.
- 'Rehabilitation' should begin in parallel with the medical treatment as soon as possible.
- Arrange early counselling and psychological support for the child, their parents and family members.
- Start physiotherapeutic procedures to prevent contractures of paralysed muscles, chest infections and pressure sores.
- Train all systems of the body to function as safely and with as near normal convenience as possible.

- Aim for psychosocial and physical reintegration of the child in the community without significant loss of education.
- Ensure a teaching programme for the child and/or their parents aimed at minimising the development of complications (medical, physical and psychological) in the medium and long term.
- Offer lifelong regular hospital assessment and treatment if necessary to maintain health and rehabilitation.

Acute spinal injury

- Keep the spine in a neutral position (with pillow arrangements). For cervical spine injury, immobilise with a cervical collar or sandbags at the side of the head for about 6 weeks, followed by bracing for 6 to 8 weeks. In children under 6 years of age, the sagittal diameter of the skull exceeds that of the chest, forcing the neck into flexion. A cut-out should be made in the board or the mattress to recess the occiput.
- Children with an unstable fracture of the spine but with intact neurology can be adequately braced in a Minerva cast for cervical spine injuries and a body cast for thoracolumbar injuries. Alternatively, or later, surgery can be undertaken, but only in a specialist centre (if available).
- Minerva and body casts should not be applied to children with sensory loss, because of the risk of pressure sores.
- A hard cervical collar for the quadriplegic patient and a Jewett brace for the paraplegic child are likely to provide adequate support until healing occurs.

Temperature control

The patient may not be able to control their body temperature, becoming pyrexial in a hot environment or hypothermic in a cold environment.

Cardiovascular and peripheral vascular system problems

- Spinal shock (autonomic areflexia) may cause bradycardia with hypotension.
- Care is needed with IV hydration, as circulatory overload and pulmonary oedema can easily occur.
- Hypoxia, hypothermia and tracheal suction can aggravate the bradycardia.
- Postural hypotension is most profound during the state of spinal areflexia. Early mobilisation can result in a significant drop in blood pressure which may affect spinal cord blood flow and adversely affect neurological recovery.
- Following the return of autonomic reflex activity, patients with cord lesions above T6 can develop autonomic dysreflexia (sudden onset of pounding headaches, flushing, blotchiness of the skin above the level of the injury, conjunctival congestion associated with sweating, and high blood pressure). The commonest causes are urinary retention and constipation. Treat this condition by placing the patient in the upright position (usually sitting) and if they are over 12 years of age the administration of sublingual glyceryl trinitrate (300 micrograms). If urinary retention is the cause, catheterisation following the liberal instillation of urethral lubricant with local anaesthetic will rapidly reduce the blood pressure and relieve the symptoms.

Respiratory system

- Children with injuries above C4 are unlikely to be able to breathe spontaneously.
- Children with lesions below C4 (most children with activity in the biceps) are able to breathe independently using their diaphragm, provided that no major chest injury is present.
- Encourage deep-breathing exercises and postural drainage, assist coughing and monitor oxygen saturation if possible.

Gastrointestinal system

- In the acute phase after a spinal cord injury, all patients are at risk of developing paralytic ileus. The resulting abdominal distension can embarrass the diaphragm and further impede diaphragmatic breathing. Avoid oral intake in the first 48–72 hours following injury and until bowel sounds are audible.
- The risk of gastrointestinal bleeding from stress ulcers is high. Therefore administer H_2-blockers such as ranitidine, 2–4 mg/kg twice daily up to a maximum of 150 mg twice daily, or antacids, for the first 3 to 4 weeks following injury.
- A regular bowel regime consisting of suppositories at fixed and regular intervals not exceeding 24 hours should be instituted initially by a nurse or parent, and later by the child (see below for details).

Hypercalcaemia

- This occurs in 10–20% of children, especially in quadriplegia and complete spinal cord injuries. The onset is insidious in the first few weeks following injury. Nausea, anorexia and vomiting can mimic an acute abdomen. Polydipsia, polyuria, dehydration, lethargy and occasionally psychosis can occur.
- Adequate hydration and furosemide are the first-line treatment.

Management of nutrition
What food should be given?

If the child is malnourished, give them 200 kcal/kg/day (see Section 5.10.A and 5.10.B). The daily number of kilocalories should be divided by the number of meals given during the day, usually four meals per day.

F100 can be used to correct malnutrition (see Section 5.10.B).

Commercial F100

This special milk is prepared in a sachet. All that the family has to do is open the packet and dilute the contents in 2 litres of water.

Home-made F100

When commercial milk is not available, F100 can be prepared from the recipe shown in Table 4.2.D.1.

The basic diet is composed of F100 meals. However, when the patient is gaining weight quickly other foods can be introduced. For example, the usual food eaten in the area can be used, but this should be enriched with the addition of oil and vitamin and mineral mix, and sometimes dried skimmed milk.

Example of calculation:

A child who weighs 20 kg should receive
200 kcal × 20 = 4000 kcal per day.

They will receive 4 meals per day, therefore 1000 kcal per meal.

Doses of supplemental nutritional aids
These are as follows (*see* Section 5.10.A and 5.10.B):
- **Zinc:** 2 mg/kg/day, or for children over 5 years of age, 40 mg once a day (of the elemental formula).
- **Vitamin C:** 45 mg/day.
- **Iron:** one ferrous sulphate tablet of 200 mg once weekly for children over 5 years of age.

TABLE 4.2.D.1 Recipe for preparing 1 litre of high-energy food

Food item	Quantity
Dried skimmed milk (DSM) or oiled full cream milk	80 grams (900 mL)
Vegetable oil	60 grams (20 mL)
Sugar	50 grams
Water (boiled)	Add water to make 1 litre of preparation
CMV (minerals and vitamin mix)*	20 mL (should be added after the water)

*The CMV should be added when the preparation of milk is ready. Whisk to prevent the oil from separating. This keeps for 12 hours.

Subsequent nursing and medical management and education of the child and their family
Early questions that a child with spinal cord injury and their family may ask

Will my child always remain paralysed?
This will depend on how much the spinal cord has been damaged. If paralysis below the level of the injury is not complete (e.g. if the child has some feeling and control of movement in their feet) there is a better chance of some improvement.

Usually the greatest improvement occurs in the first months. The more time that goes by without improvement, the less likely it is that any major improvement in feeling or movement will occur.

After 1 year, the paralysis that remains is almost certainly permanent. As gently as you can, help both the child and their parents to accept this fact. It is important that they learn to live with the paralysis as best they can, rather than waiting for it to get better or going from clinic to clinic in search of a cure.

Immediately after a spinal cord injury, the paralysed parts are in 'spinal shock', and are hypotonic. Within a few days or weeks the legs may begin to stiffen, especially when the hips or back are straightened. Also, when it is moved or touched, a leg may begin to 'jump' (a rapid series of jerks, or 'clonus').

This stiffening and jerking is an automatic reflex called 'spasticity'. It is not controlled by the child's mind, and often happens where spinal cord damage is complete. It is **not** a sign that the child has begun to feel where they are touched or is recovering control of movement. Some children with spinal cord injury develop spasticity, while others do not.

If the spinal cord injury is above the level of the top edge of the hipbone (above the second lumbar vertebra), spasticity is likely. If the injury is below this level, paralysis is usually floppy (no muscle spasms).

Severe spasticity often makes moving and control more difficult. However, the child may learn to use both the reflex jerks and spastic stiffness to help them to do things. For example:
- When the child wants to lift their foot, they hit the thigh, triggering the jerks that lift the leg.
- In lower back injuries, the spasticity or stiffness of the legs may actually help the child to stand for short periods.

Will my child be able to walk?
This will mainly depend on how high or low in the back the injury is.

If the child's injury is in the lower back and if their arms are strong and they are not overweight, there is a chance that they may learn to walk with crutches and braces. However, they will probably still need a wheelchair to go long distances.

It is best not to place too much emphasis on learning to walk. Many children who do learn to walk find it so slow and tiring that they prefer to use a wheelchair.

It probably makes sense to give most paraplegic children a chance to try walking. However, do not make the child feel guilty if they prefer a wheelchair. Let the child decide which is the easiest way for them to move about.

For independent living, other skills are more important than walking, and the family and child should place greater emphasis on these skills, such as dressing, bathing, getting in and out of bed, and toileting. Self-care in toileting is especially important, and is made more difficult because of the child's lack of bladder and bowel control.

What are the prospects for my child's future?
The likelihood of a child with **paraplegia** leading a reasonably normal life are good, provided that:
- Three major medical risks are avoided:
  - skin problems (pressure sores)
  - recurrent urinary tract infections
  - contractures (shortening of muscles, causing deformities); these are not life-threatening, but they can make moving about and doing things much more difficult.
- The child is helped to become more self-reliant:
  - home training and encouragement to master basic self-help skills such as moving about, dressing and toileting
  - education: learning of skills that make keeping a household, helping other people, and earning a living more achievable.

It is more difficult for children with **quadriplegia** to lead a normal life because they are more dependent on physical assistance.

In well-resourced countries, many children with paraplegia manage to lead full rich lives, earn their own living, get married, and play an important role in the community.

With effort and organisation, the same potential for leading a normal life can exist in all countries.

Can anything be done about loss of bladder and bowel control?

Yes it certainly can. Although normal control rarely returns completely, the child can often learn to be independent in their toilet, and to stay clean and dry (except for occasional accidents). Often they will need to learn to use a urinary catheter, and learn to bring down a bowel movement with a finger or suppository (see below).

What about sexual relationships and having children?

Many people with spinal cord injuries marry or have fulfilling sexual relationships. Women with spinal cord injuries can become pregnant and have babies.

Helping the child and their family to adjust to and accept the injury

Perhaps the biggest problem is that one day the child is physically active and able, and the next they are suddenly paralysed and (at first) unable to do much for themselves. They have lost all feeling and control in part of their body, which feels like a 'dead weight'. This is very hard for both the child and their family to accept. Both have enormous and partially justified fear and uncertainty about the future. The child may become deeply depressed, or angry and uncooperative. They may refuse even to sit in a wheelchair because this means accepting that they are unable to walk.

There are no easy ways to address the child's fear and depression, but here are some suggestions that families have found helpful.

Recognise that **the child's fear, depression and anger are natural responses**, and that with love, understanding and encouragement they will gradually overcome them.

Be honest with the child about their disability. Do not tell them 'We will find a cure for you' or 'Soon you will get well and be able to walk again.' Very probably this is untrue, and misleading the child in this way only makes it more difficult for them to accept their disability and begin to shape a new life. Also, as the promised 'cure' fails to materialise, the child will become more uncertain, distrustful and afraid. In the end, it will be much easier if you gently tell them the truth.

Provide opportunities to **keep the child's mind active by playing, working, exploring, and learning through stories, games, and studies**. But at the same time **respect and be supportive of the child when they feel sad and frightened**. Let the child cry, comfort them when they do so, but do not tell them not to cry. Crying helps to relieve fear and tension.

Start the child with **exercises, activities and relearning to use their hands and body** as soon as possible. Start with what the child can do, and build on that.

Try to arrange for the child to **watch, talk with and get to know other people with spinal cord injury**.

Invite the child's friends to come and visit, play with him or her, and let the child know that they are eager for the day he or she will be back in school.

Encourage the child to do as much for him- or herself as possible, even if it takes a little longer.

As far as possible **avoid the use of 'tranquillisers'** or other inappropriate medication. The child needs an alert mind and the ability to move actively all day.

To prevent or reduce the harmful effects of the complications of spinal cord injury, **special precautions need to be taken early and continued throughout life**.

Early care

Early care following spinal cord injury is best provided in hospital. Family members should stay with the child to make sure that he or she is kept clean and turned regularly, so that bed sores and pneumonia are avoided. Busy hospital staff with little experience of treating spinal cord injuries sometimes allow severe bed sores to develop, which may be life-threatening for the child.

The damage that has already been done to the spinal cord cannot be corrected with surgery or medicine.

Preventing pressure sores (bed sores)

When sensation has been lost, pressure sores can easily form on the skin over bony areas, especially on the hips and bottom. The time of greatest risk of sores developing is in the first weeks after the injury. This is because the child must stay very still, and has not yet learned to move or turn over their body. Prevention of pressure sores is extremely important, and needs understanding and continuous care, both by the child and by those caring for them.

Early prevention of pressure sores

- Lie the child on a soft mattress or a thick firm foam rubber pad.
- Place pillows and pads to keep the pressure off bony areas.
- Change their position (turn over from front to back and side to side) every 2 to 3 hours. To avoid pressure sores, lying on the abdomen is the best position.
- Keep the skin and bedclothes clean and dry.
- Give the child healthy food rich in vitamins, iron and protein.
- Move and exercise the child a lot to promote healthy flow of the blood.
- Check their skin daily for the earliest signs of pressure sores, and keep all pressure off areas where sores might be developing until the skin is healthy again.

Avoiding contractures

In the first weeks following a spinal cord injury, when the child is in a lying position, joint contractures (muscle shortening) can easily develop, especially in the feet and elbows. Pillows and pads should be placed to keep the feet supported, the elbows straight, and the hands in a good position. Gentle range-of-motion exercises of the feet, hands and arms should begin as early as possible, taking care not to move the back until the injury has healed.

Movement and exercise

Do range-of-motion exercises for about 10 minutes for each leg. In the first weeks, do the exercises twice a day; later on, once a day may be enough. If any signs of contracture develop, spend more time and effort on those parts of the body. From the start, exercises should be both **passive** (someone else moving the child's body parts) and, whenever possible, **active** (the child moving them).

Range-of-motion exercises should begin with great care the day after the spine is injured. The exercises will help to improve the flow of blood (which reduces the likelihood of bed sores), prevent contractures, and build the strength of the muscles that still work. Range-of-motion exercises should be **continued throughout life**, when possible as a part of day-to-day activity.

Cautions

- Until any breaks or tears in the spine have healed (this takes 6 weeks or more), exercise must be very gentle and limited, with smooth motions and no jerking.
  - Especially at first, take great care that exercises do not move the position of the back and neck (depending on the site of injury). Start with the feet, ankles, hands, wrists and elbows.
  - If exercises trigger severe muscle spasms or jerking, do not do them until the break in the spine has healed.
- Do not use force in trying to get the full range of motion, as joints can easily be damaged.
- Try to keep the full range of motion of all parts of the body, but **work most with those joints that are likely to develop contractures**, especially:
  - paralysed parts that tend to hang in one position, such as the feet
  - joints that are kept straight or bent by spasticity or by muscle imbalance.

Maintaining a healthy position

The position that the body is in during the day and night is also important to prevent contractures.

Contractures that cause 'tiptoeing' of the feet can develop easily, especially when there is spasticity. Keep the feet in a supported position flexed at 90 degrees to the lower leg, not in the extended position, for as much of the time as possible when lying down and when sitting.

Teach the child to check that their feet are in a good position. Even for the child who may never walk, maintaining the feet in a flexed position makes moving from chair to bed, toilet or bath easier.

Another common problem for children with spasticity is that the knees pull together and in time contractures prevent the legs from separating. To prevent this, when the child lies on their side, they should learn to place a pillow between the legs, and to keep it there most of the time.

A common problem with wheelchair users is that they slump forward. In time this can deform the spine. In a wheelchair with a straight-up back a person with spinal cord injury slumps like this in order to balance. A chair can be designed (or adapted) so that it tilts back. This provides balance for a better position.

A special cushion also helps to prevent the child's bottom from sliding forward (and also helps to prevent pressure sores). If possible, use a cushion mad of 'micropore' foam rubber (foam containing very tiny air bubbles). Rubber-coated coconut fibre also works well.

Early physical development

The goal is for the child to become as independent as possible in doing what they want and need to do. However, even before the skills of daily living are relearned, the child needs to **learn to protect the body where functions that used to be automatic have been lost**. The protective functions that may be lost or changed include the following:

- adjustment of the blood pressure to changes in body position

- sensation (including pain) that protects the body from injuries (e.g. bed sores)
- the sense of body position and ability to keep balance
- muscle strength and coordination.

A sudden fall in blood pressure in the brain when the person rises from lying to sitting, or from sitting to standing, can cause dizziness or fainting. This is a common problem in spinal cord injury because the blood pressure adjustment mechanism is partly lost. The body can be helped to gradually readapt, but precautions are needed. (These same precautions are the same for anyone who has been kept lying down for a long time.) Before beginning to sit, raise the head of the bed – a little more and a little longer each day. If the child starts to feel dizzy or faint when sitting, tilt their back and lift their feet. Lifting exercises help the body to relearn to adjust blood pressure, and also prevent bed sores and strengthen the arms.

The loss of sensation **in parts of the body can lead to pressure sores and other injuries**, such as burns and cuts. This is because the body no longer feels pain, so does not warn the child to change position or move away from danger.

It is important that the child learns to protect him- or herself by changing positions often and avoiding injuries. This includes the following:

- learning to roll over
- turning at least every 4 hours when lying or sleeping
- lifting from a sitting position every 15 minutes
- washing daily
- examining the whole body every day for signs of injuries or sores
- learning to protect him- or herself from burns and other injuries.

Keeping clean is very important for people with reduced sensation, especially if they lack bladder and bowel control. Take care to bathe them daily. Wash and dry the genitals, the bottom, and between the legs as soon as possible each time they get wet or dirty.

If redness, rash or sores develop, wash more often and keep the sore area dry. Keep the legs spread open and exposed to the air. When they must be covered, use soft absorbent cotton cloth.

For treatment of specific fungal, yeast and bacterial infections of the skin, see Section 5.18.

Loss of the sense of body position affects a person's sense of balance, as does **loss of muscle control**. The child needs to develop new ways to sense the position of their body and keep their balance.

Start with the child sitting on a bench, if possible, in front of a mirror, and help them to progress through the following stages:

1 Place both hands on the bench.
2 Place both hands on the knees.
3 Lift one arm sideways, forward and back.

After doing this in front of a mirror, ask the child to do it without the mirror.

- As the child begins to develop better balance, start doing different movements with first one and then both arms, such as lifting weights or playing ball.

- Some children may experience so much difficulty with balance that they have to start in a wheelchair or a chair with a high back and arm supports.

Redeveloping muscle strength and coordination. All muscles that still work need to be as strong as possible to make up for those that are paralysed. Even imagining movements helps to re-educate the brain about body posture. The most important muscles are those around the shoulders, arms and stomach.

Self-care

With the help and encouragement of family, friends and rehabilitation workers, the child can learn to become as independent as possible in meeting their basic needs, including moving about, eating, bathing, dressing, toileting, and in time other skills for daily living.

Progress toward self-care, especially at first, may be slow and frustrating. The child will need a great deal of understanding and encouragement. To make activities easier both for the child and for their helper, it is important that **they avoid becoming overweight**.

Useful methods and techniques have been devised for helping to relearn basic skills. Much depends on determination, imagination and common sense. Start with movements like rolling over and sitting up in bed.

Keeping active

Many of the 'complications' of spinal cord injury occur because the person spends a lot of time either lying down or sitting. To stay healthy, the body needs to keep active. Lack of movement and activity causes poor flow of the blood. This can lead to pressure sores, swollen feet, painful or dangerous blood clots (thrombosis), especially in the legs, increasing weakness of bones (osteoporosis) with the risk of fracture, bladder or kidney stones, increased risk of urinary tract infections, and general physical weakness and poor health.

It is important for both body and mind that people with a spinal cord injury keep physically active. Children should be allowed to do as much for themselves as they can, including pushing their own wheelchair, bathing, transferring, washing their clothes, helping to clean the house, and helping with work.

Active participation in games and sports can also be encouraged. Swimming, basketball and archery can be done well using only the upper body.

To keep the leg bones growing well and to prevent them from becoming weak and breaking easily, even children who may always have to use a wheelchair should if possible stand for a short time every day. This can be done by strapping the child to a 'standing board', or by making some kind of standing frame. Standing also helps to prevent constipation.

Management of bowel movements

When a person's spinal cord is damaged, they almost always lose control over when they will open their bowels. This makes it difficult to stay clean, which can be inconvenient and embarrassing. Although they can never regain complete control over the muscles that hold in or push out the stool, **they can learn to help the stool come out, with assistance, at certain times of day**. This kind of 'bowel programme' can greatly increase the person's self-confidence and freedom to take part in school, work and social activities.

People with spinal cord damage often have problems with constipation. Some constipation can be an advantage when a person lacks bowel control. However, sometimes it can lead to serious problems, such as impaction or dysreflexia. It is therefore important to prevent serious constipation by adopting the following measures:

- Drink plenty of water.
- Eat foods that are high in fibre (e.g. bran, wholegrain cereals, fruits, vegetables, cassava, beans, nuts).
- Stick to a scheduled bowel programme.
- Keep active.

Planning a bowel opening programme

Any bowel programme will work better if the child:

- does the programme every day (or every other day) and at the same time, even if they have had an accidental bowel movement shortly before, or have diarrhoea
- does the programme at the same time of day as they normally had bowel movements before their injury
- performs the task after a meal; often the bowels move best after a meal or a hot drink
- if possible, performs the task on a toilet or pot; the bowels work better in a sitting position than when lying down
- is patient; the bowels sometimes takes days or even weeks to change their pattern.

Types of bowel programme in spinal injury

Different people require different types of bowel programme, depending on whether their bowels are 'automatic', 'flaccid' or 'pull back'.

- **Automatic bowel** usually occurs in people who have muscle spasms in their legs, and an 'automatic bladder'. The muscle or 'sphincter' in the anus remains shut until there is a stimulation of the bowel to make it open, so that the stool can come out. An automatic bowel will 'move' in response to a suppository or stimulation by a finger.
- **Flaccid bowel** usually occurs in children with low spinal cord damage who have limp (not spastic) legs and bladder. The sphincter muscle in the anus is also limp, so the person tends to 'ooze' or 'dribble' faeces. A limp bowel does not respond to finger stimulation.
- **A bowel that pulls back** is neither automatic nor limp. When you insert a finger in the anus, the stool moves back up instead of coming out.

Management of an automatic bowel

1. Start with a suppository (Dulcolax or glycerine) prior to digital evacuation of the bowel. Glycerine suppository sizes are as follows: for an infant, 1 gram; for a child aged < 12 years, 2 grams; for a child aged > 12 years, 4 grams. With a finger covered with a glove or plastic bag, and then vegetable oil or Vaseline, push the suppository about 2 cm (1 inch) up the anus. Do not push it into the stool, but push it against the wall of the bowel. It is possible to try this same activity without a suppository; often finger stimulation alone is enough to stimulate a bowel action.
2. Wait for 5–10 minutes. Then help the child to sit on a toilet or pot. If they cannot sit, have them lie on their left side (on top of toilet paper or newspaper).
3. Put an oiled finger into the anus for a distance of about

2 cm. Gently move the finger in circles for about 1 minute, until the anus relaxes and the stool pushes out.

4 Repeat the finger action three or four times, or until no more stool is felt.

5 Clean the bottom and anus well and wash your hands.

Management of a flaccid bowel

Since the bowel does not push, the stool must be taken out with a finger. This is best done after each meal, or at least once a day.

- If possible, the child should be sitting on a toilet or pot, or lying on their left side.
- With a gloved and oiled finger, remove as much stool as you can.
- Since a limp bowel tends to ooze stool, the child should be given foods that make the stool firm or slightly constipated (**do not give the child stool-loosening foods**).

Management of a bowel that 'pulls back'

For this kind of bowel, the bowel programmes described above do not usually work. Finger stimulation makes the bowel act in the opposite direction and pull the stool back in. The child will have 'accidents' during the day. Often it is more effective to first put some anaesthetic jelly (e.g. lidocaine) up the anus. If you cannot obtain the jelly, you can mix some liquid injectable lidocaine with Vaseline or any other jelly. Wait for several minutes, and then proceed to the automatic bowel management.

Other important issues

- Children can almost always learn to do their own 'bowel programme'.
- Do not use enemas or strong laxatives regularly. They stretch the bowel, injure its muscles, and make following a regular programme more difficult. A mild laxative (senna or Dulcolax; *see* Section 5.12.C) may be taken occasionally when needed. However, drinking more liquid and eating food high in fibre is usually sufficient.
- If there is bright red blood in the stool, a blood vessel was probably torn during the management described above. Be more gentle! If there is dark old blood and the stools are black and tar-like, and the child is generally unwell, the parents should seek hospital advice urgently.
- A small amount of liquid stool (diarrhoea) may be a sign of 'impaction', which is a ball of hard stool stuck in the bowel. Only liquid stool can leak around it. Do not give medicine that is used to stop diarrhoea, as this could make the impaction worse. Try to remove the stool with a finger, or use stronger laxatives on a temporary basis (*see* Section 5.12.C).

A bowel management programme may at first seem difficult and messy, and is initially very embarrassing for the child. However, it soon becomes an easy habit. It is very important both for the child's health and for their social well-being. Do it regularly at the same hour of the day, and do not miss a day.

Constipation is almost always a potential problem, and can cause haemorrhoids, anal fissures and mucosal tears. For management of an acute episode, *see* Section 5.12.C. If constipation is regularly a problem, consider giving regular senna tablets (7.5 mg sennoside): aged 6–12 years, 1–2 tablets once daily; for 12–18 years, 2–4 tablets once daily or liquid (7.5 mg sennoside in 5 mL); for children under

6 years of age, 2.5–5 mL once daily; and for children over 6 years of age, 5–10 mL or 1–2 tablets once daily.

Locomotor system

- There is a high risk of contractures of muscles, limitation of the range of movement in the joints of the paralysed limbs, excess spasticity and fractures of long bones which are preventable.
- Passive movements and good positioning in bed and early splinting (if necessary) should prevent contractures.

Urinary system

- Urinary retention occurs during the stage of spinal areflexia, and is usually permanent in children with lower motor neuron lesions.
- Reflex micturition gradually develops in children with upper motor neuron lesions, usually from the sixth week onwards.
- Extra fluid intake should be encouraged.
- Up to the age of 2 to 3 years, 4-hourly gentle suprapubic pressure will empty the bladder.
- Children above the age of 3 years are best managed with intermittent catheterisation until effective reflex micturition occurs and the residual urine is consistently below 60 mL.
- Children with lower motor neuron lesions are likely to require intermittent catheterisation for the rest of their life. Initially this should be done by an attendant or parent. However, with teaching and training, a child with good hand function can learn to do clean intermittent self-catheterisation. Intermittent catheterisation is the safest method of bladder drainage.
- The use of indwelling urethral catheters is not recommended after the first 48–72 hours, but may sometimes be appropriate (see below).
- Antibiotics should be reserved for urinary tract infections with systemic manifestations.

Most children with spinal cord injury do not have normal bladder control. This can be inconvenient, embarrassing, and causes social and emotional difficulties. In addition, the loss of control can cause skin problems and **dangerous urinary tract infections**. For these reasons, it is important to learn ways to stay clean, dry and healthy. Most of the methods are not difficult, so children should be able to do this themselves, and this in turn will help them to feel more self-reliant.

The main goals of urine system management are as follows:

1 to prevent urinary infection
2 to promote self-care in staying as dry as possible.

Prevention of urinary tract infections is extremely important. **Infections of the urinary system (bladder and kidneys) are very common in spinal cord injury, and are one of the main causes of early death.** Therefore any method that is used for self-care or staying dry must also help to prevent urinary tract infections. Make every effort to prevent infection from entering the bladder. **Keeping clean is essential.** It is also important to empty the bladder regularly and **as completely as possible**. If some urine remains in the bladder, bacteria will grow in it and cause infection.

The ideal method of urinary control empties the bladder completely and in a clean, regular, easy and self-reliant way.

Types of bladder problems

Automatic bladder: A child with paralysis whose legs have 'reflex spasms' (uncontrolled stiffening or jerking) may have reflex spasms in their bladder. As the bladder fills with urine, the walls of the bladder stretch and cause a reflex spasm. As the bladder squeezes, the muscles that hold back the urine relax, letting the urine flow out. This is called an 'automatic bladder' because it empties automatically when it gets full.

Flaccid bladder: When a child's paralysed legs are limp (due to lower motor neuron damage) and do not have spasms, usually the bladder is also limp or flaccid. No matter how much urine fills the bladder, it will not squeeze to empty. The bladder stretches until it cannot hold any more urine. The urine then begins to drip out and overflow incontinence develops. The bladder does not completely empty, and because some urine remains in the bladder, there is an increased likelihood of infection.

The most simple methods of bladder management work well with an automatic bladder but do not work with a limp bladder. Therefore **it is important to try to establish which type of bladder the child has**.

For the first few days or weeks after the spinal cord injury occurred, the bladder is almost always flaccid. Urine either drips out or does not come out at all. Then, as the 'spinal shock' wears off, people with higher back injuries (above the second lumbar vertebra) usually develop an automatic bladder. In people with lower back injuries the bladder usually remains flaccid.

During the first weeks after the spinal cord injury, usually a Foley catheter is kept in the bladder all the time. However, after about 2 weeks it is a good idea to test how the bladder works by removing the catheter and trying one of the methods described below. If the child is often wet, try another method for that type of bladder.

Methods for managing the automatic bladder

Triggering programme: This method usually causes the bladder-emptying reflex to work when the person is ready to pass urine. It can be done using a urinal, toilet, potty or jar. **This is the first method to try**, because nothing is put into the bladder. It is easy, so a child can do it unaided.

1 Tap the lower belly (over the bladder) firmly with your hand for about 1 minute. Stop and wait for the urine to flow.
2 Tap again. Repeat several times until no more urine flows.

If possible, once a week after triggering, use an in–out catheter to see how much urine is left. If there is less than a cupful (150 mL), continue the triggering programme. It there is more than a cupful on several occasions, the bladder is not emptying well enough, and another method should be tried (see below).

Periodic use of a catheter: This method allows the bladder to be emptied completely before it becomes too full. Sometimes it can be used to prepare the body for triggering. Put a clean or sterile standard catheter into the bladder every 4–6 hours to empty the urine, and then remove the catheter. If the child drinks more liquid than usual, put in the catheter more frequently to keep the bladder from stretching too much.

To reduce the risk of urinary tract infections, **regular frequent use of the catheter is more important than using a sterile catheter**. It is a mistake to stop using the catheter only because you have not had an opportunity to boil it (e.g. when travelling, or at school). Just wash out the catheter with clean drinkable water after use, and keep it in a clean jar or towel. **Do not go too long without catheterising, and do not stop catheterising altogether.** It is important not to leave a large amount of urine in the bladder.

How to insert a catheter

Healthcare workers and parents can easily be taught to put in a catheter. With a little practice, children with paraplegia can also learn to do this. A mirror can help girls to see the perineal area.

- The best catheter size is usually #8 or #10 for a small child, and #14 or #16 for a large child.
- Vigilance about cleanliness (i.e. boiling the catheter and wearing gloves) is important when using a fixed (Foley) catheter. However, for periodic use of a regular (in and straight out) catheter, a clean rather than sterile technique is more practicable (and therefore may be safer). Wash the catheter well with clean water after each use, and keep it in a clean container. Wash your hands well before using it.

The procedure for insertion of a catheter is as follows:
1 If possible, boil the catheter for 15 minutes, or at least wash it well and keep it clean.
2 Bathe the child well (at least daily). Wash well under the foreskin or between the vaginal lips and the surrounding areas.
3 Wash your hands with soap. After washing, touch only things that are sterile or very clean.
4 Put very clean cloths or towels under and around the area.
5 Put on sterile gloves, or rub your hands well with alcohol or surgical soap.
6 Cover the catheter with a lubricant (slippery cream) such as KY Jelly that dissolves in water (do not use oil or Vaseline).
7 Pull back the foreskin or open the vaginal lips.
8 Holding the foreskin back or the vaginal lips open, gently put the catheter into the urethra. Twist it as necessary, **but do not force it**. Hold the penis straight at this angle.
9 Push the catheter in until urine starts to flow out, then push it in 3 cm further.
10 If using a regular catheter, each time the child passes urine they should tighten their stomach muscles or gently massage the lower abdomen to empty all urine. Then take out the catheter, wash it well, boil it, and store it in a clean jar or towel.

To avoid introducing infections when using a catheter, it is important to be very clean and to use only a catheter that is sterile, boiled or very clean.

Using a fixed (Foley) catheter: With this method, the catheter is left in all the time to drain the urine from the bladder continuously. A Foley catheter is often used immediately after injury, and in some cases for many months or years. The catheter connects to a collection bag that can be attached to the leg and worn under the clothes. The catheter should be changed using a sterile technique once weekly or more frequently if there is a urinary tract infection (see below).

In many areas this is the easiest method because other

supplies are difficult to obtain. However, a Foley catheter can cause many problems, including the following:

- bacteria entering the bladder, causing a **high risk of infection**
- **continuous bladder irritation**, which can cause bladder stones to form.

If you have tried other methods unsuccessfully or no other equipment is available, a Foley catheter may be the only option. To prevent complications from occurring **it is very important that the Foley catheter is used carefully**:

- Always wash your hands thoroughly before touching the catheter.
- Clean the skin around the catheter with soap and water at least twice a day, and after each bowel movement.
- Do not disconnect the collection bag except to empty and wash it. Wash out the collection bag with soap or diluted bleach and water once a day.
- If the catheter must be clamped, use a sterile plug, **never a glass ampoule (small bottle)**, as this may break and cause injury.
- **Keep the collection bag below the level of the bladder** to keep the urine from flowing back into the bladder via gravity.
- Tape the catheter to the leg when the child is in a wheelchair.
- Check regularly to make sure that the urine is emptying and that the catheter is not blocked. Make sure that there are no sharp bends or folds in the tubing.
- When turning, lifting or moving the child, remember to move the bag, too. Do not let it pull at the catheter or stay under the child.
- If the catheter becomes blocked, take it out, squirt boiled water through it, and put it back. Alternatively, use a new catheter. Use a sterile or very clean syringe.

Condom catheter for male children: This is a practical method for male children and adolescents who cannot control their urine flow. It can be used in combination with triggering, to avoid accidental wetting.

A condom catheter is a thin rubber bag that fits over the penis. It has a tube that connects to a collection bag. Condom catheters are available in different sizes. If they are too costly or not available, a regular condom can be attached to the collection tube with a rubber band or tape. Alternatively, a thin, very clean plastic bag or the finger of a rubber glove (or a 'finger cot') can be used.

To hold the condom on the penis, stretchy adhesive tape can be used.

Important precautions for condom catheter use include the following:

- Ensure that it is not too tight, otherwise it could stop the blood flow and seriously harm the penis. Avoid the use of non-stretch tape.
- If the penis has erections, try to put on the condom when it is erect.
- Remove the condom once a day and wash the penis well.
- If possible, remove the condom at night, and use a bottle or urinal to catch the urine.
- Check the condom and penis often, to ensure that everything is all right.
- If the penis becomes injured, swollen or looks sore, remove the condom until it is healthy again.

Methods for the limp bladder

If the person's bladder is flaccid, it never empties by reflex. The bladder will constantly contain some urine unless an effective emptying method is used.

Girls can use a Foley catheter. This is often the simplest method, but it can lead to urinary tract infections. Alternatively, try an 'intermittent' (in-and-out) programme, using a regular catheter every 4–6 hours. If there is leaking in between catheter times, use diapers, rags or a thick sanitary pad to catch the urine. Change them often and wash the skin often to protect the skin and prevent sores.

Boys can use an intermittent catheter every 4–6 hours.

Other suggestions for the flaccid bladder

- **The push method:** Strain to push the urine out by tightening the abdominal muscles. This method is recommended by many professionals, but it can cause problems. If the muscles do not relax to let the urine flow out, pushing on the bladder can force urine back into the kidneys, causing kidney infection and damage. Therefore **the push method should only be used if the urine flows out easily with gentle pressure, or if no other method is possible**.
- However, it is best to also use a regular catheter at least three times a day. This is because the bladder may not have emptied completely, which makes infection more likely.

Management of urinary tract infections (*see* Section 5.6.A)

Children with spinal cord injury have a high risk of urinary tract infections, for the reasons discussed above. Long-term or untreated infections and kidney problems are a common cause of early death. Preventive measures are essential, but even when precautions are taken, some urinary tract infections are still likely to occur. Therefore it is very important to recognise the signs and provide effective treatment.

Clinical signs

When a person who has normal sensation has a urinary tract infection, pain is felt when they pass urine or when they pass urine more frequently, including at night. The person with spinal cord damage may not feel this pain or be able to have frequency or nocturia, and therefore has to use other signs to know when they have an infection. The child may learn to recognise certain unpleasant feelings, or may only know that they do not feel as well as usual. Parents and healthcare workers should learn to listen to the child and be aware of changes in behaviour or other signs that might mean that an infection is probably present.

Possible signs of a urinary tract infection include the following:

- cloudy urine, possibly with mucus, pus or blood specks
- dark or red urine
- strong-smelling or bad-smelling urine
- increased bladder spasms (cramps)
- increased wetting or changes in bladder function
- pain in the back or loins
- body aches
- general discomfort
- increased muscle spasms
- fever

- dysreflexia (headache, 'goose-bumps' when sweating, high blood pressure).

Treatment

At the first signs of infection, the child should drink even more water than usual. Antibiotics may also be necessary. However, avoid frequent use of antibiotics because they may become less effective as bacterial resistance develops.

If the child has had urinary infections before, they can start with the last medicine that was effective (for details of antibiotic treatment, *see* Section 5.6.A).

If a medicine seems to help, continue taking it for at least 1 week, or for 4 days after the last clinical signs have disappeared. Do not change from one medicine to another unless the medicine is not working or causes serious side effects.

Prevention of urinary tract infections in patients with spinal injury

- Drink plenty of liquid (for normal daily fluid intake that should always be maintained, *see* Section 9, Appendix), with higher intake if there is a high ambient temperature. An intake of at least 2 litres (eight 250-mL glasses) a day is required for a teenager.
- Eat apples, grapes or cranberries, or drink juice made from these fruits, or take vitamin C tablets to make the urine more acidic. It is more difficult for bacteria to grow in acidic urine. (*Note:* the fruit and juice of oranges, lemons and other citrus fruits do not have this effect, and in fact make the urine **less** acid.)
- Keep hands, catheter and collection bags very clean before, during and after the child's bladder programme.
- Encourage the child not to lie in bed all day, but to remain active.
- Do not clamp the Foley catheter or plug it with anything unless absolutely necessary, in which case always use a sterile plug.
- Adhere strictly to the bladder programme, and do not allow urine to remain in the bladder.
- Ensure that the catheter does not become bent or twisted so that the flow of urine is blocked.
- If you are using an in–out catheter, put it in regularly, at least every 4 to 6 hours. For prevention of infections, frequency of catheter use is even more important than cleanliness. It is safer to put in the catheter without boiling it, than not to put it in. If infections are common, catheterise more often.

Sexuality and fertility

- Discuss the situation with sensitivity as soon as the child reaches early adolescence.
- Advice about contraception is necessary for girls, as fertility is not affected, regardless of the level and severity of the spinal cord injury.
- Boys with upper motor neuron lesions will have reflexogenic but not psychogenic erections. Male fertility is significantly affected. However, male adolescents should be reassured that the results of assisted fertility (if available) are good.

Psychosocial integration, education, vocational training and employment

Continuing education, vocational training and employment must be pursued as the child grows older.

Skin problems

Sensory impairment or loss, impairment of vasomotor regulation of skin blood flow associated with paralysis, double incontinence, possible anaemia and urinary tract infections all render the skin of patients with spinal cord injuries vulnerable to breakdown and infections. **Skin breakdown is preventable.**

In the acute stage, regular turning of the child together with adequate management of the bladder and bowels and vigilance in maintaining cleanliness will prevent skin breakdown.

In the rehabilitation stage, training of the parents and the child in self-care, hygiene and the provision of adequate seating can all assist.

Pressure sores

Pressure sores, or 'bed sores', form over bony parts of the body when a person lies or sits on that part of the body for too long without moving. Where the skin is pressed against the bed or chair, the blood vessels are squeezed shut so that the blood cannot transport air to the skin and underlying tissue. If too much time passes without the person moving or rolling over, the skin and underlying tissue in that spot may become injured or die. First, a red or dark patch appears. Then, if the pressure continues, an open sore can form. The sore may start on the skin and work inwards, or it may start at a deep level, near the bone, and gradually work its way to the surface.

Risk factors for pressure sores

When a healthy person lies or sits in one position for a long time, it begins to feel uncomfortable, or even painful, so they move or roll over, and the formation of pressure sores is prevented. The people who are most likely to develop pressure sores are those who are unconscious or who have no **sensation** in parts of their body, and who therefore do not feel the warnings of pain or discomfort when their body is being damaged. This includes people with spinal cord injury.

Commonest sites of pressure sores

Pressure sores can form over any bony area. The sites where they are most likely to develop are shown in Figure 4.2.D.1.

Risks and complications associated with pressure sores

If pressure sores are not very carefully managed, they can become large and deep. Because they contain dead skin and tissue, they can easily become infected. If a sore reaches the bone, which often happens, the bone can also become infected. Bone infections can be very difficult to cure, may last for years, and may keep recurring even after the original pressure sore has healed.

Infections in deep pressure sores often spread to the blood and then affect the whole body, causing fever and general illness, including bacteraemia and septicaemia.

Incidence of pressure sores

In patients who have lost sensation in parts of their body, **pressure sores are very common.** Most people with spinal cord injuries in developed countries, and nearly all people with such injuries in resource-limited countries, develop pressure sores. **Often the sores start to develop in hospital shortly after the injury, due to inadequate nursing care. Therefore it is important that the families of patients with spinal cord injuries, and those patients**

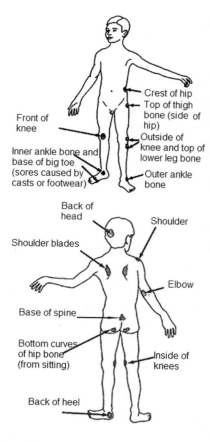

Crest of hip
Top of thigh bone (side of hip)
Front of knee
Outside of knee and top of lower leg bone
Inner ankle bone and base of big toe (sores caused by casts or footwear)
Outer ankle bone

Back of head
Shoulder
Shoulder blades
Elbow
Base of spine
Bottom curves of hip bone (from sitting)
Inside of knees
Back of heel

FIGURE 4.2.D.1 Sites where pressure sores are most likely to develop, with the most high-risk areas (in the hip region) labelled in bold type.

themselves, learn as early as possible about the prevention and early treatment of pressure sores, and put this knowledge into practice.

Prevention of pressure sores

It is important that both the child and their family are taught about the risk of pressure sores developing, and how to prevent them. The following actions are important:

- Avoid staying in the same position for very long. When lying down, turn from side to side or from front to back at least every 2 hours (or up to 4 hours if padding and cushioning are adequate). When sitting, lift the body up and change position every 10 to 15 minutes.
- Use thick soft padding, pillows or other forms of cushion arranged so as to protect bony areas of the body.
- Use soft clean dry bed sheets, and try to avoid them wrinkling. Change the bedding or clothing every day and also each time it becomes wet or soiled. A child who stays wet will develop pressure sores, especially if the wetness is caused by urine.
- Bathe the child daily. Dry the skin well by patting it, not rubbing it. It is probably best not to use body creams or oils, or talc, except on the hands and feet to prevent cracking, as these products soften the skin and make it weaker. **Never use heat-producing oils, lotions or alcohol.**
- Examine the whole body carefully every day, checking in particular those areas where pressure sores are most likely to develop. If any redness or darkness is present,

take extra care to prevent all pressure over this area until the skin returns to normal.
- Good nutrition is important for preventing pressure sores. Make sure that the child gets enough to eat (but do not let them become overweight). Give them plenty of fruits, vegetables, and protein-containing foods (beans, lentils, eggs, meat, fish and milk products). If the child looks pale, check for signs of anaemia (see Section 5.11.A), and make sure that they are given iron-rich foods (meat, eggs and dark green leafy vegetables) or take iron tablets (ferrous sulphate), as well as foods rich in vitamin C (oranges, lemons, tomatoes, etc.).
- As far as possible, the child should learn to examine their own body for pressure sores every day, and eventually learn to take responsibility for all the necessary preventive measures themselves.

Other precautions

- To avoid pressure sores or other injuries developing on feet that have lost sensation, use well-fitted, well-padded sandals or shoes.
- Changing positions is important. When a child has recently had a spinal cord injury, they must be turned regularly, taking great care not to bend their back. Using a sheet under the body can help with turning.
- As the child gets stronger, hang loops and provide other aids, if necessary, so that they can learn to turn themselves.

At first it is important that the person turns, or is turned, at least **every 2 hours day and night**. Later, if there are no signs of pressure sores, the time between turns can gradually be lengthened to 4 hours. To avoid the child (or the person turning them) sleeping through the night without turning, an alarm clock can be very helpful.

When the child begins to sit or to use a wheelchair, there is a new serious danger of pressure sores developing. The child must now get into the habit of taking the pressure off their bottom at least every 30 minutes.

If their arms are strong enough, the child can lift up their whole body and hold it up for a minute or two. This allows the blood to circulate in the bottom.

If the chair has no arm rests, or if they can be removed, the child can lie sideways over a pillow on a high bed. They can rest for 15 to 30 minutes like this.

To prevent pressure sores, it is essential that the person who has lost sensation lies and sits on a soft surface that reduces pressure on bony areas. It is best for them to lie on a flat surface with a thick spongy mattress. A **thick foam rubber mattress** often works well. However, some foam is so spongy that it sinks completely under a person's weight, so that the bony area is not protected from the hard board underneath. A firm sponge with very small air bubbles (microcell rubber) works well, but is expensive.

A 'waterbed' (a bag-like mattress filled with water) or air mattress also works well.

In some countries, an excellent mattress material is made from rubber-coated coconut fibre. Urine can be washed out of the material by pouring water through it. Because this material is costly, a rehabilitation programme in Bangladesh has adopted the practice of cutting a square out of a cheap mattress and replacing it with a square of the coconut fibre sponge.

Careful placement of pillows, pads or soft folded

blankets can also help to prevent pressure sores. Such measures are especially important in the first weeks or months after a spinal cord injury, when the person must lie flat and be moved as little as possible. Pillows should be placed to avoid pressure on bony areas, and to keep the person in a position that is healthy and that helps to prevent contractures.

Chair and wheelchair cushions

For the child who has lost sensation in their bottom, the type of seat cushion used is very important, especially if the paralysis makes it difficult for them to lift up or change positions. All patients with spinal cord injury should use a good cushion. Sitting directly on a canvas seat or a poorly padded wooden seat will cause pressure sores.

Good cushions can be made of 'microcel' rubber, which is fairly firm. It works best if it is cut and shaped to reduce pressure on bony areas.

A useful low-cost way to make a fitted cushion is to build a base out of many layers of thick cardboard glued together, and then cover it with a 2 or 3 cm thick layer of sponge rubber.

Wet the cardboard and sit on it wet for 2 hours, so that it moulds to the shape of the bottom. Then let it dry, and varnish it.

Before making a specially fitted cushion, you can make a 'mould' of the patient's bottom by having them sit in a shallow container of soft clay, mud or plaster. Note the bony hollows and form the seat to fit them.

Air cushions made from bicycle tyre inner tubes are excellent for the prevention of pressure sores, and for bathing on a hard surface. Use one, two or more tubes, depending on the size of the tube and the size of the child. Bind loops of the tubes together with thin straps of inner tube. Then pump in enough air to ensure that the whole of the child's bottom is held up by air. (This idea was suggested by wheelchair rider-builders at Tahanang Walang Hagdanan (House With No Stairs), Quezon City, Philippines.)

Treatment of established pressure sores

Be alert for the first signs of a pressure sore by examining the whole body every day. Teach the child to do this using a mirror.

If early signs of a pressure sore (redness, darkness, swelling or open skin) are observed, change body positions and use padding to protect that area from pressure.

For larger areas (such as the bones near the base of the spine), you can try using a small (motor scooter) inner tube to keep the weight off the sore area. Put a towel over the tube to soak up sweat, as sweaty skin against the rubber can also cause sores.

Warning: For small areas such as the heels, never use a ring or 'doughnut' of cloth to keep the weight off the sore, as this can cut off the blood supply to the skin inside the ring and make the sore worse.

If a pressure sore has already formed:
- Keep the pressure off the sore area completely and continuously.
- Keep the area completely clean. Wash it gently with clean or boiled water twice a day. Do **not** use alcohol, iodine or other strong antiseptics.
- Make sure that the child has a healthy diet. If a large amount of liquid is lost from the sore, a lot of protein and iron will be lost with it. These must be replaced to

allow quicker healing. The child should also take iron tablets if signs of anaemia are present, and they should eat foods rich in protein (beans, lentils, eggs, meat, fish and milk products).
- Do not rub or massage areas where pressure sores might be forming, as this could tear weakened tissue and make the sore inside larger.

If the sore is deep and contains dead tissue within it:
- Clean the sore three times a day.
- Each time you clean the sore, try to scrape and pick out more of the dead rotten tissue. Often you will find that the sore is much larger inside than you first thought. It may go deep under the edges of the skin. Little by little remove the dead tissue until you come to healthy red flesh (or bone).
- Each time you have cleaned out the dead tissue, wash the sore out well with soapy water. Use liquid surgical soap if possible. Then rinse with clean (boiled and cooled) water. A syringe without a needle can help with irrigation.

If the sore is infected (signs of this include pus, foul smell, a swollen hot red area around the sore, or the presence of fevers and chills):
- Clean out the sore three times a day as described above.
- If possible, take the person to a clinical laboratory where a sample from the sore can be removed and cultured to find out what organisms are causing the infection and what is the most appropriate medication to treat it.
- If this is not possible, try treating the patient with penicillin, cloxacillin or flucloxacillin.

If the sore does not get better, or if liquid or pus keeps draining from a deep hole, the bone may be infected, so tell the parents to take their child to the hospital.

Honey and sugar

Once a pressure sore is free of dead tissue, filling it two to three times a day with honey or sugar helps to prevent infection and speeds up healing. This treatment, which was used by the ancient Egyptians and was recently rediscovered by modern doctors, works remarkably well. It is now being used in some hospitals in the UK and the USA.

To make it easier to fill the sore, mix honey with ordinary sugar until it forms a thick paste. This can easily be pressed deep into the sore. Then cover the sore with a thick gauze bandage.

It is important to clean out and refill the sore at least twice a day. If the honey or sugar becomes too diluted with liquid from the sore, it will feed the bacteria rather than kill them.

The amount of honey that is needed on the wound depends on the amount of fluid that is being produced by the pressure sore. If there is a lot of fluid it will dilute the honey and make it less effective. The frequency of dressing changes required will depend on how rapidly the honey is being diluted. If there is no exudate, dressings need to be changed twice weekly to maintain the antibacterial properties of the honey as it enters the pressure sore. If the sore is producing a lot of fluid, the dressing will need to be changed twice a day.

To achieve the best results the honey should be applied to a dressing (cotton plus cellulose) which can absorb this prior to application. If applied directly to the wound, the honey tends to run off and be less effective. Honey will not soak easily into absorbent dressings. Soaking is helped by warming the honey to body temperature and/or adding 1 part of water to 20 parts of honey to make the honey more fluid. If the pressure sore is producing a lot of fluid, the absorbent dressing can be secured in place using cling film taped over it to help to keep the honey on the wound.

Alginate dressings impregnated with honey are a good alternative to cotton/cellulose dressings, as the alginate is converted into a honey-containing soft gel. Any holes in the wound need to be filled with honey in addition to using a honey-impregnated dressing. As infection may be present in the tissues underlying the edges of the pressure sore,

honey dressings need to extend beyond the inflamed area surrounding the sore.

Further reading

Betz RR and Mulcahey MJ (eds) (1996) *The Child with a Spinal Cord Injury.* Rosemont, IL: American Academy of Orthopedic Surgeons.

Grundy D and Swain A (2002) *ABC of Spinal Cord Injuries,* 4th edn. London: BMJ Books.

Werner D (1996) *Disabled Village Children: a guide for community health workers, rehabilitation workers and families.* Palo Alto, CA: Hesperian Foundation.

El Masri WS (2006) Traumatic spinal cord injury: the relationship between pathology and clinical implications. *Trauma,* **8**, 29–46.

4.2.E Facilities for children with special needs and learning difficulties

Introduction

The most valuable asset is healthcare staff who can spend time with these children and their families, and preferably who are also able to visit them at home.

For children presenting at the hospital with established disabilities, the challenge is to ensure that they make the best use of their abilities and do not develop further disabilities.

TABLE 4.2.E.1 Equipment for assessment

Equipment for physical examination	Equipment for skills assessment
Tape measure	20 brightly coloured wooden cubes, 2.5 cm in diameter
Auroscope	Threading beads of various sizes, and string
Ophthalmoscope	20 culturally appropriate pictures of common domestic objects, some of which have similar sounding names in the local language
Tendon hammer	Soft ball, approximately 10 cm in diameter
128-Hz tuning fork	Denver Developmental Screening Test
Simple audiometer	

Aids for disabled children

This section outlines the types of aids that should be available for disabled children in all hospitals. There are many conditions which can cause disability, and **the aim of the aids listed is to minimise disability and maximise independent function**. It should be noted that some positions which may appear desirable (e.g. the upright walking posture in a child with excessive extensor tone) may adversely affect the child's ultimate mobility. The advice of a trained paediatric physiotherapist is invaluable.

David Werner's book, *Disabled Village Children*, is an excellent source of ideas and advice.

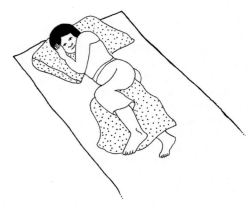

FIGURE 4.2.E.1 Lying aids.

General principles

- 'Look first at my strengths and not at my weaknesses': the preservation of best function is primarily achieved by education of the child and their carers, but aids and appliances can be very useful.
- Always consider the developmental stage of the child.
- An understanding of the home environment of the child is essential (e.g. in some regions a donkey may be a more useful mobility aid than a wheelchair once the child leaves hospital).
- The prevention of secondary disabilities (e.g. contractures or pressure sores) is a major priority in the care of disabled children.
- Always consider the purpose of the aid that you think will help, and ask yourself the following questions:
  - How will this aid help this child to function in their daily life?
  - Will the use of this aid reduce this child's abilities to do other things?
  - Will the use of this aid improve the way the child feels about him- or herself?
  - Who will review this aid to ensure that it is still helping the child and is still the right size for the growing child?
  - Who will maintain this aid to ensure that it still works?

Developmental aids

These are primarily used with children with delayed development, but may also be useful for children who have suffered a neurological insult, whether or not they are showing signs of recovery. Most children function better if they can experience a variety of positions and can be part of activities with others.

Lying aids

Many children who are ill or who are recovering from illness spend most of their time lying on their back or on their side. Lying on their front helps to develop trunk and arm strength and stretches muscles in the hips, knees and shoulders. **A pillow under the chest** helps to release the arms and hands for play.

A **wedge** is a more substantial version of the same idea, and can be made from material such as stiff foam plastic. Some children who need to have their legs separated because of adductor spasm will need a leg separator or pillow, also made of similar material.

Sitting aids

The type of sitting aids used will depend on the particular difficulties and developmental stage of the child. Most children with cerebral palsy benefit from being seated in a position in which their ankles, feet and hips are at 90 degrees and their legs are kept apart (abducted). There are many varieties of seats available. For a young child, a **corner seat** is often helpful. Special seating can also be fun (e.g. the 'steam engine').

Children with spasticity also often benefit from a slight tilt backwards. The position and amount of head support needed depend on the amount of head control and extensor tone.

Standing aids

These may be useful for children who are showing improvement in their motor skills and can be expected to learn to stand independently, but are also useful for children who may never stand independently, because the standing position aids the circulation and also bone growth and strength, particularly of the hip joints. Some children find standing frames difficult to get used to at first, and may need encouragement to use them.

Walking aids

There are a wide variety of these aids available. Perhaps the most useful is a walking frame that goes behind the child and which can have a variety of attachments depending on the child's balance and arm strength. Some **parallel bars** are also useful and will need to be set at different heights depending on the size of the child.

A selection of **underarm crutches, elbow crutches** and **tripod sticks** will be useful. These can often be made locally, and will need to be of various sizes.

Note that underarm crutches can cause nerve damage if the child hangs off the crutches when attempting to walk.

Wheelchair technology

This is beyond the scope of this book. The general principles listed at the beginning of this section apply. Remember that a wheelchair is not the only solution for an otherwise immobile child. If the child has no sensation in their buttocks as a result of spinal cord damage, they will be at risk of developing pressure sores if they remain seated in the same position for long periods of time. They can learn ways of taking the pressure of their buttocks. If pressure sores have developed, getting around the hospital may be better using a **gurney**.

Eating and drinking aids

Utensils with thick handles and cups with handles on both sides may be easier to use for children who find gripping difficult. It may be helpful to put a non-slip material underneath a bowl or plate to stop it sliding while the child is eating (a damp cloth works very well). Eating and drinking aids must be easy to wash. Assessments by occupational and speech and language therapists (if available) are invaluable for children with complex feeding difficulties.

Toileting aids

For details, *see* Section 4.2.D.

Communication aids

Children who are unable to communicate verbally because of deafness and/or inability to use their oro-motor muscles will often be able to use a **communication board** or book with pictures of objects, people and actions. If the child is unable to point using a finger, hand, toe or foot, they may well be able to 'eye point'. An attentive carer will be aware that the child is eye pointing, and the use of a communication aid may 'unlock' the child who had previously been assumed to be unable to communicate beyond indicating pleasure or distress. More technological solutions are available using computers with specialised software which enables children to 'speak', but the basic principle of being able to select a pictorial representation of an object or an idea is the same.

Aids to prevent common secondary problems developing in hospital
Preventing foot drop

One of the commonest preventable complications in children with weak legs is the development of foot drop. This should not happen in your hospital. Regular exercises to move the ankles through their full range of movement should be done at least twice a day. The use of tight or heavy bed covers should be avoided, as they may hold weak feet in a bad position. It is best for the feet to rest with the ankles at 90 degrees. This is easily ensured by positioning a roll of blanket or similar material so that the feet are braced in this position.

Preventing knee and hip contractures

Regular exercises that take the joints through as full a range of movement as possible are the mainstay of prevention. If possible, the child should spend some time each day lying on their front with their hips and knees extended.

Preventing scoliosis

This is achieved by symmetrical positioning of the child so that attention must be paid to both lying and sitting positions. With excessive and asymmetrical muscle tone it is often difficult to prevent scoliosis, and once it has developed, it often gets worse, particularly at times of rapid growth.

Preventing pressure sores

Pressure sores develop anywhere in the body where skin is kept under pressure for too long. This commonly happens in areas where sensation has been lost, and will develop more quickly if the circulation is poor. There is no substitute for good nutrition and regular moving and turning of the child. The skin should regularly be gently cleaned and dried, and moisturising lotion used. Prevent bony areas from pressing on each other and on the mattress by using pillows or foam wedges, for example, between the knees or under the heels (see Section 4.2.D).

Further reading

Werner D (1999) *Disabled Village Children: a guide for community health workers, rehabilitation workers and families.* Palo Alto, CA: Hesperian Foundation.

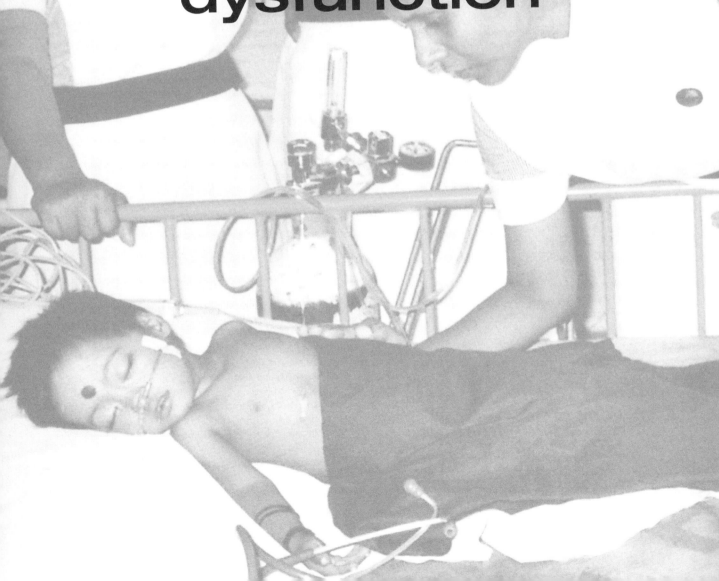

The child presenting with a system or organ dysfunction

5.1 Upper airway disorders

5.1.A Acute upper airway infections: croup and epiglottitis

BOX 5.1A.1 Minimum standards
- Dexamethasone/prednisolone.
- Nebulised 1 in 1000 adrenaline.
- Choking management skills.
- Intubation.
- Cricothyrotomy or tracheostomy.
- Antibiotics: cefuroxime, chloramphenicol, ceftriaxone, ceftazidime.
- *Haemophilus influenzae* immunisation.
- Measles immunisation.

Introduction

Obstruction of the upper airway (larynx and trachea) is potentially life-threatening. The cardinal feature is stridor (a harsh noise during inspiration), which is due to narrowing of the air passage in the oropharynx, subglottis or trachea. If the obstruction is below the larynx, stridor may also occur during expiration. **Like the wheeze in asthma, the loudness of the stridor does not indicate the severity of the obstruction.** There may also be hoarseness and a barking or seal-like cough. The severity of the obstruction is best assessed by the degree of sternal and subcostal recession, and the respiratory and heart rate. Increasing agitation or drowsiness, or central cyanosis, indicates severe hypoxaemia and hypercapnia and the need for urgent intervention.

The major causes of severe stridor are viral croup (caused by measles or other viruses), foreign body, retropharyngeal abscess, diphtheria, and trauma to the larynx.

Differential diagnosis of upper airway obstruction

1 Collapse of airway due to muscle tone loss or build-up of secretions due to poor cough reflex:
- Depressed conscious level from any cause.
- Drug or alcohol intoxication or overdose.
- Bulbar palsy.
- Myopathy.

2 Airway inflammation and oedema:
- Infective:
  - Upper respiratory tract infection in an infant.
  - Viral croup.
  - Bacterial tracheitis.
  - Epiglottitis.
  - Severe tonsillitis.
- Non-infective:
- Recurrent croup.
- Anaphylaxis.

3 Space-occupying lesion or structural abnormality:
- Intranasal, pharyngeal or in upper trachea:
  - Adenoidal hypertrophy.
  - Foreign body.
  - Retropharyngeal abscess.
  - Tumour.
  - Extrinsic haematoma (e.g. post thyroidectomy).
- Congenital pharyngeal, laryngeal or upper tracheal abnormalities:
  - Choanal atresia.
  - Laryngomalacia.
  - Subglottic stenosis.
  - Laryngeal web or haemangioma.

For diagnosis of a space-occupying lesion or structural abnormality, a specialist ENT examination under anaesthetic may be needed (if available).

Croup

Croup is a condition characterised by inspiratory stridor, hoarse voice, barking cough and a variable degree of respiratory distress.

This definition embraces several distinct disorders.

- **Acute viral laryngotracheobronchitis (viral croup).** This is the commonest type of laryngotracheal infection (representing over 95% of cases). Peak incidence is in the second year of life, and most hospital admissions are between 6 months and 5 years of age. The stridor is usually preceded by fever (< 38.5°C) with coryza, and symptoms tend to be worse at night. If narrowing is minor, the stridor will be present only when the child hyperventilates or is upset. As the narrowing progresses, the stridor becomes both inspiratory and expiratory, and is present even when the child is at rest. Children under 3 years in particular may develop features of increasing obstruction and hypoxaemia with marked sternal and subcostal recession, tachycardia and agitation. If the infection extends distally to the bronchi, wheeze may also be audible.

- **Recurrent or spasmodic croup.** Some children have repeated episodes of croup without preceding fever and coryza. The symptoms are of sudden onset at night, and often persist for only a few hours. The condition is associated with atopic disease (e.g. asthma, eczema, hay fever). The episodes can be severe, but are more commonly self-limiting.

- **Bacterial tracheitis or pseudomembranous croup.** This dangerous condition is one of the important complications of measles but may occur without that antecedent. Infection of the tracheal mucosa with *Streptococcus pneumoniae*, *Staphylococcus aureus* or *Haemophilus influenzae* B results in copious purulent secretions and mucosal necrosis. The child appears toxic with a high fever, with marked signs of respiratory obstruction. In the UK, over 80% of these children need intubation and ventilatory support to maintain an adequate airway. The croupy cough and the absence of drooling help to distinguish this condition from epiglottitis. Clinical and radiological signs of segmental collapse and consolidation related to bronchial occlusion are usual. The cough is often persistent and ineffective in clearing the secretions, the illness has a prolonged course, and the restoration of normal mucosa usually takes several weeks. The condition is much less common than the two preceding ones.

TABLE 5.1.A.1 Severity of croup

Sign	Mild	Moderate	Severe
Upper airway noise	Hoarse voice, barking cough, mild stridor intermittently on inspiration only	As before, with stridor constant and also some on expiration	Stridor usually decreases as exhaustion occurs
Effort of breathing	Mild increase, some intercostal recession	Further increase in effort, nasal flare, tracheal tug, accessory muscle usage	Major increase in effort gives way to exhaustion and poor but gasping effort
Efficacy of breathing	Not distressed by effort. No cyanosis, SaO_2 may be normal	Distressed by effort. Cyanosis not usually visible but SaO_2 is low	Cyanosis visible if haemoglobin is in normal range, SaO_2 is very low
Conscious level	Alert, usually still playing	Anxious and distressed. Not playing, little interaction, drowsy	Conscious level severely reduced, causing respirations to slow, reflex gasps and apnoeas
Cardiovascular	Mild increase in heart rate	Rapid heart rate	Severe tachycardia progresses to bradycardia and hypoxic cardiac arrest

Emergency treatment of croup

- These children (and their parents) may be very frightened. **Do not alarm them further by putting instruments in the child's throat, by giving painful injections or by trying to place an IV cannula.** Crying increases their oxygen demand and may increase laryngeal obstruction **and even cause total airway obstruction.** Keep the child on their parent's lap and explain the condition and the treatment. Tell the mother to alert the nurses or doctors if the child breathes more quickly or has marked sternal recession. **These are danger signs for hypoxaemia.**
- Ensure adequate oral fluid intake.

Many children who are admitted to hospital have hypoxaemia. Humidified oxygen should be given through nasal cannulae or a face mask held just in front of the child's face by the parent. **Do not use nasopharyngeal catheters to give oxygen, as these can precipitate dangerous paroxysms of coughing and total airway obstruction.**

Milder cases of croup should not routinely be given oxygen, as this can frighten the child.

- Croup can be a very painful condition. Even if the child does not have a high temperature, prescribe regular paracetamol, but do not force the child to take this.
- There is very good evidence that steroids help. Children with mild, moderate or severe croup all benefit from steroids. Give 0.6 mg/kg dexamethasone once or twice a day. This should be given orally, **as it works just as well as if given parenterally. If the child vomits, repeat it or give the same dose intramuscularly.** An expensive but effective treatment is nebulised budesonide 2 mg in 2 mL; it may be repeated 30–60 minutes later.
- Nebulised adrenaline (5 mL of 1 in 1000 adrenaline nebulised, preferably with oxygen) will bring rapid and effective relief for severe croup. The relief lasts only for about 1 hour, but it can be repeated (although the effect diminishes), and this treatment gives the steroids time to start working. **Arrange for the child to be seen quickly by an anaesthetist.** Monitor the oxygen saturation with a pulse oximeter.
- A few children need intubation. This should be done under general anaesthetic. **If there is doubt about the diagnosis, or difficulty in intubation is anticipated, an ENT surgeon capable of performing a tracheostomy should be present.** In intubated children, 1 mg/kg prednisolone every 12 hours reduces the duration of intubation.
- Severely ill or toxic children and those with measles croup should receive an antibiotic effective against *Streptococcus pneumoniae*, *Haemophilus influenzae* and *Staphylococcus aureus*. If available, cefuroxime 150 mg/kg/day in four doses IV or ceftriaxone 80 mg/kg IV or IM once daily. An alternative is chloramphenicol 25 mg/kg IV 6-hourly.

Inhaled foreign body (*see* Section 5.2.C)

Suspect the diagnosis if there has been a sudden onset of cough and stridor in a well child. Ask the parents and child whether there has been any access to peanuts or other food, toys or other small objects that could have been put in the mouth.

Management

If the foreign body is causing symptoms of stridor, coughing and respiratory distress, emergency management of choking is required (*see* Section 1.12 on Basic Life Support, which describes acute choking management).

In addition, call an ENT surgeon for laryngoscopy (if available). A laryngeal foreign body may present very acutely with cyanosis or loss of consciousness. Therefore urgent direct laryngoscopy may be necessary.

In the absence of an ENT surgeon, tracheostomy or cricothyrotomy may be necessary (*see* Section 8.2 for cricothyrotomy procedure).

Acute epiglottitis

This is a severe infection caused by *Haemophilus influenzae*. Peak incidence is at 2–3 years of age. It is less common than croup, but important, as **the diagnosis needs to be made fast because rapid progression of stridor in the ill toxic child may be fatal within hours if not promptly treated.** Cough is not a prominent feature, and the stridor has a soft quality, often with an expiratory component. The child tends to drool and assume an upright posture.

Unlike croup, epiglottitis is always severe and progression is rapid. It is always a medical emergency. Fortunately, since the introduction of *Haemophilus influenzae* type B (HiB) vaccine the disease has become much less common in those countries where the vaccine is used.

Do not:	Do:
Examine the throat	Reassure the child and their parents, and calm the child
Lie the child down	Attach a pulse oximeter
X-ray the neck	Give oxygen if SpO$_2$ is < 94% using a face mask held close to **but not on** the child's face by the parent with the child sitting on their lap
Perform invasive procedures	Call an anaesthetist and an ENT surgeon
Use a nasopharyngeal tube to give oxygen	Arrange examination under anaesthesia
	Arrange for high-dependency care to be available

Management

- Elective intubation under general anaesthetic is the treatment of choice. Often a much smaller diameter than the usual endotracheal tube for the child's age will be needed because the airway is so swollen internally. The endotracheal tube still needs to be the right length for the child's age. This is why children's endotracheal tubes should not be pre-cut to size. The diagnosis is confirmed by laryngoscopy under general anaesthetic just prior to intubation ('cherry-red epiglottis'). **An ENT surgeon must be present if possible.**
- While the child is anaesthetised, the following procedures should be performed: blood cultures, throat swab and IV line.
- Recommended antibiotic therapy is chloramphenicol

TABLE 5.1.A.1 Contrasting features of croup and epiglottitis

Feature	Croup	Epiglottitis
Onset	Over days	Over hours
Preceding coryza	Yes	No
Cough	Severe, barking	Absent or slight
Able to drink	Yes	No
Drooling saliva	No	Yes
Appearance	Unwell	Toxic, very ill
Fever	38.5°C	38.5
Stridor	Harsh, rasping	Soft
Voice muffled	Hoarse	Reluctant to speak
Need for intubation	1%	80%

50 mg/kg IV immediately, then 25 mg/kg IV 6-hourly. If available, cefuroxime or cefotaxime 50 mg/kg IV 6-hourly or ceftriaxone 80 mg/kg once daily IV or IM should be effective.
- Following intubation the child will be able to breathe humidified air spontaneously, ideally with nasal continuous positive airway pressure (CPAP) (*see* Section 1.25 and 8.3). Sedation (discuss with anaesthetist) may be required in order to prevent self-extubation, but the child will then usually require assisted ventilation. Most children will be ready for extubation after 48 hours.

An alternative is to fix the child's arms to their thorax using a bandage to stop them pulling out the endotracheal tube but the stress to the child caused by this may have a deleterious effect on recovery. If possible, have a relative sit with the child to reassure them.

Angioneurotic oedema

See Section 5.1.B on anaphylaxis.

There are usually areas of painless swelling obvious in other areas of skin and mucous membranes. The eyes, lips and tongue are particularly likely to be affected. Stridor is caused by laryngeal oedema.

Management

- Give adrenaline, 10 micrograms/kg IM.
- Give adrenaline, 5 mL of 1 in 1000 nebulised with 100% oxygen.
- Give 100% oxygen.
- Give hydrocortisone, 4 mg/kg IV over 15 minutes or IM and repeat 8 hourly as required.
- Give chlorphenamine, 250 micrograms/kg IV or orally (maximum dose 2.5 mg) or
  - 6 months to 6 years 2.5 mg and repeat up to 4 times in 24 hours
  - 6–12 years 5 mg and repeat up to 4 times in 24 hours
  - 12–18 years 10 mg and repeat up to 4 times in 24 hours.
- Give Ringer-lactate or Hartmann's solution or 4.5% albumin (if available), 10–20 mL/kg, if the child is shocked.
- Intubation or even tracheostomy may be required (contact the ENT team).

Airway/inhalational burns (*see* Section 7.3.I.b)

Such burns are caused by inhalation of hot gases or toxic vapours. They may be associated with extensive skin burns. **Be aware that airway obstruction may develop even if it is not obvious on first assessment.**

Management

- **Admit the child to a high-dependency unit** (if available).
- Give hydrocortisone, 4 mg/kg IV 6-hourly.
- Give Ringer-lactate or Hartmann's solution or 4.5% albumin boluses (10–20 mL/kg) for shock as required.
- Intubation or tracheostomy may be necessary if indicated by assessment.

Diphtheria (*see* Section 6.1.C for further details on management)

Diphtheria is characterised by gradual onset of stridor in a child (usually 2 to 3 years old) with neck oedema and ulcerating lesions of the tonsillar bed forming a grey membrane. Bleeding may occur at the site and down the nose. The diagnosis may be confirmed by throat swab and **urgent Gram stain**. There will usually be no evidence of DTP vaccination.

5.1.B The child with anaphylaxis

> **BOX 5.1.B.1 Minimum standards**
> - ABC of resuscitation.
> - Adrenaline.
> - Oxygen.
> - Salbutamol by nebuliser or spacer.
> - Hydrocortisone.
> - Antihistamine.

Consider the diagnosis of anaphylaxis if any of the following symptoms are present when there is a history of previous severe reaction, rapidly progressive or increasingly severe symptoms, a history of asthma, eczema or rhinitis (atopy).

This situation is potentially life-threatening and may result in a change in conscious level, collapse, or respiratory or cardiac arrest.

Introduction

Anaphylaxis is an immunologically mediated reaction to ingested, inhaled or topical substances, which may progress to life-threatening shock and/or respiratory distress.

Common causes include allergies to penicillin, anaesthetic agents, blood transfusion, **radiographic contrast media**, and certain foods, especially nuts.

Management

See **Figure 5.1.B.1.**

Remove the source of allergen if possible (e.g. take down the blood giving set if blood transfusion is the cause).

The key to anaphylaxis treatment is intramuscular adrenaline.

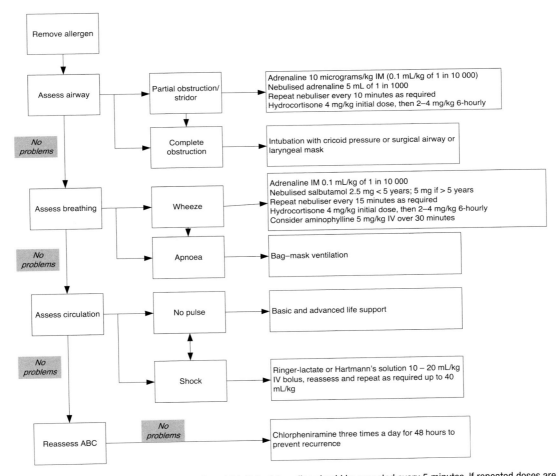

FIGURE 5.1.B.1 Pathway of care for anaphylaxis in a child. Note: Adrenaline should be repeated every 5 minutes. If repeated doses are ineffectual, use an IV infusion of adrenaline (see below)

Airway: assessment and resuscitation

- If there is no problem with the airway, assess **B**reathing.
- If stridor is present there is obstruction (usually at the larynx):
  - Give 10 micrograms/kg adrenaline IM, then 5 mL adrenaline 1 in 1000 nebulised.
  - Give 100% oxygen.
  - Consider intubation, and call for anaesthetic and ENT assistance.
- If there is stridor with complete obstruction, intubate or create a surgical airway (*see* Section 8.2).

Breathing: assessment and resuscitation

- If there is no problem with breathing, assess the **C**irculation.
- If there is no breathing, give five rescue breaths using a bag-valve-mask with 100% oxygen and assess the circulation.
- If the child is wheezing, give 10 micrograms/kg adrenaline IM and salbutamol (either by nebuliser 2.5 mg if under 5 years of age or 5 mg if over 5 years, (nebulised with 100% oxygen) or 1000 micrograms (5 puffs) of a metered dose inhaler via a spacer and repeated as required).

Circulation: assessment and resuscitation

- If there is no problem with the circulation, observe the child.
- If there is no pulse, start basic life support, assess the rhythm and treat.
- If the child is shocked, give 10 micrograms/kg adrenaline IM and 20 mL/kg IV bolus of Ringer-lactate or Hartmann's solution. It may be necessary to give adrenaline IV if shock is present (see below for dosage).

Reassess ABC and continue to give 100% oxygen

- If there is airway deterioration, repeat IM adrenaline 10 micrograms/kg with or without intubation.
- If the child is still wheezy, repeat IM adrenaline 10 micrograms/kg and hydrocortisone 4 mg/kg IV by slow Injection. Consider giving aminophylline 5 mg/kg by slow IV injection over 20–30 minutes followed by a 1 mg/kg/hour IV infusion or salbutamol 4–6 micrograms/kg IV slow injection followed by an IV infusion of 0.5–2.0 micrograms/kg/minute.
- If the child is still shocked, repeat IM adrenaline 10 micrograms/kg and give a further bolus of 10 mL/kg Ringer-lactate or Hartmann's solution. If there is a poor response then give a further 10 mL/kg and consider

TABLE 5.1.B.1 Features of anaphylaxis

Severity	Symptoms	Signs
Mild	Burning sensation in mouth	Urticarial rash
	Itching lips, mouth and throat	Angio-oedema
	Feeling of warmth	Conjunctivitis
	Nausea and abdominal pain	Red throat
Moderate	Coughing and wheezing	Bronchospasm
	Loose stools	Tachycardia
	Sweating	Pallor
	Irritability	
Severe	Difficulty with breathing	Severe bronchospasm
	Faintness or collapse	Laryngeal oedema
	Stridor	
	Vomiting	Shock
	Uncontrolled defecation	Respiratory arrest
		Cardiac arrest

giving an adrenaline infusion (see below). Intubation and ventilation may be needed if there is a poor response as now a total of 40 mL/kg of crystalloids have been given by bolus.
- If there is no problem, observe the child.
- If there are no symptoms other than rash or itching:
  - Give oral antihistamine (chlorphenamine, 250 micrograms/kg).
  - Give oral steroids (0.5–1 mg/kg oral prednisolone).

Adrenaline

Adrenaline is given intramuscularly unless there is intractable shock or cardiac arrest, in which case it should be given IV or by the intra-osseous route.

If repeated IM injections of adrenaline are not effective or last only a short time, start giving adrenaline IV. For treatment of children in severe shock:

- Place 1 mg (1 mL of 1 in 1000 adrenaline) in 50 mL of Ringer-lactate solution.
- Then give 2–5 mL (40–100 micrograms) in a child (depending on size) and 1 mL (20 micrograms) in an infant under 1 year of age. Give IV **slowly** using a peripheral vein or ideally a central vein, if possible with ECG monitoring.
- Repeat as required.
- An infusion of adrenaline at 0.05–2.0 micrograms/kg/minute may be needed (preferably via a central vein and using a syringe pump).

5.1.C The child with tonsillitis, otitis media, mastoiditis or retropharyngeal abscess

---

BOX 5.1.C.1 Minimum standards
- Antibiotics: penicillin/amoxicillin/erythromycin.
- Quinolone antibiotic ear drops.
- Adrenaline nose drops.
- Wicking.

Tonsillitis

Tonsillitis is a common childhood disorder. The bacteria most commonly involved are beta-haemolytic streptococci, *Streptococcus pneumoniae* and *Haemophilus influenzae*, and around 50% of attacks are viral.

Classic symptoms include pyrexia and sore throat.

Swallowing solid food is difficult, and fluid intake must be encouraged. Painful cervical lymphadenopathy is the rule, and referred earache from the IXth cranial nerve is common. Febrile convulsions may occur in younger children, who may also present with acute abdominal pain without any throat symptoms, due to mesenteric lymphadenitis.

Examination
- Tender lymphadenopathy beneath and/or behind the mandible.
- Red enlarged tonsils with or without purulent exudate.

Differential diagnosis
Diphtheria and infectious mononucleosis (*see* Section 6.1.C for diphtheria and later in this section for infectious mononucleosis).

Treatment
- Give paracetamol (20 mg/kg 4- to 6-hourly) for pain relief. Bear in mind that attacks are often viral, and often antibiotics are not needed.
- Penicillin is still an effective antibiotic, and in **serious cases** in hospital give penicillin 12.5 mg/kg four times daily orally. If the child is allergic to penicillin, erythromycin may be used.
- Rarely there is acute partial airway obstruction due to massive tonsillar enlargement. In this case use IV benzylpenicillin 25 mg/kg 6-hourly and IV hydrocortisone 4–8 mg/kg initially, and then a further dose 4 hours later if needed at 4 mg/kg.

Recurrent tonsillitis
- If the number of attacks increases with age rather than decreasing, tonsillectomy is appropriate if it is safe to perform in the healthcare facilities available.
- As a rule of thumb, six attacks per year for 2 years over the age of 5 years could indicate a case for tonsillectomy.
- It is often said that peritonsillar abscess (quinsy) is an indication, but one attack of quinsy is not enough to warrant the operation.

Indications for tonsillectomy
In the past, tonsillectomy was performed all too often. Sleep-related upper airway obstruction (*see* Section 5.1.D) is a good reason for undertaking tonsillectomy, and about 10% of tonsil operations are currently done for this reason.

Peritonsillar abscess (quinsy)
This is a complication of tonsillitis, and it presents with a unilateral swelling of the soft palate, deflecting the uvula to the opposite side, with associated trismus. Surgical drainage is often necessary as well as IV penicillin as described above.

Acute suppurative otitis media (ASOM)
Acute suppurative otitis media is a mucosal infection of the middle ear and mastoid air cells, arising via the Eustachian tube. *Streptococcus pneumoniae* and *Haemophilus influenzae* are the bacteria most commonly involved, and about 50% of cases are caused by viruses.

The symptoms are hearing loss, earache and fever. Pain is due to the bulging tympanic membrane from accumulated pus. Rupture leads to otorrhoea with rapid symptom improvement. Localising signs may be absent in infants, who may present with fever and systemic illness. On examination the tympanic membrane is red and bulging.

Treatment
- **Many cases of otitis media are incorrectly diagnosed:** any child who is crying or has a fever will tend to have pink eardrums. Earache often presents at night. This is usually due to Eustachian tube obstruction occurring when the child is sleeping, from accumulated mucus in the postnasal space resulting in a negative pressure in the ear, which wakes the child up with discomfort. Paracetamol, plus sitting up and drinking, will open the Eustachian tube and thus relieve the symptoms. Antibiotics are unnecessary.
- In true otitis media with bulging eardrums, treat the child as an outpatient and **always give an antibiotic as described below. It is not safe to withhold antibiotic treatment**. Give oral amoxicillin 40 mg/kg twice a day for 7–10 days. If amoxicillin is not available give co-trimoxazole (trimethoprim 4 mg/kg/sulfamethoxazole 20 mg/kg twice a day) for 7–10 days.
- Paracetamol relieves pain and reduces fever.
- Ephedrine nose drops (0.5%) given 8-hourly for a maximum of 5 days may help to open the Eustachian tube and speed resolution.
- If the eardrum is perforated, the ear must be kept dry until the resulting perforation has healed. This is achieved by teaching the parent to undertake wicking as follows. Roll a clean soft absorbent cotton cloth or strong tissue paper into a wick. **Never use a cotton-tipped applicator, or flimsy paper that will fall apart in the ear, or a stick of any kind.** Place the wick in the ear and remove it after a few seconds, when it is wet. Repeat until the ear is dry. Wicking should be undertaken at least three times daily, usually for 1 to 2 weeks, until pus is no longer present. **The parent must not leave anything in the ear after wicking, must not put oil or any other fluid in the ear, and should prevent the child from going swimming or putting their head under water until the ear has been dry for at least 2 weeks.**
- Check that the child has recovered at follow-up 1 week later. If ear pain or discharge persists, treat the child for 5 more days with the same antibiotic and continue wicking the ear. Follow up in 5 days.

Chronic otitis media
If pus has been draining from the ear for 2 weeks or longer and there is perforation of the ear drum, the child has a chronic otitis media infection.

Treatment
- Treat as an outpatient.
- Keep the ear dry by wicking (*see* above).
- Instil topical antibiotic ear drops (always without steroids, which must not be used in children) three times daily for 2 weeks. Drops containing quinolones (norfloxacin, ofloxacin, ciprofloxacin) are more effective than other antibiotic drops; 0.3% ciprofloxacin drops (5 drops twice daily) have been most researched.
- Oral antibiotics are not indicated unless there is an acute otitis media.
- Topical antiseptics and steroids should not be used.

Follow-up after 1 week

If the ear discharge persists despite ear wicking and ciprofloxacin drops, consider IV antibiotic treatment with antibiotics that are effective against *Pseudomonas* (such as gentamicin, azlocillin and ceftazidime), in addition to wicking. Do not give oral antibiotics for a chronically draining ear.

If chronic suppurative otitis media (CSOM) continues despite the above treatment, do not forget the possibility of TB.

Secretory otitis media

This may lead to recurrent attacks of acute suppurative otitis media (ASOM) because the exudate acts as a culture medium for repeated infections. **Occasionally, myringotomy with grommet insertion is necessary.** The alternative treatment is long-term low-dose oral antibiotics (trimethoprim 2 mg/kg once daily (maximum dose 100 mg) at night for 3 months). Eustachian tube function may also be improved by adenoidectomy.

Acute mastoiditis

This is a complication of ASOM. The mucosa of the mastoid system is always inflamed in ASOM. Mastoiditis occurs when the mucosal inflammation spreads to the adjacent bone, causing osteitis, and eventually the outer cortex of the mastoid is breached, leading to a subperiosteal abscess behind the ear. The symptoms are similar to those of ASOM, but the signs include a forward displaced pinna with a tender fluctuant swelling in the post-auricular sulcus.

Complications

Not only is the outer cortex of the mastoid involved, but also the bone adjacent to both the middle and the posterior cranial fossa can be affected, occasionally leading to **extradural abscess, meningitis and brain abscess. Facial nerve paralysis** may occur from the pressure of pus on an exposed facial nerve.

Treatment

- Give IV benzylpenicillin 50 mg/kg IV 6-hourly **plus** chloramphenicol 50 mg/kg 8-hourly IV OR plus flucloxacillin 50 mg IV 6 hourly both for 5 days and then orally (penicillin 25 mg/kg four times daily and chloramphenicol 50 mg/kg 8-hourly) for another 5 days. Alternatively, give ceftriaxone 100 mg/kg IV/IM for 10 days. If there is no improvement within 24–48 hours or the child's condition deteriorates, surgical drainage is necessary.
- The key is to provide drainage for the mastoid system. **If it is not possible to do a full-scale mastoidectomy (due to lack of equipment or expertise)**, a dramatic improvement, in conjunction with intravenous antibiotics, may be obtained by incising the abscess (avoiding the mastoid tip in the small child where the facial nerve may be exposed) and opening into mastoid air cells.
- If signs of meningitis or a brain abscess (indicated by a reduced level of consciousness, a fit or localised neurological signs) are seen or suspected, give high-dose IV antibiotics as for meningitis (*see* Section 5.16.B) and refer the child immediately to an appropriate specialist.

Glandular fever/infectious mononucleosis

This is caused by the Epstein–Barr virus and may be similar in presentation to diphtheria.

Diagnosis

There are atypical lymphocytes on blood, monospot and Paul-Bunnell tests (usually but not always positive).

Management

- **Do not give ampicillin, amoxicillin or Augmentin** for throat infections until glandular fever has been excluded (there is a risk of severe skin reaction). Antibiotics are unhelpful in glandular fever. Treatment is symptomatic.
- Give IV maintenance fluids if swallowing problems are causing dehydration.
- Give IV hydrocortisone 4 mg/kg 6-hourly if signs of airway obstruction occur.
- Intubation/tracheostomy is rarely indicated.

Retropharyngeal abscess

Most common in infants and young children, retropharyngeal abscess (RPA) is an abscess located behind the posterior pharyngeal wall (the retropharyngeal space).

RPA is usually caused by a bacterial infection originating in the nasopharynx, tonsils, sinuses, adenoids or middle ear, and can also result from a penetrating injury or a foreign body. It may result from suppuration of retropharyngeal lymph nodes from infected tonsil, adenoid, tooth or penetrating foreign body. The most common causative organisms are beta-haemolytic streptococci, *Staphylococcus aureus*, *Haemophilus parainfluenzae* and anaerobic organisms.

RPA is a relatively uncommon illness, and therefore may not receive prompt diagnosis in children presenting with stiff neck (limited neck mobility or torticollis), some form of palpable neck pain (which may be in 'front of the neck' or around the larynx), malaise, difficulty swallowing, high fever, stridor, trismus, dribbling of saliva, croupy cough or enlarged cervical lymph nodes. Early diagnosis is essential. Infection in the retropharyngeal space can pass down behind the oesophagus into the mediastinum, producing an extremely dangerous mediastinitis.

Peroral surgical drainage of the abscess by incision under anaesthetic (or without anaesthetic in an emergency) is often required. An ENT specialist (if available) must be called urgently.

Surgery may be required urgently to relieve obstruction, but not all patients with retropharyngeal abscesses require surgery. One study found that of 162 paediatric patients with retropharyngeal abscess, 126 required surgery initially, and of the 36 patients who were initially treated conservatively with high-dose antibiotics, 17 required surgery. Surgery is best undertaken using general anaesthesia undertaken by an experienced anaesthetist, as there is risk of rupture of the abscess during intubation. In patients who present with severe airway obstruction, tracheostomy may be required before surgical drainage.

High-dose IV antibiotics, such as ampicillin plus flucloxacillin plus metronidazole, cefuroxime or ceftriaxone plus metronidazole, or clindamycin plus metronidazole, are required in order to control the infection, and can be used to reduce the size of the abscess prior to surgery.

Chronic retropharyngeal abscess is usually secondary to tuberculosis of the cervical spine or spread from an infected lymph node, and the patient needs to be started on anti-TB treatment as soon as possible.

A CT scan (if available) is the definitive diagnostic test.

A lateral X-ray of the neck will usually show swelling of the retropharyngeal space, with the following:

- increased prevertebral soft tissue shadow
- air and fluid level in the pre-vertebral area
- concavity or straightening of the cervical vertebral column
- the air column is pushed forward.

If the retropharyngeal space is more than half of the size of the C2 vertebra, it may indicate retropharyngeal abscess.

A chest X-ray will also be valuable to exclude pneumonia and to show the size of the mediastinum.

Mediastinal tumours (see Section 5.14)

These often present with the slow onset of stridor in a child with other symptoms and signs (e.g. pallor, lethargy) may be precipitated or aggravated by mediastinal radiotherapy used for treatment of malignant causes.

Management

- X-ray the chest and mediastinal inlet.
- Intubation may be required as a temporary measure.
- Treat the primary cause.

5.1.D The child with sleep-related upper airway obstruction

> **BOX 5.1.D.1 Minimum standards**
> - Appropriate surgery (especially tonsillectomy and adenoidectomy).
> - Steroids: topical nasal and, for acute use, oral.

Introduction

The incidence of sleep-related upper airway obstruction depends on the method of diagnosis (it affects 1–3% of preschool children). It is associated with both enlargement of the tonsils/adenoids and reduced tone or diameter in the upper airway.

Groups at risk are children with any of the following:

- Pierre-Robin sequence
- craniofacial syndromes
- Down's syndrome
- cerebral palsy
- neuromuscular disease
- sickle-cell disease
- Prader–Willi syndrome.

Presenting features

- Snoring: this occurs in more than 10% of healthy 4- to 5-year-olds, and in most cases is benign.
- Sleep disturbance and restlessness.
- Apnoeic episodes followed by inspiratory gasps.
- Sleeping with the head extended.
- Subcostal and sternal recession during sleep.
- Mouth breathing and halitosis.
- Daytime hyperactivity, poor concentration and irritability (young children).
- Daytime sleepiness (older children).
- Pulmonary hypertension.
- Heart failure.

These features may be associated with developmental delay, impaired cognitive function and behavioural disorders. The disorder is insidious – the child may appear completely normal when awake, and the problem is most or only apparent during rapid eye movement (REM) sleep.

Investigations

A sleep observation or study is most useful. This can be done either by direct observation of the child during sleep with the chest and face exposed, or by video recording at home during sleep by the parents, looking for the following:

- chest wall recession
- snoring
- sleep position
- nocturnal restlessness.

It is also useful to monitor oxygen saturation (SpO_2) during sleep. An abnormal result would be a lowest level of less than 87% or more than three dips below 90% during the night.

Also consider the following investigations:

- barium swallow: to assess bulbar function and exclude tracheal compression
- upper airway endoscopy: to assess the structure and dynamics of the upper airway
- lateral X-ray of the post-nasal space: to assess the size of the adenoids.

Measurement of oxygen saturation (SpO_2)

Methodological issues that affect this measurement include the following:

- the instruments used (e.g. functional vs. fractional haemoglobin)
- exclusion of motion artefact
- averaging
- altitude
- inclusion of apnoeic pauses.

Normal data

In children outside infancy, a normal oximetry recording should have the following:

1. a median SpO_2 level of $\geq$ 95%
2. no more than four desaturations of $\geq$ 4% per hour
3. no abnormal clusters of desaturation defined as $\geq$ 5 in a 30-minute period.

Widely used criteria for abnormality in nocturnal oximetry recordings are falls of more than 4% below baseline and desaturations below 90%. The measure that correlates best with poor academic performance is the lowest level of SpO$_2$ (nadir) during the night (normal value is > 87.5%).

Adverse effects of hypoxaemia
These include the following:
- poor weight gain
- developmental delay
- poor cognitive function
- pulmonary hypertension
- cyanotic apnoeic episodes.

Treatment
- Time: the airway enlarges with growth.
- Obstruction is worse with infections and may need a rescue course of steroids (e.g. prednisolone 0.5 mg/kg once daily for up to 7–10 days).
- Topical steroids/decongestants.

- Tonsillo-adenoidectomy.
- Nasal CPAP.
- Nasopharyngeal tube (in infants).
- Tracheostomy.

Nasal CPAP (see Section 1.25)
This is an effective non-invasive treatment, but it is associated with the following potential problems:
- compliance
- side effects:
  - skin sores
  - nose bleeds
  - conjunctivitis
  - aerophagy.

Reference
British Lung Foundation. *OSA in Children*. A leaflet for the parents of children with obstructive sleep apnoea. www.blf.org.uk/Conditions/Detail/OSA-in-children#overview.

5.2   Lower airway disorders

5.2.A Bronchiolitis

> **BOX 5.2.A.1   Minimum standards**
> - Oxygen.
> - Oxygen saturation monitor.
> - Bag-valve-mask system.
> - Cannulae for thoracostomy.
> - Antibiotics.
> - Nasal CPAP.

Introduction
Wheezing is a whistling noise heard during expiration. The child who has cough or difficulty breathing **and** wheezing will fit into one of the following categories:
- bronchiolitis (mainly less than 1 year old)
- asthma (over 1 year old)
- pneumonia with wheezing (any age).

In pneumonia with wheezing in children over 1 year of age and in asthma, a bronchodilator provides important symptomatic relief. An aerosol and large-volume spacer (which may be improvised) is the best way of administering a bronchodilator (see below). Bronchodilators are not routinely effective in bronchiolitis, but may be tried in some cases.

    A lower respiratory viral infection, typically most severe in young infants, occurs in annual epidemics, and is characterised by airways obstruction and wheezing. Respiratory syncytial virus is the most important cause. Secondary bacterial infection may occur and is common in some settings. Episodes of wheeze may occur for months after an attack of bronchiolitis, but will eventually stop. Some babies who have had bronchiolitis go on to have asthma, but both bronchiolitis and asthma are common conditions, and a causal relationship has not been established.

Clinical features of bronchiolitis
- Infants are coryzal, have a troublesome cough and may feed poorly or even be unable to suck and feed. There may be vomiting.
- The nose is often obstructed by secretions.
- On examining the chest, there may be hyperinflation, chest wall indrawing, nasal flaring, grunting, wheeze and fine crackles at the lung bases.
- Young infants may present with apnoeic/hypoxaemic episodes which may be recurrent and life-threatening.
- There may be hypoxaemia, with SaO$_2$ less than 94%, with or without cyanosis.
- Some infants will have such severe respiratory distress that there is gasping; this is pre-terminal.

Treatment
Only supportive treatment (e.g. oxygen, gentle suction of the nose, and fluids) is of benefit. Antibiotics and bronchodilators have no role. However, in the most severe cases and unless you are **certain** that pneumonia is not present,

it is safer to give antibiotics and a trial of a bronchodilator (stop the bronchodilator if it is not helping).

Non-invasive respiratory support to help to overcome small airway obstruction (nasal CPAP and continuous negative extrathoracic pressure (CNEP)) may be valuable (*see* Section 1.25 and Section 8.3). CNEP may be more effective because of the nasal blockage that accompanies bronchiolitis.

- Give oxygen by nasal cannulae to keep SaO_2 in the range 94–98%. Check that the nasal cannulae are in the correct place, and check frequently that they are not blocked by secretions.
- Nasal clearance. Gentle nasal suction should be used to clear secretions in patients in whom nasal blockage is thought to be causing respiratory distress. This may be aided by saline nasal drops or spray.
- Ensure that daily maintenance fluids are achieved. If this is not possible by mouth, use nasogastric feeding. This should be considered in any patient who is unable to maintain oral intake or hydration (use the mother's expressed breast milk if possible and if tolerated).
- If the patient is vomiting despite nasogastric feeding, or severe respiratory distress is present, give fluids IV.
- If there are signs of pneumonia, give antibiotics (*see* Section 5.3.A).
- If fever (≥ 39°C or ≥ 102.2°F) is causing distress, give paracetamol. High fever is the exception rather than the rule in bronchiolitis, and should make you suspect bacterial infection.

Failure to improve

If the condition worsens suddenly, consider pneumothorax, although this is uncommon. Tension pneumothorax associated with major respiratory distress and shift of the heart requires immediate relief by needle thoracocentesis (i.e. placing a needle to allow the air that is under pressure to escape) (*see* Section 8.3). If needle thoracocentesis is helpful, insert a chest tube with an underwater seal until the air leak closes spontaneously and the lung expands (*see* Section 8.3). **The signs of pneumothorax in severe bronchiolitis may be difficult to detect clinically. However, needle thoracocentesis in the absence of a pneumothorax may cause one, so if you are unsure, take a chest X-ray.** Even on a chest X-ray, the diagnosis may be very difficult due to the areas of hyperlucency in bronchiolitis caused by air trapping.

If respiratory failure develops, nasal continuous positive airways pressure (CPAP) or continuous negative extrathoracic pressure (CNEP) may be of benefit (*see* Section 8.3).

If apnoeic episodes develop (this is most likely in premature infants), give bag-valve-mask resuscitation, then nasal CPAP or CNEP. Sometimes **intubation and ventilation may be needed in a high-dependency ward (if available)**; if so, contact an anaesthetist urgently.

Infection control

Bronchiolitis is infectious and easily transmitted to other infants and young children in hospital. Babies in the neonatal unit are particularly at risk. The following strategies may reduce the risk of cross-infection (*see* Section 1.2):

- hand washing between patients
- the wearing of gloves and aprons
- ideally isolate the affected patient, but close observations are needed
- restrict visiting by anyone with symptoms of upper respiratory tract infection.

5.2.B Asthma

> **BOX 5.2.B.1 Minimum standards**
> - Inhaled bronchodilators (with spacers).
> - Inhaled steroids.
> - Prednisolone/hydrocortisone.
> - Nebulised bronchodilators.
> - Oxygen.
> - Salbutamol, magnesium sulphate, adrenaline and aminophylline.
> - Pulse oximetry.

Introduction

Asthma is a condition characterised by episodic or recurrent symptoms of cough, prolonged expiration with wheeze, chest tightness and shortness of breath without fever (although some episodes are precipitated by an upper respiratory tract infection which may have an accompanying fever). It is due to variable and reversible airway obstruction associated with chronic airway inflammation. Asthma has become more prevalent over the last 20 years, along with the other atopic conditions such as allergic rhinitis and eczema. This is particularly so in well-resourced countries, where it is reported to occur in up to 10–15% of children.

Young children (under 5 years of age) often have 'asthma-like' symptoms (cough, wheeze and shortness of breath) in response to respiratory infections, but with no demonstrable problem between infections. This tendency often stops in the early school years. In these children, treatment of episodic symptoms with acute asthma therapies ('relievers') may still provide relief of symptoms, but 'preventers' (i.e. inhaled steroids) will not usually be of benefit unless the child has continuous symptoms or is likely to be atopic (e.g. due to a personal or family history of asthma, eczema or allergic rhinitis). In the youngest children (less than 2 years old) with severe episodes or symptoms continuing between infections (interval symptoms), it is necessary to consider other diagnoses, such as bronchiectasis, tuberculosis, foreign body and cystic fibrosis.

Diagnosis of asthma between episodes

The diagnosis is clinical, and is based on a **history** of the following:

- recurrent cough (mostly dry, becoming productive with exacerbations), wheeze, shortness of breath or chest tightness
- symptoms worse at night, and on exertion

- symptoms worsened by respiratory infections, inhaled irritants (e.g. cigarette smoke), cold air, animal fur, excitement or upset
- a personal or close family history of eczema, rhinitis or asthma.

Examination may identify any of the following:
- no abnormalities
- slow growth
- overinflation of the chest, Harrison's sulci
- wheeze, particularly on forced expiration
- rhinitis or eczema.

Investigations

Investigations are not usually needed, but may help to support the diagnosis or exclude other conditions:

1 Chest X-ray. This is normal or shows overinflation (flat diaphragms and hyperlucency, particularly when severe or acute), or increased perihilar linear markings.

2 Peak flow (in children aged 7–8 years or over). This may show the following:
   - more than 15% variability from morning to night (keep a peak flow diary)
   - a fall after 5–10 minutes of hard exercise
   - a rise after a dose of inhaled bronchodilators (e.g. salbutamol)
   - **spirometry will show FEV1:FVC of less than 85% and concavity in the flow-volume loop, which is at least partially reversed by a dose of inhaled bronchodilators.**

Skin prick tests, or IgE RASTs, do not aid the diagnosis, and only infrequently help in the management.

Symptoms that resolve with bronchodilators with or without steroids support the diagnosis, but bear in mind that conditions other than asthma may also show reversibility.

Ongoing management

- Avoid allergic/irritant factors (e.g. smoke, chemical fumes, house dust mites, animal fur). Discourage cigarette smoking and acquiring new pets at home.
- Do not prevent the child from exercising, but pre-dose them 5–10 minutes beforehand with a dose of inhaled beta-2 agonist bronchodilators (e.g. salbutamol).

Use of 'reliever' medication

- Occasional symptoms (e.g. on 2 to 4 days per week) may be managed with only the use of a bronchodilator (a 'reliever'), and do not usually need a 'preventer' (see below).
- Use inhaled drugs where possible, except in acute severe or life-threatening attacks, when the IV route may be used.

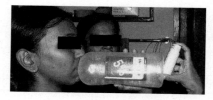

FIGURE 5.2.B.1 'Spacer' made from a large plastic bottle in use with an inhaler.

- Use an aerosol spray (metered-dose inhaler) with a spacer (first choice):
  - A commercial medium- to large-volume spacer (e.g. Volumatic, AeroChamber), or a large (2-litre) plastic bottle with the aerosol sealed into one end, and the open end held closely over the nose and mouth (see Figure 5.2.B.1).
  - Use 200–1000 micrograms of salbutamol (2–10 sprays); more may be needed in younger children, or if the patient is acutely breathless (and repeated).
  - Each spray or puff should be inhaled individually in turn with 4 to 5 breaths, rather than filling the spacer device with multiple sprays.
  - For children under 5 years of age, attach a face mask (e.g. inverted adult mask) to the mouthpiece of a spacer.

Clean the spacer with soapy water and leave it to dry naturally to reduce static electrical charges on the inside. Alternatively, use a nebuliser to deliver salbutamol (this is less portable).

Children with asthma should always have immediate access to their usual reliever inhaler device. Children over 7–8 years of age may keep their device with them.

Use of 'preventer' medication

More frequent symptoms, regular nocturnal symptoms or daily use of a bronchodilator should be treated with regular medication aimed at controlling airway inflammation (a 'preventer'), such as inhaled steroids. Use inhaled (preferably through a spacer) beclomethasone propionate or budesonide, 200–400 micrograms twice daily.

- Rinse the mouth (if feasible) after each dose of inhaled steroid.
- Aim for rapid control of symptoms, and then tail down the dose over a period of months.
- Gaining control may be helped by a short course (7–10 days) of systemic steroid (e.g. prednisolone 500 micrograms/kg once daily after food or milk, maximum daily dose 40 mg).
- Continue with bronchodilator use for symptom relief (but avoid regular use).

For frequent or severe symptoms, consider:
- whether the diagnosis is correct
- aggravating factors (e.g. rhinitis, stress, gastro-oesophageal reflux)
- whether the medication is being taken, and whether it is being taken correctly
- increasing the inhaled steroid dose (beclomethasone to 400–800 micrograms twice daily) **or**
- **adding leukotriene antagonists (e.g. montelukast), which are useful in preschool children, or a long-acting inhaled drug (e.g. salmeterol) or**
- oral methylxanthines (e.g. theophylline 5 mg/kg three to four times a day)
- **as a last resort**, use of alternate-day oral prednisolone (start at 500 micrograms/kg on alternate days and reduce rapidly to 100 micrograms/kg on alternate days, to the nearest 1 mg or 5 mg tablets). Stop as soon as possible.

Children on inhaled or oral steroids should have regular

checks of their growth and be watched for steroid side effects (e.g. oral thrush)

The control of asthma should be regularly reviewed (e.g. 3-monthly) and medication stepped up or down depending on the symptoms and on peak flow measurements **or spirometry** *in* those over 7 years of age. Families should be given written instructions and helped to change the treatment themselves, with support.

Management of an episode of acute asthma

Initial treatment of a mild to moderate acute attack of asthma is as follows:

- Reassure the child and their parents, and avoid upset as this may exacerbate respiratory distress.
- Give a regular inhaled beta-2 agonist bronchodilator, such as salbutamol aerosol 200–1000 micrograms (2 to 10 sprays each of 100 micrograms, with each spray given after every four to five breaths) via a spacer every 30 minutes to 2-hourly until the child is better.
- If the child does not respond to the spacer, give 2.5 mg salbutamol for children under 5 years and 5 mg salbutamol for those over 5 years via a nebuliser 2- to 4-hourly (use oxygen to drive the nebuliser if possible).
- Give systemic steroids: oral prednisolone 1 mg/kg (maximum dose of 40 mg) for 3–5 days, depending on the duration of symptoms; administer with food or milk to avoid gastric irritation.
- Treat or remove any exacerbating factors (see the 'Diagnosis' section above).
- Give antibiotics only if there are signs of pneumonia, especially a persistent fever.

Very severe or life-threatening asthma

Features of severe or life-threatening asthma include the following:

- being too breathless to feed, drink or talk
- marked recession/use of accessory muscles
- respiratory rate of more than 50 breaths/minute
- pulse rate of more than 140 beats/minute
- poor chest movement or silent chest
- exhaustion, agitation or reduced conscious level (due to hypoxia or hypercapnia)
- hypoxaemia (SaO_2 less than 90% in air or cyanosis) (this is a very late sign).

Treat immediately (use the 'ABC' approach):

- Give **100% oxygen** via a face mask with reservoir bag held by the parent or nurse close to the child's face at 10–15 litres/minute to keep SaO_2 in the range 94–98%.
- Give salbutamol inhaled from a nebuliser, 2.5 mg nebules for children under 5 years and 5 mg for those over 5 years, and repeated as required (drive the nebuliser with oxygen at 6–8 litres/minute rather than compressed air). Sometimes nebulisers may be needed continuously (described as 'back to back', i.e. as each nebule finishes, repeat with another).
- If a nebuliser is not available, use inhaled salbutamol via a spacer (but now without a valve that needs opening with each breath; *see* Figure 5.2.B.1, in which the home-made 'spacer' has no valve) as described above in acute asthma. That is, give salbutamol aerosol 1000 micrograms (10 sprays each of 100 micrograms,

with each spray given after every four to five breaths) via the spacer every 5–10 minutes initially and then, once there is some improvement, 10 sprays over four to five breaths each, every 10–30 minutes until the child is better. Children under 4 years of age are likely to require a face mask connected to the mouthpiece of a spacer for successful drug delivery. Inhalers should be sprayed into the spacer in individual sprays and inhaled immediately by tidal breathing.

- If nebulised or inhaled beta-agonist bronchodilators are not available or are not effective and the child is deteriorating, give an intramuscular injection of adrenaline: 10 micrograms/kg (0.01 mL/kg of 1 in 1000 solution, up to a maximum of 300 micrograms), measured accurately with a 1-mL syringe (**ensure that the needle is not in a vein before injecting**). If there is no improvement after 15 minutes, repeat the dose once.
- **In addition to the bronchodilator treatment, give systemic steroids either as** IV/IM hydrocortisone 4 mg/kg 4- to 6-hourly (preferable) or as **oral** prednisolone (see above) until recovery. Start the steroids as soon as possible. A soluble preparation dissolved in a spoonful of water is preferable in those unable to swallow tablets. Use a dose of 20 mg for children aged 2–5 years. Repeat the dose of prednisolone in children who vomit, and give IV (or IM if a venous cannula cannot be inserted) hydrocortisone (4 mg/kg repeated 4-hourly) in those who are unable to retain orally ingested medication. Treatment for 3–5 days is usually sufficient, but the length of the course should be tailored to the number of days necessary to bring about recovery. Weaning is unnecessary unless the course of steroids exceeds 14 days.

If two to three doses of inhaled bronchodilator and systemic steroids do not result in improvement, or if life-threatening features are present, use:

- IV beta-2-agonist salbutamol (loading dose 5 micrograms/kg over 10–15 minutes in children under 2 years of age and 15 micrograms/kg over 2 years of age). If resources allow (i.e. only where high-dependency or intensive care is available), this can be followed by 1–2 micrograms/kg/minute (maximum of 5 micrograms/kg/minute) adjusted according to response and heart rate, and with monitoring of serum potassium levels as this electrolyte falls when salbutamol is given IV (see below)
- **or** IV magnesium sulphate 40 milligrams/kg (maximum of 2 grams) over 20 minutes
- **or** both of the above
- an alternative to the above treatments is to give aminophylline (loading dose 5 mg/kg over 20 minutes, followed by 1 mg/kg/hour by IV infusion in children aged 1–12 years and 500 micrograms/kg/hour in patients aged over 12 years or under 1 year). Do not give the loading dose if the child has already received any form of aminophylline or caffeine in the previous 24 hours. Side effects include nausea, vomiting, tachycardia or tachyarrhythmia and seizures, and consequently this treatment is less preferred.

Severe and life-threatening hypokalaemia may occur with IV salbutamol, potentiated by steroids. If possible, monitor the ECG continuously and check potassium levels 12-hourly. ECG signs of hypokalaemia are ST depression, T-wave

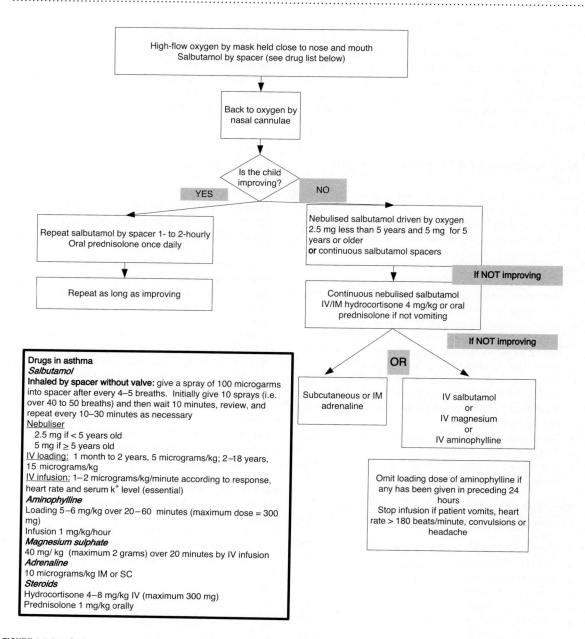

FIGURE 5.2.B.2 Pathway of care for very severe or life-threatening asthma.

reduction and prominent U waves. Ensure that maintenance potassium intake is given in the infusion fluid.

If there is a poor response to the above treatment, or the child's condition worsens suddenly, obtain a chest X-ray to look for evidence of pneumothorax. In the presence of hyperinflation from asthma, detection of a pneumothorax on the chest X-ray may be difficult.

Monitor the above clinical features regularly, and also monitor oxygen saturation, by pulse oximeter if available. Keep SaO2 in the range 94–98% by administering oxygen, either by face mask or by nasal cannulae. Use oxygen to drive nebulisers.

If the above measures do not result in improvement, or the child is tiring and gasping, this may progress to a respiratory arrest. Positive airway pressure would be the usual next step. Some respiratory support can be given by the use of a bag-valve-mask system to increase tidal breaths, but beware of aspiration (insert a nasogastric tube).

Transcutaneous pCO2 monitoring is valuable in severe asthma.

In cases that do not respond to the above measures, obtain a chest X-ray and consider mechanical ventilation (slow rate, long expiration). A blood gas measurement showing respiratory acidosis can be valuable at this time, but remember that invasive procedures can worsen respiratory distress.

If intubation and ventilation become essential, ketamine induction followed by inhalational anaesthetic gases (e.g. halothane) may assist bronchodilatation.

Indications for intubation and ventilation (if available) in severe asthma include the following:
- increasing exhaustion
- progressive deterioration in clinical condition
- oxygenation decreasing and/or oxygen requirement increasing

- pCO$_2$ increasing (if measurable from arterial/capillary gas)
- sudden deterioration – and always consider the possibility of a pneumothorax.

Follow-up care

Once the child has improved sufficiently to be discharged home, prescribe inhaled salbutamol through a metered-dose inhaler with a suitable commercially available or home-made spacer (*see* Figure 5.2.B.1), and instruct the parents in how to use this.

Following any acute episode, review asthma control and management, including correct use of medications and the need for a step up in 'preventive' treatment.

5.2.C The child with an inhaled foreign body

> **BOX 5.2.C.1 Minimum standards**
> - Chest X-ray.
> - Antibiotics.
> - Physiotherapy.
> - Bronchoscopy.

Introduction

Any small object that can get through the trachea or large bronchi, such as a seed, a peanut or an eraser from the top of a pencil, can lodge in the lower airway. If the object is too small to cause life-threatening choking it will enter the lower respiratory tract and cause subacute respiratory symptoms after an initial coughing bout.

Diagnosis

There may be a clear history from the parent or child of an episode of coughing or choking, followed by difficulty in breathing.

- On examination of the child's chest, look to see whether there is less chest expansion on one side when breathing in.
- Feel the trachea. It may be pushed away from the midline by air trapping on the side affected by the foreign body.
- This may also be seen on a chest X-ray (if available) (*see* Figure 5.2.C.1), ideally an expiratory and inspiratory film.

An inhaled foreign body in a young child can go down the right or left side. In older children and adults, a foreign body on the right side is more common. There may be a harsh wheezing noise heard on the side of the chest where the foreign body has lodged.

Treatment

Air may be trapped in the lungs beyond the point where the foreign body has lodged, or this part of the lung may become infected. Give the child antibiotics. Chloramphenicol, 25 mg/

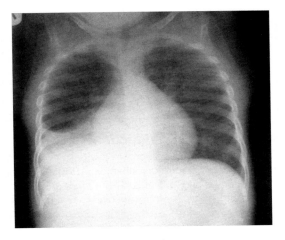

FIGURE 5.2.C.1 Chest X-ray of a child with a foreign body occluding the right middle and right lower lobe bronchi. The right upper lobe of the lung shows air trapping due to a 'ball-valve' effect. The foreign body is not visible because it is not radio opaque.

kg every eight hours, is a good first choice, but add flucloxacillin or cloxacillin 25 mg/kg six hourly if there is a suspicion of or proven infection with *Staphylococcus aureus*. If there is evidence of severe pneumonia use the antibiotic combination in Section 5.3.A for severe pneumonia. Removal of a foreign body is a specialised procedure that must be carried out using a bronchoscope. Treat the infection until the child can be transferred to a hospital where this procedure can be performed. Some gentle physiotherapy may help, but take care not to dislodge the foreign body, as this will cause infection and obstruction in another part of the lung.

If the foreign body is not removed there will be subsequent bronchiectasis and recurrent chest infections (*see* Section 5.3.B).

For the management of choking, *see* Section 1.12.

5.3 Lung disorders

5.3.A Pneumonia

Acute respiratory infection

There are two categories of acute respiratory infection (ARI).
- **Acute upper respiratory infection (AURI):** above the vocal cords and epiglottis. These infections include colds, tonsillitis and otitis media. They are not life-threatening, but may lead to disability (e.g. otitis media is a leading cause of deafness in resource-limited countries) and complications (e.g. rheumatic fever following streptococcal pharyngitis).
- **Acute lower respiratory infection (ALRI):** below and including the vocal cords and epiglottis. These infections include croup (and other infectious causes of upper airway obstruction), pneumonia and bronchiolitis. Acute upper airway obstruction is described in Section 5.1.

Importance of acute respiratory infection

Pneumonia is responsible for around two million deaths annually in children under 5 years of age. In resource-limited countries, most of these infections are bacterial, and the most common causative bacteria are *Streptococcus pneumoniae* and *Haemophilus influenzae*. **In severely malnourished children, *Klebsiella pneumoniae* and *Staphylococcus aureus* are the most common causative organisms.**

Immunisation

Pneumococcal conjugate vaccine has been introduced to the primary immunisation schedule in many well-resourced countries, and reduces the incidence of X-ray-proven pneumonia in infants by around one-third. The HiB vaccine (against encapsulated *Haemophilus influenzae* type B) will not protect against unencapsulated *H. influenzae*, which causes some cases of pneumonia in resource-limited countries. Nevertheless, the HIb vaccine is very effective against other very serious infections caused by *H. influenzae* (e.g. meningitis, epiglottitis), and should be given to all infants in every country. Unfortunately, around 34 million children do not receive routine immunisations, and most of these are **living** in resource-**limited** countries.

Management of the child with acute upper respiratory infection
Coryza or pharyngitis

These are common self-limiting viral infections that require only supportive care. Antibiotics should not be given. Wheeze or stridor may occur in some children, especially infants. Most episodes end within 14 days. Cough lasting 30 days or more may be caused by tuberculosis, asthma or pertussis.

Presentation

These infections present with cough, running nose, fever and sore throat, but **not** with fast breathing, chest indrawing, stridor or danger signs for pneumonia (see below). Wheezing may occur in young children (*see* Section 5.2.A).

Treatment

- Treat the child as an outpatient.
- Soothe the throat and relieve the cough with a safe remedy, such as a warm sweet drink.
- Relieve high fever (≥ 39°C or ≥ 102.2°F) with paracetamol if it is causing distress.
- Give normal fluid requirements plus extra breast milk or fluids if there is a fever. Small frequent drinks are more likely to be taken and less likely to be vomited.
- Clear secretions from the nose before feeds using a cloth which has been soaked in water and twisted to form a pointed wick.
- Do not give any of the following:
  - antibiotics (they are not effective for viral illnesses and do not prevent pneumonia)
  - remedies containing atropine, codeine or codeine derivatives, or alcohol (which may be harmful)
  - medicated nose drops.

Advise the mother to feed the child normally, to watch for fast or difficult breathing, and to return if either develops or if the child is unable to drink or breastfeed.

Inform the mother that the child has mucus in the upper airways that 'drops' in the lungs, so the child coughs in order to remove it, and this means that the cough in itself is not dangerous.

Management of the child with acute lower respiratory infection (ALRI)

Children at greatest risk of dying from an ALRI have the following risk factors:
- age under 1 year
- malnutrition

- pneumonia as a complication of infection with measles, pertussis, malaria or HIV.

Diagnosis of ALRI

In many hospitals in resource-limited countries, special tests (e.g. blood culture, microbiology of respiratory secretions, X-rays) may be limited or unavailable. However, because the prevalence of bacterial pneumonia is high, the diagnosis must usually be made clinically. This will not be 100% accurate, so a few children may receive antibiotics unnecessarily (i.e. clinical diagnosis has less than 100% **specificity**). However, it is more important not to miss children who do need antibiotics (i.e. clinical diagnosis should have a good **sensitivity**). Clinical diagnosis may be as accurate as an X-ray and more helpful in deciding whether treatments such as oxygen are indicated. The clinical features will also help to decide how severe the child's infection is and what treatment is appropriate.

The following clinical features should be recorded:

- The presence of **cyanosis**, which is best seen in the lips or tongue. It may be missed if the lighting is poor or if the child is anaemic (e.g. due to co-infection with malaria), and it can be difficult to detect in black children. Cyanosis is a late sign of respiratory problems, and if possible oxygenation should be assessed with a pulse oximeter. Normal saturation at sea level (SaO_2) is greater than 94%.
- Inability of the child to drink.
- The presence of chest wall indrawing (an inward motion of the lower chest wall when the child breathes in).
- The presence of grunting (expiratory braking).
- The presence of hyperinflation (asthma or bronchiolitis).
- Elevated respiratory rate. Respiratory rate is measured over 1 minute, using a suitable timing device. The respiratory rate in children varies with age. Table 5.3.A.1 lists the abnormal values for respiratory rate for various age groups.

TABLE 5.3.A.1 WHO definition of abnormally fast breathing

Age	Abnormally fast breathing
< 2 months	≥ 60 breaths/minute
2–12 months	≥ 50 breaths/minute
12 months to 5 years	≥ 40 breaths/minute

Remember that conditions such as severe anaemia, dehydration and high fever are accompanied by a raised respiratory rate.

A high fever in a child with breathing difficulties may be due to pneumonia, bacterial tracheitis or even epiglottitis. If the airway is clear, the most likely diagnosis is pneumonia. Although high fever and respiratory signs are the usual way for pneumonia to present, pneumonia should always be considered in the list of causes of abdominal pain and neck stiffness.

Clinical examination (or chest X-ray) cannot reliably differentiate between a viral pneumonia and a bacterial one, so all cases are treated with antibiotics.

Features of pneumonia include the following:

- fever, cough, breathlessness and lethargy
- pleuritic chest pain, abdominal pain and neck stiffness (these indicate pleural involvement)

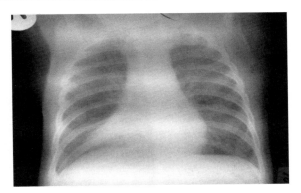

FIGURE 5.3.A.1 Right middle lobe pneumonia. Note the loss of the right heart border.

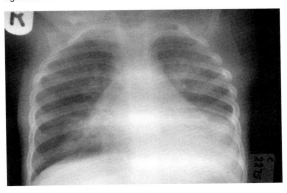

FIGURE 5.3.A.2 Left lower lobe pneumonia. Note that the silhouette of the diaphragm cannot be seen on the left. The right middle lobe is also affected.

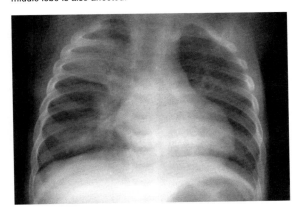

FIGURE 5.3.A.3 Right upper lobe pneumonia. Note that the horizontal fissure is pulled up.

- signs of consolidation:
  - dull percussion
  - reduced breath sounds
  - bronchial breathing may be absent in an infant
- chest X-ray may show pleural effusion or empyema as well as consolidation.

Auscultation should always be undertaken, **but only after first checking for cyanosis, observing the breathing pattern and the other signs as described above.** Important clinical signs include evidence of the following:

- consolidation or effusion/empyema
- wheeze

- bronchiolitis (hyperinflation with crackles at the lung bases)
- alveolitis (e.g. in HIV-induced *Pneumocystis* pneumonia) with end-inspiratory crackles.
- pericardial involvement (rare)
- pneumothorax (rare).

A chest X-ray may be helpful if there is any doubt about the diagnosis or if the child is seriously ill.

Figures 5.3.A.1, 5.3.A.2 and 5.3.A.3 show the appearance of lobar pneumonia affecting different lobes.

Additional features of ARLI usually include a fever and a cough. Pleuritic chest pain (which may radiate to the abdomen) may also be present in older children if the diagnosis is pneumonia.

Table 5.3.A.2 gives guidelines for the assessment and treatment of acute respiratory infection. Children with the following features should be managed differently, as described elsewhere in this book:

- stridor (*see* Section 5.1.A)
- wheeze (*see* Sections 5.2.A and 5.2.B)
- severe malnutrition (*see* Section 5.10.B)
- signs suggesting meningitis (*see* Section 5.16.B).

Diagnosis of severe pneumonia

This is diagnosed by the presence of cough or difficult breathing plus at least one of the following:

- central cyanosis

- inability to breastfeed or drink, or vomiting after every drink
- convulsions, lethargy or unconsciousness
- severe respiratory distress.

In addition, some or all of the other signs of pneumonia may be present, such as the following:

- fast breathing:
  - age < 2 months: ≥ 60 breaths/minute
  - age 2–11 months: ≥ 50 breaths/minute
  - age 1–5 years: ≥ 40 breaths/minute
- nasal flaring
- grunting (in young infants)
- lower chest wall indrawing
- chest auscultation signs of pneumonia:
  - decreased breath sounds
  - bronchial breath sounds
  - crackles
  - abnormal vocal resonance (decreased over a pleural effusion, and increased over lobar consolidation)
  - pleural rub.

Obtain a chest X-ray and SaO_2 (if available).

For children with no evidence of pneumonia but with signs suggesting a chest infection, look for ear and throat infections or infections in another system and treat accordingly.

TABLE 5.3.A.2 The management of children with different severities of acute lower respiratory tract infection (ALRI) (modified from the WHO *Pocket Book of Hospital Care for Children*, second edition 2014)

Sign or symptom	Classification	Treatment
Central cyanosis and/or $SaO_2 < 90\%$ Severe respiratory distress (e.g. head nodding, gasping, chest wall indrawing, grunting) Fast breathing as below under 'pneumonia that is not severe' Decreased breath sounds and/or bronchial breathing Crackles in the lung fields Vocal resonance and percussion suggesting consolidation and/or effusion Pleural rub Inability to drink, vomiting, reduced consciousness **Plus** signs of pneumonia in the row below	Severe pneumonia	Admit to hospital Give IV/IM appropriate antibiotics* Give oxygen Manage the airway Treat high fever if present If the child has HIV infection, refer to specific guidelines (and *see* Section 6.2.D)
Fast breathing but no chest wall indrawing: ≥ 60 breaths/minute in a child aged < 2 months ≥ 50 breaths/minute in a child aged 2–11 months ≥ 40 breaths/minute in a child aged 1–5 years Definite crackles on auscultation	Pneumonia that is not severe	Home care (but depends on home circumstances and overall clinical state of the child) Give an appropriate antibiotic* Advise the mother when to return if treatment fails on amoxicillin and more appropriate second-line treatment is needed Follow up in 2 days
No signs of pneumonia or severe pneumonia	No pneumonia Cough or coryza	Home care Advise the mother to return for follow-up in 5 days if not improving If coughing for more than 14 days, consider investigations for TB, asthma, inhaled foreign body, pertussis, HIV, bronchiectasis and lung abscess (*see* Figure 5.3.C.1).

* See details of antibiotics, routes of administration and durations for different categories of pneumonia in section 'Antibiotics' below

Oxygen

Children with severe or very severe pneumonia are likely to be hypoxaemic. However, cyanosis is a late sign of hypoxaemia.

Oxygen must always be available in sufficient quantity to provide 24-hour treatment without depending on the availability of a reliable electricity supply.

Give oxygen if the child shows any of the following:

- restlessness (if oxygen makes the child more comfortable)
- severe chest wall indrawing
- a breathing rate of more than 70 breaths/minute (in a child aged 2 months to 5 years)
- grunting (in an infant under 2 months of age)
- gasping
- if a pulse oximeter is available, SaO_2 of less than 94% (at sea level; lower values will be normal at high altitude, and normal values of SaO_2 should be known for healthy local children in your area if it is at high altitude). Aim to maintain SaO_2 in the range 94–98%.

Give oxygen until the signs of hypoxia (e.g. severe lower chest wall indrawing, high breathing rates and/or SaO_2 < 94% in air) are no longer present.

Oxygen delivery

A good source of oxygen is an oxygen concentrator. This is a durable piece of equipment, but it requires a continuous supply of mains electricity to provide oxygen. It works on the 'molecular-sieve' principle, removing nitrogen from room air. The alternative is cylinder oxygen, but cylinders must be replenished regularly and need to be available at all times, which is expensive and may give rise to transport difficulties. **A combination of the two supplies of oxygen is essential.** An oxygen generator which can provide oxygen and fill cylinders when the electrical power is available (e.g. Diamedica equipment). The concentrator or cylinder should be connected to a low-flow meter. The use of a flow splitter will allow up to four children to receive oxygen from one source. The oxygen should be delivered to the child using nasal cannulae. **These should be only 2–3 mm long, to avoid nasal irritation.**

Figure 5.3.A.4 shows the delivery of oxygen through nasal cannulae.

A mask should be used to give high-flow oxygen during resuscitation.

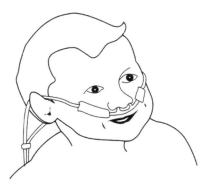

FIGURE 5.3.A.4 Nasal cannulae for delivering oxygen. The cannula has been taped to the child's cheeks, close to the nostrils. The tubing is run under the child's shirt to stop them pulling it, and leads to the low-flow meter and oxygen concentrator or cylinder. A flow splitter may be used.

Nurses should check frequently that the nasal cannulae are not blocked with mucus and are in the correct position, and that all connections are secure.

Antibiotics

Children who are vomiting or who require IV fluids should have their antibiotics given intravenously (preferably), or intramuscularly **if vascular access is difficult to achieve or maintain**, for the first 48 hours. Some antibiotics, such as gentamicin, are always given IV or IM. Certain antibiotics are reserved for specific circumstances, such as high-dose co-trimoxazole for suspected *Pneumocystis jirovecii* pneumonia, and flucloxacillin or cloxacillin for pulmonary abscess or bacterial tracheitis where *Staphylococcus aureus* is likely to be responsible. These are described at the end of the section on antibiotics.

For severe pneumonia:

- Give ampicillin 50 mg/kg IM/IV or benzyl penicillin 50 000 units/kg that is 30 mg/kg IM or IV every 6 hours plus gentamicin 7.5 mg/kg IM or IV once a day for 5 days. Then, if the child responds well, complete treatment with oral amoxicillin (25 mg/kg three times a day, maximum 500 mg, or 1 gram in severe cases) plus IM or IV gentamicin 7.5 mg/kg once daily for a further 5 days.
- Alternatively, if the above are not available, give chloramphenicol (25 mg/kg IM or IV every 8 hours) until the child has improved. Then continue orally four times a day for a total course of 10 days.
- **Or** use ceftriaxone (80 mg/kg IM or IV once daily) or cefotaxime (50 mg/kg IV 6-hourly) for 10 days.
- If the child does not improve within 48 hours, switch to gentamicin (7.5 mg/kg IM or IV once a day) and cloxacillin (50 mg/kg IM or IV every 6 hours), as described below for possible staphylococcal pneumonia.

For pneumonia that is not severe:

- Treat the child as an outpatient.
- Give amoxicillin 40 mg/kg twice a day for 5 days.
- Give the first dose at the clinic, and teach the mother how to give the other doses at home.
- In infants aged 2–12 months who have some of the signs suggestive of non-severe pneumonia without a high fever but **with** wheeze, the most likely diagnosis is bronchiolitis. This is caused by a virus, and in the absence of signs suggesting the development of secondary bacterial infection (severe pneumonia), antibiotics are not necessary (*see* Section 5.2.A). The WHO recently published the following conclusion: **Antibiotics are not routinely recommended for children aged 2 months to 5 years with non-severe pneumonia (that is, fast breathing with no chest indrawing or danger signs) with a wheeze but no fever (temperature below 38°C), as the cause is most likely to be viral.**

Symptomatic and supportive treatment for children with all degrees of pneumonia

Nurse the child in a thermoneutral environment (lightly clothed in a warm room at around 25°C).

Fever:

- Remember that fever may not be simply due to the child's pneumonia. Consider other diagnoses, such as malaria.
- If the child has fever (≥ 39°C or ≥ 102.2°F) that appears

to be causing distress, give paracetamol oral or rectally, 10–15 mg/kg 4- to 6-hourly.

- Remove by gentle suction under direct observation any thick secretions in the throat which the child cannot clear.
- Ensure daily maintenance fluids appropriate for the child's age, but avoid over-hydration.
- Encourage breastfeeding and oral fluid intake.
- If the child cannot drink, insert a nasogastric tube and give maintenance fluids in frequent small amounts. If the child is taking fluids adequately by mouth, do not use a nasogastric tube, as it increases the risk of aspiration pneumonia. Encourage eating as soon as food can be taken. When the child is recovering, nutritional rehabilitation may be necessary.

Failure to start to improve within a few days

If the child has not improved after 2 days, or if their condition has worsened, re-examine them thoroughly, looking for signs of pleural effusion/empyema and other causes of fever. If possible, obtain a chest X-ray. This may show a pleural effusion or empyema (see Section 5.3.B) into which antibiotics cannot penetrate, or it may show the characteristic pneumatocoeles (lung abscesses) of staphylococcal pneumonia.

Also consider *Mycoplasma pneumoniae* or *Bordetella pertussis* infections. **Pertussis should be recognisable because of the characteristic nocturnal emetic cough and the whoop in the child over 2 years of age.**

Prescribe **erythromycin** if either of these infections is suspected. It should be given orally as follows:

- 125 mg 6-hourly (children aged 1 month to 2 years)
- 250 mg 6-hourly (children aged 2–8 years)
- 500 mg 6-hourly (children over 8 years of age).

Pneumonia that does not respond to standard antibiotics within 2 weeks
Tuberculosis

A child with persistent fever for more than 2 weeks and signs of pneumonia should be evaluated for tuberculosis. If another cause of the fever cannot be found, tuberculosis should be considered and treatment for tuberculosis, following national guidelines, may be initiated and response to anti-tuberculous treatment evaluated (see Section 6.1.N).

Children who are HIV-positive or in whom HIV is suspected

Some aspects of antibiotic treatment are different in children who are HIV-positive or in whom HIV is suspected. Although the pneumonia in many of these children has the same aetiology as in children without HIV, pneumocystis pneumonia (PCP), often at the age of 4–6 months, is an important additional cause which must be treated when present (see Section 6.2.D). While confirming the diagnosis, give ampicillin plus gentamicin as described above for severe pneumonia.

Staphylococcal pneumonia

Staphylococcal pneumonia is suspected if there is rapid clinical deterioration despite treatment, a pneumatocoele or necrotising pneumonia with effusion on chest X-ray, numerous Gram-positive cocci in a smear of sputum, or heavy growth of *Staphylococcus aureus* in cultured sputum or empyema fluid.

- Treat with cloxacillin (50 mg/kg IM or IV every 6 hours) and gentamicin (7.5 mg/kg IM or IV once a day) for at least 7 days.
- When the child improves, continue cloxacillin/flucloxacillin orally four times a day for a total course of 3 weeks. Note that cloxacillin can be substituted by another anti-staphylococcal antibiotic, such as oxacillin, flucloxacillin or dicloxacillin.

Severe dehydration

This may be a problem in pneumonia, arising from high fever and poor fluid intake (see also Section 5.12.A for the treatment of diarrhoea and Section 5.5.A for the management of shock).

Look for signs of dehydration or shock (tachycardia, weak pulse, poor peripheral circulation, and capillary refill time prolonged by more than 3 seconds).

- **If the child is shocked:** Site an intravenous line and give a bolus of crystalloid – for example, Hartmann's solution, Ringer-lactate or colloid 10–20 mL/kg (10 mL/kg in a neonate).
- **If the child is not shocked but is clinically dehydrated** (see Section 5.12.A): Give oral rehydration solution (ORS), 15–20 mL/kg/hour for 2 hours orally or via nasogastric tube. Encourage breastfeeding.

Management of ALRI in special circumstances
Management of the child under 6 months of age

Young infants with severe ALRI/pneumonia may not cough, but rather they may present with apnoea, poor feeding or hypothermia. Remember that in infants under 2 months of age, the abnormal respiratory rate cut-off is higher (> 60 breaths/minute). For infants aged 2–12 months the cut-off is > 50 breaths/minute.

- Some chest wall indrawing is normal during REM (dream) sleep.
- **All infants with severe ALRI/pneumonia should be admitted to hospital for treatment.**
- Bronchiolitis is a frequent cause, and usually involves hypoxaemia due to ventilation to perfusion mismatch. Oxygen is usually required. Additional respiratory support (see Section 5.2.A) may also be necessary, especially if there is apnoea or severe respiratory distress leading to exhaustion.
- Grunting (a short expiratory noise at the start of expiration) is **common and usually an indication for oxygen**.
- **Avoid using chloramphenicol in infants under 2 months of age** (there is a risk of development of 'grey baby syndrome'). Use benzylpenicillin or ampicillin plus gentamicin instead.
- Respiratory infection in neonates may rapidly develop into septicaemia, shock and death, so it is essential to act quickly (see Section 3.4).

Further reading

World Health Organization and UNICEF (2013) *Ending Preventable Child Deaths from Pneumonia and Diarrhoea by 2025: the integrated Global Action Plan for Pneumonia and Diarrhoea (GAPPD)*. http://apps.who.int/iris/bitstream/10665/79200/1/9789241505239_eng.pdf

5.3.B Pleural effusion, empyema and bronchiectasis

> **BOX 5.3.B Minimum standards**
> ■ Oxygen.
> ■ Pulse oximeter.
> ■ Chest drain.
> ■ Antibiotics.
> ■ Physiotherapy.
> ■ Chest X-ray/ultrasound.

Pleural effusion

A pleural effusion is a collection of fluid between the chest wall and the lung. A small effusion of clear fluid is common in children with pneumonia. Effusion should be suspected when one side of the chest sounds very dull to percussion and the breath sounds are very quiet. It can also be seen as usually unilateral shadowing on the X-ray. Usually this fluid will quickly disappear once the infection has been treated. However, if treatment is started late, or the child is unlucky, this clear fluid can become infected, too. This leads to pus accumulating in the chest cavity (an empyema).

On examination, the chest is dull to percussion and breath sounds are reduced or absent over the affected area. A pleural rub may be heard at an early stage before the effusion is fully developed. A chest X-ray shows fluid on one or both sides of the chest.

An ultrasound examination may be helpful for identifying the size of the effusion and guiding drainage.

When empyema is present, fever persists despite antibiotic therapy, and the pleural fluid is cloudy or frankly purulent.

Treatment

If a pleural effusion is suspected, X-ray the chest if possible. If this confirms your suspicions, perform a diagnostic tap as follows:

1 In the case of young children, the child should sit on the mother's lap, facing her. The mother then holds the child tightly in a bear hug. Older children can sit or lie on a bed, but it is important to explain carefully to them what is being done and have an assistant to hold the child steady.

2 Percuss out the area of dullness, put on sterile gloves and clean the skin with alcohol.

3 Gently inject some local anaesthetic (1% lidocaine) under the skin, down to the rib, using an orange (25-gauge) or blue (23-gauge) needle.

4 Then take a fresh 20-gauge needle or butterfly needle connected to a syringe and press the needle though the chest wall just below the level where the percussion note becomes dull. **Remember to go just above the rib (to avoid the intercostal blood vessels)** and aspirate all the time. Ultrasound support is ideal if available.

5 When fluid appears, aspirate a diagnostic specimen and send this for microscopy, protein, glucose, cell count, Gram and Ziehl–Neelsen stain (low yield for acid-fast bacilli), and culture for bacteria and tuberculosis. Remember that a clear fluid aspirate can suggest another diagnosis, such as tuberculosis or lymphoma (especially if bloodstained).

6 Aspirate as much fluid as possible during the procedure to allow the child to breathe more comfortably. A three-way tap connected to the catheter can be helpful. **Ensure that air cannot enter the pleural space.** If clear fluid (straw coloured or brown) is aspirated, remove sufficient fluid to relieve distress and then remove the needle.

If more than a few millilitres of fluid containing pus (opaque) are aspirated, and this does not easily pass down the needle, a chest drain will be required. This must be a sterile procedure, and is performed as follows:

1 Select a drain, the largest that will comfortably pass through the intercostal space into the cavity by holding the tip of the tube in the forceps. Do not use the stylet, as this can damage the lung.

2 Position the child and locate the effusion in the same way as for the diagnostic tap.

3 Use sufficient local anaesthetic (1% lidocaine).

4 Make an incision in the skin and part the underlying muscle with artery forceps.

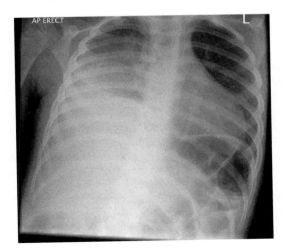

FIGURE 5.3.B.1 Chest X-ray of right-sided empyema. Note that this 5-year-old boy had a 1-week history of fever and shortness of breath. There was dullness to percussion and reduced air entry at the right lung base.

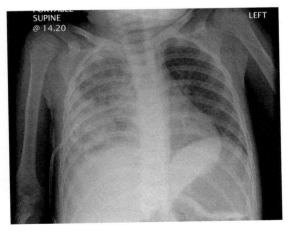

FIGURE 5.3.B.2 Chest X-ray in the same child after placement of a right-sided chest drain.

5 Avoid the neurovascular bundle on the inferior part of the rib by keeping the incision and passage of the drain on top of the rib.

6 When the pleura is reached, puncture it with the forceps and thread the chest drain through the pleural hole.

7 Ensure that all of the drainage holes of the catheter are inside the chest.

8 Fix the drain with a gauze dressing, tape and a suture.

9 Connect to an underwater seal. If the drain has been placed correctly, fluid will flow out and the fluid level will 'swing' with respiration.

Give ampicillin or cloxacillin/flucloxacillin 50 mg/kg IV or IM every 6 hours plus gentamicin 7.5 mg/kg IM/IV once daily. After at least 7 days IV/IM antibiotics, and providing the child is improving, continue flucloxacillin/cloxacillin orally 50 mg/kg 6 hourly for a total of 3 weeks from the onset of the antibiotics.

If the patient does not improve despite adequate chest drainage and antibiotics consider HIV and/or TB.

Figures 5.3.B.1 and 5.3.B.2 show the chest X-ray in a child with empyema, and the effect of placing a chest drain.

Lung abscess
Diagnosis
A lung abscess is a collection of pus in the lung. This can result from an untreated foreign body, aspiration of other material (e.g. vomit), infection with *Staphylococcus aureus*, or as a complication of bronchiectasis. When examining the child, the findings may be similar to those in the child with pneumonia, though they will often have been ill for longer. A chest X-ray (if available) will be helpful. Ultrasound scanning can show whether the abscess lies close to the posterior chest wall.

Treatment
Antibiotics are the most important form of treatment, and a long course (4–6 weeks) must be given. Give ampicillin or flucloxacillin/cloxacillin 50 mg/kg IV/IM every 6 hours

plus gentamicin 7.5 mg/kg IM/IV once daily. Continue, as in empyema, for up to 3 weeks. If you are certain that the abscess lies close to the posterior chest wall, it can be aspirated in the same way as an empyema (see above).

A chest drain must never be placed in a pulmonary abscess, as this can create a fistula.

Surgical management may be required for a large abscess, especially if haemoptysis or a deterioration despite appropriate antibiotic therapy occur.

If the child has been ill for weeks, ensure good nutrition.

Bronchiectasis
Diagnosis
Bronchiectasis occurs when the bronchi become baggy and full of mucus and pus. Bronchiectasis may follow infection such as tuberculosis, pertussis and measles. It may be due to congenital problems such as cystic fibrosis (see Section 5.3.C) and rarer lung diseases in which there are abnormal cilia or abnormal cilial activity, or an inhaled foreign body that has not been removed (see Section 5.2.C).

Sometimes a child who has had lobar pneumonia does not recover fully, and develops bronchiectasis in the affected lobe. There are other rare causes, such as some viral infections.

Children with bronchiectasis usually cough and produce sputum every day. Their symptoms may become much worse at times due to secondary infection. The child may have finger clubbing, a hyperinflated chest and coarse crackles in many parts of the lung. Look for thickened bronchi and areas of consolidation on the chest X-ray.

Treatment
Bronchiectasis cannot be cured, although **occasionally symptoms can be improved by removing the lung lobe that is most severely affected**. The child and their parents must understand that daily treatment with chest physiotherapy and frequent courses of antibiotics will be needed. The use of physiotherapy is described in Section 8.3.

5.3.C Cystic fibrosis

> **BOX 5.3.C.1 Minimum standards**
> - Diagnostic testing.
> - Pancreatic enzyme supplements.
> - Fat-soluble vitamins (A, D and E).
> - Daily chest physiotherapy.
> - Early use of antibiotics, including flucloxacillin, amoxicillin, chloramphenicol, ciprofloxacin, gentamicin and ceftazidime.

Introduction
Pathophysiology
In the cells lining the airways of patients with cystic fibrosis (CF), chloride ions cannot leave the cell to enter the bronchial lumen. The cell cytoplasm has a high salt content, and water moves from the airway lumen into the cell by osmosis. The mucus within the lumen then becomes dehydrated.

Sticky mucus interferes with the action of the respiratory cilia, and this leads to bacterial colonisation of the airway, with chronic inflammation and neutrophil damage. There are also viscid secretions in the biliary tract, pancreas and reproductive system, causing poor fat digestion and very low fertility in male patients.

Cystic fibrosis is an autosomal-recessive genetic disorder that affects the lung, digestive system, sweat glands, liver, pancreas and reproductive system. Most deaths from cystic fibrosis are caused by respiratory failure. In well-resourced countries, many patients now survive well into adulthood.

Incidence
The incidence of cystic fibrosis in countries such as the UK and the USA is around 1 in 2500 live births, and around 1 in 25 of the population are carriers. Very little is known about

the frequency of the disorder in resource-limited countries. Diagnosis relies on the sweat test, which is difficult to perform where laboratory facilities are limited. The incidence of cystic fibrosis among black South Africans is thought to be between 1 in 700 and 1 in 14000, with between 1 in 14 and 1 in 60 of the general population being carriers. In some well-resourced countries there is routine screening of newborn infants from heelprick blood samples.

The CF gene

The CF gene is on chromosome 7. The commonest mutation causing disease is DF508, and it occurs all over the world. (It is as common in cystic fibrosis patients in North Africa as it is in those in Northern Ireland.) Over 1000 other mutations have been found, many of which are rare. The gene product is a protein which sits on the apical membrane of epithelial cells and regulates the movement of chloride ions. As cystic fibrosis is a recessively inherited condition, two abnormal genes, one from each parent, are required for the disease to occur, and then this protein is defective and chloride transport is disrupted.

Presentation

Meconium ileus

In the newborn period, babies may present with a triad of:
- failure to pass meconium in the first 24 hours
- abdominal distension
- vomiting.

This picture may also occur in surgical conditions (e.g. Hirschsprung's disease, imperforate anus), and any sick newborn infant may develop non-specific abdominal distension. Around 15% of babies with cystic fibrosis present with meconium ileus (i.e. difficulty passing thick, sticky meconium, leading to small bowel obstruction).

Presentation in older children

This includes the following:
- malabsorption (pale, greasy stools)
- failure to thrive
- rectal prolapse
- chronic and recurrent chest infections
- partially digested material with a high fat content may block the ascending colon (distal intestinal obstruction syndrome).

Differential diagnosis

The differential diagnosis of chronic cough and failure to thrive includes the following:
- pulmonary tuberculosis
- bronchiectasis (especially following measles, which may also cause chronic diarrhoea)
- HIV infection.

Figure 5.3.C.1 shows a flow diagram for investigation of the child with chronic cough and failure to thrive, in areas where pulmonary tuberculosis and HIV infection are prevalent.

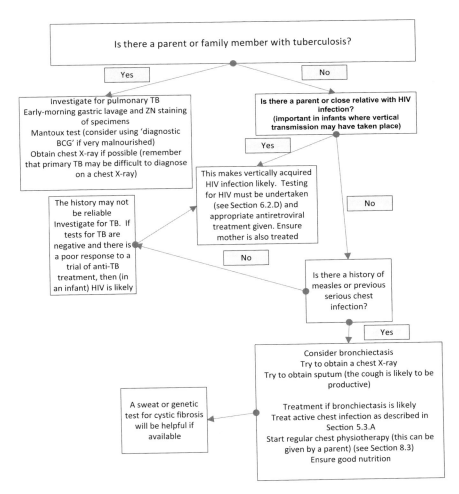

FIGURE 5.3.C.1 Differential diagnosis of the child with chronic cough and failure to thrive.

Diagnosing cystic fibrosis
The sweat test

This detects the high levels of chloride and sodium in sweat that occur in cystic fibrosis patients. The principle of the test is to allow pilocarpine to diffuse into the skin of the forearm using an electric current (pilocarpine iontophoresis), which stimulates sweating via cholinergic receptors in sweat glands. The sweat is collected on filter paper and the weight, chloride and sodium concentrations are calculated. At least 100 mg of sweat are needed. Values highly suggestive of cystic fibrosis are concentrations of chloride and sodium of greater than 60 mmol/litre, with a higher concentration of chloride than sodium. False-negative and false-positive results are usually a consequence of faulty test technique, which is why there is a need for a specialised laboratory and experienced technician, which should be available in at least one hospital in every country.

Genetic tests

These can be performed on very small amounts of blood, collected as a dried blood spot on filter paper. It is possible to send dried blood spots to a genetics laboratory for analysis. A negative genetic test does not rule out cystic fibrosis (only common genes are tested).

Management

Treatment of children with cystic fibrosis in resource-limited countries has been identified as a priority area by the WHO. For practical reasons, children with cystic fibrosis can be seen regularly in a clinic alongside children with bronchiectasis. It is important that the child's parents understand that cystic fibrosis cannot be cured. However, these children can lead active lives with minimal symptoms initially, provided that daily treatment is given and deteriorations are treated promptly.

Pancreatic enzyme supplements

Most children with cystic fibrosis will require pancreatic enzyme supplements (e.g. Creon, Solvay Healthcare, or Pancrease, Janssen-Cilag). Young infants are given half a capsule per milk feed. Older children may need over 10 capsules per meal. The capsules contain protease, lipase and amylase. The lipase is the most important component for preventing malabsorption. Most brands contain 5000–10 000 units of lipase per capsule. The correct dose of pancreatic enzyme supplements is not necessarily related to age, but rather it is the amount required to control symptoms of steatorrhoea and achieve normal growth. The maximum dose (expressed as units of lipase) is 10 000 units/kg/day.

Fat-soluble vitamins

The child should be given extra fat-soluble vitamins. Appropriate doses are vitamin E, 50 mg once daily in infants and young children (aged 0–5 years), 100 mg/day in older children (aged 5–12 years), and 200 mg/day in patients over 12 years of age. Vitamin E may be given as vitamin E suspension 100 mg/mL or as 50 mg tablets. Multivitamin drops, such as Abidec, which contains vitamin A 4000 units/6 mL and vitamin D_2 400 units/6 mL, are also required.

Abidec should be given as follows:

- 0.3 mL/day for newborn infants
- 0.6 mL/day for infants aged 1–12 months
- 1.2 mL/day for children over 1 year of age.

Remember that an adequate calorie intake is vital. **Do not restrict fat in the diet.**

Chest physiotherapy

Routine daily chest physiotherapy should be started as soon as the diagnosis is suspected. The most common method is percussion and postural drainage. In young infants this can be performed with the child across their parent's lap, whereas in preschool children a foam 'wedge' helps the child to achieve the correct position for postural drainage. The percussion element of the treatment involves firm 'clapping' movements with the flat of the hand against the child's chest. Older children and teenagers should be encouraged to take a more active part in their physiotherapy. A technique incorporating periods of diaphragmatic breathing followed by a forced expiration or 'huff', causing coughing, is suitable at this age.

(For physiotherapy techniques, *see* Section 8.3)

Antibiotics

Children with cystic fibrosis have intermittent or chronic infection with *Staphylococcus aureus* in the first 2 to 3 years of life. *Haemophilus influenzae* is also seen in the early years and should be treated as a pathogen. In most children, chronic infection with *Pseudomonas aeruginosa* becomes established sooner or later. Later still, a variety of opportunistic organisms colonise the lungs. If the results of sputum or 'cough swab' cultures are available, these will allow you to choose an appropriate antibiotic. If not, the likely organisms in the age groups described above will be a rough guide. Ideally, the child's respiratory microorganisms should be monitored on a frequent and regular basis so that the appropriate antibiotic can be given promptly.

Antibiotic prophylaxis

In well-resourced countries, a continuous prophylactic oral antibiotic is often given to children with cystic fibrosis, up until 2 years of age. An antibiotic active against *S. aureus*, **usually flucloxacillin**, is chosen. In resource-limited countries this may not be an option, either because the diagnosis is made late or because continuous antibiotics are too expensive. However, flucloxacillin (125 mg twice daily) should be prescribed if possible for children under 2 years of age. Once mucoid *Pseudomonas aeruginosa* has become established, respiratory deterioration occurs, so in well-resourced countries various antibiotic regimes are used to reduce the bacterial burden in the lungs and slow down lung damage. Oral ciprofloxacin, inhaled nebulised colistin or intravenous ceftazidime and tobramycin are variously used. Up-to-date details on antibiotic treatment for cystic fibrosis can be found on the website of the charity the Cystic Fibrosis Trust (www.cysticfibrosis.org.uk).

Treatment of exacerbations

If the cough worsens or the child produces more sputum, a full course of antibiotics should be started and continued for at least 2 weeks. Longer courses of antibiotics are given than in most other conditions. The following antibiotics are suitable.

Flucloxacillin

TABLE 5.3.C.1 Oral flucloxacillin doses

Age (years)	Dose	Number of doses/day
< 1 year	125 mg	4
1–6 years	250 mg	4
7–12 years	500 mg	4
> 12 years	500–1000 mg	4

Amoxicillin or ampicillin

TABLE 5.3.C.2 Oral amoxicillin or ampicillin doses

Age (years)	Dose	Number of doses/day
< 1 year	125 mg	4
1–7 years	250 mg	4
> 7 years	500 mg	4

Flucloxacillin, combined with amoxicillin, has good activity against *S. aureus* and *H. influenzae*.

An alternative is chloramphenicol, which is active against *S. aureus* and *H. influenzae*. Its activity against *P. aeruginosa* is poor. Children with cystic fibrosis may receive many courses of antibiotics in their lifetime, and it is important to limit the number of courses of chloramphenicol that they receive, because of the risk of aplastic anaemia. However, because chloramphenicol is cheap and readily absorbed when given orally, it is justified to use it sparingly in cystic fibrosis. The oral dose of chloramphenicol is 12.5 mg/kg 6-hourly.

If *P. aeruginosa* has been identified in sputum, or infection is suspected, use one of the following antibiotics.

Gentamicin

Dose: 7.5 mg/kg, once daily for 2 weeks.

Monitor gentamicin levels if possible. Peak is 5–10 micrograms/mL and trough is < 1 microgram/mL.

Patients with cystic fibrosis often have more rapid renal clearance and have lower levels for a given dose than other patients. If possible, combine gentamicin with another antipseudomonal antibiotic, such as ceftazidime.

Ciprofloxacin

Dose:
Age < 1 year: 7.5 mg/kg/dose.
Age 1–3 years: 62.5 mg.
Age 3–7 years: 125 mg.
Age 7–12 years: 250 mg.

All age groups should have two doses of ciprofloxacin daily, and a course will last 2 weeks.

Ceftazidime

Dose: 50 mg/kg, three times daily, given over 30 minutes for 2 weeks.

Other manifestations and complications of cystic fibrosis

In addition to those features mentioned above under clinical presentation, the following may occur:

- haemoptysis (not usually a major problem)
- pneumothorax (usually small because of chronic pleural thickening)
- bronchiectasis
- biliary cirrhosis, portal hypertension and oesophageal varices
- diabetes mellitus (requiring insulin)
- infertility (in men)
- women may become pregnant but will need careful management of their chest problems
- 'meconium ileus equivalent' (obstructed bowel occurring in older children)
- arthropathy.

With the best care or in those rare patients with mild disease, survival is possible into the fourth decade. Careful management will improve the quality of life greatly for children in resource-limited countries. Sadly, most patients with cystic fibrosis, in any part of the world, ultimately die of respiratory failure.

5.4 Cardiac disorders

5.4.A Congenital and rheumatic heart disease

BOX 5.4.A.1 Minimum standards
- Electrocardiograph.
- Chest X-ray.
- Prostaglandin E.
- Oxygen.
- Beta-blockers.

Introduction

Congenital heart disease occurs in 5–8 in 1000 live births.

Every country should have immediate access to a hospital that can surgically correct the easily curable acquired or congenital heart defects. The reality is very different with more than 90% of countries without access to such facilities.

Investigations or treatments, which are likely to be unavailable or irrelevant in the absence of a specialist cardiac centre are highlighted.

TABLE 5.4.A.1 Percentage frequency of common congenital heart defects in the UK

Ventricular septal defect (VSD)	32%
Persistent ductus arteriosus (PDA)	12%
Pulmonary stenosis	8%
Atrial septal defect (ASD)	6%
Coarctation of the aorta	6%
Tetralogy of Fallot	6%
Aortic stenosis	5%
Transposition of the great arteries	5%
Hypoplastic left heart syndrome	3%
Atrioventricular septal defect (AVSD)	2%

Cardiac defects may present as any of the following:
- cyanosis in the newborn period
- cyanosis in the older infant
- cardiovascular collapse in the newborn period
- cardiac failure in infancy
- an asymptomatic murmur.

This section explains how to recognise the presence of congenital heart disease in each of these clinical scenarios, and provides enough information to make a working diagnosis. Management decisions can then be made when modern imaging techniques are not immediately available.

The cyanotic newborn

Is there a cardiac problem?

When a child is referred as a 'blue baby', first check to see whether there is genuine central cyanosis. Examine the lips and tongue for blue discoloration, and confirm the clinical impression by measuring the oxygen saturation (less than 94% is abnormal). If there is central cyanosis this may have a cardiac or respiratory cause.

TABLE 5.4.A.2 Features that distinguish cardiac from respiratory cyanosis in the neonate

Cardiac cyanosis	Respiratory cyanosis*
Mild tachypnoea but no respiratory distress	Respiratory distress
May have cardiac signs on examination	Chest X-ray: abnormal lung fields
Arterial blood gas: $pO_2\downarrow$, $pCO_2\downarrow$ or normal	Arterial blood gas: $pO_2\downarrow$, $pCO_2\uparrow$ or normal
Fails hyperoxia test	Passes hyperoxia test

*A respiratory cause for cyanosis is more likely in infants born preterm.

The hyperoxia test is performed as follows:
1. Ensure that there is good IV access.
2. Monitor oxygen saturations continuously.
3. Give 100% oxygen for 10 minutes.
4. Take an arterial blood gas sample in the right arm (preductal).
   - If pO_2 is lower than 20 kPa (150 mmHg), a cardiac cause of cyanosis is likely (the test is 'failed').
   - If pO_2 is higher than 20 kPa, a respiratory cause of cyanosis is likely (the test is 'passed').
   - Although pulse oximetry cannot reliably be used in place of an arterial blood gas, a resting saturation of less than 80% and a saturation of less than 90% after 10 minutes in 100% oxygen suggests cyanotic heart disease requiring early intervention.
   - **Note: Oxygen administration could cause closure of the arterial duct, precipitating profound hypoxaemia in some types of cyanotic congenital heart disease.**
   - Prostaglandin E (which opens the duct) should therefore be available at the time of the test and should be given if oxygenation deteriorates.

Persistent pulmonary hypertension of the newborn (PPHN) may often mimic cyanotic heart disease using these clinical criteria. However, PPHN is usually distinguished by a history of fetal distress, resuscitation is often needed at birth, and there may be neurological signs. Improvements in oxygenation may be possible after intubation and ventilation, and saturations in the right arm may be significantly higher than those in the feet, suggesting right-to-left shunting across the arterial duct.

What type of cardiac defect is present?

Cyanotic cardiac defects can be divided into three broad categories, as described below.

Once cyanotic congenital heart disease is suspected, attempt to place the defect in one of the three categories. This may be done using Table 5.4.A.3, which describes the typical findings in each physiological category. These guidelines assist the clinician but are not infallible, and the nature of the defect is sometimes only clear after echocardiography.

Cyanotic heart diseases

Low pulmonary blood flow

In defects where there is low pulmonary blood flow the physiology is the same regardless of the precise anatomy of the defect. Deoxygenated blood returning from the systemic veins cannot flow through the right side of the heart to the lungs. The pulmonary blood supply is therefore via the arterial duct. The deoxygenated blood from the right side of the heart shunts to the left side of the heart (via either an atrial or a ventricular septal defect), and the left ventricle receives both deoxygenated blood from the right heart and oxygenated blood from the pulmonary venous return. Blood entering the aorta is therefore not fully oxygenated, and the child appears cyanosed. If the duct closes, the infant becomes profoundly cyanosed and is unlikely to survive unless pulmonary blood flow is rapidly restored. This is **duct-dependent pulmonary circulation**, an example of which is shown in Figure 5.4.A.1.

Complete transposition of the great arteries (TGA)

Here the aorta arises from the right ventricle and the pulmonary artery arises from the left ventricle (*see* Figure 5.4.A.2). Systemic venous return enters the right side of the heart and is recirculated to the systemic arteries. Pulmonary venous return enters the left side of the heart and is recirculated to the lungs. Oxygenated blood and deoxygenated blood are therefore separated in two parallel circuits. Oxygenated blood enters the systemic circulation only when there is mixing between the two circuits. Mixing occurs at atrial level (across the foramen ovale) and at ductal level (while

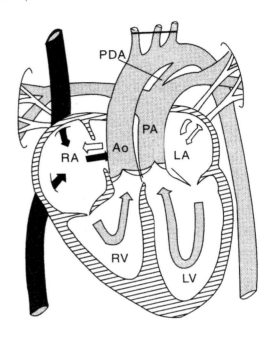

FIGURE 5.4.A.2. Transposition of the great arteries. For explanation of abbreviations, see legend to Figure 5.4.A.1.

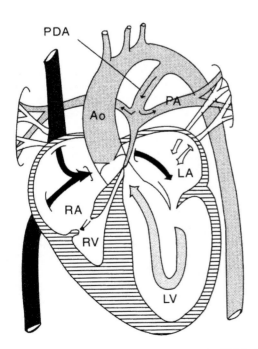

FIGURE 5.4.A.1 The circulation in pulmonary atresia with intact ventricular septum. PDA, patent ductus arteriosus; Ao, aorta; PA, pulmonary artery; LA, left atrium; LV, left ventricle; RV, right ventricle; RA, right atrium.

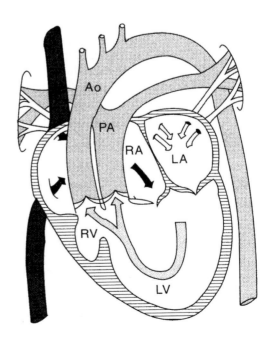

FIGURE 5.4.A.3 The circulation in double-outlet left ventricle. For explanation of abbreviations, see legend to Figure 5.4.A.1.

the duct remains open). Systemic oxygen saturation reflects the amount of mixing (which in turn depends on the size of these communications). If the atrial communication is small, oxygenation may therefore be duct dependent.

Common mixing lesions

In common mixing lesions, oxygenated pulmonary venous blood and deoxygenated systemic venous blood mix in one of the cardiac chambers. An example is shown in Figure 5.4.A.3. The systemic output is therefore only partly oxygenated. The relative amounts of pulmonary and systemic

blood in the mixture determine the oxygen saturation and the mode of presentation. If pulmonary blood flow is high, cyanosis is minimal, and the child usually presents at about 2 months of age in heart failure. If pulmonary blood flow is low (the complex lesion may coexist with pulmonary stenosis), cyanosis is severe and is often detected early.

Once the defect has been placed in one of these categories, immediate management decisions can be made. Although it is not imperative to reach a more specific diagnosis, an anatomical diagnosis can sometimes be made using clinical information and simple investigations.

TABLE 5.4.A.3 Features that help to distinguish the three types of cyanotic congenital heart defect

	Low pulmonary blood flow	Complete TGA	Common mixing lesion
pO_2 at rest SaO_2 at rest	Often $\leq$ 35 mmHg < 80%	Often $\leq$ 35 mmHg < 80%	Often $\geq$ 45 mmHg 80–90%
pO_2 hyperoxia test SaO_2 hyperoxia	Often $\leq$ 50 mmHg < 90%	Often $\leq$ 50 mmHg < 90%	75–200 mmHg 90–100%
Chest X-ray	Reduced pulmonary vascular markings	Normal or increased pulmonary vascular markings with or without narrow mediastinum	Normal or increased pulmonary vascular markings

TABLE 5.4.A.4 Conditions with low pulmonary blood flow

Critical pulmonary stenosis
Pulmonary atresia with intact ventricular septum
Tetralogy of Fallot (with severe right ventricular outflow tract obstruction)
Pulmonary atresia with ventricular septal defect
Absent right atrioventricular connection

Pulmonary atresia with intact ventricular septum and critical pulmonary stenosis

These two conditions are similar pathologies with either complete or almost complete closure of the pulmonary valve. Both are often associated with hypoplasia of the right ventricle. There is either no murmur or a soft murmur at the lower left sternal border (tricuspid regurgitation). The chest X-ray usually shows a normal heart size. The precordial leads on the ECG usually show decreased right ventricular voltages (small R waves in leads V1 and V2) and dominant left ventricular voltages (prominent S waves in leads V1 and V2 and prominent R waves in leads V5 and V6).

Tetralogy of Fallot and pulmonary atresia with ventricular septal defect

These two pathologies are also similar, but in Fallot's tetralogy the right ventricular outflow tract is patent, albeit narrow, generating a high-pitched ejection systolic murmur at the upper left sternal border. In both defects, the cardiac silhouette on the chest X-ray has a concavity on the left heart border where there is usually a convexity produced by the right ventricular outflow tract and pulmonary artery. The ECG shows dominant right ventricular voltages (normal neonatal RS progression).

Absent right atrioventricular connection (also known as tricuspid atresia)

There is often a long harsh systolic murmur (this may arise from a restrictive ventricular septal defect or pulmonary stenosis). The precordial leads on the ECG show decreased

right ventricular voltages and dominant left ventricular voltages. The QRS axis is characteristically directed to the left and superiorly between 0 and –90 degrees.

Complete transposition of the great arteries

There is usually no murmur. The ECG shows dominant right ventricular voltages (normal neonatal RS progression). Therefore, if a newborn is severely cyanosed and otherwise appears clinically normal, actively look for a narrow mediastinum on the chest X-ray to help to make the diagnosis.

Management of defects with low pulmonary blood flow or complete TGA

- Do not give oxygen after the hyperoxia test, as it may precipitate ductal closure.
- Start IV prostaglandin E (PGE) to maintain ductal patency. There are two formulations, namely prostaglandin E1 (PGE1) and prostaglandin E2 (PGE2). Commence PGE1 at 25 nanograms/kg/minute or PGE2 at 5 nanograms/kg/minute.
- PGE infusion is made up by adding 30 micrograms/kg of prostaglandin to 50 mL of 5% dextrose (if the pump runs at 1 mL/hour this is equivalent to 10 nanograms/kg/minute).
- If saturations are initially very low and fail to improve 10 minutes after starting PGE, intubate and ventilate the baby in air and increase the PGE dose to 50 nanograms/kg/minute. The dose can be increased further to a maximum of 100 nanograms/kg/minute if there is still no response. Prostaglandin sometimes causes vasodilation, so fluid boluses may be required at high doses of PGE in order to maintain blood pressure.
- PGE often causes hypoventilation and apnoea (particularly at doses of PGE2 above 10 nanograms/kg/minute). If oxygen saturations initially improve with PGE and then start to fall, assess respiratory effort. If respiration is shallow or slow, intubate and ventilate in air.
- If oxygen saturations start to fall after PGE is started, and respiratory effort appears adequate, increase the

PGE dose stepwise until a response is seen. At doses over 10 nanograms/kg/minute watch very carefully for hypoventilation.

- Arrange for an urgent paediatric cardiology review and transfer the child to a cardiac centre.
- Defects with poor pulmonary blood flow usually require a systemic to pulmonary artery shunt (modified Blalock–Taussig shunt) to provide a stable pulmonary blood supply. Where special interventional expertise is available it may be possible to implant a coronary stent in the duct to maintain patency and avoid surgery.
- TGA often requires enlargement of the interatrial communication by balloon atrial septostomy, followed by an arterial switch operation if surgical expertise is available.
- For critical pulmonary valve stenosis or pulmonary atresia, early intervention to open the pulmonary valve is required. This can be done by the transcatheter route if interventional expertise is available.

Management of common mixing lesions

- Monitor the child on the neonatal unit.
- Arrange for an echocardiogram as soon as possible to define the anatomy.
- If oxygen saturations fall progressively to less than 70%, commence PGE and arrange for an urgent paediatric cardiology review.
- Once the anatomy is defined it may be possible to discharge the baby without further treatment (after paediatric cardiology advice has been obtained).

The older infant with cyanosis

Is there a cardiac problem?

When an older infant presents with cyanosis, cardiac pathology is likely if:

- Respiratory distress is not severe.
- There is no carbon dioxide retention.
- Respiratory pathology is not evident on the chest X-ray.
- The cardiovascular examination is abnormal (see below).

What type of cardiac defect is present?

The cyanotic defects that commonly present after the neonatal period are tetralogy of Fallot and cyanotic defects with high pulmonary blood flow. They may escape detection at birth because cyanosis is initially only mild. In tetralogy of Fallot, there is right ventricular outflow tract obstruction and a large ventricular septal defect (VSD) (right ventricular hypertrophy and aortic override are the other components of the tetralogy). The right ventricular outflow tract obstruction limits blood flow to the pulmonary arteries, causing deoxygenated blood to shunt right to left across the VSD, resulting in cyanosis. With time, the right ventricular outflow tract obstruction usually becomes more severe, causing further reductions in pulmonary blood flow, more right to left shunting, and increasing cyanosis.

Cyanotic defects with high pulmonary blood flow

In cyanotic defects with high pulmonary blood flow (mostly common mixing defects), pulmonary flow increases as pulmonary vascular resistance decreases over the first few weeks of life, resulting in progressively worsening cardiac failure.

TABLE 5.4.A.5 Cyanotic defects with high pulmonary blood flow

Truncus arteriosus
Total anomalous pulmonary venous connection
Double-outlet left ventricle
Absent right atrioventricular connection with large ventricular septal defect (tricuspid atresia)
Pulmonary atresia with large or multiple aorto-pulmonary collateral arteries
TGA with large ventricular septal defect

Findings in defects with high pulmonary blood flow

- May present with cardiac failure at 2–6 weeks of age.
- Active praecordium.
- Murmur usually present (may be systolic, diastolic or continuous).
- Increased pulmonary vascular markings on chest X-ray.

Management of cyanotic defects with high pulmonary blood flow

Define the anatomy by echocardiography. Manage cardiac failure medically (see Section 5.4.B). Surgical correction or pulmonary artery banding will be necessary in most cases.

Findings in tetralogy of Fallot

- May present with increasing cyanosis.
- May present with an ejection systolic murmur at the upper left sternal border.
- Reduced pulmonary vascular markings on chest X-ray, and concavity on the left heart border where there is usually a convexity produced by the right ventricular outflow tract and pulmonary artery.
- Children are often asymptomatic, but there may be sudden periods of increased cyanosis known as hypercyanotic spells.

Characteristics of hypercyanotic spells

- Spells often occur on waking from sleep or after feeding.
- The infant becomes restless and agitated.
- There is increased cyanosis and pallor.
- Respiration is often rapid and shallow.
- In severe spells, crying is followed by limpness or loss of consciousness.
- Spells usually last 1–5 minutes, but may last longer when severe.
- The ejection systolic murmur shortens or becomes inaudible.

Management of tetralogy of Fallot

The anatomy should be confirmed by echocardiography, preferably within a few weeks of presentation, and surgical correction should be carried out between 6 and 12 months of age (although it can be carried out later).

Hypercyanotic spells may be life-threatening. If a child starts to have such spells, discuss this with a paediatric cardiologist immediately, as it is an indication for urgent surgery.

If hypercyanotic spells are more than a few minutes in duration, treat them urgently as follows:

- Knee–chest position.
- Give oxygen by face mask.
- Give an IV bolus of Ringer-lactate or Hartmann's solution

10–20 mL/kg, as during spells children are often relatively hypovolaemic.

- Give IV or IM morphine, 100 microgram/kg (or IV ketamine 1 mg/kg).
- Give IV propranolol at an initial dose of 20 micrograms/kg with a maximum of 100 micrograms/kg (have isoprenaline ready in case of excessive β–blockade).
- Adrenaline may make spells worse.
- General anaesthesia and artificial ventilation are needed in intractable cases.
- If cyanosis persists, consider an emergency aorto-pulmonary shunt.

Neonatal cardiovascular collapse

Is there a cardiac problem?

When a child presents in shock in the first month of life, the working diagnosis is often dehydration or sepsis. The following features help to distinguish cardiac causes of poor systemic output from non-cardiac causes:

- collapse in the first 2 weeks of life
- poor feeding, lethargy and tachypnoea prior to collapse
- hepatomegaly
- pulmonary oedema and cardiomegaly on chest X-ray
- lack of response to intravascular volume expansion.

What type of cardiac defect is present?

Left heart obstruction is the most likely cardiac cause of cardiovascular collapse with low systemic output in the first 2 weeks of life:

TABLE 5.4.A.6 Left heart obstruction

Critical aortic stenosis
Hypoplastic left heart syndrome (HLHS)
Coarctation of the aorta
Interrupted aortic arch

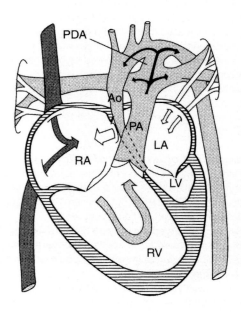

FIGURE 5.4.A.4 Hypoplastic left heart. For explanation of abbreviations, see legend to Figure 5.4.A.1.

Hypoplastic left heart syndrome

In hypoplastic left heart syndrome all of the left heart structures are small (see Figure 5.4.A.4). There is insufficient forward flow through the left ventricle and the aortic valve to support the systemic circulation. Pulmonary venous return cannot pass through the left heart, so it crosses the atrial septum and enters the right atrium, mixing with systemic venous return. Mixed pulmonary and systemic venous blood enters the right ventricle and is pumped to the pulmonary arteries and also across the arterial duct to supply the systemic circulation. Ductal flow passes to the descending aorta and retrogradely around the aortic arch to supply the head and neck vessels and the coronary arteries. Ductal flow is not fully oxygenated, so there is a degree of central cyanosis. When the duct closes, the cardiac output falls precipitously, the infant becomes shocked, and cardiac failure develops. This is duct-dependent systemic circulation. The haemodynamics are the same in **critical aortic stenosis**.

Coarctation of the aorta

Coarctation of the aorta consists of a narrowing in the descending aorta close to the aortic end of the arterial duct. Contractile tissue may extend from the duct into the aorta so that when the duct closes it draws in the adjacent section of aorta, causing obstruction. Flow to the head and neck vessels is maintained, but flow to the lower body distal to the coarctation site is dramatically reduced. The infant becomes shocked and acidotic. Cardiac failure develops secondary to high systemic afterload. This is also an example of the systemic circulation depending on ductal patency (although systemic blood flow may not directly depend on a right-to-left shunt through the duct). In **interrupted aortic arch**, perfusion to the lower part of the body depends on right-to-left ductal flow and presentation is similar to that with coarctation.

The following features help to distinguish between the lesions:

- If all of the pulses are weak or absent, consider HLHS or critical aortic stenosis.
- If the right arm pulses are palpable and the femoral pulses are weak or absent, consider coarctation or interrupted aortic arch (note, however, that all pulses may initially be impalpable if the cardiac output is poor).
- If four limb blood pressures demonstrate significantly lower blood pressures in the legs than in the right arm (a gradient of more than 20 mmHg), consider coarctation or interrupted aortic arch.
- Coarctation often presents towards the beginning of the second week of life.
- HLHS often presents in the first 2 days of life.
- In HLHS, the ECG shows reduced left ventricular voltages (small R waves in leads V5 and V6).

Other cardiac causes of cardiovascular collapse in the first few weeks of life are supraventricular tachycardia (SVT) (see Section 5.4.C) and cyanotic congenital heart disease with duct-dependent pulmonary blood flow (when the duct closes, the ensuing profound hypoxaemia causes acidosis and cardiovascular collapse). SVT should be evident on the ECG and cyanotic heart disease should be suspected when the oxygen saturation remains low after instituting the management described below for left heart obstruction.

Emergency management of low systemic output secondary to left heart obstruction

1. Check the ECG (to exclude SVT as a cause of collapse).
2. Obtain peripheral IV access if not already established (if IV access is difficult, intra-osseous access should be obtained).
3. Give a fluid bolus of 10 mL/kg Ringer-lactate or Hartmann's solution if not already given.
4. Intubate and ventilate if there is significant respiratory distress (high PEEP, 8–10 cmH$_2$O).
5. Once ventilated, commence prostaglandin E$_1$ or E$_2$ at 100 nanograms/kg/minute (give for 30 minutes, then reduce to 25 nanograms/kg/minute, reducing again to 10 nanograms/kg/minute when stabilised). If the initial clinical condition is not poor, commence PGE$_2$ at a lower dose of 10 nanograms/kg/minute, which should avoid PGE-related apnoea and the need for ventilation.
6. Admit the child to the paediatric ICU.
7. Check blood sugar levels, full blood count, urea and electrolytes, coagulation, calcium levels and magnesium levels, and correct abnormalities.
8. Take blood cultures and treat with IV antibiotics, as sepsis cannot be excluded.
9. Check arterial blood gas (using the right arm if possible).
10. Give IV furosemide 1 mg/kg if the chest X-ray shows pulmonary oedema.
11. Insert central venous access and an arterial line.
12. Reassess whether further intravascular volume is needed (give if the central venous pressure is low).
13. Give dopamine 5–10 micrograms/kg/minute if perfusion remains poor or the blood pressure remains low.
14. Give adrenaline 0.1–0.2 micrograms/kg/minute if perfusion remains poor or the blood pressure remains low (by central venous access only).
15. If acidosis is profound and not improving with other measures, give IV sodium bicarbonate 4.2%.
16. Ask for an urgent paediatric cardiology review and advice.

Asymptomatic murmurs

When a child presents with an asymptomatic murmur, first examine them for cyanosis and measure the oxygen saturation. If there is desaturation, refer the child for an echocardiogram, as cyanotic congenital heart disease requires a detailed anatomical assessment. Tetralogy of Fallot is the most likely diagnosis. If cyanosis is excluded, the child may have an innocent cardiac murmur or one of the following defects.

TABLE 5.4.A.7 Initially asymptomatic heart lesions

Left-to-right shunts	Left or right heart obstruction
Small to moderate-sized VSD	Pulmonary stenosis
Small to moderate-sized PDA	Aortic stenosis
Atrial septal defect (ASD)	Coarctation of the aorta
Partial AVSD	

Innocent murmurs are characterised as follows:
- The Still's murmur is a vibratory short systolic murmur heard at the lower left sternal border or apex.
- The venous hum is a soft continuous murmur heard best below the clavicles, and is abolished by pressure over the jugular vein or lying down with the neck flexed.
- The pulmonary flow murmur is a soft ejection systolic murmur at the upper left sternal border, and may be confused with an ASD or mild pulmonary stenosis.
- The neck bruit is an ejection systolic murmur that is maximal above the clavicle and may be confused with aortic stenosis.

The cardiac defects are characterised as follows:
- In **coarctation**, the right arm blood pressure is often elevated, the femoral pulses are weak or impalpable, and there is brachiofemoral delay.
- The **patent ductus arteriosus (PDA)** has a continuous murmur that is loudest in the left infraclavicular region.
- The **ventricular septal defect (VSD)** has a harsh pansystolic murmur that is loudest at the lower left sternal border radiating to the lower right sternal border.
- **Aortic stenosis, pulmonary stenosis, atrial septal defect (ASD)** and **partial atrioventricular septal defect (AVSD)** all have an ejection systolic murmur at the upper left sternal border.
  - In **aortic stenosis** the ejection systolic murmur is harsh and may be heard at the upper right and left sternal border. The murmur radiates to the carotid arteries and there is often a carotid thrill. There may be an ejection click at the apex if the stenosis is at valvar level.
  - In **pulmonary stenosis**, the ejection systolic murmur is harsh and radiates to the back. There may be an ejection click along the left sternal border if the stenosis is at valvar level.
  - In an **atrial septal defect (ASD)** there is a soft ejection systolic murmur at the upper left sternal border from increased flow across the pulmonary valve. There is sometimes a fixed widely split second heart sound, and there may be a mid-diastolic murmur at the lower left sternal border (from increased flow across the tricuspid valve) when the left-to-right shunt is large.
  - In **partial atrioventricular septal defect (AVSD)** there is an abnormal atrioventricular valve and a defect in the atrial septum. There may be a blowing pansystolic murmur at the lower left sternal border or apex from atrioventricular valve regurgitation. The ejection systolic murmur may mimic an ASD, but the defect is distinguished by a superior QRS axis on the ECG.

Unless the murmur is clearly innocent, perform an ECG and chest X-ray.

Right ventricular hypertrophy (RVH) is indicated by an R wave in lead V1 > 98th centile for age (^{3} 20 mm is always abnormal), a neonatal RS progression beyond the neonatal period (dominant R waves in lead V1 and dominant S waves in lead V6) or an upright T wave in lead V1 before the teenage years.

Left ventricular hypertrophy (LVH) is indicated by T inversion in leads V5 and V6, loss of the Q wave in lead V6 or the amplitude of the R wave in lead V6 plus S wave in lead V1 > 98th centile for age (^{3} 50 mm is always abnormal). RVH may indicate significant right heart obstruction or high pulmonary artery pressure (secondary to a large left-to-right shunt or pulmonary vascular disease). LVH may indicate significant left heart obstruction. Cardiomegaly and increased pulmonary vascular markings on the chest X-ray may indicate a large left-to-right shunt.

Any child who is thought to have an anatomical defect on the basis of the clinical examination, or any child with an abnormal ECG or chest X-ray, should if possible be referred to a paediatric cardiologist for an echocardiogram and opinion. If there is evidence of a significant left-to-right shunt (see Section 5.4.B) in a VSD or PDA, the referral should be as soon as possible, as there is still a risk of pulmonary vascular disease even when the child does not present in heart failure.

Rheumatic fever

For the diagnosis and treatment of rheumatic fever, see Section 5.13.

Long-term consequences of rheumatic fever

After an attack of acute rheumatic fever there may be permanent valve damage. Rheumatic heart disease occurs when acute valve inflammation is followed by scarring and fibrosis, resulting in various degrees of shortening, thickening, rigidity, deformity, retraction and fusion of the valve cusps. The commonest valve lesions are mitral regurgitation, mitral stenosis and aortic regurgitation.

Rheumatic heart disease is most severe and progressive in (1) children who initially have severe carditis in (2) children who have recurrent attacks of acute rheumatic fever. The prognosis is more favourable if recurrences are prevented (residual cardiac disease may disappear or improve and valve damage only worsens in a few cases). It is therefore crucial to maintain continuous antibiotic prophylaxis to prevent further valve damage, particularly as children are prone to develop a recurrence after the initial attack (below).

Mitral regurgitation

Mitral regurgitation is the commonest valve lesion in children with rheumatic heart disease. Patients are often asymptomatic during childhood as symptoms are caused by left ventricular failure which may take as long as two decades to develop. However, cases may present before adolescence and mitral regurgitation may be rapidly progressive in regions where the incidence of rheumatic fever is high and recurrent rheumatic fever is common. Mitral regurgitation may be diagnosed by the presence of a blowing apical pansystolic murmur radiating to the left axilla. There may also be a third heart sound and a short low frequency mid-diastolic murmur from increased transmitral flow.

Features of severe mitral regurgitation:
- Easy fatigue (caused by low cardiac output)
- Shortness of breath on exertion (caused by pulmonary oedema)
- Hyperdynamic apical impulse and pansystolic murmur
- Apical impulse displaced laterally and inferiorly
- The chest X ray demonstrates cardiomegaly and left atrial enlargement (a double density on the right heart border and elevation of the left main bronchus)
- The ECG demonstrates left atrial enlargement (broad bifid P waves in lead II and a prominent negative component to the P in V1) and left ventricular hypertrophy
- Signs of pulmonary hypertension (see below).

If there are features of severe mitral regurgitation, the child should be urgently referred for a paediatric cardiology opinion as surgery is likely to be necessary. Ideally all children

with mitral regurgitation should be evaluated by echocardiography annually, as progressive left heart dilation may result in irreversible left ventricular dysfunction if referral is delayed until symptoms develop. Medical treatment should be given for heart failure (captopril is particularly useful) but children who are unwell enough to require this often need either a mitral valve repair or a mitral valve replacement with a mechanical valve or bioprosthesis.

Mitral stenosis

If there is effective antibiotic prophylaxis, mitral stenosis usually develops slowly over 5–10 years and is often not sufficiently severe to cause symptoms in childhood. The reality in countries where there is inadequate prophylaxis and recurrent attacks of rheumatic fever are common is that mitral stenosis may progress much more rapidly and symptoms may be evident 6 months to 3 years after the first attack. Mild stenosis does not cause symptoms, moderate stenosis causes shortness of breath on exertion and severe stenosis causes easy fatigue, shortness of breath at rest, orthopnoea, paroxysmal nocturnal dyspnoea and haemop-tysis. Mitral stenosis may be diagnosed by the presence of a low frequency mid-diastolic murmur maximal at the apex. The murmur may be accentuated by exercise and is often accompanied by a loud first heart sound and a diastolic opening snap. The murmur becomes longer as the severity of the stenosis increases. In severe cases there are also signs of pulmonary hypertension.

Signs of pulmonary hypertension:
- Left parasternal heave
- Loud second heart sound
- Early diastolic murmur of pulmonary regurgitation at the upper left sternal border
- Elevated JVP and hepatomegaly if there is right heart failure.

The chest X ray and ECG often show left atrial enlargement when there is moderate mitral stenosis. Radiographic signs of pulmonary oedema may be evident when stenosis is severe. ECG changes of right ventricular hypertrophy and right axis deviation are present when there is pulmonary hypertension. Symptoms should be treated with diuretics and a low-sodium diet. Digoxin is only indicated in rare cases where there is atrial fibrillation secondary to left atrial enlargement. Symptomatic children and children with signs of pulmonary hypertension should be referred for paediatric cardiology review as surgery is often necessary. The options for treatment are open or closed mitral commissurotomy, mitral valve replacement and percutaneous catheter balloon mitral commissurotomy.

Aortic regurgitation

Aortic regurgitation is less common than mitral regurgitation and frequently occurs in combination with mitral valve disease. Affected children usually remain asymptomatic for many years as symptoms only become evident when left ventricular dysfunction develops secondary to chronic left ventricular volume overload. Severe symptomatic aortic regurgitation may however become established within 1–2 years of the initial attack of rheumatic fever if recurrence is not prevented. Once symptoms appear deterioration is often rapid. Symptoms include exercise intolerance, shortness of breath on exertion and chest pain in a few severely affected cases. Examination reveals a blowing decrescendo early diastolic murmur maximal at the mid to lower left sternal border. The murmur is loudest sitting forward with the breath held in expiration.

Signs of moderate to severe aortic regurgitation:

- The murmur lengthens and may be throughout diastole
- Hyperdynamic apex
- Apical impulse displaced laterally and inferiorly
- Wide pulse pressure
- Collapsing pulses
- Visible pulsations in the suprasternal notch and neck vessels
- Systolic murmur at the upper right sternal border (from increased aortic valve flow).

If patients are symptomatic or have signs of severe aortic regurgitation they should be referred for paediatric cardiology assessment as surgery may be necessary. Marked cardiomegaly on the chest X ray or multiple ventricular ectopics on the ECG should also prompt referral. Ideally all children with aortic regurgitation should have an echocardiogram at least annually as it is important to assess left ventricular dilation and function to ensure that surgery is carried out before irreversible left ventricular dysfunction develops. Exercise tolerance may be improved by captopril treatment and medical treatment for heart failure may be necessary in severe cases. Surgical options include aortic valve reconstruction, aortic valve replacement with an aortic homograft or mechanical valve and transferring the patient's own pulmonary valve to the aortic position (Ross procedure).

5.4.B The child with heart failure and cardiomyopathy

BOX 5.4.B.1 Minimum standards
- Electrocardiograph.
- Chest X-ray.
- Furosemide.
- Spironolactone.
- Anticoagulant.

Introduction

Heart failure occurs when the heart is unable to pump enough blood to meet the metabolic needs of the body. The term is often used to indicate the clinical changes that occur when the cardiac pump cannot meet the workload it is presented with. This may occur either because the pump is weak (due to a primary abnormality of the cardiac muscle) or because the workload imposed on the heart is higher than normal. The latter is the case in congenital heart disease, where heart failure occurs because the heart is pumping against a high resistance (in the case of obstructive lesions) or because it is volume loaded (commonly in left-to-right shunting cardiac lesions).

Left-to-right shunting cardiac defects are the commonest cause of heart failure in infancy identified in well-resourced countries.

In resource-poor countries most heart failure is related either to severe anaemia or to fluid overload when treating infections or severe malnutrition, particularly with IV fluids or during blood transfusion (see below).

The physiology of left-to-right shunts

A large defect between the ventricles or great arteries allows free communication between the left and right sides of the heart. Left and right heart pressures therefore equalise, and pulmonary artery pressure is maintained at systemic level. The pulmonary vascular resistance then determines the pulmonary blood flow. In the newborn period the pulmonary vascular resistance is high, which limits the pulmonary blood flow and therefore the left-to-right shunt across the defect. Over the first 6 weeks of life, the pulmonary vascular resistance gradually falls, allowing pulmonary blood flow and the left-to-right shunt to increase. This gives rise to heart failure, which usually appears after 4 weeks of age. If the pulmonary arteries are exposed to high pressure and flow for a prolonged period, pulmonary vascular disease develops. This normally becomes significant between 12 and 18 months of age. High pulmonary vascular resistance secondary to pulmonary vascular disease reduces the left-to-right shunt, and symptoms of heart failure gradually resolve. Eventually, pulmonary resistance becomes so high that flow across the defect becomes right to left, and cyanosis develops (Eisenmenger's syndrome). The pulmonary artery pressure remains high throughout, and it is only the amount of flow through the lungs that changes.

Is heart failure present?

TABLE 5.4.B.1 Diagnosis of heart failure secondary to **congenital heart disease in infancy**

Symptoms	Signs
Easily tired	Failure to thrive
Poor feeding	Tachypnoea
Breathlessness (particularly during feeds)	Increased respiratory effort
	Tachycardia > 160 bpm
Sweaty (particularly during feeds)	Sweating
	Pallor
	Hepatomegaly
	Gallop rhythm

What type of cardiac defect is present?

Heart failure in the first few weeks of life is a medical emergency.

The following causes should be considered:

- supraventricular tachycardia
- complete atrioventricular block
- high-output cardiac failure
- left heart obstruction.

Perform an ECG to detect supraventricular tachycardia and heart block. Check the haemoglobin level, as severe anaemia may cause high-output cardiac failure. Also examine the baby for cranial and hepatic bruits, as cranial and hepatic arteriovenous malformations are a potential (although very rare) cause of high-output cardiac failure.

If these tests are negative, refer the child to a paediatric cardiologist, as a left heart obstructive lesion is likely and there may be duct-dependent systemic circulation. Consider the use of prostaglandin to keep the ductus arteriosus open until the referral can be achieved (*see* Section 5.4.A).

Heart failure in infancy presenting after the first few weeks of life may be caused by any of the following:

- the left-to-right shunting lesions listed in Table 5.4.B.2
- cyanotic congenital heart defects with high pulmonary blood flow
- the same causes that present in the first few weeks of life
- myocarditis or cardiomyopathy.

TABLE 5.4.B.2 Common left-to-right shunting lesions that cause heart failure

Large ventricular septal defect (VSD)
Atrioventricular septal defect with large ventricular component (AVSD)
Large persistent ductus arteriosus (PDA)

Examine the child for cyanosis and measure the oxygen saturation. It should be possible to detect those children with cyanotic defects immediately (note, however, that children with AVSD are sometimes mildly desaturated). Next, attempt to detect the children with left-to-right shunts, looking for the following features which are present in significant shunts:

- hyperdynamic precordial impulse
- apical impulse displaced laterally and inferiorly
- apical mid-diastolic murmur (from increased flow across the mitral valve)
- loud second heart sound (from increased pulmonary artery diastolic pressure)
- cardiomegaly and increased pulmonary vascular markings on the chest X-ray
- signs of heart failure and pulmonary oedema on the chest X-ray in severe cases.

If these examination findings are not present and there is no evidence of SVT or a hyperdynamic circulation (see above), a left heart obstructive lesion should be considered. **Some of these are eminently treatable conditions** and if they are suspected the child should be referred for paediatric cardiology review without delay.

If there is evidence of a large left-to-right shunt, refer the child to a paediatric cardiologist within a few weeks. These signs must not be missed, as a remediable cardiac defect is rendered inoperable by delay.

Although it is not imperative to make a more specific diagnosis, the following clinical features discriminate between the three most common left-to-right shunts:

- The persistent arterial duct has a continuous murmur that is maximal in the left infraclavicular area.
- A large ventricular septal defect has a quiet pansystolic murmur that is maximal at the lower left sternal border radiating to the lower right sternal border. There may also be a soft ejection systolic murmur at the upper left sternal border from increased flow across the pulmonary valve.
- An atrioventricular septal defect with a large ventricular component may have a blowing pansystolic murmur at the lower left sternal border or apex from atrioventricular

valve regurgitation. The ECG shows a characteristic superior QRS axis (between −30 and −180 degrees).

Heart failure in later infancy and childhood

In addition to the symptoms seen in early infancy (easily tired, poor feeding, breathlessness particularly during feeds, excess sweating particularly during feeds), older children may have decreased exercise tolerance, shortness of breath on exertion and when lying flat.

The signs of heart failure are cyanosis or $SaO_2 < 94\%$, basal lung crepitations, failure to thrive, tachypnoea > 50 breaths/minute for children aged 2–12 months, tachypnoea > 40 breaths/minute for children aged 12 months to 5 years and the cut-offs for tachycardia are > 120 bpm aged 1–5 years and > 100 bpm after age 5 years.

There is usually increased respiratory effort, sweating, pallor and hepatomegaly.

In older children the hepatomegaly may be tender, a gallop rhythm may be heard and a raised jugular venous pressure may be observed.

In addition to the congenital heart defects described in Section 5.4.A the following causes of heart failure should be considered:

- Severe anaemia
- Severe malnutrition
- Excessive intravenous fluids
- Rheumatic fever
- Myocarditis
- Cardiomyopathy
- Infective endocarditis
- Constrictive pericarditis (rare and most often caused by tuberculosis) (*see* Section 6.1.N).

Anaemia is a common and often severe problem in poorly resourced settings (*see* Section 5.11.A). When the haemoglobin falls below 7 g/dl cardiac output must increase to maintain oxygen delivery and heart failure frequently develops with a haemoglobin < 5 g/dl). The treatment is careful blood transfusion, but the increase in intravascular volume may precipitate worsening heart failure. Blood must therefore be infused slowly in small boluses and an exchange transfusion may be needed if there is clinical deterioration. Furosemide 1 mg/kg IV may be given during transfusion (*see* Section 5.11.A).

Protein-calorie malnutrition is also an important cause of cardiac failure in disadvantaged countries (*see* Section 5.10.B) with specific contributions from certain vitamin deficiencies (*see* Section 5.10.A). Although cardiac failure is unusual at presentation, it may occur after several days of refeeding. Rapid refeeding can cause a hypermetabolic state, demanding an increase in cardiac output which cannot be met by the malnourished heart which has a decreased cardiac reserve. The problem is exacerbated by coexisting anaemia, blood transfusion, inappropriate intravenous fluid administration and high sodium diets.

The other common causes of cardiac failure are dealt with individually in the sections below.

Management of heart failure

Monitor heart and respiratory rates, respiratory distress and oxygenation regularly during treatment of acute heart failure. It is necessary to both control the symptoms of failure and to determine and treat the underlying cause.

- Treat severe anaemia if present, be careful with IV fluids and ensure adequate nutrition.
- Nasogastric feeding if there is inadequate oral intake.
- For older children nurse sitting up with legs dependent
- Treat hypoxaemia with oxygen to keep $SaO_2 > 94\%$.
- In an emergency where there is pulmonary oedema, give furosemide 1 mg/kg IV which should produce a diuresis within 2 hours. If the initial dose is ineffective, give 2 mg/kg IV and repeat after 12 hours if necessary.
- For chronic heart failure give oral furosemide 1 mg/kg once a day, twice a day or three times a day.
- Spironolactone 1 mg/kg once a day or twice a day in combination with furosemide, matching the dose frequency, to enhance diuresis and prevent furosemide-related hypokalaemia.
- If furosemide is used without spironolactone, oral potassium 3–5 mmol/kg/day, should be given (supplemental potassium is not required if furosemide is given for less than 4 days).

If more than twice daily diuretics are required, consider using captopril. Captopril should be commenced in hospital with a 100 microgram/kg test dose. The dose should then be increased gradually over a number of days 100–300 microgram/kg 2–3 times a day to a maximum total dose of 4 mg/kg daily. After the test dose and each increment monitor the blood pressure carefully, as hypotension is common. Reduce the dose if significant hypotension occurs. Monitor urea and electrolytes daily while building up the dose, as renal failure is a well-recognised side effect. Stop spironolactone when the captopril dose is greater than 500 micrograms/kg per day as both drugs cause potassium retention. Do not give captopril if there is left heart obstruction.

Cardiomyopathy and myocarditis

Myocarditis and dilated cardiomyopathy both cause impairment of myocardial contractility. This results in a dilated poorly functioning heart. Children present with heart failure, sometimes in association with shock. They may also more rarely present with ventricular arrhythmias.

The unexpected onset of heart failure in a previously well child should suggest the diagnosis. However, in the first 3 months of life, heart failure associated with cardiomegaly is more likely to be caused by congenital heart disease than by heart muscle disease. Echocardiography is therefore particularly important in this age group, to discriminate between the two potential causes of heart failure.

In addition to the features of heart failure listed earlier in Table 5.4.B.1, signs may include lateral displacement of the apex beat and an apical pansystolic murmur from mitral regurgitation. The chest X-ray often demonstrates cardiomegaly. It is not essential to identify whether the child has cardiomyopathy or myocarditis, as the management of both conditions is the same. However, the latter may be suggested by a preceding viral illness or evidence of acute myocardial damage with elevated blood levels of creatinine kinase or troponin. Myocarditis may be confirmed by identifying enterovirus by polymerase chain reaction (PCR) or serology.

In most cases, the cause of the cardiomyopathy remains unknown. However, it is important to perform a 12-lead ECG in all cases of cardiomyopathy, as it may reveal two particular conditions that are reversible causes of poor heart function:

- Incessant tachyarrhythmias may cause cardiomyopathy. In cardiomyopathy there is often sinus tachycardia, which appears on the ECG as a heart rate faster than that expected for the child's age, with each QRS complex being preceded by a P wave that is positive in both lead I and lead aVF. If the QRS complexes are not preceded by P waves, or P-wave morphology is unusual, the rhythm is not sinus rhythm and a tachyarrhythmia must be suspected. Sometimes the tachyarrhythmia heart rate is only marginally higher than that expected for the child's age, but many months of mild tachycardia have resulted in poor function. If the arrhythmia is successfully controlled with anti-arrhythmic drugs or radiofrequency ablation, the heart function should normalise.
- Anomalous origin of the left coronary artery from the pulmonary artery (ALCAPA) presents with severely impaired cardiac function at around 3 months of age. The ECG will show transmural anterolateral myocardial infarction in most cases. If the coronary artery is reimplanted in the aortic root the function will usually recover.

Post-intervention management is aimed at supporting the heart while function spontaneously recovers. It includes the following:

- Furosemide and spironolactone (see above, under heart failure)
- Captopril (see above, under heart failure)
- Digoxin:
  - 5 micrograms/kg orally twice a day (in children under 5 years old).
  - 3 micrograms/kg orally twice a day (in children over 5 years old).
  - Plasma levels should be in the range 0.8–2.0 micrograms/litre (check the level after 5 days, and at least 6 hours after giving a dose).
- Aspirin 3–5 micrograms/kg once a day if function is poor, to prevent thromboembolism.
- Anticoagulation if cardiac function is very poor:
  - Heparin IV, initially 20 U/kg/hour, titrated to APTT 2–3 times normal.
  - Warfarin if anticoagulation is needed long term.
- Intubation and ventilation if pulmonary oedema is severe.
- Inotropic support (dobutamine 5–10 micrograms/kg/minute, dopamine 5–10 micrograms/kg/minute, milrinone maximum dose of 0.7 micrograms/kg/minute). Ventilation and inotropic drugs should be a last resort if the child is deteriorating despite other measures, as it can be difficult to wean them off intensive care support once these steps are taken.
- Once the child is stabilised, introduce carvedilol at a dose of 50 micrograms/kg (maximum dose 3.125 mg) twice a day, doubling the dose at intervals of at least 2 weeks up to an upper limit of 350 micrograms/kg (maximum 25 mg) twice a day. Use echocardiography to check that cardiac function has not deteriorated before each dose increment, and monitor blood pressure for 4 hours after every dose increment. Carvedilol promotes myocardial remodelling.

Bacterial endocarditis

Endocarditis should always be suspected in a child with

a cardiac defect when there is a fever without a focus. Infection develops on injured areas of endothelium or on abnormal or damaged heart valves. In some cases the onset may be sudden with obvious signs of sepsis and cardiac fail-ure (secondary to valve damage). However, in most cases the onset is insidious and the diagnosis is unclear. There may be fever, malaise, fatigue, arthralgia, anorexia and weight loss. It may occur in a child previously thought to have a normal heart but with an undiagnosed congenital heart defect or undiagnosed episode of rheumatic fever.

Signs of endocarditis:
- Pyrexia
- Microscopic haematuria
- Splenomegaly
- Changing heart murmur
- Petechiae
- Neurological abnormalities (caused by cerebral abscess or infarction)
- Splinter haemorrhages, Janeway lesions, Osler's nodes and Roth's spots (characteristic but rare).

The diagnosis is made by isolating bacteria from the blood. At least three sets of blood cultures must be obtained from different puncture sites. If possible, antibiotics should be witheld until multiple blood cultures have been obtained and should only be started when the diagnosis is clear or there is a pressing clinical urgency. Blood cultures will be negative in 10–15% of cases. Echocardiography helps to make the diagnosis if vegetations are seen, but a negative echocardiogram does not exclude the diagnosis.

Organisms most commonly isolated in endocarditis:
- *Streptococcus viridans* (commonest overall)
- *Staphylococcus aureus* (most cases of fulminant endocarditis)
- Coagulase-negative staphylococci (if the patient has a central venous line or is immunocompromised e.g. with HIV).

If the organism is *Streptococcus viridans*, IV benzylpenicillin 25 mg/kg 6 hourly and gentamicin 7.5 mg/kg once daily are given for two weeks, followed by a further two weeks of oral amoxycillin. If the organism is *Staphylococcus aureus*, IV flucloxacillin 25 mg/kg 6 hourly is given for 4 weeks, coupled with IV gentamicin 7.5 mg/kg once daily (or sodium fucidate) 6–7 mg/kg 8 hourly for the first two weeks. Vancomycin 10 mg/kg 6 hourly is used in place of flucloxacillin if the organism is a coagulase negative Staphylococcus or the patient is allergic to penicillin.

The effectiveness of treatment is monitored by symptoms and inflammatory markers (WBC, ESR and CRP). Surgery is necessary when the organism cannot be eradicated, when there is evidence of embolisation, where there is a large mobile vegetation at risk of embolisation or when there is severe cardiac failure from valve damage.

5.4.C The child with a cardiac arrhythmia

> **BOX 5.4.C.1 Minimum standards**
> - Electrocardiograph.
> - Defibrillator.
> - Adenosine.
> - Beta-blockers.
> - Flecainide.
> - Amiodarone.
> - Atropine.

Supraventricular tachycardia

Supraventricular tachycardia (SVT) is the commonest tachyarrhythmia in childhood.

It may present with poor systemic output and heart failure in infancy, or palpitations and dizziness in later childhood. SVT can be distinguished from sinus tachycardia because the rate is usually more rapid (200–300 beats/minute) than can be explained by the child's level of activity, fever, agitation or pain. The ECG in most cases shows narrow QRS complexes without a preceding P wave. The commonest cause of SVT in childhood is an accessory pathway, which is an abnormal bundle of muscle fibres bridging from the atrium to the ventricle. In accessory pathway-mediated tachycardia, depolarisation passes down from the atrium to the ventricle through the atrioventricular node, and then returns back up to the atrium using the accessory pathway. If the electrical wavefront then passes down the atrioventricular node again and once again returns up to the atrium via the accessory pathway, SVT has initiated. Some, but not all, accessory pathways are evident on the resting ECG because forward conduction across the accessory pathway in sinus rhythm causes a slurred stroke just before the QRS complex, known as a delta wave. The condition is often known as the Wolff–Parkinson–White (WPW) syndrome. The best method of treating this condition is by radiofrequency ablation of the abnormal pathway by means of a catheter passed into the atria, but this is a skilled technique that is only available in specialist centres.

Some patients have a different type of SVT, where the electrical wavefront loops back on itself to form a 'short circuit' entirely within the atrioventricular node. This is less often seen in early childhood, but becomes more common towards adolescence. A totally different mechanism of tachycardia occurs when there is an abnormally rapid atrial discharge (atrial flutter or atrial ectopic tachycardia). This is relatively rare in childhood.

Management of SVT

1 Record a 12-lead ECG in tachycardia,
2 While attempts are made to terminate the tachycardia, record a rhythm strip (this can often be easily run off a standard defibrillator).
3 In the infant, try to terminate the SVT by facial immersion in ice-cold water.
4 To terminate symptomatic or prolonged attacks of SVT in the older child, try vagal manoeuvres such as ice-cold packs on the face, the Valsalva manoeuvre or carotid sinus massage.
5 If tachycardia persists, obtain IV access (via a large antecubital vein if possible) and give a rapid bolus of

adenosine 100 micrograms/kg followed by a rapid crystalloid flush.

6 If the SVT is not terminated, give larger doses of adenosine, doubling the dose until a maximum dose of 400 micrograms/kg is reached.

7 If adenosine terminates the tachycardia transiently, and then SVT re-initiates, anti-arrhythmic drug treatment needs to be initiated straight away to prevent constant recurrence of the arrhythmia.

8 If adenosine successfully terminates the tachycardia, it is not compulsory to initiate anti-arrhythmic treatment. As SVT is not dangerous beyond infancy, anti-arrhythmic drugs are only given if the child wants to avoid further attacks (this decision is usually influenced by the frequency and duration of attacks). In infancy, SVT may cause serious haemodynamic compromise. In view of this, all infants who present with SVT should be started on anti-arrhythmic medication, which should be continued until the child's first birthday.

9 If adenosine does not terminate the tachycardia at all, carry out synchronised DC cardioversion, after anaesthesia, intubation and ventilation with 0.5 joules/kg, rising to 2 joules/kg in steps if the first shocks are unsuccessful.

10 In rarer cases, adenosine causes only transient block of the atrioventricular node, revealing rapid atrial activity in the form of P waves or sawtooth flutter waves. When atrioventricular nodal conduction returns after a few seconds, the tachycardia is re-initiated. These tachycardias require either anti-arrhythmic drug treatment to be initiated straight away or DC cardioversion.

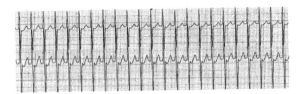

FIGURE 5.4.C.1 Supraventricular tachycardia (SVT).

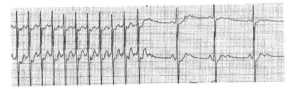

FIGURE 5.4.C.2 Termination of supraventricular tachycardia (SVT).

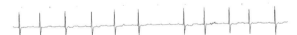

FIGURE 5.4.C.3 Administration of adenosine during atrial tachycardia shows underlying rapid P waves.

Ventricular tachycardia

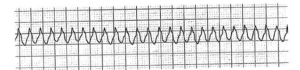

FIGURE 5.4.C.4 Ventricular tachycardia.

Ventricular tachycardia (VT) is normally diagnosed when there is a broad complex tachycardia. However, the latter is more often seen in childhood when there is SVT with bundle branch block. In view of this, adenosine should be given if a child presents with regular broad complex tachycardia. If the adenosine terminates the tachycardia, this proves that SVT was the correct diagnosis. If there is irregular broad complex tachycardia, do not give adenosine (this pattern indicates a dangerous arrhythmia). If the tachycardia persists even after high-dose adenosine, ventricular tachycardia is likely. Not all childhood ventricular tachycardia is dangerous. If the child is haemodynamically stable, attempts can be made to terminate the tachycardia with anti-arrhythmic drugs (see below). If there is haemodynamic compromise, immediate DC cardioversion is required.

Direct current (DC) cardioversion

Sedate or anaesthetise the child unless they are in extremis. Use paediatric paddles if the child weighs less than 10 kg. Place one paddle over the apex of the heart in the mid-axillary line and the other immediately below the clavicle just to the right of the sternum. If there are only adult paddles and the child weighs less than 10 kg, place one on the back and one over the lower chest anteriorly. The first shock should be 0.5 joules/kg, and subsequent shocks should be increased stepwise to a maximum of 2 joules/kg.

Anti-arrhythmic drugs

This is only a guide, and other types of drug within a class can be given.

First choice

Beta-blockers (oral doses given)

Infants: propranololol 1 mg/kg/dose three times a day.

Children (when cannot swallow tablets): atenolol 1–2 mg/kg once a day.

Older children (when can swallow tablets): bisoprolol 0.2–0.4 mg/kg once a day (tablets come as 2.5 mg, so use multiples of this amount).

Second choice

Flecainide (oral doses given)

Under 12 years of age: initially 2 mg/kg/dose twice a day. It is possible to increase to 3 mg/kg/dose if tachycardias persist (maximum of 8 mg/kg/day).

Over 12 years of age: 50–100 mg twice a day (maximum of 300 mg a day).

It is preferable to measure the flecainide level after 5 days just before the next dose is due to be administered, to check that the plasma level has not exceeded 800 micrograms/litre.

Avoid feeds for 30 minutes before or after giving oral flecainide, as the absorption of the drug is significantly affected by milk and dairy products.

Third choice

Beta-blocker and flecainide together

If the tachycardia does not respond to the above drugs in the acute setting, or the child's haemodynamic status is borderline, IV amiodarone is the safest option.

IV amiodarone

Give a loading dose of 5 mg/kg over 2 hours (dilute with 5% dextrose only). Then continue infusion at a rate of

5–20 micrograms/kg/minute (maximum of 1.2 grams in 24 hours).

Consider stopping the infusion 4–8 hours after the SVT has resolved.

If tachycardia recurs after stopping amiodarone, give a further loading dose and recommence infusion, continuing for at least 1 day after tachycardia resolution.

As amiodarone has a large number of side effects, consider switching to either a beta-blocker or flecainide once the tachycardia has been controlled and the child is haemodynamically stable.

Make up the amiodarone infusion as follows:
15 mg/kg in 50 mL of 5% dextrose (1 mL/hour = 5 micrograms/kg/hour: such a slow infusion will need an electrically driven syringe pump).

Amiodarone is incompatible with sodium chloride. Therefore do not make up with and do not flush lines with this solution.

Amiodarone can be given through a peripheral line, but serious tissue damage may be caused by the drug if extravasation occurs, so central access is preferred. If peripheral access is used, dilute the infusion to a concentration between 600 micrograms/mL and 2 mg/mL. This dilution will be more appropriate in situations where electrically driven syringe pumps are not available, but the infusion needs close monitoring.

Congenital complete heart block

- Consider this in any newborn who has a consistent bradycardia without apparent cause, such as terminal respiratory failure or very severe shock.
- P waves are dissociated from QRS complexes on the 12-lead ECG.
- Perform an echocardiogram to exclude structural heart disease.
- Check for anti-Ro and anti-La antibodies in the child's mother (the underlying cause in the majority of cases).
- Monitor the heart rate for 24–48 hours.
- Assess perfusion and blood pressure, and examine for signs of heart failure.
- Arrange for a permanent pacemaker if there is inadequate cardiac output, heart failure, structural heart disease or the heart rate is < 50 beats/minute.
- Atropine 20 micrograms/kg or isoprenaline infusion 0.02–0.2 micrograms/kg/minute can be used for emergency treatment of severe bradycardia with inadequate cardiac output.

5.5 Shock

5.5.A Shock

Introduction

'Shock' occurs when the circulatory system fails to deliver adequate amounts of primarily oxygen, but also nutrients, to the tissues, and fails to remove unwanted metabolites from the tissues for excretion.

Pathology at cell level

At a cellular level, the end result of shock is anaerobic metabolism (oxygen-depleted metabolism). This is an inefficient mechanism and requires much more energy than aerobic metabolism (the normal oxygen-dependent system). In addition, anaerobic metabolism builds up excess toxic acid products in the cells which cannot be removed by the failed circulation. Cellular function deteriorates and there is a downward spiral of increasing loss of homeostasis, the onset of disseminated intravascular coagulation, and after a short while so much cell death occurs in vital organs that recovery is impossible and the patient dies.

In the early stages of shock the body has mechanisms to try to combat this process. The circulatory system is under the control of the sympathetic nervous system. This system regulates the flow of blood in health and in disease to all organs so as to respond to demands on different organs. In health, more blood is sent to muscles if a person is exercising, more to the digestive system if they are eating, and more to the skin if their body is too warm.

In shock, the sympathetic nervous system attempts to protect the vital organs by diverting blood away from muscle, skin and the digestive system and directing it to the heart, brain and kidneys. This gives rise to some of the earlier signs of shock, such as cold peripheries, increased capillary refill time, cerebral anxiety or agitation, tachycardia to increase cardiac output, and reduced urine output as the kidneys conserve fluid.

Later signs such as depressed consciousness, weak pulses, falling blood pressure and acidotic breathing show that the body's compensation mechanisms are failing. It can be seen that it is vital to recognise and treat shock in the patient as soon as possible, as this will give the best chance of patient recovery.

Clinical diagnosis of shock

The signs of shock are listed below, although not all of them are present in all types of shock.
- **Tachycardia** (best measured with a stethoscope).

- **Weak pulse** (ideally central – brachial, femoral or carotid, but difficult to gauge).
- Low blood pressure (this is a **late sign** and very difficult to measure in young children).
- Extreme central pallor (severe anaemia).
- Raised respiratory rate (due to acidosis).
- **Cold skin with poor circulation.**
- **Prolonged capillary refill time (CRT) > 3 seconds.**
- Increased skin sweating in some cases.
- Agitation and anxiety (this is an early sign).
- **Reduced conscious level.**
- Reduced urine output (this is an early sign).

The WHO diagnosis of shock includes all of the above signs that are highlighted in bold type.

The problem is that shock is quite difficult to diagnose in the early stages, as some signs also occur as a result of medical causes other than shock. The diagnosis in the early stages depends on the following:

- tachycardia, which is a very useful sign of shock, but also occurs with fever and with anxiety or fear
- anxiety and/or agitation
- prolonged capillary refill time, which also occurs in dehydration and is influenced by environmental temperatures and by how hard the nail bed or sternum is pressed
- cold skin, which is also dependent on environmental temperature
- reduced urine output, which is also dependent on fluid intake.

It is vital that if any of these early signs are noted in a patient that they are not dismissed as some unrelated cause, but are seriously considered as likely to be indicating the development of shock.

This is why it is so useful to have regular vital signs (pulse, respiration, conscious level, temperature and blood pressure) observations on patients, so that abnormal trends can be detected early.

It is also important to note that shock is not diagnosed on the basis of one physical sign alone, but on the basis of several signs occurring together. For example, a tachycardia alone does not diagnose shock, but if you note a tachycardia, you should look for cold limbs, prolonged capillary refill time, or a history suggestive of a cause of shock, such as a fever, severe diarrhoea or bleeding.

Pathological mechanisms that can cause shock

The circulatory system is complex, so there are many causes of shock. The organs, systems and pathologies that can be the primary cause of the shock include the heart itself, the blood vessels, restriction to the flow of blood, failure of the oxygen-carrying capacity of the blood, and loss of blood or fluid from the body. The main mechanisms of shock can be summarised as follows:

- loss of fluid or blood: **hypovolaemic shock** (e.g. diarrhoea, blood loss)
- failure of the heart pump: **cardiogenic shock** (e.g. dysrhythmias, cardiomyopathy, myocarditis, malnutrition)
- abnormal function of vessels supplying nutrients and oxygen to tissues: **distributive shock** (e.g. sepsis, anaphylaxis)
- inadequate capacity of the blood to release oxygen:

dissociative shock (e.g. severe anaemia, carbon monoxide poisoning)
- restriction of circulation to the tissues: **obstructive shock** (e.g. some congenital heart diseases, tension pneumothorax, cardiac tamponade, pulmonary embolus).

In an individual with shock, often several of these mechanisms may coexist. Therefore the clinician must consider which emergency treatments will be effective **and which will be harmful** for any particular patient. One of the most difficult situations is in the anaemic malnourished child with sepsis, where fluid is required to expand the circulating volume, but the heart is already failing and cannot cope with a rapid fluid infusion (*see* Section 5.10.B).

Basic management of shock

Shock is managed according to the following principles:

- High concentrations of oxygen are safe and must be given regardless of the cause of shock.
- Airway and breathing stability or support must be established promptly first (the only exception is to control exsanguinating external bleeding in trauma or major obstetric haemorrhage concurrently with airway and breathing; *see* Sections 7.3.A, 2.5.D.i and 2.5.D.iv).
- Frequent reassessment, at least after every therapeutic manoeuvre, is vital to avoid both under-infusing and over-infusing fluids.
- The underlying pathology must be treated to arrest the pathological process.

The clinical diagnosis of the cause of shock is not easy or definitive. Shock is a spectrum of conditions and mechanisms, and it is a clinical challenge.

Immediate resuscitation is needed to maintain oxygenation and perfusion of vital organs. Once this is under way, the cause of shock needs to be found and treated.

Diagnosis depends on history, clinical examination, and response to treatment given. It is often possible to identify the cause of shock with a good history and a careful examination.

Investigations
- Haemoglobin measurement is essential.
- Blood glucose measurement is essential, as some signs of shock are the same as signs of hypoglycaemia.
- Plasma electrolyte measurements are helpful, especially sodium and bicarbonate.
- Lactate measurement is helpful (if available).
- Central venous pressure (CVP) measurement is useful, if skilled staff are available to undertake the procedure and measurement (not an emergency procedure, but helpful if in high-dependency care).

Choice of intravenous fluid
Fluid infused into the circulation should approximate to plasma in its electrolyte content, osmolality and pH.

Dextrose-only fluids
It is clear that although glucose or dextrose is necessary to prevent or manage hypoglycaemia, fluids containing only dextrose should **never** be used for IV fluid replacement

TABLE 5.5.A.1 Diagnostic pointers to the clinical causes of shock (each is discussed in the sections indicated)

Diarrhoea and/or vomiting with signs of severe dehydration	Gastroenteritis (*see* Section 5.5.B and Section 5.12.A), volvulus, intussusception (*see* Section 5.19)
Fever, non-blanching (purpuric) rash	Meningococcal septicaemia (*see* Section 5.5.C and Section 6.1.G), dengue haemorrhagic fever (*see* Section 6.2.B)
Urticaria, wheeze, oedema, exposure to allergen	Anaphylaxis (*see* Section 5.1.B)
Trauma	Blood loss, tension pneumothorax, internal bleeding, spinal cord transection (*see* Section 7.3.A)
Major obstetric haemorrhage in children who are pregnant	Blood loss: ruptured ectopic pregnancy, antepartum haemorrhage, postpartum haemorrhage (*see* Section 2)
Burns	Fluid loss from burns (*see* Section 7.3.I.b)
Pallor, tachycardia, severe malaria, severe acute malnutrition	Severe anaemia, often with malnutrition (*see* Section 5.10.B) and malaria (*see* Section 6.3.A.d)
Fever, signs of shock and a very sick child	Septicaemia (*see* Section 5.5.C) and malaria (*see* Section 6.3.A.d)
Baby < 4 weeks old: cyanosis, with no response to oxygen, very weak pulses	Congenital heart disease (*see* Section 5.4.A)
Very fast pulse, heart failure	Arrhythmia (*see* Section 5.4.C) and cardiomyopathy (*see* Section 5.4.B)
Dehydration, polyuria, polydipsia, high glucose levels	Diabetic ketoacidosis (*see* Section 5.8.A)
History of sickle-cell disease or diarrhoeal illness and low haemoglobin levels	Haemolysis with severe anaemia (*see* Section 5.11.C)

or maintenance, or for the emergency management of shock.

The reason for this is that the dextrose is rapidly metabolised, so the effect of a dextrose-only IV fluid on the child's body is as if pure water had been given. The outcome of this treatment would be severe hyponatraemia, which could quickly lead to brain damage or death.

In addition, this pure water is rapidly moved out of the circulation and into the cells, and the state of shock is then worse than before the infusion.

Sodium-containing fluids

The fluid traditionally infused into the circulation for the management of shock has been 'normal saline' (0.9% sodium chloride, NaCl). This fluid has increasingly been shown to be potentially dangerous, especially in the sick patient. An infusion of normal saline causes a hyperchloraemic acidosis (a high chloride concentration leading to an acidosis), which in the shocked patient, who is already acidotic, causes a deterioration in the health of cells in vital organs, even though perfusion of the cells has been improved by the increased circulating volume.

There are sodium-containing alternatives to normal saline which are safer as they approximate more closely to human serum in content (*see* Table 5.5.A.2), although they are a little more expensive. We recommend the use of either of these alternatives (**Ringer-lactate and Hartmann's solution** are widely available) for all fluid replacement. Recognising that not all hospitals will have access to these solutions immediately, there may sometimes be no alternative but to start fluid replacement with normal saline. However, if more than 20 mL/kg needs to be given, one of the safer alternatives should be used in these very sick children if at all possible.

Note that hospitals and clinics will need to have access to some 0.9% NaCl (normal saline), usually in 5 mL or 10 mL ampoules. This will be used for dissolving or diluting drugs for IV injection. If a specific fluid is indicated as the diluent for a particular drug (e.g. 0.9% NaCl, 5% dextrose, water for injection), **this fluid must be used**. If drugs are infused using the wrong fluid, their effect on the patient may be altered.

Clinicians should try to ensure that their hospital facility does have access to these safer infusion fluids, such as Ringer-lactate or Hartmann's solution.

TABLE 5.5.A.2 Comparison of electrolytes, osmolality and pH levels in IV fluids with those in human serum

Fluid	Na^+ (mmol/litre)	K^+ (mmol/litre)	Cl^- (mmol/litre)	Ca^{2+} (mmol/litre)	Lactate or bicarbonate (mmol/litre)	Osmolarity (mOsm/litre)	pH
Human serum/plasma	135–145	3.5–5.5	98–108	2.2–2.6	22–30	276 to 295	7.35–7.45
Ringer-lactate or Hartmann's solution	131	5.0	111	2.0	29	279	6.0
0.9% 'normal' saline	154	0	154	0	0	310	5.4

Initial management of shock

Even though it may be clear on initial inspection that the child is in shock, the first priority must still be to call for help, manage the airway, manage breathing and then manage the circulation.

Call for help.

Airway

At this stage also stop any obvious exsanguinating bleeding.

Assess the airway by the simple technique of asking the child 'Are you all right?'

Any vocalisation such as a reply or crying indicates an open airway and some ventilation. In the absence of a response, formally open the airway with a head tilt/chin lift or a jaw thrust manoeuvre (*see* Section 1.12), and assess breathing by looking, listening and feeling for its presence.

Stop any obvious exsanguinating bleeding by applying external pressure (or in the case of postpartum haemorrhage, *see* Section 2.5.D.iv).

Breathing

All children with suspected shock must receive high-flow oxygen.

In the absence of spontaneous breathing, give assisted ventilation with a bag-mask (*see* Section 1.13).

Circulation

Intravenous access with a short wide-bore venous cannula, or placement of **an intra-osseous line** (*see* Section 8.4.B), is vital. More than one line is preferable, as rapid fluid resuscitation may be needed, although always start treatment as soon as the first access has been achieved and insert the second line when possible. Take blood samples for the

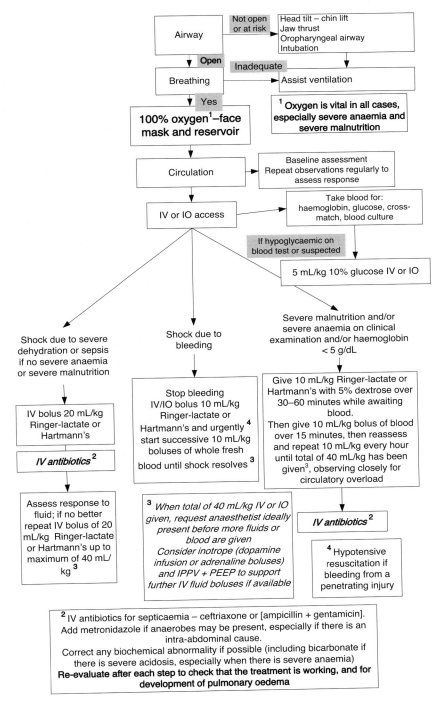

FIGURE 5.5.A.1 Pathway of care for the child with shock that is not cardiac in origin.

following investigations: full blood count, glucose levels, electrolytes, blood culture (and, if relevant, cross-matching and malarial parasite test).

Nutritional status

While starting to give fluid, assess the child's nutritional status (*see* Section 5.10.B). Look for visible severe wasting or **marasmus**. The WHO recommended criteria are as follows: 'Look at the arms, legs and chest. The marasmic child does not look just thin, but appears to be all skin and bone. The skin looks too large for the body, there is no fat on the child and you will see the outlines of the ribs. There is also severe muscle wasting of the arms, legs and buttocks. The head may appear relatively large because of wasting of the body.' Use the mid upper arm circumference (MUAC) (*see* Section 9) to assess marasmus, as the urgency of the child's need for treatment precludes a weight and height measurement.

Look also for kwashiorkor. Check for oedema of both feet. Look at the bare feet. Press the top of the foot gently with your thumb for a few seconds. Oedema is present if a definite dent is left in the tissues. Look and feel to determine whether the child has oedema of both feet.

Some assessment of weight will be necessary to calculate the amounts of fluid and antibiotics to be given. If the child is not malnourished, use the following formula:

$$\text{weight in kg} = 2\ (\text{age in years} + 4).$$

If the child is malnourished, this formula can still be used, but perhaps a percentage such as 25–50% subtracted from the result.

Severe anaemia

In very anaemic children (with either obviously pale palms or haemoglobin levels of less than 3–4 grams/dL), crystalloid alone will worsen oxygen delivery to the tissues. These children need blood, either packed cells or a partial exchange transfusion, in addition to initial **slow** fluid resuscitation (*see* Section 5.10.B, Section 5.11.A and Section 8.4.B).

The next step is to **give fluid intravenously**. In most cases this should be a crystalloid such as Hartmann's or Ringer-lactate solution, but give normal saline (0.9%) if this is all that is available. In children, the volume of fluid to be given is usually 20 mL/kg, which is 25% of the child's circulating volume (10 mL/kg in severe anaemia or severe malnutrition while awaiting blood for transfusion). Shock is not usually clinically evident until 25% of the circulation has been lost, so any child with signs of shock must have lost at least this amount of fluid from the circulation.

The concept of **targeted crystalloid fluid resuscitation** is important if the cause of hypovolaemic shock in a child is haemorrhage from a penetrating injury. Here the initial boluses of IV crystalloids required to treat shock should only be given to keep the vital organs (especially the brain, heart and kidneys) perfused before life-saving surgery and blood transfusion can be undertaken. Fresh blood is particularly useful to combat the coagulopathy that occurs in major blood loss if specific coagulation components such as platelets are unavailable.

Giving too large a volume of IV fluids can increase the blood pressure and thus increase bleeding by disrupting early clot formation. IV crystalloid also dilutes the red cells in the circulation, but whether or not this could reduce oxygen-carrying capacity requires further research.

We suggest that when giving boluses of crystalloid or blood to patients in shock due to bleeding, only the amount needed to keep the blood pressure at a level sufficient to perfuse the vital organs should be given. There is no clear evidence to indicate the precise blood pressure that should be achieved in a child in shock due to haemorrhage from penetrating injury. **Adequate perfusion of vital organs may best be indicated by the following: in the child over 2–3 years of age, a radial pulse that can be palpated and a conscious level of A or V on the AVPU scale (i.e. the child is either awake or will respond by opening their eyes when spoken to). In children under 2–3 years of age the radial pulse may be difficult to feel, and in children with shock due to haemorrhage the presence of a palpable brachial pulse may be the best available indicator at present.**

In this situation, therefore, and to maintain a palpable radial or brachial pulse, start with IV boluses of 10 mL/kg of crystalloid, or ideally blood, and reassess after each bolus.

The next very important step is to reassess the patient's vital signs to see whether the fluid has helped, and to ensure that circulatory overload has not given rise to a situation where more IV fluids may produce very dangerous heart failure (see below for clinical signs of this).

During this reassessment, give IV antibiotics, as shock without obvious fluid loss is probably sepsis (*see* Section 5.5.C).

At this point, some children will need more crystalloid fluid, while others will not, or they will need other fluids (e.g. plasma expanders such as albumin or blood). Many will need additional treatments. The next two sections (Sections 5.5.B and 5.5.C) deal with two of the commonest causes of shock in children, and the reader is referred to the sections indicated in Table 5.5.A.1 for details of the various other causes of shock.

5.5.B The child with shock from dehydration

> **BOX 5.5.B.1 Minimum standards**
> - Oral rehydration solution (ORS), including ReSoMal.
> - Crystalloid infusion fluids (preferably Hartmann's solution or Ringer-lactate solution, but normal saline may be used if it is the only available alternative).
> - Blood transfusion.
> - Antibiotics.
> - Furosemide.
> - MUAC tapes.

Dehydration

- Dehydration is loss of water, sodium and other essential electrolytes.
- The most common cause in resource-limited countries is gastroenteritis (from a number of different organisms; *see* Section 5.12.A).
- Most cases can be treated with low-osmolarity oral rehydration solution (ORS) administered by mouth or nasogastric tube.
- In children with severe malnutrition, use a solution with lower sodium content, such as ReSoMal.
- It is important to also consider diabetic ketoacidosis (*see* Section 5.8.A) and surgical causes of dehydration, such as intussusception and volvulus (*see* Section 5.19).

Dehydration classification

Dehydration is classified by estimating the percentage of body water lost according to clinical criteria (except in malnutrition, where clinical signs are more difficult to interpret; see below).

'No dehydration'

If there is less than 3% weight loss there are **no clinical signs**.

'Some dehydration'

If there is 3–9% weight loss, the following signs are seen:
- increased thirst
- drinks eagerly
- dry mucous membranes
- loss of skin turgor, tenting when pinched
- sunken eyes
- sunken fontanelle in infants
- restless or irritable behaviour
- decreased capillary refill time (> 3 seconds)
- decreased urine output.

'Severe dehydration'

If there is ≥ 10% weight loss, the following signs are seen:
- more pronounced signs than those seen in moderate dehydration
- lack of urine output
- lack of tears when crying
- inability to drink or drinking poorly (because of reduced conscious level)
- lethargy

plus
- **hypovolaemic shock**, including:

— rapid and weak low-volume pulse (radial pulse may be undetectable) (use a stethoscope for measuring heart rate)
— altered consciousness or coma
— low or undetectable blood pressure
— cool and poorly perfused extremities
— severe nail bed or sternum decreased capillary refill time
— peripheral cyanosis
— rapid deep breathing (from acidosis).

It is important to realise that the above classification is made only to guide the start of treatment. **Levels of dehydration are a continuous spectrum, not three separate and distinct categories.** The only way to be absolutely certain about the percentage dehydration of a child is to compare an accurate weight measured just before the onset of the diarrhoeal illness with an accurate current weight. It is very unlikely in most cases that the former weight will be available. In the case of the shocked patient, immediate treatment takes precedence over weighing the child (estimate the child's weight from the formula:

$$\text{weight (kg)} = 2 \text{ (age in years +4)}$$

for previously well children before puberty, or read it from a weight/age chart (*see* Section 9)).

However, if the clinical situation is not so critical, the weight of the child on presentation is very helpful for subsequent management, and should be measured and recorded as a daily routine.

Emergency treatment of severe dehydration: principles of treatment

- Recognise and treat shock.
  — Give a fluid bolus, 20 mL/kg IV of Hartmann's or Ringer-lactate solution (0.9% saline, or 'normal' saline, can be used if there is no alternative; *see* Section 5.5.A).
  — A second bolus may be needed if the child does not respond (*see* the 'shock' pathway in Figure 5.5.A.1).
  — It is unusual to need more than two boluses in cases of dehydration due to gastroenteritis alone, unless they are due to cholera (*see* Section 5.12.A). Consider other causes, such as septicaemia, diabetic ketoacidosis (check blood sugar levels), volvulus or intussusception (check whether vomit is bile-stained, and whether there is fresh blood in stools; *see* Section 5.19).
  — If septicaemia is suspected, treat with IV antibiotics.
- Think of the most likely cause of the dehydration.
- Estimate the level of dehydration (see above) to calculate the fluid deficit, maintenance needs and ongoing losses (see below).

Shock recognition and treatment

Children with shock associated with dehydration will have a high and increasing heart rate, weak pulse, poor skin circulation time with prolonged capillary refill time (> 3 seconds), depressed conscious level, and low or even unmeasurable blood pressure.

These children require immediate resuscitation (ABC) and emergency treatment.

Call for help (summon an anaesthetist if possible).

Airway (in cases of reduced conscious level)

Use an opening manoeuvre if the airway is not open or if it is partially obstructed. Keep the airway open. If there is immediate improvement but the airway closes without active opening support, consider airway adjuncts to support the airway.

Suction if necessary under direct vision, but not routinely.

If the child is deeply unconscious (P or less on the AVPU scale), the airway may need to be secured by intubation using experienced senior help (if available).

Breathing

Give 100% oxygen (using a mask with reservoir and a flow rate of at least 6 litres/minute) regardless of SpO_2 (this increases oxygen delivery as well as improving tissue oxygenation). For inadequate ventilation or depressed conscious level (check with the AVPU scale) with hypoventilation, respiration should be supported with oxygen via a **bag and mask**, and experienced senior help should be summoned (if available).

Circulation

- Obtain vascular access to give IV boluses quickly. Insert an IV cannula and send blood for a full blood count, urea and electrolytes, cross-matching (if the patient is anaemic) and clotting. If peripheral veins are difficult to access, the **external jugular vein** or **long saphenous vein cut-down** are good alternatives, as is an **intra-osseous infusion** (*see* Section 8.4.B). If a skilled operator is available, an internal jugular or femoral vein central line is ideal, as it can also allow central venous pressure (CVP) measurements (if available).

Some assessment of weight will be necessary to calculate the amounts of fluid and antibiotics to be given. If the child is not malnourished, use the formula:

weight (kg) = 2 (age in years +4).

If the child is malnourished, this formula can still be used but perhaps a percentage such as 25–50% subtracted from the result.

Children with normal nutrition

- **If the child is not malnourished**, give an initial **rapid** bolus of 10–20 mL/kg of Ringer-lactate or Hartmann's solution, but give normal saline (0.9%) if this is all that is available. It is essential that the bolus is given as rapidly as possible. **Do not use 5% glucose or 0.18% saline/4% glucose solutions for resuscitation, which can be dangerous (risk of hyponatraemia and cerebral oedema).** Boluses should be manually pushed in using a 20- to 50-mL syringe (with a three-way tap and linked to an IV giving set).
- When this bolus of fluid has been given, review the child's condition, looking to see whether there has been any improvement in pulse rate, conscious level,

respiratory rate, capillary return and limb warmth, and blood pressure.

- A further 10–20 mL/kg bolus will be required if signs of shock remain. Once a **total** of 40 mL/kg of boluses has been given IV, complications such as pulmonary oedema are more likely to occur. In a child with shock from severe dehydration caused by diarrhoea, it would be unusual to need more than 40 mL/kg to improve the child's circulation, unless cholera was the cause. In severe cases, where more than a total of 40 mL/kg is considered essential, intubation, ventilation, CVP monitoring and inotrope support might be indicated (if available), but **the diagnosis should be reviewed as this need is unusual in straightforward gastroenteritis.** Reconsider the diagnosis. For example:
  - surgical abdominal pathology, such as intussusception, peritonitis or volvulus (bile-stained vomiting, abdominal distension or tenderness) (*see* Section 5.19)
  - additional pathology, severe anaemia, septicaemia or a cardiac problem.

Children with severe malnutrition or severe anaemia

- **If the child is malnourished and/or has severe anaemia, fluid must be given much more carefully.** Give 15 mL/kg IV over 1 hour. The recommended solution is Ringer-lactate or Hartmann's solution, each with 5% glucose (insert 50 mL of 50% dextrose into a 500-mL bag of the bolus fluid, ideally after first removing 50 mL from the bag: not essential), but give normal saline (0.9%) if this is all that is available, also with 5% dextrose. At the same time, insert a nasogastric tube and give ReSoMal, 10 mL/kg/hour. Monitor carefully for signs of over-hydration: reassess the respiratory and heart rates every 15 minutes. It is also wise to give IV antibiotics in this situation, as it can be very difficult to distinguish septic shock from dehydration shock in children with malnutrition.

Nutritional status

- **While starting to give fluid, assess the child's nutritional status** (*see* Section 5.10.B). Look for visible severe wasting or **marasmus**. Follow the WHO criteria: 'Look at the arms, legs and chest. The marasmic child does not look just thin, but appears to be all skin and bone. The skin looks too large for the body, there is no fat on the child and you will see the outlines of the ribs. There is also severe muscle wasting of the arms, legs and buttocks. The head may appear relatively large because of wasting of the body.'
- Use the mid upper arm circumference (MUAC) (*see* Sections 5.10.B and 9) to **assess marasmus**, as the urgency of the child's need for treatment precludes a weight and height measurement.
- **Look also for kwashiorkor.** Check for oedema of both feet. Look at the bare feet. Press the top of the foot gently with your thumb for a few seconds. Oedema is present if a definite dent is left in the tissues. Look and feel to determine whether the child has oedema of both feet.

Severe anaemia

In very anaemic children (with either obviously pale palms or haemoglobin levels less than 3–4 grams/dL), crystalloid alone may worsen oxygen delivery to the tissues. These children need blood, either packed cells or a partial exchange transfusion, in addition to initial **slow** fluid resuscitation (*see* Section 5.10.B and Section 8.4.B).

- **If after 1 hour** the child is improving but still severely dehydrated, stop the IV fluids, but continue nasogastric ReSoMal 10 mL/kg/hour for up to 5 hours (*see* Section 5.10.B for further details).
- A child with a haemoglobin level of less than 5 grams/dL will also need a transfusion of 10 mL/kg of packed cells over 4 hours, watching continuously for evidence of pulmonary oedema. If pulmonary oedema develops, furosemide 1 mg/kg IV may be required, but if possible pulmonary oedema of severity requiring diuretics should be avoided by a slow and vigilant approach to therapy in these very sick children.
- Keep the patient warm, but do not overheat them, as this will cause peripheral vasodilatation and reduce the blood supply to vital centres. Hypothermia will exacerbate poor peripheral perfusion, acidosis and coagulation abnormalities.
- Elevate the patient's legs (raise the foot of the bed).
- A central venous pressure (CVP) line is potentially helpful for avoiding under-transfusion or fluid overload. Insertion should not delay initial resuscitation, but if peripheral access is inadequate this route may be used for volume replacement. If disseminated intravascular coagulation (DIC, a clotting disorder) has become established, CVP insertion is hazardous, must be undertaken by an expert, especially via the subclavian vein.
- If the child has a reduced level of consciousness or has a convulsion, particularly if they are an infant or a young child, hypoglycaemia may be present. Always measure the blood glucose concentration in this situation. However, if blood glucose measurement is not possible, always treat as for presumed hypoglycaemia and, in addition to the IV fluids given above, give 5 mL/kg of 10% glucose IV or, if there is no IV access, by intra-osseous needle.

While treating shock, reassess the child, ideally continuously, until signs of shock have resolved.

When signs of shock have resolved

When shock has resolved and the patient's level of consciousness has returned to normal, the remaining estimated fluid deficit MUST be taken by mouth or by gastric tube, especially if there is malnutrition and/or anaemia (due to the danger of a large IV fluid volume). Use WHO Plan B (*see* Appendix to Section 5.12.A).

- Check the serum sodium concentration, and if it is higher than 155 mmol/litre, reduce it **slowly** with oral rehydration solution over 48 hours. Too rapid a reduction in sodium levels leads to cerebral oedema.
- Further tests might include abdominal X-ray or ultrasound scanning, if there is concern about a distended abdomen.
- A surgical opinion is needed if there is bile-stained vomiting or abdominal signs.

Fluid requirements

WHO Plans A, B and C for gastroenteritis in children (*see* Appendix to Section 5.12.A) include estimates of total fluid requirements, and assume that most children will be drinking by 4 hours into treatment and thus able to 'self-regulate'. For patients for whom this is not the case, the following guidelines can be used.

Estimating fluid requirements

The amount of fluid needed in a 24-hour period must be calculated. It is the sum of:

estimated fluid deficit + maintenance requirements + ongoing losses.

Deficit

If an accurate recent pre-illness weight is available, subtract the current weight to estimate lost fluid (1 kg = 1 litre of fluid).

For example, a child who weighed 9.2 kg is seen with diarrhoea and a weight of 8.3 kg. The estimated fluid loss in this case is (9.2 − 8.3) kg = 0.9 kg = 900 mL deficit, i.e. 10% dehydrated.

If no recent reliable weight is available:
1 Estimate the degree of dehydration.
2 Weigh the child or estimate their weight from their age as follows:

$$weight (kg) = 2 [age (years) + 4].$$

3 Use the formula: percentage dehydration × weight (kg) × 10 = deficit (in mL).

For example, a child whose weight is estimated to be 10 kg is 10% dehydrated. The estimated fluid loss in this case is 10 × 10 × 10 = 1000 mL (i.e. 40 mL/hour if replaced over 24 hours).

Maintenance

The estimated maintenance fluid requirements based on body weight for a child are shown in Table 5.5.B.1.

TABLE 5.5.B.1 Fluid requirements per day

Body weight	Volume of fluid needed per day	Volume of fluid needed per hour
First 10 kg of body weight	100 mL/kg	4 mL/kg
Second 10 kg	50 mL/kg	2 mL/kg
Subsequent kg	20 mL/kg	1 mL/kg

Ongoing losses

Estimated ongoing fluid losses are shown in Table 5.5.B.2.

TABLE 5.5.B.2 Estimates of ongoing fluid losses in gastroenteritis

For each diarrhoea stool	Age < 2 years: give 50–100 mL
	Age ≥ 2 years: give 100–200 mL
For each vomit	2 mL/kg oral rehydration solution: give small frequent volumes (e.g. 5 mL every minute for a child) via a spoon, syringe or cup
For nasogastric tube aspirates	Replace volume for volume with either oral rehydration solution or Hartmann's or Ringer-lactate solution with 5% or 10% glucose or normal saline with 5% or 10% glucose and 5 mmol/litre of potassium chloride

Over-hydration

Signs of over-hydration, especially if there is cardiac failure (e.g. in severe malnutrition) are as follows:

- tachycardia, increased respiratory rate, oedematous (puffy) eyelids, crepitations at lung bases, enlarged liver and raised jugular venous pressure (JVP)
- pulmonary oedema on chest X-ray.

Management

- Stop giving IV fluids or oral rehydration solution, but give breast milk or plain water and food.
- Do not give a diuretic unless there is pulmonary oedema

(crepitations in lungs), in which case give furosemide 1 mg/kg IV.

Reassess:

- ABC.
- The state of intravascular rehydration.
- Plasma electrolytes (if possible).
- Urine output and urine electrolytes.
- Glucose levels.

Reduce fluid intake and continue to monitor, responding to changes in the child's condition as described above.

5.5.C The child with septic shock

> **BOX 5.5.C.1 Minimum standards**
> - High-dependency care.
> - Ringer-lactate or Hartmann's solution (or 0.9% saline if no other crystalloid is available).
> - Urgent blood transfusion.
> - Antibiotics: cefotaxime, flucloxacillin, gentamicin, metronidazole and penicillin.
> - Dopamine and adrenaline.
> - MUAC tapes.

Introduction

Septic shock develops when a number of different mechanisms of shock operate in the context of an invasive bacterial infection (an exception is dengue, which is caused by a viral agent; *see* Section 6.2.B). These mechanisms are as follows:

- **hypovolaemic:** there is abnormal capillary permeability, fever and accompanying vomiting and diarrhoea
- **distributive:** there is loss of the normal sympathetic nervous system control of vascular tone, so that blood is lost from vital organs into non-vital areas
- **cardiogenic:** there is impaired cardiac function secondary to hypovolaemia and the toxic effects of the pathogen.

These multiple factors make septic shock difficult and complex to treat, and they contribute to a high mortality rate in these conditions.

The bacteria that cause septic shock include *Meningococcus*, *Staphylococcus*, *Streptococcus pneumoniae* and *Streptococcus pyogenes*, together with Gram-negative organisms such as *E. coli* which particularly affect **patients who are at risk due to lower immunity**, such as the newborn, those with HIV/AIDS, and the malnourished.

Diagnosis of septic shock

The early recognition and treatment of septic shock is key to a good outcome, so a high degree of vigilance for this condition is necessary.

In a child who has an infection, with a fever (although the **at-risk** group mentioned above may have a normal or subnormal temperature), the development of a change in

mental status, such as irritability, drowsiness, lack of interaction or reduced or absent eating or breastfeeding is often the first feature to alarm parents, and is the result of the effect of poor cerebral perfusion and possible accompanying hypoglycaemia on the child's brain.

The signs which should then be sought include the following:

- tachycardia (best measured with a stethoscope)
- weak pulse (ideally central – brachial, femoral or carotid, but difficult to gauge)
- reduced urine output (this is an early sign)
- cold skin with poor circulation, or sometimes peripheral skin vasodilatation
- prolonged capillary refill time (CRT) > 3 seconds
- agitation and anxiety
- increased skin sweating in some cases
- extreme central pallor (in cases with severe anaemia)
- raised respiratory rate (due to acidosis)
- reduced conscious level (**this is a serious and dangerous sign**)
- low blood pressure (this is a **late sign** and difficult to measure in young children; the correct-sized cuff is needed).

Difficulties in managing septic shock

In well-resourced countries or well-resourced areas of countries with specialist paediatric intensive care units (PICUs) or high-dependency units, some cases of septic shock are still difficult to manage and some children die.

In resource-limited countries the following additional difficulties need to be taken into account:

- **Severe malnutrition:** this makes the diagnosis of septic shock more difficult, as the child's malnourished body does not respond with the same physical signs as that of a well-nourished child. In addition, malnourished children may have poor myocardial function and almost always have severe anaemia. This will result in cardiac failure and probable death if rapid infusions of large and repeated boluses of fluid (an important part of septic shock management) are given (*see* Section 5.10.B).
- **Severe anaemia:** as shock is a failure of oxygen delivery to the tissues, clearly anaemia will make this worse. Rapid crystalloid fluid infusion will dilute the blood further and worsen the heart failure which may be present in severe anaemia. These children need early **fresh**

whole blood transfusion, where the red blood cells will improve oxygen-carrying capacity, and the plasma will support the circulation and supply coagulation factors. If only stored blood is available, it should be packed to provide predominantly red blood cells. In the absence of a suitable centrifuge, hanging the bag vertically allows the red cells to fall to the bottom of the pack and these can be transfused first.

- **HIV/AIDS:** again diagnosis may be difficult, as physical signs and laboratory tests may be unreliable. A low threshold for treatment of suspected sepsis with broad-spectrum antibiotics is recommended (*see* Section 6.2.D).

- **Lack of PICU or high-dependency care facilities:** even in children with good nutrition, no severe anaemia and no other long-term debilitating condition, the amount of fluid infusion required to successfully treat some cases of septic shock is sufficient to induce heart failure and pulmonary oedema. If facilities are available, intubation and ventilation, IV infusion of inotropic drugs such as dopamine and adrenaline, invasive cardiovascular monitoring, renal dialysis and other aspects of paediatric intensive care are required. The absence of these facilities limits the treatment that can be offered to children with septic shock.

Initial management of septic shock

Even though it may be clear on initial inspection that the child is in shock, the first priority must still be to call for help, manage the airway, manage breathing, and then manage the circulation.

Call for help.

Airway

Assess the airway by the simple technique of asking the child 'Are you all right?'

Any vocalisation such as a reply or crying indicates an open airway and some ventilation. In the absence of a response, formally open the airway with a head tilt/chin lift or a jaw thrust maneouvre (*see* Section 1.12), and assess breathing by looking, listening and feeling for its presence.

Breathing

All children with suspected shock must receive high-flow oxygen.

If possible, this should be given through a mask with a reservoir to achieve the higher concentrations. In the absence of spontaneous breathing give assisted ventilation with a bag-mask (*see* Section 1.13).

Circulation

Some assessment of weight will be necessary to calculate the amounts of fluid and antibiotics to be given. If the child is not malnourished, use the following formula:

weight in kg = 2 (age in years + 4).

If the child is malnourished, this formula can still be used, but perhaps a percentage such as 25–50% subtracted from the result.

Intravenous access with a short wide-bore venous cannula, or placement of **an intra-osseous line** (*see*

Section 8.4.B), is vital. More than one line is preferable, as rapid fluid resuscitation may be required, and other drugs may need to be given simultaneously, but start IV treatment as soon as the first line is in place before seeking additional IV access (unless sufficient staff are available). Take blood for the following investigations: full blood count, glucose levels, electrolytes (including calcium and lactate levels if possible), blood grouping and blood cross-matching in all cases. Treat hypoglycaemia if it is identified (*see* Section 5.8.B).

Nutritional status: severe malnutrition

While starting to give fluid, assess the child's nutritional status (*see* Section 5.10.B). Look for visible severe wasting or **marasmus**. Follow the WHO criteria: 'Look at the arms, legs and chest. The marasmic child does not look just thin, but appears to be all skin and bone. The skin looks too large for the body, there is no fat on the child and you will see the outlines of the ribs. There is also severe muscle wasting of the arms, legs and buttocks. The head may appear relatively large because of wasting of the body.' Use the mid upper arm circumference (MUAC) (*see* Section 9) to **assess marasmus**, as the urgency of the child's need for treatment precludes a weight and height measurement.

Look also for kwashiorkor. Check for oedema of both feet. Look at the bare feet. Press the top of the foot gently with your thumb for a few seconds. Oedema is present if a definite dent is left in the tissues. Look and feel to determine whether the child has oedema of both feet.

Severe anaemia

In very anaemic children (with either obviously pale palms or haemoglobin levels of less than 3–4 grams/dL), crystalloid alone will worsen oxygen delivery to the tissues. These children need blood, either packed cells or a partial exchange transfusion, in addition to initial **slow** fluid resuscitation (*see* Section 5.10.B, Section 5.11.C and Section 8.4.B).

First fluid

The next step is to **give fluid and antibiotics intravenously.**

Malnourished and/or severely anaemic children

- **If the child is malnourished and/or anaemic (haemoglobin concentration < 5 grams/dL), fluid must be given much more carefully.** Give 10 mL/kg IV over 30–60 minutes. The recommended solution is Ringer-lactate solution or Hartmann's solution, each with 5% glucose (insert 50 mL of 50% dextrose into a 500-mL bag of the bolus fluid), but give normal saline (0.9%) if this is all that is available, also with 5% dextrose. For antibiotic treatment, see below.

- Give a bolus of 10 mL/kg of fresh blood (if available) or stored blood over 15 minutes as soon as possible.

- Assess the child and **if they are not in clinical heart failure**, give another 10 mL/kg bolus of fresh or stored blood over 15 minutes.

  - **If the child is in heart failure**, give 10 mL/kg of blood as packed red cells over 2–3 hours, or use a partial exchange transfusion as follows: using a cannula in a large vein, withdraw 5–10 mL of the patient's anaemic blood (depending on the child's size) and infuse 10–20 mL, respectively, of new blood over 5 minutes and repeat 10 times.

- If the child is not improving after having been given the above treatment and antibiotics (see below), further clinical interventions must be determined by the individual situation.

Normal nutrition

- **If the child is not malnourished,** infuse a crystalloid such as Hartmann's or Ringer-lactate solution as quickly as possible, but give normal saline (0.9%) if this is all that is available. In well-nourished children, the initial bolus volume of fluid to be given is usually 20 mL/kg, which is 25% of the child's circulating volume. Shock is not usually clinically evident until 25% of the circulation has been lost, so any child with signs of shock must have lost at least this amount of fluid from the circulation. For example, a child weighing 12 kg would need 240 mL of crystalloid. This fluid should be given as quickly as possible, usually over 5–10 minutes. It is easily given by pushing the fluid in using a 50-mL syringe.

Antibiotics

- While giving the first bolus of IV fluid, also give IV antibiotics if sufficient staff are available to avoid introducing delays with the first fluid bolus. The choice of antibiotics will depend on the clinical clues as to the infecting organism. In the presence of a purpuric rash (and in a non-endemic dengue area), meningococcus is the likely organism. Otherwise *Streptococcus* or *Staphylococcus* or Gram-negative organisms are candidates. A third-generation cephalosporin such as ceftriaxone or a combination of gentamicin and a penicillin would be advisable. Flucloxacillin should be added if *Staphylococcus* is suspected (e.g. if there are boils or a known abscess). In newborn infants or children with suspected intra-abdominal sepsis, Gram-negative organisms are likely. Metronidazole should be given to cover anaerobic organisms if clinically appropriate.

Reassessment

- The next very important step before a second IV bolus is given is to **reassess the patient's vital signs** to see if the fluid has helped. Check the pulse rate, capillary return, limb temperature and blood pressure, and pay particular attention to the child's mental status. Observe the parent–child interaction. Is the child more or less responsive to the parent? Look for signs of heart failure (i.e. raised jugular venous pressure, enlarged liver, and crackles in the lung bases).
- If the child still shows the signs of shock, give further fluid. If there are signs of fluid overload with or without heart failure, stop the IV fluid.

Further fluid

- If there has been a little improvement or no improvement, give **a further bolus of 10–20 mL** of fluid. Reassess the child after each 10 mL/kg of fluid, checking the pulse rate, capillary return, limb temperature, blood pressure and alertness, and looking for signs of heart failure, raised jugular venous pressure, enlarged liver, and crackles in the lung bases.
- Once a total of 40 mL of fluid have been given, there is an increasing risk that you will cause fluid overload with pulmonary oedema, which will make the child worse, not better. The problem is that there may still be leakage of fluid out of the circulation (into which you have been infusing the crystalloid or other fluid), which makes

the tissues oedematous but leaves the circulation still hypovolaemic and the tissues under-perfused.

Inotropes

- One response to this situation is to give an infusion of a drug that stimulates the heart to pump harder and supports the circulation (an inotrope). **Dopamine is a very potent drug and must be given carefully.** It should be given into a peripheral vein or intra-osseously at a starting dose of 5 micrograms/kg/minute. The dose can be increased in steps up to 20 micrograms/kg/minute if lower doses do not help.

Dopamine infusion

- Make up 0.3 mg/kg of dopamine in 500 mL of Ringer-lactate or Hartmann's solution or normal saline. This will give 0.1 microgram/kg/minute if run at a rate of 1 mL/hour. Use an 100-mL paediatric burette in the infusion line for this fluid. The burette can then be filled with a further 100 mL and a further dose of dopamine added when necessary. To give 5.0 micrograms/kg/minute, give 50 mL/hour of this dilution for a child. Do not forget that the fluid that you are using for the infusion must be included in your calculations of total fluid given. If higher doses of dopamine are needed, a more concentrated solution of dopamine should be used or too much fluid will be given.
- If dopamine is not available or is not having any significant effect in the larger doses, then adrenaline, which is more potent than dopamine, may be tried.

Intermittent adrenaline infusions

- Dissolve 0.1 mL of 1 in 1000 adrenaline or 1 mL of 1 in 10 000 adrenaline in 10 mL of 0.9% saline and give 1 mL IV in a child (100 microgram) or 0.2 mL in an infant (20 micrograms). Check the response (in particular of blood pressure), and repeat after 15–30 minutes if it helps to improve perfusion. Then intermittently give further doses as required (1 mL of this solution contains 100 micrograms).
- It must be emphasised that in the absence of paediatric intensive care, the above infusions of inotropic (circulation-supporting) drugs are an attempt to save a child in extremis, and may not be effective.
- Once the infusion of inotropes has been started and the child's vital signs reassessed, fluid may cautiously be continued, reassessing frequently and stopping the infusion if signs of heart failure appear.
  - If there is a skilled operator (an anaesthetist or surgeon) available, the placing of a central venous line would be very helpful for monitoring the venous pressure (around + 8 mmHg is a good target) and for infusing the dobutamine or adrenaline centrally.
  - Once 60 mL/kg have been given in total along with inotropes, further fluid is unlikely to be beneficial unless skilled ventilation is available.
  - In this situation, provided that adequate facilities and expertise are available, positive pressure ventilation through an endotracheal tube (usually with positive end-expiratory pressure) can assist the circulation and help to manage the effects of any pulmonary oedema.

Reviewing the full blood count and biochemistry

- Blood tests were taken at the beginning of treatment, but it is useful to check the blood tests again (taking the blood from a vein with no IV in place).
  - Check the haemoglobin level to see whether there is now a need for a blood transfusion (fresh blood would be best). Studies have shown that the haemoglobin concentration should ideally be above 10 grams/dL when treating shock in children.
  - Check the blood glucose level and treat with 2 mL/kg of 10% dextrose in a neonate and 2–5 mL/kg of 10% dextrose in an older infant or child if the level is less than 2.5 mmol/litre. Also add glucose to any infusion fluid.
  - Check the calcium level, and if the concentration of ionised calcium is less than 1 mmol/litre, give 0.3 mg/kg of 10% calcium gluconate IV slowly (over 30 minutes, as calcium can cause cardiac arrest if given too quickly).
- Consider giving 0.5–1 mmol/kg of sodium bicarbonate (0.5–1 mL/kg of 8.4% sodium bicarbonate) over 15 minutes IV for refractory acidosis that is not responding to fluid resuscitation and effective ventilation.

Steroids

- There is some evidence that IV steroids can be helpful in some cases of septic shock. If the suspected organism is meningococcus or the child has previously been on a prolonged course of steroid treatment (e.g. for nephrotic syndrome), IV hydrocortisone can be given at a dose of 1–2 mg/kg/day in divided doses or as a continuous infusion. Occasionally higher doses up to 50 mg/kg/day have been used.

Further treatment

- Many children with septic shock may respond to the above treatments. For those who have not done so, paediatric intensive or high-dependency care is needed. If this is available, contact should be made with the PICU team as soon as it becomes clear that the child has septic shock. Advice on their care can then be given by experts and arrangements made, if possible, for the child to be 'retrieved' by the intensive care team coming to stabilise and transfer them.

5.6 Renal disorders

5.6.A Medical renal disorders

BOX 5.6.A.1 Minimum standards

- Accurate weight-measuring scales.
- Fluid input and output charts.
- Urine microscopy, culture and sensitivity.
- Antibiotics: trimethoprim, cephalosporins, amoxicillin, nitrofurantoin, gentamicin, penicillin.
- Blood biochemistry: urea, creatinine, sodium, potassium, chloride, bicarbonate.
- Urinary electrolytes.
- Full blood count.
- Ultrasound scan.
- Blood pressure measurement.
- Furosemide and chlorothiazide.
- Nifedipine or amlodipine, hydralazine, propranololol or atenolol, captopril or enalapril.
- Prednisolone, levamisole and cyclophosphamide.
- IV albumin.
- Analgesia: morphine.
- IV Ringer-lactate solution, Hartmann's solution, phosphamide and 5% albumin.
- IV glucose 10% and insulin.
- Sodium bicarbonate, calcium gluconate, calcium resonium and calcium carbonate.
- Antihypertensive drugs.

Introduction

Common renal investigations: plasma or serum biochemistry

Electrolytes

Sodium (Na^+) and potassium (K^+) assays are essential for the logical management of children with kidney dysfunction. Bicarbonate (HCO_3^-) is also extremely helpful, but more difficult to measure.

Problems with fluid and electrolyte balance are common in ill children. They can occur in a wide variety of clinical situations and with a wide range of underlying diagnoses. A methodical approach to history taking and clinical examination is therefore essential, and interpretation of biochemical results must always be done in the context of the clinical situation.

TABLE 5.6.A.1 Maintenance water, sodium and potassium requirements

	Age Preterm	Term	1 year	5 years	12 years
Sodium (mmol/kg/24 hours)	5	3	2	2	1
Potassium (mmol/kg/24 hours)	5	3	2	2	1
Water (mL/kg/24 hours)	200	150	100	75	50
Fluid (mL/kg/hour)	8	6	4	3	2

Dehydration and hypovolaemia

Fluid within the body is distributed between the intracellular fluid (ICF) and extracellular fluid (ECF) compartments, the ECF being composed of the intravascular and interstitial components. Differential solute composition of the ICF and ECF compartments is maintained by cell membrane pump activity and solute size and electrical charge. Fluid movement is regulated by a balance between osmotically active solutes and hydrostatic pressure.

It is useful when clinically assessing the fluid volume status of a patient to try to consider which compartment has insufficient or excess volume.

The effects of ECF volume depletion are usually shared between the intravascular and interstitial compartments, and are seen as hypovolaemia and dehydration, respectively. However, assessment can be complex. For example, in a condition like nephrotic syndrome, on examination there may be weight gain and oedema. However, since there is hypoalbuminaemia, and albumin is the primary intravascular osmotic component, the intravascular fluid volume may be low but the total ECF volume is high. Conversely, in acute renal failure there can be weight gain and oedema in a situation where both the total ECF and the intravascular volume are high. In heart failure, oedema can be present with high, normal or low intravascular volume, depending on other additional pathologies. In summary, oedema can occur with high, normal or low intravascular fluid volume, which makes the clinical history and a full examination vitally important for understanding the individual patient.

Often, in dehydration, sodium and water have been lost in an approximately normal ratio and therefore the deficit should be replaced as Ringer-lactate or Hartmann's solution. Normal saline can be used if these two solutions are unavailable, but it is less satisfactory because large volumes cause the patient to develop a hyperchloraemic acidosis, due to the larger chloride load in normal saline than there is in plasma.

Practical point

When prescribing rehydration fluids:

A Make an assessment of volume deficit and replace this as Ringer-lactate or Hartmann's solution.
B Calculate maintenance fluids and insensible losses.
C Initially estimate, and then measure, ongoing losses and replace them appropriately in volume and content.

Fluid prescription should consist of A + B + C.

Aim to treat cardiovascular collapse or 'shock' quickly over the first 1–2 hours. Infuse Ringer-lactate or Hartmann's solution to restore the circulating blood volume, reviewing to assess the response (see Section 5.5.A), and thereafter use a slow replacement rate so that the total deficit is replaced over at least 24 hours.

In hypernatraemic dehydration, after an acceptable cardiovascular state has been restored, aim to reduce plasma sodium levels slowly over 24–48 hours by altering the sodium concentration of the infusion fluid appropriately, and repeatedly monitoring the rate of fall of the plasma sodium and urinary sodium concentration.

Fluid and electrolyte disorders

Good management depends on measurement of input and output, plus **repeated:**

- clinical examination
- biochemical data on urine and blood
- weight measurements.

Hyponatraemia

Hyponatraemia is defined as a plasma sodium concentration of less than 130 mmol/litre, and it occurs when there is:

- sodium loss in excess of water loss
- **or** water gain in excess of sodium gain.

The total body sodium level may be high, low or normal, and therefore initial and ongoing clinical assessment of the extracellular fluid volume is essential.

Hypernatraemia

Hypernatraemia is defined as a plasma sodium concentration greater than 150 mmol/litre, and occurs when there is:

- water loss in excess of sodium loss
- **or** sodium gain in excess of water gain.

Again, the total body sodium level may be high, low or normal.

TABLE 5.6.A.2 Clinical estimation of ECF volume deficit in dehydration

Mild 3–5% weight loss	Thirsty Mucous membranes dry Decreased skin turgor
Moderate 5–10% weight loss	Increased severity of the above Depressed fontanelle Sunken eyes Tachycardia
Severe 10–15% weight loss	Increased severity of the above Drowsiness, confusion or coma 'Shock' Cool peripheries Prolonged capillary refill time Hypotension

Hypernatraemic dehydration: water loss in excess of sodium loss

Because sodium is the principle ECF osmole, the ECF volume is relatively well maintained, and signs of dehydration and hypovolaemia are less apparent.

Creatinine

Plasma creatinine concentration is the best available, most clinically useful and relatively inexpensive guide to glomerular renal function. It is easily, quickly and cheaply measured on a small blood sample. Individual measurements are of use in determining whether renal function is within the normal range. Sequential measurements are useful for following deterioration or improvements in renal function over a short time scale of hours or days, or over a long time scale of months or years. Although formulae can be used, the following guidelines allow the glomerular filtration rate (GFR) to be estimated in most clinical situations.

The plasma creatinine concentration depends on the bulk of the patient's muscle (where it is produced) and the patient's height, so on average men have higher values than women, and older children have higher values than babies, except in the first few days of life (see Table 5.6.A.3).

For example, a creatinine concentration of 150 mmol/litre in a well-nourished 5-year-old girl would be three times the upper limit of normal, indicating a GFR of one-third normal. The same creatinine concentration in a very undernourished girl with little muscle bulk would imply a GFR considerably lower than one-third.

TABLE 5.6.A.3 Upper limit of normal plasma creatinine concentrations

Subject	Plasma creatinine concentration (micromol/litre)	Plasma creatinine concentration (mg/dL)
Well-nourished average man	100	1.15
Well-nourished average woman	75	0.85
Well-nourished average 10-year-old child	60	0.70
Well-nourished average 5-year-old child	50	0.65
Well-nourished average baby or toddler	40	0.45
Baby aged 3 days to 3 weeks	Variable	
Baby in first 2 days of life	Maternal	

Urea

Although useful for managing children with renal failure, urea concentration is an inaccurate way of measuring renal function because it is also highly dependent on hydration, and on carbohydrate and protein intake.

Urine biochemistry

Concept of fractional excretion

Clearance of any substance which is filtered by the glomeruli and then reabsorbed by the tubules can be compared to the clearance of creatinine which is filtered and then excreted largely unmodified by the tubule. The fractional excretion is that fraction of substance x that has been filtered at the glomerulus that actually reaches the urine.

$$\text{Fractional excretion (FE) } x \text{ \%} = \frac{\text{urine } x}{\text{filtered } x} \times 100$$

Fractional excretion of sodium

Normally, most of the filtered sodium (Na^+) is reabsorbed; the majority of this reabsorption occurs in the proximal tubule. When plasma sodium is normal and the patient is not shocked, physiologically fractional excretion of sodium can vary. However, calculating FE Na can give useful clues in pathological states.

The normal renal response to intravascular fluid volume reduction is to excrete urine with a low sodium content. It does this by a number of mechanisms, including reduction of glomerular filtration rate (GFR) and aldosterone-stimulated sodium reabsorption, which requires intact tubules.

Fractional excretion of sodium (FE Na) is calculated from the urine (U) and plasma (P) concentrations (check that P and U creatinine values are expressed in the same units), using the following formula:

FE Na (%) = U/P sodium × P/U creatinine × 100.

TABLE 5.6.A.4 Interpretation of excretion of sodium in pathological processes

	FE Na	Interpretation
Shock	< 1%	Tubules functioning = pre-renal failure
	> 1%	Acute tubular necrosis (ATN)
Hyponatraemia	< 1%	Salt loss or water overload (appropriate renal response)
	> 1%	Renal salt wasting (tubular disease)
Hypernatraemia	< 1%	Renal concentration defect
	> 1%	Salt overload (may be abuse)

Urine collection and examination

Collecting urine from babies can be time consuming, but is important in establishing a diagnosis.

Methods of urine collection

- Clean catch into a sterile pot.
- Sterile collecting pads are cheaper and easier to use than an adhesive bag.
- For toddlers it is fine to use a potty or equivalent which has been thoroughly washed in hot water and detergent (using antiseptics or bleach, or scalding with boiling water, are unreliable).
- Suprapubic or catheter urine sampling is useful in ill children when antibiotics need to be started without delay.

Stick testing of urine and protein measurement

- Dipstick testing for blood, protein and glucose is useful and reliable.
- Stick testing for nitrite to identify urinary tract infections (UTIs) is useful when positive to rule in UTIs, but unreliable when negative because it remains negative in 50% of cases.
- Stick testing for white cells to diagnose UTIs is unreliable because they may occur without white cells, and because white cell numbers also increase in the urine of febrile children without UTIs.

Laboratory measurement of protein in urine

Urine protein should be < 20 mg protein/mmol creatinine in an early-morning sample of urine.

In nephrotic syndrome there is typically > 500 mg protein/mmol creatinine.

Microscopy of urine

Microscopy of unspun fresh urine can provide a cheap and reliable way of rapidly diagnosing UTIs (by identifying bacteria directly, rather than by counting white cells), and of diagnosing schistosomiasis.

Red blood cells can be identified as being due to glomerulonephritis (when they are small, fragmented and of varied and distorted shapes), or due to other causes, such as trauma, stones or bladder inflammation (when they are all similar, and typically biconcave).

A standard light microscope with a magnification of × 400 is sufficient. Using a counting chamber (or a microscope slide with a scratched surface) and cover slip ensures that the microscope is focused at the correct plane, otherwise it is not possible to tell when microscoping a normal urine. A counting chamber with a mirrored surface is not essential, but makes identification of bacteria easier. Phase contrast makes identification even easier. A highly reliable, almost pocket-sized microscope (McArthur) is available with phase contrast.

Urinary tract imaging techniques

All renal imaging techniques are relatively expensive, and many will have limited availability.

Ultrasound scanning

Useful information can only be obtained from ultrasound scanning by a skilled operator using an adequate machine. It demonstrates anatomy, but not function. It is ionising radiation free, and, when available, is now the first choice for initial imaging of most renal conditions in children. It is excellent at demonstrating cysts, stones and dilatation, and has a similar sensitivity to the intravenous urogram (IVU) for demonstrating long-standing or extensive scarring. Nephritis causes echo brightness of the kidneys. Tumours and cysts are easily seen, usually before they are visible by other modalities. Stones can be easily identified, but may be misinterpreted by the inexperienced because the whole stone is not seen; a bright line identifies where the ultrasound hits the front edge of the stone, and an acoustic shadow is thrown behind it. Nephrocalcinosis can be detected easily as white renal pyramids long before it can be seen on X-rays.

Ultrasound scanning during the acute phase of the UTI will often show dilation of the ureters. It is therefore suggested that this investigation should be undertaken 2–3 weeks after the infection. Any dilation of the ureters should then be regarded as significant.

Micturating cystogram (MCUG)

This is still the most reliable way to assess vesico-ureteric reflux (VUR), but unfortunately depends on invasive urethral catheterisation, and depending on the equipment used it may require a relatively high dose of radiation. It should be reserved for use when the result will affect management. (Reflux is less commonly found in Afro-Caribbean children.)

This investigation is very important to confirm posterior urethral valves, one of the commonest obstructive uropathies seen in Afro-Caribbean children. The age of presentation is variable. When it presents in the neonatal period there is usually severe renal involvement.

Plain abdominal X-ray

This demonstrates radio-opaque stones, but these and nephrocalcinosis are usually easier to see on an ultrasound scan.

Urinary tract infections (UTIs)
Background

UTIs are very common. The risk of UTI is increased in babies with anatomical nephro-urological abnormalities, those with obstruction, those with VUR, and in girls. Management of VUR is controversial (see Section 5.6.B). Recent studies have shown that about 10% of girls and 3% of boys will have had a UTI diagnosed by the age of 16 years in the UK. Most children with UTIs have no underlying renal tract problem and suffer no serious consequences. However, UTI may be the first indicator of underlying renal tract abnormality, and may be associated with acquired renal scarring. Distinguishing the small group of children with important findings in this common condition remains a challenge, and the question of how intensively to investigate children after UTI remains controversial.

Large scars may cause renal failure, but even small ones can cause hypertension, often in later childhood or in adulthood. **To prevent serious sequelae of hypertension, children with scars should have lifelong blood pressure monitoring, as symptoms do not occur until serious irreparable disease is present.**

Infants are the most vulnerable to scarring, and most children who will acquire scarring will have started to do so by the age of 4 or 5 years. Animal studies and case series suggest that a UTI in a vulnerable individual may cause permanent scarring rapidly, in a matter of a very few days.

Diagnosis
Symptoms

Older children may present with typical 'cystitis' symptoms, typically due to bladder and urethral irritation, such as frequency and dysuria. Loin pain suggests likely upper renal tract involvement, but some children have few or no symptoms. Younger children (under 2 years of age) often only have non-specific symptoms such as anorexia, failure to thrive, unexplained fever or prolonged jaundice. Therefore all young children with an unexplained illness, particularly with a fever, should have a UTI excluded.

Urine testing

A diagnosis is usually made by culture of a pure growth of one species of bacteria (most commonly *E. coli*) at a concentration of more than 10^5/mL. Any concentration of bacteria in a suprapubic urine sample suggests infection. White blood cells (> 50/microlitre) are usually considered helpful in making the diagnosis, but UTIs can occur without any white cells (sometimes because they lyse in minutes), and urinary white blood cells can be found in children with fever who have some other cause and do not have a UTI.

As stated above, the organism most commonly involved is *E. coli*. If unusual organisms such as *Pseudomonas* are cultured at the first episode of UTI, it is mandatory to rule out an underlying urinary tract abnormality.

Microscopy

Microscopy of freshly voided unspun urine is a quick, reliable and cheap way to diagnose UTIs if a × 400 microscope is available, and it enables an immediate diagnosis to be made. This allows the best-guess antibiotic to be started at once. Infected urines need to be cultured to obtain antibiotic sensitivities. Infected urine will contain many bacteria, up to thousands per high-power field, depending slightly on the depth of urine under the cover slip. The bacteria will all look the same, and are typically rods of identical length. Occasionally, UTIs are caused by streptococci, which are seen as long chains of dots. Separate small dots that appear to be swimming are not streptococci, but are phosphate crystals (the shimmering movement is due to Brownian motion). Most but not all children with UTIs will also have > 50 white blood cells/microlitre, or at least 1 per 10 high-power fields.

If no bacteria are seen in about 5 high-power fields, the urine is not infected; the samples therefore need no further testing and can be discarded. Urine samples containing less than 1 bacterium per high-power field, or mixtures of rods and cocci, are likely to have been contaminated. Because this can be identified quickly, further samples can and should be collected until a clearly uninfected or infected one is obtained.

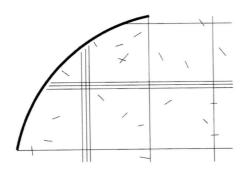

FIGURE 5.6.A.1 Rods seen in 10 high-powered fields.

Imaging

Imaging after the first UTI is controversial. Young children and infants warrant more intensive investigation, as do those with a family history of renal disease.

Ultrasound scanning

This should be undertaken for all children after their first recognised UTI in order to identify structural abnormalities, and to try to identify scars. The likelihood of detecting a scar is much greater if it is large, involving multiple renal segments, or several years old, so that it will have had time to shrink and distort. Negative scans in young children (under 4 years) therefore need to be interpreted with caution.

Ultrasound scanning during the acute phase of the UTI will often show dilation of the ureters. It is therefore suggested that this investigation be undertaken 2–3 weeks after the infection. Any dilation of the ureters should then be regarded as significant.

Micturating cystogram (MCUG)

It is probably ideal to perform an MCUG on very young children who have had a definite UTI. It is recommended that an MCUG be performed on all those under 1 year of age, because about a third will have an anatomical abnormality detected, usually vesico-ureteric reflux (VUR). However, there is not universal agreement about this, as there is a high percentage of normal results.

Posterior urethral valves may present with a UTI, especially in parts of the world where there is little or inadequate antenatal scanning. Thus in baby boys who have had a UTI, a good view of the urethra is essential.

Children with VUR are at risk of developing scars with UTI. Therefore finding VUR should make you suspect that the child may have a scar that was not identified by ultrasound.

Management of VUR is controversial (*see* Section 5.6.B). Prophylactic antibiotics may reduce the recurrence of infection; awareness and rapid treatment of infection is important. Most VUR is self-resolving and the aim of medical treatment is to keep free of UTI while allowing natural resolution (over a period of years). The possibility of VUR should be considered and, if possible, tested for if scarring is identified on ultrasound scanning.

Most VUR resolves with time; the lower the grade, the more likely it is that resolution will occur (80–90% resolution of grade 1–2 over 5 years).

Treatment of UTIs

Encourage a high fluid intake to produce dilute urine and reduce the symptoms of dysuria.

Treat the child for 7 days initially with:
- oral trimethoprim (4 mg/kg twice daily)
- or cephalexin (10 mg/kg three times daily)
- or amoxicillin (1 month to 1 year 62.5 mg: 1–5 years 125 mg: 5–18 years 250 mg, all three times daily)
- or nitrofurantoin (3 months to 5 years: 750 micrograms/kg 4 times daily, 12–18 years: 50 mg 4 times daily).

Intravenous antibiotics may be necessary for very unwell children (particularly under 2 years of age) for as long as they are unable to tolerate oral medication. This may include **gentamicin** 7.5 mg/kg as a loading dose and then 7.5 mg/kg once daily only after confirmation that the plasma creatinine concentration is normal. If there is renal failure, no more should be given after the single dose, unless blood levels are available to guide the dosage. If necessary, change the antibiotic according to the laboratory sensitivity testing, when and if it is available.

Use of prophylactic antibiotics is controversial. Use may reduce recurrence of UTI and should be considered when there is VUR. A night-time dose of trimethoprim (2 mg/kg) or cephalexin (12.5 mg/kg maximum 125 mg) or nitrofurantoin

(1 mg/kg) may be used. Do not use amoxicillin for prophylaxis, because resistant organisms are likely to emerge.

In many resource-limited countries where there may be inadequate procedures for ensuring that antibiotics are used appropriately and where disposal of body fluids containing antibiotics may contaminate drinking water supplies, UTIs are resistant to trimethoprim but remain sensitive to cephalosporins and amoxicillin. Ideally, where available, cultures for antibiotic sensitivity should be undertaken.

Hypertension
Background
There is a steady increase in blood pressure with age, and definitions of hypertension are arbitrary. However, in most children with hypertension the blood pressure becomes very much higher than normal (unlike the majority of adult hypertension patients, whose blood pressure is only moderately elevated, causing a skewed frequency distribution curve). Primary hypertension is rare in children, and in more than 80% of them hypertension is secondary, and in at least 75% it is renal in origin. Diagnosis of the underlying cause is therefore very important in management. Children are

relatively intolerant of hypertension, so they are at major risk of sequelae, especially encephalopathy, blindness and death.

Measurement
Blood pressure is best measured with a simple sphygmomanometer, as automatic blood pressure machines may be unreliable. It is more reliable to use the largest cuff that will fit on to the upper arm, rather than using 'formulae' that relate the cuff size to the child's size. A cuff that is too large will not significantly underestimate the blood pressure, but one that is too small will overestimate it. In children, it is best to use systolic blood pressure; it is just as important as diastolic pressure for diagnosis and treatment, and is easier and more reliable to measure. In most children, palpating the reappearance of the pulse at the wrist is as accurate as using a stethoscope at the antecubital fossa, or a Doppler (if available) may be used at the wrist to detect the reappearance of the pulse. High values should be confirmed with the child relaxed to reduce the effects of anxiety. Measurements should be repeated several times if they are abnormal. Table 5.6.A.5 shows the upper limit of normal blood pressure ranges according to age.

TABLE 5.6.A.5 Mean, upper limit of normal and dangerous levels of systolic blood pressure in children of different ages

Value	1 month	1 year	5 years	10 years	15 years
Mean (mmHg)	75	85	95	105	115
Upper limit of normal (mmHg)	80	90	100	110	125
Needing urgent treatment (mmHg)	100*	120	130	140	150

*In infants, the likeliest cause of hypertension is coarctation of the aorta.

TABLE 5.6.A.6 Oral hypotensive drugs* for children, with maximum doses

Class of drug	Example	Maximum dose (mg/kg/day)
Calcium-channel blocker	Nifedipine	1
Vasodilator	Hydralazine	10
Beta-blocker	Atenolol	1
Angiotensin-converting-enzyme (ACE) inhibitor†	Captopril	5

* These are often given in combination to achieve a powerful effect with fewer side effects.

† ACE inhibitors must be started by giving a very low test dose first and building up slowly. They must be used with great care if renal artery stenosis is suspected.

Causes and diagnosis
It is important to find the underlying cause of the hypertension to guide management. Sometimes the cause is clear from the history, examination or urine testing, and sometimes it requires diagnostic imaging. Ultrasound is the most useful screening technique, but is quite operator dependent. Hypertension can be caused by renal scarring that is difficult to detect with ultrasound.

Treatment
If the hypertension is known to be of recent onset, as in acute glomerulonephritis, it is safe to reduce the blood pressure quickly. Usually salt and water overload is a major factor; if so, restrict sodium and give furosemide 1–2 mg/kg (the oral route is as effective as the intravenous one).

In other cases, treat the blood pressure slowly because cerebral arterial vasoconstriction may have occurred to protect the brain parenchyma from the impact of the

hypertension, and made the cerebral blood flow dependent on a high blood pressure being sustained.

A rapid fall in blood pressure may cause cerebral infarction and blindness. Reduction over 2 days or more allows the vascular tone to return to normal. **Slow control may be achieved by introducing oral hypotensive drugs slowly at well below the maximum dose.**

Glomerular disease
Glomerular disease is characterised by proteinuria with or without haematuria. It may be caused by a primary glomerular disease or be secondary to a systemic illness, and it can cause a wide spectrum of clinical pictures, including the following:
- nephrotic syndrome
- acute glomerulonephritis
- chronic glomerulonephritis
- asymptomatic proteinuria or haematuria.

TABLE 5.6.A.7 Renal and arterial causes of hypertension in childhood

Diagnosis	Notes	Renal ultrasound
Reflux nephropathy	Also called pyelonephritis (*see* UTI)	Focal scars or shrunken kidney
Glomerulonephritis Post-infective Other causes	Typically have proteinuria and glomerular haematuria. Typically after a streptococcal infection, sore throat/skin infection. Give a 10-day course of penicillin May have evidence of Henoch–Schönlein purpura or lupus; if not, renal biopsy is needed	Echo bright
Inherited polycystic disease Infantile type (recessive) Adult type (dominant)	Kidneys large at birth, typically severe hypertension, renal failure in early life Seldom causes renal failure in childhood, but may cause hypertension. Screen blood pressure of children of affected parents	Huge, homogeneous, echo bright Discrete cysts develop through childhood
Narrowed arterial supply Coarctation of the aorta Renal artery stenosis	Check femoral pulses; may need surgical treatment or balloon angioplasty Requires long-term medical treatment. May occur with neurofibromatosis; screen for this	May be small, and difficult to diagnose without expensive imaging

Nephrotic syndrome

Background and clinical features

The clinical picture is of proteinuria, hypoalbuminaemia and oedema.

It must be differentiated from other causes of hypoalbuminaemia, such as protein malnutrition (*see* Section 5.10.B) and protein-losing enteropathy (*see* Section 5.12.D).

It is traditionally classified as early-onset (congenital, diagnosed at under 6 months of age) and later-onset types.

Early onset

Children with congenital nephrotic syndrome frequently do not survive, many of them dying early of protein malnutrition, infection or thrombosis unless they are aggressively treated.

Those with severe proteinuria, including the recessively inherited Finnish type, tend to fare worst. Diffuse mesangial sclerosis is a similar condition, but is usually less acute. Congenital syphilis can cause neonatal nephrotic syndrome which may respond to penicillin treatment. Some early nephrotic syndromes are self-resolving, but this is uncommon.

Treatment is often difficult. Early-onset nephrotic syndrome is generally not responsive to steroids. Treatment may be supportive, including frequent albumin infusions, and in the most severe cases may require early unilateral or even bilateral nephrectomy, leading to dialysis and transplantation. Reduction of proteinuria by the use of ACE inhibitors or indomethacin may be attempted, but very careful monitoring is required.

Later onset

Most children with nephrotic syndrome presenting in childhood (after the age of 1 year and before the teenage years) are steroid responsive, losing their proteinuria within 1 to 2 months of treatment. They share clinical characteristics (*see* Table 5.6.A.8). Children with steroid-resistant nephrotic syndrome may have a range of diagnoses, including focal segmental glomerulosclerosis, Henoch–Schönlein purpura, lupus and mesangiocapillary glomerulonephritis. There is a strong association with infections, especially malaria and hepatitis B, as well as hepatitis C and HIV.

Acute management

It is reasonable to attempt to induce a remission with steroids, unless the clinical picture virtually excludes the possibility of steroid sensitivity.

- Use prednisolone 60 mg/m^2 daily (*see* Section 9 to convert from body weight to surface area) for up to 6 weeks (about 95% of children who are going to respond do so within 1 month). Monitor carefully for the development of hypertension on steroids.
- Limit fluid retention by imposing a tight dietary sodium restriction.
- Prevent secondary pneumococcal infection with prophylactic penicillin V (125 mg twice daily up to 5 years of age, and 250 mg twice daily thereafter).
- Avoid the sequelae of hypovolaemia (thrombosis).
- Intravascular hypovolaemia is a high risk and should be monitored clinically by the appearance of cold peripheries and sometimes abdominal pain. There may be initial paradoxical hypertension, and hypotension may not occur until late. The best laboratory test is a urinary sodium concentration of less than 15 mmol/litre, especially if combined with a urine osmolality of over 800 osmol/kg. Blood tests are seldom helpful.
- Treatment of hypovolaemia should be with 1 gram/kg

TABLE 5.6.A.8 Clinical characteristics of steroid-sensitive and steroid-resistant nephrotic syndrome

Feature	Steroid-sensitive nephrotic syndrome	Steroid-resistant nephrotic syndrome
Gender	Male > female	Varies with condition
Age	1–3 years	Usually older
Blood pressure	Normal	Often elevated
Speed of onset	Rapid (days or weeks)	Usually weeks or months
Haematuria	Microscopic	Often macroscopic
Plasma creatinine concentration	Normal or low unless hypovolaemic	May be elevated

of IV 20% albumin over 4 hours, preferably with 2 mg/kg of IV furosemide given halfway through. If shocked, give 10 mL/kg of 4.5% albumin.
- Avoid the use of furosemide in the acute situation without adequate volume replacement.

Subsequent management if steroid-sensitive

This is ideally based on daily home monitoring of the morning urine protein level by stick testing. A common definition of a relapse is ++ proteinuria for 7 consecutive days, or +++ for 3 days, and it should be responded to by reintroducing salt restriction, penicillin V and prednisolone.

Protocols for doses and duration of use of prednisolone and steroid-sparing agents vary. The following is a proposed example:

First presentation: give prednisolone 60 mg/m^2 daily (see Section 9), and if the patient responds (by loss of proteinuria), complete 6 weeks of 60 mg/m^2 daily, followed by 40 mg/m^2 on alternate days for a further 6 weeks.

Subsequent relapse: restart 60 mg/m^2 daily until there is no proteinuria for 3 days, then give 40 mg/m^2 on alternate days for a further 4 weeks.

Frequent relapses: give prophylactic low-dose (e.g. 200 micrograms/kg) alternate-day prednisolone. Titrate the dose up until either relapses are prevented, or steroid side effects develop.

If steroid prophylaxis causes unacceptable side effects, add prophylactic levamisole 2.5 mg/kg on alternate days (approximately 50% of cases will benefit), which can be used relatively long term.

If levamisole is ineffective, consider giving cyclophosphamide 2.5–3 mg/kg daily for 12 weeks, monitoring weekly with white blood cell count, and reducing the dose if the absolute neutrophil count falls below 1×10^9/litre, or stopping if it falls below 0.5×10^9/litre. Or give 6 × monthly cyclophosphamide infusion (600 mg/m^2). Note that this is potentially dangerous in resource-limited circumstances where infections are frequent.

Subsequent management if steroid resistant

Persistent haematuria and hypertension at the first presentation may be early warning signs of steroid resistance. Steroids should be used with caution, as the hypertension may be aggravated.

There is a wide range of conditions that may induce steroid-resistant nephrotic syndrome. These include infective agents, autoimmune diseases, some drugs and poisons, and unknown causes. The cause may be apparent from the history and examination and other tests, but **in most cases the diagnosis relies on the accurate interpretation of a kidney biopsy**.

The infective causes include hepatitis B, HIV, Schistosoma mansoni, leprosy, tuberculosis and malaria. These conditions should be sought in those parts of the world where they are likely to be found, and treated appropriately. Hepatitis B typically causes a membranous nephropathy which tends to improve spontaneously. Post-streptococcal glomerulonephritis may cause nephrotic syndrome, but it is seldom the presenting feature. Although it is not the only cause of this clinical picture, **it is sensible to treat any child who develops nephrotic syndrome after an acute nephrotic illness with 10 days of oral penicillin V, 1–6 years 125 mg, 6–12 years 250 mg, 12–18 years 500 mg per dose 6-hourly.**

The autoimmune causes of nephrotic syndrome include Henoch–Schönlein purpura and IgA nephritis, lupus, mesangiocapillary glomerulonephritis, and some cases of membranous nephropathy. The commonest cause of steroid-resistant nephrotic syndrome in many parts of the world is focal segmental glomerulosclerosis (FSGS), the pathophysiological mechanism of which is unknown. In some of these conditions (including lupus, mesangiocapillary glomerulonephritis and FSGS), some children do respond to steroids. However, many children with steroid-resistant nephrotic syndrome do not respond to any treatment at all. Most of those who do only respond to more powerful immunosuppressants, such as cyclophosphamide or cyclosporine. Some conditions have been treated with plasmapheresis, but in most conditions the evidence for this is purely anecdotal. These treatments are difficult to use because they are expensive, and they require close monitoring for side effects. Even under ideal medical conditions with considerable resources, many cases still progress to end-stage renal failure.

Protein in the diet

Children with nephrotic syndrome may lose huge quantities of protein in their urine. If they are on a low-protein diet they will quickly lose muscle mass as the body proteins are utilised to synthesise plasma albumin. A relatively high-protein diet will be muscle sparing, but will make no significant difference to the plasma albumin concentration.

Glomerulonephritis

Glomerulonephritis (GN) strictly refers to inflammation of the glomeruli with cellular proliferation, although it is often used to include other glomerulopathies such as FSGS and membranous nephropathy, both of which typically cause steroid-resistant nephrotic syndrome.

The commonest cause of childhood glomerulonephritis varies widely across the world. In resource-limited countries, acute post-streptococcal glomerulonephritis is the commonest type. In wealthier countries this is now becoming more unusual, and IgA nephropathy predominates.

Post-streptococcal glomerulonephritis

This is caused by antibodies produced in response to specific strains of streptococci. These bacteria typically cause throat and skin infections. The antibodies then form complexes and are deposited within the glomeruli along with C3. Because it takes time for antibody production to occur, the signs and symptoms of nephritis do not usually begin to appear until 10–20 days after the start of the infection.

The inflamed glomeruli leak blood and protein, so the first symptom is usually the child passing smoky or frankly bloody urine. The glomerular filtration rate usually falls slightly, so the plasma creatinine concentration is typically slightly elevated. Also the tubules reabsorb sodium and water excessively, which causes water retention out of proportion to the fall in glomerular filtration rate. This leads to swelling, which is most easily noticed around the eyes and face, and in the legs, but which does not pit as easily as oedema does in the nephrotic syndrome. The water retention also leads to hypertension. Most children with acute post-streptococcal glomerulonephritis do not lose enough protein into the urine to cause nephrotic syndrome as well, although some do, producing a mixed nephrotic–nephritic picture.

A presumptive diagnosis is made by examination of the urine for the presence of protein (using stick tests) and glomerular red cells and casts (by microscopy; see Section 8.S), in a child with a history of a recent sore throat or skin infection. Culture of a specific strain of *Streptococcus* from a throat or skin swab may confirm the diagnosis.

It is not reliable to make a diagnosis from a single titre of an anti-streptococcal antibody such as the ASOT or the anti-DNase B, because many children have an elevated level from previous exposure to other strains of streptococci. Confirmation requires a significant rise between two titres taken at least 10 days apart.

If plasma complement levels (C3 and C4) can be measured, they may give a clue to the underlying diagnosis but are not confirmatory. In post-streptococcal glomerulonephritis the plasma C3 concentration is reduced, and often stays subnormal for up to 6 weeks before rising back to normal. The plasma C3 level is usually low in mesangiocapillary glomerulonephritis, and the C3 and C4 levels are often both low in lupus, and these conditions may present clinically identically to post-streptococcal glomerulonephritis.

Treatment

If post-streptococcal glomerulonephritis is suspected, immediately start penicillin V, 1–6 years 125 mg, 6–12 years 250 mg, 12–18 years 500 mg per dose four times daily for 10 days, to eradicate the organism. There is always a delay in obtaining bacteriological confirmation, either from culture or from paired titres, so it is best to start the penicillin at once, and use these tests as retrospective confirmatory evidence.

It is essential to measure the child's fluid intake and losses accurately as well as daily weighing, and restrict the amounts of sodium and water allowed. This should be to balance the losses, or to cause net fluid reduction if the child is significantly fluid-overloaded. The insensible loss is about 300 mL/m² daily, but will be higher in a hot dry climate. (Estimate the surface area from Table 9.16 in Section 9.) **Salt restriction is far more important than water restriction**, and is sometimes all that is required for a child to maintain fluid balance. This is because the tubules retain sodium avidly, so any salt that is eaten will be retained in the body and cause hypernatraemia. This drives an intense thirst, and it then becomes almost impossible to stop the child drinking. By contrast, a tight salt restriction will minimise the thirst, which aids management.

If the plasma albumin concentration is normal or only slightly reduced, it is safe to give an oral dose of furosemide, 1–2 mg/kg. This will increase the urinary excretion of sodium and water, and thus improve fluid overload and hypertension. It will also increase potassium loss, which is helpful if the fall in glomerular filtration has led to hyperkalaemia. It may be repeated as needed. However, if the child has a very low plasma albumin concentration from a mixed nephrotic–nephritic picture, giving furosemide may precipitate hypovolaemia. Because of this, either give intravenous albumin combined with furosemide (see section on acute management of nephrotic syndrome), or give furosemide under close observation and be prepared to give albumin if hypovolaemia occurs. Cold peripheries and abdominal pain (from splanchnic vasoconstriction) are important signs of this.

The raised blood pressure is frequently fully controlled by salt and water restriction and furosemide, but in some cases hypotensive agents are also needed (see Table 5.6.A.5). Under such acute conditions it is safe to reduce the blood pressure rapidly.

In children with post-streptococcal glomerulonephritis, the kidneys usually make a full recovery, and progression to renal failure is rare. Therefore most of these children will have no sequelae, provided that their fluid and electrolyte balance and blood pressure are carefully managed.

IgA nephropathy (Berger's disease)

The typical presentation is of a child aged 5–15 years who develops an acute upper respiratory tract illness, and simultaneously has heavy haematuria that lasts for several days. Urine microscopy reveals distorted 'glomerular' red cells (see above). Usually the urine then clears completely, but the haematuria may return with subsequent illnesses. Some children with IgA disease have a more insidious illness with little or no macroscopic haematuria.

The diagnosis is suggested in children who present with recurrent heavy glomerular haematuria. There may be a family history. The plasma IgA concentration may be elevated in affected children, but this test is a poor discriminator. In children with a less obvious clinical picture the diagnosis can only be made on a kidney biopsy. Antibody staining will show granular deposits of IgA in glomeruli that have mesangial proliferation. Histologically, IgA disease is identical to Henoch–Schönlein nephritis.

The best prognostic indicator in IgA nephropathy is the amount of proteinuria that persists between the acute episodes of haematuria. Most children have heavy haematuria but little or no proteinuria between attacks, and virtually all of these grow out of the condition, usually without any sequelae. Often the ones with the most dramatic haematuria recover particularly well. The children with a more insidious onset are more likely to have persistent proteinuria, and to continue with the condition into adulthood, eventually developing end-stage renal failure by middle age. There is no good evidence for treatments to prevent this happening. However, adequate blood pressure control is important in slowing the progression of renal disease.

Rarely, IgA disease first presents as a severe rapidly progressing glomerulonephritis. The picture is one of an acute nephritis in which the creatinine level rises rapidly and inexorably. It is therefore clinically indistinguishable from any other rapidly progressive glomerulonephritis, other than by renal biopsy. Treatment options include various immunosuppressive drugs and plasmapheresis. These have not been subjected to controlled trials, are expensive and may lead to serious complications.

Haematuria

- Urine test sticks are highly sensitive and detect the smallest traces of blood.
- **For most conditions that can cause haematuria, the clinical significance is best predicted by the quantity of protein present, so always test for that, too.**
- **The most important test for determining the cause of haematuria is to check the shape of the red cells, ideally under phase-contrast microscopy** (see above).

Macroscopic glomerular haematuria

The presence of distorted red cells may be due to any

form of glomerulonephritis, as listed above. The history of a simultaneous infection may suggest IgA nephropathy, while a recent infection points to post-streptococcal glomerulonephritis. The presence of a rash, or joint involvement, or abdominal pain might suggest Henoch–Schönlein or lupus nephritis as causes, but most other types can only be diagnosed on renal biopsy.

Macroscopic non-glomerular haematuria

The presence of red cells with a normal biconcave appearance indicates bleeding into the urine, and excludes glomerulonephritis as a cause. This may be due to trauma, but this would have to be major, because the renal tract is physically well protected. Minor trauma will only cause bleeding if the kidney is enlarged with cysts, as in adult-type (dominantly inherited) polycystic kidney disease, or if it is vulnerable due to being ectopically positioned. Urinary tract stones can also cause bleeding.

The cystitis caused by a urinary tract infection or by *Schistosoma mansoni* may cause frank haematuria. These can be distinguished on phase-contrast microscopy of a fresh sample, when either bacteria or ova are easily visible.

Although bleeding into the urine can be due to a malignancy, this is rare in childhood, and is then usually from a Wilms' tumour. Frank haematuria in a newborn suggests a renal vein thrombosis, which may be unilateral or bilateral, and the affected kidney is usually easily palpated.

Trauma, stones, an ectopic kidney, adult polycystic disease, a Wilms' tumour and renal vein thrombosis can each be identified by their characteristic appearance on ultrasound scanning. In cases for which no cause has been found, cystoscopy should be considered.

Microscopic glomerular haematuria

Blood may be detected in urine that looks completely clear. Rarely, the red cells appear normal on microscopy; these children should be investigated as for frank non-glomerular haematuria. Most children with microscopic haematuria have distorted 'glomerular' red cells. In this group, management depends on how much proteinuria they have. Those with massive nephrotic-level proteinuria should be assessed and managed in the same way as for other children with nephrotic syndrome. Those with moderate proteinuria are likely to have a form of glomerulonephritis. The vast majority of children will not have any proteinuria with their microscopic haematuria. Investigation of this group is unlikely to identify a cause. If the renal ultrasound scan is normal, these children should be monitored annually with just a urine stick test and blood pressure measurement. If the blood disappears, follow-up may be discontinued. If it persists without proteinuria or hypertension developing, continue the annual reviews. If proteinuria or hypertension appears, the child needs to be investigated accordingly.

Haemolytic uraemic syndrome (HUS)

HUS is a common cause of established (parenchymal) acute renal failure (see above). Children with HUS fall broadly into two groups, according to their pathophysiological mechanisms. It is important to divide them clinically into diarrhoea-associated HUS (D + HUS) and diarrhoea-negative HUS (D – HUS).

D + HUS

This is the common type, and it occurs in otherwise normal children, often in outbreaks or clusters of cases. It is triggered by a toxin that is produced by some colonic bacteria, including *Shigella* and some strains of enteropathic *E. coli*. Infection is from ingestion of contaminated food or fluids. Public health measures to identify a source of the organism are important in preventing and limiting outbreaks. Typically the child has several days of bloody diarrhoea, and then becomes pale and mildly jaundiced (from haemolytic anaemia), may bruise and have petechiae (from thrombocytopenia), and develops oligo-anuria. A blood film shows fragmented red blood cells and a low platelet count.

Antibiotics are not of benefit, and may worsen the condition by causing the acute release of more bacterial toxin. Blood transfusion may be needed (usually when the haemoglobin level falls below 6 grams/dL). Platelet transfusion may exacerbate the condition, and should only be used in the face of uncontrolled bleeding. There is no evidence that any specific medication is of benefit. Management is as for other children with acute renal failure (see above). Mortality from this condition has decreased with active management of fluid and electrolyte imbalance and dialysis.

In a minority of cases, D + HUS can affect other organs, sometimes severely. Effects can include bowel perforations, pancreatitis with diabetes mellitus, and cerebral involvement, with fits, coma and death.

The long-term outcome for children who survive the acute episode of D + HUS is relatively good. Most appear to fully recover renal function, although up to 25% have persistent hypertension or proteinuria. Few develop end-stage renal failure.

D – HUS

This variant is very rare, and is often associated with a functional or actual deficiency of factor H, so a minor trigger (such as a minor viral illness) can precipitate the typical clinical and haematological HUS picture, but without a diarrhoeal prodrome. Typically, D – HUS patients fare much worse long term than D + HUS patients.

Confusing findings

Blood may be present on stick testing without any red cells visible on microscopy. This indicates acute haemolysis such as may occur in glucose-6-phosphate dehydrogenase (G6PD) deficiency or malaria.

Large quantities of urate make the urine brick red. Although families may think the colour resembles blood, it is easily distinguished visually. Porphyria is a very rare cause of confusion. Ingestion of red vegetables, especially beetroot, causes red urine. Rarely, but this possibility must not be forgotten, a parent may place their own blood in a child's urine, leading to unnecessary investigations. This condition is called fabricated or induced illness (FII).

Urinary tract stones
Background

There is wide geographical variation in the frequency of stone disease, and there have been major changes in prevalence with time within populations. The incidence appears to be influenced by a wide range of factors, such as climate, race, diet, dehydration, infections and socio-economic status.

Causes

There are three broad causes of urinary tract stones (which may coexist in individual children).

Proteus urinary tract infections

The mechanism is twofold. The infection results in turbid urine containing cells and debris, and secondly *Proteus* splits urea to form ammonia, which raises the urinary pH. Because calcium ammonium phosphate is relatively insoluble in alkaline urine, it will co-precipitate readily on to the urinary debris under these conditions to form thick sludge initially, and subsequently a stone. This explains why these stones take up the shape of the tract they form in ('staghorns' in the pelvi-calyceal system, 'date stones' in the lower ureter, and round stones in the bladder). Preschool boys are affected much more than any other groups.

Relative dehydration and possibly dietary factors

The mechanisms of stone formation are probably similar to those for infection stones, with chemicals normally found in the urine reaching relatively high concentrations due to low urine volumes, and high dietary intake and consequent excretion rates of relatively insoluble chemicals.

Rare inherited metabolic conditions

These result in excessive urinary excretion of poorly soluble chemicals. Calcium stones are most commonly caused by isolated hypercalciuria (without hypercalcaemia), and more rarely by hypercalciuria combined with hypercalcaemia in hyperparathyroidism. Cystine stones are seen due to an inherited (dominantly or recessively) failure of the proximal tubules to reabsorb this amino acid. Oxalate stones may be due to excessive gut absorption of oxalate when the calcium is unavailable to precipitate it, such as with steatorrhoea. Rarely it is also produced and excreted in excess due to a recessive liver enzyme deficiency.

Presentation and diagnosis

Children may pass a stone or present with severe colicky abdominal pain (typically in one loin), often with frank haematuria. Ultrasound scanning is a sensitive imaging tool, showing the front edge as a bright line, with an acoustic shadow thrown behind it, rather than showing the whole stone. Nephrocalcinosis associated with hypercalciuria is seen as white (echo-bright) renal pyramids.

A plain abdominal X-ray will show radio-opaque stones, and is thus useful for distinguishing the type. Similarly, the appearance of a passed stone or fragment may aid identification. Infection and dehydration stones are usually grey, and only moderately X-ray dense, and take up the shape of the collecting system. Calcium (white) and cystine (yellow) stones are very X-ray dense, may grow up to 2 cm or more in diameter, and are typically smooth, and round or oval wherever they form. Oxalate stones are yellowish-buff coloured and typically grow to 5 mm, with irregular spiky edges. A high oxalate load will result in many small stones rather than large individual ones.

If the type of stone is not clear from the history, chemical measurements can be made and compared with urinary creatinine measurements on an untimed 'spot' urine sample collected during the morning (but not the overnight sample).

The **upper normal limits** of the ratio of the chemical x to creatinine concentrations, both in mmol/litre, are as follows:

- calcium:creatinine ratio of < 0.8
- cystine:creatinine ratio of < 25
- oxalate:creatinine ratio of < 0.18.

These ratios will be normal in children with infection stones, or those secondary to dehydration.

Treatment
Removal of stones

Small stones may be passed spontaneously. Ureteric colic may be excruciatingly painful and should be treated with powerful opiate analgesia (*see* Section 1.15). Spasmolytics such as hyoscine butylbromide (age 6–12 years: 5–10 mg IV or orally; age > 12 years: 20 mg IV or orally) are sometimes used, but are often not effective. Larger stones may need surgical removal by open surgery or cystoscopy. Percutaneous nephrostomy or lithotripsy may be used where specialist facilities exist.

Preventing recurrences

Infection stones should not recur in the absence of infection. Stones due to metabolic causes and those related to dehydration are all helped by a consistently high fluid intake, but it is probably even more important to avoid episodes of acute dehydration (e.g. with vomiting or diarrhoea) than increasing daily fluid intake.

Chlorothiazide up to 10 mg/kg twice daily reduces urinary calcium excretion; its dose can be titrated in hypercalciuria to keep the urinary calcium:creatinine ratio in the normal range. Furosemide should be avoided because it increases urinary calcium excretion.

Children with hyperparathyroidism may require parathyroidectomy.

In cystinuria, it is essential to maintain a lifelong high fluid intake. Alkalinising the urine increases the solubility of cystine. Give oral sodium bicarbonate supplements (start with 1 mmol/kg daily) until the urine pH is usually ≥ 7 on home testing with strip test paper.

With oxalate stones due to malabsorption, treat the underlying bowel problem. Inherited hyperoxaluria typically leads to renal failure and widespread calcification of soft tissue.

5.6.B The child with vesico-ureteric reflux

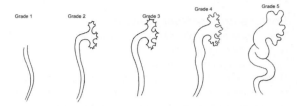

FIGURE 5.6.B.1 The different grades of vesico-ureteric reflux (VUR) according to the International Reflux Study Group classification.

Introduction

Vesico-ureteric reflux (VUR), which is the abnormal flow of urine from the bladder into the upper urinary tract, occurs in about 1 in 100 members of the general population and is more common in girls. Reflux nephropathy is a cause of hypertension and chronic renal failure in children and young adults.

Renal scarring is an acquired phenomenon that usually occurs during the first few years of life, and rarely after the age of 5 years.

Grades of VUR (International Reflux Study Group classification)

These are as follows:
- Grade I: partial filling of an undilated ureter.
- Grade II: total filling of an undilated upper urinary tract.
- Grade III: dilated calyces but sharp fornices.
- Grade IV: blunted fornices and degree of dilatation greater than in lower stages.
- Grade V: massive hydronephrosis and tortuosity of the ureters.

Figure 5.6.B.1 illustrates the different grades of VUR.

Clinical presentation
- VUR almost always occurs in conjunction with an associated UTI.
- It is rarely a cause of flank pain.
- Fever is the single most important symptom for differentiating children with upper tract infections (pyelonephritis) from those with lower tract infections (cystitis).

Investigations

The minimal acceptable standards of investigation would include the following:
- ultrasonography (useful for detection of dilatation, but not for demonstrating scars or reflux)
- micturating cystourethrogram

- investigations in siblings: VUR occurs in up to 30% of siblings, and families should be made aware of this.

Medical management
- Spontaneous resolution occurs most often in the first 2–3 years after diagnosis and then at the rate of 10–15% per year.
- The main goal is the prevention of ascending UTI and renal scarring.

The following measures should be used to prevent UTI:
- Proper wiping techniques (girls should be taught to wipe their bottoms backwards, and to avoid using soap on the vulva if possible; they should be discouraged from wearing nylon knickers).
- Frequent voiding.
- Avoidance of constipation.
- Low-pressure voiding.
- Continuous antibiotic prophylaxis, usually maintained for 2 years. Trimethoprim, 2 mg/kg/day, is the usual prophylactic agent. If breakthrough infections that are resistant to this occur, a suitable alternative prophylactic such as nitrofurantoin (1 mg/kg/day) or nalidixic acid (7.5 mg/kg twice daily) may be used.

In children of all ages the preferred initial treatment is medical, but they need regular follow-up. The need for surgery is becoming increasingly uncommon, but re-implantation of the ureters is occasionally necessary if the VUR is not resolving, is bilateral, in late presentations and in children, or with higher grades of VUR and with antenatally detected hydronephrosis.

5.6.C Acute renal failure

Types of acute renal failure

Acute renal failure (ARF) may be caused by a wide variety of insults to the renal tubule cells. Each type of ARF has a different management. It is therefore important to distinguish them clearly.

Pre-renal failure

This is caused by poor perfusion and hypovolaemia secondary to gastroenteritis, septic shock, haemorrhage, burns, nephrotic syndrome or cardiac failure.

Established (intra-) renal failure

Established renal failure most commonly results from more extreme or more prolonged versions of the same insults that cause pre-renal failure, leading to acute damage to the kidney cells. Other causes include haemolytic–uraemic syndrome and drug toxicity and acute rapidly progressive glomerulonephritis. The prognosis for recovery depends on the underlying cause, whether only the tubule cells are damaged, and whether the glomeruli are also involved.

Post-renal failure

Acute complete obstructions of the renal tract causing failure of urine production are rare, but include posterior urethral valves, obstruction of a single kidney, bilateral stones and trauma.

Diagnosis and initial management of ARF
Pre-renal ARF

Pre-renal failure is essentially a reversible renal dysfunction due to the kidneys being under-perfused, but where the perfusion is still sufficient to prevent necrosis of the renal tissue.

The clinical diagnosis is made by recognising the signs of shock, the commonest of which are a delayed capillary refill time, cool peripheries, a weak pulse, and usually a low blood pressure. However, the blood pressure may also be unexpectedly high because of the powerful renin drive in response to hypovolaemia. An important feature is that the child may complain of abdominal pain (induced by splanchnic ischaemia as blood flow is diverted from the gut to more vital organs).

Laboratory support of the clinical diagnosis is made by measuring the fractional excretion of sodium (FE Na; *see* Section 5.6.A). This requires measurement of the sodium and creatinine concentrations in a sample of blood and urine. If the FE Na is less than 1% this indicates that the renal tubule cells are still alive, and able to respond to shock by reabsorbing sodium avidly. This therefore confirms a diagnosis of pre-renal failure. No other tests, including

measurements of osmolality, urinary sodium concentration alone, or urine microscopy, can reliably differentiate pre-renal from established renal failure. Ultrasound scanning is useful to exclude obstruction, but cannot differentiate pre-renal from established renal failure.

Treatment

This consists of urgent volume expansion followed by furosemide. Percentage dehydration should be estimated, and rehydration should be with Hartmann's or Ringer-lactate solution, plasma, 4.5% albumin or other similar isotonic fluid or plasma substitute. Give 10–20 mL/kg as rapidly as possible initially, and repeat if necessary. If urine output does not commence after adequate volume replacement and furosemide, consider whether this is actually established renal failure, and **do not continue repeating fluid boluses**. Thereafter give Hartmann's or Ringer-lactate solution to fully correct the fluid deficit within 2–4 hours. The deficit can be estimated by multiplying the child's weight by the estimated percentage dehydration. For example, a 6 kg infant estimated to be 10% dehydrated is deficient of approximately 600 mL. According to the above guidelines he would receive 60–240 mL of plasma or plasma substitute very rapidly, and the rest of the 600 mL as Hartmann's or Ringer-lactate solution over a few hours.

Once rehydration has started, give furosemide 2 mg/kg orally or IV. **If there is a urine output response to furosemide this will usually indicate that the renal failure can recover.** If the blood pressure remains markedly depressed after rehydration, it may be due to cardiogenic shock, so consider administering inotropes (*see* Section 5.5.C).

Established ARF

Established failure is due to acute parenchymal damage to the kidneys. In most cases the causes are exactly the same as for pre-renal failure, but an increased severity or duration of the insult has led to death of some of the renal cells. Therefore the pertinent history and clinical signs are usually the same as for pre-renal failure. Other cases are due to directly toxic effects of drugs such as gentamicin, or poisons to the tubular cells. Some forms of glomerulonephritis may lead to ARF (*see* Section 5.6.A), as may the arteriolar disease, haemolytic–uraemic syndrome.

The laboratory diagnosis of established renal failure due to under-perfusion or an ischaemic insult can be made reliably by calculating the FE Na from a measurement of the sodium and creatinine concentrations in a plasma sample and a spot urine sample. The FE Na is typically greater than 2% because the damaged tubules are usually unable to reabsorb sodium avidly. Again, attempts to use other laboratory criteria are unreliable. The history, clinical examination and laboratory confirmation of glomerulonephritis and haemolytic–uraemic syndrome are described in Section 5.6.A.

The most vulnerable region of the kidney is the highly metabolically active mass of proximal tubule cells. If these cells alone die from the insult, this causes acute tubular necrosis (ATN), which will fully recover in 2–4 weeks if the child is maintained in good health during that period of renal failure (likely to require dialysis). More severe insults may result in damage to some or all of the glomeruli as well, which are in the renal cortex. Glomerular damage is irreversible, and acute cortical necrosis may therefore result in chronic or end-stage renal failure.

Fluid repletion and furosemide administration will not result in recovery of renal function. If an FE Na is not available to distinguish between pre-renal and established ARF, it is sensible to give a trial of fluid bolus and furosemide. Management consists of correcting the dehydration, as for pre-renal failure, and thereafter careful maintenance of fluids (usually restriction) and electrolyte balance and nutrition (restricting potassium intake) while it is hoped that some recovery of tubule cells will lead to recovery of kidney function. **This is likely to require dialysis.** If recovery is going to happen it is likely to have begun by 4 weeks, but can occur up to 2 or even 3 months later. There are no reliable imaging techniques for determining whether the child has recoverable ATN or irrecoverable cortical necrosis, but renal biopsy if available may distinguish between these.

Post-renal ARF

Post-renal causes are due to obstruction to all of the urinary flow, and are uncommon. This will not occur if the flow from just one kidney is blocked (unless a single kidney is present). Causes in a child with two kidneys include congenital urethral valves, or a bladder stone obstructing the urethra. Causes in a child with a single kidney include a ureteric stone, or a pelvi-ureteric junction narrowing (which is congenital, but often blocks intermittently and presents late).

All of these pathologies cause severe acute colicky abdominal pain. This is well localised in older children to either unilateral pain with ureteric obstruction, or lower abdominal pain with bladder neck obstruction. An ultrasound scan will reveal stones and dilatation of the urinary tract proximal to the site of the obstruction.

Treatment

The treatment of post-renal ARF is to remove or bypass the obstruction. For a bladder neck stone obstruction, catheterise the child. Giving pain relief with an opiate analgesic may allow time for an obstructing urethral stone to pass, or for the intermittent blockage from a pelvi-ureteric junction narrowing to clear. If not, the stone may need to be removed cystoscopically or by ureterolithotomy, or the upper renal tract can be drained by insertion of a percutaneous nephrostomy under ultrasound guidance. Once removal of the obstruction has allowed the renal function to recover, procedures such as surgical repair of the pelvi-ureteric junction may be performed.

Ongoing management of persistent ARF
General management

The management of ARF consists of the provision of good general care for an acutely ill child, plus the specific management of fluid and electrolyte balance, blood pressure, and the adjustment of some drug dosages. In many instances the limitations that need to be imposed to keep in metabolic balance compromise the care that can be given in other areas.

The safe management of these children requires the maintenance of meticulous fluid balance. To achieve this it is necessary to accurately measure all intake and losses. For babies, stool and urine losses are best estimated by weighing their clean and dirty nappies. Insensible

water losses need to be estimated. This is done most reliably by assuming it to be $300\,\text{mL/m}^2$ in temperate conditions, and higher in hotter climates and at low humidity (for estimation of body surface area, see Table 9.16, Section 9). The best guide to the overall changes in fluid balance is to weigh the child twice daily.

Nutrition, fluid and electrolyte balance

Adequate nutrition is important for recovery, but may be difficult to provide. If a child is old enough and well enough to eat solid food they are relatively easy to manage because they can obtain their requirements with little water. Aim to provide their normal calorie intake from carbohydrates and fats, and limit their protein intake to about 1 gram/kg/day to minimise uraemia. It is necessary to limit the salt intake to prevent sodium retention and hypernatraemia, which leads to insatiable thirst and hence fluid overload. It may be necessary to provide some of the sodium as bicarbonate to prevent acidosis, typically at a starting dose of 1 mmol/kg/day (note that 1 mL of an 8.4% sodium bicarbonate solution contains 1 mmol, and 1 gram of powder contains 12 mmol).

Dietary potassium must be restricted (avoid in particular bananas, tomatoes, coconut, citrus fruits or juices, and chocolate) to decrease the risk of hyperkalaemia. Dietary phosphate must be restricted (restrict milk and dairy products but not breastfeeding) to reduce the risk of hyperphosphataemia.

Giving calcium carbonate with the food (e.g. 0.5–2 grams with each meal) will bind the intestinal phosphate and reduce hyperphosphataemia as well as reducing the tendency to hypocalcaemia.

Young infants who normally take milk, and children who are too ill to eat solid food, or who have gastrointestinal involvement, will need either nasogastric tube feeding or intravenous nutrition. The enteral route should always be used if possible. However, adequate nutrition has to be delivered in a relatively large fluid volume. If the child has polyuric renal failure, or has high non-renal water losses (e.g. from diarrhoea or drain fluids), this can be achieved. However, if the child is oligo-anuric it is very difficult (and often impossible) to give sufficient nutrition without causing fluid overload, which can lead to hypertension and pulmonary oedema. Concentrated fat-based oral feeds can be made up from ingredients such as double cream. **Specialist parenteral nutrition solutions will be required if they are to be used for a child in renal failure.**

The need for dialysis

Although severe fluid and electrolyte restriction is possible for short periods of time while awaiting spontaneous recovery of renal function, it is not possible to both provide adequate nutrition and maintain stable water and chemical balance over a prolonged period in a child with oligo-anuria. If such a child does not start to regain renal function, they will die unless they are dialysed.

The main indications for starting dialysis (where available) are as follows:

- Hyperkalaemia: this is discussed below.
- Fluid overload causing pulmonary oedema and/or hypertension.
- Severe metabolic acidosis: this is another important reason for dialysis (if available). Treatment with sodium bicarbonate is limited because this may lead to massive

sodium overload, and thus to dangerous levels of hypernatraemia, and to greater fluid retention. Fluid overload is worsened if hypoglycaemia occurs (this needs to be treated with IV glucose solutions) and if other fluids are required (e.g. platelets).

- Uraemia: clinical symptoms are apparent at concentrations above 40 mmol/litre, but uraemia is not as acutely life-threatening as hyperkalaemia or pulmonary oedema. It needs to be reduced by providing more non-protein calories.

Hyperkalaemia

Hyperkalaemia causes life-threatening arrhythmias, especially in acute renal failure, where other metabolic changes may exacerbate the risk (e.g. hypocalcaemia). Aim to keep the plasma potassium concentration below 6.5 mmol/litre in older children and below 7.0 mmol/litre in neonates (who appear to tolerate hyperkalaemia better).

There are three pharmacological approaches to managing children with hyperkalaemia.

1 **Reduce the risk of it causing arrhythmias.** Reduce the effect of hyperkalaemia by increasing the plasma calcium concentration. Give 0.5 mL/kg (0.1 mmol/kg) of calcium gluconate 10% IV.

2 **Remove potassium from the body.** Give calcium resonium 1 gram/kg orally or rectally, and repeat with 0.5 grams/kg 12-hourly. This ion-exchange resin exchanges potassium for calcium. It is not well tolerated. If volume status and urine flow permit, furosemide will increase urinary potassium excretion.

3 **Push potassium into the cells.** This last option only results in a temporary improvement, because as soon as the treatment stops the potassium moves back out of the cells. Essentially this approach is only a holding treatment while a more effective therapy such as dialysis is prepared:

- Give a beta-2-adrenergic agonist, such as salbutamol. Nebulise 2.5 mg for children under 25 kg, and 5 mg for larger children, or give 4 micrograms/kg IV. This works rapidly, but the potassium will move back out of the cells within a few hours.

- Alternatively, infuse a high concentration of glucose. Monitor the plasma glucose concentration and be prepared to infuse insulin beginning at a dose of 0.05 units/kg/hour if it exceeds 12 mmol/litre. It is unsafe to mix the glucose and insulin and infuse them together in children, as this may cause hypoglycaemia. This necessitates close monitoring, an inevitable fluid load, and only lasts while it is continued.

- Bicarbonate infusions push potassium into the cells. A dose of 2.5 mmol/kg may be infused over 15 minutes. If a solution of 8.4% is used, containing 1 mmol/mL, it will increase the plasma sodium concentration by approximately 5 mmol/litre very quickly, which may be hazardous. It is better to use a solution of 1.26% which is isonatraemic, but this requires that a volume of 17 mL/kg be infused, adding to fluid overload.

Acute peritoneal dialysis

Indications

Children with acute renal failure can be considered for peritoneal dialysis if their biochemical control is not safe despite careful treatment (see section on management of acute renal failure above). Although the specific indications for initiating peritoneal dialysis vary from case to case, the commonest reason is a high and rising plasma potassium concentration (e.g. above 6.5 mmol/litre in an older child, or above 7 mmol/litre in a neonate). Others indications include a urea concentration above 40 mmol/litre, a phosphate concentration above 3.5 mmol/litre, or acidosis with a bicarbonate concentration below 12 mmol/litre, as well as hypertension or pulmonary oedema due to fluid overload.

The primary underlying reason for needing to proceed to dialysis is usually anuria or severe oliguria. This is because even a moderate urine flow will prevent fluid overload if the intake is restricted, and because it 'makes space' for biochemically appropriate replacement fluid. Even poor-quality urine contains potassium, so replacement with potassium-free fluid allows a net loss. Also, urinary sodium losses can be replaced with IV sodium bicarbonate to counter acidosis, and a high infused glucose concentration will reduce catabolism and so minimise urea, potassium and phosphate production. Take advantage of all fluid losses; diarrhoeal losses will 'make space' just as effectively as urine losses.

Practical techniques
PD Catheter

Ideally, a catheter with side holes should be inserted so that its tip lies in or near one of the iliac fossae. The ideal catheter is a cuffed silastic Tenckhoff which has a series of side holes and an end which is cut off straight, but these are expensive and need to be inserted through a peel-away sheath (usually in the midline below the umbilicus). It is possible to dialyse adequately using other more readily available catheters that have side holes, such as chest drains. These are usually inserted over a metal trocar, and have a tapered tip with an end hole that is considerably smaller than the diameter of the tube lumen, which can lead to difficulties with blockage with omentum (see below).

Insertion of catheter

- This must be a strictly aseptic technique performed either under general anaesthetic, or under sedation/systemic analgesia (see Section 1.15) and local anaesthetic. The catheter may be placed directly percutaneously or with a subcutaneous tunnel or with full surgical procedure.

- If the catheter is not tunnelled, to prevent fluid leakage it is essential that it is inserted through the skin with a very tight fit; using a larger skin hole and stitching it closed will inevitably result in leakage in time. Cut a skin slit that is obviously smaller than the tube, and stretch it with a surgical clip or stitch holder.

- Before introducing the catheter, insert an IV cannula through the skin cut and fill the abdomen with about 40 mL/kg of Ringer-lactate solution or 0.9% saline until the abdominal wall is fairly tense.

- To insert the catheter through a tight hole requires some force, and this is best done by pushing the catheter and trocar tip into the dilated skin slit as far as possible, and then suddenly advancing it with a sharp force through the tense abdominal wall. Grip the catheter and trocar tightly about 3 cm from its tip to act as a stop as it pops into the abdomen (the risk of causing damage is greatly reduced by the presence of sufficient instilled fluid).

- To further minimise the risk of trauma, it is better to

enter the upper quadrant lateral to the rectus sheath, and aim towards the opposite iliac fossa, than to use an infra-umbilical approach. Be aware of the possibility of an enlarged spleen or liver.

- Once sited, test to check that fluid flows rapidly in and out, before securing with a skin stitch and sterile dressing.

Problems with omentum

It is common for omentum to wrap around the end of the catheter, and for some to enter the end hole. This slows or stops drainage because the omentum is sucked further into the lumen, but has little effect on filling because the omentum is washed back towards the catheter tip, and the fluid exits through the side holes. Deal with it as follows:

- The omentum can often be forced out by rapidly injecting up to 50 mL of dialysis fluid, Ringer-lactate solution or 0.9% saline into the catheter under pressure.
- If this fails, withdraw the catheter from the abdomen using full aseptic technique. If the omentum has become detached, simply reinsert the catheter, and resume dialysis.
- If (as usually happens) the catheter comes out with the omentum attached, detach it, and gently pull more omentum out, tie round it with an absorbable suture near to the skin surface, cut off the excess, and return the omentum into the abdomen, using the stitch to obtain easy purchase, and replace the catheter.

Fluid and cycles

- Run the dialysis fluid in through a giving set with a burette, and with the bag held about 1 metre above the patient, and leave it to dwell for 30 minutes. Allow it to drain by gravity through a Y-connector into a sealed bag for about 10–15 minutes; by then, it should have drained about as much as was instilled, and the flow should have stopped.
- The osmolality of the dialysis fluid determines the amount of water that is drawn off (ultra-filtered) during each peritoneal dialysis cycle, and this is adjusted by varying the glucose content. Typical glucose concentrations available are 1.36% (standard) and 3.86% (high-osmolality) bags. Start with 1.36% glucose.
- Add heparin, 1000 units/litre, to the fluid initially to prevent any blood from the insertion clotting the catheter. Discontinue it once the effluent fluid looks clear.
- Start with 10 mL/kg cycles of dialysis fluid for the first 2 days. Using this small volume minimises the risk of a peritoneopleural leak of dialysate.
- The first cycle balances are unreliable because there is always a sump of fluid left, but after that the ultra-filtrate required is the volume of fluid that needs to be removed to correct any overload, plus an amount equivalent to the urine that would normally be passed (so just a little less than the normal fluid intake).
- If there is too little ultra-filtrate, increase the glucose concentration of the dialysate by giving some cycles of 1.36% glucose and some of 3.86% glucose. Continue to review the fluid balance, and vary the proportion of cycles of each strength as necessary.
- Increase the cycle volume by 10 mL/kg every 2 days until tolerance occurs, or a maximum of 40 mL/kg. As the cycle volume increases, it is not necessary to dialyse so intensively. Either continue with 30-minute dwells,

but just for part of the day (e.g. 8 hours overnight), or lengthen the dwells, eventually moving to chronic ambulatory peritoneal dialysis (CAPD), in which the fluid is left in the peritoneum all the time, and exchanged four to six times per day.

Biochemical control

The sodium, calcium and magnesium content of the dialysis fluid is similar to that of plasma, and the fluid contains lactate, which is converted to base, so is equivalent to bicarbonate. Cycling therefore tends to keep the plasma concentrations stable. Peritoneal dialysis fluid contains no potassium, urea or creatinine, so these are removed.

- Urea equilibrates rapidly, so is cleared well, allowing the child to have a normal protein intake.
- Creatinine is removed slowly, so peritoneal dialysis never restores the plasma levels to normal. This is useful because creatinine is not toxic, and its plasma concentration continues to provide a measure of intrinsic renal function and renal recovery.
- Sometimes the dialysis required to control fluid or urea excretion is sufficient to cause hypokalaemia. If so, reduce the potassium dialysis clearance by adding up to 3 mmol/litre potassium chloride to the dialysate bags (do not use more than this; if the potassium concentration is still too low, give extra orally or intravenously).

Peritonitis

Infection is the major hazard of peritoneal dialysis, and produces a cloudy dialysis effluent in the drainage bag due to white blood cells. Prevention is crucial, by scrupulous hand washing and avoiding touching the open tubing ends while changing peritoneal dialysis bags, and by changing connections as infrequently as possible.

- Monitor constantly by inspecting the clarity of the effluent fluid.
- Undertake daily microscopy for white blood cells (there should be < 50 white blood cells/mL; see Section 8.5).
- If the effluent fluid is cloudy, and microscopy confirms the presence of large numbers of white blood cells (over 100, but typically several hundred), culture a sample of fluid, and start treatment at once by adding heparin (to stop blockage of the tube holes with fibrin) and antibiotics to peritoneal dialysis bags and revert to continuous cycling if not still doing that. Start with vancomycin and ceftazidime, and adjust according to the culture and sensitivity results. Concentrations of antibiotics that may be added to peritoneal dialysis fluid are as follows:
  - vancomycin, 25 mg/litre
  - ceftazidime, 125 mg/litre
  - ampicillin, 125 mg/litre
  - flucloxacillin, 250 mg/litre
  - gentamicin, 8 mg/litre.
- Continue continuous cycling until a count of < 50 white blood cells/mL is obtained for two samples taken 12 hours apart. Then return to previous dialysis cycles, adding peritoneal dialysis antibiotics for 14 days.
- If accidental contamination occurs, such as touching the open dialysis catheter during a bag exchange, or a fluid leak from a connection or punctured bag, add vancomycin and either ceftazidime or gentamicin to the dialysis fluid for the next 12 hours.
- Fungal peritonitis is difficult to clear. It is best to remove

the catheter and treat systemically until the peritonitis resolves.

The urine output must be measured throughout the procedure.

Analgesia for the procedure and throughout the dialysis is likely to be required.

Chronic renal failure
Background

Chronic renal failure (CRF) is more frequent in boys than in girls. Its commonest cause is congenital renal abnormalities such as dysplasia associated with severe antenatal vesico-ureteric reflux, and often also with posterior urethral valves. It can also follow almost any form of acute renal failure.

It is relatively easy to improve the quality of life of children with milder forms of CRF by simple treatments, especially in the case of older children. In its more severe forms, CRF is very difficult to treat effectively, requiring expensive drugs and intensive laboratory monitoring.

Very young children with CRF are particularly difficult to manage, as they usually have marked anorexia and failure to thrive. Successful treatment requires a massive family and medical input, highly expensive drugs, and a complex medical infrastructure of a kind that has only limited availability worldwide at present. **Each country should have a specialised centre that can provide care for such children.**

Progression of CRF

CRF tends to worsen progressively through childhood. This is mainly because dysplastic or damaged kidneys may not grow in parallel with body growth, and renal function becomes outstripped by demand. Deterioration is likely to be quicker if the child has hypertension, or has recurrent urinary infections with continuing reflux, both of which require active treatment.

Management
Water, sodium and potassium

Children with dysplastic kidneys usually have **polyuric renal failure** in which they lose water and salt, and often potassium, in an uncontrolled way. Consequently, they have a persistent thirst, and can become dehydrated extremely rapidly if they vomit persistently. They need IV fluids early, particularly if there is an episode of gastroenteritis.

Hyperkalaemia due to severe CRF occurs relatively late in children with polyuria.

Supplementing with sodium bicarbonate or salt, as needed, can improve well-being and growth. For each of these, start by adding about 1 mmol/kg per day. For bicarbonate, increase daily until the plasma concentration is in the normal range. The total extra sodium needed is best judged by measuring lying and standing blood pressures to detect postural hypotension; a fall in plasma sodium concentration is a very late event. Note that:

- For bicarbonate, 1 mmol is equivalent to 84 mg, so 1 gram contains about 12 mmol bicarbonate. For intravenous use, 8.4% bicarbonate solution contains 1 mmol/mL.
- For sodium chloride (salt), 1 mmol is equivalent to 57 mg, so 1 gram contains about 18 mmol sodium. For intravenous use, each litre of 0.9% saline contains 150 mmol

(*see* Table 5.5.A.2 in Section 5.5.A on 'shock' for details of electrolyte concentrations in other more physiological infusion crystalloids, such as Ringer-lactate and Hartmann's solution), and strong sterile sodium chloride solutions can be used to increase the sodium concentrations of standard IV fluids (e.g. a 30% solution contains 5 mmol sodium/mL).

Children with **oliguric renal failure** are more difficult to manage because they require salt and water restriction to prevent hypertension, and potassium restriction to prevent hyperkalaemia.

When dialysis is available, indications to begin this treatment are often multiple, and include an intolerable diet or fluid restriction, and symptoms such as poor growth and lethargy as important factors, rather than just specific biochemical parameters.

Calcium and phosphate

CRF can lead to abnormalities of the plasma calcium and phosphate concentrations, and these can cause rickets and hyperparathyroidism (renal osteodystrophy), which can result in bone pain, limb deformities, and fractures (especially slipped femoral capital epiphyses). The primary problem is phosphate retention due to a reduced glomerular filtration rate. This causes a high plasma phosphate concentration, which in turn leads to a low plasma calcium level by mass action, and by suppressing the enzyme 1-alpha-hydroxylase, thus lowering the concentration of circulating activated 1-alpha-hydroxyvitamin D. A primary lack of 1-alpha-hydroxylase enzyme from destruction of kidney tissue is rare except in very severe CRF.

Treatment is therefore aimed at reducing the phosphate intake, either directly by dietary restriction (reducing the intake of meat and dairy products), or by **giving calcium carbonate** with meals. This binds with the phosphate in the gut, and prevents its absorption. The dose needed is very variable. Start at about 50–100 mg/kg, divided among the day's meals, and titrate the dose (if biochemical monitoring is available) to keep plasma phosphate levels at the lower end of the normal range. This commonly also results in a rise in plasma calcium levels into the normal range. Because of this, it is seldom necessary to treat mild CRF with 1-alpha-hydroxyvitamin D_3. If it is needed, in more severe CRF, start with about 20 nanograms/kg once daily, and titrate the dose up until the plasma calcium concentration is normalised. It is extremely potent, and using it without regular monitoring can easily lead to severe hypercalcaemia, which can result in permanent calcification of tissues, including the renal medullae.

Anaemia

Severe CRF leads to anaemia because the kidneys fail to produce enough erythropoietin. Treatment by repeated transfusions is unsatisfactory because blood is often scarce, carries infective risks, is always expensive, and eventually leads to iron overload. Recombinant erythropoietin (if available) should be used, after adequate iron levels have been achieved (folate and vitamin B_{12} supplementation is seldom required, but levels should be checked if possible).

Growth

Many factors lead to growth failure in children with CRF.

In older children, attention to fluid and electrolyte intake, prevention of acidosis with bicarbonate supplements, and control of the bone biochemistry help considerably. Control of uraemia by encouraging a diet containing about 1 gram of protein/kg daily and a high carbohydrate intake will also contribute to good growth.

In young children, the problems are much greater. They are often extremely anorexic; most babies with severe CRF virtually do not feed, and only survive if tube fed for months or even years. Many also vomit excessively. Even when supplemented with tube feeds, very young children with CRF often remain small.

Transplantation

Renal transplantation (if it is available) from a living or deceased donor gives the best quality of life for children with end-stage renal failure.

5.7 Liver disorders

5.7.A Acute liver failure

BOX 5.7.A.1 Minimum standards
- Vitamin K.
- IV glucose 10%.
- Oxygen.
- Lactulose.
- Blood transfusions and clotting factors.
- Ranitidine/antacids.
- Antibiotics and antifungal treatment.
- High-carbohydrate diet.
- N-acetylcysteine.
- Measurements of prolonged blood clotting times.

TABLE 5.7.A.1 Clinical features of ALF

1.	Nausea and vomiting is a frequent early feature.
2.	Bruising, petechiae and bleeding secondary to deranged clotting (INR > 4 is associated with 90% mortality).
3.	Jaundice with tender hepatomegaly or a liver that is enlarged but reducing in size in days.
4.	Encephalopathy latterly complicated by features of raised intracranial pressure.
5.	Metabolic alkalosis from failure of the urea cycle associated with a low serum potassium concentration.
6.	Failure to maintain normoglycaemia.

Introduction

In contradistinction to fulminant liver failure in adults, acute liver failure (ALF) in children may not be accompanied by encephalopathy, which tends to be a late feature, or if it occurs early in the course suggests a metabolic cause.

Prolonged prothrombin time (PT) or international normalised ratio (INR) indicates coagulopathy due to the absence of liver-synthesised coagulation factors, and is the basis of the definition of ALF. However, coagulopathy in the presence of liver dysfunction can also result from vitamin K deficiency (usually due to prolonged cholestasis) and consumption of coagulation factors due to disseminated intravascular coagulation (DIC).

Definition

Based on the above, ALF is present in children when coagulopathy accompanies liver disease but is not due to DIC or a lack of vitamin K (see Table 5.7.A.1). Administration of IV or IM vitamin K (300 micrograms/kg for children aged 1 month to 12 years: 10 mg for those over 12 years of age) ensures that remaining coagulopathy is due to failed production (liver failure) or excess consumption (DIC). Markers that suggest DIC, rather than ALF, include a low platelet count, compatible blood film (fragmented cells, schistocytes) and a serum bilirubin that is predominantly unconjugated.

Diagnosis of ALF

- The history may establish a recent episode of shock including severe dehydration, sepsis or heatstroke, evidence of ingestion of toxic mushrooms or drugs (including those bought over the counter or obtained from any non-conventional source), or exposure to infection such as *Salmonella typhimurium* (see Table 5.7.A.2).
- The possibility of bloodborne or other parenteral infection with hepatitis B up to 6 months previously should be explored.
- Examination may show features of acute portal hypertension with liver tenderness suggesting Budd–Chiari syndrome or a veno-occlusive disease, or lymphadenopathy suggesting malignancy.
- Urine should be tested for bilirubin, urobilinogen and reducing substances.
- Stools should be examined for colour.
- **Tests to establish many of the causes of ALF require sophisticated laboratory facilities which may not be available.**
- The cause may be diagnosed from local epidemiology.
- A blood film and an INR or prothrombin ratio should be measured.
- A full septic screen, **excluding lumbar puncture because of coagulopathy**, should be performed (including fungal cultures and chest X-ray).

TABLE 5.7.A.2 Causes of acute liver failure

Type	Cause
Infective Viral	Hepatitis A, B, C or D, HIV, parvovirus, herpes virus, enterovirus, adenovirus, echovirus varicella, yellow fever, Lassa fever, Ebola virus, Marburg virus, dengue
Bacterial, protozoal	Leptospirosis, typhoid, malaria
Metabolic	Wilson's disease, tyrosinaemia, urea cycle disorders, galactosaemia, mitochondrial disorders, haemochromatosis, Niemann–Pick disease type C
Drugs	Paracetamol, anti-TB drugs, halothane, carbamazepine, sodium valproate
Toxins	*Amanita phalloides*, heatstroke, shock (all causes)
Autoimmune	Anti-smooth-muscle antibodies and anti-liver-kidney microsome (LKD) antibodies, antibody-positive giant cell hepatitis with haemolytic anaemia
Vascular	B Budd–Chiari syndrome, veno-occlusive disease (may follow bush tea ingestion)
Cryptogenic	Non-A, non-B hepatitis

Complications of ALF

These include the following:

- Encephalopathy and raised intracranial pressure, convulsions.
- Hepatorenal syndrome.
- High-output cardiac failure.
- Hepatopulmonary syndrome.
- Acid–base disturbance; initially alkalosis with hypokalaemia, followed by metabolic acidosis from multi-organ failure.
- Gastrointestinal bleeding, including early development of oesophageal varices.
- Pancreatitis.
- Bone-marrow aplasia.
- Sepsis, particularly Gram-negative and fungal, pulmonary (including aspiration) and septicaemia.

Fluids in ALF

- Fluids in ALF should be restricted to two-thirds of normal maintenance (*see* **Section 9 Appendix**).
- When albumin needs to be infused, the dose is 5 mL/kg of 20% albumin, and for fresh-frozen plasma the dose is 10–20 mL/kg.
- Do not give any potassium if the patient is anuric.
- Treat hypoglycaemia in the usual way (*see* **Section 5.8.B**).

Management of children with ALF

- **In the absence of liver transplantation, conservative management relies on liver recovery, which will occur in many cases of ALF, taking place before irrecoverable damage occurs in another organ, particularly the brain. The best possible high-dependency care may improve the likelihood of this occurring.**
- Refer the child to a specialised centre if one exists in that country. Undertake frequent reviews and clinical observations and high-dependency nursing.

TABLE 5.7.A.3 Four grades of hepatic encephalopathy

Grade I
Irritable, inappropriate behaviour
Lethargy
Mildly depressed awareness
Tremor or flap (slow wave in outstretched extended hand)
Grade II
Aggressive outbursts, bad language
Unable to stay still
Pulling at IV cannulae, plaster, etc.
Grade III
Mood swings
Irritable, odd behaviour
Not recognising parents
Photophobia
Grade IVa
Mostly sleeping, but rousable
Incoherent, sluggish pupils
Hypertonia with or without clonus and extensor spasm
Grade IVb
Absent reflexes
Irregular gasps with imminent respiratory failure
Bradycardia
Unresponsive to painful stimuli

- Blood tests for coagulation, electrolytes, blood glucose levels and blood count should be performed frequently (ideally 8-hourly).
- Hypoglycaemia and hypokalaemia must be detected and corrected.
  - Maintain blood glucose levels in the range 4–9 mmol/litre using a restricted fluid volume (two-thirds of maintenance) consisting of a minimum concentration of 10% glucose (given IV or orally); 20% glucose is the preferred solution, but is irritant to peripheral veins and is best given into a central vein or, better still, if tolerated, orally or via a nasogastric tube.
  - A metabolic alkalosis resulting from a failure of the urea cycle may cause hypokalaemia as a result of a shift of potassium into the cells. This hypokalaemia can worsen encephalopathy, and should be corrected enterally or IV.
- Children with encephalopathy should be nursed with their head elevated at 30 degrees above the horizontal and without neck flexion (to decrease intracranial pressure and minimise cerebral irritability). Children with agitated encephalopathy of grade II or III represent a major management problem, as they may pull out monitoring equipment and IV lines. **Sedation will worsen their encephalopathy.**
- Strict fluid balance is essential.
  - Allowance should be made for a hot climatic environment by giving 10–20% extra fluid, and 10% extra fluid should be given for each degree of fever.
  - Strict monitoring of urinary output and fluid balance is required. Aim for a urine output of not less than

0.5 mL/kg/hour (determined by weighing nappies or measuring output).

— Daily weights are useful if the child can be moved, and will allow greater precision in fluid balance.

- If possible and appropriate, insert a central venous line and aim to provide a central venous pressure (CVP) of 6–10 cmH$_2$O if necessary to give a normal blood pressure. Increased CVP may be required to compensate for an increased cardiac output, or to treat the reduced cardiac performance that is seen as liver failure progresses.
  — Patients who require inotropes despite adequate central venous filling are developing multi-organ failure and have a very poor prognosis.
- Stop oral protein initially, and during recovery gradually reintroduce 0.5–1 gram/kg/day in oral or nasogastric feeding.
- A high-energy intake, predominantly of dietary carbohydrate, should be promoted to prevent protein catabolism with an increased serum ammonia level. In the absence of products such as Maxijul, uncooked cornstarch may be used as a source of carbohydrate. It may be given up to 2-hourly to provide predicted energy requirements, and may also help to maintain normoglycaemia.
- Lactulose, 5–10 mL two to three times a day, is given to produce two to four soft and acid stools per day (it should be omitted if diarrhoea occurs).
- Maintain normothermia by environmental measures (but NOT with paracetamol, aspirin or ibuprofen).
- Give one dose of IV or IM vitamin K (300 micrograms/kg for children aged 1 month to 12 years: 10 mg for those over 12 years of age) to attempt correction of prolonged clotting time.
- If there is frank bleeding (gastrointestinal or other), consider giving fresh blood, fresh-frozen plasma or cryoprecipitate at 10 mL/kg IV.
- A prophylactic H$_2$-blocking agent (e.g. ranitidine 2 mg/kg twice daily orally or IV) is given with oral antacid (e.g. sucralfate 250 mg four times a day for children aged 1 month to 2 years, 500 mg four times a day for those aged 2–12 years, 1 gram four to six times a day for those aged 12–18 years) to prevent gastric and/or duodenal ulceration.
- Treat any confirmed sepsis aggressively.
  — Broad-spectrum antibiotics, such as a cephalosporin plus amoxicillin, or penicillin plus gentamicin, should be used prophylactically.
  — Systemic fungal infection may require IV amphotericin (250 micrograms to 1 mg/kg/day) or oral fluconazole (10 mg/kg once daily).
  — Give prophylactic oral nystatin mouthwashes (100 000 IU (1 mL) four times a day).
- Manage hypotension with IV colloids and possibly dopamine and nor-adrenaline infusions if central venous access has been obtained (see Section 5.5.C).

Paracetamol overdose

If paracetamol overdose is suspected or confirmed, N-acetylcysteine must be started immediately, whatever the time between the alleged overdose and the visit to the hospital. Histories after overdose are often misleading,

with multiple administrations and other drugs not immediately admitted. N-acetylcysteine is given IV at 150 mg/kg over 15 minutes as a loading dose, then 100 mg/kg over 12 hours, then 100 mg/kg/day as a continuous infusion until the INR is normal.

Prognosis for ALF

The most important prognostic parameter for ALF is metabolic acidosis. Even in the presence of a very prolonged INR, a patient who is not acidotic will have an 80% chance of survival. A plasma pH of < 7.25 (if blood gas measurement is available) indicates a 95% risk of mortality.

Other factors that predict a poor outcome are grade III or IV hepatic encephalopathy and oliguric renal failure (usually occurring 3–4 days after onset).

Risk factors

- Age < 2 years.
- INR ≥ 4 (associated with a mortality of > 90%).
- Serum bilirubin concentration > 350 micromol/litre.
- Grade III or IV encephalopathy.
- Non-A non-B hepatitis.
- Drug-induced ALF.

Poisoning or toxic reactions associated with the development of ALF

These include the following:

- paracetamol
- mushrooms, particularly *Amanita phalloides* and similar species
- carbon tetrachloride
- copper
- iron
- halothane and other volatile anaesthetic agents
- sodium valproate
- carbamazepine
- phenytoin
- phenobarbitone
- isoniazid
- cytotoxic drugs
- irradiation.

Galactosaemia

- A defect of galactose-1-phosphate uridyl transferase is revealed in the perinatal period when affected infants are first exposed to milk feeding.
- Infants present with vomiting, hepatitis, liver failure and DIC, often with septicaemia.
- Symptoms settle within 2–3 days when feeding with milk is discontinued.
- Hypoglycaemia is seen in the majority of cases.
- Cataracts may be detected.
- Fanconi's nephropathy explains the presence of galactose in the urine giving the characteristic 'Clinistix negative, Clinitest positive' side-room test pattern when the infant is receiving feeds.
- Management consists of the removal of galactose from the diet and standard management of liver failure and sepsis.

5.7.B Chronic liver disease

Introduction

The liver is anatomically strategically positioned between the gastrointestinal tract and the systemic circulation to perform its nutritional homeostatic role. Through the portal system, it filters organic and inorganic substances, microorganisms and their breakdown products, including endotoxins. It also stores and processes nutritional substrates and coordinates nutritional status through endocrine carrier proteins. The liver is therefore the major organ of nutritional homeostasis.

It can be helpful in diagnostic and prognostic terms to think of clinically evident liver dysfunction as having degrees of severity in three simultaneous dimensions: cholestasis, portal hypertension (with hypersplenism) and synthetic function (although homeostasis of ammonia and blood glucose levels may fit better into this synthetic group). The clinical features are summarised in Table 5.7.B.1.

Clinical symptoms and signs of chronic liver disease (CLD)

TABLE 5.7.B.1 Clinical features of CLD

Clinical feature	Cholestasis	Portal hypertension	Cell dysfunction
Jaundice	Conjugated	−	Mixed if severe
Pruritis	+	−	−
Leuchonychia	+	−	−
Fat-soluble vitamin deficiency	+	−	−
Xanthomas	+*	−	−
Splenomegaly	−	+	−
Cutaneous shunts	−	+	+
Other cutaneous stigmata	−	+	+
Hypersplenism	−	+	−
Hepatopulmonary syndrome	−	+	+
Oesophageal varices	−	+	−
Ascites	−	+	+
Encephalopathy	−	+	+
Dependent oedema	−	−	+
Malnutrition	+	+	+

*Not in familial intrahepatic cholestasis.

Jaundice

Accompanied by dark urine and pale stools, jaundice is characteristic of cholestatic liver disease. The urine of infants should not contain significant colour or stain the nappy, and yellow urine strongly suggests bile obstruction. Yellow sclerae suggest cholestatic jaundice but are difficult to detect in small infants, and children with deep skin pigmentation may have some scleral pigmentation. There is no substitute for personal examination of stool and urine, as the history can be misleading. White stool, or stools the colour of cream cheese or uncooked pastry, are clearly abnormal, whilst pale yellow, pale green or pale brown stools may also raise concern about liver function. Comparison with a stool colour chart (www.yellowalert.org/file_download.aspx?id=7358) can be extremely helpful if there is doubt.

Hepatomegaly

Healthy infants may have up to 2 centimetres of liver edge palpable below the costal margin, but the texture is soft. An abnormally hard texture or irregular inferior margin strongly suggests established liver disease with fibrosis/cirrhosis. Changed liver conformation with prominence in the mid-line but an impalpable right lobe suggests collapse, regeneration and the development of cirrhosis. Tenderness of a smoothly enlarged liver suggests a rapid recent increase in liver size (e.g. in acute hepatitis and also congestive cardiac failure).

Splenomegaly

Newborns may normally have a palpable spleen tip. Later palpable spleen suggests splenomegaly, possibly from portal hypertension, but as children get older a larger spleen can be accommodated beneath the ribs, so the sign becomes less sensitive.

Coagulopathy

With cholestasis, coagulopathy results from a failure of absorption of sufficient vitamin K. In infants this may present as haemorrhagic disease of the newborn, who should not normally suffer spontaneous bleeding. Routine vitamin K is given to newborns in some countries. Fresh blood from sites such as the umbilicus or nares should always prompt a search for evidence of vitamin K malabsorption or liver disease even when jaundice seems trivial.

In liver disease and coagulopathy unresponsive to vitamin K, but without consumptive coagulopathy, liver synthetic failure must be present. **The degree of coagulopathy is the most sensitive index of liver impairment in children.**

Hypoglycaemia

Hypoglycaemia may suggest a metabolic disease as a cause of liver dysfunction or profound failure of liver function.

Encephalopathy

More common in acute liver failure (see Section 5.7.A), chronic hepatic encephalopathy may be insidious, with educational failure, poor impulse control, bizarre behaviour and absences noted intermittently over months or years. Improvement may be associated with a low-protein diet reduced to 1 gram/kg/day, with lactulose to give acid stools and change the gut flora in favour of organisms that are less likely to produce the amines associated with encephalopathy.

Ascites

This is seen in advanced CLD, being a function of the balance between plasma oncotic pressure, which is mostly contributed by serum albumin, and hydrostatic pressure from portal hypertension.

Cutaneous manifestations

Pruritus, liver palms, cutaneous shunts, clubbing, white nails and xanthomas are well-recognised signs.

Hepatopulmonary syndrome

Progressive cyanosis occurs without lung disease, associated with low pulmonary artery pressure. Exertional dyspnoea is a frequent early feature. Type 1 implies pulmonary capillary vasodilatation and improves at least in part with inspired oxygen, whereas type 2 implies fixed intrapulmonary shunts without a response to oxygen.

Other presentations

Chronic liver disease may be present without detectable symptoms or signs. For example, chronic viral hepatitis B can be present for decades, proceeding to cirrhosis without any external evidence.

TABLE 5.7.B.2 Laboratory features of CLD

Laboratory feature	Cholestasis	Portal hypertension	Cell dysfunction
Serum bilirubin	Conjugated	Normal	Normal or mixed
Serum albumin	Normal	Normal	Low
Serum cholesterol	High[†]	Normal	Low
Prothrombin time/ratio	Normal[‡]	Normal[*]	Prolonged if severe

[*] Implies minor prolongation seen in portal vein thrombosis.

[†] Except in familial intrahepatic cholestasis types 1 and 2.

[‡] If there is adequate vitamin K.

Investigations into CLD

Consider liver dysfunction according to the following three categories (see Table 5.7.B.2):

- **cholestasis:** impairment of bile flow with a consequent reduction in intraluminal bile salt concentration and associated conjugated hyperbilirubinaemia and malabsorption
- **portal hypertension (PHT)** with associated hypersplenism and the effects of portosystemic shunting
- **hepatocellular impairment** (cell dysfunction) with failure of synthetic and homeostatic function, such as hyperammonaemia and hypoglycaemia.

Clinical findings (see Table 5.7.B.1) can be interpreted according to this classification, although some (e.g. ascites) are represented in more than one category. Serum albumin concentration reflects liver synthetic function but also depends on nutritional status and losses (e.g. via the gastrointestinal tract or kidneys). Thus it is necessary to consider all clinical features supported by basic laboratory parameters when possible to evaluate the severity of liver disease.

A precise diagnosis of the various causes of CLD is often not possible without specialised and expensive investigations, yet use of the above clinical assessment may allow a general if unconfirmed diagnosis.

Outcome of CLD

Although CLD can often only be cured in specialised centres in countries where transplantation is available (costs are over $120 000 per case), much can be done to relieve suffering in children with CLD, and most notably Wilson's disease can be treated successfully for US$1–2 per day depending on the patient's size and age.

Cholestatic CLD: diagnosis and management

Cholestasis is most frequently seen as a complication of the neonatal hepatitis syndrome. The commonest defined diagnosis is **biliary atresia**, an obliterative inflammatory condition of the intra- and extrahepatic biliary system exclusive to the perinatal period. Infants typically present with jaundice, pale stools and dark urine. If left untreated, biliary atresia progresses to biliary cirrhosis and death from complications of decompensated liver function within 2 years in 95% of cases. It is the commonest individual cause of severe liver disease in childhood in all populations, occurring in 1 in 9000 to 1 in 16 000 live births.

Causes of cholestatic CLD that are rare and difficult to treat include the following:

- **Alagille syndrome:** a condition characterised by

TABLE 5.7.B.3 Basic investigations in liver disease

Investigation	Role
Serum bilirubin, total and conjugated	Conjugated bilirubin is elevated in cholestasis
	Unconjugated bilirubin is elevated in hepatocellular injury
Urine bilirubin	Present in cholestasis
Serum aspartate aminotransferase, alkaline phosphatase, gamma-glutamyl transpeptidase	Elevated in hepatocellular injury plus cholestasis
Serum sodium, potassium, urea, creatinine, albumin and glucose	Hepatocellular injury
Full blood count, prothrombin time or INR	Coagulopathy in liver failure and in cholestasis from vitamin K malabsorption
Hepatitis A antigen, toxoplasma, rubella, herpes, CMV, syphilis antibodies	Congenitally acquired infection
Serum total protein and immunoglobulins	Abnormal in autoimmune disease
Alpha fetoprotein	Elevated in liver tumour
X-ray of spine, cardiac	Alagille syndrome, dextrocardia rarely in biliary atresia
Ultrasound scanning	Biliary, portal and parenchymal abnormalities
Eye review for Kayser–Fleischer rings and embryotoxon	Wilson's disease, Alagille syndrome

cholestasis of variable severity associated with syndromic features.

- **Progressive familial intrahepatic cholestasis (PFIC):** a series of clinical syndromes of cholestasis representing impairment of bile salt transport or handling that may present as neonatal giant-cell hepatitis or drug- or viral-induced cholestasis.
- **Neonatal sclerosing cholangitis:** a rare condition which may mimic biliary atresia, although stools may show variable pigmentation.

The consequences of cholestasis include **pruritus**. This is a particularly troublesome symptom, resulting in disruption for the whole household, especially at night. Persistent scratching can be complicated by secondary infection of broken skin and bloodstaining of clothes and bedclothes. Early onset, before 7 months of age, implies profound cholestasis and a poor prognosis. Treatment is often difficult. First-line management is with **cholestyramine**, at a starting dose of 1 gram/day for under 1 year olds, 2 grams (sachets)/day for children under 6 years, or 4 grams (sachets)/day for those over 6 years, up to 6 sachets/day according to response, but not given within 4 hours of vitamins or other medicine, Second-line treatment is **rifampicin**, 2–4 mg/kg (maximum 300 mg) twice daily, and third-line treatment is **ursodeoxycholic acid**, 5–10 mg/kg two to three times a day up to 15 mg/kg two to three times a day.

Fat-soluble vitamin deficiencies (A, D, E and K) are frequently encountered in cholestasis unless patients receive prophylactic treatment. Clinical features of **rickets**, such as splayed epiphyses, especially swollen wrists, rickety rosary and craniotabes should be sought regularly. Metabolic bone disease should, if possible, be screened for by measurements of serum phosphate, calcium and parathormone levels and regular wrist X-rays. Prothrombin time or INR should be measured to ensure adequate vitamin K repletion.

Vitamin A replacement is 5000–10 000 units per day or 100 000 units by deep IM injection every 2 to 4 months. Vitamin D deficiency may be refractory to oral calciferol (vitamin D_2) tablets or cholecalciferol (vitamin D_3), but 10 000–25 000 units (250 micrograms) for 1–12 years and

10 000–40 000 for 12–18 years per day of either may help. More water-soluble preparations such as 1-alpha-calcidol, 15–30 nanograms/kg for 1 month to 12 years and 250–500 nanograms for 12–18 years once daily, are more effective. **They may also cause hypercalcaemia.** Vitamin E deficiency is associated with hypotonia, peripheral neuropathy, developmental delay and haemolysis, and is the most frequently encountered vitamin deficiency in liver disease. The dose of vitamin E for all age groups is initially 100–200 mg/day adjusted according to response up to 200 mg/kg once daily, to increase until normal plasma levels are maintained. Vitamin K replacement for infants orally is 1 mg/day, and for children it is 5–10 mg/day.

Nutritional management applies to all three categories of CLD, and is discussed below.

Portal hypertension (PHT): diagnosis and management

The complications of portal hypertension can be divided into:

- those related to the increased pressure (e.g. enteropathy, hypersplenism)
- those related to the anatomy of any collateral circulation (e.g. bleeding varices, haemorrhoids)
- those related to the effects of substances bypassing the liver by porto-systemic shunting (e.g. hepatic encephalopathy, hepatopulmonary syndrome, porto-pulmonary syndrome, hepatorenal syndrome). In this group complications may increase as shunting increases and portal pressure then falls.

The aetiology of PHT has conventionally been divided into the following:

- **pre-hepatic causes**, including portal vein thrombosis and other congenital and acquired portal vein anomalies, including arterioportal fistulae
- **hepatic causes**, including all causes of cirrhosis, especially cystic fibrosis and other biliary diseases, congenital hepatic fibrosis, and causes of non-cirrhotic portal hypertension, including portal vein sclerosis

- **post-hepatic causes**, including hepatic venous outflow obstruction such as Budd–Chiari syndrome, various causes of veno-occlusive disease and problems of inferior vena caval flow or right heart function; particularly difficult to detect are constrictive pericarditis and IVC webs.

Treatment of bleeding varices

BOX 5.7.B.2 Minimum standards: oesophageal varices

- Vitamin K.
- Blood transfusion (ideally fresh blood) and blood-clotting factors (if available).
- Propranololol.
- Antacids (aluminium hydroxide or magnesium carbonate).
- Ranitidine.

Acute management

1 Advise the parents not to panic, but to stay with the child.
2 Unless the CLD is very advanced, or the child is vitamin K deficient, the bleed will probably stop spontaneously, although the child may be shocked by that time.
3 Give oxygen by face mask.
4 Gain IV access and obtain cross-matched blood if possible. Resuscitation with 10–20 mL/kg boluses of Ringer-lactate or Hartmann's solution is appropriate in the acute situation while waiting for blood for transfusion.
5 Give IV vitamin K slowly over 5 minutes 250–300 microgram/kg up to a maximum of 10 mg (or 1 mg for children under 1 year; 3 mg for those aged 1–4 years; 5 mg for those aged 5–12 years; 10 mg for those over 12 years). Repeat according to the results of clotting studies.
6 Start antacids (see below).
7 Arrange skilled endoscopy with sclerotherapy or banding (if available).

Prevention

- Propranololol is beneficial as primary and secondary prophylaxis for variceal bleeding, particularly when given early in the course of PHT. Give 500 micrograms/kg orally twice daily (adjust according to the heart rate; aim to reduce the rate by up to 25%). Around 30% of patients who receive propranololol have side effects, including wheeze and systemic vasoconstriction.
- Antacids. If there is a tendency to diarrhoea, use aluminium hydroxide (children aged 6–12 years: 5 mL three to four times a day between meals; children over 12 years: 10 mL three to four times a day). If there is a tendency toward constipation, use magnesium carbonate in the same dosage. The two may be used in combination.
- Avoid aspirin, ibuprofen and other gastric irritants.
- H$_2$-receptor antagonists are of no proven value but are often used (ranitidine 1 mg/kg for 1–6 months, 2–4 mg/kg 6 months to 12 years, 150 mg 12–18 years ALL twice daily).

Hepatocellular liver disease: diagnosis and management
Chronic viral hepatitis B, C and D
Hepatitis B

Millions of children worldwide are infected with hepatitis B virus (HBV), and many ultimately die in adulthood from its complications, particularly decompensated cirrhosis and hepatocellular carcinoma. The population prevalence may exceed 10%, making HBV a major international public health problem. Spread may occur vertically at the time of birth or shortly afterwards, but also horizontally, especially in poor communities. Unlike HIV infection, surface contact with very small amounts of infected blood (e.g. as a result of sharing toothbrushes) can result in infection. A neonate exposed to HBV for the first time has more than a 90% risk of becoming chronically infected, a child has a 25% risk, and an adult has a 10% risk.

Risk factors associated with the development of cirrhosis and hepatocellular carcinoma include eAg+, a high level of HBV DNA, and male gender. Once infected, children have about a 15% probability per annum of reducing a high-risk state to a low-risk state as defined by eAg/antibody status.

Vaccines based on the antigenicity of the S Ag are highly efficacious in generating antibody response and providing protection. Protocols that involve three subcutaneous immunisations given at 0, 1 and 6 months give adequate antibody levels in 95% of individuals. In neonates, vaccination with the same dose, or half the dose for economy, at birth, 1 month, 3 months and 1 year achieves similar protection. Up to 5% of individuals will not mount an antibody response despite repeated vaccination, but it is not clear whether they all fail to develop immunity. As implied above, all neonates of HBV-positive mothers should receive a course of vaccine, irrespective of the mother's eAg/antibody status, as infants of S Ag+/e Ab+ mothers may develop fatal liver failure.

The WHO has recommended universal HBV vaccination. If such a policy was to be implemented it is highly likely that HBV would become a rare disease of children within less than 10 years, with a corresponding reduction in cirrhosis and hepatocellular carcinoma in one generation, representing one of the current great unseized opportunities of international public health.

Hepatitis C

Hepatitis C virus (HCV) was responsible for at least 90% of post-transfusion hepatitis in early US studies. Around 5% of sexual partners may become infected. Around 4–5% of infants of viraemic mothers may become infected. The risk is related to the level of maternal viraemia, with HIV-positive mothers having the highest HCV viral loads and the highest risk of transmission. HCV is also a small but significant risk for healthcare workers.

Following exposure, viraemia in HCV occurs within 7 days, with antibody positivity appearing from 21–28 days. Less than 10% of affected individuals adequately remove the virus, and the remainder progress to chronic liver disease. The rate of progression to cirrhosis is unclear, but factors such as liver iron content, alcohol consumption and other viral infections (including hepatitis A) contribute. Around 5% of adults with HCV develop cirrhosis each year. The median timescale for developing cirrhosis in HCV is probably of the order of four decades.

Hepatocellular carcinoma is a recognised complication of HCV and cirrhosis, following the latter by 5–15 years typically. Treatment is becoming rapidly more effective, including that for the more resistant genotypes I and IV. Children should be treated after the age of 5 years in order to avoid the neurotoxic effects of interferon.

Wilson's disease

This is an autosomal-recessive disorder caused by the accumulation of copper in the liver, brain, eyes, kidney and bone. The prognosis depends on the speed of diagnosis. Treatment with a low-copper diet and penicillamine is highly successful if started well before the onset of liver failure.

Drugs and the liver

Drugs are a major cause of liver dysfunction. Over 600 drug hepatopathies have been documented; common examples are given below. Drug clearance may be reduced in liver disease, and liver disease increases the risk of drug injury to the liver.

Acute/subacute hepatocellular toxicity is caused by paracetamol, aspirin, ibuprofen, iron, isoniazid, sodium valproate, carbamazepine, methotrexate and ketoconazole.

Cholestasis is caused by rifampicin, penicillins, erythromycin, oestrogens and anabolic steroids.

Progressive fibrosis is caused by azathioprine.

HIV and the liver

HIV is known to be associated with worsening of hepatitis due to other conventional causes and cholangiopathy, probably related to ascending infection with low-grade organisms such as Cryptosporidium or cytomegalovirus (CMV) infection (see Section 6.2.D). Hepatitis due to a conventional cause, especially CMV, may be particularly severe or progressive when associated with a low CD4 count.

Metabolic liver diseases

These are rare and difficult, if not impossible, to treat without liver transplantation or expensive diets. Advice from a specialist unit should be sought.

The management of nutrition in CLD

Malnutrition is a serious consequence of CLD. Thin limbs and a prominent abdomen are frequently seen, and malnutrition will be evident in anthropometric measurements. Triceps skinfold thickness tends to become reduced earlier in the course of progressive disease, followed by a reduction in mid upper arm circumference (MUAC). Stunting tends to occur later, unless severe rickets is present. Weight is affected by fluid balance abnormalities and organomegaly, and is therefore an insensitive indicator of nutritional state. Lean body mass, and skeletal muscle in particular, is prone to depletion as a result of progressive liver disease.

Anorexia is attributed to organomegaly or pressure effects of ascites, but may be equally due to a congested gastric mucosa or reduced gastrointestinal motility of portal hypertension or central effects of unidentified toxins. Malabsorption of long-chain fats, including those with polyunsaturated fatty acids (PUFAs), is dependent on intra-luminal bile acid concentration. Cholestasis may result in the intra-luminal bile acid concentration falling below that required for micelles to be formed. The resulting steatorrhoea creates faecal energy loss, but also risks essential fatty acid deficiency, with possible neurodevelopmental consequences, particularly in early life. Protein malabsorption may also result from functional pancreatic insufficiency with failure of protease activation by bile acids. Malabsorption may also result from bacterial overgrowth or other unspecified effects of portal hypertension; for example, congestion of the gut may cause impaired active or passive absorption.

Thus malnourished children with liver disease have high energy expenditure for their size. Target energy intake should be estimated from what the child's current weight for age should be.

Breast milk contains more PUFAs than typical formula milks. PUFAs are long-chain fats that are dependent on intraluminal bile acids for absorption, and are essential for normal cell membranes and for myelination, particularly in infancy. **Breastfeeding is therefore important in children with CLD.**

Treatment with intensive enteral feeding and **high-dose enteral or parenteral vitamins** can improve the quality of life of children who have malnutrition from their liver disease. In the absence of specialist feeds, a modular feed may be prepared using protein powder, carbohydrate polymer, MCT oil and long-chain fat oil, preferably with essential fatty acids from walnut oil or another similar source, to provide 4% of fat. Up to 4 grams/kg/day of protein, and 100–140 kcal/kg/day of energy, of which two-thirds is from carbohydrate and one third is from lipid as MCT, is an ideal target range.

Commercial liver formulas are extremely expensive, and their effect on the outcome of the liver disease is unproven. In the absence of the supplements described above, proprietary baby formula can be enriched with locally available oils and starches to give 140 kcal/kg/day, with half of the total formula energy as lipid and half as starch. Remember that if commercial formula is given at an increased concentration to increase protein intake, the electrolyte intake will increase proportionally, with a risk of sodium overload and fluid retention.

5.8 Endocrine disorders

5.8.A Diabetes

> **BOX 5.8.A.1 Minimum standards**
> - ABC resuscitation skills and equipment.
> - Oxygen.
> - IV 0.9% saline or Plasma-Lyte 148.
> - Insulin.
> - Potassium.
> - Mannitol or 3% saline.
> - ECG monitoring.

Diabetic ketoacidosis

Diabetic ketoacidosis (DKA) is the commonest endocrine emergency that may occur in individuals with previously diagnosed diabetes, but should be suspected in any child with:

- dehydration (diarrhoea is not the only cause)
- abdominal pain
- ketone smell on the breath
- acidosis
- acidotic breathing
- unexplained coma.

A child with DKA may die from inhalational pneumonia, hypokalaemia, severe metabolic acidosis or cerebral oedema. Cerebral oedema is unpredictable, occurs more frequently in younger children and those newly diagnosed with diabetes, and has a mortality of around 80%.

These guidelines are intended for the management of children who are more than 3% dehydrated and/or vomiting and/or drowsy and/or clinically acidotic.

Children who are 3% dehydrated or less and not clinically unwell usually tolerate oral rehydration and subcutaneous insulin.

Every unit should have a written policy for the care of children with DKA. The following guidance is adapted from that provided by the British Society for Paediatric Endocrinology and Diabetes (BSPED) (www.bsped.org.uk/clinical/docs/DKAGuideline.pdf).

Emergency management of children who are over 3% dehydrated and clinically unwell
General resuscitation: A, B, C

- **Airway:** ensure that the airway is patent, and if the child is comatose consider inserting an oropharyngeal airway. If they are comatose or suffering from recurrent vomiting, insert a nasogastric tube, aspirate and leave on open drainage.
- **Breathing:** give 100% oxygen. Give bag-and-mask ventilation if the child is apnoeic or hypoventilating.
- **Circulation:** insert an IV cannula and take blood samples (see below). Only if the child is shocked (tachycardia with poor capillary filling or hypotension) give 10 mL/kg 0.9% saline or Plasma-Lyte 148 solution as quickly as possible, and repeat as necessary up to a maximum of 30 mL/kg. Note that normal (0.9%) saline causes a hyperchloraemic acidosis because of its excess of the chloride anion. In patients who are acidotic because of diabetes, Plasma-Lyte 148 may be preferable, as it does not contain such a high concentration of chloride ions.

Confirm the diagnosis

- History: polydipsia, polyuria.
- Clinical signs: acidotic respiration, dehydration, drowsiness, abdominal pain/vomiting.
- Biochemical investigations: high blood glucose levels on finger-prick or venous blood test, presence of ketones or glucose in the urine.

Investigations

- **Weigh the child.** If this is not possible because of their clinical condition, use the most recent clinic weight as a guideline, or an estimated weight from centile charts.
- Blood glucose concentration.
- Urea and electrolytes (if plasma bicarbonate is not available, measure **arterial blood gas**).
- Packed cell volume (PCV) and full blood count.
- Blood culture.
- Urine microscopy, culture and sensitivity.
- Set up a cardiac monitor to observe T waves (hypokalaemia causes flat T waves and may cause cardiac dysrhythmias; hyperkalaemia causes peaked T waves).
- Other investigations (e.g. chest X-ray, CSF, throat swab, etc.) if indicated if the child is febrile, as there may be an underlying infection.

Assessment

Assess and record the following in the child's notes, so that comparisons can be made by others later:

- Degree of dehydration:
  - < 3%: dehydration is only just clinically detectable.
  - 3–5%: dry mucous membranes, reduced skin turgor.
  - 5–8%: as above with sunken eyes, poor capillary return.
  - > 8%: with shock – severely ill with poor perfusion, thready rapid pulse, reduced blood pressure.
- Conscious level:
  - Assess the AVPU score (**A**lert, responds to **V**oice, responds to **P**ain, **U**nresponsive).
  - Institute hourly neurological observations. If less than **A**lert on admission, or there is any subsequent deterioration, record the Glasgow Coma Scale score (*see* Section 7.3.C) and transfer the child to a

high-dependency-care unit (if available). Consider instituting cerebral oedema management.

- Full examination, looking in particular for evidence of the following:
  - **Cerebral oedema: irritability, slow pulse, high blood pressure** and papilloedema. Examine the fundi: papilloedema is a late sign.
  - Infection: look for a focus. **DKA can cause a leucocytosis but not a fever.**
  - Ileus.
- Observations to be carried out (ensure that full instructions are given to the nursing staff):
  - Strict fluid balance and urine testing of every sample for glucose.
  - Hourly capillary blood glucose measurements.
  - Twice daily weights.
  - Initially hourly or more frequent neurological observations.
- **Report immediately to the medical staff (even at night) symptoms of headache or any change in either conscious level or behaviour.**
  - Report any changes in the ECG trace, especially T-wave changes.

Management

By this stage, the circulating volume should have been restored if shock was initially present. If not, give a further 10 mL/kg of 0.9% saline or Plasma-Lyte 148 over 30 minutes. Avoid overzealous fluid replacement, as this may be a risk factor for cerebral oedema.

Estimating fluid requirements

The amount of fluid that the child needs over a 24-hour period must be calculated. It is the sum of:

estimated fluid deficit + maintenance requirements + ongoing losses.

Deficit

In DKA the deficit must be replaced more slowly than in gastroenteritis, over 48 hours rather than 24 hours. Even in very severe dehydration, use no more than 10% dehydration as the maximum in your calculations. Document the fluid balance carefully.

Determine the degree of dehydration, and **never estimate more than 10% dehydration in this situation**.

Weigh the child, or else estimate their weight from their age as follows:

weight (kg) = 2 × [age (years) + 4]).

Use the following formula: **percentage dehydration × weight (kg) × 10 = deficit (in mL)**.

For example, a child whose weight is estimated to be 10 kg is 10% dehydrated.

Their estimated fluid loss is 10 × 10 × 10 = 1000 mL (40 mL/hour if replaced over 24 hours **or** 20 mL/hour **if replaced over 48 hours, which is safer in DKA**.

Maintenance

TABLE 5.8.A.1 Estimated maintenance fluid requirements based on child's body weight

Body weight	Volume of fluid needed per day	Volume of fluid needed per hour
First 10 kg of body weight	100 mL/kg	4 mL/kg
Second 10 kg of body weight	50 mL/kg	2 mL/kg
Subsequent kg	20 mL/kg	1 mL/kg

Ongoing losses

For each diarrhoea stool	< 2 years old: give 50–100 mL > 2 years old: give 100–200 mL
For each vomit	2 mL/kg oral rehydration solution (ORS): give small frequent volumes (e.g. 5 mL/minute in a child) via a spoon, syringe or cup
For nasogastric tube aspirates	Replace volume for volume with either ORS or 0.9% saline or Plasma-Lyte 148 containing 5% or 10% glucose

Type of fluid

Initially use 0.9% saline or Plasma-Lyte 148. Once the blood glucose concentration has fallen to 14 mmol/litre, change the fluid to 0.9% saline or Plasma-Lyte 148 containing, in addition, 5% glucose and 20 mmol KCl per 500-mL bag.

Expect the sodium concentration to rise initially as the glucose level falls and water is removed from the circulation.

Cerebral oedema may be related to a plasma sodium concentration that falls or does not show the expected rise as glucose levels fall.

Electrolytes
Bicarbonate

Bicarbonate is rarely, if ever, necessary. Continuing acidosis usually indicates insufficient resuscitation. Bicarbonate should only be considered in children who are profoundly acidotic (pH < 7.0) and shocked with circulatory failure. Its only purpose is to improve cardiac contractility in severe shock. The maximum volume of 8.4% sodium bicarbonate for half-correction of acidosis is calculated according to the following formula, and given over 60 minutes:

Volume (mL) of 8.4% sodium bicarbonate = 1/3 × weight (kg) × base deficit (mmol/litre) divided by 2.

If no **blood gas measurement** is available, do not give bicarbonate unless the child is in **profound shock**.

Potassium

- Commence potassium immediately unless anuria is suspected, or there are peaked T waves on the ECG, or the serum potassium concentration is higher than 7.0 mmol/litre.
- Potassium is mainly an intracellular ion, and there is always massive depletion of total body potassium, although initial plasma levels may be low, normal or even high. Potassium levels in blood will fall once insulin is commenced.
- Add 20 mmol KCl to every 500 mL unit of IV fluid given.
- Check urea and electrolytes 2 hours after resuscitation

is commenced and then at least 4-hourly thereafter, and alter potassium replacements accordingly (more potassium is sometimes needed).

- Use a cardiac monitor to observe frequently for T-wave changes, and alert nursing staff to any changes that might be seen, and advise them when to call for medical help.
- **If potassium-containing fluids are not available, start insulin (see below) after 1–2 hours of rehydration, and arrange transport to a unit that can provide this (if available).**

Insulin

Once fluids are running, calculation of the insulin infusion rate may be undertaken at leisure, as the blood glucose levels will already be falling. Continuous low-dose IV infusion is the preferred method.

However, **if a syringe pump is not available or not safe to use** after at least 1 hour of rehydration treatment give subcutaneous boluses of short-acting insulin 1- to 2-hourly at 0.1 unit/kg/dose. Give half the dose if the blood glucose level is falling too fast.

There is no need for an initial bolus, and some evidence that insulin should not be given during the first hour of IV fluid treatment.

If an infusion system is available and safe to use, make up a solution of 1 unit/mL of human soluble insulin (e.g. Actrapid) by adding 50 units (0.5 mL) of insulin to 49.5 mL of 0.9% saline in a syringe pump. Attach this using a Y-connector to the IV fluids that are already running. Do not add insulin directly to the fluid bags. The solution should then run at 0.1 unit/kg/hour (0.1 mL/kg/hour).

Once the blood glucose level is down to 14 mmol/litre, change to 5% glucose in 0.9% saline (add 50 mL of 50% glucose to a 500 mL bag of saline) and potassium as above. Do not reduce the insulin infusion until the pH is > 7.3 and the glucose concentration is < 14 mmol/litre, when it may safely be reduced to 0.05 mL/kg/hour.

If the blood glucose level falls below 7 mmol/litre, consider adding extra glucose to the infusion.

If the blood glucose level rises out of control, re-evaluate the patient (check whether there is sepsis or some other condition). Then:

1 Check that the insulin syringe pump is connected and working.
2 Make up a fresh solution of insulin, preferably using a new source of insulin in case the original one is denatured, and consider starting the whole protocol again.

Frequent sips of oral rehydrating fluid or nasogastric fluid up to 5 mL/kg/hour may be used as a substitute in the immediate initial period while arranging transport. Once the blood glucose level is < 14 mmol/litre, more glucose may be required (e.g. fruit juice if tolerated).

Remember that **you must have glucose ready to treat hypoglycaemia (5 mL/kg of 10% dextrose).**

Continuing management
Output

- Urinary catheterisation should be avoided, but may be useful in a critically ill child with impaired consciousness. With or without catheterisation, documentation of fluid balance, if necessary by weighing nappies, is of paramount importance.

- Measure accurately and test all urine samples for glucose and ketones.
- Record all fluid input (even oral fluids).
- If a massive diuresis continues, fluid input may need to be increased.
- If large volumes of gastric aspirate continue, replace them IV with 0.45% saline plus 10 mmol/litre KCl.

Laboratory results

Check biochemistry, blood pH and laboratory blood glucose levels 2 hours after the start of resuscitation, and at least 4-hourly thereafter.

Review the fluid composition and rate according to each set of electrolyte results. If acidosis is not correcting, resuscitation may have been inadequate, in which case consider giving more 0.9% saline or Plasma-Lyte 148. Consider sepsis as a cause of persistent acidosis. Consider antibiotic treatment.

Insulin management

Continue to give IV fluids until the child is drinking well and able to tolerate food. Do not expect ketones to have disappeared completely before changing to subcutaneous insulin. **Discontinue the insulin infusion 60 minutes after the first subcutaneous injection in order to avoid rebound hyperglycaemia.**

Cerebral oedema in DKA
Signs and symptoms of cerebral oedema
These include the following:
- headache
- irritability
- seizures
- increasing blood pressure and slowing pulse
- confusion
- reduced conscious level
- small pupils
- possible respiratory impairment.

Management
- Exclude hypoglycaemia as a cause of neurological symptoms.
- Give mannitol 500–1000 mg/kg immediately (2.5–5 mL/kg 20% mannitol over 15 minutes). Alternatively, give 3% saline 5 mL/kg over 5–10 minutes. Give this as soon as cerebral oedema is suspected.
- **Restrict IV fluids to two-thirds maintenance, and replace the deficit over 72 hours rather than 48 hours.**
- **Keep Na+ levels > 135 mmol/litre. Keep the head in the midline and 30 degrees elevated.**
- **Avoid fever > 38.0°C.**
- Repeated doses of mannitol or strong saline (at the dose stated above, every 2–4 hours) should be used to control intracranial pressure.

Care of the newly diagnosed diabetic child
After treatment of DKA in the newly presenting but well diabetic child, the process of education and treatment should commence. It is not feasible to stabilise the child's control or to teach all aspects of diabetic care while they are an inpatient, so ideally (if resources permit) this should take place at home, although some authors advocate a prolonged initial admission for this process.

Ensure that the parents and the child (if he or she is able to do so) understand or can perform the following:

- insulin administration
- urine testing for ketones
- blood testing
- dietary measures
- other general issues.

Insulin

Draw up the specified dose of insulin correctly. As a rough guide, a new patient will need approximately 0.5 unit/kg/day.

The frequency and choice of insulin depends entirely on local resources. This may mean twice daily medium-acting insulin alone (60% in the morning, 40% in the evening), or medium-acting insulin mixed together with short-acting soluble insulin (usually in a 30% short/70% long ratio). If newer analogue fast-acting insulins are available, these may be given before every meal in an initial dose of 1 unit for every 20 grams of carbohydrate eaten, with a longer-acting insulin (40% of the total daily dose) given before bedtime.

It is very rarely possible to achieve adequate control with a single daily dose of insulin except in very small children. However, once-daily medium-acting or pre-mixed insulin should be seen as a minimum fallback position if availability of insulin is a problem. Likewise, although it is common practice to use human or genetically modified insulins, pork or beef insulin may be substituted if necessary.

Further modification of the dose will take place as an outpatient, as more insulin will be needed after the initial period and with growth and puberty.

Urine testing

Test the urine for sugar using stick tests. Clinitest tablets for reducing substances are too cumbersome for routine use, but may be used as a substitute if they are the only option. Suggest stick testing about twice daily at home. Emphasise the value of testing the first morning urine to estimate overnight control.

Test the urine for ketones using Ketostix or tablets. This only needs to be routinely done if the urine contains 3% glucose or more, and in times of intercurrent illness when the persistence of ketonuria should prompt the seeking of medical attention for incipient DKA.

The importance of accurate recording of the results in a control book, if possible, should be emphasised, to aid decision making at follow-up.

Blood testing

If resources allow, all parents should be able to test the blood glucose level, at least in an emergency, and ideally also for routine monitoring of control. The parent or carer (and also the child, if appropriate) should be taught the following:

- how to use a lancet (or automatic finger-pricking device) to draw blood from the side (**not the pulp**) of the finger
- how to ensure that an adequate sample is placed on the strip
- how to read the strip visually (a meter may be used if resources allow)
- if this method of monitoring control is chosen, the importance of providing test results at staggered times through the day (ideally one or two tests per day) should be explained; **the need for accurate recording of the values in a diary should be emphasised** (ascertain the parents' literacy and numeracy levels)
- the instantaneous nature of the result obtained and the detection of hypoglycaemia with blood testing should be highlighted, and compared with urine testing.

Diet

The parents or carers and the child should **ideally meet a specialist diabetic dietitian** and discuss the concept of carbohydrate balance and how the diet is spread through the day. The diet must be adequate for growth and nutrition, and should contain around 50% of energy as complex carbohydrate. It is not advisable to allow 'free' fatty foods, as they may accentuate later macrovascular complications.

Explain the importance of fairly close adherence to the advised diet, and that the diet may need to be revised from time to time as the child grows and their pattern of activity changes.

The parents or carers and the child should understand the influence of food intake on blood sugar levels. Diabetic carbohydrate 10-gram 'portions' are often used with analogue short-acting insulin boluses before meals (if available), but need considerable expertise to be taught effectively.

Sweet unrefined sugars should ideally only be taken before exercise or as occasional treats, although ideally the insulin dose should be varied to take this into account.

General care

- **It is essential that the parents or carers and the child (if he or she is old enough) understand how inadequate glycaemic control may predispose to micro- and macrovascular complications in the longer term. These are not uncommon findings in teenagers in Africa, due to their appalling glycaemic control in earlier childhood.**
- **It is also important that the parents or carers ensure that a supply of insulin is always available, as the commonest cause of DKA is lack of insulin at home in resource-limited environments.**
- The parents or carers and child (if appropriate) should understand how exercise, diet and insulin interact to influence blood sugar levels.
- The symptoms of hypoglycaemia should be explained. It is important that the parents or carers understand the possible signs of an attack and what can be done to terminate the 'hypo'. They should know how to use rapid-acting sweet sugary gel, non-'diet'/'lite' sugary drinks or tablets during the early stages of the attack. Ideally, a 1-mg glucagon pack (if available) should be given to each family prior to discharge, and the parents should be shown how to prepare and give the prepacked injection in an emergency to terminate a severe hypoglycaemic attack with unconsciousness or fits. If a 'hypo' is treated, a more complex carbohydrate snack should be given to prevent immediate recurrence.
- The family should be given the address of any local support groups for individuals with diabetes and their families (if such groups exist). If possible, give the parents and child a folder containing relevant booklets on diabetes.
- The family should ideally have access to medical advice and treatment 24 hours a day if they are worried about their child's immediate health, or can be seen at the next outpatient clinic for less urgent problems.

Ideal checklist for use at discharge

- Dextrose gel: 1 box of plastic tubes or 50 grams of dextrose tablets.
- Disposable syringes and needles, ideally 0.3-mL low-volume syringes with as small a needle as can be located (down to 31-gauge are available).
- Insulin.
- GlucaGen Novo 1 mg pack.
- Glucose testing blood sticks, finger-pricking device, plus lancets **or** urine sticks.
- Control book and pen.
- Ketostix.
- Sharps disposal bin.
- Appointment at next diabetic clinic.

Outpatient care

The patient should be reviewed at regular intervals (as frequently as resources allow). Ideally, at least once a year the child should have the following reviewed:

- their knowledge of diabetes and emergency management
- growth
- blood pressure

- state of injection sites
- foot examination and discussion of foot care
- fundoscopy (at diagnosis, for cataracts; after 5 years of diabetes or in teenagers, for retinopathy)
- microalbumin/creatinine ratio in the first morning urine sample for detection of renal complications (after 5 years of diabetes or in teenagers)
- **glycosylated haemoglobin** for monitoring long-term control (ideal control is a level of < 55 mmol/mol).
- **thyroid disorders and coeliac disease are both more likely to occur in children with diabetes. Although, ideally, antithyroid antibodies and antigliadin antibodies could be checked** at the time of diagnosis of diabetes, and every 4 years thereafter, they are expensive tests and in resource-limited environments it is better to undertake a careful clinical assessment for additional thyroid or coeliac disease at annual outpatient appointments.

Transfer to adult services should take place in a planned manner, ideally at a joint handover clinic.

5.8.B The child with hypoglycaemia

> **BOX 5.8.B.1 Minimum standards**
> - Oral glucose solutions.
> - IV 10% and 50% glucose.

Introduction

Hypoglycaemia is an important cause of morbidity and mortality that needs to be recognised, as the complications are potentially preventable.

Definition

Hypoglycaemia is now widely defined as a blood glucose concentration of less than 2.5 mmol/litre (45 mg/dL) at any age. The measurement should ideally be made in a laboratory with appropriate quality control. Testing with reagent strips is less accurate, particularly within the critical range.

Presentation and aetiology

Hypoglycaemia may present at any age from birth into adulthood. Symptoms are varied and rarely specific, particularly in infants. In neonates, fits and apnoeic attacks may be important clues. In infants and children the most important presentation, because of the risk of complications, is also fits and encephalopathy (*see* Table 5.8.B.1). The common causes are listed below.

In infants and children in well-resourced countries, ketotic hypoglycaemia, endocrine disorders and metabolic disorders usually predominate. By contrast, in resource-limited countries, malnutrition and infections such as malaria (and its treatment) are more common.

Treatment
Glucose dosage

There is insufficient scientific data to be definite about the

quantity of glucose to give parenterally to a hypoglycaemic child. 5 mL of 10% glucose was the standard dose for a time but there is evidence that this much glucose can raise the plasma glucose to a level high enough to produce an insulin surge which then results in another hypoglycaemic episode. Of course, in a diabetic child who has become hypoglycaemic because of insufficient calories or too much insulin, this will not occur, so in these circumstances 5 mL of 10% glucose is safe.

- When testing for hypoglycaemia is not possible, treat any critically ill child presenting with suspicious symptoms such as fits, with encephalopathy, or with a condition known to be associated with hypoglycaemia, such as severe malnutrition or malaria.
- If the child is conscious and able to eat and drink, give them food or sugary fluids or glucose orally (0.5–1.0 gram/kg).
- Otherwise, give 2–5 mL/kg 10% glucose IV over 3 minutes. **Never use stronger glucose solutions IV.** Continue with 0.1 mL/kg/minute 10% glucose to maintain the blood sugar concentration in the range 5–8 mmol/litre.
- If hypoadrenalism/pituitarism is suspected, give hydrocortisone as described in Section 5.8.C.
- In hypoglycaemic children with diabetes or suspected hyperinsulinaemia, if IV access is not possible and glucagon is available, give IM 100 micrograms/kg (maximum of 1 mg as a single dose).

Longer-term management

- Provide appropriate endocrine management (*see* Section 5.8.C).
- Avoid periods of fasting. Give glucose orally when at risk during intercurrent infections, or IV if the child is comatose or vomiting, and during anaesthesia.

Diagnosis of the cause of hypoglycaemia

If the blood sugar level is less than 2.5 mmol/litre, it is important to establish a cause. Transfer 1 mL of blood into a fluoride tube, if possible also 1 mL heparinised blood, and the first urine after the hypoglycaemic episode to send for metabolic analysis, in particular for ketones.

- Is there ketosis? If so, look for signs of hypopituitarism and/or growth hormone deficiency.
- If feasible, check the cortisol growth hormone level and insulin levels in blood taken at the time of hypoglycaemia.
- If the blood lactate level is raised, consider organic acidaemia or a defect of gluconeogenesis.
- If ketosis is absent, consider hyperinsulinism (high birth weight) or disorders of fatty acid oxidation.

Prevention

As the symptoms are non-specific, measure blood glucose levels if possible in any suspected situation. If hypoglycaemia is suspected and blood glucose measurement is not possible, treat with glucose and observe the response. **If the response is clearly related to giving glucose, assume that hypoglycaemia was present.**

In the neonate, every effort should be made to avoid those factors that will exacerbate hypoglycaemia, including delayed feeding and hypothermia (*see* Section 3.4).

TABLE 5.8.B.1 Common symptoms and signs of hypoglycaemia

In childhood	In neonates
Convulsions	Convulsions
Reduced conscious level	Reduced conscious level
Anxiety	Jitteriness, tremor
Sweating, pallor	Cyanotic episodes
Palpitations	Apnoeic episodes
Headache	
Behaviour abnormalities	
Visual disturbances	
Slurred speech	
Ataxia	
Hunger	

Some causes of hypoglycaemia
Neonates

- Birth asphyxia.
- Small for gestational age.
- Preterm birth.
- Sepsis.
- Malnutrition.
- Hypothermia.
- Infant of diabetic mother.
- Liver disease, endocrine and metabolic disorders (see below).

Infants and children
Endocrine disorders

- Diabetic on treatment.
- Persistent hyperinsulinaemic hypoglycaemia of infancy (formerly nesidioblastosis) and other congenital and inherited hyperinsulinaemic syndromes.
- Islet-cell tumours.

- Hypopituitarism.
- Growth hormone deficiency.
- Adrenal insufficiency (any cause).

Metabolic disorders

- Disorders of glycogen metabolism, gluconeogenesis or fatty acid oxidation, organic acidaemias, etc.
- Ketotic hypoglycaemia ('accelerated starvation').
- Liver disease: any severe acute liver disease.
- Malnutrition.
- Infections: malaria, especially when treated with quinine.
- Any severe illness.

Poisoning

- Alcohol.
- Salicylates.
- Insulin.

Drugs

- Oral hypoglycaemic agents.

How to give glucose in suspected hypoglycaemia

If the patient is conscious, give sugary drinks or foods such as jam, candy or honey.

If the patient is unconscious:

1. Insert an IV or IO line and draw blood for emergency laboratory investigations.
2. Check blood glucose levels with a glucose monitoring stick. If low (< 2.5 mmol/litre (45 mg/dL) in a well-nourished child or < 3 mmol/litre (54 mg/dL) in a severely malnourished child) or if blood glucose cannot be measured because no stick test is available, treat as for hypoglycaemia anyway.
3. Give 2–5 mL/kg of 10% glucose solution rapidly by IV or IO injection or 2.5 mL/kg of 10% glucose in the neonate.
4. Recheck the blood glucose level after 20 minutes. If it is still low, repeat 2–5 mL/kg of 10% glucose solution. Continue if necessary with an infusion of a glucose containing fluid such as 5 mL/kg/hour of 10% glucose in 0.45% saline until the child is capable of drinking. Monitor the blood glucose until stable.
5. If venous or intra-osseous access is impossible in an unconscious patient, give sublingual sugar (*see* below for technique).
6. Feed the child as soon as they are conscious.
7. If is it not possible to feed the child without risk of aspiration, give:
   - milk or sugar solution via a nasogastric tube (to make sugar solution, dissolve 4 level teaspoons of sugar (20 grams) in a 200-mL cup of clean water)
   - IV fluids containing 5–10% glucose (dextrose).

Note: 50% glucose solution is the same as 50% dextrose solution or D50.

If only 50% glucose solution is available: dilute 1 part of 50% glucose solution to 4 parts of sterile water, or dilute 1 part of 50% glucose solution to 9 parts of 5% glucose solution. **For example, 10 mL of 50% solution with 90 mL of 5% solution gives 100 mL of an approximately 10% solution.**

Note: For the use of blood glucose stick tests, refer to the instructions on the box. Generally, the strip must be stored in its box, at 2–3°C, avoiding sunlight or high humidity. A drop of blood should be placed on the strip (it is necessary to cover all of the reagent area). After 60 seconds, the blood should be washed off gently with drops of cold water and the colour compared with the key on the bottle or on the blood glucose reader. (The exact procedure will vary with different strips.)

Sublingual sugar (sucrose) for treatment of hypoglycaemia

Sublingual sugar may be used as an immediate 'first-aid' measure when managing hypoglycaemia in an unconscious child in situations where IV or IO administration of glucose may be impossible or delayed.

1 Give ½ to 1 teaspoonful of sugar, moistened but not dissolved with 1–2 drops of water and insert under the tongue (sublingually) and between the lower jaw and the gums (in the buccal area). Children should be monitored for early swallowing, which leads to delayed absorption, and in this case another dose of sugar should be given. If sublingual sugar is given, repeat the doses at 20-minute intervals. This is a useful technique in the community where facilities for parenteral glucose may not be available. However, note that sublingual and buccal absorption is not as effective as gastrointestinal absorption of sugar.

2 Recheck the blood glucose level after 20 minutes, and if the level is still low (< 2.5 mmol/litre or < 45 mg/dL), repeat the IV glucose (5 mL of 10% glucose/kg) or repeat the sublingual sugar.

3 Prevent further hypoglycaemia by feeding where possible. If IV fluids are being given, prevent hypoglycaemia by adding 10 mL or 20 mL of 50% glucose to 90 mL or 80 mL, respectively, of Ringer-lactate solution or 0.9% saline to give a 5% or 10% glucose solution, respectively.

5.8.C Other endocrine disorders

Adrenal crisis

BOX 5.8.C.1 Minimum standards
- ABC resuscitation skills and equipment.
- Hydrocortisone and fludrocortisone.
- IV saline 0.9%.
- IV glucose 10%.

Diagnosis

An adrenal crisis is most likely to be encountered in a neonate with congenital adrenal hyperplasia (CAH) or hypopituitarism (look for virilisation in the female with CAH, and micropenis and cryptoorchidism in the male with hypopituitarism). It may occur in older children with adrenal destruction secondary to autoimmune processes or tuberculosis.

Suspect adrenal crisis in a severely ill child with:
- acidosis
- hyponatraemia
- hypotension
- hyperkalaemia
- hypoglycaemia.

Children receiving long-term steroid therapy

Replacement steroids given as hydrocortisone up to 10 mg/m²/day replicate natural secretion and are free of side effects if adequately monitored.

Therapeutic doses of steroids for asthma, rheumatoid arthritis, etc. will produce adrenal suppression in a manner related to the dose and duration of treatment. Short 5-day courses of prednisolone therapy will produce measurable adrenal suppression that almost never requires action. Longer courses up to 1 month should be tapered off over a 2-week period to allow recovery of the pituitary adrenal axis.

More prolonged treatment with high-dose steroids may produce profound hypoadrenalism for months after cessation of treatment. In this case, taper the steroid dose to the equivalent of 5 mg/m²/day of prednisolone. Then convert this to an equivalent dose of hydrocortisone given in the morning (1 mg prednisolone is equivalent to approximately 3 mg hydrocortisone). Then reduce the hydrocortisone by 2.5 mg/week until the child is on approximately 6 mg/m²/day, when it is probably safe to stop treatment after 2 weeks. **If possible, check the 9 a.m. pre-dose cortisol level** and stop treatment if this exceeds 150 nmol/litre at any time. Severe stress, infection or injury will require increased steroid cover **during the next 6 months**.

Children on physiological replacement treatment or prolonged pharmacological doses of steroids should ideally carry some warning identification for medical staff, advising against the abrupt cessation of steroids, and stating the emergency stress dose of oral (usually three times replacement dose) or parenteral treatment for operative cover or at times of illness associated with vomiting (hydrocortisone, 12.5 mg for infants, 25 mg for children, 50 mg for older children and 100 mg for adults, given as an immediate IV/IM dose and then 4- to 6-hourly IV).

Management of adrenal crisis

- Treat airway, breathing, shock and hypoglycaemia (see Section 5.8.B).
- Continue 0.9% saline to correct the deficit and for maintenance (see Section 5.8.A).
- Give hydrocortisone IV 6-hourly as follows: 12.5 mg dose for neonates and infants, 25 mg for children aged 1–5 years, 50 mg for children aged 6–12 years, and 100 mg for adolescents aged 13–18 years.
- If the diagnosis is established, continue maintenance hydrocortisone, 8–12 mg/m²/day in three divided doses (12–15 mg/m²/day for CAH) and, if salt loss is demonstrated in the context of CAH or adrenal destruction, fludrocortisone 150–250 micrograms/m²/day in one dose. Infants may also require oral sodium chloride, 1 gram/10 kg/day (60 mg = 1 mmol).

Hypoglycaemia

For a discussion of neonatal hypoglycaemia, see Section 3.4.

Thyroid disorders

BOX 5.8.C.2 Minimum standards
- Thyroxine.
- Carbimazole.
- Propranolol.
- Iodine supplements.

Neonatal thyrotoxicosis

Mothers who have active thyrotoxicosis or who have become hypothyroid as a consequence of treatment of thyrotoxicosis may still pass thyroid-stimulating antibodies to the fetus during the last trimester. The neonate (or fetus) will show the following:
- hydrops in severe cases
- tachycardia with heart failure: **this may occur at up to 1 week post delivery**, especially if the mother is on anti-thyroid drugs
- thinness/light for dates
- diarrhoea
- hyperkinesis
- possibly craniosynostosis.

Management
- If hyperthyroidism is detected antenatally, treat the mother with low-dose carbimazole, 5–15 mg/day (use the lowest dose possible for control).
- Treat the infant with:
  - propranololol, 1 mg/kg three to four times orally daily
  - carbimazole, initially 250 micrograms/kg 3 times a day
  - aqueous iodine oral solution (5% iodine plus 10% potassium iodide), 130 mg/mL of total iodine, 1 drop 0.05–0.1 mL every 8 hours until thyroid control is achieved.
- Stimulating antibodies will clear by 3 to 6 months of age, and treatment can be stopped.

Congenital hypothyroidism

Between 1 in 2000 and 1 in 10 000 babies are born with a maldescended or absent thyroid gland. There are rarer cases of dyshormonogenesis (dominant and recessive – more common as a consequence of consanguineous relationships) associated with neonatal goitre and very rare central isolated thyroid-stimulating hormone (TSH) deficiency.

Untreated early hypothyroidism results in cretinism.

Many countries screen for this condition in the first month of life, looking for elevated TSH (except in TSH deficiency) and/or low thyroxine or free thyroxine levels. Different screening laboratories will produce different assay results.

In general, TSH in high double figures (mU/litre) is unequivocally raised and will be confirmed by a total thyroxine concentration of less than 50 nmol/litre or a free thyroxine in single figures (pmol/litre).

In resource-limited countries, X-ray of the knee or wrist to detect delayed bone age in infants and young children is helpful for diagnosis where TSH or thyroxine assays are unavailable.

An untreated affected child will develop, in the following order:
- jaundice
- constipation
- hoarse cry
- umbilical hernia
- coarse features
- mental retardation
- poor growth.

Therefore clinical awareness is important in order to identify possible cases of hypothyroidism in babies with the common symptoms of jaundice and constipation. Prolonged jaundice should lead to investigations, including those for hypothyroidism (see Section 3.4).

Management
Give thyroxine, 10–15 micrograms/kg once daily, titrated to maintain TSH in the normal range with normal growth and development. The adult dose is around 2–3 micrograms/kg.

Iodine deficiency
This most commonly occurs in inland mountainous areas. The clinical features vary among different ethnic groups, with deafness, mutism, mental impairment and poor growth being common, and goitre being universal. The disorder may be prevented by adding potassium iodide to cooking salt (10 mg/kg salt) or providing it as supplemented sweets and bread. Iodide as an oily suspension can be given intramuscularly every 3 years.

Acquired hypothyroidism
This is usually part of an autoimmune process (which may be familial), and may be associated with diabetes mellitus. It is much more common in older girls, who will usually have the following:
- goitre
- lethargy
- poor growth rate with excess weight gain
- pallor
- constipation
- hair loss/dry skin
- delayed puberty.

The diagnosis is confirmed by raised blood TSH levels and, if possible, demonstration of antithyroid peroxisomal antibodies.

Management
Thyroxine is given to suppress TSH to the normal range and allow normal growth and pubertal development.

Doses of thyroxine
Neonate: initially 10–15 microgram/kg once daily (maximum 50 micrograms daily) then adjusted in steps of 5 micrograms/kg every 2 weeks or as clinically indicated; usual maintenance dose 20–50 micrograms daily.

Child 1 month–2 years: initially 5 microgram/kg once daily (maximum 50 micrograms daily) then adjusted in steps of 10–25 micrograms daily every 2–4 weeks or as clinically indicated; usual maintenance dose 25–75 micrograms daily.

Child 2–12 years: initially 50 micrograms once daily then adjusted in steps of 25 micrograms daily every 2–4 weeks or as clinically indicated; usual maintenance dose 75–100 micrograms daily.

Child 12–18 years: initially 50 micrograms once daily then adjusted in steps of 25 micrograms daily every 3–4 weeks or as clinically indicated; usual maintenance dose 100–200 micrograms daily.

Thyrotoxicosis

This is much more common in older girls, often those with a family history of thyroid disease. It should be suspected if the following are present:

- fine tremor
- weight loss
- psychiatric disturbance
- exophthalmos (rare in children)
- tachycardia with a wide pulse pressure
- loose stools
- goitre with bruit.

The diagnosis is confirmed by suppressed TSH (level is undetectable) with raised thyroxine level.

Management

Treatment is with low-dose carbimazole. In neonates to children aged 12 years initially 250 micrograms/kg 3 times a day (maximum 30 mg/day) and adjusted as necessary until euthyroid. In children aged 12 to 18 years initially 10 mg 3 times a day adjusted as necessary. Carbimazole should be continued for at least 2 years, after which withdrawal should be attempted. If relapse occurs, the options include further medical therapy, surgery by an experienced thyroid surgeon, or radio-iodine in a specialised centre.

Thyroid mass
Smooth goitre

An isolated smooth goitre with or without a bruit may occur in:

- iodine deficiency
- acute and subacute thyroiditis (viral, bacterial, lymphocytic or other), which is usually tender
- ingestion of goitrogens (e.g. cabbage, kale or other brassicas)
- familial dyshormonogenesis
- idiopathic pubertal goitre
- thyrotoxicosis (Graves' disease, thyroiditis, thyroid hormone resistance)
- Hashimoto's thyroiditis.

If thyroid function is normal, no treatment is necessary; otherwise treat as described above. In iodine-deficient areas where thyroid investigations are not available, treat with oral aqueous iodine as described above.

Nodules require investigation by fine-needle aspiration and histology.

Nodular goitre

Nodular goitre may occur in:

- Hashimoto's thyroiditis
- adenoma (hot, cold, euthyroid)
- lymphoma
- non-thyroidal masses (lymph nodes, branchial cleft cyst, thyroglossal cyst)
- isolated simple cyst
- carcinoma
- histiocytosis.

Disorders of sexual development (DSD)

Uncertainty regarding a child's gender is a distressing emergency for the family.

Most of these children are well unless associated with congenital adrenal hyperplasia (CAH) and salt loss (see above) or other major congenital abnormalities.

Avoid the urge to decide the appropriate sex of rearing of the child until the results of diagnostic tests are available.

Support the parents during this difficult time.

- DSD may be the result of excess androgens in females (the commonest situation, usually secondary to CAH of the 21-hydroxylase deficiency variety), lack of androgens (or the receptor) in males, or (rarely) mixed gonadal DSD with the presence of ovarian and testicular tissue. Minimum investigations are chromosome analysis and plasma for 17-hydroxyprogesterone (**which is** elevated in the commonest form of CAH). **If a baby with a DSD becomes unwell with hypotension, hyponatraemia and hyperkalaemia, assume an adrenal crisis and treat as described above.**
- Further investigation requires highly specialised tests (i.e. blood, radiology and ultrasound, fibroblasts, laparoscopy or laparotomy). Treatment of non-CAH DSD is also complex, but can often be deferred to allow appropriate transfer of care to a specialist centre. In specialist centres there need to be close working relationships between the different specialists. It is not appropriate for surgeons to operate without involving endocrinologists in working up these patients, and **it is essential that the members of the multidisciplinary team work closely together in the management of these cases.**

Congenital adrenal hyperplasia (CAH)

Congenital adrenal hyperplasia (CAH) is an autosomal-recessive condition, and therefore is more common in consanguineous relationships. Many forms exist, as several enzymes involved in the synthesis of cortisol and aldosterone may be deficient; partial cases also occur within each subtype.

Salt-losing 21-hydroxylase deficiency is by far the commonest type. Most forms result in over-masculinisation of the female (although under-masculinisation of the male can also occur in defects near the start of the biosynthetic pathway). Salt loss occurs in several forms (see above), although the second commonest deficiency (11-beta-hydroxylase) causes salt retention and hypertension.

Females usually present as DSD (see above) and males with salt loss, which usually occurs after the first week of life (see above for acute and long-term management). In non-salt-losing forms there will be incomplete early puberty (see below).

Once the diagnosis is established, treat with mildly suppressive doses of hydrocortisone, 12–15 mg/m^2/day in three divided doses and, if salt loss is demonstrated, fludrocortisone, 150–250 micrograms/m^2/day in one dose. Infants may also require oral sodium chloride, 1 gram/10 kg/day (60 mg = 1 mmol).

Addison's disease and Cushing's syndrome

Addison's disease (hypoadrenalism)

Hypoadrenalism may present as an emergency (see above) or be suspected if there is:

- unexplained lethargy
- failure to thrive
- pigmentation of scars and skin
- vitiligo or other signs of autoimmune disease
- a strong family history of hypoadrenalism or unexplained sudden death
- hyponatraemia and hyperkalaemia
- syndrome of candidiasis and hypoparathyroidism pre-dating the hypoadrenalism (HAM or APECED syndrome).

If confirmed by a low 9 a.m. cortisol level (< 150 nmol/ litre), treat as outlined above for adrenal crisis.

Cushing's syndrome (hyperadrenalism)

Cushing's syndrome is usually the result of iatrogenic corticosteroid administration (> 12 mg/m²/day hydrocortisone or the equivalent; see above). Over-secretion of adrenal steroids is rare. Signs of corticosteroid excess include the following:

- poor (zero) growth rate
- red cheeks
- striae
- glucose intolerance
- excess weight gain (central)
- muscle weakness
- hypertension.

Adrenal carcinoma or adenoma may produce Cushing's syndrome. There is often accompanying virilisation and an abdominal mass. The child is usually young, in contrast to the older child with Cushing's disease secondary to an ACTH-secreting pituitary adenoma.

The diagnosis is supported by a **detectable midnight cortisol level (> 50 nmol/litre) or raised urinary free cortisol excretion. The 9 a.m. cortisol level fails to be reduced to undetectable levels in response to dexamethasone 0.3 mg/m² given as a single dose the previous night.**

Treatment usually requires specialist surgery.

Hypogonadism and delayed puberty

- Hypogonadism may be secondary to central gonadotrophin deficiency (hypogonadotrophism: LH/FSH low) or peripheral gonadal failure (hypergonadotrophism: LH/FSH high).
- Suspect congenital central hypogonadism in a male neonate with undescended testes and micropenis (shaft length < 2.5 cm). Hypopituitarism may also be present.
- If hypogonadism remains undetected, failure of or incomplete pubertal development will occur.
- Delayed puberty is often familial, but may be induced by emotional or nutritional deprivation.
- There is delayed maturation of gonadotrophin secretion.
- Treat if the delay is severe enough to cause psychological damage.
- Give a brief course of testosterone esters (100 mg by deep IM injection (Sustanon) at 1-month intervals three times in boys) or oral oestrogen (5–10 micrograms/day

for 3 months in girls). This allows puberty to be induced and also reduces the risk of later osteoporosis.

- If the hypogonadism is likely to be permanent, continue and gradually increase testosterone to 250 mg/month or oestrogen to 25–50 micrograms/day over a 2½-year period (the latter eventually as a combined oral contraceptive medication to allow withdrawal bleeding).

TABLE 5.8.C.1 Causes of delayed puberty

Low LH/FSH + low testosterone/oestrogen	High LH/FSH + low testosterone/oestrogen
Chronic ill health	Gonadal trauma/infection
Constitutional/familial	Gonadal dysgenesis or Turner's syndrome (XO)
Starvation, low body mass index	Klinefelter's syndrome (XXY)
Genetic (e.g. Kallmann's syndrome, Prader–Willi syndrome)	Some cases of DSD
Prolactinoma (rare)	Autoimmune ovarian damage
Hypopituitarism, hypothyroidism	Galactosaemia
Thalassaemia	

Precocious puberty

- In precocious puberty, early sexual maturity (at less than 8 years of age in females, or less than 10 years of age in males) is usually accompanied by a growth spurt and relatively tall stature for age.
- In central gonadotrophin activation, there is development of full puberty (i.e. breasts and pubic hair with eventual menstruation, or testicular enlargement plus pubic hair and penis development).
- In secondary cases there is excess peripheral sex steroid production/ingestion. Some aspects of puberty will be exaggerated, whereas other tissues will be normal, or may regress (e.g. large penis and pubic hair plus small hard testes in androgen excess in CAH, large breasts but no pubic hair in oestrogen-secreting tumour).
- Idiopathic central precocity is commonest in females, and may be familial.
- Male gonadotrophin activation may be a sign of a CNS tumour.
- Investigation and treatment are complex and specialised, and include suppression of gonadotrophin secretion in central precocious puberty, and surgical removal or suppression/blocking of the peripheral source of sex steroid production in peripheral causes.

Growth hormone deficiency and short stature

Growth hormone deficiency (GHD) may be idiopathic, familial, part of hypopituitarism or isolated.

In the neonatal period, isolated GHD or hypopituitarism may cause hypoglycaemia (see Section 3.4). After excluding or treating hypoadrenalism (see above), growth hormone may be required to maintain **normoglycaemia and normal growth but such treatment requires expert input**.

Growth hormone is essential for normal growth, and GHD should be suspected in the child who is:

- short in relation to their peers and in comparison with their parents
- growing slowly
- relatively heavy for their height.

Outside the neonatal period, treatment is rarely urgent. Growth hormone is administered as a subcutaneous injection. It is expensive and difficult to store.

The causes of severe short stature include the following:

- secondary to chronic ill health or under-nutrition; these patients are often thin
- secondary to chronic emotional trauma; these patients are often thin
- endocrine (hypothyroid, hypopituitary, GHD, Cushing's syndrome); these patients are often relatively heavy
- syndromic (e.g. Turner's syndrome, etc.); these patients are usually dysmorphic, but some may have few external features, so it should be suspected in all short females outside their genetic range
- disproportionate with short limbs (bony dysplasias, rickets)
- metabolic (storage disorders, osteogenesis); these patients have longer limbs than back.

Short stature in the latter three causes is extremely difficult and expensive to treat.

Hypopituitarism

In the neonate there will be hypoadrenalism with or without GHD leading to hypoglycaemia. Suspect hypopituitarism in any male neonate with cryptoorchidism and micropenis.

Onset later in life may signal an intracranial lesion such as craniopharyngioma (which may be visible as a calcified mass on plain lateral skull X-ray or CT scan; MRI scans show a cystic cavity at the base of the brain). Symptoms outside the neonatal period include the following:

- poor growth/short stature (secondary to GHD)

- lethargy
- hypotension
- hypothermia
- hypothyroidism (see above)
- hypogonadism (see above)
- visual field defects, headache and/or raised intracranial pressure if secondary to tumour.

Treatment is outlined in the sections on individual hormone deficiencies above.

Diabetes insipidus

Isolated diabetes insipidus is rare, but it can occur as part of hypopituitarism or secondary to infiltration of the posterior pituitary by tumour or destruction by infection. Suspect it in any case of:

- dehydration with dilute (colourless) urine
- polyuria and polydipsia not due to diabetes mellitus
- secondary daytime wetting without an obvious cause
- familial history.

It is important to request a fluid balance diary at home, and for carers to allow access to water alone between meals as the only fluid permitted. This will help to identify the many behavioural causes of polydipsia, and will avoid the need for awkward and unnecessary tests of urinary concentrating capacity.

Diagnosis is confirmed by the simultaneous presence of hyperosmolar serum (> 290 mOsm/litre) and dilute urine (< 300 mOsm/litre or specific gravity < 1005).

Treat by allowing free access to water and, if possible, replacement of antidiuretic hormone **with** a long-acting analogue, DDAVP, which can be given intramuscularly, by nasal spray or orally. The dose is titrated to keep **the** specific gravity **of the urine** in **the range** 1005–1010 and/or the serum osmolarity normal. Try to allow one period of diuresis before each dose is due, to prevent dangerous hyponatraemia from over-treatment.

5.9 The child or adolescent with a mental health problem

BOX 5.9.1 Minimum standards
- Knowledge, skills and tests that exclude organic medical causes.
- Effective child protection systems.
- Fluoxetine.
- Resperidone, chlorpromazine and flupenthixol.
- Supportive family therapy.

Introduction

Around 10–20% of all children have one or more mental or behavioural problems (World Health Report 2001). The rates are higher in urban areas and increase in adolescence. One in ten young people suffers from mental illness or symptoms

of mental distress severe enough to cause some level of impairment, yet less than one in five receives the treatment that they need.

Prematurity, poor nutritional status, low birth weight, organic brain damage and physical handicap often bring about biological stressors. A disadvantaged socio-economic status of families contributes negatively to the mental health of children. Child development suffers where there is persistent marital discord, parental psychiatric ill health and/or a history of substance abuse. Protective factors include stable care, an adaptable and engaging personality, problem-solving abilities and a supportive network of family and friends.

The aggregate disease burden of these disorders has

not been estimated, and it is complex because many of these disorders can be precursors to much more disabling disorders during later life. Mental health disorders of childhood and adolescence are very costly to society in both human and financial terms.

Psychiatric disorders that arise in adolescence are different from those in children and similar to those in adults. The vulnerability of adolescence relates to difficulty in establishing an identity, during which there may be alienation from the parents. There is also intense emotional interaction with friends, which makes adolescents especially vulnerable to the effects of peer pressure, and issues of sexuality. Emotional disorders include anxiety states, depression, hysteria and specific phobias.

Conduct disorders occur in about the same proportion, and include conditions that range from oppositional defiant behaviour to persistent patterns of aggression and rule breaking. About 20% of the teenagers may present with a mixture of disorders.

The link between adverse family environmental factors and mental health disorders in children and adolescents is fundamental and must be explored as part of the assessment and treatment.

Acute psychiatric emergencies: suicide and deliberate self-harm

In well-resourced countries there has been a persistent rise in fatal suicide attempts, especially in young males. A history of substance abuse, conflict with the law and personal and mental illness are important factors. **The possibility of abuse within (most likely) or outside the family must be at the forefront of a search for why this occurred, as there may be other children 'at risk'.** The method of suicide depends on the means available. Males are more likely to use violent means than females. Overdoses of drugs or poison, hanging and immolation are common methods of suicide.

Suicide is extremely rare in pre-pubescent children, but the frequency rises sharply during the teenage period. Again a search for evidence of abuse must be undertaken.

Deliberate self-harm is a non-fatal act in which a child or young person deliberately ingests noxious substances in excess of therapeutic doses, or causes self-injury. It is best interpreted as a 'cry for help'. Again, the possibility of abuse must be considered in all cases.

Assessment and questions to be asked

- **Are there any indicators or clinical signs of physical or sexual abuse?**
- **Have there been any previous attempts at suicide?**
- Is there a risk of suicide or of a repeated attempt?
- Was a suicide note left?
- Was there pre-planning?
- How likely was the young person to be found?
- What was the method used?
- How lethal was the method used?
- Did the young person know how toxic the substance was?
- What quantity of the substance was taken?
- Was it impulsive in the context of a conflictual relationship?
- Was it to attract sympathy or seek attention (e.g. following a disciplinary crisis or the loss of a friend)?

- Is there a psychiatric disorder?
- What is the family and developmental history, including educational functioning?
- How well does the child solve problems and cope with difficulties?
- How effective and who are the social/parental supports, including adequacy of supervision?

It is important to clarify to the family (preferably in the presence of the child) that information given by the child is confidential.

High-risk factors

- Undiagnosed and unmanaged abuse.
- The risk of repetition is higher in the next 4 weeks after the attempt. It also increases if there is a history of previous self-harm attempts.
- Male gender.
- Lack of support, and easy access to a means of committing suicide (e.g. a firearm or drugs belonging to other family members in the home).
- Presence of depressive illness, with loss of sleep, appetite, depressed mood, agitation, and in particular continued suicidal ideas (hopelessness, inability to enjoy life, asking 'What's the point?').

Treatment

- Treatment of the medical consequences of self-harm is the priority (see Section 7 especially Section 7.4).
- Assessment of the child and their family should be undertaken when the child is free from the after-effects of the drug overdose/self-inflicted injury.
- It is important to take the young person's suicidal ideas seriously and not to expose them to sarcasm or ridicule in discussions. Assessment should include consideration of a mental illness and also of the family and social circumstances of the young person and the context in which the self-harm occurred.
- Nothing predicts behaviour better than past behaviour. Those with a low risk of repetition can be offered support during subsequent crises, and arrangements made to assist the child and their family in developing coping strategies. A psychologist, social worker or trained psychiatric nurse (if available) can assist the family in this way.
- **If there is abuse, the child must be protected from further harm by arranging the involvement of social services and the police (as appropriate in the setting).**
- Children at high risk of death need a major input, although inpatient facilities are generally sparse and often unavailable. Depending on resources (or lack of them) the physician needs to improvise and involve social agencies and the family (particularly the extended family if there are immediate parental problems) to provide appropriate supervision, support and treatment.
- Those with a history of substance abuse will need specific counselling.
- The presence of mental illness merits specific treatment (psychological therapies and/or medication) and intervention (see below). Issues that triggered the self-harm should be addressed if possible. Relationship difficulties should be borne in mind.

Depressive disorders

Depression is a recurring illness characterised by episodes of dysfunction. It is common, and has a lifetime prevalence in adults of 15–20%. It has been reported in 1% of preschool children, 2% of school-age children and 5–8% of adolescents; girls are twice as likely to suffer from depression as boys. The incidence is rising, or else depression is being recognised more, with each successive generation. It is detected at a younger age and there has been a parallel increase in suicide in the paediatric age group.

Sadness, unhappiness and misery are common childhood experiences (usually in reaction to adverse family circumstances), but when sadness is extreme in intensity and duration, it may be due to a depressive illness. Depression or depressive illness always needs urgent attention.

The presentation of depression varies with the age of the child. Infants and preschool children cannot express feelings of sadness in language. In this age group, depressive symptoms must be inferred from apathy, withdrawal from caregivers, delay or regression of developmental milestones, and failure to thrive that has no organic cause.

School-aged children are cognitively able to internalise family conflict, criticism or failure to achieve. They display low self-esteem and guilt, but depression is often mainly expressed in somatic complaints (headaches, stomach aches, disturbed sleep and appetite), anxiety (school phobia, excessive separation anxiety), irritability (temper tantrums and other behavioural problems) and academic decline.

Common symptoms in adolescents resemble adulthood depression, with more anger than sadness, hostility mainly towards family, sleep and appetite often normal, drug abuse, academic decline and suicide attempts. A depressed mood (dysphoria) is accompanied by loss of emotional involvement (withdrawal), feelings of guilt and unworthiness, and an inability to cope effectively. A 'depressive disorder' refers to an observable depressed mood, tearfulness, suicidal thoughts, disturbance of sleep and appetite, and a lack of energy.

When the above symptoms persist or occur despite an absence of adverse environmental causes, and functioning is impaired, a diagnosis of depressive illness can be considered. It is worth noting that around 40% of children with conduct (behaviour) disorders have associated mood disturbances, and that children presenting with depression may have other problems, such as anxiety or substance abuse.

Assessment

Assessment should include the child or adolescent and their family or other people who know the young person well. This may be impossible for the teenager who has no family, or for the older teenager who refuses to have their parents involved.

At the beginning of the assessment it is helpful to clarify the bounds of confidentiality. The parents and the child need to understand that what each of them says will not be freely shared without consent. However, it should also be made clear that there are limits to confidentiality in situations in which the law requires reporting, such as abuse, and also in situations where the child's safety is at serious risk – for example, of suicide.

Assess the degree of dysfunction and distress that the symptoms are causing the child and their family.

Assessment requires a detailed history, mental state examination, play and observation of the child–parent interaction. A full medical examination and neuropsychological testing to rule out neurological or learning disorders and to assess the child's developmental capabilities should be undertaken. Psychological assessment tests such as a strength and difficulty questionnaire may be helpful.

Risk factors

- A family history of depression predisposes to depression, and the children of depressed parents are three times more likely to develop depression themselves. Early onset in the parents is associated with a higher risk for the children.
- Family and social environmental risk factors include family conflicts, rejection, lack of communication, lack of expression of love, poor family support systems, abuse (physical, emotional or sexual), and parents who are excessively controlling.
- Adverse life events, such as the death of a parent or other loved one, parental divorce, exposure to suicide, relationship problems and academic failure can precipitate depression.
- Negative emotions such as low self-esteem, self-criticism, negative interpretation of life events and a feeling of lack of control can all contribute.
- The process of puberty can precipitate depression.

Issues in management

The diagnosis of a depressive illness (as opposed to transient sadness, which is very common) should be made **only** after careful history taking and information from the family, school and (if possible) close friends. **Almost all 'depression' in children or adolescents is related to environmental factors, and a diagnosis of depressive illness should only be made when it is certain that environmental factors are not responsible.**

In addition, and in older adolescents, **bipolar disorder** may present for the first time, and a history of symptoms of hypomania should always be undertaken. If such symptoms are elicited, a daily symptom diary may be helpful. There are specific drug treatments for bipolar disorder which include mood stabilisers, and the support of an adult psychiatrist can be very helpful.

Medical conditions that can present with depressive illness must be excluded, using appropriate investigations, in particular vitamin or mineral deficiencies (full blood count), thyroid dysfunction (TSH levels), tuberculosis (chest X-ray) and HIV infection.

If possible, address any stressful factors in the child's environment.

Management of sadness

The opportunity to discuss their difficulties with a sympathetic and helpful listener can itself be very useful to a depressed child or adolescent. The depressed child will tend to blame him- or herself, and there should be an attempt to enable the child to deal with issues without such negative feelings.

It is important to explore sensitively any factors in the child's life that may have led to the episode of self-harm, and to put the problems right as far as possible, while recognising that some situations cannot be changed.

Work to help the young person to understand him- or herself, identify feelings, change maladaptive patterns of behaviour and improve relationships can be very helpful, and will provide useful skills for them later on in their life.

Consider the mental health of other members of the family, which may be having a significant effect on the child or adolescent. Helping the parents may help the child. Postnatal depression occurs in about 10% of mothers, and tends to recur with each pregnancy. Family therapy and support can also be very helpful.

Regular exercise (e.g. involvement in sport) can be very useful for some people with depression. It is also important to get enough sleep and to eat as healthy a diet as possible. Formal 'talking therapies' such as cognitive–behavioural therapy can be helpful, but they require specialist training and are not widely available, even in well-resourced countries.

Management of depressive illness

It is vital that the child or adolescent is informed that their symptoms and the effects of the symptoms on their behaviour and educational function are not due to anything they have done or are doing wrong. The young person and their family need to learn how to distinguish between the normal range of feelings and those, including sadness, that suggest the onset or presence of the depressive disorder.

In more severe forms of depressive illness, particularly in adolescents, antidepressants can be helpful, but in general their use is best avoided.

Antidepressant medication

The antidepressants of first choice for adolescents aged 12–18 years are selective serotonin reuptake inhibitors (SSRIs) such as fluoxetine, which can be effective but are expensive. They should be prescribed following baseline measurements of blood pressure and heart rate, physical examination for extrapyramidal symptoms, etc. The suggested baseline laboratory investigations are complete blood count, liver function tests, pregnancy tests for girls, and ECG. The common side effects of SSRIs are dizziness, sweating, diarrhoea, headaches, fatigue, restlessness, initial insomnia, and weight loss or gain. Uncommon side effects may include delayed micturition, blurred vision, skin rashes, etc., and should be explained to the patient and their family.

Usually fluoxetine is best tolerated if given in the morning after breakfast, but in situations in which it causes drowsiness it can be taken in the evening. Changes in symptoms do not occur for at least 3–6 weeks. Follow-up must be insisted upon while the young person is on medication.

Suicidal feelings must be explored routinely at onset and at follow-up.

Fluoxetine: the starting dose in children aged 12 to 18 years is 10 mg daily, and the dose may be increased to 20 mg daily after 1–2 weeks. There is little information about the use of fluoxetine in children under 12 years of age.

Abrupt discontinuation of SSRIs may induce withdrawal symptoms, some of which mimic a relapse of a depressive episode (e.g. tiredness, irritability and severe somatic symptoms).

Once the patient has been free of symptoms and back to normal life for at least 8 weeks, fluoxetine should be continued for 6 months, then gradually reduced and stopped over a period of 6–12 weeks. The speed of reduction should be decided with the patient, taking into consideration any symptoms of withdrawal.

Tricyclic antidepressants have major side effects, including cardiovascular complications. They are also very dangerous in overdose. Therefore they must not be used.

Monoamine oxidase inhibitors (MAOIs) must not be used because of their dangers when taken with certain foods.

Hysterical conversion disorder

This is a subgroup of somatoform disorders. It refers to loss or alteration of physical functioning without organic cause. The child presents with physical symptoms which result in disability in the absence of consistent physical signs or evidence of a physical illness. The most frequent symptoms are pseudo-seizures, loss of sensation and loss of limb function. These are common in post-pubertal female adolescents. They usually arise when the adolescent is facing a predicament that they cannot resolve. This may be related to academic, family, interpersonal, sexual, abuse, religion or societal issues.

As well as a thorough history and interview, the assessment should include a full physical examination to assess symptoms that do not correlate with known neurological pathways (e.g. a gait that is inconsistent and varying). It is important to keep an open mind about the possibility of a physical problem which has not yet manifested itself, and reconsider this regularly.

Pseudo-seizures may occur in adolescents who also have epileptic seizures, and it may be difficult to distinguish between them and provide the correct treatment. A blood test taken within 20 minutes of an episode to measure serum prolactin levels (if facilities for this are available) can be useful for differentiating between pseudo-seizures (prolactin levels are normal) and epileptic seizures (prolactin levels are raised).

Once a psychiatric disorder has been diagnosed, the emphasis should move from medical investigations to amelioration of presenting symptoms and appropriate psychological intervention. The latter should incorporate 'face-saving' formulae to allow the young person to come to terms with the absence of physical disease, but the presence of an illness which is 'real' as far as the young person is concerned. Whatever the cause, the disability and the impact on the young person's life are real, and may be more difficult to manage than a physical illness with similar symptoms. This aspect of the disorder must be carefully explained to the family as well, in case they believe that the young person is faking an illness.

Drugs and alcohol: use and abuse

Drug use and availability have changed radically in the last decade or two. The substances abused depend on availability and supply. As children get older, the proportion who have ever tried drugs increases. Which drugs are illegal and which are socially acceptable vary between countries and among different groups of people in the same country, and the use of drugs by children and adolescents is influenced by this. A child's abuse of drugs is contextual – that is, it depends on societal norms, family history, etc. Parental criminality or substance abuse increases the risk. Reliable data on drug abuse in children are scarce and not validated. However, there is increasing acceptance that the rates of drug use are increasing, particularly in inner-city areas among children who are deprived (e.g. 'street children').

Volatile substance abuse is common in children, but seldom persists into adulthood. Solvents are easily available (e.g. butane gas, lighter fuel, paint thinners, aerosols, etc.), and are most commonly abused through a plastic bag to maximise the effects.

Stimulants such as cocaine and amphetamines are taken in powder form, intranasally or injected. They produce elevation of mood, energy, a reduction in appetite and hallucinations.

Drugs may be used for pleasure, or to remove (however briefly) the pain of daily life. Many drug users live in very difficult conditions and/or have mental health problems in addition to their drug habit. Prostitution is often associated with drug use, trapping (mainly women) in a vicious cycle. There is also a strong association of substance abuse with conduct disorder. In conduct disorders there is a repetitive and persistent pattern of behaviour in which societal norms or rules are violated (e.g. fighting, bullying, cruelty to people and animals, destruction of property, stealing and deceit). Many drug abusers will take up crime to pay for their drugs.

Assessment

It is important to establish the extent, frequency and severity of drug abuse or dependence. In addition, information needs to be elicited concerning behavioural patterns, social competency, educational functioning, peer relationships and psychiatric status.

Physical examination should include a check for fresh injection marks, old scars or the physical sequelae of drug use.

Management

There are very few, if any, specialised treatment centres for children who abuse drugs. Treatment outcome will vary according to the chronicity and/or the substances abused. For example, only a limited impact is made on alcohol or marijuana abuse, whereas heroin or cocaine treatment programmes are more successful in reducing the use of these drugs.

Methadone as part of a well-controlled and structured treatment system is the most common approach to managing long-term opiate dependence. However, it is rarely available in resource-limited settings. The initial dose for children over 15 years of age is 10–20 mg daily, increasing by 10 mg/day until there are no signs of withdrawal or toxicity (the usual dose is 40–60 mg/day). Opiates can give rise to nausea and vomiting. Withdrawal symptoms include restlessness, irritability, and increased bowel activity with abdominal pain. Methadone treatment is not appropriate for those with a short history of opiate dependence.

Schizophrenia

This is a serious mental illness characterised by abnormalities of thinking, perception and emotion, usually first diagnosed in late adolescence, although rarely the onset can be seen in childhood. Consider the diagnosis if two or more of the following symptoms are present for 1 month or longer:

- delusions: beliefs which are unshakeable
- hallucinations: 80% of affected children have auditory hallucinations; visual hallucinations are more likely to be due to an organic medical disorder such as a brain tumour or poisoning
- disorganised (incoherent) speech

- grossly disorganised or catatonic behaviour
- negative symptoms (flat affect).

The onset is usually insidious. Many children have pre-existing problems with social withdrawal, disruptive behaviour, developmental delay and language problems, and then go on to develop more florid symptoms such as hallucinations. Mood disorders may present with schizophrenic-like symptoms, and making the diagnosis may be difficult.

Assessment

Any diagnosis is dependent on detailed history taking and examination, and schizophrenia is no exception. To evaluate the progress, it is important to define the baseline symptoms, functioning and problems in various aspects of the young person's life (i.e. education, family and social functioning).

Before a definitive diagnosis of schizophrenia is made, **organic medical conditions must be excluded** by the following tests. However, it has to be accepted that in resource-limited settings many of these tests will not be available: blood tests for haemoglobin, indices such as MCV (to rule out vitamin B_{12} deficiency), thyroid function, liver and renal function, heavy metals such as lead, mercury and arsenic, HIV indicators, the Wassermann reaction for syphilis, urine test for toxicology, an EEG to help to rule out temporal lobe epilepsy, and a CT scan of the brain.

Management

Children and adolescents with schizophrenia present a challenge as they are seriously ill, and often their social and educational progress is seriously disrupted. Treatment is difficult, and all management should be under the supervision of a psychiatrist (if available). Treatments aim to reduce the frequency of relapses and disability.

It is important to work closely with the family. Negative symptoms such as blunting of emotions, impoverished thinking and lack of motivation are particularly distressing to relatives. Furthermore, highly expressed emotions and negative feelings increase the risk of relapse. The family will need support and help to manage their child's symptoms. The techniques for reducing highly expressed emotions require specialist training.

Pharmacological treatment to control symptoms is the important initial management. Psycho-educational, social, cognitive and family intervention programmes are important in long-term management. Oral neuroleptics provide the patient with a sense of control. Any adverse effects will quickly become apparent, but the medication must be administered daily and the patient may not always be compliant. Depot neuroleptics provide a way of enhancing compliance.

Atypical antipsychotic drugs are now the treatment of choice (if available), as they have less extrapyramidal side effects. Risperidone can be given to children over 12 years of age, starting at 2 mg per day and increasing by 1 mg per week to a maximum daily dose of 8 mg. Side effects include postural hypotension, weight gain, hyperglycaemia and mild extrapyramidal signs.

Standard antipsychotic drugs are more likely to be available in resource-limited settings. Standard antipsychotic treatment for acute schizophrenic symptoms is usually initiated with chlorpromazine. For children aged

12–18 years, start with oral treatment with 25 mg three times a day or 75 mg at night, and then gradually increase the doses until there is control of symptoms, usually achieved with a maximum dose of 100–300 mg daily. Premature changes in drug choice should be avoided, as the response time may be 30 days or more.

Poor response may be due to an inadequate dose or poor compliance.

Depot medication is suitable for long-term treatment (flupenthixol by deep IM injection into the outer buttock or lateral thigh with a test dose of 20 mg, then after 7 days 20–40 mg repeated 3- to 4-weekly according to the response. The usual maintenance dose is 50 mg every 4 weeks to 300 mg every 2 weeks,

Side effects include extrapyramidal signs (Parkinsonism, dystonia, restlessness and tardive dyskinesia), hypotension and less commonly neuroleptic malignant syndrome (hyperthermia, fluctuating consciousness, muscle rigidity and autonomic dysfunction).

Post-traumatic stress disorder (*see also* Section 1.23)

Introduction

Nearly all children and adolescents who have experienced catastrophic situations will initially display symptoms of psychological distress, including intrusive flashbacks of the stress event, nightmares, withdrawal and inability to concentrate, among others. **Most children and adolescents will regain normal functioning once their basic survival needs are met, safety and security have been regained, and developmental opportunities have been restored, within the social, family and community context.**

Post-traumatic stress disorder (PTSD) is a relatively new diagnostic category first officially created by DSM-III in 1980. Around 25–35% of those exposed to traumatic events develop PTSD. Individual differences in response to trauma depend on the following:

- stressor severity and degree of exposure to the stressor
- exposure to previous traumatic events
- the child's perception of the event
- the child's appraisal of the threat to their survival, and the degree of human accountability
- for younger children, the response and functioning of adults, particularly close family, around them can be important.

Anxiety disorders, abnormal grief reaction, somatic complaints and impairment in educational functioning can all occur.

Diagnostic criteria

The child has experienced an event that is outside the range of normal experience and that is life-threatening to them or to those close to them. There is persistent re-experiencing of the traumatic event – that is, distressing recollections, dreams or flashbacks.

There is avoidance of the stimuli associated with the trauma, and a range of signs of physiological arousal occur, such as difficulty in sleeping, irritability or poor concentration.

In younger children, repetitive play related to the trauma may be present. They may have frightening dreams that have no obvious content, and may regress in their development.

Assessment

It must first be established that the child has experienced a traumatic event that preceded the onset of the symptoms. The traumatic event may not necessarily lead to development of PTSD. Instead, the child may develop acute stress disorder or sadness.

When assessing the child, the interviewer will need to take account of the child's maturation, and their verbal facility and functioning. Details of the traumatic event, the child's perception of the event, and their response immediately and later, should be evaluated.

The differential diagnoses include obsessive-compulsive disorder, schizophrenia and anxiety disorder. Flashbacks may need to be distinguished from intrusive and unwanted thoughts that are unrelated to the traumatic event, which occur in obsessive-compulsive disorder.

Management of trauma-affected children (*see also* Section 1.23)

If possible, reuniting the child with their parents or other close relatives and restoring normal comforting routines is helpful.

Some children will require more specialised interventions to address their suffering and help to restore their flow of development. Immediately after traumatic events, activities and opportunities that allow children to talk about or otherwise express painful experiences and feelings (e.g. by physical and artistic expression) are most beneficial if facilitated by people whom the children know and trust, and have continued contact with.

The goals of psychological treatment are reduction of symptoms, development of coping skills, and helping the individual to gain a sense of well-being and control. Education and gradually increasing goal setting help the child to relax, solve problems and gradually achieve mastery over fearful thoughts. The help of a clinically trained psychologist or psychiatrist may be needed to plan the treatment.

Trauma counselling should never be provided unless an appropriate and sustained follow-up mechanism is guaranteed.

The psychosocial well-being of adults, particularly parents and caregivers, has a direct impact on that of children, and should therefore be addressed through concurrent parent-focused psychosocial interventions. The participation of children, and adults, in decisions that affect their lives has a positive effect on their mental health, empowers them, and helps them to regain control over their own lives.

Panic attacks

These are common in children and adolescents, and can mimic physical illnesses. Hyperventilation, sometimes with tetany, is a key feature, as well as the fear of 'going crazy' or dying. The best way of controlling such attacks is to explain the physiological features of panic to the child and their family, and to teach proper breathing techniques (namely to breathe slowly at a rate normal for the child's age).

Preventive intervention

The promotion of mental health through a healthy lifestyle brought about by health education and life skills training has the potential to equip a young person for their journey through life. There is material available in the public domain on life skills training (e.g. on the WHO/UNICEF websites) which has been used in many resource-limited and middle-income countries.

Autism and autistic spectrum disorders

This is a group of disorders with similar features, although an individual child may not display all of them, and the severity may vary. Autism becomes evident before 3 years of age, but children with other conditions that form part of the autistic spectrum may present later (e.g. at school age).

Autistic behaviour may occur as an isolated problem, or it may be a component of a number of childhood developmental disorders. It is important to consider these when assessing a child, in case intervention may help. Sensory deficits, particularly deafness, which may be hard to identify in a young child, are especially important in this respect. Children with hydrocephalus, metabolic disorders (e.g. phenylketonuria), hypothyroidism, fetal alcohol syndrome, tuberous sclerosis, neurofibromatosis, Down's syndrome and other chromosomal disorders may exhibit features of autism.

Autistic children characteristically have difficulties with the following:
- social interaction and reciprocity
- language development and communication skills
- imagination and play
- rigid thinking
- restrictive and repetitive stereotypical patterns of behaviour, activities and interests.

Social interaction
Autistic children may make little or no eye contact. They may not be able to share experiences or to understand the feelings of others, or recognise clues to their feelings from their behaviour (e.g. that people who are crying are sad).

Language and communication
Young children with autism may not point to get attention or to show another person something. They may never develop any useful language, or they may have unusual speech with abnormal intonation, jumbled words, incomprehensible sounds, or repetition of the same words again and again (echolalia).

Cognitive function
Children with autism may have global cognitive impairment or general impairment but considerable skill in some areas (e.g. numbers, art).

Rigid thinking and ritualistic behaviour
Autistic children often have very structured repetitive play (e.g. organising objects in a certain pattern). They may persist much longer than usual in putting things in their mouths, or they may hold on to objects, moving and feeling them in their hands, for long periods. Routine is very important, and they are often very upset by any disruption, which may lead to outbursts of temper.

Management
There is no cure as yet for autism. Management focuses on encouraging the child to learn as much as possible and to develop behaviour that helps him or her to live happily within the family and community.

Support for the family in caring for these children, who can be very challenging, is essential. Education for the family and community about the difficulties of autistic children, so that their behaviour is not misinterpreted as naughtiness, or caregivers criticised inappropriately, is also very important. Healthcare professionals and teachers experienced in the care of children with autism can give a great deal of assistance to families.

Vigilance for other problems, especially with hearing or vision, which if undiagnosed will add to the child's difficulties, should be maintained.

For some children with autism who have severe aggressive behaviour and only under expert supervision consider risperidone:
- **Child over 5 years and 15–20 kg:** 250 micrograms daily increased if necessary after at least 4 days to 500 micrograms daily; thereafter increased by 250 micrograms daily at 2-week intervals to maximum of 1 mg daily
- **Child over 5 years and over 20 kg:** 500 micrograms daily increased if necessary after at least 4 days to 1 mg daily; thereafter increased by 500 micrograms daily at 2-week intervals; max. daily dose 2.5 mg if under 45 kg; maximum daily dose 3 mg if over 45 kg.

Review effectiveness and side effects after 3–4 weeks; stop if no response at 6 weeks.

Asperger's syndrome

Asperger's syndrome has some features in common with autism, in that affected individuals also have difficulties with social interaction, especially in understanding the usual patterns of social behaviour of their community. They often develop very deep and detailed knowledge about subjects that interest them, and become experts who can contribute to society, but they may also become isolated if others do not share or understand their interests.

Asperger's syndrome is usually identified later than autism, often when children are at school, and are recognised as different from their peers. They may be bullied and very lonely, as they long to have friends and 'fit in', but do not have the social skills to enable them to do so.

Like autism, there is no cure for Asperger's, but teaching from as early an age as possible about appropriate behaviour can help these children. Education for their families and communities, so that they understand that the child has a condition which makes it hard for him or her to pick up social clues, and is not just being difficult, along with appreciation of any special talents, is essential. If it is acceptable to the child or adolescent, written information to give to people to explain what they find hard may be useful.

Attention deficit hyperactivity disorder (ADHD)

Children with ADHD characteristically have difficulties with the following:
- inattention
- hyperactivity
- impulsivity.

These features must be present before the age of 6–7 years, evident in more than one situation (e.g. at home and at school), and interfere with the child's social or educational functioning.

These characteristics may persist into adult life, resulting in inattentive and disorganised or impulsive risk-taking behaviour.

Inattention
Children with ADHD cannot concentrate for very long, especially on tasks they have been given which have no immediate reward (e.g. schoolwork).

Hyperactivity
These children are always on the move. Young children with ADHD may run, jump, climb, make a lot of noise and never settle to anything. School-age children and adolescents have difficulty sitting still, and may be constantly tapping their feet, wriggling and fidgeting.

Impulsivity
Children with ADHD do not think before they act. They may have accidents or get into trouble for recklessness.

Other problems
Children with ADHD can be exhausting. They are often in trouble because they are so active and may have poor relationships with other children and adults, and low self-esteem. They may sleep badly, struggling to get to sleep or waking frequently, and be poor eaters because they cannot sit still for long enough to finish a meal.

Causes
There is no known cause of ADHD. Some of the contributory factors include the following:
- genetic: parents or siblings affected
- living conditions: ADHD is more common in children from disadvantaged backgrounds
- depression in the child's mother
- these factors may all interact.

In addition to occurring alone, the features of ADHD may be seen in young people with neurological conditions such as head injuries, fetal alcohol syndrome, encephalitis and meningitis, epilepsy, hypothyroidism and some syndromes, such as fragile X syndrome, Williams' syndrome and tuberous sclerosis.

Comorbidities
Children with ADHD often have additional problems, such as mild cognitive impairment, delayed language development, poor coordination, reading difficulties and mood disorders.

Assessment
- Developmental history, especially any delay and when noted.
- Pregnancy and birth, including any exposure to drugs or alcohol.
- Family history of similar problems, maternal depression and social circumstances.
- Educational progress: both intelligent children and children with specific learning difficulties who are bored can be disruptive.
- The parents' expectations of the child and their response to his or her behaviour.
- Medical history and examination for neurological problems, including any medication being taken by the child that might affect his or her behaviour.

- Careful observation of the child in several settings, including home and school.

Management
There is no cure for ADHD, but careful management can help these children and their families a great deal.
- Look for any health problems that might be contributing to the condition and could be treated (e.g. large tonsils and adenoids preventing undisturbed sleep).
- Explain to the child and their family that they have a disorder that affects their behaviour, and that they are not just a naughty child.
- The most useful management is behavioural.
- Drugs may be helpful in severe cases.

Behavioural management
Children with ADHD do best where there are as few distractions as possible around them, and where there are clear rules about the conduct that is expected, with praise or reproof given immediately if merited. When doing tasks such as schoolwork, they are best on their own or in a small group, sitting near to the person in charge. They often have low self-esteem. Giving praise when they do well, with frequent small rewards, is very helpful.

Drugs
The most widely used drugs for ADHD are stimulants such as methylphenidate (Ritalin), which can be given to children aged over 6 years in a dose of 5 mg once or twice daily, increasing by 2.5–5 mg weekly up to a maximum daily dose of 60 mg. If methylphenidate has not made any difference after 3 weeks at full dose it should be stopped. Slow-release preparations are also available and can be given less frequently. If effect wears off in the evening (with rebound hyperactivity) a dose at bedtime may be appropriate (establish need with trial bedtime dose). Careful supervision is needed, and ideally children who require these drugs should be treated by a professional experienced in their use.

Some useful websites
Patel V, Jenkins R, Lund C, the PLoS Medicine Editors (2012) *Putting Evidence into Practice: The PLoS Medicine Series on Global Mental Health Practice. PLoS Medicine*, **9**, e1001226. www.plosmedicine.org/article/citationList.action;jsessionid=54EC3D8B00FC6B7057A6FD681B26F071?articleURI=info%3Adoi%2F10.1371%2Fjournal.pmed.1001226

National Institute for Health and Clinical Excellence (2005) *Depression in Children and Young People.* www.nice.org.uk/guidance/QS48

Royal College of Psychiatrists *Fact Sheets for Children and Young People.* www.rcpsych.ac.uk/healthadvice/parentsandyouthinfo.aspx

World Health Organization. *Child Mental Health Atlas.* www.who.int/mental_health/resources/Child_ado_atlas.pdf

National Institute for Health and Clinical Excellence (2006) *Methylphenidate, Atomoxetine and Dexamfetamine for Attention Deficit Hyperactivity Disorder (ADHD) in Children and Adolescents.* www.nice.org.uk/guidance/TA98

Eapen V, Graham P and Srinath S (2012) *Where There Is No Child Psychiatrist: a mental healthcare manual.* www.rcpsych.ac.uk/publications/books/rcpp/9781908020482.aspx

5.10 Nutritional disorders

5.10.A Vitamin or mineral deficiencies

BOX 5.10.A.1 Minimum standards
- Adequate diet.
- Vitamins A, B, C, D and K.
- Folic acid.
- Zinc.
- Iodine.

Vitamin A deficiency (VAD)

Significance
- Vitamin A deficiency is the single most important cause of childhood blindness in resource-limited countries.
- It makes a significant contribution to morbidity and mortality from common childhood infections, even at subclinical levels of deficiency.
- A Cochrane review indicates that regular vitamin A supplementation reduces mortality by 24%.

Prevalence
- Vitamin A deficiency is endemic in at least 60 countries worldwide, especially in Africa, South and South-East Asia, some areas of South America and the Western Pacific.
- Around 250 million preschool children are at risk.
- It causes 250 000–500 000 cases of blindness per year.

Good food sources are red palm oil, mango, pawpaw, dark green leafy vegetables, unskimmed milk, eggs and liver.

Aetiological factors
- Persistent inadequate intake of vitamin A exacerbated by insufficient consumption of dietary fat, leading to ineffective absorption.
- Frequent infections, especially measles, gastroenteritis and respiratory infections, resulting in decreased food intake, malabsorption, increased urinary loss, and increased utilisation of vitamin A by the body resulting in depletion of liver stores. The decrease in vitamin A levels in the body in turn predisposes children to infection, and so a vicious cycle is set up.
- Vitamin A deficiency is common in the context of poverty, social under-development, hostile living environments, water shortage and food scarcity, and individual factors such as lack of breastfeeding, inappropriate weaning practices and increased physiological needs during periods of rapid growth.

Clinical effects
- Night blindness (decreased ability to generate rhodopsin in the retinal rod photoreceptors essential for vision in dim light).
- Compromised integrity of epithelial surfaces due to loss of mucus-producing goblet cells, leading to 'dry eye' (conjunctival xerosis), Bitot's spots, corneal xerosis, corneal ulceration, and irreversible damage to the eye (keratomalacia).
- Depressed immunity (both innate and adaptive immunity), which results in increased susceptibility, duration and severity of common infections (e.g. acute respiratory infection, diarrhoea, measles).
- Poor growth, apathy and slow development.

TABLE 5.10.A.1 Signs of vitamin A deficiency in the eyes

Sign	Description
Night blindness	Inability to see in dim light (e.g. at dawn or dusk). Often occurs in the later part of pregnancy
Conjunctival xerosis	The conjunctiva looks dry and slightly rough instead of smooth and shiny
Bitot's spots	White foamy patches on the conjunctiva. Not always present
Active corneal lesions:	
At this stage the condition can worsen within a few hours and complete or partial blindness can result	
Corneal xerosis	The cornea looks dry and cloudy
Ulcers on the cornea	Often on the edge of the cornea
Keratomalacia	The cornea is cloudy and soft like jelly. Rare

Assessment of vitamin A status
There are no simple tests for vitamin A deficiency, but it is likely to affect communities where vitamin-A-rich food is scarce and infection and/or malnutrition rates are high.
- Vitamin A deficiency becomes a public health problem when the following are prevalent in the child population:
  - night blindness (> 1%)
  - Bitot's spots (> 0.5%)
  - corneal xerosis with or without ulceration (> 0.01%)
  - corneal scarring (> 0.05%).

Prevention
- Encourage the use of local foods rich in vitamin A.
  - Provide dietary education about vitamin-A-rich foods (e.g. dark green leafy vegetables, carrots, mango, papaya, eggs, orange fruits, liver, red palm oil, fatty fish).
  - Treat the siblings and mother. Mothers are especially vulnerable to vitamin A deficiency, and should be supplemented in the first month of lactation.

- Give regular supplementation every 4 to 6 months as described in Table 5.10.A.2.
- Prevent recurrent infections by recommending the use of impregnated nets, deworming, using clean water and breastfeeding.

TABLE 5.10.A.2 Vitamin A supplements to prevent vitamin A deficiency

Target group	Immunisation contact	Vitamin A dose
Infants under 6 months who are not breast fed or breast fed infants whose mothers have not received vitamin A supplements.		50 000 IU
Infants aged 6–11 months	Measles vaccine contact	100 000 IU
Children aged 12–59 months	Booster doses Special campaigns Delayed primary immunisation doses	200 000 IU every 4 to 6 months

Regular vitamin A supplementation is advised for all children in resource-limited countries. It has been shown to reduce all causes of mortality, and especially mortality from diarrhoea.

If a child has malnutrition, severe diarrhoea or measles, give one high-dose vitamin A capsule, according to Table 5.10.A.3, unless they have received a dose in the previous month.

Treatment

If there are any eye signs, give vitamin A as indicated in Table 5.10.A.3.

TABLE 5.10.A.3 Doses of vitamin A for treatment of clinical deficiency

Age	Day 1	Day 2	Two weeks later
< 6 months	50 000 IU	50 000 IU	50 000 IU
6–12 months	100 000 IU	100 000 IU	100 000 IU
> 12 months	200 000 IU	200 000 IU	200 000 IU

If there are ulcers or the eyes look soft or cloudy, instil atropine 0.1%, three times a day for 3–5 days, and a topical antibiotic. Cover the affected eye with a saline-soaked bandage.

Deep IM injection of vitamin A (retinyl palmitate) 50 000 IU for children under 2 years of age, and 100 000 IU for those over 2 years, should be given if severe stomatitis, persistent vomiting or malabsorption are present.

Vitamin B$_1$ deficiency: beriberi

- This may occur in areas of severe nutritional deprivation where little more than polished rice is consumed. It is uncommon in Africa, as the staple is maize or wheat, which contains vitamin B$_1$.
- It affects adults, children and breastfed infants of thiamine-deficient mothers.
- It is often mistaken for oedematous malnutrition (kwashiorkor), nephritis, cerebral malaria, encephalopathy or septicaemia.
- It causes wet (cardiac) or dry (neurological) beriberi:
  - cardiac failure with breathlessness, oedema and tachycardia
  - peripheral neuritis, with tingling and burning of feet, and reduced tendon reflexes
  - acute encephalopathy and coma.
- An aphonic form is characterised by a noiseless cry due to laryngeal nerve paralysis.

Beriberi is rapidly fatal.
- The initial dose is 50–100 mg thiamine hydrochloride. IM or orally. This is particularly effective in heart failure (facilities for treating anaphylaxis must be available).
- Continue with 10 mg/day for children under 2 years of age, 25 mg/day for those aged 2–12 years, and 50 mg/day for those over 12 years for 3–4 days.
- Patients with beriberi often have other B vitamin deficiencies.
- Good food sources of vitamin B$_1$ are pork, whole grain cereals, legumes, nuts and liver.

Nicotinic acid (niacin) deficiency: pellagra

Nicotinic acid is synthesised from the essential amino acid tryptophan, and pellagra is found where the diet is deficient in either nicotinic acid or tryptophan. It is common where maize is the staple diet, as in many parts of Africa. Maize is deficient in tryptophan, and the nicotinic acid is bound and unavailable.

Clinical features
- Dermatosis of parts of the skin exposed to sunlight, namely the neck (Casal's necklace), face and hands, usually seen in children over 5 years.
- Diarrhoea and malabsorption.
- Encephalopathy, which is rare in children.

Treatment
- Nicotinic acid:
  - 10 mg three times daily for 7 days in children under 2 years of age
  - 25 mg three times daily for 7 days in children over 2 years. In severe cases give 100 mg IV.
- Treat other B vitamin deficiencies at the same time (thiamin and riboflavin).
- Improve the diet with protein and green vegetables, peanuts, wholegrain cereals, meat, fish, chicken and liver.

Vitamin C deficiency: scurvy

This usually presents at the age of 4–10 months. Cow's milk is low in vitamin C.
- Vitamin C is needed for collagen formation (in bones, cartilage, teeth and capillary walls).
- It is important for the healing of wounds.
- It increases iron absorption.
- It is found in citrus fruits, vegetables and breast milk.

Very little vitamin C is present in cow's milk, especially if it is heated.

- Vitamin C deficiency is found in severe malnutrition and in children fed on very poor diets in institutions.

Clinical features

- Spontaneous haemorrhages, especially from gums, and defective bone, cartilage and dentine formation.
- Local tenderness and swelling of the legs (due to subperiosteal haemorrhages), which may present as irritability when the child is picked up or moved.
- Pseudo-paralysis of the limbs.
- Haemorrhagic and spongy changes in the gums.
- Petechiae and ecchymoses around the eyes.
- Microscopic haematuria may be present.
- The anterior ends of the ribs swell.
- Mild anaemia.
- Increased risk of fractures.
- Poor healing of fractures and wounds.
- Characteristic X-ray appearance: loss of trabeculae in long bones gives a ground-glass appearance, dense lines of calcification in the epiphysis next to the epiphyseal plate and calcification of subperiosteal haemorrhages.

Treatment

- **By mouth**
  - Child 1 month–4 years 125–250 mg daily in 1–2 divided doses
  - Child 4–12 years 250–500 mg daily in 1–2 divided doses
  - Child 12–18 years 500 mg–1 g daily in 1–2 divided doses.
- A subsequent improvement in diet is needed, with plenty of fresh fruit and vegetables.

Vitamin D₃ deficiency: rickets

Vitamin D deficiency causes the following:
- rickets (failure of mineralisation of growing bone)
- hypocalcaemic tetany in infancy
- osteomalacia in adults.

Nutritional rickets is most prevalent in North Africa, the Middle East and Pakistan. Asian and Afro-Caribbean children are also at risk in the UK and other countries where there is limited sunshine. Vitamin D deficiency is unusual in African children over 18 months, as at this age they can walk and therefore go out into the sunshine. Older children in Africa with rickets must be investigated for causes of rickets other than vitamin D deficiency, such as dietary calcium deficiency or inherited forms of hypophosphataemic rickets.

Biochemistry

- Vitamin D increases Ca^{2+} absorption from the gut, reabsorption of Ca^{2+} from the kidney, and a phosphate diuresis.
- Vitamin D deficiency reduces Ca^{2+} and increases parathyroid hormone (which increases phosphate loss by the kidney), resulting in low Ca^{2+} and low phosphate levels. Subsequently there is a rise in alkaline phosphatase and then the X-ray features of rickets occur.

Aetiology

- Prolonged breastfeeding, especially if the mother is vitamin D deficient.
- Lack of vitamin-D-containing foods such as oily fish, eggs, butter and margarine.
- Lack of sunlight exposure (UV light) (black- and brown-skinned children living indoors or in countries where there is little sunlight are particularly at risk).
- An infant's diet contains only small amounts of vitamin D, so fortification of foods and vitamin D supplementation is recommended.
- If a child presents with rickets and has normal exposure to sunlight, consider a hypocalcaemic diet (reported in South Africa and Nigeria). Cereals can bind calcium and prevent its absorption.
- Rarely, there is a metabolic disorder such as familial hypophosphataemic rickets. Where consanguinity is common, renal tubular disorders can produce this.
- Vitamin D deficiency also occurs in chronic renal and liver failure.

Clinical features

- 1,25-Dihydroxyvitamin D crosses the placenta, and the neonate generally has sufficient levels for the first few months of life.
- Disturbance of the normal growth of the epiphyseal plate leads to the formation of inadequately calcified new bone at the diaphysis edge of the plate (so-called osteoid tissue). The proliferating zone on the epiphyseal side of the plate enlarges excessively, producing a swelling of the plate. Osteoid tissue may also form subperiosteally. There is also demineralisation of the skeleton. The following features result from these abnormalities:
  - epiphyseal swelling (especially distal radii at the wrists, and also the ankles and knees)
  - craniotabes (soft areas of the skull bones, especially of the occiput, which when pressed gently are easily depressed)
  - rickety rosary (enlarged costochondral junctions)
  - delayed fontanelle closure
  - curvature of the shafts of the tibia and femur (may occur in severe cases)
  - bossing of the frontal and parietal skull bones due to osteoid formation
  - pigeon chest (pectus carinatum)
  - Harrison's sulci
  - deformities of the thoracic and lumbar spine can produce kyphoscoliosis and lumbar lordosis
  - pelvic bone deformities in female children can lead to subsequent birthing difficulties due to damage to the inlet and outlet of the birth canal
  - delayed dentition
  - delayed gross motor development with generalised muscle weakness and hypotonia
  - growth retardation
  - occasionally, especially in infants, symptoms of hypocalcaemia.

Diagnosis

- Very elevated plasma alkaline phosphatase activity.
- Usually normal, but possibly slightly low, plasma calcium levels.
- Very low plasma phosphate levels.

- Lowered plasma levels of 25-hydroxyvitamin D_3, but often this cannot be tested for.
- The best sites to radiologically assess for rickets are those where there is rapid bone growth, namely the wrists and knees.
  - Typical X-ray appearance: cupping and fraying of the distal ends of the long bones, such as the ulna and radius.
  - There is widening of the metaphyseal plate due to osteoid formation.
  - The periosteum may be raised.
  - There may be abnormal curvature of bones and generalised under-calcification.

Prevention measures
- Exposure to sunlight and foods such as egg yolk, milk and fortified margarine.
- Vitamin D_2 (ergocalciferol) supplementation, 400–600 IU daily.

Treatment
- Vitamin D_3 (colecalciferol) or vitamin D_2 (ergocalciferol) by mouth daily for 4 weeks: child aged 1–6 months 3000 IU, 6 months–12 years 6000 IU and 12–18 years 10 000 IU.
- If hypocalcaemia is present, calcium supplements may be added in the early stages of treatment.

Vitamin K deficiency
- Vitamin K is a cofactor for the hepatic synthesis of clotting factors (prothrombin, and factors VII, IX and X).
- Sources are green leafy vegetables, meat, liver, cheese, and synthesis by gut flora.
- Deficiency may occur as a result of the lack of bile salts and the malabsorption of fats after the use of broad-spectrum antibiotics, or in the breastfed newborn whose gut is not yet colonised with bacteria and therefore does not produce vitamin K.
- Treat bleeding due to vitamin K deficiency with 250–300 microgram/kg (max 10 mg) IV; neonates 1 mg. Repeat doses every 8 hours if needed.
- Prevent haemorrhagic disease of the newborn by giving 1 mg vitamin K to all newborn infants either orally or IM (preterm 400 microgram/kg maximum dose 1 mg).

Folic acid deficiency
- The most important issue here is that women who are deficient in folic acid at the time of conception and in early pregnancy are at increased risk of having a baby with a neural tube defect (spina bifida or anencephaly).
- Relative deficiency occurs in haemolytic anaemias and in preterm infants (see Section 3.3 and Section 5.11.C).
- Deficiency occurs in malabsorption syndromes such as coeliac disease and blind loop syndromes.
- Anticonvulsants such as phenytoin may interfere with the metabolism of folic acid.
- Consequences of folic acid deficiency include the following:
  - fetal abnormalities
  - megaloblastic anaemia, neutropenia and thrombocytopenia.
- Sources of folic acid include green leafy vegetables, oranges and other fruit, legumes, nuts, liver and yeast.

Treatment
- All women who are anticipating pregnancy should be taking an additional 400 micrograms of folic acid per day before and throughout pregnancy.
- To treat deficiency, give infants 500 micrograms/kg once daily and children over 1 year of age 5 mg once daily.
- Treat for up to 4 months and exclude concomitant vitamin B_{12} deficiency, which if untreated could result in neuropathy.
- For haemolytic anaemia, treat with 2.5–5 mg orally once a day for children aged 1 month to 12 years, and 10 mg once a day for those over 12 years of age.
- Neonates 50 micrograms once daily or 500 micrograms once weekly.
- Give preterm infants 100–200 micrograms orally per day.

Iodine deficiency
Iodine deficiency in pregnancy causes maternal hypothyroidism and cretinism in the newborn.

- It is one of the commonest causes of disability worldwide.
- Clinical features of cretinism range from mild neuro-muscular incoordination and cognitive deficit to severe mental retardation, spasticity and deafness, and severe stunting of growth.
- Iodine deficiency is endemic in mountainous regions far from the sea (e.g. the Andes, the Himalayas, Central Africa, Papua New Guinea) and areas where iodine is eluted from the soil by repeated flooding (e.g. Bangladesh).
- The prognosis is poor even after early recognition and treatment with thyroid hormone.
- Prevention is by salt iodination or a single oral dose of iodine in pregnancy.

Zinc deficiency
- Zinc is an essential trace element required for maintaining cells, bone growth and immune function (it scavenges for free radicals).
- Deficiency often occurs in children living in resource-limited settings, and arises from either insufficient intake of zinc-containing foods or insufficient absorption.
- Foods high in zinc are of animal origin, such as meats, fish and dairy products.
- Dietary fibre and phytates found in cereals and legumes bind zinc and reduce its absorption.
- Zinc deficiency is difficult to diagnose, as serum zinc levels do not reflect total body zinc levels.
- Zinc deficiency is associated with stunting of growth, impaired immunity and increased risk and severity of diarrhoea and respiratory infections.
- Zinc deficiency is a feature of the rare disease acrodermatitis enteropathica, in which children present with peri-oral and peri-anal rashes.

Therapeutic zinc supplementation is now recommended as an adjunct to oral rehydration therapy for treatment of diarrhoea. Routinely giving 10 mg per day to children under 6 months of age and 20 mg per day to those over 6 months of age for 10–14 days can reduce diarrhoea duration and severity and the likelihood of subsequent infections for 2 to 3 months.

Zinc supplements of 2 mg/kg/day should be an essential component of the mineral mix used in the management of severe malnutrition.

Useful website

World Health Organization (1997) *Vitamin A Supplements: a guide to their use in the treatment and prevention of vitamin A deficiency and xerophthalmia*, 2nd edn. http://whqlibdoc.who.int/publications/1997/9241545062.pdf

5.10.B Severe malnutrition

BOX 5.10.B.1 Minimum standards
■ Scales (accurate to 5 gram), metre length board, MUAC tapes, care charts.
■ ReSoMal.
■ Vitamin and mineral mixtures.
■ Antibiotics.
■ IV 10% glucose.
■ Antihelmintic drugs.
■ F-75 and F-100 feeds.
■ Barrier skin cream.
■ Sources of heat (blankets, hat, warm room, clothes).

Introduction

Severe acute malnutrition (SAM) is characterised by oedema or wasting, often with anorexia and infection. The main immediate causes of death are infections, septic shock, hypoglycaemia, electrolyte imbalance, dehydration, hypothermia, cardiac failure and severe anaemia. Every physiological and metabolic function is impaired, so the children affected are extremely fragile, similar to the premature neonate.

In 2009 the WHO and UNICEF defined SAM for children aged 6–60 months as follows:

1 using new weight for length/height charts (see procedures) a cut-off of below minus 3 standard deviations
2 **and** the mid upper arm circumference (MUAC) less than 115 mm.

Two clinical pictures are seen, with much overlap between them.

● Marasmus (wasting) affects all ages, but young infants are particularly at risk. It is usually due to insufficient intake of growth nutrients after breastfeeding stops. It can also be due to chronic illness. The baby is extremely thin, with loss of subcutaneous fat, resulting in skin wrinkles and folds. Weight for length or height is less than 70% of the median (*see* Section 9), or the MUAC is less than 115 mm.
● Kwashiorkor (oedematous malnutrition) usually occurs in children aged 2–4 years. It is an acute illness that suddenly appears over a few days. It is thought to be due to a deficit in the antioxidant nutrients. It presents with sodium retention and oedema of various degrees (from pedal to generalised), and skin lesions that are like severe sunburn in a fair-skinned person. There is fatty liver, with low circulating levels of all hepatic export proteins. The hair may be de-pigmented (this has no relation to the prognosis, and should be ignored clinically), and the hair pulls out very easily and painlessly (which **is** related to the prognosis).

In severe malnutrition, biochemical abnormalities include the following:

● low urea
● severe hypoproteinaemia
● hypokalaemia and hypophosphataemia
● hypomagnesaemia
● hypoglycaemia (see below)
● anaemia (frequently present).

Principles of treatment

Early identification and treatment is important, and children are often missed on the general admission wards or in outpatients because they are not measured. Screening using MUAC is helpful for identifying children if length measurement is not easily performed, or weight for height is not charted.

Treatment is much more successful if standard treatment protocols are followed than if clinical judgements are made on individual patients. This is because the illness itself changes the clinical presentation, signs and symptoms of common complications.

Inpatient versus outpatient community management of acute malnutrition (CMAM)

Traditionally, care has been provided for all children in inpatient hospital units, ideally in a defined malnutrition ward. However, carers are less likely to be prepared to attend these until the child is unwell, so patients tend to present late. They also want the child to be discharged as soon as they are clinically stable, so often leave before nutritional deficits have been restored and the child has recovered. This predisposes to higher post-discharge mortality, which is rarely identified by the inpatient programme.

There has been a change to management of the malnourished child who is not unwell, through CMAM programmes. This is sometimes referred to as community-based therapeutic care (CTC). These programmes separate children into those with complications or severe oedema (complicated malnutrition), and those with uncomplicated malnutrition, Children with uncomplicated malnutrition have a reasonable appetite, and on formal testing are able to eat a portion of ready-to-use therapeutic food (RUTF). Children with fever, poor appetite, diarrhoea or dehydration, or who are not fully alert or have generalised oedema are identified and referred to inpatient care (a stabilisation centre), where initial management is delivered.

If a CMAM programme is operating in your area, children with complicated malnutrition will be sent to the hospital, and you may be able to direct those with uncomplicated malnutrition to the CMAM programme after hospital admission for an illness, or if they present with complicated malnutrition, once they are stabilised and on phase II feeds (see later).

This subsection will deal with the care of children managed in an inpatient hospital unit.

Inpatient management

The inpatient treatment of severe malnutrition is divided into two phases, which are separated by a transition phase.

Phase I (initial treatment)

Specific objectives: return of normal homeostasis and treatment of complications.

- The immediate treatment of life-threatening complications: hypoglycaemia, hypothermia, heart failure, septic shock, infections and infestations, severe dehydration and very severe anaemia.
- The prevention of hypoglycaemia and hypothermia.
- Nutritional treatment based on a maintenance diet (total 100 kcal/kg/day), divided into frequent meals (eight meals per 24 hours).

Transition phase: the diet is gradually increased over 4–5 days.

Phase II (rehabilitation or catch-up growth)

Specific objectives: promotion of rapid weight gain (10–20 g/kg/day) and preparation for discharge.

- A nutritional treatment based on a high energy intake (160–200 kcal/kg/day) divided into six meals a day.
- Emotional and physical stimulation.

The treatment in phase II can be given as ready-to-use therapeutic food (RUTF) in the community, or through an Outpatient Therapeutic Programme (OTP), either administered through a hospital clinic, or preferably in community-based clinics. If RUTF or an equivalent (such as a high-energy biscuit) is not available, children continue on F-100 until nutritional cure is achieved. This is usually defined as achieving 85% of median weight for height.

Ongoing nutritional support

After discharge from this therapeutic programme, it is good practice to link the child to a supplementary feeding programme, which gives a food ration to the family for up to 4 months following discharge. This is a means of ensuring food security for the vulnerable child. Programmes with this safety-net provision often discharge children at 80% of median weight for height.

Admission criteria

- Weight for height less than 70% of the median.
- Oedema (exclude nephritic syndrome and other clinical conditions).
- MUAC of less than 110 mm if the child is over 65 cm in length.

Assessment of nutritional status and recovery

For practical procedures relating to nutrition measurement, see Section 9.

Discharge criteria

These depend upon the quality of the follow-up services. If adequate follow-up services and a Supplementary Food Programme (SFP) are available, the discharge criteria are as follows:

- weight for height of more than 80% of the median for 3 days (85% if there is no SFP)
- **and** no oedema for 10 days
- **and** no medical complications.

Medical and nutritional history and examination

The pro-forma history and examination sheet (see Appendix, Section 9) should be filled in by the admitting physician or an experienced nurse.

Key points in the history

- Recent intake of foods and fluids.
- Usual diet before current illness.
- Whether breastfeeding or not.
- Duration and frequency of diarrhoea and vomiting.
- Type of diarrhoea (watery/bloody).
- Appetite.
- Family circumstances.
- Previous attempts at treatment, local drugs and/or traditional medicines given.
- History of chronic cough or contact with TB.
- History of contact with measles.
- Potential HIV infection (including mother's status and whether parents are alive).

Key points on examination

- Oedema.
- Dehydration (this is very difficult to diagnose, and impossible in the oedematous child).
- Shock (often gives the appearance of dehydration in a child with oedema).
- Severe palmar pallor.
- Eye signs for vitamin A deficiency (dry eyes, Bitot's spots, corneal ulceration, keratomalacia) (see Section 5.10.A).
- Signs of local infection (ear, throat, skin, pneumonia).
- Signs of HIV (adenopathy, oral candida, chronic ear discharge) (see Section 6.2.D).
- Fever.
- Hypothermia (oral temperature < 35.5°C, axillary temperature < 35°C).
- Mouth ulcers, *Candida* or other oral problems.
- Skin changes of kwashiorkor (hypo- or hyperpigmentation, desquamation, ulceration, exudative lesions resembling burns, often with secondary infections such as *Candida*).

Children with vitamin A deficiency are likely to be photophobic and will keep their eyes tightly closed. Examine their eyes carefully to prevent corneal rupture.

Laboratory tests

Laboratory tests are not needed to guide or monitor treatment. Electrolytes and haemoglobin are difficult to interpret and can easily be misleading. If haemoglobin is measured this should be done on admission only, and a transfusion should be given at this time if essential. The patient should not be given a blood transfusion after the first 48 hours following admission. The haemoglobin level nearly always falls after admission due to haemodilution with expansion of the circulation during mobilisation of oedema and export of sodium from inside the cells in marasmus. At this time, with expansion of the circulation, there is such a grave danger of precipitating heart failure that a transfusion should rarely be given, even for very severe anaemia.

In endemic areas, a malaria smear or rapid test is useful if malaria treatment is not given as part of the routine management of all severely malnourished children.

In regions where HIV is prevalent, HIV testing (serology using two tests in children over 1 year of age, or serology and PCR for children under 1 year) is informative for ongoing care, initiating co-trimoxazole prophylaxis, and determining eligibility for antiretroviral (ARV) therapy. The mother of a seropositive child is invariably HIV infected, and mothers of seropositive children should be offered an HIV test. Services vary, but would normally include counselling prior to voluntary HIV testing. Where testing is routinely offered, uptake is usually high. CD4 counts are not usually required for the initial management of severe acute malnutrition, as this follows the standard protocols, but may be relevant when considering initiating ARV therapy (see Section 6.2.D).

Details of treatment

In Phase I (initial phase) the aim is to restore nutritional imbalances and metabolic function and treat complications. Phase II (catch-up growth) is a period of rapid weight gain. There is a 'transition phase' between these phases.

TABLE 5.10.B.1 Phases of malnutrition treatment

Phases of treatment		
Phase 1 (1–7 days)	**Transition phase (3–4 days)**	**Phase 2 (usually 14–21 days)**
Treat dehydration		Correct nutrient deficiencies
Treat hypoglycaemia		
Treat hypothermia		
Treat infection	Treat helminths	
Do not give iron	Do not give iron	Correct iron deficiency
Correct electrolyte problems		
Diet is maintenance intake	Diet is moderate intake	Diet is high intake
Stimulate the child	Stimulate the child	Stimulate the child
		Provide physical activities
		Prepare for discharge

- There are **routine measures** that are systematically implemented for all malnourished children, and additional routine treatments that are often included.
- **Specific treatments:** these include emergency management of life-threatening complications and of specific diseases.
- **General points:** on admission, severely malnourished children should be separated from those with infections and kept in a warm room (25–30°C) without draughts. Washing should be minimal and when possible with warm water, and the child immediately dried. The mother should be encouraged to stay with her child.

Intravenous infusion and blood transfusion

Intravenous infusions are to be avoided whenever possible in all severely malnourished children. The risk of precipitating heart failure is very high because of their atrophic heart muscle and high intracellular sodium and electrolyte imbalance.

- The only indication for IV infusion in severely malnourished children is unconsciousness due to circulatory collapse or shock. This is a condition which is difficult to diagnose.
- The only indication for blood transfusion is when anaemia is present on admission and is life-threatening.
- Cannulas should not have IV fluids running after the prescribed treatment has been given. If flushed for IV treatment, they should be removed when not required.

Nasogastric tube feeding is recommended in cases of:

- anorexia with an intake of less than 70 kcal/kg (70% of phase I feed prescribed)
- severe dehydration with inability to drink
- inability to drink and eat because of weakness or clouded consciousness
- painful or severe mouth lesions (herpes, cancrum oris)
- repeated, very frequent vomiting.

Try to not tube-feed for more than 3–4 days. Always explain the reason to the mother.

Try to breastfeed or feed by mouth every time, and top up by nasogastric tube.

Dehydration with severe malnutrition

Dehydration from diarrhoea is common in severely wasted children (with marasmus) on admission. The treatment of dehydration is not the same as in the non-malnourished child (with the exception of cholera).

This section does not apply to mild diarrhoea occurring during transition from one phase to another, which is a common event.

Signs of dehydration in malnutrition

The normal signs used to assess dehydration are all unreliable in severe malnutrition.

Assume that all children with acute watery diarrhoea have some dehydration.

The interpretation of the signs relies on the history. The specific signs are as follows:

- history and observation of frequent **watery** diarrhoea
- history of recent sinking of the eyes; the eyes appear 'staring'
- history of not passing urine for 12 hours
- history and observation of thirst.

Reduced skin turgor and sunken eyes (that are long-standing symptoms) are features of malnutrition itself. It is not possible to adequately determine the degree of dehydration in the severely malnourished child.

The appearance of dehydration in children without watery diarrhoea or in those with oedema can be caused by a toxic shock with dilatation of the blood vessels. These patients should not be treated as if they have dehydration, but as cases of septic shock (see later).

Note that low blood volume can occur with oedema.

Oral treatment of dehydration in malnutrition

Standard WHO oral rehydration solutions (ORS) have too high a sodium content and too low a potassium content for children with severe malnutrition.

ReSoMal (rehydration solution for malnutrition; see below) is a special solution for this situation.

TABLE 5.10.B.2 Composition comparison of ReSoMal, standard WHO ORS and reduced-osmolarity WHO ORS

Composition	ReSoMal (mmol/litre)	Standard ORS (mmol/litre)	Reduced-osmolarity ORS (mmol/litre)
Glucose	125	111	75
Sodium	45	90	75
Potassium	40	20	20
Chloride	70	80	65
Citrate	7	10	10
Magnesium	3	–	–
Zinc	0.3	–	–
Copper	0.045	–	–
Osmolarity (mOsm/litre)	300	311	245

Children with watery diarrhoea in an adequate clinical state

At admission, give one dose of ReSoMal orally or by nasogastric tube and start to feed the child with the phase I diet. Feed smaller amounts more frequently if they are vomiting. Further ReSoMal can be given after each stool or vomit.

- Give a 50-mL dose for children less than 2 years or less than 85 cm in length.
- Give 100 mL for children over 2 years or over 85 cm in length.

Children with watery diarrhoea in a poor clinical state

Start rehydration with ReSoMal immediately. Give 10 mL/kg/hour for the first 2 hours, and then 5 mL/kg/hour until rehydration is complete.

This rate is slower than for normally nourished and dehydrated children.

Completed rehydration

The rehydration is completed when the child is alert, no longer thirsty, and has passed urine. There should be less sunken eyes and fontanelle and improved skin turgor. **(Note that loss of sunken eyes in a severely wasted patient or the worsening of oedema can be a sign of over-hydration.)**

The diet should now be given.

Monitoring

ReSoMal at 70 mL/kg weight per day is usually enough to restore hydration. However, be careful, as **rehydration can quickly lead to fluid overloading, causing cardiac failure or sudden death**. Malnourished children do not excrete excess sodium well. The clinical state of the child should be reassessed every 30 minutes during the first 2 hours, and then every hour. The best way to monitor the child is by regularly measuring their weight; this gives 'fluid balance' directly and accurately, without having to measure any stool or vomit. The ReSoMal should be stopped immediately if:

- the body weight increases by 10% or more
- the respiratory rate or pulse rate increase
- the jugular vein becomes engorged
- oedema appears or the eyelids become puffy
- the liver enlarges by more than 2 cm (mark its position on the skin with marker pen at the onset of rehydration).

Note: It is common for malnourished children to pass many small unformed stools. This must not be confused with profuse watery stools, and does not require fluid replacement.

Feeding and rehydration

- Breastfeeding should continue during rehydration.
- Phase I diet should start immediately when the child is alert.
- If the child has had severe dehydration, feeding should start as soon as the child is alert and the severe dehydration has been treated (2–3 hours).

Rehydration solutions

If no commercial ReSoMal is available, a solution can be made. (Note that this is double the quantity of water normally used, i.e. 2 litres, so the solution is effectively half strength.)

To 2 litres of boiled filtered water add:

- 1 sachet of ORS (3.5 grams sodium chloride, 2.9 grams trisodium citrate dihydrate, 1.5 grams potassium chloride, 20 grams glucose)
- 50 grams of sugar
- 40 mL of combined mineral mix* (or commercial CMV if available).

* See below for the recipe for the electrolyte/mineral solution. If this cannot be made up, use 45 mL of potassium chloride solution (100 grams of KCl in 1 litre of water) instead.

Formula for concentrated electrolyte/mineral solution

This is used in the preparation of starter and catch-up feeding formulas and ReSoMal. Sachets containing pre-mixed electrolytes and minerals are produced by some manufacturers. If these are not available or affordable, prepare the solution (2500 mL) using the ingredients shown in Table 5.10.B.3.

TABLE 5.10.B.3 Electrolyte and mineral mixture

Constituent	Grams	Concentration/20 mL
Potassium chloride (KCl)	224	24 mmol
Tripotassium citrate	81	2 mmol
Magnesium chloride	76	3 mmol
Zinc acetate	8.2	300 micromol
Copper sulphate	1.4	45 micromol

Water: make up to 2500 mL.

If available, also add selenium (0.028 grams of sodium selenate) and iodine (0.012 grams of potassium iodide) per 2500 mL.

- Dissolve the ingredients in cooled boiled water.
- Store the solution in sterilised bottles in the fridge to slow down deterioration. Discard if it turns cloudy.
- Make fresh solution each month.
- Add 20 mL of the concentrated electrolyte/mineral solution to each 1000 mL of milk feed.

If it is not possible to prepare this electrolyte/mineral solution, and pre-mixed sachets are not available, give potassium, magnesium and zinc separately. Make a 10% stock solution of potassium chloride (100 grams in 1 litre of water) and a 1.5% solution of zinc acetate (15 grams in 1 litre of water).

Emergency IV treatment of severe dehydration with shock in severe malnutrition

IV infusion should be administered only in the case of circulatory collapse severe enough to reduce consciousness. **Alert children should never be given an infusion.**

The main signs are as follows:
- cold hands and feet with increased capillary refill time > 3 seconds
- weak or absent radial pulse
- diminished consciousness.

Severe dehydration and septic shock are difficult to differentiate in children with severe malnutrition. They both present with signs of hypovolaemic shock. The following points help to differentiate them:

- Eyelid retraction associated with a history of diarrhoea is a sign of severe dehydration. The child with septic shock has eyelids that droop.
- If the child is unconscious (or asleep) without having the eyelids together (a sign of excess adrenaline), either dehydration or hypoglycaemia is present.
- Superficial veins are always constricted in severe dehydration, but may be dilated in septic shock.

Treatment protocol for life-threatening dehydration with shock in severe malnutrition

Immediate treatment should be given as follows:
1. Give 15 mL/kg IV over 1 hour. The recommended solution is Ringer-lactate or Hartmann's solution, each with 5% glucose.
2. At the same time, insert a nasogastric tube and give ReSoMal at 10 mL/kg per hour.

3. Monitor carefully for signs of over-hydration, reassessing respiratory rate and heart rate every 15 minutes.
   - **If after 1 hour the child is improving but still severely dehydrated**, continue nasogastric ReSoMal 10 mL/kg/hour for up to 5 hours.
   - If after 1 hour the child has not improved (i.e. radial pulse is still weak), assume that they have septic shock and treat it accordingly (see below for treatment of septic shock). Since hypoalbuminaemia is likely also to be present, 4.5% albumin 5–15 mL/kg IV over 1 hour may also be helpful in intractable shock but this approach requires urgent research.

Electrolyte problems in SAM

All severely malnourished children have deficiencies of potassium and magnesium that may take 2 weeks or more to correct. Oedema is partly a result of these deficiencies. **Do not treat oedema with a diuretic.** Excess body sodium exists even though the plasma sodium levels may be low. **Giving high sodium loads could kill the child.**

Treatment
- Give extra potassium (3–4 mmol/kg daily).
- Give extra magnesium (0.4–0.6 mmol/kg daily).
- The extra potassium and magnesium are present in commercial F-75 and F-100 feeds, but if making from ingredients locally should be added to the feeds during their preparation. See Table 5.10.B.3 for a recipe for a combined electrolyte/mineral solution. Add 20 mL of this solution to 2.5 litres of feed to supply the extra potassium and magnesium required.
- Prepare food without adding salt.

Infections in SAM: treatment and prevention

All malnourished children must be assumed to have an infection. Because of the lack of an inflammatory response, clinical signs of infection may be entirely absent in a malnourished child with severe systemic infection. If untreated, this may cause mortality, morbidity and poor weight gain.

All children with severe acute malnutrition should routinely be given broad-spectrum antibiotics.

Protocol for treatment
Specific infections
Children with specific infections should receive the appropriate antibiotic according to local guidelines.

No specific infection and no suspected septic shock

The principle is to have a first-line treatment and a second-line treatment.

- **First-line treatment** is routinely given on admission to all severely malnourished children **without** complications such as septic shock, hypothermia, hypoglycaemia or a specific infection (skin, eyes). This is usually oral amoxicillin or co-trimoxazole.
- **Second-line treatment** is given after 48 hours to children who do not respond to the first-line treatment, and to all children with complications. This usually includes a parenteral antibiotic, although absorption of oral ciprofloxacin and chloramphenicol is excellent, so these can

be used orally once the child is stabilised. Some units routinely give metronidazole 7.5 mg/kg orally 8-hourly for 7 days in addition to the above.

The choice of the antibiotics used in first-line and second-line treatment is based on local guidelines, which are ideally informed by local resistance patterns. Factors such as route of administration, availability and cost of the drugs are all relevant. It should be a broad-spectrum antimicrobial agent, such gentamicin 7.5 mg/kg IV once daily for 7 days, **in combination** with either ampicillin (50 mg/kg 6-hourly for 2 days IV) then oral amoxicillin (15 mg/kg/dose 8-hourly for 5 days) **or** ciprofloxacin (10 mg/kg 12-hourly IV or orally for 7 days). If the child fails to improve after 48 hours, add chloramphenicol 25 mg/kg 8-hourly (IV or oral) or ceftriaxone 100 mg/kg daily IV (or IM if this is not possible). These doses are correct for children over 1 year of age, but all doses should be checked against local guidelines, and for infants.

Septic shock: recognition

Septic shock is a very common cause of deaths in these patients. The signs are as follows:

- clouding of consciousness
- rapid respiratory rate:
  - 50 breaths/minute for children aged 2–12 months
  - 40 breaths/minute for children aged 12 months to 5 years
- rapid pulse rate
- cold hands and feet with visible subcutaneous veins and prolonged capillary refill time > 3 seconds
- signs of dehydration but without a history of watery diarrhoea
- hypothermia or hypoglycaemia
- poor or absent bowel sounds
- an abdominal splash when the child is shaken.

It can be very difficult to distinguish between severe dehydration and septic shock.

Suspected septic shock: treatment

- A broad-spectrum IV antibiotic treatment (ceftriaxone) is started immediately.
- Warm the child to prevent or treat hypothermia (see hypothermia below).
- Feeding and fluid maintenance should be undertaken by nasogastric tube or orally.
- Close monitoring of the vital signs (pulse, respiration and conscious level) is essential.

Circulatory collapse

- Give high-flow oxygen through a face mask with reservoir.
- Give IV infusion as described in the case of circulatory collapse due to severe dehydration. However, as soon as the radial pulse becomes strong and the child regains consciousness, discontinue the infusion and start the diet orally or by nasogastric tube.

Hypothermia: prevention and treatment

Malnourished children have a low metabolic rate. The thermoneutral temperature is 28–32°C. At 24°C they can become hypothermic. Those with infection or extensive skin lesions are at particular risk. A hypothermic malnourished child should always be assumed to have septicaemia.

Signs

The signs of hypothermia are a core temperature (oral) < 35.5°C (with a low-reading thermometer). If the axillary temperature is < 35°C or does not register, assume hypothermia.

Routine prevention

- Cover all children with clothes and blankets. They should wear a warm hat (most heat is lost from the head).
- Ensure that the mother sleeps alongside her child. **Do not leave a child alone in bed at night.**
- Keep the ward doors and windows closed to avoid draughts.
- Avoid wet nappies, clothes or bedding.
- Do not wash very ill children. Others can be washed quickly, ideally with warm water, and dried immediately.
- Make sure that the child is fed, so that metabolic heat can be produced. Ensure that feeds occur during the night.
- **Avoid medical examinations which leave the child feeling cold.**

Emergency treatment of hypothermia

- Immediately place the child on the mother's bare chest or abdomen (skin to skin) and cover both of them. Give the mother a hot drink to increase her skin blood flow.
- If no adult is available, clothe the child thoroughly (including the head) and put them near a lamp or radiant heater.
- Immediately treat for hypoglycaemia (see below) and then start normal feeds.
- Give second-line antibiotics.
- Monitor the temperature every 60 minutes until it is normal (> 36.5°C).

Hypoglycaemia: prevention and treatment

Severely malnourished children easily develop hypoglycaemia. This is associated with serious infection. If available, test blood glucose levels (< 2.5 mmol/litre), or if they are not measurable assume that hypoglycaemia is present.

Signs

The main signs of hypoglycaemia are as follows:

- lethargy, limpness, loss of consciousness or convulsions
- drowsiness/unconsciousness with the eyelids partly open, or retraction of the eyelids
- low body temperature
- convulsions.

Sweating and pallor do not usually occur in this situation.

Routine prevention

- Give frequent small feeds, day and night.
- Feeding should start while the child is being admitted.
- Treat any infections.

Emergency treatment

If hypoglycaemia is suspected:

- **If the child can drink:** give therapeutic milk or 50 mL of glucose 10%, or 50 mL of drinking water plus 10 grams of sugar (one teaspoon of sugar in 3.5 tablespoons of clean water). Follow this with the first feed as soon as possible. If achievable, divide the first feed into four and give half-hourly. If not, give whole feeds every 2 hours during the day and night for at least the first day.

- **If the child is unconscious or has convulsions:** give 5 mL/kg body weight of glucose 10% IV or by the intra-osseous (IO) route, or if neither of these routes is possible give 5 mL/kg of glucose 10% or sugar solution as described above by nasogastric tube.

Continue frequent feeding to avoid a recurrence.
Give second-line antibiotics.

If there are convulsions other causes must be excluded, including cerebral malaria, meningitis, encephalitis, thiamine deficiency and hypernatraemic/hyponatraemic dehydration (especially in hot dry climates).

If blood glucose levels are available and are low, repeat the finger or heel prick after 60 minutes.

Congestive heart failure

This is a common and dangerous complication that usually occurs several days after admission. The heart muscle is atrophic (effectively there is a cardiomyopathy). During early recovery from severe malnutrition, sodium can be mobilised from the tissues before the kidney recovers sufficiently to excrete the excess. All blood transfusions must be done as soon as possible (in the first 2 days after admission), and should be rarely indicated.

Heart failure is usually caused by inappropriate treatment, including the following:

- misdiagnosis of dehydration with consequent inappropriate 'rehydration'
- very severe anaemia
- overload due to blood transfusion
- a high-sodium diet, using conventional oral rehydration solution, or excess ReSoMal
- inappropriate treatment that involves 're-feeding diarrhoea' with rehydration solutions.

Signs

Excess weight gain is the most reliable sign, and daily weights should be taken for all malnourished children. Differentiate pneumonia and heart failure by weighing the child. If their weight has increased, particularly if by more than 5%, consider heart failure. If they have lost weight, consider pneumonia.

First sign: fast breathing:
- 50 breaths/minute for children aged 2–12 months
- 40 breaths/minute for children aged 12 months to 5 years.

Later signs:
- lung crepitations
- respiratory distress
- rapid pulse rate
- engorgement of the jugular vein
- cold hands and feet
- cyanosis or hypoxaemia diagnosed by pulse oximetry if available ($SaO_2 < 94\%$ in air at sea level)
- liver enlarged by > 2 cm from baseline.

Emergency treatment of congestive cardiac failure
- **Give high-flow oxygen.**
- Stop all oral intake and IV fluid.

- The treatment of heart failure takes precedence over feeding of the child.
- No fluid at all should be given until the cardiac function improves, even if it takes 24–48 hours.
- Give a diuretic IV, usually furosemide (1 mg/kg). This is the only situation in which diuretics should be used: **diuretics should never be given to reduce oedema in malnourished children.**

Measles: prevention and treatment
Measles is especially dangerous in severe malnutrition.

Routine prevention
All children over 6 months of age who are admitted with malnutrition should be vaccinated against measles. This is often done weekly, but if measles is being transmitted locally, it should be done on admission. A second dose of vaccine in a previously immunised child is not harmful. A second dose should be given once recovered or at the normal time, where the prior vaccination state is uncertain or the child was not vaccinated before admission.

Treatment of measles
If a case of measles is admitted:
- Isolate the individual and any suspected cases.
- Review the vaccination status of all patients in the ward, and ensure that all are immunised.
- Give two doses of vitamin A separated by 1 day.
- Treat for measles (see Section 6.2.E) as well as for malnutrition.

Micronutrient deficiencies
All children with acute malnutrition will have these deficiencies. Commercial F-100 and RUTFs contains all of the required micronutrients in the correct amounts.

If not using these, give a daily multivitamin supplement, and add a mineral mix to the feeds. This should contain potassium, zinc, copper, magnesium and ideally selenium. Premixed sachets are available, or a solution can be made. It is important to **avoid** adding iron to milk-based feeds during the first 2 weeks, and until the child is gaining weight (RUTFs contain iron within the food, and this is safe to use for stable children and in CMAM programmes). After 2 weeks, iron is added to the F-100 feeds. In goitrous regions, potassium iodide should be added to the mineral mixture (12 mg/2500 mL), or else the child should be given Lugol's iodine, 5–10 drops per day.

Vitamin A: prevention and treatment
Routine preventive treatment
Oral vitamin A is particularly important for the severely malnourished child, and one dose should be given routinely to each child admitted with malnutrition.

TABLE 5.10.B.4 Vitamin A dosage: preventive treatment

Weight	Dose at admission
< 6 kg	50 000 IU once
6–10 kg	100 000 IU once
> 10 kg	200 000 IU once

Treatment of xerophthalmia

If a child shows signs of vitamin A deficiency (xerophthalmia) or has measles, three doses of vitamin A treatment should be given.

TABLE 5.10.B.5 Vitamin A dosage in xerophthalmia

Weight	Dose on day 1	Dose on day 2	Dose on day 3
< 6 kg	50 000 IU	50 000 IU	50 000 IU
6–10 kg	100 000 IU	100 000 IU	100 000 IU
> 10 kg	200 000 IU	200 000 IU	200 000 IU

If the eyes show signs of inflammation or ulceration, give the following additional care to the affected eye(s) to prevent corneal rupture and extrusion of the lens:

- Instil chloramphenicol or tetracycline eye drops, 2- to 3-hourly as required for 7–10 days.
- Instil atropine eye drops, one drop three times daily for 3–5 days.
- Cover with sterile saline-soaked eye pads.
- Bandage the eye(s).

Note that **children with vitamin A deficiency are likely to be photophobic and have their eyes closed. It is important to examine their eyes very gently to prevent corneal rupture.**

Treatment of anaemia

The majority of malnourished children have anaemia. This is due to the many deficiencies they have (iron, folic acid, riboflavin, pyridoxine, ascorbic acid, vitamin E, copper) and their inability to metabolise iron. **Iron should not be given until 2 weeks after the start of treatment.**

Routine treatment
Folic acid

Give 5 mg of folic acid on the day of admission, then 1 mg/day thereafter (in F-100 already).

Iron

Iron should **never be given during Phase I or during the transition phase.** In malnourished patients, iron is not properly metabolised and is therefore dangerous. The free iron enhances the production of free radicals that can damage cell walls. Excess free iron encourages systemic infection.

Oral iron supplementation should start **14 days after admission.** This is best added to the F-100 milk diet at a dose of one crushed tablet of ferrous sulphate (200 mg) to 2 litres of therapeutic milk. Alternatively, it can be given as ferrous sulphate 3 mg/kg/day orally, which should be continued until anaemia has resolved clinically, or ideally on blood test. It is present in adequate amount in RUTF.

Emergency treatment of very severe anaemia

Blood transfusion in malnourished children is potentially dangerous because it can precipitate heart failure. There are only two indications for considering blood transfusion, namely:

- the child with a haemoglobin concentration of < 4 grams/100 mL, especially if in shock

- the child with signs of heart failure due to anaemia (at immediate risk of death).

Give 10 mL/kg body weight of packed cells (or whole blood) slowly by partial **exchange** transfusion. Ideally, and if this can be achieved, use a carefully and continuously observed cannula in an artery or central vein. It is also possible in a vein in the antecubital fossa. First 2.5 mL/kg of anaemic blood is removed and then when 5 mL/kg of appropriately screened and cross-matched blood has been transfused, 2.5 mL/kg is again taken and the cycle is repeated. The child is closely monitored for signs of congestive heart failure.

If partial exchange is not possible and heart failure is present, give 10 mL/kg, ideally as packed cells, otherwise as whole blood. Transfuse over 4 hours and give IV furosemide 1 mg/kg at the start of the transfusion. Monitor carefully for worsening heart failure.

Intestinal parasites
Routine treatment

Routine deworming treatment is given to all children over 1 year of age, but only in phase II or the transition phase.

For children over 1 year of age, give mebendazole 100 mg (1 tablet) twice daily for 3 days. Some countries use albendazole 200 mg (for children aged 12–24 months) or 400 mg (for those over 24 months of age) once.

Dermatosis of kwashiorkor

Shedding of the skin in scales or sheets, desquamation, exfoliation, cracking of the skin surface, and ulceration of the genital or perianal areas are all common.

There can be widespread weeping skin lesions that resemble burns.

Zinc deficiency is usual in this situation, and oral zinc supplements improve the skin (give 2 mg/kg/day of elemental zinc).

Treatment

- Leave the exposed area open to dry during the day.
- Apply barrier cream (zinc and castor oil ointment) or petroleum jelly or tulle gras to the raw areas, and gentian violet or nystatin cream to the skin sores twice a day.
- These children should be on broad-spectrum antibiotics.
- Do not use plastic pants or disposable nappies for these children.

Continuing diarrhoea

See also Section 5.12.B.

Diarrhoea should subside during the first week of treatment. In the rehabilitation phase, loose or poorly formed stools are normal and do not need treatment provided that weight is increasing.

Treatment
Giardiasis

Giardiasis and mucosal damage are common causes of continuing diarrhoea. Where possible, examine the stools by microscopy.

If cysts or trophozoites of *Giardia lamblia* are found, give metronidazole (7.5 mg/kg 8-hourly for 7 days). If not detected but clinically *Giardia* is possible, give metronidazole anyway.

Lactose intolerance

Diarrhoea is only rarely due to lactose intolerance. Only treat for lactose intolerance if the continuing diarrhoea is preventing general improvement. Starter F-75 is a low-lactose feed. In exceptional cases:

- Substitute milk feeds with yoghurt or a lactose-free infant formula.
- Reintroduce milk feeds gradually in the rehabilitation phase.

Osmotic diarrhoea

This may be suspected if the diarrhoea worsens substantially with hyperosmolar F-75, and ceases when the sugar content and osmolarity are reduced. In these cases:

- Use a lower osmolar cereal-based starter F-75 (for the recipe, *see* Table 5.10.B.7) or, if available, use a commercially prepared isotonic starter F-75.
- Introduce catch-up F-100 gradually.

Malaria: treatment and prevention

In endemic areas, all malnourished children should have a rapid malaria smear or rapid test on admission. Where this is not possible, all malnourished children should receive antimalarial treatment according to local guidelines for the area. The parasitaemia is usually much lower than in normal children. In initially smear-negative children, there can be a recrudescence during nutritional replacement treatment, so consider malaria in children who develop fever.

Children and mothers should sleep under impregnated nets in the wards.

Tuberculosis

In patients treated for malnutrition, tuberculosis (TB) can be a cause of failure to gain weight. In malnourished children, the diagnosis of tuberculosis is particularly difficult and misdiagnosis is common.

How to diagnose pulmonary TB

The signs of TB in malnourished children are often not specific (e.g. anorexia, failure to thrive). Asymmetric chest signs or asymmetric lymph nodes are usually TB. Pneumonia in malnourished children affects both lungs, and HIV gives symmetrical lymphadenopathy.

Consider TB as a possible diagnosis in children who fail to gain weight during admission.

Sputum is rarely available. The Mantoux test can be negative in malnutrition. Undertake a chest X-ray if possible. A family history is often helpful. BCG offers protection against TB, but does not protect completely against infection.

Treatment (*see* Section 6.1.N)

Children with TB should not be isolated, for the following reasons:

- Young children are not a source of transmission (as it is rarely a cavitating disease).
- Treatment quickly eliminates the risk of transmission.
- An isolated child is stigmatised and neglected in resource-limited settings.

Usually paediatric TB is acquired from a sputum-positive adult, so the TB infected carer is a much higher infection risk to the ward. Take note of the carer on the ward with cough, as they should have a chest X-ray.

Malnutrition and AIDS

Basically, the initial stabilisation phase and nutritional treatment of HIV-infected patients is the same as for any other severely malnourished patient (*see* Section 6.2.D). They follow the same dietary and initial medical treatments. Many HIV-positive patients will respond well to the nutritional treatment and gain weight.

However, in units where HIV is prevalent, and particularly where there are programmes that offer additional nutritional support, co-trimoxazole, ARV treatment, PMTCT, and counselling on future pregnancies, there are excellent reasons why a carer would choose to have their child identified during admission as infected with HIV. Moreover, where this is routinely offered, such a policy is not found to be stigmatising.

The presentation of HIV-infected children is similar to that of the uninfected, so cannot be easily identified clinically, although there are some conditions that are more common. HIV-infected children are less likely to present with kwashiorkor than with marasmus. They are more likely to have oral candida, discharging ears, lymphadenopathy, chronic cough, persistent diarrhoea and dermatosis. They may have a family member with HIV, or be orphaned. They may present in infancy, while still breastfeeding, which is an uncommon time for presentation with severe acute malnutrition otherwise.

HIV testing should follow counselling, and be voluntary. It is usually done using two rapid ELISA serological tests. In infants under 1 year of age, serology reflects maternal status rather than infection in the infant. To diagnose infection in infants, a PCR test is required. All children identified as infected with HIV (or where PCR is not available as having indeterminate status) should be commenced on prophylactic co-trimoxazole. This has been shown to reduce long-term mortality.

In an HIV-infected infant, or one possibly infected with HIV and presenting with malnutrition, it is not sensible to stop breastfeeding during admission, as this will deprive the infant of an important source of nutrition. For children who are PCR negative, but exposed to HIV, the decision is less clear, although it will depend on the mother's likely viral load (check whether she is on ARV treatment), the food security of the family, the mother's ability to provide an alternate breast milk substitute, and her choice. There will usually be guidelines depending on local factors.

If the HIV-infected child is not responding well to malnutrition treatment, this may be because of unidentified infection. Non-typhoidal salmonella (NTS) is more common, as are organisms resistant to commonly used antibiotics. TB is a recognised co-infection, although it may be difficult to identify. Some children do not start gaining weight until ARV drugs are started.

It is not known when it is best to initiate ARV therapy in severe acute malnutrition, although it is generally accepted that children should be on phase II feeds. Some children do not meet the criteria for treatment clinically if they respond well to nutritional support with rapid weight gain. CD4 testing is helpful for determining who would benefit, as not all HIV-infected children have severe immunodeficiency, because HIV can be related to malnutrition through food insecurity as well as illness. However, long-term follow-up of infected malnourished children has identified them as being at high risk of mortality, suggesting that earlier ARV treatment might be of greater help in reducing this.

On discharge it is important to ensure that the child is linked into HIV and nutrition support programmes which the family can access, that carers are aware of the ongoing needs of the child, and that the wider family is offered HIV testing.

Dietary treatment of severe malnutrition
Dietary treatment in Phase I
Objectives
The aim of this phase is progressive restoration of the electrolyte, metabolic and physiological balance by the frequent feeding of special formula milk.

Principles
Severely malnourished children are usually anorexic, and have thin bowel walls, damaged metabolism, and too much sodium in their bodies. Initially they require a low-salt and low-protein diet and are unable to tolerate large amounts of food because their **capacity is reduced**. Therefore initially a diet high in carbohydrate with low levels of sodium and iron and very modest protein content is given. This diet leads to restoration of metabolic and physiological function, but is insufficient for weight gain.

- Feeding should start quickly after admission.
- It should be divided into many small meals to stay within the absorptive and metabolic capacity of the child and to prevent hypoglycaemia and hypothermia.
- The child should be encouraged to eat, but not be forced to do so. Feeding a malnourished child requires time and patience. Use a cup, bowl, spoon or syringe to feed very weak children. If the child takes less than 70% of the prescribed diet, they should be fed by a nasogastric tube.
- Always continue breastfeeding, and encourage the mother to breastfeed. After the breastfeed give the scheduled amounts of starter formula first (see below).

The following guidelines are also useful:
- Give frequent small feeds of low osmolarity and low lactose content.
- Night feeds are essential.
- Give oral or nasogastric feeds (never parenteral preparations).
- Give 100 kcal/kg/day.
- Protein: give 1–1.5 grams/kg/day.
- Liquid: give 130 mL/kg/day to all children, whether or not oedema is present.

TABLE 5.10.B.6 A recommended schedule

Days	Frequency	Volume/kg/feed	Volume/kg/day
1–2	2-hourly	11 mL	130 mL
3–5	3-hourly	16 mL	130 mL
6 onwards	4-hourly	22 mL	130 mL

TABLE 5.10.B.7 Volumes of F-75 per feed

Child's weight (kg)	2-hourly (mL/feed)	3-hourly (mL/feed)	4-hourly (mL/feed)
2.0	20	30	45
2.2	25	35	50
2.4	25	40	55
2.6	30	45	55
2.8	30	45	60
3.0	35	50	65
3.2	35	55	70
3.4	35	55	75
3.6	40	60	80
3.8	40	60	85
4.0	45	65	90
4.2	45	70	90
4.4	50	70	95
4.6	50	75	100
4.8	55	80	105
5.0	55	80	110
5.2	55	85	115
5.4	60	90	120
5.6	60	90	125
5.8	65	95	130
6.0	65	100	130
6.2	70	100	135
6.4	70	105	140
6.6	75	110	145
6.8	75	110	150
7.0	75	115	155
7.2	80	120	160
7.4	80	120	160
7.6	85	125	165
7.8	85	130	170
8.0	90	130	175
8.2	90	135	180
8.4	90	140	185
8.6	95	140	190
8.8	95	145	195
9.0	100	145	200
9.2	100	150	200
9.4	105	155	205
9.6	105	155	210
9.8	110	160	215
10.0	110	160	220

Mix the milk, sugar, oil and electrolyte/mineral solution to a paste, and then slowly add the warm boiled water. Make up to 1000 mL. If available, use an electric blender or hand whisk.

What food to give
The special milk for phase I is called F-75. If it is not available, F-100 should be diluted to the same calorie strength as F-75 and given in its place. Alternatively, it can be made from ingredients using the recipe in Table 5.10.B.7 above.

TABLE 5.10.B.8 Homemade recipes for re-feeding formulas F-75 and F-100

	F-75[ab] (starter)	F-75[c] (starter: cereal-based)	F-100[d] (catch-up)
Dried skimmed milk (grams)	25	25	80
Sugar (grams)	100	70	50
Cereal flour (grams)	–	35	–
Vegetable oil (grams)	27	27	60
Electrolyte/mineral solution (mL)	20	20	20
Water: make up to (mL)	1000	1000	1000
Contents per 100 mL			
Energy (kcal)	75	75	100
Protein (grams)	0.9	1.1	2.9
Lactose (grams)	1.3	1.3	4.2
Potassium (mmol)	4.0	4.2	6.3
Sodium (mmol)	0.6	0.6	1.9
Magnesium (mmol)	0.43	0.46	0.73
Zinc (mg)	2.0	2.0	2.3
Copper (mg)	0.25	0.25	0.25
% energy from protein	5	6	12
% energy from fat	32	32	53
Osmolality (mOsm/litre)	413	334	419

[a] A comparable starter formula can be made from 35 grams of whole dried milk, 100 grams of sugar, 20 grams of oil, 20 mL of electrolyte/mineral solution, and water to make 1000 mL. If using fresh cow's milk, take 300 mL of milk, 100 grams of sugar, 20 mL of oil, 20 mL of electrolyte/mineral solution, and water to make 1000 mL.

[b] Isotonic versions of F-75 (280 mOsmol/litre) are available commercially, in which maltodextrins replace some of the sugar, and in which all of the extra nutrients (potassium, magnesium and micronutrients) are incorporated. These are of lower osmolarity and therefore less likely to cause osmotic diarrhoea.

[c] Cook for 4 minutes. This may be helpful for children with dysentery or persistent diarrhoea.

[d] A comparable catch-up formula can be made from 110 grams of whole dried milk, 50 grams of sugar, 30 grams of oil, 20 mL of electrolyte/mineral solution, and water to make 1000 mL. If using fresh cow's milk, take 880 mL of milk, 75 grams of sugar, 20 mL of oil, 20 mL of electrolyte/mineral solution, and water to make 1000 mL.

F-75 contains:
- 75 kcal/100 mL
- 0.9 grams of protein/100 mL (around 5% of kcal provided by protein)
- 2 grams of fat/100 mL (around 32% of kcal provided by fat)
- 13 grams of carbohydrate/100 mL (around 62% of kcal provided by carbohydrates).

What quantity of food to give

Give 100 kcal/kg/day. The daily number of kcal should be divided by the number of meals given during the day (usually eight meals per day).

F-75: 133 mL = 100 kcal.

Example

A child of 6 kg should receive a diet of 100 kcal/kg/day. The child will be given eight meals of F-75.

Number of kcal/day: 100 kcal × 6 kg = 600 kcal. Quantity of F-75 per day: 800 mL (798 exactly). Quantity per meal: 800/8 = 100 mL.

Do not exceed 100 kcal/kg/day in this initial phase. Diarrhoea should gradually decrease and oedematous children should **lose weight** as the oedema disappears. If diarrhoea continues, see above.

Dietary treatment in the transition phase (for 48 hours)
What food to give

In the transition phase, full-strength F-100 is given in the same volume that was calculated for F-75 in phase I. There is no other change made in the transition phase. F-100 contains:
- 100 kcal/100 mL
- around 2.6 grams of protein/100 mL (10% of kcal provided by protein)
- around 5.6 grams of fat/100 mL (50% of kcal provided by fat)
- around 9.8 grams of carbohydrate (40% of kcal provided by carbohydrate).

There are two forms of F-100.

Commercial F-100

This therapeutic milk is prepared in a sachet. All that the nurse has to do is open the packet and dilute the contents in 2 litres of potable (boiled) water. The commercial F-100 has a lower osmolarity to reduce 're-feeding' diarrhoea in the severely malnourished children.

Home-made F-100
This can be made from ingredients using the recipe shown in Table 5.10.B.8 above.

Dietary treatment in phase II
Objectives
The aim is catch-up growth of the child with rapid weight gain (10–20 g/kg/day). Usually the appetite has returned.

Principles
The child has re-established their physiological balance and should get enough food to gain weight as quickly as possible. They are given a high-energy diet with normal protein content.

- The intake is increased in quantity (to about 200 kcal/kg/day).
- Reduce meal frequency from eight to six meals per day.
- There should be no limit on the quantity of food given. The child is allowed to eat as much as they want, but must never be forced to eat.
- Breastfeeding continues. Breast milk must always be offered **before** the high-energy food is given.
- Aim for weight gain of more than 10 grams/kg/day.
- Remain alert for heart failure.

What food to give
The basic diet is composed of F-100 meals. However, when the child is gaining weight quickly, other foods can be introduced – for example:

- enriched porridges (1 mL contains 1 kcal/gram) as one to two meals a day
- enriched biscuits (useful for overnight feeding if phase II is conducted in a day-care centre) or RUTF (see below)
- local meal: composed of the usual food eaten in the area; this should be enriched in the pot with the addition of oil and CMV and sometimes DSM.

Quantity of food to give
Dispense and offer 200 kcal/kg of F-100 per kg of body weight per day.

Example of calculation
A child who weighs 9 kg should receive 200 kcal × 9 = 1800 kcal per day. The child will receive six meals per day, and each meal should provide 1800 kcal/6 = 300 kcal.

The diet is composed of six meals of F-100. The enriched porridge or family meal is given **in addition** if the child wishes to take it.

- F-100 (1 mL of F-100 = 1 kcal): the child should receive 300 mL of F-100 per meal.

Older children and adolescents, when they are gaining weight rapidly, often do not want the milk and demand 'solid food'. This usually slows the rate of recovery. The solid food should always be enriched.

When developing local recipes the weight gain should be compared with that of children taking F-100 alone. If the weight gain is similar, the recipe for the porridge is adequate.

Ready-to-use therapeutic foods (RUTFs)
RUTFs have been developed to provide the same nutritional content as F-100, but in a peanut-butter-type paste that is not susceptible to pathogens growing in it, due to its low water content. These are usually based on a mix of groundnuts, vegetable oil, dry skimmed milk, sugar and micronutrient mix. If this is available, children can be introduced to this when on phase II feeds, and if they have a good appetite, could be followed up after 1–2 weeks in an outpatient- or community-based malnutrition programme. This is referred to as an Outpatient Therapeutic Programme (OTP), CMAM or CTC (see Further Reading at the end of this subsection).

Individual child monitoring
Phase I
A daily medical and nutritional round of all the children in phase I should be done. The children should be carefully monitored every day for:

- oedema
- weight
- appetite: how the child is eating and the quantity eaten
- clinical state: consciousness, diarrhoea, vomiting, skin, etc.
- behaviour: apathetic, alert, crying, etc.
- temperature
- liver size, heart rate and heart sounds.

This information should be recorded every day on an individual chart.

When to pass to the transition phase
Children usually remain in phase I for 1–7 days. The child can pass to the transition phase when:

- they regain appetite
- they are lively and interested
- serious medical complications are under control
- oedema is decreasing (although it may be still present).

If after 5–7 days the child is not ready for the transition phase, they should be completely re-examined and investigated.

After 2 days in the transition phase without experiencing any problem, the child is ready to move to phase II. Oedema should be significantly improved, and the child must be stable, before progressing to phase II.

Phase II
The monitoring in phase II includes the following:

- a daily round by the nurse, who checks the general state of the child, including whether there is oedema, nausea or vomiting, and how the child is eating
- a physician round undertaken weekly if the child is stable
- measurement of the child's weight twice a week if they are well
- measurement of their height monthly or in each OTP clinic review.

This information should be recorded on the individual chart.

If a child develops a complication in phase II, such as re-feeding diarrhoea or vomiting that requires passage of a nasogastric tube, rehydration solutions, transfusion, etc., they should be returned to phase I and subsequently the transition phase again. The above treatments must never be given to children while in phase II and taking very large amounts of F-100 diet.

When the child can be discharged
Children remain in phase II until they meet the criteria for recovery. The average total length of stay is around 4 weeks

in traditional inpatient care, and longer if very severe complicated malnutrition, HIV, TB, or underlying disease or disability is present.

Figure 5.10.B.1 shows an example of a typical growth recovery chart.

When the child has reached their target weight and is in a good clinical state, they will be either referred to a supplementary feeding programme or sent directly home with arrangements made for follow-up. Children with long-term illness should be transferred to an appropriate community service.

Failure to gain weight

If the child fails to gain weight they should be investigated. Weight gain is defined as poor if it is less than 5 grams/kg/day, moderate if it is 5–10 grams/kg/day, and good if it exceeds 10 grams/kg/day. The following are the most common reasons for failure to gain weight:

- Food prescription or food preparation (kitchen) is incorrect and the child has not received the right quantity of the right food.
- The child does not eat the amount of food prescribed (e.g. because they dislike the food, or the food is being eaten by other people).
- Suspect hidden acute infections (e.g. urinary tract infection, acute respiratory infection, otitis media, mouth candidiasis, giardiasis).
- There are chronic hidden infections (tuberculosis, HIV).
- Re-examine, do stool and urine microscopy, and take a chest X-ray.
- Look for poor feeding techniques, and check that night feeds are occurring.

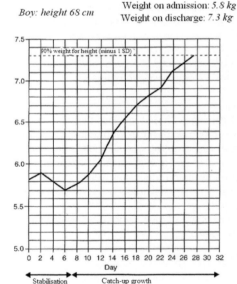

Boy: height 68 cm

Weight on admission: *5.8 kg*
Weight on discharge: *7.3 kg*

FIGURE 5.10.B.1 Weight catch-up chart for a boy weighing 5.8 kg on admission to hospital.

Emotional and physical stimulation

The severely malnourished child is nearly always psychosocially deprived. The illness itself makes the child unresponsive, and so they do not cry or complain. Because mothers use a cry as the signal to give attention, these children do not receive the attention they need to stimulate them. The neglect is not wilful on the part of the mother, but rather it is a failure of the two-way communication between the mother and her child.

Because they do not cry or complain, these children are often also neglected by nurses and staff. This greatly compounds the problems associated with being in a strange environment. It is essential to stimulate these children, particularly the unresponsive ones. The ward should be made as much like home as possible and children should sleep alongside their mothers.

- **In phase I** it is essential that the mother (or other carer) is present, feeds the child, comforts them, holds them, plays with them, and talks and sings to them.
- **In phase II** it is important to stimulate the child to move, and to play with other children. A play area should always be present. Staff should be identified who have a responsibility for providing (local) toys and encouraging play.

The daily organisation of the activities

To organise the treatment of malnourished children, a schedule of activities (e.g. care, distribution of meals) must be established. An example is given below.

TABLE 5.10.B.9 Daily organisation of activities

Time (24-hour clock)	Children in phase I and transition phase	Children in phase II (day care)
02.00	Milk distribution	
05.00	Milk distribution	
07.00	Team changeover (day shift)	
07.30	Temperatures	Arrival of children
08.00	Milk distribution and drugs	Milk distribution and drugs
09.00	Weight, oedema assessment	Weight, oedema assessment
09.30	Mother's meal	Medical round
10.00	Medical round	Milk distribution
11.00	Milk distribution	Mother's meal
12.00		Milk distribution and drugs
13.00	Dressings	Dressings
14.00	Milk distribution and drugs	
15.00		Porridge distribution
16.00	Mother's meal	Mother's meal
17.00	Milk distribution	Milk distribution
18.00	Medical round	Departure home with porridge and enriched biscuits for the night
19.00	Team changeover (night shift)	
20.00	Milk distribution and drugs	
21.00	Close windows, wrap child	
23.00	Milk distribution	

Inappropriate practices

- Too much sodium, energy and protein given during phase I of treatment.
- No distinction made between phases I and II.
- Failure to monitor food intake.
- Lack of feeding at night.
- Lack of blankets and hats.
- No daily schedule organised.
- Diuretic given to treat oedema.
- Anaemia treated from time of admission with iron supplements.
- Intravenous fluids given for indications other than circulatory collapse.
- Use of high-sodium diet and standard oral rehydration solution.
- Routine antibiotics not given.
- No vitamin A given.
- No measles vaccine given.

Problems with the management of severe malnutrition

A high level of care is needed. The treatment of a severely malnourished child requires intensive protocol-based care, like that for a premature neonate, with close monitoring, some complex medical care (severe or chronic infections), a diet well enriched in nutrients (F-100, etc.), and an emotionally stimulating, rich and physically warm environment.

The resources are almost always limited. The limited financial resources lead to difficulty in obtaining therapeutic milks and other fortified food, drugs and materials.

However, if staff follow the protocols advocated by the WHO, and described above, outcomes can improve. Staff need to be confident that they can follow the guidelines approved for their unit, and if they are unable to do so, be able to address these deficits in care provision. Nursing staff are often better at following the guidelines than doctors, who may try to individualise treatment as they would for other children. The recording charts, weight charts and pro forma are tools that greatly help in the management of these children.

Analysis has shown that the main reasons for death are inappropriate medical interventions, such as fluid overload from ORS, blood transfusion, and the use of diuretics in oedema. Another reason is failure to adhere to the guidelines, due to either a lack of resources, or a lack of understanding of the differences in the care needs of this group of children. A significant and often unrecognised cause of death and relapse is inadequate discharge planning, or premature discharge.

However, perhaps the greatest problem is posed by the limited human resources on the malnutrition ward, with an insufficient number of skilled personnel, and constant movement of staff as soon as they are trained. The greatest resource that a unit can have is a motivated, trained and experienced staff, who have the basic resources to deliver the care described in this subsection.

Further reading

Briend A, Lacsala R, Prudhon C *et al*. (1999) Ready-to-use therapeutic food for treatment of marasmus. *Lancet*, **353**, 1767–8.

Bunn JEG (2009) Severe acute malnutrition and HIV in African Children. *HIV Therapy*, **6**, 595–611.

Jackson AA (2010) Severe malnutrition. In: Weatherall DJ, Cox TM and Firth JD (eds) *The Oxford Textbook of Medicine*. Volume 1, 5th edn. Oxford: Oxford University Press.

Sadler K, Kerac M, Collins S *et al*. (2008) Improving the management of severe acute malnutrition in an area of high HIV prevalence. *Journal of Tropical Pediatrics*, **54**, 364–9.

Valid International (2006) *Community-Based Therapeutic Care: a field manual*. Oxford: Valid International. Available at www.validinternational.org

Waterlow JC (1992) *Protein-Energy Malnutrition: body composition and body water*. London: Edward Arnold.

World Health Organization (1999) *Management of Severe Malnutrition: a manual for physicians and other senior health workers*. Geneva: World Health Organization. www.who.int/nutrition/publications/severemalnutrition/en/manage_severe_malnutrition_eng.pdf

World Health Organization (2014) *Pocket Book of Hospital Care for Children: guidelines for the management of common illnesses with limited resources*. Second edition. Geneva: World Health Organization. www.who.int/maternal_child_adolescent/documents/child_hospital_care/en/

World Health Organization (2003) *Guidelines for the Inpatient Treatment of Severely Malnourished Children*. Geneva: World Health Organization. www.who.int/nutrition/publications/severemalnutrition/guide_inpatient_text.pdf

5.11 Haematological disorders

5.11.A Anaemia

Introduction
Definition of anaemia
Table 5.11.A.1 gives the World Health Organization (WHO) definition of haemoglobin concentrations below which anaemia is present at sea level.

TABLE 5.11.A.1 Lower limit of normal haemoglobin concentrations

Age of child	Haemoglobin concentration (grams/dL)	Haematocrit (%)
6 months to 4 years	11	33
5–11 years	11.5	34
12–14 years	12	36

The problem of anaemia
- It is widespread in disadvantaged countries.
- It is common in young children under 5 years of age.
- More than one cause of anaemia is usually found in each anaemic child.
- Genetic causes of anaemia are common.
- It has significant deleterious effects on growth, health and development.

Main causes of childhood anaemia in resource-limited settings
- Low birth weight:
  — results in low iron and folate stores (0–2 years age group).
- Dietary:
  — diets tend to be low in iron
  — delayed weaning
  — poor maternal iron intake in breastfed infants
  — weaning on to non-fortified cow's milk.
- Infections:
  — malaria (haemolysis)
  — hookworm (*Ancylostoma duodenale* and *Necator americanus*) (*see* Section 6.3.C)
  — whipworm (*Trichuris* species)
  — congenital infection (CMV, rubella)
  — HIV.
- Genetic:
  — haemoglobinopathies (HbSS, thalassaemias)
  — glucose-6-phosphate dehydrogenase deficiency.
- Malignancy:
  — leukaemia
  — other types of malignancy.

The child with iron-deficiency anaemia
Clinical features of anaemia
- Often asymptomatic until haemoglobin concentration is < 8 grams/dL.
- Breathless on exertion when haemoglobin concentration is < 6 grams/dL.
- Pallor:
  — nail beds (the best site)
  — palmar creases
  — mucous membranes.
- Suboptimal growth, delayed puberty.
- Congestive heart failure.

Investigations
The tests in **bold** listed below should **always be done before a transfusion** (to exclude causes other than iron deficiency):
- **Haemoglobin concentration** (cyanmethaemoglobin method or **HemoCue B**).
- Haematocrit or PCV (microcentrifuge).
- **Blood film:**
  — **malarial parasites**
  — red blood cells: hypochromia, microcytosis, anisocytosis target cells (iron deficiency, thalassaemia)
  — sickle cells
  — macrocytes (folate, vitamin B_{12} deficiency)
  — white blood cells: hypersegmented neutrophils (folate, vitamin B_{12} deficiency).
- Mean corpuscular volume (MCV) and reticulocyte count as the two principal criteria for the initial classification of anaemia.
- **Haemoglobin electrophoresis:** sickle cell, thalassaemia.
- Stool test: parasitic ova, blood.

Management of anaemia
- Establish the diagnosis, cause and severity of iron-deficiency anaemia.
- Treat malaria (oral route) (*see* malaria guidelines in Section 6.3.A.d).
- Give empirical antihelmintic therapy in endemic areas (*see* Section 6.3.C).
- Give haematinics:

— folic acid: up to 5 years of age, 2.5 mg once daily; above 5 years, 5 mg once daily
— iron (*see* Table 5.11.A.2).

Iron medication

TABLE 5.11.A.2 Dosage of iron medications for iron-deficiency anaemia in childhood

Age or weight (6 mg/kg elemental iron)	Ferrous sulphate 200 mg (60 mg/kg elemental iron)	Ferrous fumarate 60 mg per 5 mL (12 mg elemental iron/mL)
2–4 months (4–6 kg)	–	2 mL
4–12 months (6–10 kg)	–	2.5 mL
1–3 years (10–14 kg)	½ tablet	4 mL
3–5 years (14–19 kg)	½ tablet	5.5 mL
> 5 years (> 19 kg)	1 tablet	–

- Preterm infants should start prophylactic iron (5 mg/day) from 4–6 weeks of age until mixed feeding is established.
- Treatment with iron injections may increase mortality (meningitis) and morbidity (respiratory infections, malaria) in infants.

Antihelmintic drugs (see Section 6.3.C)

- Albendazole (the drug of choice if available):
  - 400 mg as a single dose (200 mg if child is less than 2 years of age).
- Mebendazole (most effective against hookworm and whipworm):
  - For children over 1 year of age, 250 mg as a single dose (or 500 mg if the child is over 2 years). May be repeated after 2 or 3 weeks.

Blood transfusion (see also Section 1.7)

Only undertake this if it is essential.

- Warm the blood first under the mother's clothing, in contact with the skin, especially if it is to be given to an infant.
- Do not use blood that has been stored for more than 35 days at 2–6°C or out of the fridge for more than 2 hours, or that is visibly spoiled (plasma must not be pink, and red cells must not be purple or black), or from a bag that is open or leaking.
- Check that the blood is the correct group and that the patient's name and number are identical on both label and form.
- Use a needle/catheter that is 22 gauge or larger, to prevent clotting.
- If there are signs of heart failure, give 1 mg/kg of furosemide IV at the start of transfusion unless hypovolaemic shock is also present.
- Record the baseline temperature and pulse rate.
- Each transfused unit must be completely used within 4 hours of removal from the fridge.
- Ideally, in infants or those with heart failure, control the flow with an in-line burette.
- Record observations every 30 minutes, looking for heart failure (shortness of breath) and transfusion reactions (fever and malaise).

- Record the quantities given.

Indications for transfusion

- Severe anaemia (haemoglobin concentration < 4 grams/dL).
- Impending or overt cardiac failure if the haemoglobin concentration is < 6 grams/dL.
- Hyperparasitaemia in malaria if the haemoglobin concentration is < 6 grams/dL.
- Children in congestive cardiac failure due to severe anaemia (consider partial exchange).
- Acute severe blood loss with shock that is unresponsive to 40 mL/kg of volume resuscitation given in 10 mL/kg aliquots, or where massive haemorrhage is continuing.

Volume of transfusion

- Use packed red cells where possible.
- Give whole blood: 20 mL/kg or:
  - required volume (mL) = weight (kg) × 4 × desired rise in haemoglobin (grams/dL) **or**
- Packed red cells: 10–15 mL/kg **or**
  - required volume (mL) = weight (kg) × 3 × desired rise in haemoglobin (grams/dL).
- In all cases, rate = 5–10 mL/kg/hour (usually over 3–4 hours unless shocked).
- Consider giving furosemide 1 mg/kg IV immediately in advance of transfusion to avoid precipitating cardiac failure (unless there is hypovolaemic shock) in cases of very severe anaemia.

Treatment of severely anaemic child with septic shock

The first priority will still be to call for help, and manage the airway, followed by breathing and then the circulation.

Call for help.

Airway

Assess the airway by the simple technique of asking the child 'Are you all right?'

Any vocalisation, such as a reply or crying, indicates an open airway and some ventilation. In the absence of a response, formally open the airway with a head tilt/chin lift or a jaw thrust manoeuvre (*see* Section 1.12), and assess the breathing by looking, listening and feeling for its presence.

Breathing

All children with suspected shock must receive high-flow oxygen.

If possible, this should be given through a mask with a reservoir to achieve the higher concentrations. In the absence of spontaneous breathing, give assisted ventilation with a bag-mask (*see* Section 1.13).

Circulation

Intravenous access with a short wide-bore venous cannula, or placement of **an intra-osseous line** (*see* Section 8.4.B), is vital. Severely anaemic children cannot tolerate rapid boluses of fluid as they are likely to be in heart failure and may also be malnourished. The fluid they need most is blood. When transfusing severely anaemic children we usually give packed cells, but in **suspected septic shock**, fresh whole blood has the following advantages:

- It increases oxygen-carrying capacity.
- Plasma content improves circulating volume better than crystalloids.
- Clotting factors and platelets are beneficial in septic shock.

While awaiting the blood, which should be transfused at 20 mL/kg, give 10 mL/kg of Hartmann's solution or Ringer-lactate solution, and then reassess the child. If fresh whole blood is not available, give stored blood, but it should be packed, or if the child is in heart failure, consider partial exchange transfusion. Give antibiotics IV. A third-generation cephalosporin or a combination of gentamicin and a penicillin would be advisable. Flucloxacillin should be added if *Staphylococcus* is suspected (e.g. if there are boils or a known abscess). In suspected intra-abdominal sepsis, metronidazole should be added to cover anaerobic organisms.

Transfusion reactions

See Section 1.7.

Prevention of iron-deficiency anaemia

- Improve iron intake in infants:
  - breastfeeding for at least 6 months
  - give breastfeeding mothers iron
  - include vitamin-C-rich foods (citrus fruit juices) and/or meat, fish, beans and leafy vegetables by 6 months with cereals
  - low-birth-weight babies should receive oral iron 2 mg/kg daily from the age of 4 weeks, for 6 months.
- Prevent infections:
  - diarrhoea (breast milk)
  - measles (vaccination)
  - prevention and prompt treatment of malaria
  - routine deworming of children under 5 years every 3–6 months
  - malaria prophylaxis in sickle-cell patients.

5.11.B Sickle-cell disease

BOX 5.11.B.1 Minimum standards
- Facility for haemoglobin estimation and electrophoresis.
- Analgesia: paracetamol, NSAIDs, opiates.
- Blood transfusion.
- Oxygen.
- Penicillin prophylaxis.
- Pneumococcal (PCV and Pneumovax), hepatitis B and *Haemophilus influenzae* vaccines.
- Oral rehydration solution (ORS).
- Antimalarial drugs.
- Iron chelation: desferrioxamine, deferasirox or deferiprone.

Introduction

Genetic basis

Sickle-cell disease is a recessively inherited disorder of haemoglobin synthesis. It occurs due to a point mutation at position 6 on chromosome 11 resulting in the substitution of valine for glutamic acid on the beta-globin chain. Those affected inherit two copies of the altered beta-globin gene and are therefore homozygous for HbS (HbSS). Alternatively, a single HbS may be inherited with another beta-chain mutation such as beta thalassaemia (HbSB+ or HBSB°) or HbC (HbSC).

A child who inherits two of the same trait genes, one from each parent, will be born with the disease. However, a child of two carriers has only a 25% chance of receiving two trait genes and developing the disease, and a 50% chance of being a carrier. Most carriers lead completely normal healthy lives.

The HbS mutation is common. It is estimated that up to 5% of the world population are healthy carriers of sickle gene, and this can rise to 25% in West Africans. Although the HbS mutation is most common in Africa, it occurs widely across many groups. It is estimated that each year 300 000 children are born with homozygous sickle-cell disease worldwide.

Prognosis

In well-resourced countries, the life expectancy of individuals with sickle-cell disease has been continuously improving, and historic data suggest that it is now well beyond the fifth decade of life, with the overwhelming majority of children surviving into adulthood. The pattern of the disease and its complications is also changing in well-resourced countries, with a shift from being a fatal paediatric illness to a chronic disease associated with episodic painful crises and progressive deterioration and organ damage in later life.

However, in resource-limited countries, sickle-cell disease is still associated with a very high mortality and morbidity, particularly during childhood. Sickle-cell disease remains a major cause of mortality in children under 5 years of age, with estimates as high as 50–90% in some rural areas of Africa. The major causes of death are infection, especially malaria and invasive pneumococcal infection, and severe profound anaemia. For those who live with the condition, sickle-cell disease is the cause of a great burden of suffering for those affected and their families.

Pathogenesis

The clinical manifestations of sickle-cell disease are due to vaso-occlusion and chronic haemolysis, often in response to triggers such as illness, hypoxia or dehydration.

The presence of abnormal HbS leads to the production of a haemoglobin tetramer ($\alpha2/\beta S2$) that is poorly soluble when deoxygenated, and polymerises readily into a rope-like fibre within the red blood cell. This leads to red cell distortion into the classic sickle shape, a reduction in red cell deformability, and red cell destruction through haemolysis, with consequent shortening of the red cell lifespan, and anaemia.

Vaso-occlusive episodes occur when blood vessels become clogged with sickle cells, causing pain, tissue oxygen deprivation and organ damage alongside altered cell adhesion and abnormal erythrocyte–endothelium interaction. In addition to vaso-occlusion, there is a chronic intravascular haemolysis leading to a compensated anaemia with functional nitric oxide (NO) dysregulation with chronic vascular endothelial damage. This means that polymerisation alone does not account for the pathophysiology of sickle-cell disease. Changes in red cell membrane structure and function, disordered cell volume control, and increased adherence to vascular endothelium also play an important role.

Clinical presentations

In children, the most common presentation of sickle-cell disease is with an acute crisis, usually as a painful episode. More recently, as more countries adopt a newborn screening programme, children may be diagnosed with sickle-cell disease before their first crisis.

Presentation includes the following:
- newborn screening
- a painful vaso-occlusive crisis
- infection and overwhelming sepsis
- severe anaemia
- acute chest syndrome (ACS)
- stroke.

Newborn screening programmes

The goal of any newborn screening programme for sickle-cell disease is to identify affected children as early as possible and thus reduce the morbidity and mortality of sickle-cell disease, especially from bacterial infections, through the early introduction of antibiotic prophylaxis. In well-resourced countries, the preferred option is the universal screening programme rather than selective screening of high-risk infants only.

Methodology of newborn screening

The methodology of screening can vary, but in principle involves the collection of a dried neonatal blood spot sample for transport and testing by haemoglobin electrophoresis, thin-layer isoelectric focusing, or HPLC. A second confirmatory test may be taken 1–2 weeks later for repeat testing by isoelectric focusing, HPLC, PCR techniques or DNA analysis by a reference laboratory. The tests used must have the capability to distinguish between HbF, HbS, HbA and HbC. As several of the sickle-cell disease syndromes can have similar results on electrophoresis or isoelectric focusing, examining the peripheral blood smear remains useful.
- Haemoglobin electrophoresis is the standard method for separating HbS from other haemoglobin variants.
- Thin-layer isoelectric focusing is a more complicated technique, which can distinguish some haemoglobins not seen on standard electrophoresis, as the bands are more sharply seen.
- High-performance liquid chromatography (HPLC) is a very precise and fully automated technique for identification and quantification of haemoglobins.
- Sickle solubility test. A positive sickle solubility test will detect the presence of HbS but will not identify whether the person is a carrier or has sickle-cell disease.

Results and patterns in the newborn period

Finding	Pattern	Interpretation
HbF and HbA	FA	Normal baby
HbF, HbA and HbS	FAS	Sickle-cell trait
HbF, HbS and HbA	FSA	Sickle-cell beta+ thalassaemia
HbF and HbA	FS	Sickle-cell disease (HbSS or HbS beta⁰ thalassaemia)

In countries with limited resources, the combination of haemoglobin electrophoresis and a sickle solubility test will confirm the diagnosis of sickle-cell disease for most older children once the beta-chain production is fully developed beyond the newborn period.

Diagnosis

- Haemoglobin electrophoresis demonstrates the absence of HbA and either HbS (SS) or HbS and another haemoglobin such as HbC (SC).
- A positive sickle solubility test denotes the presence of sickle haemoglobin, but does not indicate whether the person is a carrier (Hb AS) or Hb SS.
- A full blood count shows severe (SS) to mild anaemia (SC).
- Examination of the peripheral blood shows sickled erythrocytes.

General principles of the management of an acute sickle crisis

Most children do not develop symptomatic disease in the first few months of life until adult haemoglobin production is established. The principles of managing any acute crisis are based on searching for, and actively treating, any precipitants (see Table 5.11.B.1). Any child presenting with an acute crisis should be considered at risk of sudden and life-threatening deterioration, and clinicians are advised to have an anticipatory approach.

Crisis precipitants include the following:
- infection
- dehydration
- extremes of temperature.

TABLE 5.11.B.1 Precipitants of sickle crises

Problem/precipitant	Approach
Fever and/or evidence of infection Child should be considered functionally asplenic and immunocompromised	Treatment dose of appropriate antibiotics
	Use of appropriate antimalarial drugs
	Use of antipyretic drugs
Dehydration	Rehydration
Extremes of temperature and cold	Warmth and rest

Clinicians should be alert to signs suggesting the possibility of a sudden acute deterioration during a crisis. The following **trigger list may be helpful for identifying children at increased risk of sudden or rapid deterioration:**
- uncontrolled pain despite strong opiate analgesia
- increasing pallor, breathlessness or exhaustion
- marked fever (> 38°C)
- significant tachycardia, tachypnoea or hypotension

TABLE 5.11.B.2 Management of an uncomplicated acute painful episode

Treatment	Comment
Antibiotics and antimalarial drugs (see later)	Any fever should prompt the search for infection and active treatment. Oral antibiotic dosages should be administered at higher dose as per the immunocompromised child
Hydration	Dehydration occurs readily in children with sickle-cell disease, due to impairment of renal concentrating power. Fluids should be given at 150% maintenance (orally or IV)
Analgesia	Assess pain using an age-appropriate visual analogue scale (VAS) (see below). Use the VAS to assess response to analgesia with the goal of minimal pain allowing successful mobilisation. Manage pain with prompt administration of the most appropriate choice and dose from the analgesic ladder. Take into account previous drugs and dosages given at home. Children in severe pain may need early use of opiates orally or IV. **Do not use pethidine**
Severe anaemia	Consider transfusion if the haemoglobin concentration is very low (e.g. < 5 grams/dL) or has fallen by > 2 grams/dL from a known baseline level, or the child is clearly clinically compromised
Oxygen	Provide oxygen if the saturations in air are below 95%. Falling saturations in air or a rising oxygen requirement should prompt re-evaluation and the search for an emerging complication of the crisis

- chest pain with or without signs of consolidation
- desaturation in air or a rising oxygen requirement to maintain saturations above 94%
- abdominal pain with or without distension
- severe diarrhoea and vomiting
- sudden profound pallor with or without jaundice
- parents reporting an enlarged spleen
- any abnormal neurological signs, including painless loss of function, headache and fitting.

The acute painful sickle episode

- This is also referred to as a painful or vaso-occlusive crisis, and is the most common presentation of sickle-cell disease in childhood, resulting from blockage of small vessels. The mainstay of treatment is effective and prompt pain control (*see* Section 1.15), alongside management of any precipitants.
- Approximately 40% of children with sickle-cell disease will have an episode of 'hand–foot syndrome' or dactylitis during early childhood, and this number rises to 50% of children under 2 years old who go on to develop symptomatic disease. Typically children present with vaso-occlusion and infarction of the metacarpals or metatarsals, which is evident as an overlying soft tissue reaction with swelling, redness and marked tenderness affecting either one or all of the hands and feet.
- By later childhood the most common sites of bony sickle-related pain include the long bones, thighs, hips, spine, ribs, shoulders and upper humerus, as well as the bones of the cranium, joints and muscles.

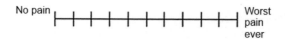

No pain ┣━┼━┼━┼━┼━┼━┼━┼━┼━┫ Worst pain ever

FIGURE 5.11.B.1 Visual analogue scale.

Hydration and fluids in sickle-cell disease

Dehydration occurs readily in children with sickle-cell disease, due to impairment of renal concentrating power.

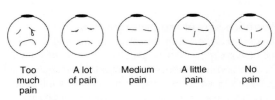

| Too much pain | A lot of pain | Medium pain | A little pain | No pain |

FIGURE 5.11.B.2 Faces scale.

Diarrhoea and vomiting are thus of particular concern. Rehydration calculations are therefore based on the assumption that children with sickle-cell disease have a higher fluid requirement than unaffected children.

Fluids can be delivered by the oral, nasogastric or IV route (or a combination of these) and titrated against clinical response. Generally it is safe to start with hyperhydration (150% of normal), although this may be reduced to normal hydration in children who are less unwell.

TABLE 5.11.B.3 Fluids in sickle-cell crises

Body weight (kg)	Fluids (mL/kg/day)
First 10 kg	150
11–20 kg	75
Subsequent kg over 20	30

Infection

Infection is a common precipitating factor in painful or other types of sickle crises. All children with sickle-cell disease (regardless of type) should be considered to be immunocompromised.

Bacteria

Patients with sickle-cell disease are immunodeficient due to functional asplenia.

Functional asplenia occurs irrespective of spleen size in sickle-cell disease well before the age of 1 year in the majority of sufferers. Clinicians should therefore consider all patients to have increased susceptibility to infection,

TABLE 5.11.B.4 Antibiotic choices in sickle-cell crises

Drug	Rationale and comment
Augmentin	Good activity against *Pneumococcus*
	Haemophilus resistance is low
	Suitable for use with clarithromycin for pneumonia
	Does not mask *Salmonella* osteomyelitis
Clarithromycin	Good activity against *Haemophilus*
	Pneumococcal resistance is low
	Suitable for use with augmentin for pneumonia
	Does not mask *Salmonella* osteomyelitis
Cefuroxime	Suitable for severe pneumonia with or without clarithromycin
	Masks *Salmonella* osteomyelitis
Ceftriaxone and other third-generation cephalosporins	For suspected sepsis
	First-line treatment for suspected osteomyelitis (with clindamycin)
	Second-line treatment for *Yersinia* if there is glucose-6-phosphate dehydrogenase (G6PD) deficiency
Ciprofloxacin	For use in patients on desferrioxamine with suspected *Yersinia* infection
	Stop iron chelation if suspected

particularly with the encapsulated organisms listed below, all of which can cause life-threatening sepsis:

- *Pneumococcus*
- *Salmonella* species
- *Haemophilus*.

Any suspected bacterial infection should be managed with prompt institution of IV antibiotics to cover these organisms. Suggested choices are listed in Table 5.11.B 4 (note that these may vary according to region and local sensitivities).

Persistent localised bone pain, swelling or fever should raise suspicion of osteomyelitis, which may require surgical treatment, and 6 weeks of antibiotic therapy

Specific infections
Osteomyelitis

This infection can be very difficult to distinguish from vaso-occlusive bone pain, which is commonly associated with localised swelling and joint effusions. Osteomyelitis should be considered in any child with persistent and localised pain who is systemically unwell.

The diagnosis of osteomyelitis in sickle-cell disease is more likely in the presence of:

- swinging pyrexia (fevers may not be persistent)
- severe systemic upset
- unusual swelling or pain
- positive blood cultures.

Few if any investigations are absolutely conclusive in making the diagnosis. Treatment is complex and may involve surgical intervention (rare) and a prolonged course of IV antibiotics (6 weeks). The oral route can be used to complete a course of antibiotics once the child is systemically well (i.e. fevers have settled) and any tests such as CRP have returned to normal. Antibiotic choices are broad, but may include the following:

- first line: IV ceftriaxone and clindamycin (consider flucloxacillin if no clindamycin available).
- second line: IV clindamycin.
- alternatives: meropenem, imipenem or ciprofloxacin.

Malaria

Studies confirm that sickle-cell trait (HbAS) is protective against severe complicated malaria, including cerebral malaria and severe anaemia related to malaria in children.

By contrast, malarial infection in homozygous sickle-cell disease (HbSS) can be rapidly fatal, and requires prompt recognition and urgent treatment. Although children with sickle-cell disease are not at greater risk of complicated malaria infection, once infected they have a higher mortality, especially related to severe anaemia. In addition to drug treatment, transfusion may be required.

Prevention should be emphasised (*see* Section 6.3.A.d).

Meningitis

Bacterial meningitis is more common in children with sickle-cell disease than in unaffected children, especially in the youngest age groups. The most frequent infecting organism is pneumococcus. Clinicians should maintain a high index of suspicion for this complication and treat it empirically.

Gastroenteritis/diarrhoea

Severe diarrhoea may precipitate sickling and crisis, including stroke. Hydration must therefore be maintained vigorously using ORS or IV fluid where necessary. Education relating to hand hygiene, clean water and prompt treatment should be given.

Children who are systemically unwell with a diarrhoeal illness may also be at higher risk of sepsis related to Gram-negative infection, and may require IV antibiotic treatment in addition to vigorous rehydration under such circumstances.

Children with diarrhoea who are also on the iron chelation medication desferrioxamine are at high risk of *Yersinia* or *Klebsiella* infection, and require prompt treatment with ciprofloxacin, alongside discontinuation of the desferrioxamine until they recover.

Viral infection

Children with sickle-cell disease are at particular risk of profound anaemia secondary to parvovirus B19 infection, which may trigger an aplastic crisis.

Children with sickle-cell disease should also be protected from blood-borne viral infection, specifically HIV and hepatitis B infection. Routine immunisation against HBV must be undertaken in view of the probability that a child with sickle-cell disease may at some stage be a recipient of blood products or be started on a long-term transfusion programme.

Severe anaemia in sickle-cell disease

Children with sickle-cell disease are known to have a compensated anaemia, but are also at risk of events that may precipitate a sudden and potentially fatal drop in their haemoglobin levels. The main conditions to consider are as follows:

- acute sequestration events
- aplastic crisis
- infection with malaria.

Acute sequestration events

Sequestration events are characterised by pooling of red cells in an organ, most commonly the spleen, lungs and liver, and are associated with a sudden and potentially life-threatening fall in haemoglobin level, with shock and collapse alongside rapid (and often painful) expansion of the organ affected.

Sequestration events are often precipitated by infection or sepsis that requires vigorous antibiotic treatment. There is a high mortality. Any child who appears to be deteriorating during an acute painful crisis should be re-examined to exclude undiagnosed sequestration.

Treatment includes administration of antibiotics to manage any precipitating infection, and blood transfusion in children with cardiovascular compromise, or who have a haemoglobin level of < 5 grams/dL, or where there has been a sharp fall in haemoglobin level by > 2 grams/dL.

Urgent blood transfusion in children with sickle-cell disease is not uncommon, but does carry some risks. Clinicians should be cautious about over-transfusing beyond a target of 8 grams/dL (usually a maximum of 20 mL/kg) or at a higher rate than 5 mL/kg/hour, due to the risks of hyperviscosity associated with a sudden increase in haematocrit.

Aplastic crisis

Transient red cell aplasia caused by parvovirus B19 (with an associated reticulocytopenia) can lead to a sudden severe worsening of the patient's anaemia. Ask about any recent viral prodromal illness, but classical erythema infectiosum ('slapped cheek syndrome') is uncommon. Second infections with parvovirus are extremely rare, as immunity to parvovirus is lifelong. Review other family members with sickle-cell disease, because they too may be infected with parvovirus.

The differential diagnosis of a sudden fall in haemoglobin level includes sequestration crisis, and therefore abdominal palpation is mandatory in any acutely anaemic child to exclude this diagnosis.

Treatment includes use of blood transfusion in children who are cardiovascularly compromised, if the haemoglobin level is < 5 grams/dL, or if there has been a sharp fall in haemoglobin level by > 2 grams/dL.

See above for the risks of urgent blood transfusion.

Acute chest syndrome (ACS)

This is a major cause of morbidity and mortality in sickle-cell disease. It is strictly defined by evidence of new pulmonary infiltrates involving at least one complete lung segment consistent with the presence of alveolar consolidation, but excluding atelectasis. Clinically, patients have chest pain, a temperature of more than 38.5°C, tachypnoea, wheezing, or cough usually associated with arterial desaturation.

It is important to recognise that patients can be in the process of developing ACS and be severely ill before these strict criteria are met. Signs of lung consolidation, usually bilateral, generally start at the bases, but may be unilateral and impossible to distinguish from infection.

Chest X-ray signs may lag or be misleading. Early treatment may prevent further deterioration, so **prompt action on clinical suspicion is essential**.

Acute sickle chest syndrome is likely to be multifactorial in origin, with infection, thrombosis of pulmonary arteries and fat embolism all resulting in potentially similar clinical patterns. The diagnosis of this potentially life-threatening crisis must therefore be considered if there is a combination of desaturation in air, tachypnoea, pain and a high fever.

Management of ACS

- Anticipatory clinical approach.
- Effective analgesia to prevent basal atelectasis.
- Careful observations, including regular pulse oximetry.
- Chest X-ray:
  - upper lobe consolidation without basal changes suggests pneumonia rather than ACS.
- Start dual IV antibiotics: treat pneumonia aggressively as it is often clinically indistinguishable.
- High-flow oxygen.
- Hyperhydration.
- Arterial gases in air if the oxygen requirement is rising.
- CPAP (if available) and saturations falling to the low 90s in air.
- Exchange transfusion (if available) if PaO$_2$ in air is < 8 kPa or the child is deteriorating.
- May require ventilation.
- There is no role for diuretics.

Neurological involvement in sickle-cell disease

Sickle-cell disease is associated with several central nervous system complications and events, as outlined below. The most significant event is stroke, mainly infarction. The treatment approach is outlined in the next section.

Neurological complications of sickle-cell disease

- Infection: meningitis and malaria.
- Stroke: ischaemic stroke, subarachnoid haemorrhage and transient ischaemic attacks (TIAs).
- Silent infarcts.
- Convulsions.
- Neurocognitive decline: reduction in IQ, attention deficits.

Stroke in sickle-cell disease

Stroke is a potentially devastating complication of sickle-cell disease, most commonly occurring in (but not limited to) individuals with homozygous disease (HbSS). The most common event is infarctive stroke, but haemorrhagic stroke can also occur with increasing frequency as children progress towards adulthood. Stroke can occur in any age group, but is most common in children under 10 years.

Predictive factors for stroke include a history of transient ischaemic attacks, a recent episode of acute chest syndrome, hypertension, or a low haemoglobin F percentage and/or low baseline haemoglobin levels. Any child with sickle-cell disease can have a stroke (even if they are apparently not 'high risk').

Precipitating factors for stroke include a recent history of fever, infection, dehydration and acute chest syndrome. However, some children will have a stroke without any identifiable precipitating event or risk factor.

Symptoms and signs of stroke can be broad, and range from the 'classic' presentation of a focal neurological deficit such as a hemiplegia (painless loss of function) to behavioural changes, severe headache, altered consciousness, convulsions or coma.

Historic data from the USA suggest that 11% of children with sickle-cell disease have a stroke episode by the age of 20 years. More recent data from well-resourced countries speculate that this figure is coming down with the advent of transcranial Doppler (TCD) screening to identify children at high risk of stroke and the aggressive use of regular long-term blood transfusion programmes as a primary prevention strategy.

Stroke is a major cause of mortality and morbidity in sickle-cell disease. On the long-term transfusion programme the risk of stroke falls to approximately 10%.

Treatment of acute stroke

Prompt treatment of an ischaemic stroke can potentially arrest a stroke in evolution. Children with a suspected stroke require:

- rehydration with fluids
- antibiotic treatment of any suspected infection, including malaria or meningitis
- treatment of any convulsions (see Section 5.16.D and E)
- exchange transfusion to reduce the circulating sickle percentage as rapidly as possible to less than 25%; this procedure is usually performed in a staged manner over 24–48 hours
- there is no role for aspirin in stroke related to sickle-cell disease.

In the absence of accessible exchange transfusion, it may be reasonable to consider a cautious top-up blood transfusion to maximise oxygen-carrying capacity and reduce the HbS percentage through a dilutional effect. Extreme care must be taken to avoid over-transfusion and the risk associated with increasing blood viscosity thus further contributing to the stroke. In either situation, the haematocrit should not exceed 0.4.

Most children make a good motor recovery from an initial stroke, but may be left with intellectual defects. If untreated, most of these children will suffer a second cerebrovascular accident, usually within 2–3 years of the first episode, as a result of which many of them will die and most will be seriously impaired. Transient ischaemic attacks may presage a more major event.

Secondary prevention of stroke

Because of the risk of a subsequent stroke, all children should be considered for the long-term transfusion programme to reduce their recurrence risk (although the risk is never fully eradicated). Most children require a top-up transfusion every 4 weeks for life, and this is a heavy burden for patients and their families.

The treatment goals of secondary prevention of stroke using the transfusion programme are as follows:

- to reduce and then maintain the pre-transfusion HbS% at below 30%
- to maintain the pre-transfusion haemoglobin level in the range 9–9.5 grams/dL
- in order to achieve these goals, the post-transfusion target is usually set no higher than 12.5 grams/dL
- to monitor and treat iron overload.

Note that there is no role for co-administration of desferrioxamine during transfusions.

Risks of the long-term transfusion programme include the following:

- transmission of bloodborne viral infection
- allo-immunisation to foreign red cell antigens
- iron overload.

In more well-resourced settings, some children may be able to receive alternatives to long-term top-up transfusions as outlined above. These alternatives include the use of manual or automated **exchange transfusions** to maintain a low HbS% without incurring iron overload states. These children may be able to go for longer periods between blood transfusions, although the risk of exposure to blood does not change.

Unfortunately, recent trials have indicated that there is little role for drugs such as hydroxyurea as an effective alternative to transfusion in the primary or secondary prevention of stroke.

Transcranial Doppler (TCD) and primary prevention of stroke

The use of annual TCD monitoring in more well-resourced countries is having a significant impact on the reduction of the incidence of stroke events in children with no prior apparent risk of stroke, and is now a routine screening tool in sickle-cell disease care.

Children are identified as at high risk of stroke if the recorded velocities on TCD persistently exceed 200 cm/second. The stroke risk can be significantly reduced from 40% in high-risk patients through the use of the long-term transfusion programme as outlined above. Unfortunately, once started, there is little evidence as to whether transfusions could ever be discontinued, as the data suggest that once transfusions are stopped the original stroke risk rapidly returns.

In areas where access to TCD machines and trained technicians may be limited, use of TCD may not be possible, particularly when weighing up the risks and benefits of the long-term transfusion programme.

Prevention programmes
Iron overload and transfusions

Children who are exposed to multiple and regular blood transfusions are likely to develop iron overload. The most widely available iron-chelating agent is desferrioxamine (Desferal), which is administered as a subcutaneous dose around 20–30 mg/kg over slow subcutaneous infusion (8–12 hours) for 5–7 nights per week. Many children become non-compliant with this regimen, and newer medications are available as outlined below.

TABLE 5.11.B.5 Drug treatments to reduce iron loading (iron chelation)

Drug	Advantages	Disadvantages	
Desferrioxamine	Well-understood safety profile through long-term use Cheap	Relatively poor iron chelation properties Poor patient compliance Risk of *Yersinia* infection	
Deferiprone	Oral administration Effective chelation agent	Requires close monitoring due to risk of sudden unexpected neutropenia and risk of overwhelming infection	
Deferasirox (Exjade)	Oral once-daily administration Well tolerated Highly effective iron chelation	Expensive Long-term safety profile not yet fully understood Common side effects are deranged urea and electrolytes and gastrointestinal upset Requires some monitoring	

Note: *see* Section 5.11.C for doses of newer iron chelation treatments

Prevention of infection

Prevention of infection is the mainstay of reducing mortality and morbidity in sickle-cell disease.

- All children should receive immunisation against *Pneumococcus, Haemophilus influenzae*, meningococcus and hepatitis B, in addition to any standard immunisation schedule.
- Pneumococcal immunisation should be as broad as possible, including pneumococcal conjugate vaccine **and** Pneumovax. Pneumovax should be given from the age of 2 years, every 5 years for life.
- All children should receive prophylactic penicillin V (erythromycin or clarithromycin can be used as an alternative):
  — age up to 1 year: penicillin 62.5 mg twice a day
  — age up to 5 years: penicillin 125 mg twice a day
  — age 5 years or over: penicillin 250 mg twice a day into adulthood.
- All children should be protected from malaria infection (*see* Section 6.3.A.d).
- Families should be counselled about prevention, risks and signs of infection, so that they can seek prompt treatment.

Prevention of crises

- Maintain good fluid intake, especially during gastroenteritis or other infections.
- Folic acid:
  — age up to 1 year: 1 mg daily
  — age up to 5 years: 2.5 mg daily
  — age 5 years or over: 5 mg daily into adulthood.
- Families should be taught how to feel their child's abdomen in order to identify the onset of a sequestration crisis.
- Hydroxyurea (hydroxycarbamide) may raise baseline haemoglobin levels by promoting fetal haemoglobin (HbF) production. This may reduce the frequency and severity of crises in children. However, it is myelosuppressive and should be used with caution and only where facilities for monitoring blood counts exist and the dose can be monitored carefully.

Splenectomy (and surgery) in sickle-cell disease

Splenectomy is not routinely undertaken in children with sickle-cell disease, although it does have a role in allowing the baseline haemoglobin to rise by approximately 2 grams/dL in children with evidence of hypersplenism.

Splenectomy may also be indicated in children who have had an episode of life-threatening splenic sequestration.

As with all surgical procedures in sickle-cell disease, careful risk assessment should be undertaken before a planned procedure involving a general anaesthetic, due to the risk of post-operative sickling secondary to hypoxaemia and cold. Current advice suggests that children with sickle-cell disease undergoing moderate- or low-risk surgical procedures should be considered for a pre-operative transfusion to bring their haemoglobin level up towards (but not higher than) 10 grams/dL, to maximise oxygen-carrying capacity.

Growth

Growth failure and delayed puberty are common in children with sickle-cell disease, especially in those with hypersplenism or who have had multiple acute sickle crises. Weight tends to be affected more than height, and malnutrition is a major factor in determining whether children achieve their full growth potential.

Puberty may be delayed because of hypersplenism or malnutrition because of the hyper-metabolic state and inadequate nutrition.

Dietary advice, treatment of any chronic infections and possibly splenectomy (if hypersplenism is present) may be helpful. Occasionally, children may benefit from temporary use of the monthly transfusion programme to assist them into puberty.

Priapism

Priapism is a serious but under-reported complication of sickle-cell disease. If untreated, it can lead to fibrosis of the corpus cavernosa and impotence, a risk which appears to be lower in pre-pubertal boys. The duration of an episode predicts the overall outcome. Therefore prompt recognition and management are essential.

Patients typically present with an erect painful penis, which may be precipitated by a painful sickle crisis, fever, dehydration, use of recreational drugs, or sexual activity.

Acute fulminant priapism is characterised by a prolonged and sustained episode, more than 4 hours in duration. In stuttering priapism, episodes are repetitive and may be individually brief. Patients may have a combination of both of these events.

Treatment of acute priapism is still the subject of much debate. Current best practice suggests the initial use of warm baths, exercise, hydration and gentle sedation while preparing for a more definitive intervention. Subsequent definitive treatment choices include aspiration of blood from the corpus cavernosum followed by surgical washout using saline (irrigation) or adrenergic agonists, which can be performed under conscious sedation. The goal is rapid detumescence within 4–12 hours of the procedure. Ideally, treatment should start within 2 hours of an episode. After 12 hours the patient may require surgical intervention to achieve detumescence. Exchange transfusion (the target haemoglobin concentration is approximately 10 grams/dL, with a haematocrit no higher than 0.4) may be required.

There is still considerable debate about the best treatment options for stuttering priapism, and this is the subject of an ongoing international trial (PISCES). Currently patients with stuttering priapism can be advised to try gentle exercise and warm baths. A preventative approach may be needed, and the following options are available:

- Pseudoephedrine at 30 mg/kg/day, increasing to 60 mg/kg four times a day:
  - alternatively give etilefrine 0.25 mg/kg twice a day
  - both of these drugs are part of the ongoing PISCES trial (2011).
- Hydroxyurea at 10–30 mg/kg/day.
- Use of the long-term transfusion programme.

Other problems

- Around 30% of SS children suffer from **sleep-related upper airways obstruction** with consequent hypoxaemia. Nocturnal hypoxaemia has been increasingly identified as a risk factor for acute chest syndrome (and possibly an independent risk factor for stroke) in children with sickle-cell disease, and marked improvement can occur after adeno-tonsillectomy. Treatment is as indicated for other children with upper airways obstruction (*see* Section 5.1.D).
- Chronic pain resulting from damage caused by acute vaso-occlusive crises occurs, and other pain secondary to the haemolytic process can occur.
- Avascular necrosis of the hip or shoulder can occur as young as 6 years, although it is uncommon before adolescence. The initial presentation may be with the acute vaso-occlusive crisis, but once disintegration of the femoral head occurs, the pain is of a chronic osteoarthritic type, and should be managed as such.
- Leg ulcers that can become seriously infected are common, and their prevalence rises with age. Appropriate antibiotics such as erythromycin and flucloxacillin, wound cleaning and protection together with rest and elevation of the leg are helpful. Compression stockings may also be of benefit.
- Children develop a renal tubular concentrating defect by the age of 2 years. During adolescence, proteinuria, the nephrotic syndrome or chronic renal failure may develop.
- Renal papillary necrosis may produce haematuria, urinary tract infection and renal colic. Rarely the haematuria is severe and blood transfusion is required. Renal colic is treated with copious fluids and adequate analgesia.
- Many patients are chronically jaundiced with exacerbations. There is no treatment, and reassurance should be given that this rarely represents liver failure.
- Gallstones are common, due to pigment from haemolysis. The pain can mimic an acute painful crisis. Treatment is surgical. Antibiotic treatment of cholecystitis with amoxicillin and metronidazole may be required.

5.11.C Haemolytic anaemias

> **BOX 5.11.C.1 Minimum standards**
> - Folic acid.
> - Screened blood for transfusion.
> - Splenectomy.
> - Iron chelation therapy: desferrioxamine.
> - Pneumococcal vaccine/penicillin.
> - Meningococcal vaccine.
> - *Haemophilus influenzae* type B (HiB) vaccine.

Definition

Haemolytic anaemias are disorders characterised by a reduction in the lifespan of red blood cells, and may be congenital or acquired.

Clinical features of haemolytic anaemia

These include **pallor, jaundice, splenomegaly** and **gallstones.**

The degree of splenomegaly can be a useful clue to the cause of haemolytic anaemia.

TABLE 5.11.C.1 The differences between congenital and acquired haemolytic anaemia

Congenital	Acquired
Haemoglobin defects: sickle-cell disease, thalassaemia	Infection: malaria, visceral leishmaniasis
Red cell enzyme defects: G6PD, pyruvate kinase deficiency	Alloimmune: haemolytic disease of the newborn, transfusion reactions
Red cell membrane defects: spherocytosis, elliptocytosis	Red cell fragmentation: haemolytic–uraemic syndrome
	Autoimmune infection (e.g. EBV, CMV, HIV, mycoplasma), malignancies (lymphomas, leukaemias), immune deficiencies
	Drugs
	Burns

TABLE 5.11.C.2 Degree of splenomegaly in haemolytic anaemias

With minor splenomegaly	With marked splenomegaly
G6PD deficiency	Sickle-cell disease
Autoimmune haemolytic anaemia	Beta-thalassaemia major
Haemolytic–uraemic syndrome	Hb E beta-thalassaemia
Beta-thalassaemia minor	Hereditary spherocytosis
Hb H alpha-thalassaemia syndrome	Hyper-reactive malarial splenomegaly (tropical splenomegaly)
	Visceral leishmaniasis (kala-azar)

Laboratory features of haemolytic anaemias: general

These include low haemoglobin, increased reticulocyte count, raised and predominantly unconjugated bilirubin, pink plasma after centrifuging of blood (due to free haemoglobin) in severe cases, reduced haptoglobin, and increased urinary urobilinogen.

Hereditary haemolytic anaemias
Red cell membrane defects (dominant inheritance)
Spherocytosis

This is the most common haemolytic anaemia due to a membrane defect. It may present at any time from birth to old age, and varies in severity from patients with haemoglobin concentrations of 4–5 grams/dL to asymptomatic individuals with normal haemoglobin levels. Acute haemolytic or aplastic crises may be triggered by viral infections. These usually last for 10–14 days, but may result in sudden severe anaemia requiring transfusion.

Diagnosis

- Along with a positive family history, the clinical features are mild jaundice, pallor and splenomegaly. Gallstones may occur in children.
- Laboratory features: blood film shows spherocytes, increased osmotic fragility of red cells, increased reticulocytes, negative antiglobulin (Coombs') test.

Treatment

- Folic acid 1 month–12 years 2.5–5 mg daily; 12–18 years 5–10 mg daily.
- Severely anaemic and symptomatic moderately anaemic children may benefit from splenectomy if the facilities available make this a low-risk procedure.
  - Splenectomy carries a major risk of lifelong increased vulnerability to infection with capsulated bacteria such as pneumococci, meningococci and *Haemophilus influenzae* type B. The risks and benefits need to be weighed up very carefully before splenectomy is undertaken.
  - Delay splenectomy until after the age of 5–10 years if possible.
- Administration of **pneumococcal, meningococcal and HiB vaccine** prior to splenectomy, and lifelong prophylactic oral **penicillin** thereafter (under 12 months of age,

62.5 mg twice daily; 1–5 years 125 mg twice daily; over 5 years 250 mg twice daily).

Elliptocytosis

This condition is less common than spherocytosis. It is rare in European populations, but is seen more often in West Africa. In South-East Asia there is a variant, South-East Asian ovalocytosis (SAO), which causes oval-shaped red cells and neonatal hyperbilirubinaemia, but little haemolysis later in life.

Diagnosis

- Blood film shows 25–90% of oval, elliptical or rod-shaped red blood cells.
- Homozygotes tend to have severe haemolytic anaemia from infancy.

Treatment

This is the same as for spherocytosis.

Stomatocytosis

Hereditary stomatocytosis is rare, but it can be acquired in several conditions, especially liver disease. The hereditary form may cause neonatal oedema and ascites which resolves spontaneously.

Diagnosis

Blood film shows erythrocytes with a central mouth-like slit (stomatocytes).

Treatment

This is the same as for spherocytosis, but **splenectomy is ineffective and may be harmful**, leading to a thrombotic tendency.

Metabolic defects
Glucose-6-phosphate dehydrogenase deficiency (G6PD) (X-linked)

There are two types of normal G6PD enzymes (types A and B). Worldwide, there may be 100 million people with diminished red cell G6PD activity. G6PD A deficiency is common in black children, and their G6PD function is reduced to about 10% of normal. G6PD B deficiency (G6PD Mediterranean) is less common, and the enzyme activity is reduced to 1–3%; this and the Chinese variant of G6PD deficiency are the more severe forms of the disease.

Clinical features

Severe enzyme deficiency causes chronic haemolytic anaemia and jaundice.

Haemoglobinuria may occur with less than 10% enzyme activity, and severe episodes of haemolysis occur with oxidant stress:

- favism due to ingestion of the fava broad bean or inhalation of its pollen
- oxidant drugs such as antimalarial drugs, sulphonamides, high-dose aspirin, non-steroidal anti-inflammatory drugs (NSAIDs), quinidine, quinine, nitrofurantoin, phenacetin and vitamin K analogues
- other chemicals, such as those in mothballs, can also trigger an episode.

Diagnosis

- Blood film shows 'blister' and 'bite' cells. Heinz bodies may be seen on unstained blood film.
- Enzyme assay (if available) is needed to make the diagnosis (but this may be normal if reticulocyte numbers are raised). It may be necessary to wait several weeks after an acute episode before measuring enzyme levels.

Treatment

- Avoid drugs that cause oxidant stress (i.e. chloroquine, primaquine, sulphonamides, nitrofurantoin, quinolones, dapsone, high-dose aspirin, phenacetin) or fava beans. If primaquine is necessary, this can be given weekly for 8 weeks.
- Patients usually recover spontaneously once the precipitating factors have been removed.
- Transfusion may be necessary if there is severe haemolysis.

Pyruvate kinase deficiency (autosomal recessive)

This is the second commonest enzyme defect of the glycolytic pathway, and affects mainly northern Europeans.

Clinical features

These are very variable.

- Neonates may have severe haemolysis and present with early jaundice (within 48 hours), anaemia and hyperbilirubinaemia.
- In older children, haemolysis is variable and may be asymptomatic or lead to poor growth, delayed puberty and the skeletal changes associated with chronic haemolysis, such as maxillary prominence and frontal bossing and an increased tendency to long bone fractures.

Diagnosis

- Blood film shows increased reticulocytes, Heinz bodies and mild macrocytosis.
- Enzyme assay for pyruvate kinase.

Treatment

- Folic acid (250 micrograms/kg once daily).
- Splenectomy (only if the facilities available make this a low-risk procedure).
- Transfusion if there is severe anaemia or an aplastic crisis.

Haemoglobin defects

- Abnormal variants: sickle (see Section 5.11.B), Hb C, Hb E, Hb D, etc.
- Defective synthesis: thalassaemias.
- Beta-thalassaemia major (autosomal recessive).

Beta-thalassaemia major

In this condition there is a complete or almost complete absence of the beta-globin chain synthesis. There is a high incidence of the beta-thalassaemia gene (1–15%) in southern Europe, the Middle East, India, Pakistan and South-East Asia.

Clinical features

- Anaemia, which becomes obvious by 3 months.
- Weakness and tiredness.

- Failure to thrive, intermittent fever and poor feeding.
- Cardiac failure may develop.
- Infections and splenomegaly.
- Stunted growth with skeletal changes (e.g. frontal bossing, maxillary hyperplasia, increased tendency to fractures).
- Increased skin pigmentation.
- Delayed puberty.

Diagnosis

- Blood film shows microcytosis, anisocytosis, and hypochromic and nucleated red cells.
- Haemoglobin electrophoresis: Hb F increased (10–90%), Hb A absent, Hb A_2 can be reduced, normal or occasionally elevated.
- Serum iron and ferritin levels are increased.
- Reticulocyte numbers are often lower than expected for the degree of anaemia.

Management of beta-thalassaemia major

Management is by regular blood transfusion and iron chelation therapy to reduce iron deposition in tissues, especially the heart, liver and endocrine glands (transfusion haemosiderosis).

Blood transfusion

- Monitor haemoglobin levels, growth and development, and **transfuse when the child stops developing or when the haemoglobin concentration is less than 7 grams/dL in the absence of infection.**
- **Blood should be ABO, rhesus (Dd, Cc, Ee) and Kell matched and filtered to avoid allo-immunisation and transfusion reactions.**
- Immunise against hepatitis B prior to transfusion.
- Transfuse 20 mL/kg of filtered red cell concentrate over 2–3 hours.
- To monitor, calculate the transfused red cell concentrate in mL/kg yearly. If blood consumption is > 300 mL/kg, investigate the cause.
- Increased blood consumption may be due to large spleen, large liver, autoimmune haemolytic anaemia or multiple allo-antibodies.
- To prevent bone deformities, osteoporosis and extramedullary haematopoiesis, **aim for a pre-transfusion level of not less than 9 grams/dL.**
- Pre-transfusion haemoglobin is mandatory. Post-transfusion haemoglobin is optional.
- As a rule, the haemoglobin level drops by 1 gram/week in splenectomised children, whereas in non-splenectomised patients it drops by 1.5 grams/week.
- Monitor serum ferritin levels (normal range is 7–200 micrograms/litre in children over 5 months old).

Iron chelation

- To avoid damage to the endocrine glands, liver and heart, iron chelation should be started when the **serum ferritin level is around 1000 micrograms/litre.**
  1. Desferrioxamine infusion IV or subcutaneous given slowly over 10–12 hours. The initial dose should not exceed 30 mg/kg desferrioxamine in 10 mL of water for injection, followed by maintenance doses of 20–50 mg/kg each over 10–12 hours on 3–7 nights a week.
     Too much desferrioxamine can cause growth,

hearing and eyesight problems. Give 100–200 mg vitamin C orally at the same time as desferrioxamine. This enhances iron excretion in the urine, but it should be given separately from food as it also enhances iron absorption from food. Desferrioxamine should not be given to children with cardiac dysfunction.

2. Oral chelation (Deferiprone or Deferasirox) may be used when desferrioxamine is not available or not tolerated. These drugs are much more acceptable to children than desferroxamine as they are oral rather than a long overnight infusion but they have significant side effects.

- Deferiprone by mouth: child 6–18 years 25 mg/kg 3 times daily (maximum 40 mg/kg daily).
- Deferasirox by mouth: child 2–18 years initially 10–30 mg/kg once daily according to serum-ferritin concentration. For maintenance, consult product literature.
- The most serious side effect is neutropenia.
- Monitor the neutrophil count every 2 weeks.
- If the neutrophil count is less than 1.0×10^9/litre, stop iron chelation and monitor recovery.
- If infection is present, the neutrophil count is less than 0.5×10^9/litre and there are symptoms, take blood cultures and treat with a broad-spectrum antibiotic to prevent septicaemia.
- Other side effects are joint pain, nausea, fluctuating liver enzymes and zinc deficiency.

Monitoring treatment
- Measure height and weight, plot height velocity and watch for delayed puberty.
- To avoid psychological trauma and ensure the development of secondary sexual characteristics, treat if no signs of sexual development have occurred by 16 years of age (see Section 5.8.C).
- Check the following at least twice yearly: serum ferritin (iron overload), liver function tests, calcium, phosphate, alkaline phosphatase (hypoparathyroidism, tetany).
- Undertake yearly screening for HCV and HIV infection.
- If HCV is positive, assess viraemia (serotype) if possible, perform a liver biopsy and give interferon with or without ribavirin to avoid cirrhosis and hepatoma.
- If HIV-positive, continue transfusions and give the latest available antiviral treatment.
- All blood donors should be tested for HCV and HIV.

Acquired haemolytic anaemia
Immune mediated
- Haemolytic transfusion reaction.
- Haemolytic disease of the newborn (see Section 3.4).

- Hypersplenism.
- Secondary to infection: EBV, CMV, *Mycoplasma*, rarely HIV.
- Secondary to malignancies: lymphomas, leukaemias.
- Secondary to autoimmune diseases: SLE, rheumatoid arthritis.

Diagnosis
- Anaemia with increased reticulocytes.
- Splenomegaly.
- Positive direct Coombs' test.

Management
- Most secondary cases (70–80%) are transient, lasting about 3 months.
- Infants and older children may develop the chronic form.
- Treatment may not be needed if the symptoms are not severe.
- Transfusion may be necessary if there is severe haemolysis.
- Steroids: prednisolone 2 mg/kg/day (up to 6 mg/kg/day in severe cases) can be given if treatment is needed until the rate of haemolysis declines, and then stopped gradually.

Malaria
See Section 6.3.A.d.

Secondary to organ disease
Renal failure (see Section 5.6.C).
   Liver disease (see Section 5.7.B).

Burns
See Section 7.3.I.b.

Miscellaneous
- Chemicals and drugs.
- Toxins (e.g. *Haemophilus influenzae* type B, staphylococcal, streptococcal, clostridial).
- Venoms (e.g. cobra, viper, rattlesnake, bee, wasp, yellow jacket).

Reference
British Committee for Standards in Haematology. www.bcshguidelines.com (up-to-date guidelines on spherocytosis and infection risk in people who have had splenectomy).

5.11.D Blood clotting disorders

BOX 5.11.D.1 Minimum standards
- Regional/national centre.
- Prednisolone.
- Immunisation; hepatitis B.
- Blood clotting products.
- Desmopressin and tranexamic acid.

Factor deficiencies

The incidence of haemophilia is similar worldwide, at around 1 in 5000–10 000 male births. Major advances have been made in both separating haemophilia A (factor VIII deficiency) and haemophilia B (factor IX deficiency) and delivering safe therapeutic intervention with replacement therapy. However, this is only available to the 20% of haemophiliacs who live in well-resourced countries. For those in resource-limited countries, severe haemophilia continues to be a personal and social disaster, with affected boys becoming progressively crippled during childhood from spontaneous painful intractable haemorrhages into muscles and joints. These boys commonly die in childhood or early adulthood. Severe deficiencies of the other coagulation factors (X, XI, VII, V, XIII, fibrinogen and von Willebrand factor) are also associated with severe and sometimes life-threatening or fatal haemorrhage.

- The largest barrier to providing replacement therapy is its high cost.
- There are also non-financial barriers, including insufficient knowledge even among the medical community, lack of a proper healthcare structure, and low levels of literacy.
- In the last decade the WHO and the World Federation of Haemophilia (WFH) have made considerable progress in setting up programmes in resource-limited countries.
- The WHO has identified the following as core components:
  - training of care providers and the establishing of care centres
  - identification and registration of people with haemophilia
  - improving social awareness of haemophilia
  - prevention of haemophilia
  - providing safe therapeutic products
  - developing a programme of comprehensive care.

How can delivery of haemophilia care be implemented in resource-limited countries?

- National haemophilia societies are crucial. In addition to supporting affected families, they can lobby for support from the healthcare budget.
- The WHO and WFH have visiting teams that have contributed to education and improvement through these national groups. They include international haemophilia training fellowships, workshops and twinning programmes, in order to transfer knowledge and diagnostic expertise to these embryo services.
- It is important that those planning healthcare fully appreciate that provision of laboratory diagnostic services for haemophilia and the development of safe blood transfusion services to provide safe replacement therapy will benefit a wide range of medical services.

How should the service be built and structured?

- At least one national centre should be created where the laboratory, scientific and medical expertise exists to make an accurate diagnosis, which will then allow the appropriate counselling, including genetic counselling, of the patient's family (similar to a national centre for cancer therapy with links to centres in well-resourced countries: see Section 5.14). With advances in molecular biology, carriers of haemophilia can currently be identified and antenatal diagnosis provided so that a choice can be made to prevent the birth of haemophiliac boys, particularly if treatment is not available.
- National registers should be set up for service planning.
- A clinical service involving paediatricians, dentists, orthopaedic surgeons and adult physicians needs to be set up. Safe replacement therapy, probably initially derived from donated plasma, should be developed.
- Donor screening and product treatment to remove the risk of at least HIV and hepatitis B and C infection must be provided.
- Haemophiliacs should be vaccinated at an early age against hepatitis B.

What treatment should be given in the absence of replacement therapy?

Spontaneous haemorrhages into muscles and joints can be extremely painful and will lead to progressive crippling deformities. The acute episode must be managed with bed rest. For bleeds such as those in the knees, splinting with a back slab to restrict movement may help. Analgesia for the pain is also required (see Section 1.15). Opiates may be needed to obtain adequate pain relief. Bleeding with loss of first dentition may be severe enough to warrant blood transfusion.

In mild to moderate cases, desmopressin (DDAVP) can be helpful.

- **By intravenous infusion over 20 minutes:** Child 1 month–18 years 300 nanograms/kg as a single dose immediately before surgery or after trauma; may be repeated at intervals of 12 hours if no tachycardia.
- **Intranasally:** Child 1–18 years 4 micrograms/kg as a single dose. For pre-operative use, give 2 hours before procedure.

Avoid drugs that impair haemostasis, such as aspirin and non-steroidal anti-inflammatory drugs (NSAIDs) (e.g. ibuprofen).

Platelet deficiencies: idiopathic thrombocytopenic purpura (ITP)

- Isolated thrombocytopenia usually follows a viral infection 1–3 weeks previously.
- Boys and girls are equally affected, and the peak incidence is in those aged 2–4 years.

- There is a 90% probability of complete remission, but those presenting over the age of 10 years are more likely to have chronic ITP.
- ITP that persists for 6 months is defined as chronic.
- Children with chronic ITP are more likely to have an underlying cause (e.g. autoimmune disease).
- Bleeding manifestations include petechiae, purpura, epistaxes, haematuria, gastrointestinal haemorrhage and (rarely) intracerebral haemorrhage. The child has no hepatosplenomegaly and is usually well.
- Other causes of thrombocytopenia must be excluded. If there is any doubt, a bone-marrow aspirate will show normal haematopoiesis with increased numbers of megakaryocytes in ITP.

Management

- Treatment is based on symptoms, **not platelet count**, and many patients require no treatment.
- Petechiae on the head and neck, and gastrointestinal and oral bleeding, are indicators for prednisolone (1–2 mg/kg/day after food in two divided doses for no more than 14 days or 4 mg/kg for no more than 4 days; reduce over 5 days and stop irrespective of the platelet count if the patient is asymptomatic). Prednisolone does not alter the course of the disease. The time to remission is very variable.
- Tranexamic acid can be useful in the treatment of mucosal bleeding. Give 10 mg/kg IV slowly over 10 minutes in children 6–18 years (maximum 1 gram) followed by 25 milligrams/kg orally (maximum 1.5 gram) three times daily for 2–8 days.
- Hormonal treatment can benefit girls with menorrhagia. In addition Tranexamic acid 1 gram orally 3 times daily for up to 4 days can help (initiate when menstruation starts).
- Chronic ITP with serious bleeding into the gastrointestinal tract or brain may require splenectomy. However, in resource-limited countries there is a high risk of infection following splenectomy, and long-term penicillin prophylaxis and pneumococcal vaccination are required.

Reference
Grainger JD, Rees JL, Reeves M *et al.* (2012) Changing trends in the UK management of childhood ITP. *Archives of Disease in Childhood*, **97**, 8–11.

5.12 Gastrointestinal disorders

5.12.A Acute diarrhoea

> **BOX 5.12.A.1 Minimum standards**
> - Reduced-osmolarity ORS.
> - ReSoMal for children with severe malnutrition.
> - IV fluids: Hartmann's or Ringer-lactate solution with glucose 5% or 10% to prevent hypoglycaemia.
> - Potassium: oral and IV.
> - ABC resuscitation for shock.
> - Antibiotics: co-trimoxazole, amoxicillin, nalidixic acid, ciprofloxacin, cefotaxime, chloramphenicol, erythromycin, metronidazole, tetracycline, vancomycin, doxycycline.

Important issues

- Shock management, rehydration therapy and continued feeding are key strategies.
- Antibiotics are **not** given routinely, but they are indicated in bloody diarrhoea (probable *Shigella* infection) and suspected cholera.
- Antidiarrhoeal drugs and anti-emetics should never be given and can be dangerous in children.
- Zinc supplementation speeds recovery and helps to prevent further episodes.

Introduction

Diarrhoeal diseases are a leading cause of childhood morbidity and mortality in resource-limited countries. In 2001, an estimated 1.5 million children under 5 years of age died from diarrhoea, 80% of them in the first 2 years of life. Around 50% of these deaths are due to watery diarrhoea and occur either because of lack of access to oral rehydration solution (ORS) or because of incorrect case management. About one-third of deaths are caused by persistent diarrhoea and the remainder (approximately 15%) are caused by dysentery.

This section is primarily aimed at the management of the infant and child under 5 years as they are the most seriously affected. There are particular problems in managing children with severe co-morbidities: these include significant malnutrition and anaemia (Hb below 6 G/dL *see* Sections 5.10.B and 5.11.A). In these children, assessment is more difficult and there is likely to be an abnormal response to a fluid load because of poor cardiac function. Modifications to the management plans for these children largely involve slower shock management and rehydration, the careful use of blood transfusion and diuretics and very frequent re-assessment.

ORS has been a simple and effective solution, reducing morbidity and mortality in diarrhoeal illness. The new low-osmolarity ORS reduces by 33% the need for supplemental

IV fluid therapy after initial rehydration compared with the previous standard WHO ORS solution. The new ORS also reduces the incidence of vomiting by 30% and stool volume by 20%.

In addition, zinc supplementation has been shown to significantly reduce the severity and duration of diarrhoea.

Definition

Diarrhoea is the passage of loose or watery stools, usually at least three times in a 24-hour period. However, it is the consistency of the stools rather than the number that is most important. Mothers usually know when their children have diarrhoea, and may provide useful working definitions in local situations. The volume of fluid lost through the stools in 24 hours can range from 5 mL/kg (near normal) to 200 mL/kg, or more. Dehydration occurs when these losses are not replaced adequately and a deficit of water and electrolytes develops. The concentrations and amounts of electrolytes lost also vary. The total body sodium deficit in young children with severe dehydration due to diarrhoea is usually about 70–110 millimoles/litre of water deficit. Potassium and chloride losses are in a similar range.

The most common causes of diarrhoea are rotavirus, enterotoxigenic *E. coli* (ETEC) and, during epidemics, *Vibrio cholerae* O1 or O139.

Classification of diarrhoea

- **Acute watery diarrhoea** (including cholera): this lasts from several hours to days. The main danger is dehydration, and malnutrition also occurs if feeding is not continued. If there is a current epidemic, cholera is likely and causes severe dehydration with a positive stool culture for *Vibrio cholerae* O1 or O139.
- **Acute bloody diarrhoea**, or dysentery (blood is mixed in with stool): the main dangers are intestinal damage, sepsis and malnutrition. Other complications, including dehydration, may also occur.
- **Persistent diarrhoea:** this is defined as passage of three or more loose watery stools in a 24-hour period, which lasts for 14 days or longer. The main danger is malnutrition and serious non-intestinal infection; dehydration may also occur (*see* Section 5.12.B).
- **Diarrhoea with severe malnutrition** (marasmus or kwashiorkor): the main dangers are severe systemic infection, dehydration, heart failure and vitamin and mineral deficiency (*see* Section 5.10.A).
- **Diarrhoea associated with a recent course of broad-spectrum oral antibiotics.**

Assessment of the child with diarrhoea

- Fever, vomiting and loose stools are the common symptoms of acute gastroenteritis.
- If possible, rule out other serious illness (e.g. meningitis, malaria, bacterial sepsis).
- Assess for degree of dehydration, bloody diarrhoea, persistent diarrhoea, malnutrition and serious non-intestinal infections.

History

Specific points to enquire about in the history include the following:

- duration of diarrhoea
- presence of blood in the stool
- local knowledge or reports of a cholera epidemic
- recent use of antibiotics
- the presence of fever, cough or other important problems (e.g. convulsions, measles)
- usual feeding practices
- the type and amount of fluids (including breast milk) and food taken during the illness
- drugs or other remedies taken
- immunisation history.

Physical examination

First assess the patient for shock and treat this urgently as a priority if it is present. Children with shock will have reduced consciousness, a high and increasing heart rate, weak pulse, poor skin circulation time with prolonged capillary refill time (> 3 seconds), and low or even unmeasurable blood pressure.

Children with shock require immediate resuscitation (ABC), including high concentrations of oxygen (if available) and an IV bolus of 10–20 mL/kg of either Ringer-lactate or Hartmann's solution given as rapidly as possible (*see* Section 5.5.B). If IV access is not possible (often the veins are collapsed), consider the intra-osseous route (*see* Section 8.4.B). If shock is not relieved by 20 mL/kg, give another bolus of 10–20 mL/kg, but watch very carefully for fluid overload and in particular pulmonary oedema (this is most likely if the patient is also severely anaemic and will be shown by increasing breathlessness, crepitations may be heard).

The examination includes measurement of vital signs together with clinical correlation. The degree of dehydration is graded according to signs and symptoms that reflect the amount of fluid lost (*see* Table 5.12.A.2). Infants with acute diarrhoea are more apt to dehydrate than are older children, because they have a higher body surface area to weight ratio, have a higher metabolic rate, and are dependent on others for fluid. Although the most accurate assessment of fluid status is acute weight change, the patient's premorbid weight is often not known.

In severe dehydration, prolonged skin retraction time and decreased perfusion are more reliably predictive of dehydration than a sunken fontanelle or the absence of tears. A good correlation has been reported between capillary refill time and fluid deficit. However, fever, ambient temperature and age can affect capillary refill time as well. **In severe dehydration, shock and death soon follow if rehydration is not started quickly.**

Children with some dehydration or severe dehydration should be weighed without clothing when estimating their fluid requirements. If weighing is not possible, the child's age may be used to estimate their weight:

- Weight = (age in years + 4) × 2 for children less than 10 years old.
- For an infant up to 1 year old, birth weight doubles by 5 months and triples by 1 year.

Treatment should never be delayed because facilities for weighing are not rapidly available.

In addition:

- Look for an abdominal mass or abdominal distension.
- In an infant less than 1 week old, diarrhoea is sometimes a sign of neonatal sepsis (*see* Section 3.4). In an infant, blood in the stool may be due to an intussusception (*see* Section 5.19).

Remember other diagnoses, including typhoid, antibiotic-associated colitis and (rarely) inflammatory bowel disease (*see* Section 5.12.D).

Investigations

Laboratory investigations are rarely needed at the outset. Serum electrolytes, especially sodium or potassium concentrations, are useful in severe dehydration and for monitoring progress, if available. Stool cultures should be undertaken if at all possible in dysentery (bloody diarrhoea), but are not needed to initiate treatment in the usual case of acute watery diarrhoea. Stool microscopy can be useful for diagnosing *Giardia lamblia, Cryptosporidium* and amoebic dysentery.

Principles of case management

There are five essential elements of the management of all children with diarrhoea:

- **Resuscitation from shock, if present:** Give IV boluses of Hartmann's solution or Ringer-lactate solution. This needs to be done rapidly (caution is required in malnutrition and anaemia; *see* Section 5.10.B). Improvement in conscious level is a good indicator of response to circulatory shock treatment.
- **Rehydration therapy:** this should be done more slowly, so as not to cause rapid metabolic change.
- **Maintenance therapy:** this is to replicate the normal fluid needs and any ongoing extra losses.
- **Zinc supplementation.**
- **Continued feeding.**

Calculating fluid requirements

WHO Plans A to C for gastroenteritis in children (*see* Appendix to this section) include estimates of total fluid requirements, and assume that most children will be drinking by 4 hours into treatment and thus able to 'self-regulate'. For patients for whom this is not the case, fluid management can be undertaken using the following guidelines.

Estimating fluid requirements

The amount of fluid that the child needs over a 24-hour period needs to be calculated. It is the sum of:

estimated fluid deficit + maintenance requirements + ongoing losses.

Deficit

If an accurate recent pre-illness weight is available, subtract the current weight to estimate lost fluid (1 kg = 1 litre of fluid).

For example, a child who weighed 9.2 kg is seen with diarrhoea and weighs 8.3 kg:

estimated fluid loss is (9.2 − 8.3) kg = 0.9 kg = 900 mL deficit, i.e. 10% dehydrated.

If no recent weight is available, or the recorded weight is considered to be unreliable, assess the degree of dehydration as described in Table 5.12.A.2.

Weigh the child (or estimate their weight from their age as follows: weight (kg) = 2 × [age (years) + 4]) if over one year.

Then use the following formula: percentage dehydration × weight (kg) × 10 = deficit (in mL).

For example, a child whose weight is estimated to be 10 kg is 10% dehydrated.

Their estimated fluid loss is 10 × 10 × 10 = 1000 mL (40 mL/hour if replaced over 24 hours).

Maintenance

TABLE 5.12.A.1 Estimated maintenance fluid requirements based on body weight for a child

Body weight	Fluid needed per day	Fluid needed per hour
First 10 kg of body weight	100 mL/kg	4 mL/kg
Second 10 kg of body weight	50 mL/kg	2 mL/kg
Subsequent kg	20 mL/kg	1 mL/kg

Ongoing losses

For each diarrhoeal stool:
- < 2 years of age: give 50–100 mL or 10 mL/kg
- ≥ 2 years of age: give 100–200 mL or a cup or small glass if drinking or tolerating NG fluid.

For each vomit: use 2 mL/kg ORS, and give small frequent volumes (e.g. 5 mL/minute in a child) via a spoon, syringe or cup. Gradually increase the amount given and closely supervise this.

For nasogastric tube aspirates: replace volume for volume with either ORS or Ringer-lactate solution with 5% or 10% glucose **or** Hartmann's solution with 5% or 10% glucose.

Signs of over-hydration

- Oedematous (puffy) eyelids.
- Heart failure (especially in severe malnutrition), chronic malnutrition or protein-losing enteropathy: look for tachycardia, tachypnea, crepitations at the lung bases, hepatomegaly or gallop rhythm (*see* Section 5.4.B).
- A chest X-ray may be helpful in showing pulmonary plethora or oedema.

Stop giving ORS, but give breast milk or plain water, and food.

Do not give a diuretic unless there is pulmonary oedema (lung crepitations), in which case give furosemide 1 mg/kg IV.

Treatment phases in dehydration with shock

In the shock phase, the circulating volume must be improved sufficiently to perfuse vital organs, this will be identified by an improvement in conscious level, falling heart rate and stronger pulse volume.

- In the rehydration phase, the fluid deficit should be replaced and clinical hydration achieved.
- In the maintenance phase, adequate dietary and fluid intake should be maintained.
- In all phases, excess fluid losses must be replaced continuously.

TABLE 5.12.A.2 Estimated degrees of dehydration with symptoms, signs and treatment

Degree of dehydration with diarrhoea	Symptoms and signs present	Treatment
No dehydration	None Increased thirst	• Treat at home with extra fluids. WHO Treatment Plan A (see below) • Breastfeeding or standard diet must continue • Warn mother about danger signs of some or severe dehydration and when to return • Zinc supplements
Some dehydration (5–9% fluid deficit)	Two or more of the following signs: • Restless and irritable • Sunken eyes • Drinks eagerly/thirsty • Loss of skin turgor; tents when pinched and goes back slowly Any one additional sign of severe dehydration below	• Treat with WHO Treatment Plan B in hospital for at least 24 hours (if feasible) • Give ORS or ReSoMal if there is malnutrition • Breastfeeding or standard feeding to continue • Zinc supplements
Severe dehydration (10% or greater)	Two or more of the following signs • Prostration • Sunken eyes • Loss of skin turgor; tents when pinched and goes back very slowly ($\geq$ 2 seconds) • Not able to drink or drinks poorly In addition may show: • Rapid deep breathing from acidosis • Lack of urine output	• WHO Treatment Plan C • Rapid IV rehydration, giving ORS while IV cannula is put in place • Test for and treat any hypoglycaemia • Breastfeeding or standard feeding as soon as possible • Zinc supplements
Shock	As above with: • High and increasing heart rate; weak pulse volume • Poor skin circulation time (cool and poorly perfused extremities) with prolonged capillary refill time (> 3 seconds) • Low or even unmeasurable blood pressure • Very reduced conscious level or coma	• Urgent IV or intra-osseous access • Urgent IV/intra-osseous fluid bolus of 10 mL/kg Ringer-lactate or Hartmann's solution • Repeat 10 mL/kg boluses if remains shocked, up to a total of 40 mL/kg, then beware of fluid overload • Then rehydrate more slowly • Use NG or oral ORS/breast milk as soon as tolerated

A child's fluid deficit can be estimated as follows:

• Mild or no signs of dehydration: < 5% fluid deficit; < 50 mL/kg.
• Some dehydration: 5–10% fluid deficit; 50–100 mL/kg.
• Severe dehydration: > 10% fluid deficit; > 100 mL/kg.

Rehydration therapy is based on degree of dehydration.

Treatment with low-osmolarity ORS

The formula for standard ORS and the latest low-osmolarity ORS recommended by the WHO and UNICEF is given in Table 5.12.A.3. The quantities shown are for preparation of 1 litre of ORS, by adding one sachet of oral rehydration salts to 1 litre of clean water.

When prepared and given correctly, ORS provides sufficient water and electrolytes to correct the deficits associated with acute diarrhoea. Potassium is provided to replace the large potassium losses associated with acute diarrhoea, especially in infants, thus preventing serious hypokalaemia. Citrate (or bicarbonate) is provided to prevent or correct base deficit acidosis. Glucose is essential because, as it is absorbed, it promotes the absorption of sodium and water in the small intestine. This is true irrespective of the cause of the diarrhoea. Without glucose, ORS solution would be ineffective.

Healthcare workers and mothers criticised standard ORS because it did not reduce stool output or the duration of diarrhoea. Reduced-osmolarity ORS is as effective as standard ORS for preventing and treating diarrhoea, but it also reduces stool output/volume by 25%, reduces vomiting by almost 30%, and reduces the need for supplemental IV rehydration by 33%. This means that there is less need for hospital care, less disruption of breastfeeding, less use of needles and, where IV treatment is not available, less risk of dying from acute diarrhoea.

It is as effective as standard ORS in the treatment of cholera in adults, but may produce transient hyponatraemia. In children it appears to be as effective as standard ORS in cholera, but careful observations for hyponatraemia should be undertaken if possible.

Use ReSoMal instead of low-osmolarity ORS in

TABLE 5.12.A.3 Composition by weight of WHO/UNICEF oral rehydration salts to be dissolved in boiled water to produce 1 litre

Ingredient	Original standard ORS (grams/litre clean water)	New and recommended low-osmolarity ORS (grams/litre clean water)
Sodium chloride	3.5	2.6
Trisodium citrate dihydrate	2.9	2.9
Potassium chloride	1.5	1.5
Glucose anhydrous	20	13.5

TABLE 5.12.A.4 Resulting molar concentration of components of standard and reduced-osmolarity WHO oral rehydration solutions

ORS	Standard osmolarity (mEq/litre)	Reduced osmolarity (mEq/litre)
Glucose	111	75
Sodium	90	75
Chloride	80	65
Potassium	20	20
Citrate	10	10
Osmolarity	311* mOsm/litre	245 mOsm/litre

* Hyperosmolar with respect to plasma osmolality (normal = 276–295 mOsm/litre).

If using bicarbonate ORS there are 30 mmol/litre of bicarbonate instead of citrate.

children with severe malnutrition, as this product is specifically designed for such children.

Zinc supplementation

Zinc is an important micronutrient for children's overall health and development. It is lost in greater quantity during diarrhoea. Replacing the lost zinc is therefore important both for helping the child to recover and for keeping them healthy in the coming months. It has been shown that zinc supplements given during an episode of diarrhoea reduce the duration and severity of the episode, and lower the incidence of diarrhoea in the following 2–3 months. For these reasons, all patients with diarrhoea should be given zinc supplements as soon as possible after the diarrhoea has started. **Give 10 mg/kg for infants less than 6 months old and 20 mg/kg for older infants and children for 14 days.**

Treatments for different degrees of dehydration with/without shock

Dehydration does not neatly fit into discrete categories, although texts such as this one and the WHO publications show practicality in this way for clarity and guidance. Similarly, it can be very difficult to distinguish severe dehydration from dehydration with shock, and the two 'categories' overlap. The essential point to understand is that each severely ill patient must be reassessed frequently to ascertain whether the treatment protocol is having the desired effect of reversing the life-threatening signs of fluid loss. Look for the following:

- increasing awareness and response to stimuli
- gradually strengthening pulse with a decreasing rate (however, a slow weak pulse is a pre-terminal sign).

Children severely dehydrated with shock: shock treatment phase

Children with shock will have a high and increasing heart rate, weak pulse, poor skin circulation time with prolonged capillary refill time (> 3 seconds), depressed conscious level, and low or even unmeasurable blood pressure.

These children require immediate resuscitation (ABC) and emergency treatment (see also Section 5.5.B).

Airway (if patient has a reduced conscious level)

- Use an opening manoeuvre if the airway is not open or

if it is partially obstructed. Then keep the airway open. If there is immediate improvement but the airway closes without active opening support, consider using airway adjuncts to support the airway.

- Suction if necessary, but not routinely.
- If the child is deeply unconscious (P or less on the AVPU scale), the airway may need to be secured by intubation using experienced senior help (if available).

Breathing

- Give 100% oxygen (mask with reservoir and flow rate of at least 6 litres/minute) regardless of SpO_2 (this increases oxygen delivery as well as improving tissue oxygenation).
- For inadequate ventilation or depressed conscious level (as indicated by the AVPU score) with hypoventilation, respiration should be supported with oxygen via a **bag and mask**, and experienced senior help summoned (if available).

Circulation

- Obtain vascular access to give boluses quickly. Insert an IV cannula and if facilities available send blood for a full blood count, urea and electrolytes blood glucose, cross-matching (if anaemic) and clotting. If peripheral veins are difficult to access an intra-osseous infusion (e.g. EZIO) is rapid and effective. In the absence of IO equipment, the **external jugular vein** or **long saphenous vein cut-down** are good alternatives (see Section 8.B for circulatory procedures). If a skilled operator is available, an internal jugular vein central line is ideal, once an initial rapid infusion has been given, if the patient is very severely shocked and likely to need ongoing high dependency care, as it can also allow CVP measurements (if available).
- Give an initial **rapid** bolus of 10 mL/kg of Ringer-lactate or Hartmann's solution and reassess. **Do not use 5% glucose or 0.18% saline/4% glucose solutions for resuscitation, as these can cause hyponatraemia and cerebral oedema.** Boluses should be manually pushed in using a 20- to 50-mL syringe (utilising a three-way tap and link to an IV giving set).
- The re-assessment after the first bolus allows the clinician to ascertain whether the child has any contraindications to large volume resuscitation. Assess for:
  — malnutrition (this should be obvious: see Section 5.10.B) severe anaemia or cardiac problem. **Rapid fluid infusion can be fatal in malnutrition, severe anaemia or cardiac problems. Stop the rapid infusion and proceed more slowly with reference to Sections 5.10.B malnutrition, 5.11.A anaemia and 5.4.B heart failure and consider a blood transfusion.**
- Further 10 mL/kg boluses with reassessment will usually be required if shock continues. In a child with shock from severe dehydration caused by diarrhoea, it would be very unusual to need more than 30–40 mL/kg to improve the child's circulation. Reconsider the diagnosis. For example:
  — surgical abdominal pathology (e.g. intussusception or volvulus) (see Section 5.19)
  — additional pathology e.g septicaemia (see Section 5.5.C)
  — ongoing severe diarrhoea, particularly if there is a cholera epidemic.

- Once a **total** of 40 mL/kg of boluses have been given IV, complications such as pulmonary oedema may occur. If available, expert help (including CVP monitoring and facilities for positive pressure ventilation) is essential. If expert help is not available and there is ongoing severe diarrhoea, continue with fluid resuscitation until there is some improvement in conscious level.
- If a blood glucose shows hypoglycaemia (< 2.5 mmol.L) or glucose stick test has not been available, give a dose of 5 mL/kg of 10% glucose IV to any child who still has a depressed conscious level, as hypoglycaemia may be contributing to this problem. Increased alertness confirms hypoglycaemia (and see below).
- Keep the patient warm, but do not overheat them as this will cause peripheral vasodilatation and reduce the blood supply to vital centres. Hypothermia will exacerbate poor peripheral perfusion, acidosis and coagulation abnormalities.
- Elevate the legs (raise the foot of the bed).
- Give a 10 mL/kg bolus of fresh blood as soon as possible if severe anaemia is present, but watch for circulatory overload.
- Consider using broad-spectrum IV antibiotics.
- Monitor urine output.
- If the child has a reduced level of consciousness or has a convulsion, particularly if they are an infant or young child, hypoglycaemia may be present. Always measure the blood glucose level in this situation. However, if blood glucose measurement is not possible, always treat as for presumed hypoglycaemia and, in addition to the IV fluids given above, give 5 mL/kg of 10% glucose IV or, if there is no IV access, by intra-osseous needle.

As shock is being treated, reassess the child's vital signs: alertness, pulse, respiratory rate etc. after each bolus and at least every 15–30 minutes until signs of shock are improving. Increased alertness, lower pulse and respiratory rate are encouraging signs, but the easiest and most sensitive to recognise is the degree of responsiveness.

Children severely dehydrated with shock: rehydration phase

The best route for rehydration is the oral or nasogastric one, but in children who were sick enough to require rapid IV boluses, further IV fluid is likely to be needed initially.

At this stage, also, there is a need to again consider hypoglycaemia (which may have been identified earlier on stick testing). See below.

Fluid requirement for replacing in the rehydration phase

Fluid requirement falls into the three categories mentioned above:

1 Correction of deficit
   - Weigh the child again or estimate the weight as above
   - Re-assess the clinical signs of dehydration as shown in Table 5.12.A.2 and estimate the percentage of dehydration: fluid deficit in mL = weight in kg × % dehydrated × 10
   - e.g. a 6 kg child with a 5% dehydration will have 6 × 5 × 10 = 300 mL deficit.
2 Replacement of ongoing losses
   - For each diarrhoeal stool: < 2 years of age: give

50–100 mL or 10 mL/kg and ≥ 2 years of age: give 100–200 mL
   - For each vomit: use 2 mL/kg ORS
   - For nasogastric tube aspirates: replace volume for volume
   - e.g. a 6 kg child of 7 months with 5 loose watery stools will need another 300 mL as replacement.
3 Maintenance fluids (see Table 5.12.A.5).

TABLE 5.12.A.5 IV maintenance fluids

Weight	Total fluid in 24 hours	Fluid/ hour
First 10 kg of body weight	100 mL/kg	4 mL/kg
Second 10 kg of body weight	50 mL/kg	2 mL/kg
Subsequent kg	20 mL/kg	1 mL/kg

The 6 kg child will need 600 mL in 24 hours for maintenance

Total fluid in 6 kg child with 5 loose watery stools who is 5% dehydrated is 300 + 300 + 600 mL = 1200 in 24 hours. The IV would be set to run at 50 mL/hr. initially. Adjustments to the volume will have to be made in the presence of further large watery stools or vomits or nasogastric aspirate. If available, a check on the plasma electrolytes is very useful at least daily to monitor response to treatment and to guide further therapy. Clinical observations should be done at least hourly and include looking for evidence of urine output.

Choice of IV fluid

As described before, a solution such as **Ringers's lactate or Hartman's** solution is preferable to Normal (0.9%) Saline as it contains less chloride and contains potassium which is vital in diarrhoea treatment. If N saline must be used, add 10 mmol of potassium chloride to each 500 mL bag **once urine has been passed**. If Ringers's lactate or Hartman's solution are being used, add 5 mmol to each 500 mL bag **once urine has been passed**.

There is an advantage in managing these children with a urinary catheter as urine volume measurement is a useful guide to fluid need in the absence of cardiac failure but its use must be weighed against the risk of infection.

There is always a possibility of hypoglycaemia as the child is not eating (see below) so for this reason, add glucose to the infusion fluid.

To make a 5% solution of dextrose in Ringers's lactate, Hartman's solution or N saline, remove 50 mL from the 500 mL bag and replace with 50 mL of 50% dextrose

To make a 10% solution of dextrose in Ringers's lactate, Hartman's solution or N saline, remove 100 mL from the 500 mL bag and replace with 100 mL of 50% dextrose.

Start the rehydration fluid regime, review the child's vital signs at least hourly, including assessing urine output and looking for signs of fluid overload, such as puffy face or limbs or increased breathlessness. Also review if there is any change reported by the mother. Once the child is regaining a degree of responsiveness and has a gag reflex, consider introducing oral or nasogastric (enteral) fluids to replace the IV route.

Re-introduction of enteral fluid

Re-assess the child's dehydration status by checking skin pinch, level of consciousness, and ability to drink, at least every hour, in order to confirm that hydration is improving. Sunken eyes recover more slowly than other signs, and are less useful for monitoring.

As has been mentioned earlier, enteral fluid is the safest way to rehydrate the child. Enteral rehydration can be achieved when:

- The child is conscious enough to be fed by a nasogastric tube without aspiration i.e there is a gag reflex present OR
- The child is conscious enough to take sufficient fluid orally AND
- The child is not vomiting a significant volume of the fluid

The enteral rehydration fluid should be reduced osmolarity ORS (or ReSoMal if malnutrition is present). ORS should be introduced while the IV infusion is still running and the IV fluid volume reduced accordingly. Allow the child to breast feed whenever they want.

Once volumes approaching those required (see WHO Plan B in the Appendix to this section) are reached, the IV infusion can be discontinued and WHO Plan B rehydration continued alone.

All the WHO Plans for rehydration with details on prevention fluids, home fluids and advice for parents can be found in the Appendix to this section (see below).

Hypoglycaemia in diarrhoea (blood glucose < 2.5 mmol/L or < 45 mg/dL)

If the child has a reduced level of consciousness or has a convulsion, particularly if they are an infant, hypoglycaemia may be present. Always measure the blood glucose level in this situation. However, if blood glucose measurement is not possible, always treat as for presumed hypoglycaemia. Give 2–5 mL/kg of 10% glucose IV or, if there is no IV access, by intra-osseous needle. If there is no circulatory access, while further attempts are made to access the circulation, any hypoglycaemia can be temporarily managed as below, if there are sufficient staff.

Sublingual sugar (sucrose) for treatment of hypoglycaemia

- Sublingual sugar may be used as an immediate 'first-aid' measure for managing hypoglycaemia in an unconscious child in situations where IV administration of glucose may be impossible or delayed.
- Give 1 teaspoonful of sugar, moistened with 1–2 drops of water, under the tongue. More frequent repeated doses are needed to prevent relapse. Children should be monitored for early swallowing, which leads to delayed absorption, and in this case another dose of sugar should be given. If sublingual sugar is given, repeat doses at 20-minute intervals.
- Recheck the blood glucose concentration in 20 minutes, and if the level is low (< 2.5 mmol/litre or < 45 mg/dL) repeat the sublingual sugar.
- Clearly, once an IV or IO access has been established, glucose can be given into the circulation if necessary.

Electrolyte disturbances in dehydration from diarrhoeal illnesses

Knowledge of the levels of serum electrolytes rarely changes the management of children with diarrhoea. Indeed, these values are often misinterpreted, leading to inappropriate treatment. The disorders described below are usually adequately treated by oral rehydration therapy (ORT).

Hypernatraemia

Some children with diarrhoea develop hypernatraemic dehydration, especially when given drinks that are hypertonic due to their sugar content (e.g. soft drinks, commercial fruit drinks) or salt. These draw water from the child's tissues and blood into the bowel, causing the concentration of sodium in extracellular fluid to rise. If the solute in the drink is not fully absorbed, the water remains in the bowel, causing osmotic diarrhoea.

Children with hypernatraemic dehydration (serum Na^+ > 150 mmol/litre) have thirst that is out of proportion to other signs of dehydration. Their most serious problem is convulsions, which usually occur when the serum sodium concentration exceeds 165 mmol/litre, and especially when intravenous therapy is given. Seizures are much less likely to occur when hypernatraemia is treated with ORS, which usually causes the serum Na^+ concentration to become normal within 24 hours.

It is absolutely essential that intravenous rehydration does not lower the serum Na^+ too rapidly. Intravenous glucose solutions (5% glucose or 0.18% saline/4% glucose) are particularly dangerous and can result in cerebral oedema, which is usually fatal or permanently disabling.

Hyponatraemia

Children with diarrhoea who drink mostly water, or watery drinks that contain little salt, may develop hyponatraemia (serum Na^+ < 130 mmol/litre). Hyponatraemia is especially common in children with shigellosis and in severely malnourished children with oedema. It is occasionally associated with lethargy and (less often) with seizures. ORS is safe and effective therapy for nearly all children with hyponatraemia. An exception is children with oedema, for whom ORS may provide too much sodium. ReSoMal (see Section 5.10.B) may be helpful here.

Hypokalaemia

Inadequate replacement of potassium losses during diarrhoea can lead to potassium depletion and hypokalaemia (serum K^+ < 3 mmol/litre), especially in children with malnutrition. This can cause muscle weakness, paralytic ileus, impaired kidney function and cardiac arrhythmias. Hypokalaemia is worsened when base (bicarbonate or lactate) is given to treat acidosis without simultaneously providing potassium. Hypokalaemia can be prevented, and the potassium deficit corrected, by using ORS for rehydration therapy and by giving foods rich in potassium during diarrhoea and after it has stopped (e.g. bananas, coconut water, dark green leafy vegetables).

It is also essential to check blood potassium levels, especially if the child has not passed urine, prior to replacing potassium IV, in order to avoid complications of hyperkalaemia secondary to pre-renal failure.

If it is necessary to give potassium intravenously (e.g. if serum K^+ is < 2.0 mmol/litre or there are ECG signs of hypokalaemia, namely ST depression, T-wave reduction and prominent U waves), great care must be taken. In acute depletion, an infusion at the rate of 0.2 mmol/kg/hour can be used and the serum K^+ level checked after 3 hours. The potassium for injection **must** be diluted before use and thoroughly mixed before being given. **The maximum** concentration of potassium that can be given through a peripheral vein is 40 mmol/litre. The maximum infusion rate of potassium is 0.5 mmol/kg/hour. The recommended concentration is 20 mmol/litre.

Note: The injectable form of KCl usually contains 1.5 grams (i.e. 20 mmol of potassium in 10 mL), and can be given orally. The daily potassium requirement is 2.5–3.5 mmol/kg.

Supportive treatments
Dietary therapy
During diarrhoea, a decrease in food intake, lack of nutrient absorption and increased nutrient requirements combine to cause weight loss and failure to grow. In turn, malnutrition can make the diarrhoea more severe, more prolonged and more frequent, compared with diarrhoea in non-malnourished children. Therefore give nutrient-rich foods during the diarrhoea and when the child is recovering.
- Breastfed infants: continue feeding on demand.
- Bottle-fed infants: administer full-strength formulas immediately after rehydration (no longer than 4 hours). Lactose intolerance may develop and cause an exacerbation of diarrhoea with a lactose-containing formula. If this happens, temporarily reduce or remove lactose from the diet.
- Older children: continue their usual diet during diarrhoea. Recommended foods include starches, cereals, yoghurt, fruits and vegetables. Foods high in simple sugars and fats should be avoided. Excess fluid losses via vomiting or diarrhoea must be replaced with ORS (see above).

Zinc treatment
Zinc is an important micronutrient which is lost in diarrhoeal illnesses. Replacement speeds recovery and reduces severity as well as reducing the frequency of diarrhoeal illnesses in the ensuing 2 to 3 months.

Dose under 6 months of age 10 mg (½ tablet) daily for 10–14 days; dose over 6 months of age 20 mg (1 tablet) daily for 10–14 days.

Drug therapy: use of antimicrobial and 'antidiarrhoeal' drugs
Antimicrobial drugs should not be used routinely. This is because, except as noted below, it is not possible to distinguish clinically episodes that might respond, such as diarrhoea caused by enterotoxigenic *E. coli*, from those caused by agents unresponsive to antimicrobials, such as rotavirus or *Cryptosporidium*. Moreover, even for potentially responsive infections, selecting an effective antimicrobial drug requires knowledge of the likely sensitivity of the causative agent, and such information is usually unavailable. In addition, use of antimicrobials adds to the cost of treatment, risks adverse reactions and enhances the development of resistant bacteria.

Antimicrobial drugs are reliably helpful only for children with bloody diarrhoea (probable shigellosis), suspected cholera with severe dehydration, and serious non-intestinal bacterial infections such as pneumonia. Antiprotozoal drugs are rarely indicated except as described below when a definite diagnosis is available.

Antimicrobial drugs for acute diarrhoea
Neonates
Diarrhoea and vomiting may be a symptom of septicaemia. If septicaemia is suspected, parenteral antibiotics are required (see Section 3.4).

Bloody diarrhoea
- **Bacterial causes:** *Campylobacter jejuni*, *Shigella sonnei*, *Shigella flexneri* and *Shigella dysenteriae*, and less commonly *Salmonella*, *E. coli* 0157:117 and *Aeromonas*.
- May be accompanied by abdominal pain and rectal prolapse.
- As culture facilities may not be available, sick toxic children with bloody diarrhoea should be treated for shigella dysentery.
- Children with diarrhoea and blood in stool (dysentery) should be treated with ciprofloxacin as first-line treatment and ceftriaxone as second-line treatment if they are severely ill and local antimicrobial sensitivity is not known. Where local antimicrobial sensitivity is known, local guidelines should be followed:
  - ciprofloxacin: 20 mg/kg/dose twice daily for 5 days
  - ceftriaxone: 80 mg/kg IV or IM once daily for 5 days.
- Mild infections due to *Shigella sonnei* are usually self-limiting. *Shigella* in resource-limited countries is commonly resistant to co-trimoxazole and ampicillin. Nalidixic acid, ciprofloxacin, ceftriaxone **or the antibiotic of choice for the area** should be used for a 5-day course.
- In infants and young children, exclude surgical causes (e.g. intussusception) (see Section 5.19).

Salmonella
If non-typhoidal *Salmonella* is suspected in infants under 1 year of age or in immunocompromised children, blood cultures should be undertaken. If these are positive or the infant is toxic, an appropriate parenteral antibiotic should be given (e.g. chloramphenicol, ceftriaxone or ciprofloxacin) for 7–10 days. Be alert for pneumonia or metastatic abscesses in bone, brain or elsewhere. Otherwise *Salmonella* gastroenteritis is not treated with antibiotics.

Systemic *Salmonella* infection is common in malnutrition, HIV infection, sickle-cell disease and schistosomiasis.

Campylobacter jejuni (and also *Shigella* and *Salmonella*) may cause severe abdominal pain, mimicking a surgical emergency. Otherwise the disease is self-limiting and does not require antibiotics. If treatment is considered appropriate, erythromycin (12.5 mg/kg four times daily) for 5 days is the antibiotic of choice.

Other causes of diarrhoea that warrant antimicrobial treatment
- **Amoebic dysentery:** this is diagnosed by microscopy of fresh warm stool. Treatment is with metronidazole 10 mg/kg three times daily (maximum dose 2 grams) for 5–7 days.
- **Cholera:** this is usually only diagnosed during epidemics. If the child has severe watery diarrhoea, suspect cholera or enterotoxigenic *E. coli* (only diagnosed by specialist laboratories). Treatment for cholera is with tetracycline 12.5 mg/kg four times a day for 3 days in children aged over 8 years. The alternative for young children is chloramphenicol 25 mg/kg 8-hourly for 3 days. In addition to rehydration, give an antibiotic to which local

strains of *Vibrio cholerae* are sensitive. These include tetracycline, doxycycline, co-trimoxazole, erythromycin and chloramphenicol.

- **Giardiasis:** this is diagnosed by microscopy of stool, and is usually self-limiting or asymptomatic. If symptomatic in a malnourished child or the disease is prolonged, it is justified to treat with metronidazole for 5 days (as for amoebic dysentery). Tinidazole is an alternative (50–75 mg/kg once only (maximum dose 2 grams), a second dose may be given if necessary).

- *Clostridium difficile* usually occurs after a course of antibiotics for some other illness, and is associated with antibiotic-associated pseudomembranous colitis (there is a danger of bowel perforation). Antibiotics, especially clindamycin, may alter the flora of the gastrointestinal tract and allow overgrowth of *C. difficile*. The latter produces a toxin which causes damage to the gut mucosa, resulting in pseudomembranous colitis. Confirmation is by culture of *C. difficile* in the faeces. Treatment is with oral vancomycin for 7–10 days, which clears *C. difficile* from the gut. The doses are orally:
  - **Child 1 month–5 years:** 5 mg/kg 4 times daily for 10–14 days (increased up to 10 mg/kg 4 times daily if infection fails to respond or is life threatening)
  - **Child 5–12 years:** 62.5 mg 4 times daily for 10–14 days (increased up to 250 mg 4 times daily if infection fails to respond or is life threatening)
  - **Child 12–18 years:** 125 mg 4 times daily for 10–14 days (increased up to 500 mg 4 times daily if infection fails to respond or is life threatening).

Symptomatic drugs

'Antidiarrhoeal' drugs and anti-emetics have no practical benefits for children with acute or persistent diarrhoea. They do not prevent dehydration or improve nutritional status, which should be the main objectives of treatment. Some, like loperamide, have dangerous and sometimes fatal side effects. These drugs should never be given to children under 5 years of age.

Treatment of rectal prolapse

Gently push back any tissue that has come out of the anus using a surgical glove or wet cloth, or if it is oedematous and cannot be reduced, warm compresses of magnesium sulphate may reduce the oedema.

Haemolytic–uraemic syndrome

If laboratory tests are not available, suspect this syndrome when purpura, pallor, altered level of consciousness and low or absent urine output are present. If laboratory tests are available, blood smear shows fragmented red cells and decreased or absent platelets. There will be an increase in blood urea and creatinine levels (*see* Section 5.6.A).

Appendix
WHO Treatment Plan A: home therapy to prevent dehydration and malnutrition

Children with no signs of dehydration need extra fluids and salt to replace their losses of water and electrolytes due to diarrhoea. If these are not given, signs of dehydration may develop.

Mothers should be taught how to prevent dehydration at home by giving the child more fluid than usual, how to

prevent malnutrition by continuing to feed the child, and why these actions are important. They should also know what signs indicate that the child should be taken to a health worker. *These steps are summarised in the four rules of Treatment Plan A.*

Rule 1: Give the child more fluids than usual, to prevent dehydration
What fluids to give

Many countries have designated recommended home fluids. *Wherever possible, these should include at least one fluid that normally contains salt* (see below). Plain clean water should also be given. Other fluids should be recommended that are frequently given to children in the area, that mothers consider acceptable for children with diarrhoea, and that mothers would be likely to give in increased amounts when advised to do so.

Suitable fluids

Most fluids that a child normally takes can be used. It is helpful to divide suitable fluids into two groups:

Fluids that normally contain salt, such as:
- ORS solution
- salted drinks (e.g. salted rice water or a salted yoghurt drink)
- vegetable or chicken soup with salt.
  Insert

Teaching mothers to add salt (about 3 g/L) to an unsalted drink or soup during diarrhoea is also possible, but requires a sustained educational effort.

A home made solution containg 3 g/L of table salt (one level teaspoon) and 18 g/l of common sugar (sucrose) is effective but is not generally recommended because the recipe is often forgotten, the ingredients may not be available or too little may be given.

Fluids that do not contain salt, such as:
- plain water
- water in which a cereal has been cooked (e.g. unsalted rice water)
- unsalted soup
- yoghurt drinks without salt
- green coconut water
- weak tea (unsweetened)
- unsweetened fresh fruit juice.

Unsuitable fluids

A few fluids are potentially dangerous and should be avoided during diarrhoea. Especially important are drinks sweetened with sugar, which can cause osmotic diarrhoea and hypernatraemia. Some examples are:
- commercial carbonated beverages
- commercial fruit juices
- sweetened tea.

Other fluids to avoid are those with stimulant, diuretic or purgative effects, for example
- coffee
- some medicinal teas or infusions.

How much fluid to give

The general rule is: give as much fluid as the child or adult wants until the diarrhoea stops. As a guide, after each loose stool, give:

- children under 2 years of age: 50–100 mL (a quarter to half a large cup) of fluid
- children aged 2 up to 10 years: 100–200 mL (a half to one large cup)
- older children and adults: as much fluid as they want. Insert

Rule 2: Give supplemental zinc (10–20 mg) to the child every day for 10 to 14 days

Zinc can be given as a syrup or as dispersible tablets, whichever formulation is available and affordable. By giving zinc as soon as diarrhoea starts, the duration and severity of the episode as well as the risk of hydration will be reduced. By continuing zinc supplementation for 10–14 days, the zinc lost during diarrhoea is fully replaced and the risk of the child having new episodes of diarrhoea in the following 2 to 3 months is reduced.

Rule 3: Continue to feed the child, to prevent malnutrition

The infant's usual diet should be continued during diarrhoea and increased afterwards. Food should never be withheld, and the child's usual foods should not be diluted. Breastfeeding should always be continued. The aim is to give as much nutrient-rich food as the child will accept. Most children with watery diarrhoea regain their appetite after dehydration is corrected, whereas those with bloody diarrhoea often eat poorly until the illness resolves. These children should be encouraged to resume normal feeding as soon as possible.

When food is given, sufficient nutrients are usually absorbed to support continued growth and weight gain. Continued feeding also speeds the recovery of normal intestinal function, including the ability to digest and absorb various nutrients. In contrast, children whose food is restricted or diluted lose weight, have diarrhoea of longer duration, and recover intestinal function more slowly.

What foods to give

This depends on the child's age, food preferences and pre-illness feeding pattern; cultural practices are also important. In general, foods suitable for a child with diarrhoea are the same as those required by healthy children. Specific recommendations are given below.

Milk

- Infants of any age who are breastfed should be allowed to breastfeed as often and as long as they want. Infants will often breastfeed more than usual; this should be encouraged.
- Infants who are not breastfed should be given their usual milk feed (or formula) at least every three hours, if possible by cup. Special commercial formulas advertised for use in diarrhoea are expensive and unnecessary; they should not be given routinely. Clinically significant milk intolerance is rarely a problem.
- Infants below six months of age who take breast milk and other foods should receive increased breastfeeding. As the child recovers and the supply of breast milk increases, other foods should be decreased (if fluids other than breastmilk are given, use a cup, not a bottle).

This usually takes about 1 week. If possible, infants of this age should become **exclusively** breastfed.

There is no value in routinely testing the stools of infants for pH or reducing substances. Such tests are oversensitive, often indicating impaired absorption of lactose when it is not clinically important. It is more important to monitor the child's clinical response (i.e. weight gain, general improvement). Milk intolerance is only clinically important when milk feeding causes a prompt increase in stool volume and a return or worsening of the signs of dehydration, often with loss of weight.

Other foods

If the child is at least 6 months old or is already taking soft foods, he or she should be given cereals, vegetables and other foods, in addition to milk. If the child is over 6 months old and such foods are not yet being given, they should be started during the diarrhoea episode or soon after it stops.

Recommended foods should be culturally acceptable, readily available, have a high content of energy and provide adequate amounts of essential micronutrients. They should be well cooked, and mashed or ground to make them easy to digest; fermented foods are also easy to digest. Milk should be mixed with a cereal. If possible, 5–10 mL of vegetable oil should be added to each serving of cereal. (Most staple foods do not provide enough calories per unit weight for infants and young children. This is improved by adding some vegetable oil.) Meat, fish or egg should be given, if available. Foods rich in potassium, such as bananas, green coconut water and fresh fruit juice, are beneficial.

How much food and how often

Offer the child food every three or four hours (six times a day). Frequent small feedings are tolerated better than less frequent large ones.

After the diarrhoea stops, continue giving the same energy-rich foods and provide one more meal than usual each day for at least 2 weeks. If the child is malnourished, extra meals should be given until the child has regained normal weight for height.

Rule 4: Take the child to a healthcare worker if there are signs of dehydration or other problems

The mother should take her child to a healthcare worker if the child:

- starts to pass many watery stools
- has repeated vomiting
- becomes very thirsty
- is eating or drinking poorly
- develops a fever
- has blood in the stool
- does not get better in 3 days.

WHO Treatment Plan B: oral rehydration therapy for children with some dehydration

Children with some dehydration should receive oral rehydration therapy with ORS in a healthcare facility following the treatment plan described below.

Children with some dehydration should also receive zinc supplementation as described above.

TABLE 5.12.A.6 Guidelines for treating children with some dehydration: approximate amount of ORS to give in the first 4 hours

Age	< 4 months	4–11 months	12–23 months	2–4 years	5–14 years	15 years or older
Weight (kg)	< 5	5–7.9	8–10.9	11–15.9	16–29.9	30 kg or more
Volume (mL)	200–400	400–600	600–800	800–1200	1200–2200	2200–4000

How much ORS is needed?

Use Table 5.12.A.6 to estimate the amount of ORS needed for rehydration. If the child's weight is known, this should be used to determine the approximate amount of solution needed. The amount may also be estimated by multiplying the child's weight in kg by 75 mL. If the child's weight is not known, select the approximate amount according to the child's age.

The *exact* amount of solution required will depend on the child's dehydration status. Children with more marked signs of dehydration, or who continue to pass frequent watery stools, will require more solution than those with less marked signs or who are not passing frequent stools. *If the child wants more than the estimated amount of ORS, and there are no signs of over-hydration, give more.*

Oedematous (puffy) eyelids are a sign of *over-hydration*. They may be a sign of chronic malnutrition. If this occurs, stop giving ORS, but give breast milk or plain water, and food. Do not give a diuretic. When the oedema has gone, resume giving ORS or home fluids according to Treatment Plan A.

How to give ORS

A family member should be taught to prepare and give ORS. The solution should be given to infants and young children using a clean spoon or cup. Feeding bottles should *not* be used. For babies, a dropper or syringe (without the needle) can be used to put small amounts of solution into the mouth.

Children under 2 years of age should be offered a teaspoonful every 1 to 2 minutes. Older children (and adults) may take frequent sips directly from the cup.

Vomiting often occurs during the first hour or two of treatment, especially when children drink the solution too quickly, but this rarely prevents successful oral rehydration, as most of the fluid is absorbed. After this time vomiting usually stops. If the child vomits, wait 5–10 minutes and then start giving ORS again, but more slowly (e.g. a spoonful every 2–3 minutes).

Monitoring the progress of oral rehydration therapy

Check the child from time to time during rehydration to ensure that ORS is being taken satisfactorily and that signs of dehydration are not worsening. If at any time the child develops signs of severe dehydration, switch to WHO Treatment Plan C.

After 4 hours, reassess the child fully, following the guidelines in Table 5.12.A.2. Then decide what treatment to give next:

- If signs of *severe dehydration* have appeared, intravenous (IV) therapy should be started following Treatment Plan C. This is very unusual, however, occurring only in children who drink ORS poorly and pass large watery stools frequently during the rehydration period.
- If the child still has signs indicating *some dehydration*, continue oral rehydration therapy by repeating Treatment Plan B. At the same time start to offer food, milk and

other fluids, as described in Treatment Plan A (see above), and continue to reassess the child frequently.

If there are *no signs of dehydration*, the child should be considered fully rehydrated. When rehydration is complete:
- the skin pinch is normal
- thirst has subsided
- urine is passed
- the child becomes quiet, is no longer irritable and often falls asleep.

Teach the mother how to treat her child at home with ORS and food following Treatment Plan A. Give the mother enough ORS sachets for 2 days. Also teach her the signs that mean she should bring her child back.

- Use the patient's age only when you do not know their weight. The approximate amount of ORS required (in mL) can also be calculated by multiplying the patient's weight in kg by 75.
- If the patient wants more ORS than is shown above, give more.
- Encourage the mother to continue breastfeeding her child.
- For infants under 6 months who are not breast fed, if using the old WHO ORS solution containing 90 mmol/L of sodium also give 100–200 mL clean water during this period. However, if using the new reduced (low) osmolality ORS solution containing 75 mmol/L of sodium, this is not necessary.

Note: During the initial stages of therapy, while still dehydrated, adults can consume up to 750 mL per hour, if necessary, and children up to 20 mL/kg body weight/hour.

Meeting normal fluid needs

While treatment to replace the existing water and electrolyte deficit is in progress, the child's normal daily fluid requirements must also be met. This can be done as follows:

- **Breastfed infants:** continue to breastfeed as often and for as long as the infant wants, even *during* oral rehydration.
- **Non-breastfed infants** under 6 months of age: if using the old WHO ORS solution containing 90 mmol/L of sodium also give 100–200 mLs clean water during this period. However, if using the new reduced (low) osmolality ORS solution containing 75 mmol/L of sodium, this is not necessary.
- **Older children:** throughout rehydration and maintenance therapy, offer as much plain boiled water to drink as they wish, in addition to ORS.

If oral rehydration therapy must be interrupted

If the mother and child must leave hospital before rehydration with ORS is completed:
- Show the mother how much ORS solution to give to finish the 4-hour treatment at home.

- Give her enough ORS packets to complete the 4-hour treatment and to continue oral rehydration for two more days, as shown in Treatment Plan A.
- Show her how to prepare ORS solution.
- Teach her the four rules in Treatment Plan A for treating her child at home.

When oral rehydration fails

With the previous ORS, signs of dehydration would persist or reappear in about 5% of children. With the new reduced (low) osmolality ORS it is estimated that such treatment 'failures' will be reduced to 3% or less. The usual causes for these 'failures' are:

- continuing rapid stool loss (more than 15–20 mL/kg/hour), as occurs in some children with cholera
- insufficient intake of ORS due to fatigue or lethargy
- frequent severe vomiting.

Such children should be given ORS by nasogastric (NG) tube or Ringer Lactate Solution intravenously (IV) (75 mLs/kg in four hours) usually in hospital. After confirming that the signs of dehydration have improved, it is usually possible to resume ORT successfully.

Rarely, oral rehydration therapy should not be given. This is true for children with:

- abdominal distension with paralytic ileus, usually caused by opiate drugs (e.g. codeine, loperamide) and hypokalaemia
- glucose malabsorption (indicated by a marked increase in stool output, failure of the signs of dehydration to improve, and a large amount of glucose in the stool).

In these situations, rehydration should be given IV until the diarrhoea subsides; nasogastric therapy should *not* be used.

Giving zinc

Begin to give supplemental zinc, as in Treatment plan A, as soon as the child is able to eat, following the four hour rehydration period.

Giving food

Except for breast milk, food should not be given during the initial 4-hour rehydration period. However, children who are continued on Treatment Plan B for longer than 4 hours should be given some food every 3–4 hours as described in Treatment Plan A. All children older than 6 months of age should be given some food before being sent home. This helps to emphasise to mothers the importance of continued feeding during diarrhoea.

WHO Treatment Plan C: intravenous rehydration therapy for patients with severe dehydration

The preferred treatment for children with severe dehydration is initial rapid intravenous rehydration following Treatment Plan C. If possible, the child should be admitted to hospital. Guidelines for IV rehydration are given in Table 5.12.A.7.

Children who can drink, even poorly, should be given ORS by mouth until the IV drip is running. In addition, all children should receive some ORS solution (about 5 mL/kg/hr) when they can drink without difficulty, which is usually within 3–4 hours for infants and 1–2 hours for older patients.

This provides additional base and potassium which may not be adequately supplied by the IV fluid.

Monitoring the progress of intravenous rehydration

Patients should be reassessed every 15–30 minutes until a strong radial pulse is present. If it is not, the intravenous drip should be given more rapidly.

When the planned amount of intravenous fluid has been given (after 3 hours for older patients, or 6 hours for infants), the child's hydration status should be reassessed fully as in Table 5.12.A.2.

Look and feel for all the signs of dehydration

- If signs of *severe* dehydration are still present, **repeat** the intravenous fluid infusion as outlined in Treatment Plan C. This is very unusual, however, occurring only in children who pass large watery stools frequently during the rehydration period.
- If the child is improving (able to drink) but still shows signs of *some dehydration*, **discontinue** the intravenous infusion and give ORS for 4 hours, as specified in Treatment Plan B.
- If there are *no signs of dehydration*, follow Treatment Plan A. If possible, observe the child for at least six hours before discharge while the mother gives the child ORS, to confirm that she is able to maintain the child's hydration. Remember that the child will require therapy with ORS until the diarrhoea stops.

If the child cannot remain at the treatment centre, teach the mother how to give treatment at home following Treatment Plan A, give her enough ORS packets for two days and teach her the signs that mean she should bring her child back.

What to do if intravenous therapy is not available

- If IV therapy is not available at the facility, but can be given nearby (i.e. within 30 minutes), send the child immediately for intravenous treatment. If the child can drink, give the mother some ORS and show her how to give it to her child during the journey.
- If IV therapy is not available nearby, healthcare workers who have been trained can give ORS by NG tube, at a rate of 20 mL/kg body weight per hour for 6 hours (total of 120 mL/kg body weight). If the abdomen becomes

TABLE 5.12.A.7 Guidelines for intravenous treatment of children with severe dehydration

Start IV fluids immediately. If the patient can drink give ORS by mouth until the drip is set up. Give 100 mLs/kg of Ringers Lactate Solution[a] divided as follows		
Age	First give 30 mL/kg in:	Then give 70 mL/kg in:
Infants under 12 months	1 hour[b]	5 hours
Older	30 minutes[b]	Over 2.5 hours

Reassess the patient every 1–2 hours. If hydration is not improving, give the IV drip more rapidly. After six hours (infants) or three hours (older patients), evaluate the patient using the assessment chart. Then choose the appropriate Treatment Plan (A, B or C) to continue treatment

a. If Ringers Lactate Solution is not available, normal saline may be used

b. Repeat once if radial pulse is still very weak or not detectable

swollen, ORS should be given more slowly until the abdomen becomes less distended.

- If NG treatment is not possible but the child can drink, ORS should be given by mouth at a rate of 20 mL/kg body weight per hour for 6 hours (total of 120 mL/kg body weight). If this rate is too fast, the child may vomit repeatedly. In this case, give ORS more slowly until the vomiting subsides.
- Children receiving NG or oral therapy should be reassessed at least every hour. If the signs of dehydration do not improve after 3 hours, the child must be taken immediately to the nearest facility where intravenous therapy is available. Otherwise, if rehydration is progressing satisfactorily, the child should be reassessed after

6 hours and a decision on further treatment made as described above for those given IV therapy.

- If neither NG nor oral therapy is possible, the child should be taken *immediately* to the nearest facility where IV or NG therapy is available.

Further reading

World Health Organization (2005) *The Treatment of Diarrhoea: a manual for physicians and other senior health workers*, 4th revision. http://whqlibdoc.who.int/publications/2005/9241593180.pdf

World Health Organization and UNICEF (2013) *Ending Preventable Child Deaths from Pneumonia and Diarrhoea by 2025: the integrated Global Action Plan for Pneumonia and Diarrhoea (GAPPD)*. http://apps.who.int/iris/bitstream/10665/79200/1/9789241505239_eng.pdf

5.12.B Post-infectious prolonged or persistent diarrhoea

BOX 5.12.B.1 Minimum standards
- Low-osmolality ORS and ReSoMal in severely malnourished children.
- Ringer-lactate or Hartmann's solution with potassium: oral and IV.
- Antibiotics: amoxicillin, gentamicin.
- Vitamin A and zinc.
- Electrolyte and mineral mix.
- Folic acid.

Introduction
Epidemiology
- Diarrhoeal episodes that start acutely and last for 7–14 days are usually labelled as prolonged diarrhoea, and may be associated with greater morbidity and more severe nutritional consequences.
- Persistent diarrhoea is commonly defined as diarrhoea that starts acutely, but lasts for more than 14 days and is associated with growth faltering.
- Most cases are thus post-infectious in origin, and other disorders such as inflammatory bowel disease and coeliac disease are therefore excluded.
- Around 4–20% of all episodes of diarrhoea in resource-limited countries become prolonged, with associated case-fatality rates that may exceed 50% in severe cases.
- In parts of sub-Saharan Africa, the association of persistent diarrhoea with HIV infection is often the terminal event.

Risk factors for prolonged and persistent diarrhoea
Appropriate case management of acute diarrhoea is key to the prevention of prolonged episodes.

Specific pathogens: although some studies have identified an association between persistent diarrhoea and infections with organisms such as entero-aggregative *E. coli* or *Cryptosporidium*, this is by no means pathognomonic, nor is there a particular pattern of small bowel microbial colonisation or overgrowth seen in most cases. In HIV-endemic parts of Africa an association of persistent diarrhoea with cryptosporidiosis is well recognised, but may

represent a manifestation of immunodeficiency. Evidence from Bangladesh does suggest that recurrent bouts of infection with bacterial pathogens such as *Shigella* lead to prolongation of the duration of successive diarrhoeal episodes, and thus there is a link between prolonged and persistent diarrhoea as an epidemiological continuum.

Malnutrition: persistent diarrhoea is commonly seen in association with significant malnutrition, and the relationship may be bidirectional. It is widely recognised that diarrhoeal episodes, especially if invasive, may become prolonged in malnourished children. The recent evidence of micronutrient deficiencies, especially of zinc and vitamin A in malnourished children with persistent diarrhoea, may indicate impaired immunological mechanisms for clearing infections, as well as ineffective mucosal repair mechanisms.

Dietary risk factors: although many children with persistent diarrhoea are lactose-intolerant, there is no role of specific dietary allergies in inducing and perpetuating enteropathy of malnutrition or post-infectious prolonged diarrhoea. Several studies have highlighted the high risk of prolonged diarrhoea with lactation failure and early introduction of artificial feeds in resource-limited countries.

Inappropriate management of acute diarrhoea: the association of prolongation of diarrhoea with food deprivation and inappropriately prolonged administration of parenteral fluids is well recognised. Unnecessary food withdrawal, and replacement of luminal nutrients, especially breast milk, with non-nutritive agents is prolonging the mucosal injury after diarrhoea. In particular, blanket administration of antibiotics and **any administration of antimotility agents must be avoided**. Optimal management of acute diarrhoea episodes with ORS, zinc and appropriate diets is a key factor in reducing the risk of recurrence and prolongation of diarrhoeal episodes.

Principles of management of persistent diarrhoea

In general, the management of persistent diarrhoea in malnourished children (*see* Figure 5.12.B.1) represents a blend of the principles of management of acute diarrhoea and malnutrition (*see* Section 5.12.A and Section 5.10.B).

Associated malnutrition may be quite severe in affected children, necessitating appropriate and rapid nutritional rehabilitation, sometimes in hospital. Given the chronicity of the disorder, prolonged hospitalisation may be quite problematic in resource-limited countries, and whenever possible the importance of ambulatory or home-based therapy must be emphasised.

The following represent the basic principles of management of persistent diarrhoea, and a suggested therapeutic approach is shown in Figure 5.12.B.1.

Rapid resuscitation and stabilisation

- Most children with persistent diarrhoea and associated malnutrition are not severely dehydrated, and oral rehydration is adequate.
- However, acute exacerbations and associated vomiting may require brief periods of intravenous rehydration with Ringer-lactate solution.
- Acute electrolyte imbalance such as hypokalaemia and severe acidosis may require correction (*see* Section 5.6.A).
- Associated systemic infections (bacteraemia, pneumonia and urinary tract infections) are well recognised in severely malnourished children with persistent diarrhoea, and are a frequent cause of early mortality. These must be screened for at admission. In severely ill children requiring hospitalisation, it may be best to cover with intravenous antibiotics at admission (usually ampicillin, IV 25 mg/kg three times daily up to a maximum of 4 grams/day, and gentamicin, IV 7.5 mg/kg once daily) while awaiting cultures. In other instances with suspected severe pneumonia, oral amoxicillin will suffice.
- It should be emphasised that there is little role for oral antibiotics in persistent diarrhoea, as in most cases the original bacterial infection that triggered the prolonged diarrhoea has disappeared by the time the child presents.

Oral rehydration therapy

This is the preferred mode of rehydration and replacement of ongoing losses. Although in general the standard low-osmolality WHO oral rehydration solution (containing 75 mmol/litre of Na$^+$) is adequate, some evidence indicates that the hypo-osmolar rehydration fluid ReSoMal (containing 45 mmol/litre of Na$^+$) as well as cereal-based oral rehydration fluids may be advantageous in severely malnourished children. In general, replacing each stool with about 50–100 mL of ORS or ReSoMal is safe.

Enteral feeding and diet selection

- Most children with persistent diarrhoea are not lactose intolerant, although administration of a lactose load exceeding 5 grams/kg/day is associated with higher rates of stooling and treatment failure. In general,

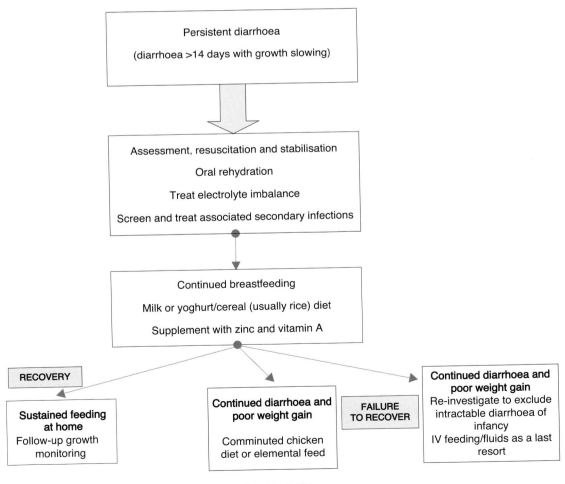

FIGURE 5.12.B.1 Management of persistent diarrhoea in malnourished children.

therefore, withdrawal of milk and replacement with specialised (and expensive) lactose-free formulations is unnecessary.

- Alternative strategies for reducing the lactose load in malnourished children with persistent diarrhoea include reducing the overall amount of milk intake, addition of lactose-free milk to cereals, and replacement of milk with fermented milk products such as yoghurt. These measures have now been extensively evaluated in successive studies of the management of persistent diarrhoea in South Asia, and found to be extremely effective.
- It is rare to find persistent diarrhoea in breastfed infants, and **it must be emphasised that breastfeeding must not be stopped under any circumstances**.
- Rarely, when dietary intolerance precludes the administration of cow's-milk-based formulations or milk, it may be necessary to administer specialised milk-free diets such as a comminuted or blenderised chicken-based diet or an elemental formulation. However, the latter may be almost unaffordable in most resource-limited countries. A choice of enteral diets and formulations is given in Table 5.12.B.2. It must be emphasised that this

is extremely rare, and most infants will recover with the approach outlined above.

- The usual energy density of any diet used for the therapy of persistent diarrhoea should be around 1 kcal/gram, aiming to provide an energy intake of at least 110 kcal/kg/day and a protein intake of 2–3 grams/kg/day (in meals given six times daily). Nasogastric feeding may be required during the first 2–3 days of care, particularly while infection is being treated.
- There should be at least 3 successive days of increasing weight before a response can be verified.
- Dietary failure is shown by an increase in stool frequency (> 10 watery stools/day) or a failure to establish a daily weight gain within 7 days.
- In selected circumstances when adequate intake of energy-dense food is problematic, the addition of amylase to the diet through germination techniques which increase the endogenous amylase content of foods may be helpful. The ready-to-use therapeutic foods (RUTFs) can be used in moderate amounts in children with severe malnutrition and persistent diarrhoea, and the diets below also offer a suitable alternative.

TABLE 5.12.B.2 Suggested composition of selected diets in children with persistent diarrhoea

Component	Khitchri (rice-lentils) (per 100 grams)	Home made version of F-75 diet (WHO) (per 1000 mL)	Comminuted chicken (per 100 grams)	Semi-elemental diet (per 100 mL)
Protein	Mung lentils, 30 grams	Dried skimmed milk, 25 grams	Protein, 8 grams	Protein, 2.25 grams (hydrolysed)
Fat	Oil, 2 grams	Vegetable oil, 27 grams	Fat, 4 grams	Fat, 1.65 grams (medium-chain triglycerides)
Minerals and micronutrients	Salt (to taste)	Vitamin mix, 140 mg Mineral mix, 20 mL	Electrolytes (sodium, 0.4 mmol; potassium, 1.3 mmol; calcium, 0.2 mmol; phosphorus, 1.5 mmol)	Electrolytes (sodium, 1.9 mmol; potassium, 2.3 mmol; calcium, 1.8 mmol)
Carbohydrate	Rice, 60 grams	Cereal flour, 35 grams Sugar, 70 grams		Caloreen, 5 grams

First diet: a starch-based reduced milk concentration (low-lactose) diet

The diet should contain at least 70 kcal/100 grams, provide milk or yoghurt as a source of animal protein, but no more than 3.7 grams of lactose/kg body weight/day, and should provide at least 10% of calories as protein. The following example provides 83 kcal/100 grams, 3.7 grams of lactose/kg body weight/day and 11% of calories as protein:

- full-fat dried milk: 11 grams (or whole liquid milk: 85 mL)
- rice: 15 grams
- vegetable oil: 3.5 grams
- cane sugar: 3 grams
- water to make up to 200 mL.

Of the children who do not improve on this first diet, more than 50% will improve when given the second diet, from which the milk has been totally removed and starch (cereals) partly replaced with glucose or sucrose.

Second diet: a no-milk (lactose-free) diet with reduced cereal (starch)

The second diet should contain at least 70 kcal/100 grams, and provide at least 10% of calories as protein (egg or chicken). The following example provides 75 kcal/100 grams:

- whole egg: 64 grams

- rice: 3 grams
- vegetable oil: 4 grams
- glucose: 3 grams
- water to make up to 200 mL.

Finely ground, cooked chicken (12 grams) can be used in place of egg to give a diet that provides 70 kcal/100 grams.

Of the children who do not improve on the first diet, more than 50% will improve when given the second diet, from which milk has been totally removed and starch (cereals) partly replaced with glucose or sucrose.

Micronutrient supplementation

Most malnourished children with persistent diarrhoea have associated deficiencies of micronutrients, including zinc, iron and vitamin A. This may be a consequence of poor intake and continued enteral losses. It is therefore important to ensure that all children with persistent diarrhoea and malnutrition receive an initial dose of vitamin A orally, or if that is not possible by deep intramuscular injection (< 6 months of age, 50 000 units; 6–12 months, 100 000 units; > 1 year, 200 000 units). They should also receive a daily intake of the following for the next 2 weeks:

- a multivitamin supplement

- folic acid, 250 micrograms/kg on day 1, then 75 micrograms/kg/day
- zinc, 3–5 mg/kg/day.
- copper, 0.3 mg/kg/day
- magnesium, 0.2 mmol/kg/day.

Although the association of significant anaemia with persistent diarrhoea is well recognised, iron replacement therapy should not be initiated until recovery from diarrhoea has started (ferrous sulphate 18 mg/kg/day, or 6 mg/kg/day of elemental iron in two divided doses).

Follow-up and nutritional rehabilitation

Given the high rates of relapse in most children with persistent diarrhoea, it is important to address the underlying risk factors and institute preventive measures. These include appropriate feeding (breastfeeding, complementary feeding) and close attention to environmental hygiene and sanitation. This poses a considerable challenge in communities deprived of basic necessities such as clean water and sewage disposal.

By the time they return home, children should be receiving a diet that provides at least 110 kcal/kg/day (including milk and fresh fruit and well-cooked vegetables).

Further reading

Bhutta ZA, Molla AM, Isani Z et al. (1991) Dietary management of persistent diarrhoea: comparison of a traditional rice-lentil based diet with soy formula. *Pediatrics*, **88**, 1010–18.

International Working Group on Persistent Diarrhoea (1996) Evaluation of an algorithm for the treatment of persistent diarrhoea: a multicentre study. *Bulletin of the World Health Organization*, **74**, 479–89.

Bhutta ZA and Hendricks KH (1996) Nutritional management of persistent diarrhoea in childhood: a perspective from the developing world. *Journal of Pediatric Gastroenterology and Nutrition*, **22**, 17–37.

Imdad A, Sadiq K and Bhutta ZA (2011) Evidence-based prevention of childhood malnutrition. *Current Opinion in Clinical Nutrition and Metabolic Care*, **14**, 276–85.

Haider BA and Bhutta ZA (2009) The effect of therapeutic zinc supplementation among young children with selected infections: a review of the evidence. *Food and Nutrition Bulletin*, **30 (1 Suppl.)**, S41–59.

Bhutta ZA, Nelson EA, Lee WS et al. (2008) Recent advances and evidence gaps in persistent diarrhea. *Journal of Pediatric Gastroenterology and Nutrition*, **47**, 260–5.

World Health Organization (1999) *Management of Severe Malnutrition: a manual for physicians and other health care workers*. Geneva: World Health Organization.

5.12.C Constipation

BOX 5.12.C.1 Minimum standards
- Movicol – osmotic laxative – softens
- Lactulose – osmotic laxative – softens
- Docusate sodium – softener and weak stimulant
- Senna or sodium picosulphate-stimulant laxative
- Glycerine suppositories – lubricant and rectal stimulant
- Small volume of phosphate enema (e.g. fleet enema)
- Sodium citrate enema (e.g. Micralax enema).

Introduction

Definition

Constipation is defined as difficulty with, delay in or pain on defecation.

Normal defecation patterns

- Breastfed babies average three stools per day and formula-fed babies two stools per day. However, the range of normal stool frequency in breastfed babies is very wide, from one stool every few days to a stool with every feed.
- Children average one stool per day after 3 years, but the normal range is from once on alternate days to three times daily.

Pathophysiology

Most children with constipation have no underlying medical cause. An episode of constipation can be triggered by inadequate food or fluid intake, an intercurrent illness, or excessive intake of cow's milk.

Constipation cycle

The child passes a hard painful stool. On subsequent occasions they try to withhold the stool in order to avoid experiencing pain (faecal holding). The stool remains in the rectum, becoming harder still, and so causing even more pain when it is eventually passed.

If this cycle is allowed to continue, eventually the rectum may become enlarged, resulting in a 'megarectum'. The child by this stage has lost the normal urge to defecate, and the large rectal mass of stool holds open the anal sphincter, which leads to soiling with liquid faeces. This is involuntary and should not be confused with encopresis, which occurs when the child voluntarily passes normal stools in unacceptable places.

Diagnosis

Diagnosis can usually be made by taking a good history.

- On examination of the abdomen, faecal masses may be palpable. These are often in the left and right iliac fossae, but sometimes suprapubically. On inspection of the anus, anal tags and fissure may be seen in chronic constipation.
- On rectal examination, hard impacted faeces may be felt. Rectal examination is usually not necessary. If there is an anal fissure, rectal examination should be done with topical lignocaine jelly (1%) and terminated if it is too painful.
- Abdominal X-ray is not a useful examination for diagnosis of constipation.

Pathological causes

The vast majority of constipation is idiopathic, but there are a few uncommon causes that are important not to miss.

Hirschsprung's disease

Suspect this when there is infancy-onset constipation and a delay of more than 48 hours in passing meconium at birth. In more advanced cases there will be abdominal distension and sometimes failure to thrive and vomiting. There may be alternating constipation and diarrhoea and surprisingly little soiling for the degree of constipation. On rectal examination an explosive gush of faeces occurs when the examining finger is withdrawn.

Anal lesions that cause pain or create an obstruction

These include anal fissures, perianal skin infections and (rarely) congenital anterior anus and anal stenosis. One cause of painful anal lesions is sexual abuse, a rare but important cause which should not be missed.

Endocrine conditions

Hypothyroidism, renal tubular acidosis, diabetes insipidus and hypercalcaemia can be associated with constipation. There should be a high level of suspicion for a metabolic or endocrine cause if constipation and failure to thrive coexist.

Neurogenic constipation

Spinal cord lesions involving sensation in the rectum will cause neurogenic constipation. These can be excluded by a normal neurological and spinal examination.

Management of idiopathic constipation

Parental understanding of the aetiology and sequence of events in developing chronic constipation is crucial to successful physical and psychological management (see Figure 5.12.C.1). Each and every element of this flow diagram should be addressed and treated if management is to be completely successful.

Explanation

A careful and thorough explanation of the problem should be given to the parent and child. Emphasise that soiling is not deliberate, and that the child needs support, not condemnation. Assess the need for psychological as well as physical treatment.

Evacuation of hard impacted faeces

1 To soften and lubricate the retained faeces, initially give a softener. This could be a macrogol such as Movicol or another softening laxative such as docusate sodium. The dose will vary according to age.

2 Alongside the softener, in order to expel the retained mass, give a stimulant laxative (e.g. sodium picosulphate).

3 If sodium picosulphate is not available, a large dose of senna can be tried, but may need to be used for longer.

4 Only if the above fails give suppositories (glycerine) once daily (infant, 1 gram; child < 12 years, 2 grams; child > 12 years, 4 grams).

5 If the oral and suppository methods are unsuccessful, if excessive abdominal pain develops and/or there is vomiting, stimulant enemas will be required. Phosphate enemas should not be used in children under 2 years of age. For children aged 2–10 years give 60 mL (half a phosphate enema) and for those over 10 years of age give 120 mL (full enema). If phosphate enemas are not available, a small-volume sodium citrate enema (micro-enema) can be used. However, the use of enemas can add to the child's fear of defecation. **The child should never be forcibly held down to receive an enema.** Give enemas **once a day** in the morning. Most children need two or three enemas to clear a faecal mass.

6 If these measures fail, the child should undergo manual evacuation of faecal mass under general anaesthetic, **but only if this is available and can be done safely.**

Maintenance laxatives to keep the stool soft, defecation pain-free and overcome faecal holding

● Softening agents such as Movicol or docusate sodium to keep the stool soft.

● Stimulant laxatives, usually senna or sodium picosulphate, to expel the soft stool. The aim is to produce

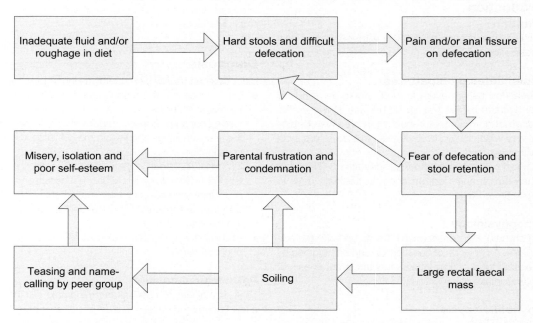

FIGURE 5.12.C.1 Sequence of events in faecal soiling.

loose stools initially and then subsequently reduce the dose to produce at least one soft stool per day. Often large doses will be required initially to overcome the child's faecal holding.

Behaviour changes

- Encourage increased fluid intake and a high-roughage diet (fruit, vegetables and cereals).
- Give positive praise and encouragement for regular toileting, and for passage of stool into the toilet.

Length of treatment

Children are likely to require several months of stimulant laxatives until their fear of defecation resolves, and often months to years of continuous or intermittent treatment with softening laxatives. A general rule of thumb is that the child will need laxatives for the same length of time that they were constipated before treatment started.

5.12.D Inflammatory bowel disease

BOX 5.12.D.1 Minimum standards
- Aminosalicylates.
- Prednisolone.
- Methylprednisolone.
- Corticosteroid enemas.
- Blood transfusion.
- Polymeric diet.
- Metronidazole.

Introduction

Inflammatory bowel disease (IBD) is uncommon in children in resource-limited countries, where abdominal tuberculosis is more common. However, in the UK about 18% of children with IBD are non-white, of whom most are of either Indian or Caribbean origin. Although IBD may present in younger children, the mean age in the UK is approximately 12 years. Crohn's disease is more than twice as common as ulcerative colitis. A family history is common.

Diagnosis

- Clinical symptoms of ulcerative colitis are almost invariably bloody diarrhoea with predefecation abdominal pain and tenesmus. Crohn's disease may have a wide variety of symptoms, especially extra-intestinal ones. Iron-deficiency anaemia is common in both.

- The interval between onset of symptoms and diagnosis is often over 6 months in Crohn's disease, and may be 2–3 months in ulcerative colitis. Denial of symptoms is common, especially in adolescents.

Investigations

- Growth parameters and investigations are a guide to the severity and duration of disease and the nutritional state of the child.
- Examination of the mouth and anus is essential.
- Stool examination is essential to exclude bacterial and parasitological causes of diarrhoea, especially before corticosteroids are prescribed.
- Normal investigations: acute-phase reactants (erythrocyte sedimentation rate or C-reactive protein), haemoglobin, platelet count, albumin; do not exclude ulcerative colitis, but normal blood tests would be very unusual in Crohn's disease.
- Children with ulcerative colitis often have little or no weight loss or growth failure.
- Children with Crohn's disease and severe involvement of the colon may present similarly to those with ulcerative colitis, but generally have larger haematological changes.

TABLE 5.12.D.1 Comparison between Crohn's disease and ulcerative colitis

Feature	Ulcerative colitis	Crohn's disease
Pathology	Mucosal disease	Transmural disease, skin lesions, strictures, fistulae
Site	Recto-colonic (rectum always involved). In children over 70% have a pancolitis	Panenteric disease is common in children: small bowel and colon, 50%; colon, 35%; ileum, 6%; upper gastrointestinal tract, 50%
Common presenting symptoms	Diarrhoea mixed with blood/mucus Pain (lower abdominal) Often no or little weight loss	Pain in the right iliac fossa Diarrhoea with or without blood Growth failure and weight loss Peri-anal and oral disease
Extra-intestinal features (finger clubbing, arthritis, skin disorders, fever)	Uncommon	Common

General investigations
Stool
- Blood, mucus.

- Microscopy for *Entamoeba histolytica*, *Schistosoma*, *Trichuris trichiura*, *Giardia lamblia*.
- Culture for bacteria.

Full blood count
- Haemoglobin level decreased.
- White blood cell count increased.
- Platelet count increased.

Acute-phase reactants
- Erythrocyte sedimentation rate raised.
- C-reactive protein raised.

Chemical pathology
- Electrolytes (if diarrhoea severe).
- Ferritin (may be spuriously raised – acute-phase reactant).
- Albumin level low.

Specific investigations
Specific investigations depend on the availability of paediatric gastrointestinal facilities.
- Sigmoidoscopy is essential.
- Flexible endoscopy of the lower and upper gastrointestinal tract should ideally be undertaken.
- Barium enema (double contrast) is required in colitis **only** if colonoscopy is not available.
- Normal macroscopic appearance of the lower or upper gut **does not exclude IBD**. **Histology is essential.**
- 'Indeterminate colitis' is a term used to describe patients whose histology is not typical of ulcerative colitis or Crohn's disease. They are usually treated initially as having ulcerative colitis.

TABLE 5.12.D.2 Specific investigations for Crohn's disease and ulcerative colitis

Feature	Ulcerative colitis	Crohn's disease
Endoscopy*	Proctoscopy Sigmoidoscopy Colonoscopy	Lower gut Upper gut*
Radiological studies	Barium enema† (double contrast)	Barium meal and follow-through
White blood cell scan (technetium labelled)‡	Screening	Screening

* Depending on availability.

† Only required if colonoscopy is unavailable.

‡ Only available in well-resourced countries.

Management of ulcerative colitis
- Initial management depends on severity.
- Follow-up: parents and older children should be taught so that they understand how to recognise and treat any relapse promptly.

Management of active colitis (see Table 5.12.D.3)
- **Mild disease:** less than four motions per day, intermittent blood, normal acute-phase reactants, no toxicity:
  - Aminosalicylates.
  - Mesalazine (1 g rectally) or corticosteroid (20 mg) enema until the bleeding stops, and then given alternate nights for 1 week.

- Corticosteroids given orally if there is no response within 2 weeks.
- **Moderate disease:** four to six motions per day, moderate blood, slight toxicity, anaemia and raised acute-phase reactants:
  - As above plus oral steroids immediately. If there is a poor response, treat as for severe disease.
- **Severe disease:** more than six bloody motions per day, nocturnal stools, toxicity, fever, anaemia and hypoalbuminaemia:
  - Intravenous pulse methylprednisolone or hydrocortisone dose for 3–5 days.
  - Antibiotics (e.g. metronidazole) (benefit is not proven).
  - Intravenous fluids and correction of electrolyte deficits.
  - Blood transfusion if required.
  - Intravenous cyclosporine (500 micrograms–1 mg/kg aged 3–18 years) or oral cyclosporine (2 mg/kg twice daily maximum 5 mg/kg aged 2–18 years) may be of value if there is no response to intravenous corticosteroids.
- **Toxic dilation:** if there is no response to intensive therapy by 12–24 hours, perform colectomy.

Relapse
Prompt commencement of rectal mesalazine or a corticosteroid enema is essential. If there is no response, give a course of oral corticosteroids.

Maintenance
- Aminosalicylic acid preparations are generally given life-long. Mesalazine 10 mg/kg 2–3 times daily 5–12 years, 2 G once daily 12–18 years.
- If relapses occur when corticosteroids are reduced, give azathioprine for up to 3–5 years.

TABLE 5.12.D.3 Drug dosages for ulcerative colitis

Corticosteroids	
Prednisolone:	2 mg/kg/day (maximum 40 mg) for 3 weeks, then reduce by 5 mg/week
Methylprednisolone:	IV 1–1.5 mg/kg/day (maximum 60 mg)
Hydrocortisone:	IV 4 mg/kg 6-hourly
Prednisolone enema or foam (20 mg in 100 mL):	50–100 mL at night
Aminosalicylates	
Sulphasalazine: (tablets 10 mg and 50 mg)	10 mg/kg 4- to 6-hourly for acute episodes. Decrease the dose by half for maintenance as soon as possible. Urine and tears will turn orange. Report sore throat
Mesalazine: (oral tablets 500 mg)	Under 40 kg body weight aged 5–12 years give 10 mg/kg 2–3 times daily; over 40 kg body weight aged 12–18 years, give 2 G once daily
Mesalazine: rectal	Aged 12–18 years, 1 gram daily
Metronidazole: (orally)	7.5 mg/kg three times daily
Azathioprine: (orally)	1.5–2.5 mg/kg once daily

- Regular monitoring of the blood count (every 1 to 2 months) is important.

Indicators for colectomy

- Toxic megacolon (see above), intractable disease and growth failure.
- The risk of cancer relates to the extent of disease and its duration. Good maintenance therapy is important for prevention. Two-yearly colonoscopy should be considered in those with pancolitis for 10 years after the commencement of disease.
- Colectomy and ileostomy would be the usual operation in resource-limited settings, and are curative symptomatically, but the patient then has the ileostomy for life.

Management of Crohn's disease

- The key to management is to maintain growth and nutrition and control symptoms.
- Most children will have recurrent relapses.
- Many will require surgery at some stage.
- Nutritional treatment and support are essential.

Polymeric diet

A polymeric diet can be any liquid nutritional preparation that is nutritionally complete. Examples would include PaediaSure/Ensure (Abbott Nutrition), Modulen IBD/Resource Junior (Nestle) and Alicalm/Fortini (Nutricia). Polymeric diet is effective in producing 70% remission in small bowel disease and 50% remission in colonic disease. The advantages over corticosteroids are the positive effect on growth and lack of side effects. The diet is given for 6 weeks, usually orally, during which time no other food is given (but the child can drink water), and then the normal diet is re-introduced.

Maintenance therapy with polymeric diet can also be used.

Drug therapy

See Table 5.12.D.3 for drug dosages in ulcerative colitis.

- Prednisolone 2 mg/kg/day (maximum 40 mg/day) is effective in small and large bowel disease. Continue this dose for 3 weeks, then reduce it by 5 mg/week and then stop. If required to maintain remission, alternate-day therapy may have fewer side effects.
- Mesalazine but not sulphasalazine can be effective for maintaining remission in ileal as well as colonic disease (dose is aged 5–12 years 10–15 mg/kg orally 2–3 times daily, aged 12–18 years 2 G once daily).
- Azathioprine is effective in long-term maintenance and has steroid-sparing effects. It may be useful for healing perianal fistulae. It takes many months to act, and it should be continued for at least 4 years. Blood counts should be undertaken every 1–2 months.
- Metronidazole may be effective in controlling perianal disease and fistulae. It may also reduce small bowel overgrowth. Ciprofloxacin is an alternative.
- Infliximab is a very expensive monoclonal antibody that inhibits tumour necrosis factor alpha (TNFα). It is used in severe Crohn's disease that is not responding to conventional treatment. It is administered IV at intervals. Because of its immunosuppressive effects there are real dangers from infection, especially **latent TB**. Other side effects include anaphylaxis, lymphoma and possibly demyelinating disorders.

Surgery

Indications for surgery include failure of medical therapy, intestinal obstruction and growth failure. Strictureplasty may be an effective method of avoiding excision of bowel when strictures are present.

Follow-up and support for IBD

Patients and their families require long-term understanding and support. Psychological therapy may be helpful in some cases.

5.12.E Upper gastroenterological disorders

Introduction

Upper gastrointestinal disorders are not common complaints in the population presenting to hospitals in resource-limited countries. It may be that symptoms are under-reported or overlooked because of more common problems, such as gastroenteritis, persistent diarrhoea, intestinal helminths and malnutrition. However, certain life-threatening conditions do occur, including obstruction of the oesophagus due to a foreign body, strictures due to caustic soda poisoning, haematemesis due to peptic ulcer or portal hypertension, and volvulus due to malrotation.

In well-resourced communities, particularly **where facilities for upper gastrointestinal paediatric endoscopy** are available, similar symptoms to those that occur in well-resourced countries present. These include recurrent abdominal pain, epigastric and substernal pain, recurrent/persistent vomiting, dyspepsia and water-brash/heartburn.

Gastro-oesophageal reflux

TABLE 5.12.E.1 Gastro-oesophageal reflux

Symptoms	Complications
Vomiting (regurgitation)	*In Infants*
Water-brash/heartburn	Apnoea
Nausea	Life-threatening event
Epigastric/retrosternal pain	*All ages*
	Failure to thrive*
	Aspiration pneumonia
	Haematemesis
	Anaemia
	Oesophageal stricture

*Particularly in children with cerebral palsy.

Gastro-oesophageal reflux (GOR) is a normal physiological condition in infants, children and adults. If GOR is associated with complications (as below) then it is termed gastro-oesophageal reflux disease (GORD). GORD is common in children with cerebral palsy.

Note: Sandifer–Sutcliffe syndrome is dystonic posturing associated with GOR.

Diagnosis

Often no investigations are needed and a diagnosis can be made by taking a good clinical history. The following investigations are helpful if they are needed and available:

- **Barium swallow:** This is often the only diagnostic facility available in resource-limited countries. It is a much less sensitive method for diagnosing reflux than pH monitoring, but will detect associated or other conditions such as oesophageal stricture, hiatus hernia, diaphragmatic hernia and malrotation.
- **Endoscopy and biopsy** (particularly looking for oesophagitis).
- pH monitoring: this grades the frequency and duration of exposure of the lower oesophagus to acid (pH < 4.0).

Management

- Simple GOR in the thriving child: reassurance is all that is needed.
- Excessive regurgitation causing failure to thrive in an infant, or mild symptoms of oesophagitis: treatment by thickening feeds with Carobel (Cow & Gate) or an alginate preparation (e.g. Gaviscon) can be tried.
- Moderate to severe GOR with oesophagitis: H_2-receptor antagonists, such as ranitidine (2–4 mg/kg twice daily, maximum 150 mg twice daily) or the proton pump inhibitor, omeprazole (700 micrograms to 3 mg/kg once daily) should be given. Motility stimulants such as domperidone (200–400 micrograms/kg every 4–8 hours) may be effective, particularly in children with cerebral palsy. However, proof of their efficacy is lacking.
- Surgery: Nissen fundoplication would be considered if, despite medical management, there **was** severe oesophagitis, failure to thrive or aspiration pneumonia. It is sometimes required in children with cerebral palsy and GOR.

Helicobacter pylori

Helicobacter pylori is a ubiquitous bacterium that commonly infects the stomach (especially the antrum) of children in resource-limited countries from an early age. Child-to-child transmission is important. In developed countries up to 40–60% of adults are infected, probably mainly during childhood. Conditions associated with *H. pylori* include the following:

- **Chronic gastritis:** often asymptomatic; not a major cause of abdominal pain in children.
- **Duodenal ulcer:** *H. pylori* has a strong association with duodenal ulcer and must be eradicated to ensure healing.

Diagnosis

Testing for *H. pylori* should only be undertaken if the child has symptoms of ulcer dyspepsia. Diagnostic tests (outlined below) are rarely available as routine in resource-limited countries.

- Serology: this is good for epidemiological studies, but has reduced sensitivity in children under 7 years of age.
- Urea breath test (13C-UBT): this is sensitive and specific, especially in children over 6 years of age.
- Faecal antigen testing: this is sensitive and specific in both children and adults.
- Endoscopy: histological demonstration and culture of *H. pylori*.

Management

Selection of optimal antibacterial agents is difficult because of the development of resistance.

Suggested regimen

1 Omeprazole
- Aged < 2 years 700 micrograms/kg to 3 mg/kg once daily up to a maximum of 20 mg.
- Aged > 2 years, body weight 10–20 kg, give 10 mg once daily up to maximum 20 mg once daily.
- Aged > 2 years, body weight > 20 kg, give 20 mg once daily up to a maximum of 40 mg once daily.
2 **plus** antibiotics, such as amoxicillin (< 1 year, 62.5 mg; 1–4 years, 125 mg; 5–12 years, 250 mg; > 12 years, 250–500 mg, three times daily)
3 **plus** clarithromycin (7.5 mg/kg twice daily) **or** metronidazole (7.5 mg/kg three times daily).

Treatment should be continued for 1–2 weeks. Strict compliance in order to avoid the development of resistance is imperative.

Duodenal ulcer

Duodenal ulcers are uncommon in children, but can be life-threatening due to haematemesis, melaena and perforation.

There is often a family history. Common symptoms include epigastric pain that typically:

- is worsened by fasting
- is improved by eating or antacids
- causes **nocturnal waking**.

Diagnosis

- **Endoscopy, including biopsy for *H. pylori*, is the optimal method.**
- Barium swallow: this is less sensitive for diagnosing acute ulceration and better at detecting scarring.

Management

- Unless facilities to diagnose *H. pylori* are available, all children should be treated for eradication of presumed *H. pylori*.
- Give H_2 antagonists or a proton pump inhibitor for 6–8 weeks: ranitidine 2–4 mg/kg twice daily (maximum 150 mg twice daily); omeprazole 10 mg for 10–20 kg (can increase to 20 mg) and 20 mg for > 20 kg once daily (can increase to 40 mg).

5.12.F Gastrointestinal bleeding

Introduction

- The causes of bleeding from the gastrointestinal tract are many, and relate to the age of the child. A good history and clinical examination are essential and will indicate specific investigations.

- In haematemesis, it is important to exclude swallowed blood due to disorders of the nose and mouth.
- In children the commonest cause of fresh rectal bleeding is an anal fissure.
- Melaena has to be differentiated from dark stools associated with medication (e.g. iron preparations) and colouring from foods.
- A large bleed from the upper gastrointestinal tract may present as red blood at the anus because of rapid transit.

TABLE 5.12.F.1 Causes of gastrointestinal haemorrhage

Site of bleeding	Clinical features/further information
Upper gut Poisoning with or treatment with salicylates Mallory–Weiss syndrome	'Coffee-ground' vomit
Oesophagitis, gastro-oesophageal reflux	*See* Section 5.12.E
Portal hypertension, oesophageal varices	*See* Section 5.7.B (liver disease) *See* Section 6.3.C.c (schistosomiasis)
Midgut Intussusception, volvulus	Infants (*see* Section 3.4 and 5.19)
Meckel's diverticulum	Often symptomless
Colorectal Infection (e.g. shigellosis, amoebiasis)	*See* Section 5.12.A and Section 6.3.B
Inflammatory bowel disease	Abdominal pain, diarrhoea, weight loss *See* Section 5.12.D
Milk protein intolerance	*See* Section 5.12.G
Polyps (single, multiple, Peutz–Jeghers syndrome)	Blood separate from normal stool
Anus Fissure	Infants, constipation, tags (*see* Section 5.12.C)
Crohn's disease	*See* Section 5.12.D
Miscellaneous Necrotising enterocolitis (*see* Section 3.4), Henoch–Schönlein purpura (*see* Section 5.13), AIDS (*see* Section 6.2.D) Any coagulation or blood malignancy disorder (*see* Section 5.11.D and Section 5.14)	

Investigations

The investigations chosen will depend on the suspected site of bleeding and the clinical features.

See appropriate sections as indicated in the tables above.

It is important to consider the following:
- Stool:
  - Direct observation: blood, mucus.
  - Microscopy: *Cryptosporidium*, *Salmonella*, *E. coli*, *Shigella*, *Campylobacter*, ova, cysts and parasites.
  - Faecal occult blood.
- Full blood count, grouping and cross-matching.
- Serum ferritin and iron levels.
- Isotope scan: diagnosis of Meckel's diverticulum (30% false negative).
- Barium studies: diagnosis of malrotation.
- Ultrasound: diagnosis of intussusception.
- Upper endoscopy: diagnosis and treatment of oesophageal, gastric and/or duodenal bleeding.
- Colonoscopy: diagnosis and treatment of colitis and/or polyps.

TABLE 5.12.F.2 Features of gastrointestinal bleeding

History/examination	Looking for:
History	
Acute/chronic, amount of blood	Severity
Endemic area	Schistosomiasis
Haematemesis	Upper gastrointestinal disorder
Nose and mouth lesions	Swallowed blood
Site of any pain	Upper or lower gastrointestinal tract
Stool: Hard/loose	Constipation/diarrhoea
Blood mixed in stool	Inflammation/infection
Blood around or separate	Anal fissure/polyp

History/examination	Looking for:
Inflammatory bowel disease, family history	*See* Section 5.12.D
Bleeding tendency	Clotting disorder, malignancy
Examination	
Nose and mouth lesions	Swallowed blood
Pallor, capillary refill, blood pressure	Anaemia, shock
Petechiae, telangiectasia	Thrombocytopenia, hereditary telangiectasia
Abdomen	Tenderness, hepatosplenomegaly
Anus	Fissure, tags, infection

5.12.G Malabsorption, including coeliac disease

Malabsorption

Malabsorption is an abnormality in absorption of food nutrients from the gastrointestinal tract.

Common causes of malabsorption and resultant failure to thrive in resource-limited countries include recurrent respiratory infection, persistent diarrhoea and HIV infection. None of these require bowel investigation. The main emphasis is on nutritional rehabilitation which regenerates the small bowel atrophy and the immune system (see management of persistent diarrhoea and severe malnutrition in Sections 5.12.B and 5.10.B, respectively). Only a limited response to nutritional support is expected in HIV infection, depending generally on the stage of disease and the response to antiretroviral (ARV) drugs.

Types of malabsorption

- **Selective:** as seen in lactose intolerance.
- **Partial:** as observed in Crohn's disease and HIV infection.
- **Total:** as seen in coeliac disease.

Pathophysiology

The gastrointestinal tract functions to digest and absorb nutrients (fat, carbohydrate, protein and fibre), micronutrients (vitamins and trace minerals), water and electrolytes. This is dependent on the proper processing of food by mechanical (chewing and gastric churning) and enzymatic (gastric, pancreatic, biliary or intestinal) means. The final products of digestion are then absorbed through the intestinal epithelial cells.

Malabsorption constitutes the pathological breakdown of the normal physiological sequence of digestion (i.e. intraluminal process), absorption (i.e. mucosal process) and transport (post-mucosal events) of nutrients.

Clinical features

Symptoms can be intestinal or extra-intestinal, and include the following:

- diarrhoea/steatorrhoea: watery, diurnal and nocturnal, bulky, frequent stools
- bloating
- flatulence
- abdominal discomfort/cramping abdominal pain
- growth retardation
- weight loss
- failure to thrive
- delayed puberty
- swelling or oedema from loss of protein
- anaemia (vitamin B_{12}, folic acid and iron deficiency)
- fatigue
- weakness
- muscle cramp
- osteomalacia and osteoporosis
- bleeding tendencies.

Diagnosis

Investigation is guided by symptoms and signs. Since a range of different conditions can produce malabsorption, it is necessary to look for each of these specifically. Tests are also needed to detect the systemic effects of deficiency of the malabsorbed nutrients (e.g. anaemia with vitamin B_{12} malabsorption).

Investigations may include the following:

- full blood count and blood film
- C-reactive protein and erythrocyte sedimentation rate
- serum albumin
- serum iron, ferritin and total iron-binding capacity (TIBC)
- serum folic acid
- serum cholesterol or triglyceride
- serum calcium, phosphate and alkaline phosphatase
- prothrombin time and activated partial thromboplastin time
- blood chemistry (electrolytes, glucose, HCO_3^-, urea and creatinine)
- serum zinc levels
- stool studies, including cultures.

TABLE 5.12 G.1 Common causes of malabsorption

	Common causes of malabsorption
Due to infective agents	Intestinal tuberculosis
	HIV-related malabsorption
	Tropical sprue
	Traveller's diarrhoea
	Parasites, such as *Giardia lamblia*, fish tapeworm, roundworm,
	hookworm (*Ancylostoma duodenale* and *Necator americanus*)
Due to structural defects	Blind loops
	Inflammatory bowel diseases (e.g. Crohn's disease)
	Intestinal hurry from surgical procedures (e.g. post-gastrectomy, gastro-jejunostomy)
	Fistulae, diverticulae and strictures
	Short bowel syndrome
Due to mucosal abnormality	Coeliac disease
	Cow's milk intolerance
	Soya milk intolerance
Due to enzyme deficiencies	Lactose intolerance (constitutional, secondary or rarely congenital)
	Sucrose intolerance
Due to digestive failure	Pancreatic insufficiencies
	Cystic fibrosis
	Chronic pancreatitis
	Bile salt malabsorption
	Terminal ileal disease
	Obstructive jaundice
	Bacterial overgrowth
Due to systemic diseases	Coeliac disease
	Hypothyroidism and hyperthyroidism
	Addison's disease
	Diabetes mellitus
	Hyperparathyroidism and hypoparathyroidism
	Malnutrition

Serological studies
The following specific tests are carried out to determine the underlying cause:
- IgA anti-transglutaminase antibodies
- IgA anti-endomysial antibodies.

Radiological studies
- Barium meal and follow-through.
- Barium enema.
- CT of the abdomen.

Specialised tests (if available)
- Biopsy of small bowel.
- Colonoscopy can be helpful in colonic and ileal disease.
- Endoscopic retrograde cholangiopancreatography (ERCP) will show pancreatic and biliary structural abnormalities.
- Glucose hydrogen breath test for bacterial overgrowth.
- Lactose hydrogen breath test for lactose intolerance.
- Magnetic resonance cholangiopancreatography (MRCP).

Management
Treatment is directed largely towards management of the underlying cause. In severe nutritional deficiency, hospital admission may be required for total parenteral nutrition (TPN). Subsequently, advice and support from a dietitian is vital.

Coeliac disease

BOX 5.12.G.1 Minimum standards
- Gluten-free diet.
- Full blood count and film.

Coeliac disease is an autoimmune disorder of the small intestine in genetically predisposed people of all ages from middle infancy onwards. It is caused by a reaction to gliadin, a gluten protein found in wheat and similar cereals. Therefore it is common among populations whose diet contains substantial amounts of wheat. Apart from people of European origin, in whom it commonly manifests, it is also frequently seen in North Africa, the Middle East, and the north of the Indian subcontinent where wheat is a staple diet. Other populations at increased risk for coeliac disease include children with Down's syndrome and Turner syndrome, type 1 diabetes and autoimmune thyroid disease, including both hyperthyroidism and hypothyroidism.

Pathophysiology
Upon exposure to gliadin, the enzyme tissue transglutaminase (tTG) modifies the immune system to cross-react with the small-bowel villous lining, causing an inflammatory reaction. This leads to villous atrophy, which interferes with the absorption of nutrients, minerals and the fat-soluble vitamins A, D, E and K.

Coeliac disease appears to be polyfactorial. Almost all people with coeliac disease have either the HLA-DQ2 or the HLA-DQ8 allele. However, additional factors are needed for coeliac disease to manifest besides the HLA risk alleles. Furthermore, around 5% of those people who do develop coeliac disease may not have typical HLA-DQ2 or HLA-DQ8 alleles.

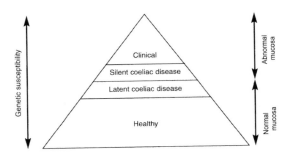

FIGURE 5.12.G.1 The spectrum of coeliac disease. Latent coeliac disease: positive anti-endomysial antibodies, normal small bowel, but risk of developing disease.

Clinical features

Clinical features may range from severe to almost non-existent. Severe coeliac disease in young children leads to the characteristic symptoms of pale, loose and greasy stools (steatorrhoea) with weight loss or failure to gain weight. Adolescents and older children with milder coeliac disease may have symptoms that are much more subtle and occur in other organs rather than in the bowel itself.

TABLE 5.12.G.2 Clinical features of coeliac disease

Under 2 years of age	Over 2 years of age
Steatorrhoea	Short stature
Vomiting	Delayed puberty
Abdominal distension	Iron-resistant anaemia
Irritability	Rickets/osteomalacia
Anorexia	Behaviour problems
Growth failure	*With or without the gut disorders that occur in younger children*

Diagnosis

The diagnosis of coeliac disease is based on two types of testing.

Serological blood tests

These are the first-line investigation and include the following:

- **IgA anti-tissue transglutaminase (tTG) antibodies:** this test is reported to have a high sensitivity (99%) and specificity (over 90%) for identifying coeliac disease. Therefore it should be done first. It is also an easier test to perform. An equivocal result on tTG testing should be followed by antibodies to endomysium.
- **IgA anti-endomysial antibodies:** this test has a sensitivity and specificity of 90% and 99%, respectively, for detecting coeliac disease.

It is important that the total serum IgA level is also checked, as coeliac patients with IgA deficiency may be unable to produce the antibodies on which these tests depend ('false-negative'). In such patients, IgG antibodies against transglutaminase (IgG-tTG) or IgG anti-gliadin antibodies (IgG-AGA) may be helpful in reaching a diagnosis.

Dudeno-jejunal biopsies

Because of the implications of a diagnosis of coeliac disease, guidelines recommend that a positive serological blood test may still be followed by a dudeno-jejunal biopsy. Similarly, a negative serology may still be followed by a recommendation for a biopsy if clinical suspicion remains high. Tissue biopsy is still considered the gold standard in the diagnosis of coeliac disease.

For this purpose, biopsies can be obtained using metal capsules attached to a suction device. The capsule is swallowed and allowed to pass into the small intestine. After X-ray verification of its position, suction is applied to collect part of the intestinal wall inside the capsule. Commonly used capsule systems are the Watson capsule and the Crosby–Kugler capsule. This method has now been largely replaced by fibre-optic endoscopy, which carries a higher sensitivity and a lower frequency of errors.

TABLE 5.12.G.3 Investigations for malabsorption

General	Specific
Full blood count plus film	Immunoglobulins IgA and IgG
Serum iron and ferritin	IgA tTG antibodies
Folate (red blood cell)	IgA anti-endomysial antibodies
Vitamin B_{12} levels	
Serum albumin	IgA anti-gliadin (AGA)
Hydrogen breath test	Small bowel biopsy:
Serum calcium, phosphate and alkaline phosphatase	• Villous atrophy • Hyperplasia of crypts • Increased inflammatory cells
Serum T_4 and TSH	

There are several ways in which these tests can be used to assist in diagnosing coeliac disease. However, all tests become invalid if the patient is already taking a gluten-free diet. Intestinal damage begins to heal within weeks of gluten being removed from the diet, and antibody levels decline over a period of months. In such cases it may be necessary to perform a re-challenge with gluten-containing food over 2–6 weeks before repeating the investigations.

A histology compatible with coeliac disease on a gluten-containing diet, followed by a clinical improvement (i.e. gain in weight and height and resolution of symptoms) once the gluten is removed from the diet is often enough to establish the diagnosis. Most guidelines do not recommend a repeat biopsy unless there is no improvement in the symptoms on the gluten-free diet. In some cases a deliberate gluten challenge, followed by biopsy, may be conducted to confirm or refute the diagnosis. A normal biopsy and normal serology after the challenge indicates that the diagnosis may have been incorrect.

In resource-limited countries where facilities for biopsies may not exist, the same model can be used with serological tests. A positive serological test on a gluten-containing diet will revert to normal with clinical improvement once the patient is on a gluten-free diet.

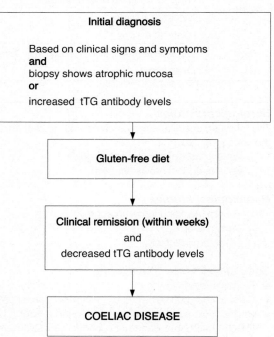

Initial diagnosis

Based on clinical signs and symptoms
and
biopsy shows atrophic mucosa
or
increased tTG antibody levels

↓

Gluten-free diet

↓

Clinical remission (within weeks)
and
decreased tTG antibody levels

↓

COELIAC DISEASE

FIGURE 5.12.G.2 Diagnosis of coeliac disease.

BOX 5.12.G.2 Gluten challenge

Do a gluten challenge if:
- the diagnosis is in doubt
- there is a possibility of another diagnosis, especially in children under 2 years of age (e.g. milk protein intolerance, persistent diarrhoea, giardiasis)
- the response to a gluten-free diet is not clear-cut
- the subject is asymptomatic (e.g. first-degree relatives).

Note: Gluten challenge should preferably be undertaken when the child is over 6 years old and before puberty, to reduce the effects on dentition and growth.

Treatment

At present, the only effective treatment is a lifelong gluten-free diet. Strict compliance allows the intestines to heal, with resolution of symptoms in most cases. Early intervention and good compliance can eliminate the heightened risk of intestinal cancer and in some cases sterility.

Dietitian input can be helpful in ensuring that the patient is aware of which foods contain gluten, which foods are safe, and how to have a balanced diet despite the limitations. The diet can be cumbersome, and failure to comply may cause relapse.

The commonly implicated cereals include wheat (and its subspecies, such as spelt, semolina and durum), barley, rye and oats.

Other cereals, such as maize (corn), millet, sorghum, teff and rice, are safe for patients to consume. Similarly, non-cereal foods such as fruits, vegetables and foods derived from animal sources (i.e. milk, fish, poultry and other meat) can be used.

Further reading
Steele R (2011) Diagnosis and management of coeliac disease in children. *Postgraduate Medical Journal*, **87**, 19–25.
European Society for Pediatric Gastroenterology, Hepatology, and Nutrition Guidelines for the Diagnosis of Coeliac Disease: http://espghan.med.up.pt/position_papers/Guidelines_on_coeliac_disease.pdf

5.13 Rheumatology

BOX 5.13.1 Minimum standards
- Penicillin.
- Aspirin.
- Prednisolone.
- Haloperidol, diazepam and lorazepam.
- Anti-endocarditis measures.
- IV gamma globulin if at all possible.
- Non-steroidal anti-inflammatory drugs (NSAIDs).
- Sulphasalazine.
- Ocular steroids and mydriatics.
- Intra-articular steroids.
- Physiotherapy and family support.

Introduction

Making a diagnosis of a rheumatic disease in a child relies primarily on clinical skill and experience, as there are few diagnostic laboratory tests. Although these diseases are rare in children, symptoms that raise the possibility of rheumatic disease are common. Rheumatic symptoms may be relatively specific, such as joint swelling, or relatively non-specific, such as fever, lethargy, pallor, anorexia, failure to thrive, muscle weakness, musculoskeletal pain, rash, headache and abdominal pain. The interpretation of these clinical features requires a meticulous approach to characterising the nature of each feature and considering the overall pattern of all the clinical features in the individual patient. The aims of this section are to assist in the recognition of common patterns of clinical features, and to provide guidance for appropriate treatment and monitoring of rheumatic disease in children.

pGALS (paediatric Gait, Arms, Legs and Spine) is a simple quick approach to joint examination and helps to discern abnormal from normal joints; this is especially useful in the context of non-specific features such as limp or fever. pGALS includes incorporates a series of simple manoeuvres to assess all joints quickly (takes approximately 2–3 minutes). It has been validated in school-aged children (although can be performed in younger children) and has been shown to be effective when performed by non-specialists in detecting significant joint abnormalities in acute paediatric practice (including in Africa). The interpretation of pGALS requires knowledge of normal musculoskeletal development and the clinical context to facilitate a differential diagnosis (www.arthritisresearchuk.org/health-professionals-and-students/video-resources/pgals.aspx).

Rheumatic fever

Rheumatic fever is an abnormal immune response to group A streptococcal infection in genetically susceptible individuals. It is most common between the ages of 6 and 16 years. Symptoms of acute rheumatic fever follow streptococcal pharyngitis after a latent period of approximately 3 weeks. The disease usually presents with joint pain, but may have an insidious onset, especially if carditis is the predominant feature. There is no definitive test, and diagnosis depends on recognition of clinical signs known as the Jones criteria.

TABLE 5.13.A.1 Jones criteria for diagnosis of rheumatic fever

Major criteria	Minor criteria
Carditis	Previous history of rheumatic fever
Migratory large-joint polyarthritis	
	Fever
Erythema marginatum	Arthralgia
Subcutaneous nodules	First-degree heart block
Chorea (onset 2–6 months after pharyngitis)	Elevated acute-phase reactants (ESR and CRP)

ESR, erythrocyte sedimentation rate; CRP, C-reactive protein.

Diagnosis: Jones criteria

The diagnosis in an individual is made by the **Jones criteria** (revised by the WHO in 2003) on the basis of the presence of either **two major criteria** (which include polyarthritis, erythema marginatum rash, subcutaneous nodules, carditis and chorea) or **one major criterion and two minor criteria** (minor criteria include persistent fever, arthralgia, raised ESR or CRP, persistent leukocytosis, abnormal ECG except if carditis is the major feature, and previous episode of rheumatic fever). Each combination must also include evidence of streptococcal infection, usually a rising titre of antistreptolysin O.

- Evidence of **streptococcal infection** (usually a pharyngitis secondary to group A beta-haemolytic streptococcus) with positive throat swab culture or, preferably, a positive serology for recent streptococcal infection. This is usually accompanied by a prolonged fever and followed by other clinical features after a 2- to 3-week period.
- **Arthritis** of the large joints. This is a reactive arthritis (rather than a septic arthritis), often affecting many joints, and it is migratory in nature. It usually responds dramatically to aspirin, up to 120 mg/kg/day in four to six divided doses by mouth after food, but do not exceed 75–80 mg/kg/day if facilities for assay of salicylate levels are not available. Alternatively, use non-steroidal anti-inflammatory drugs (NSAIDs; see below). The presence of joint pain without swelling (i.e. arthralgia alone) may still indicate rheumatic fever in the presence of the other clinical features compatible with a diagnosis of acute rheumatic fever.
- **Rash and subcutaneous nodules:** erythema marginatum is an uncommon feature. It has a 'snake-like' appearance, usually over the trunk, and occurs early in the disease, is usually transient, and disappears within a few hours. Subcutaneous nodules are not uncommon, occurring over bony prominences such as the elbows and knees.
- **Carditis:** this may range from a tachycardia with a prolonged PR interval seen on the ECG through to myocarditis with a systolic apical mitral murmur, pericarditis or cardiac failure. Cardiac inflammation may involve the endocardium (valvulitis mostly affecting the mitral and aortic valve), the myocardium (impaired cardiac function) or the pericardium in severe cases (pericarditis). Examination may reveal a pericardial friction rub, an apical pansystolic murmur from mitral regurgitation, or an early diastolic decrescendo murmur from aortic regurgitation. As the valves heal they may scar and fibrose. **Mitral regurgitation, mitral stenosis** and

aortic regurgitation are the commonest long-term consequences of acute rheumatic fever.
- **Chorea** is an involuntary movement disorder, often of the face, tongue and upper limbs. It may appear as dysarthria or clumsiness, and is associated with emotional lability. It is a late manifestation of acute rheumatic fever, and is more common in girls.

The disease may be prevented by detecting group A streptococcus in cases of pharyngitis (throat swab or rapid antigen test) and treating with penicillin (see below).

Treatment
Management of acute rheumatic fever
- Eradicate streptococcal infection (give oral penicillin V 10–12.5 mg/kg/dose (maximum dose 500 mg) three times a day for 10 days).
- Commence aspirin 90–120 mg/kg a day in four divided doses after food. Monitor serum salicylate levels (the optimal level is 15–25 mg/dL). Reduce the dose to two-thirds of the original dose when there is a clinical response.
- When the CRP and ESR decrease to normal levels, taper the aspirin dose over 2 weeks.
- Give prednisolone 2 mg/kg/day (maximum 60 mg/day) in place of aspirin if there is moderate to severe carditis or pericarditis.
- If prednisolone is given, continue treatment for 3 weeks, and then taper the dose over a further 2–3 weeks. As the prednisolone dose starts to taper, commence aspirin 50 mg/kg/day in four divided doses and stop aspirin 1 week after prednisolone is stopped.
- Treat heart failure as described in Section 5.4.B.
- Urgent valve replacement is sometimes required.

The requirement for bed rest during the acute attack is controversial; it is also very difficult to enforce on young children.

For arthralgia, give aspirin as described above or an NSAID (e.g. ibuprofen 30–60 mg/kg daily up to a maximum of 2.4 G in three to four divided doses after food). Naproxen at 20 mg/kg/day in two divided doses appears be a better alternative.

Treatment of streptococcal infection with IM benzylpenicillin (1.2 million units as a single injection, often given as 0.6 million units in each thigh) or a 10-day course of oral penicillin at high dose (12.5 mg/kg four times a day). Once there has been one episode of rheumatic fever a recurrence is likely. The recurrence risk is minimised by giving long-term penicillin prophylaxis, preferably for life. This is usually given as intramuscular injections of 1.2 million units of benzathine penicillin every 3 weeks (this drug must not be given IV). If oral penicillin is required, the highest dose generally recommended is 250 mg twice daily for all ages, as doses of oral penicillin in children below the age of 5 years need not be given because rheumatic fever does not occur in this age group. For patients who are allergic to penicillin, erythromycin in the same doses can be used.

For acute carditis, prednisolone given orally (2 mg/kg/day) for 2–3 weeks or by intravenous infusion is effective.

Chorea may respond to haloperidol, 12.5–25 micrograms/kg twice daily (maximum 10 mg a day). Extrapyramidal side effects may occur. Chorea usually becomes less of a problem within a few weeks.

Vasculitis in children

Vasculitis in childhood may be primary, including Henoch–Schönlein purpura, Kawasaki disease and the rare vasculitides, or secondary to multisystem connective tissue diseases, including juvenile dermatomyositis and systemic lupus erythematosus (SLE). In all of these diseases, skin manifestations are usually prominent, but the combination with other clinical features helps to ascertain the diagnosis.

Henoch–Schönlein purpura (HSP)
Presentation
- **Purpuric rash:** a palpable purpuric rash is most commonly seen over the buttocks and around the ankles and legs. The purpura occurs in crops and may range from small petechiae-like lesions to large ulcerating ecchymoses. Oedema and urticaria may precede the purpura, particularly at the ankles, scrotum and face.
- **Gastrointestinal pain:** abdominal pain is a prominent feature early in the disease, and is often accompanied by vomiting. Occasionally, frank gastrointestinal haemorrhage may occur.
- **Arthritis:** this typically affects the large joints of the lower limb, especially the ankles. Ankle swelling may be difficult to interpret in the presence of tissue oedema. The joint pain is usually transient. Arthritis in HSP is never erosive.
- **Renal disease:** haematuria and proteinuria are common manifestations of the disease, but are usually only detected on dipstick urine analysis. A small proportion of children (1–3%) may develop renal failure secondary to severe glomerulonephritis. Clinically significant renal disease is uncommon below 5 years of age.

Treatment
Henoch–Schönlein purpura is usually a self-limiting disease, requiring supportive care and symptomatic treatment with simple analgesia only. If the abdominal pain is severe, prednisolone (1–2 mg/kg/day) for 1 week may be helpful.

Kawasaki disease
Kawasaki disease is characterised by a combination of most of the following features in a young child (usually less than 5 years old) who is extremely irritable.
- **Fever:** an irregular spiking fever that persists for 1–3 weeks despite antibiotics is characteristic during onset.
- **Skin involvement:** rash is variable and polymorphic, ranging from diffuse erythema of the trunk and face to minimal macular lesions on the limbs. The rash in Kawasaki disease is never vesicular. Tissue oedema of the dorsal surfaces of the hands, feet and perineum is characteristic. These changes are followed within days to weeks by desquamation, usually of the finger and toe tips (periungual desquamation), but occasionally more widespread.
- **Mucositis and conjunctivitis:** inflammation of the mucous membranes of the mouth and eyes results in a characteristic appearance of red eyes (conjunctival 'injection' rather than conjunctivitis) and red swollen cracked lips.
- **Lymphadenopathy:** this usually affects the cervical lymph nodes, often unilaterally.
- **Cardiac disease:** myocarditis with heart failure or pericarditis is a rare but serious complication of Kawasaki disease. Coronary artery aneurysms may be present

from early in the disease process. Clinical manifestations are relatively non-specific, but the two-dimensional echocardiography appearances are diagnostic of the condition. However, echocardiography may be completely normal in Kawasaki disease.
- It is important to exclude infections (e.g. measles, adenovirus or streptococci), as they may present in a similar manner, despite having distinct clinical characteristics.

Kawasaki disease is a rheumatological emergency. Delays in recognition and treatment of this condition can result in the development of coronary artery abnormalities with disastrous long-term consequences, including fatalities.

Treatment
- Hospitalisation and monitoring of cardiac status.
- Aspirin, 50–75 mg/kg/day in 4 divided doses after food until the acute inflammatory phase of the disease settles, then 1–10 mg/kg/day (usually 3–5 mg/kg/day) (antiplatelet doses).
- Intravenous gamma globulin 2 grams/kg immediately on diagnosis, if available. **Every effort must be made to procure intravenous gamma globulin for the treatment of these children, as this is the only effective therapy for Kawasaki disease.** This treatment reduces the likelihood of coronary artery aneurysms if given as early as possible during the illness (several inexpensive brands of intravenous gamma globulin are now available in resource-limited countries).
- Corticosteroids (e.g. prednisolone 1–2 mg/kg/day) may have a role in controlling the acute inflammation of Kawasaki disease, but are generally not recommended.
- Follow-up clinical examination and echocardiography (if available) is recommended at 6–8 weeks, as coronary artery aneurysms may appear after the initial presentation.

Juvenile idiopathic arthritis

Juvenile idiopathic arthritis is one of the more common physically disabling chronic diseases of children. The most prominent clinical features include joint swelling, restriction of joint movement, joint pain and tenderness at the joint margins, muscle wasting and any of the features mentioned below. The most common mistake is to diagnose arthritis in the absence of objective evidence of persistent joint swelling.

Diagnosis of juvenile idiopathic arthritis
All of the following four criteria are required:
1. The presence of arthritis, defined by swelling of a peripheral joint. Loss of joint range of movement and pain on movement are sufficient for the definition of arthritis involving the hip or spine (in the absence of other causes for the pain).
2. Persistence of arthritis for more than 6 weeks.
3. Onset of arthritis before the child's 16th birthday.
4. The absence of any known cause for the arthritis.

Classification and differential diagnosis
There are a variety of different forms of juvenile idiopathic arthritis that are important to consider when advising on the prognosis and most appropriate treatment of the illness.
- **Arthritis affecting only a few joints:** oligo-arthritis

carries the best prognosis; 30% of these children may have arthritis in adulthood.

- **Arthritis affecting many joints:** polyarthritis is likely to persist into adulthood in 40% of cases.
- **Arthritis affecting few or many joints with prominent extra-articular features:**
  - **Systemic arthritis:** with fever, rash, and enlargement of the liver, spleen and lymph nodes, Pericarditis and macrophage activation syndrome are life-threatening complications. Macrophage activation syndrome presents with persistent fever, encephalopathy, liver failure and clotting abnormalities and low platelet counts. The persistence of arthritis with this illness carries the worst prognosis: over 50% of these children have arthritis as adults.
  - **Psoriatic arthritis:** often associated with a psoriatic rash, nail pitting and a family history of psoriasis. This has a similar outcome to polyarthritis.
  - **Enthesitis-related arthritis:** the clinical manifestations of enthesitis include pain, tenderness and occasionally swelling localised to the exact site of tendon insertion. Other features include back pain, red painful eyes and urethritis. There is a 60% risk of development of ankylosing spondylitis in adulthood.

Monitoring for complications and disease progress in juvenile idiopathic arthritis

There are several important complications of juvenile idiopathic arthritis, including joint failure, chronic anterior uveitis and local growth disorders, as well as the general complications of chronic inflammatory disease in children, such as anaemia, fatigue, delayed puberty and growth failure. Three of these complications, namely joint failure, chronic anterior uveitis and growth disorders, will be discussed in more detail.

Joint failure

- Inability to walk without pain and stiffness.
- Inability to write or perform activities of self-care without pain and stiffness.
- The integrity of joint cartilage and bone density is affected from the onset of the disease.
- If the inflammation remains poorly controlled, destruction of cartilage, joint space narrowing and erosion of bone will result in permanent loss of joint function.

Differential diagnosis of juvenile idiopathic arthritis

- Transient arthritides: irritable hip, reactive arthritis.
- **Septic arthritis** and **osteomyelitis**, including immunodeficiency.
- **Acute lymphoblastic leukaemia, neuroblastoma, lymphoma** and **local neoplasia.**
- Bleeding diatheses: haemophilia.
- Haemoglobinopathies: thalassaemia, sickle-cell crisis.
- Epiphyseal disorders: dysplasia, avascular necrosis, osteonecrosis, slipped upper femoral epiphysis.
- Metabolic and endocrine disorders.
- **Traumatic joint disease, including non-accidental injury.**
- Hypermobility and inherited connective tissue diseases.
- Systemic connective tissue diseases, including systemic lupus erythematosus, dermatomyositis and vasculitis.
- Idiopathic musculoskeletal pain syndromes.

TABLE 5.13.A.2 Important sites of joint contracture

Joint affected	Type of contracture	Consequence of contracture
Tibio-talar gait	Plantar flexion	Circumduction or high-deformity stepping
Knee	Flexion	Quadriceps wasting, limping gait
Hip	Flexion	Limited 'swing-phase' gait
Wrist	Flexion	Poor writing
Neck	Flexion	Poor neck rotation

- Arthritis of inflammatory bowel disease.

Note: diseases shown in bold type in the above list are emergencies, and require prompt expert management.

Initial minimal set of investigations for differential diagnosis

- Full blood count, including white blood cell differential and platelet counts.
- Plain radiographs of affected joints.
- Synovial fluid aspiration, microscopy and culture.
- Blood culture.

Eye disease

- Chronic anterior uveitis is typically insidious and asymptomatic: all children with juvenile idiopathic arthritis (but especially those with oligo-arthritis) should undergo slit-lamp eye examination to detect cells in the anterior chamber and protein 'flare'. **Delay in the diagnosis can lead to blindness.**
- Inflammation is treated with ocular topical corticosteroids (hydrocortisone 1% eye drops or ointment 0.5%) three times daily and mydriatics (3 minutes after hydrocortisone) (atropine 0.5% eye drops or 1% ointment).
- Severe chronic anterior uveitis may require systemic treatment with corticosteroids or methotrexate.

Growth disorders

- Generalised growth failure may be due to inadequate energy intake (chronic inflammatory disease increases energy demands) or the adverse effects of medication. It is usually treated with dietary energy supplements.
- Local growth disturbance: bony overgrowth of the knee with an increase in leg length, sometimes with a valgus knee deformity. Arthritis of the small joints of the hands is likely to cause premature fusion of the epiphyses and reduced growth of the affected fingers.

Treatment of juvenile idiopathic arthritis

- The first priority is to exclude the differential diagnoses, especially the emergencies of septic arthritis, acute lymphoblastic leukaemia or other malignancies, and non-accidental injury. Septic arthritis will require large doses of intravenous antibiotics (*see* Section 5.17).
- The effective treatment of juvenile idiopathic arthritis usually requires a team of trained healthcare professionals, including therapists and medical staff.
- Education of the patient and family is important, especially concerning the risks and benefits of all treatment and the natural history of the disease.
- Physiotherapy, hydrotherapy and occupational therapy

work together to maintain joint function and muscle bulk, correct joint deformities and rehabilitate affected joints.

- Drug treatment should begin as soon as the diagnosis is made, with the following:
  - **Non-steroidal anti-inflammatory drugs (NSAIDs):** Give ibuprofen up to 60 mg/kg/day up to a maximum of 2.4 g in three or four divided doses after food. Naproxen at 20 mg/kg/day in two divided doses is possibly a better alternative. Avoid using more than one NSAID at a time.
  - Intra-articular corticosteroids: Strict aseptic conditions, no-touch technique, appropriate sedation, and local or general anaesthetic must be given. Triamcinolone hexacetonide is the most effective steroid, at a dose of 1 mg/kg/large joint (e.g. knee, hip or shoulder) or 0.5 mg/kg/small joint (e.g. ankle, wrist or elbow). This technique requires an experienced operator.

For children with polyarthritis or systemic arthritis, in addition to the above, the following should be considered:

- **Methotrexate:** Begin with 500 micrograms/kg/week (up to 15 mg/week) starting dose, given orally 1 hour before food, and increased if necessary by 2.5 mg every month until 1.0 mg/kg/week (maximum 30 mg/week). Alternative dosage is 10–15 mg/m^2 once weekly starting dose and increased if necessary to a maximum dose of 25 mg/m^2 once weekly (*see* Section 9 for chart showing how to calculate m^2 from weight). The drug may be given by subcutaneous injection in severe cases. The patient should be monitored monthly for cytopenia (with full blood counts) and liver function abnormalities. Administration is sometimes accompanied by nausea, a side effect that can be improved with folic acid 1 mg once daily (not on the day of methotrexate treatment, but beginning the day after the methotrexate dose).
- **Intravenous methylprednisolone:** This may be needed for severe disease flares or for complications such as pericarditis. Give 30 mg/kg/dose (maximum dose of 1 gram) once a day for 3 days by slow intravenous infusion over a 2- to 3-hour period. Blood pressure monitoring for acute hypertension during the administration of this medication should take place every 30 minutes.
- **Sulphasalazine:** Begin with 12.5 mg/kg/day for the first week, increasing by 12.5 mg/kg/day each week until the maximum dose of 50 mg/kg/day in two divided doses is reached, or until adverse drug reactions occur. These may include a rash, nausea, abdominal pain and pancytopenia. Monitoring with 2- to 3-monthly full blood counts is a sensible precaution.
- More recently, a new group of drugs have been developed which appear to slow the progress of disease in some patients. They work by opposing tumour necrosis factor alpha, which contributes to cell damage, and are immunosuppressants. They include etanercept and infliximab. These drugs are currently very expensive.

Paediatric systemic lupus erythematous (SLE)
Pattern of clinical features in SLE
There is a malar rash and erythema of the hard palate with hair loss in a child with multiple constitutional symptoms.

Childhood SLE tends to be more severe than its adult counterpart, with a higher frequency of renal, neurological and haematological involvement. The clinical features are varied and wide-ranging (it has surpassed syphilis as the great imitator of signs and symptoms), but the more common presentations include the following:

- **Non-specific constitutional symptoms:** fever, fatigue and weight loss.
- **Skin rash:** malar erythema or discoid rash with photosensitivity. Erythema of the hard palate is common and specific. Occasionally oral or nasal ulcerations occur.
- **Haematological cytopenias:** anaemia, thrombocytopenia, lymphopenia and leukopenia.
- **Arthritis:** painful non-erosive arthralgias and overt arthritis.
- **Renal disease:** commonly nephrotic syndrome (proteinuria > 0.5 grams/day) with cellular casts. This is occasionally the sole presentation in paediatric SLE.
- **Neurological disease:** ranging from seizures to psychosis to chorea.
- **Endocrine abnormalities:** diabetes, autoimmune thyroid dysfunction, delayed menarche, lowered male virility, and reduced growth and bone mass.
- **Positive immunoserology (where available):** antinuclear antibody, anti-double-stranded DNA antibodies, antiphospholipid, anticardiolipin and lupus anti-coagulant antibodies.

Treatments
- The first step is to rule out other conditions which can mimic SLE, such as infection, malignancy, post-streptococcal nephritis, other rheumatic diseases and drug-induced lupus-like syndromes.
- For mild musculoskeletal disease, NSAIDs (e.g. ibuprofen 20–40 mg/kg/day in three daily doses) are effective.
- For rapid control of acute moderate-to-severe disease, glucocorticoids (e.g. prednisone up to 2 mg/kg per day) are useful, tapering rapidly to the lowest tolerated dose.
- Hydroxychloroquine (5–7 mg/kg/day) is now a standard adjunctive therapy for limiting joint, skin and constitutional symptoms.
- Immunosuppressive agents (e.g. azathioprine, cyclophosphamide, mycophenolate mofetil) are useful additions in moderate to severe disease.
- Other general health measures that need to be considered include the following:
  - Bone health: weight-bearing exercises with calcium and vitamin D supplementation.
  - Cardiovascular health: education on modifiable risk factors for atherosclerosis, together with advice on reducing weight, smoking and cholesterol.
  - Health education (regarding vaccination, sun protection, dietary advice, exercise and reproductive health) and psychological support.
- Routine 2- to 3-month follow-up is necessary to monitor for complications. This should involve full blood count, renal and liver profiles, ESR, urinalysis, and urine:protein creatinine ratio, together with complement and anti-dsDNA antibody levels.

Juvenile dermatomyositis (JDM)
Pattern of clinical features in JDM
There is erythema over the face, shawl area, knuckles

and knees, associated with proximal muscle weakness (which may be subtle).

Juvenile dermatomyositis is the most common inflammatory myopathy of childhood, and the diagnosis is based on the following criteria:

- **Muscle weakness:** a symmetrical, usually progressive weakness affecting proximal muscles.
- **Skin rash:** erythematous rashes occurring over the face or extremities, heliotrope rash over the eyelids, and Gottron's papules over extensor joint surfaces. More severe complications include skin ulceration and calcinosis at pressure points, causing functional disabilities. Capillary loop abnormalities seen proximal to the cuticles with an auroscope are a very characteristic sign if present.
- **Laboratory evidence of muscle disease:** this can include increased activity of muscle enzymes in the blood (creatine kinase, lactate dehydrogenase, transaminases), or results from more invasive tests, such as muscle biopsy or electromyography (if available).

Treatment

- High-dose corticosteroids are the standard treatment, namely early IV methylprednisolone 30 mg/kg per day (maximum 1 gram daily) with or without low-dose daily oral corticosteroid (500 micrograms/kg per day).
- It can be useful to add methotrexate (15 mg/m^2/week orally or subcutaneously) as a steroid-sparing agent and intravenous immunoglobulin in resistant cases (where available).
- Skin disease may also be helped by routine photoprotective agents and topical corticosteroids or tacrolimus.
- Physiotherapy and aerobic exercise are helpful for improving function and strength.

TABLE 5.13.A.3 Differential diagnosis of childhood idiopathic inflammatory myopathies

Weakness alone	Weakness with or without rash	Rash alone
Muscular dystrophies (e.g. Duchenne's, limb-girdle)	Viruses (enterovirus, influenza, coxsackie, echovirus, polio)	Psoriasis
Metabolic myopathies (e.g. glycogen- or lipid-storage disorders)	Bacterial (*Staphylococcus*, *Streptococcus*, Lyme disease)	Eczema
Endocrine myopathies (hypothyroidism, hyperthyroidism, Cushing's syndrome, diabetes mellitus)	Parasitic (toxoplasmosis, trichinosis)	Allergy
Drug-induced myopathies (e.g. glucocorticoids, hydroxychloroquine, growth hormone)	Other rheumatic conditions (SLE, mixed connective tissue disease, scleroderma, juvenile idiopathic arthritis, vasculitis)	
Neurological (myasthenia gravis, spinal muscular atrophy)	Other inflammatory conditions (coeliac disease, inflammatory bowel disease)	

5.14 Cancer in children

BOX 5.14.1 Minimum standards

- Local enthusiastic clinical lead.
- Supporting team of doctors and nurses.
- Basic diagnostic pathology and imaging (X-ray and ultrasound).
- Centre with provision for some chemotherapy and surgery.
- Access to antibiotics.
- Access to blood products.
- Access to palliative care drugs (*see* Section 1.16).

Ideal extra requirements

- Imaging with computed tomography (CT) scan.
- Access to radiotherapy.
- Indwelling long-term vascular access.

Introduction

- **More than 85% of all newly diagnosed children with cancer and 95% of deaths in children with cancer occur in low- and middle-income countries.**
- With an increasing global population, principally in resource-limited countries, the number of children will continue to increase both in terms of absolute numbers and proportionally in these countries.
- As malnutrition and infection decline, particularly in young children, the worldwide contribution to mortality from cancer will increase.
- **Only a limited proportion of all children with cancer in resource-limited countries receive curative therapy, and most do not even receive any form of palliative care.**
- **A child diagnosed with cancer who lives in one of the poorest countries has an 80% probability of dying, compared with less than 30% in the most well-resourced countries (*see* Figure 5.14.1).**

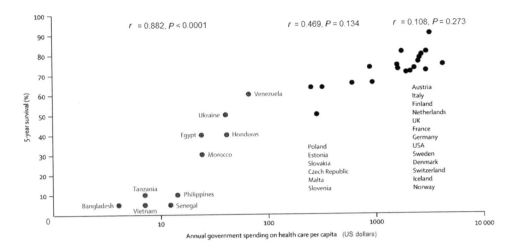

FIGURE 5.14.1 Correlation between annual government healthcare expenditure (US$) per capita and childhood cancer survival (From Ribeiro RC, Steliarova-Foucher E, Magrath I *et al.* (2008) Baseline status of paediatric oncology care in ten low-income or mid-income countries receiving My Child Matters support: a descriptive study. *Lancet Oncology.* **9**: 721–9.). Reproduced with permission from Macdonald S, Magill-Cuerden J (ed.) *Mayes' Midwifery: a textbook for midwives.* Elsevier Health Sciences; 2010. © Elsevier

Epidemiology

Globally, the reported incidence rate of cancer in children (aged < 15 years) ranges from 80 to 150 per million per year. Boys are around 20% more likely to develop cancer overall than girls. However, there are some differences between resource-limited and resource-rich countries. **The incidence rates in children from low- and middle-income countries are towards the lower end of the range, which may partly be due to both under-diagnosis and under-reporting. The ratio of boys to girls registered with childhood cancer increases with decreasing gross domestic product and with increasing infant mortality, suggesting a gender bias in diagnosing and registering cases in some resource-limited countries.**

There are clear variations in the incidence of different childhood cancers around the world – for example, a reported excess of retinoblastoma in India, Pakistan and sub-Saharan Africa. It is likely that some of this 'excess' is due to better diagnosis and recognition of retinoblastoma, which once at an advanced stage is easy to identify. On the other hand, the incidence of brain tumours and neuroblastoma is generally lower in resource-limited settings, and this may be due to varying levels of case ascertainment. In many countries, most noticeably those in sub-Saharan Africa, the HIV pandemic has been associated with a significant increase in cancers such as Kaposi's sarcoma and other tumours.

The cause of the majority of childhood cancers is unknown. Most cancers probably result from the interaction of environmental factors with a genetic predisposition. For example, African Burkitt lymphoma is related to infection with the Epstein–Barr virus (EBV) very early in life, with persistence of induced genetic rearrangements within B lymphocytes. However, the widespread use of medicinal plants which may increase the likelihood of cell transformation by EBV, chronic malnutrition that induces immunosuppression, and frequent infections that cause B-cell proliferation are all likely aetiological factors.

Problems of treating children with cancer in resource-limited countries

The problems listed below are not exclusive to resource-limited countries, and not mutually exclusive (i.e. many factors interact, compounding the difficulties in treating cancer).

- **Poverty:** national, regional, local and personal. This is often associated with low government expenditure on healthcare, absence of social care, and lack of insurance for medical illnesses.
- **Lack of suitable treatment centres and training programmes.** Existing centres lack trained staff and resources.
- **Lack of trained staff**, especially nurses, but also lack of surgeons, pathologists and paediatricians (especially paediatric oncologists).
- **Healthcare professional resources**
  Staff morale problems (*see* Section 1.1)
  Low morale may be due to low wages, overwork and dirty crowded conditions, compounded by too many patients and by becoming accustomed to low patient survival rates. Solutions may include better training and remuneration, better working and living conditions, and making staff feel valued.

  It is important that all healthcare professionals recognise that nursing care is fundamental. Nurse bonus schemes for work effectively performed can be helpful (e.g. IV antibiotics and chemotherapy correctly administered for all patients).

  Nurses often rotate every few months between departments. Try to ensure that, for paediatric oncology, a cohort of nurses remains permanently on the ward, as much of the work is very specialised (e.g. chemotherapy administration).

Paediatric oncologists

An effective service needs good leadership in a major centre. This can develop the service through training and the development of fellowship programmes. There can be support from overseas experts, perhaps with 'twinning' of hospitals from a well-resourced country to share decision making on complex cases and to supply visiting experts. Much useful work can be done in oncology with email and web conferencing to facilitate knowledge sharing in both directions. As there is an increase in the number of trained and training staff, round-the-clock expertise in paediatric oncology can be achieved with the development of on-call rotas.

- **Late presentation**
  - Patients' families are often very poor.
  - They may present to traditional healers first, leading to a delay in diagnosis and referral.
  - They often cannot afford transport.
- **High cost of treatment**
  - Expensive cytotoxic agents, counterfeit medications, quality control problems, cold chain difficulties (e.g. asparaginase is an enzyme and must be kept cool), restrictions (e.g. on oral morphine).
  - Cost of diagnostic imaging and pathology.
  - Cost of supportive care: antibiotics and other antimicrobials, blood products.
  - Cost of caring for critically ill children: high-dependency/intensive care, postoperative care.
- There is a need for multiple support networks and institutions to develop the paediatric oncology service in the face of the poverty that causes the above problems. These will include individuals and their families, non-governmental organisations (NGOs), corporate business, public social responsibilities, twinning, and public private–partnership. Government involvement is vital.
- **Inadequate provision of analgesics and other drugs**
  - For all patients, and especially where cure is not possible, palliative care is a vital part of oncology treatment. Analgesics play a large part in supportive care and procedural sedation and analgesia, as well as in palliative care. The lack of these drugs is often coupled with a poor understanding and awareness of pain management in healthcare professionals.
- **There is often an interrupted supply and insufficient quality control of all drugs.**
- **Comorbidities**
  - There is often a high prevalence of co-infections, malaria, anaemia, helminths and malnutrition which can confound the diagnosis and cause decreasing tolerance of cytotoxic therapy.
- **Untimely and inappropriate cessation of treatment (i.e. abandonment of treatment)**
  - A lack of education and knowledge about uncommon diseases among families, communities and healthcare workers leads to a lack of understanding of the need for treatment.
  - There is then a lack of financial and social support as treatment is lengthy and the parent has to stay with the child in hospital. This makes it difficult to look after other children at home, and to work, leading to loss of employment.
  - Traditional beliefs include unrealistic preconceptions about cancer and reliance on traditional medicines. In Swahili, 'the never healing sore' refers to the fact that there is no expectation of cure, and therefore no point in treatment.
  - Adolescents frequently treated on adult wards.
  - Patients may be left on wards for months because of

a lack of diagnostic facilities (e.g. children with brain tumours or osteosarcomas). It is important to search the wards for such patients and to alert colleagues to refer children to an oncologist where the diagnosis is unknown.

- **Impact on family structure**
  - The loss of parental income may result in disruption and potential disintegration of the family, and at the very least to a change in family roles, especially where both parents need to work to maintain the family income.

Management of children with cancer in resource-limited countries

The following principles and practices should guide the management of children with cancer in resource-limited settings.

- Engage in twinning – that is, developing a link between a treatment centre in a resource-limited country and one in a resource-rich country, with the objective of sharing professional and technological expertise along with other resources.
- Initially, target curative treatment for cancers that are common and have a relatively good prognosis. When curative treatment is not an option or is not offered, it is essential to provide palliative care to reduce suffering. **Both curative and palliative care must be seen as active forms of therapy.**
- If curative treatments are to be undertaken, then whenever possible they should be given in a specialist children's cancer centre (see below). There is potential for greatly increasing suffering by only offering 'half treatment' of cancer for children. It has to be done fully and professionally, or alternatively the child must be given palliative care (see Section 1.16).
- Adapt treatment protocols in accordance with local infrastructure and facilities, maintaining a balance between treatment response and cure on the one hand and treatment toxicity and mortality on the other.
- Take steps to ensure compliance with and completion of treatment. Anticipate abandonment of treatment, and address the causes, which vary from country to country.
- Maintain a database of patients using free resources such as POND4kids (www.pond4kids.org).
- Engage in the education and training of healthcare professionals, including nurses and doctors, by using free resources such as cure4kids (www.cure4kids.org) as well as conducting in-house workshops.
- Aim to be part of regional, national and international collaborative groups to derive benefit from shared expertise and uniformity of treatment and supportive care.
- Develop parent support groups and provide resources for food, lodging and transport.

In countries where there is an improving infrastructure, the following cancers may have a good or reasonable chance of cure:

- **Standard-risk acute lymphoblastic leukaemia:** children aged 2–10 years, with a white blood cell count of $< 50 \times 10^9$/litre, may have a reasonable chance of cure with induction chemotherapy (vincristine, prednisolone, asparaginase) followed by maintenance chemotherapy as described below without the use of intensification modules. However, **CNS-directed therapy with cranial radiotherapy plus limited intrathecal methotrexate or intrathecal methotrexate throughout therapy is required in all cases**.

- **Hodgkin's disease:** chlorambucil, vinblastine, procarbazine, prednisolone (ChIVPP) or mustine, vinblastine, procarbazine, prednisolone (MVPP) – six to eight courses.
- **Burkitt's lymphoma:** single-agent cyclophosphamide with intrathecal methotrexate and hydrocortisone. Alternatively, cyclophosphamide, vincristine, methotrexate, prednisolone (COMP) chemotherapy with intrathecal methotrexate and hydrocortisone.
- **Non-Burkitt/non-Hodgkin's lymphoma:** early stage – surgery plus COMP or cyclophosphamide, Adriamycin, vincristine, prednisolone (CHOP).
- **Brain tumours:**
  - Resectable low-grade gliomas: surgery alone.
  - Medulloblastoma and ependymoma (resectable/non-metastatic): surgery followed by **radiotherapy**.
- **Retinoblastoma:** enucleation (radiotherapy in some cases).
- **Neuroblastoma** (stage I and II): surgery alone.
- **Wilms' tumour:**
  - Stage I: surgery plus 10 doses of vincristine (at weekly intervals).
  - Stage II (and possibly stage III): surgery plus vincristine/actinomycin for 6 months.
- **Resectable embryonal rhabdomyosarcoma** (certain sites): surgery plus vincristine/actinomycin D (four courses).
- **Germ-cell tumours:**
  - **Mature and immature teratoma:** surgery alone.
  - **Malignant germ-cell tumours (stage I):** surgery alone.

Specialist cancer centres or units
Establishment
- Specialist cancer centres or units, and the use of standard treatment protocols (discussed below), have both been fundamental to the ever-improving survival of children with cancer in resource-rich countries.
- Cancer is a relatively rare disease and its treatment is usually complex.
- Management requires a dedicated and experienced multidisciplinary team.
- **Every country should aim to have at least one adequately equipped and funded centre, and then develop shared care or a satellite centre.**

Advantages of a specialist children's cancer centre or unit
- Development of medical, nursing and paramedical expertise.
- Improved supportive care, including pain relief for children.
- Facilities to protect cancer patients from other children suffering from contagious diseases.
- Opportunities for training and retention of staff, leading ultimately to accreditation as a principal care centre in paediatric oncology.
- Improved support, education and counselling of affected children and their families.

- Stimulus for the development of similar units in the same part of the world.
- Improved opportunities for research, including the development of treatment protocols relevant to the particular region or country.
- Development of links with national and international oncology units and organisations.

Requirements of a specialist children's cancer centre or unit
- Dedicated paediatric oncologist(s) and nursing staff supported by nutritionists, psychologists and social care workers.
- General surgeon and neurosurgeon trained in paediatric surgery.
- Access to radiotherapy and services of a radiotherapist.
- Blood and platelet banking facilities.
- Pathologist with experience of paediatric tumours with adequate histology and cytology facilities (immunohistochemistry is desirable; this can be in a centralised laboratory if it provides a service for more than one centre or country).
- Haematology, biochemistry and microbiology laboratories with good quality control.
- Diagnostic imaging: X-ray, ultrasound; CT imaging is desirable, especially for brain tumours. Families may have to pay for these, which is often a limiting factor that determines whether a child is diagnosed and treated properly. Fine-needle aspiration is important, as are lumbar punctures performed under appropriate analgesia and sedation.
- It is vital to have good supportive care, including regular supplies of medication, good stock-keeping and drug ordering (ensure that drugs are not stolen and sold on the 'black market'), IV fluid management systems to avoid tumour lysis syndrome, and good post-operative care.
- Adequate bed capacity. Most units are constantly overcrowded, with two patients per bed, and as units develop it is essential to build the capacity to cope with increasing numbers of patients.
- Computer facilities with Internet connections (for emailing to the link centre, Medline searches, patient database).
- Active involvement in auditing practice and participating in research.

Above all, there must be a keenness of all staff to work together to learn and make the unit successful.

Centre or unit database
All centres or units should keep a record of treatment, including details of patient demographics, diagnosis, treatment, side effects and survival. This will aid the identification of specific problems, the development of more effective treatment protocols for treatment and supportive care, and overall healthcare planning and development. The availability of free online and electronic resources such as POND4kids (www.pond4kids.org) makes this feasible.

Links with other centres or units and organisations
Provision should be made for communication and transportation for patients from remote areas. Satellite or shared-care centres can be developed by linking with

healthcare facilities in other areas so that appropriate care can be continued (e.g. district hospitals).

Links with centres or units in resource-rich countries (twinning)

Links with an established unit in resource-rich countries can have the following advantages:

- sharing information and experience on how to raise awareness of cancer and reduce delays in diagnosis
- helping to speed up diagnosis and make it more precise
- development of locally affordable supportive, palliative and curative care guidelines
- helping to train and retain staff
- helping to create patient data registration
- help to develop long-term sustainability
- providing support and advice for difficult problems (e.g. by email or web conferencing)
- pathology samples can be couriered for more complex testing (e.g. for immunophenotyping, special staining, VMMA, etc.)
- research collaboration.

In addition, links with international organisations are to be encouraged – for example, with the International Society of Paediatric Oncology (SIOP).

Principles of the curative treatment of children with cancer as undertaken in a specialised unit or centre
Diagnosis

- A complete history and examination.
- Investigations to confirm histology, determine the extent of the tumour (staging) and identify any tumour-related toxicity (e.g. disturbance of renal, liver and/or bone-marrow function).

Imaging

- To define the dimensions of the primary tumour and to determine the degree of tumour spread (staging).
- Good plain posterior–anterior and lateral chest X-rays are generally adequate for chest imaging, while **CT scan of the chest may be more definitive if it is available**.
- Ultrasonography affords good visualisation of the abdomen and pelvis, although **CT of the abdomen and pelvis may have advantages over ultrasonography in some patients**.
- Intravenous urography and cavagrams may also be useful in patients with abdominal tumours.
- For the brain, CT scanning is a necessary part of investigation and management. **MRI of the brain has advantages over CT**, but the availability of this technique is very limited.
- **Nuclear imaging can further assist in accurate staging (e.g. technetium bone scan for bone and soft tissue sarcomas, and metaiodobenzylguanidine (MIBG) scan for neuroblastomas).**

Biochemical markers

These are useful in the diagnosis of a limited number of tumours (e.g. urinary catecholamines in neuroblastoma, and serum alpha-fetoprotein in hepatoblastoma and germ-cell tumours).

Pathology

- Good histopathology is essential for the individual, and is the only way to compile accurate incidence figures and survival data and to identify favourable histological subgroups.
- Close involvement of the pathologist is needed before biopsy or surgery so that the surgeon can obtain an optimal specimen in the right fixative.

Multidisciplinary team meetings

Following initial clinical assessment and investigation, all children with cancer should ideally be discussed at regular multidisciplinary team meetings that may include the oncologist, radiologist, surgeon and radiotherapist. Such discussions are also recommended at the time of significant events during treatment (e.g. progression or relapse). This ensures that the child benefits from the collective knowledge of the treating team and there is consistency in treatment. However, this can be difficult as staff will be very busy and may require extra funding.

Treatment protocols

- Each unit should use a standard protocol for each tumour type, with the necessary variations for tumour stage.
- Protocols should be based on established and effective protocols used by national and international groups.
- Protocols may require modification based on the resources, drug availability, cost and the level of supportive care that can be provided by the unit.
- Such protocols are currently being developed by the SIOP Paediatric Oncology in Developing Countries (PODC) Graduated Intensity Treatment Guidelines Working Group. The first such protocol for acute lymphoblastic leukaemia was recently published.

Chemotherapy

- Late diagnosed childhood malignant tumours are almost always disseminated, requiring treatment with systemic chemotherapy.
- Cytotoxic drugs prevent cell division by a variety of mechanisms.
- Although occasionally single-agent therapy is given (e.g. for stage I Wilms' tumour), the great majority of treatment protocols employ a combination of drugs used synergistically to produce maximal cell kill with acceptable toxicity, and to prevent tumour cell resistance.

Surgery

- This is important both for obtaining diagnostic material, and as local therapy to reduce tumour bulk. Surgeons should be specially trained and have experience in oncology.
- It is preferable for surgeons to have received specific training in operating on children and in tumour surgery.
- Operating facilities must be of high quality to reduce the risk of infection.
- There must be adequate support from blood transfusion services.
- Several treatment protocols use pre-operative chemotherapy, which may reduce tumour size, and thus reduce peri-operative risks.

Radiotherapy

- Radiotherapy is used to treat regional tumour extension, including nodal disease, and as part of local tumour control to eradicate local residual microscopic (or sometimes macroscopic) disease following surgery.
- It has a particular role to play in certain brain tumours, and may also be used as curative therapy in early-stage Hodgkin's disease.
- It is also frequently used in the management of bone and soft tissue sarcomas and in the prevention of overt central nervous system disease in acute lymphoblastic leukaemia.
- Megavoltage machines have advantages over the older orthovoltage therapy in giving a more controllable beam and avoiding damage to skin and overlying tissues when administered to deep tissues.
- The whole of the original tumour volume is generally irradiated, plus a safety margin (usually 1–2 cm) of surrounding normal tissue.
- The combination of chemotherapy and radiotherapy can increase late local effects and should be avoided whenever possible.

Procedures

Bone-marrow aspiration

- This is needed in the diagnosis of leukaemia and lymphoma, and also to identify any bone-marrow infiltration with solid tumours such as neuroblastoma.
- **It is a painful procedure and must be done under analgesia and sedation (e.g. ketamine 2 mg/kg) (see Section 1.15 and Section 1.24) along with infiltration of the skin and subcutaneous tissues down to periosteal level with a local anaesthetic.**
- Aspiration is preferably performed from the posterior iliac crest, but can also be taken from the anterior crest.

Lumbar puncture

- This is needed in the diagnosis of malignant meningitis, especially with leukaemia and lymphoma, but also in certain brain tumours (e.g. medulloblastoma) and other solid tumours, particularly those affecting the head and neck.
- **Lumbar puncture is a painful procedure, and in children should be done under analgesia and sedation along with local anaesthetic wherever possible (especially if multiple lumbar punctures are needed).**

Venous access

- Venepuncture for administration of chemotherapy and blood sampling is painful and especially difficult in the young child (analgesia and sedative cover may be needed).
- Repeated venepuncture results in loss of venous access due to venous thrombosis, and may significantly compromise therapy.
- Several agents, especially vinca alkaloids, are extremely damaging to tissues when extravasated.
- Short-term percutaneous placement of medium-length or long lines under local anaesthetic may provide an alternative means of venous access.
- **The placement of a long-term central venous catheter (e.g. Broviac line, Hickman line) (if available) can be considered in children receiving intravenous chemotherapy. It should be placed by an** experienced surgeon, and its use is associated with an increased risk of infection, particularly from skin organisms such as staphylococci.

Psychological support

Cancer and its treatment are frightening experiences for many patients, and every attempt should be made to reduce the child's fears. An explanation of the diagnosis and treatment, including the likely outcome, should be given in clear understandable terms to the child's family and also to the affected child or young adult wherever appropriate. Such information is best delivered over more than one conversation, allowing the family to understand it and come back to ask questions.

All aspects of treatment and associated side effects should be clearly explained, including details of supportive care, such as infection control, the **importance of seeking a healthcare worker if a fever develops**, mouth care, pain relief, care of lines, and procedures, such as surgery, bone-marrow aspirate and lumbar puncture. These conversations need to continue throughout treatment, thus establishing a relationship with the child and their family. The family must always be fully involved in the patient's care (e.g. by donating blood when it is needed). Parents want their child's doctor to focus on a potential cure and relief of symptoms, and then they can have faith in the doctor and derive hope for the future.

Side effects of the disease and/or its treatment

TABLE 5.14.1 General side effects of chemotherapy

Acute effects
Bone-marrow suppression
• Infection
• Bleeding
• Anaemia
Nausea and vomiting
Mucositis
Alopecia
Fatigue and cachexia
Tumour lysis syndrome
Late effects
Infertility
Secondary malignancy

TABLE 5.14.2 Specific side effects of chemotherapy

Neurotoxicity	Vincristine (muscle weakness due to peripheral neuropathy, constipation, rarely encephalopathy)
Cardiomyopathy	Doxorubicin/daunorubicin
Respiratory system	Bleomycin
Urinary tract	Cisplatin (renal), ifosfamide (renal and bladder), cyclophosphamide (bladder)
Liver	Thioguanine, actinomycin D
Hearing	Cisplatin

Infection

- Neutropenia, both at diagnosis in leukaemia and following most chemotherapy, produces a risk of significant bacterial and fungal sepsis derived from the patient's own flora when the neutrophil count is $< 1.0 \times 10^9$/litre, and particularly when it is $< 0.2 \times 10^9$/litre.

- The greatest risk is from Gram-negative bowel organisms such as *E. coli, Proteus, Klebsiella* and *Pseudomonas.*
- Gram-positive organisms from the skin and mucosal surfaces, especially staphylococci, may also cause significant morbidity.
- Life-saving measures include identification of those at risk, close observation, and the empirical administration of intravenous antibiotics to patients with a neutrophil count of $< 1.0 \times 10^9$/litre who develop fever (e.g. $> 38°C$ for 2 hours or $> 38.5°C$ on one occasion).
- The antibiotic regimen should be determined by each centre depending on the prevailing flora and the cost and availability of antibiotics.
- First-line therapy for febrile neutropenia should generally be with a combination of a broad-spectrum beta-lactam antibiotic and an aminoglycoside.
- If the temperature fails to remit, or if Gram-positive organisms are isolated, therapy with vancomycin or teicoplanin is recommended.
- For microbiologically proven septicaemia, antibiotics should be given for 5–7 days, the choice of drug depending on the antibiotic sensitivity of the isolated organism.
- Newer very broad-spectrum antibiotics, such as the carbapenems and quinolones, are best avoided as they are expensive and may promote fungal colonisation and bacterial resistance if commonly or repeatedly used.
- If systemic fungal infection is proven or suspected (e.g. if fever fails to remit after 4–5 days of antibiotics), then intravenous amphotericin, despite its renal toxicity, is still the drug of choice and is widely available. Newer lipid-based formulations of amphotericin are less toxic but very expensive.
- *Pneumocystis carinii* pneumonia, especially in patients with leukaemia, requires prophylaxis with co-trimoxazole (calculated as a dose of 150 mg/m²/day of trimethoprim given twice a week).
- Viral infections are generally tolerated, but chickenpox and measles cause life-threatening infections in immunosuppressed patients. Whenever possible, children must be isolated from direct contact with these infections. **Immunoglobulin therapy, including zoster immune globulin, may be life-saving but is rarely available.**
- High-dose aciclovir is the treatment of choice for zoster infections, but is expensive and not yet widely available globally.

Bleeding and anaemia
- Adequate blood banking facilities with availability of blood component therapy such as packed red blood cells and platelets (*see* Section 1.7) are a fundamental part of therapy. Red blood cell transfusion should be reserved for symptomatic anaemia, or when the haemoglobin falls to a very low level (e.g. < 6 grams/dL).
- Platelets should be reserved for patients with florid petechiae or overt bleeding, or to cover procedures such as lumbar puncture, when a platelet count of $> 40 \times 10^9$/litre is essential.
- Prophylactic platelet transfusions in response to specific platelet counts are not recommended.

- In the presence of fever, bleeding may occur at higher platelet counts than would normally be expected.

Nausea and vomiting
- Nausea and vomiting are a very unpleasant side effect of chemotherapy and can lead to poor compliance with therapy and additional complications, such as metabolic disturbance, dehydration and oesophageal tears.
- Chemotherapeutic agents vary in their potential to produce vomiting, from very low (e.g. vincristine and etoposide) to very high (e.g. cisplatin). Anti-emetic therapy should be given wherever possible, preferably prophylactically, but certainly to patients with established retching and vomiting.

Anti-emetic agents
- **Metoclopramide:** this is effective in high dose, but a greater risk of extrapyramidal side effects exists in children. Give 100 micrograms/kg for 1/12 to 1 year, 1–3 years 1 mg, 3–5 years 2 mg, twice daily and 5–9 years 2.5 mg, 9–18 years 5 mg thrice daily orally or slowly (over 2 minutes) by IV injection. Over 60 kg children can have 10 mg three times daily. **Avoid the IM route.**
- **Chlorpromazine:** orally or IV (the IV route can cause severe hypotension), child 1–12 years 500 micrograms/kg every 4–6 hours, maximum 75 mg daily. For 12–18 years 25–50 mg every 3–4 hours until vomiting stops.
- **Prochlorperazine:** orally or IV slowly over 10 minutes, 250 micrograms/kg 1–12 years every 8–12 hours (only if the child weighs over 10 kg or is over 1 year of age). 12–18 years 5–10 mg three times daily.

The following drugs are generally available but have a high incidence of side effects, including drowsiness. They may be more effective when combined with steroids.
- **Benzodiazepines:** the main effect is sedation and amnesia. These drugs are useful for anticipatory nausea.
- **Steroids:** the main effect is in combination with other agents (prednisolone 0.5 mg/kg every 12 hours).
- **$5HT_3$ antagonists (e.g. ondansetron): these are the most effective anti-emetics, especially when combined with steroids. However, they are expensive.**

Ondansetron dosage
Six months–18 years either 5 mg/m² or 150 micrograms/kg (max single dose 8 mg) IV before chemotherapy then repeated every 4 hours for two further doses, then give orally. Oral dose < 10 kg $= 2$ mg 12 hourly, > 10 kg $= 4$ mg 12 hourly for up to 5 days.

Oral mucositis
- This is a common side effect of many cytotoxic agents and also radiotherapy.
- **Scrupulous simple oral hygiene should be maintained. This can be achieved by regular thorough tooth brushing two to three times a day together with use of a mouthwash such as chlorhexidine if available.**
- Oral fluconazole and oral acyclovir may be of benefit in oral mucositis with secondary infection from candida and herpes infection, respectively.

Alopecia

This is inevitable with most chemotherapy, but usually entirely reversible on completion of treatment. Some children are not upset by the appearance of alopecia, but for those who are distressed by it, a light but attractive head covering may be acceptable.

Nutrition

Maintenance of adequate nutrition is essential. 'Cancer wasting' or cachexia is a well-recognised complication of paediatric tumours, and is subsequently associated with a decreased tolerance of chemotherapy and its side effects, and possibly an increase in cancer mortality.

Poor nutritional status may result from any of the following:

- stress
- pain
- increased metabolism (due to tumour or infection)
- anorexia
- altered sense of taste and smell
- chemotherapy-induced nausea and mucositis (e.g. stomatitis, oesophagitis)
- radiotherapy-induced mucositis and dry mouth (xerostomia)
- surgery-induced pain, bowel obstruction and appetite suppression.

In addition to this, an unacceptably high number of children in resource-limited countries who do not have cancer are malnourished. The effect of cancer and its treatment can be even more deleterious for such children.

Each child should have a nutritional assessment, including measurement of height or length, weight, mid upper arm circumference and triceps fold thickness (using callipers). Height and weight should be plotted on a standard percentile chart (see Section 9).

Nutritional support should be given to children who consistently show a decrease across percentile lines. It may also be indicated in children with baseline malnourished status. A high-calorie diet with adequate protein should be given to all children with cancer, supplemented if necessary with specific additives to provide additional calories and protein.

If sufficient food cannot be taken orally, enteral feeding via a nasogastric tube (particularly overnight) should be considered. Total parenteral nutrition should be avoided, as it is expensive and associated with a high risk of complications, including infection and metabolic disturbance.

Tumour lysis syndrome (TLS)

This is a life-threatening complication that occurs when the rapid lysis of tumour cells, usually resulting from chemotherapy, leads to the release of excessive quantities of cellular contents into the systemic circulation, resulting in a metabolic disturbance characterised by the following:

- hyperkalaemia
- hyperphosphataemia
- hyperuricaemia
- hypocalcaemia.

This metabolic derangement may lead to acute oliguric renal failure and cardiac arrhythmias.

TLS can occur spontaneously in tumours with a very high proliferative rate, as well as following initiation of treatment. It can be classified as laboratory TLS (with no clinical manifestations) or clinical TLS (with life-threatening clinical abnormalities).

Management of TLS

- Most importantly, anticipate and recognise patients who are at high risk of tumour lysis, i.e. those with leukaemia and lymphoma (particularly T-cell or Burkitt's phenotype, and those with a high white cell count $> 50 \times 10^9$/litre, hepatosplenomegaly or mediastinal mass, or high LDH).
- Intravenous hydration with potassium-free fluids, at least 2.5–3.0 litres/m^2/day, should be commenced prior to treatment and then continued for the first few days of treatment. Ensure that there is adequate urine output (≥ 1 mL/kg/hour).
- Regular allopurinol, 100 mg/m^2 dose every 8 hours, should be commenced prior to treatment and then continued for the first few days of treatment.
- Clinical and laboratory monitoring should be undertaken, including daily weight, input and output review, and assessment of blood biochemistry, with measurement of uric acid levels up to four times a day if needed.

Infertility

- This mainly occurs in males and is a consequence of specific cytotoxic agents, especially the alkylating agents such as cyclophosphamide, or radiation to the gonads. Girls may suffer from ovarian failure causing a premature menopause after certain therapies.
- Families should receive counselling about infertility, and hormonal treatment may be offered.
- Sperm storage for adolescent boys before the start of treatment can be considered if this service is available.

Second tumours

- Chemotherapy results in a small but important risk of second tumours, especially acute myeloid leukaemia.
- This is particularly associated with alkylating agents such as cyclophosphamide (especially if used with radiotherapy), anthracyclines and topoisomerase-2 inhibitors (e.g. etoposide).

Treatment of individual tumour types

A detailed discussion of the presentation and management of every type of tumour is beyond the scope of this book.

Acute lymphoblastic leukaemia (ALL)

Approximately one-third of all children under 15 years of age with cancer have acute leukaemia, and 75–80% of these have acute lymphoblastic leukaemia, making it the most common childhood cancer in well-resourced countries.

Presentation

- Myelosuppression.
- Anaemia, infection (which can be life-threatening) and thrombocytopenia (bruising, bleeding, petechiae).
- Lymphadenopathy and hepatosplenomegaly.
- Bone pain and limp.

Diagnosis

- Full blood count.
- Blood film can be diagnostic for patients with very high white cell counts.
- Bone-marrow aspirates (these are always required).

- Morphology (e.g. FAB system), cytochemistry and immunocytochemistry (if available).
- Lumbar puncture: CSF cell count and cytospin for lymphoblasts.
- Chest X-ray (T-cell leukaemia).
- Ultrasound scan of the abdomen for assessment of the liver, spleen and kidneys.

Treatment

Rapid tumour lysis, which can sometimes be spontaneous, is a major risk, particularly for patients with high white cell counts leading to biochemical disturbances. **Intravenous fluids, allopurinol and close monitoring of renal function are required at the start of treatment.** The treatment of acute lymphoblastic leukaemia is divided into a number of phases, as described below.

Induction

The aim is to get the patient into remission (defined as the presence of < 5% blasts in bone marrow). Four weeks of oral prednisolone or dexamethasone with weekly vincristine injections will result in a 90% remission rate, *although the addition of a third drug, asparaginase (9–12 doses every 48 hours), is associated with improved long-term survival. If asparaginase is not available or is too expensive, anthracyclines (e.g. doxorubicin) can be substituted.*

CNS-directed therapy

This is needed in all patients to prevent CNS relapse. Standard therapy is to give five to six doses of intrathecal methotrexate together with cranial irradiation (18 Gy). For standard-risk (not high-risk) patients, irradiation can be replaced with intrathecal methotrexate at regular intervals throughout the treatment period, although some units may find radiotherapy easier to administer than repeated lumbar punctures.

Intensification therapy

The administration of periods of more intensive therapy (e.g. with drugs such as cyclophosphamide, daunorubicin and cytosine) has been associated with increased survival, although this treatment carries the risk of severe myelosuppression and should be used with caution unless a high level of supportive care is in place.

Continuation (maintenance) therapy

This essential part of treatment generally lasts for 2 to 3 years. Most regimens employ daily oral mercaptopurine and weekly oral methotrexate with vincristine and a short course of steroid given every month.

Prognosis

With current therapy in specialised centres one can expect at least 50% of standard-risk patients (i.e. those with a white cell count at diagnosis of < 50 × 10⁹/litre, and aged 2–10 years) to survive.

Acute myeloid leukaemia (AML)

This accounts for 15–20% of acute leukaemias in children.

Presentation

The presentation is the same as for acute lymphoblastic leukaemia, with more likelihood of tissue infiltration:
- gum hypertrophy: monocytic leukaemia

- skin involvement: myeloblastic leukaemia
- disseminated intravascular coagulation: promyelocytic leukaemia.

Diagnosis

See above section on acute lymphoblastic leukaemia.

Treatment

This is less successful than for acute lymphoblastic leukaemia. *Induction therapy is based on 8–10 days of intensive chemotherapy with drugs such as daunorubicin, etoposide, thioguanine and cytosine. Remission rates of over 80% can be achieved, but these regimens are associated with severe and prolonged myelosuppression, with a significant risk of toxic death. This risk should be carefully considered before curative therapy is attempted. Consolidation therapy is again based on intensive and life-threatening chemotherapy. The risk of CNS relapse is less than with acute lymphoblastic leukaemia. Lumbar puncture with triple intrathecal chemotherapy (methotrexate, hydrocortisone and cytosine) should be given with each course of chemotherapy.*

Prognosis

Less than 50% of these children will be expected to survive long term, with a high risk of toxic death following intensive chemotherapy.

Non-Hodgkin's lymphoma (NHL)

Childhood NHLs are a heterogeneous group of usually diffuse lymphocytic or lymphoblastic neoplasms arising from both B and T cells. Burkitt's lymphoma, a B-lineage NHL, is the most common childhood malignancy reported from tropical Africa, and is also prevalent in South America and in parts of South-East Asia.

Presentation

Lymphomas can arise in any area of lymphoid tissue, and therefore the presenting features are protean. Patients often have marrow involvement and sometimes CNS disease.
- Burkitt's lymphoma is an aggressive tumour, usually affecting the head and neck, but also arising from several abdominal organs. **Progression in size of Burkitt's lymphoma can be rapid, given its 48-hour doubling time.** Head tumours usually present with extensive involvement, with swelling of the jaw and tooth loosening, gum expansion, bleeding, ulceration and exophthalmos.
- The majority of non-Burkitt B-cell lymphomas are disseminated at diagnosis, often with diffuse abdominal disease.
- T-cell NHL presents with thymic and/or nodal involvement, often with signs of airway or superior vena cava obstruction.

Diagnosis

The diagnosis is frequently suggested on clinical examination (e.g. classical features of Burkitt's or T-cell lymphoma). The diagnosis is supported by appropriate imaging (X-ray, ultrasound). Bone-marrow aspiration and lumbar puncture should be performed. Biopsy is necessary if the diagnosis cannot be made on a bone-marrow aspiration.

Treatment
Burkitt's lymphoma

This is an extremely chemosensitive tumour, and a high remission rate can be achieved with a single course of cyclophosphamide. **Repeated courses of cyclophosphamide may be successful in some early-stage patients, but the success of therapy is further improved, particularly for patients with advanced disease, by the use of multi-agent chemotherapy using combinations such as COMP (cyclophosphamide, vincristine, methotrexate and prednisolone), for example, given over a 6-month period. This should be accompanied by administration of intrathecal methotrexate and hydrocortisone.** As with acute lymphoblastic leukaemia, biochemical disturbance as a result of rapid tumour lysis is a major risk, and intravenous fluids, allopurinol and close monitoring of renal function are required.

Non-Burkitt B-cell NHL

Repeated courses of multi-agent chemotherapy with COMP or CHOP (cyclophosphamide, Adriamycin, vincristine and prednisolone) are often successful, especially for early-stage disease. For advanced disease, more intensive regimens such as the French LMB protocols may result in a high success rate, although the toxicity of these regimens is potentially high.

T-cell NHL

In contrast to B-cell NHL, therapy for T-cell disease is usually based on leukaemia-type therapy (with intensification modules and continuing chemotherapy). CNS-directed therapy with cranial irradiation or moderate-dose methotrexate with ongoing intrathecal methotrexate should be used.

Prognosis
Burkitt's lymphoma

The prognosis varies according to the stage of disease, although overall at least 85–90% of patients will be cured with modern therapy in well-resourced countries. Where ability to give chemotherapy is restricted, simpler therapy can yield 50–60% survival rates. However, CNS disease is associated with a poor outcome.

Non-Burkitt B-cell NHL

The prognosis is poorer than with Burkitt's lymphoma, and depends on the stage of disease and the intensity of treatment. In low-stage disease a survival of at least 75% is expected. The prognosis is worse with extensive disease, particularly with bone-marrow or CNS involvement.

T-cell NHL

With modern leukaemia-type therapy, survival rates are around 65–70% or higher.

Hodgkin's lymphoma
Presentation

Unlike NHL, Hodgkin's lymphoma tends to be confined to the lymph nodes or spleen, although spread to other sites, such as the lungs, liver and bone, may occur. Most children present with a primary painless neck mass, although any nodal group may be involved. Patients are staged according to the Ann Arbor system, which incorporates an A and B

designation for the absence or presence, respectively, of fever, night sweats and weight loss.

Diagnosis

Diagnosis is generally made by lymph-node biopsy. Essential staging investigations include chest X-ray and abdominal ultrasound. Bone-marrow aspirate and trephine should be performed on patients with evidence of advanced disease.

Treatment

In the past, radiotherapy was widely utilised, often using extensive radiation fields (e.g. the 'mantle' or 'inverted Y' techniques) to cover all known sites of disease. Radiation is still used in localised disease, but generally chemotherapy is preferred for most patients, using regimens such as ChlVPP (chlorambucil, vinblastine, procarbazine and prednisolone) or MVPP (with nitrogen mustard replacing chlorambucil). Six to eight courses are given every month. Such chemotherapy may be given on an outpatient basis, and is relatively non-toxic, although the risk of infertility in boys is high. Some of the toxicity can be avoided by alternating ChlVPP or MVPP with ABVD (doxorubicin, bleomycin, vinblastine and dacarbazine), although this may have the potential to cause cardiotoxicity.

Prognosis

Hodgkin's lymphoma generally carries a good prognosis. For patients with stage I and II tumours, over 80% are expected to be cured. Even with advanced disease, over 50% of patients would be expected to survive.

Brain tumours

These are a heterogeneous collection of several tumours that together represent around 25% of all childhood cancer patients in Europe and North America. The proportion in resource-limited countries is much lower, at least partly due to under-diagnosis as a result of limited availability of neuroimaging (CT and MRI), neurosurgery and neuropathology.

Presentation

About 60% of childhood brain tumours arise in the posterior fossa, and usually present with signs and symptoms of raised intracranial pressure due to obstruction of CSF pathways. A variety of other presenting features may occur, depending on the site and rate of progression of the tumour. These include irritability, behavioural disturbance, cranial nerve palsies, long tract signs (particularly truncal ataxia), endocrine abnormalities, visual disturbance and seizures.

Diagnosis

Modern imaging with **CT scanning, or preferably MRI (if available)** has revolutionised the management of brain tumours, and should be performed if CNS tumours are suspected. Some tumours have characteristic appearances on imaging (e.g. diffuse brainstem glioma and optic nerve glioma), although most tumours require histological confirmation. Imaging of the spine and examination of the spinal fluid is required to assess for CNS spread in high-grade bone tumours (e.g. medulloblastomas, high-grade gliomas).

Treatment

For most tumours, modern neurosurgery (*see* Section 5.16.K) is vital to management. Prompt relief of raised intracranial pressure is often required, and may be life-saving. This is achieved with dexamethasone, which when used peri-operatively has also been shown to significantly reduce operative mortality.

Surgery may also be required to relieve hydrocephalus (e.g. with ventricular peritoneal shunting). The aim of definitive surgery is to provide a histological diagnosis and usually to shrink the tumour as much as possible. Tumour resection is required for most tumours, including all posterior fossa tumours (except the brainstem), tumours of the cerebral hemispheres and craniopharyngiomas. Some tumour types may be cured with surgery alone (e.g. cerebellar low-grade astrocytoma), although others (e.g. medulloblastoma) require **adjuvant radiotherapy**.

Generally a large dose of radiotherapy is given to the tumour bed, while some tumours (e.g. medulloblastoma) require whole CNS radiotherapy due to the high risk of CSF dissemination. To date chemotherapy has had relatively little impact on the treatment of brain tumours, although it can be used to try to delay radiotherapy in the very young.

Radiotherapy to the whole brain and spine has a very high risk of sequelae, particularly in young children. These include neuropsychological disability, growth failure (growth hormone deficiency and poor spinal growth) and hypothyroidism.

The following is a brief guide to the management and prognosis of individual tumour types.

Medulloblastoma
Prognosis
The prognosis is around 60% for children with non-metastatic disease and 30% for those with disseminated disease. Children with medulloblastoma aged less than 3 years have a much worse prognosis than older children. Radiotherapy may be curative, but most centres do not advocate this, as radiation therapy to the developing brain is associated with a very high incidence of severe handicap. Prolonged chemotherapy can be used to try to delay radiotherapy, but even then survival is only around 20%.

Cerebellar low-grade astrocytoma
Treatment
Surgical resection is performed, and post-operative radiotherapy is not required if the resection has been complete.

Prognosis
The prognosis is at least 80% following total resection.

Supratentorial low-grade astrocytoma
Treatment
Surgical resection is performed for accessible lesions, although many of these tumours (e.g. those involving the hypothalamus and optic pathways) are not fully resectable. In these cases, focal radiotherapy should generally be given, particularly in patients with progressive disease.

Prognosis
The prognosis is variable, mainly depending on the site of the tumour.

High-grade glioma
Treatment
Surgical resection (as complete as possible) is performed, and post-operative focal radiotherapy is required.

Prognosis
Overall, the prognosis is very poor, at around 15%. Patients who undergo complete resection and have Grade 3 (anaplastic astrocytoma) tumours have a much better chance of survival than those who undergo subtotal resection and have Grade 4 tumours (glioblastoma multiforme).

Ependymoma
Treatment
Surgical resection (as complete as possible) is performed, and post-operative focal radiotherapy is required.

Prognosis
The prognosis is around 30–50%, mainly depending on the degree of tumour resection.

Brainstem glioma
Treatment
Focal exophytic tumours are treated with surgery followed by focal radiotherapy.

Prognosis
The prognosis is around 30–50%, mainly depending on the degree of tumour resection.

Diffuse (malignant) brainstem gliomas
Treatment
Palliative radiotherapy may possibly be used.

Prognosis
These tumours are fatal (less than 5% survival).

Craniopharyngioma
Treatment
Surgical resection is performed, although there is a high peri-operative mortality rate. *Radiotherapy is sometimes used for recurrent tumours.*

Prognosis
The prognosis is variable. All patients suffer from pan-hypopituitarism, which requires hormone replacement therapy.

Neuroblastoma
This biologically unusual tumour can arise from any part of the sympathetic nervous system, although around 60% originate from the adrenal gland. Localised stage I and stage II disease and the unique stage IV S disease of infancy have a good outlook, although for the 80% of patients who present with advanced tumours the prognosis is very poor.

Presentation
A large proportion of patients present with an abdominal (adrenal) or pelvic mass, often extending across the midline. Para-spinal masses that extend into the spinal canal causing cord compression, and thoracic primaries that cause airway obstruction, also occur. Most patients (65%) present with metastatic disease that often causes bone pain and limp, with marrow infiltration mimicking leukaemia, skin infiltration or orbital masses causing proptosis or peri-orbital bruising.

Diagnosis
Ultrasound of the abdomen *(or CT of the abdomen, if*

available), chest X-ray *(or CT of the chest for thoracic tumours, if available)*, abdominal X-ray (calcification is often a feature of primary tumours), **24-hour urine collection or spot urine sample for catecholamine metabolites** (secreted in 85% of cases), bone-marrow aspirate and trephine (bilateral) are all helpful. **MIBG scan and technetium bone scan are performed to investigate metastasis to the bones.** Although the diagnosis can be made without tumour biopsy for patients with classic features of stage IV disease, histological confirmation is required for localised tumours and for advanced disease where the diagnosis is in doubt.

Treatment and prognosis

Patients with stage I and II disease should be treated with surgical excision, which if complete is associated with an 80% or higher survival rate. *For stage III patients, the prognosis is around 40%, with treatment including multi-agent chemotherapy with drugs such as cyclophosphamide, vincristine, Adriamycin, etoposide and platinum, followed by surgical excision of the tumour.* Stage IV disease has a very poor prognosis, and it is essential to provide palliative care to reduce the suffering of these patients.

Retinoblastoma

Although rare in many countries, retinoblastoma is a common paediatric cancer in many areas, including sub-Saharan Africa, Pakistan and India. Two forms are identified, namely an autosomal-dominant heritable form that may affect one or both eyes, and a sporadic (non-heritable) form that is always unilateral.

Presentation

Most children present within the first few years of life with a white mass in the pupil or with a squint. In patients with a family history, routine surveillance may detect an early lesion. Delayed presentation may result in a protruding fungating orbital mass.

Treatment and prognosis

Enucleation of the involved eye is the standard therapy, and is curative in about 75% of patients with localised disease. *Very small tumours may also be effectively treated with a cobalt plaque, local irradiation, light coagulation or cryotherapy. External beam radiotherapy may be curative in early cases, but cataract formation usually results. Extensive spread outside the orbit is usually fatal. Relatively simple chemotherapy (e.g. with carboplatin, vincristine and etoposide) appears to be effective in reducing large tumours, sometimes facilitating preservation of vision and possibly preventing metastatic spread.*

Wilms' tumour (nephroblastoma)

This tumour occurs in nearly all parts of the world, and is one of the most curable of all childhood cancers. Approximately three out of four cases occur in children under 5 years of age.

Presentation

Most patients present with a large and generally painless flank mass with or without haematuria and hypertension. The diagnosis may be confused with the abdominal distension associated with malnutrition and with other flank masses, such as neuroblastoma and splenomegaly associated with malaria or haemoglobinopathy.

Diagnosis

The presence of a renal tumour can be confirmed by ultrasonography, which should also assess the presence of inferior vena cava involvement. Alternatively, intravenous urogram (with injection into the feet to perform a cavagram) can be used, as can **CT scan (with contrast) (if available)**. The diagnosis can be made on the basis of clinical presentation and imaging findings. Histopathological confirmation is not mandatory, but is advisable, particularly in those under 6 months of age. A chest X-ray should look for evidence of lung metastases.

Treatment

The SIOP approach of up-front chemotherapy (4 weeks of vincristine and actinomycin D for non-metastatic tumours, and 6 weeks of the two drugs plus Adriamycin for metastatic tumours) followed by surgery is more suited to resource-limited countries. The duration and type of further chemotherapy after surgery depend on the local staging of the tumour and the response to initial treatment. For stage I tumours, further vincristine and actinomycin may be given for 4 weeks or 6 months depending on the histological response. For stage II disease, vincristine and actinomycin should be given for 6 months, a regimen which may also be used for stage III tumours with the possible addition of radiotherapy. *For stage IV tumours and for so-called 'unfavourable (anaplastic)' histology groups, all three drugs should be given for 6–12 months. Radiotherapy to the abdomen should only be given if residual bulky disease is present after surgery. Patients with pulmonary metastases at diagnosis should receive lung irradiation (20 Gy), particularly if the lung metastases persist after pre-nephrectomy chemotherapy.*

Prognosis

For patients with stage I and II tumours (favourable histology), at least 80% should be cured. Stage III and IV tumours have survival rates of around 60–70% and 50–60%, respectively. However, the prognosis is poor for patients with unfavourable histology.

Liver tumours

The two main types of liver tumour are hepatoblastoma and hepatocellular carcinoma (HCC). Although both are rare in Europe and North America, in several parts of the world, such as East Africa and New Guinea, HCC is a relatively frequent childhood malignancy. In children with HCC, as in adults, there is a clear and possibly causative association with hepatitis B infection both in the presence and in the absence of coexisting cirrhosis.

Presentation

Hepatoblastoma generally presents in children under 3 years of age, whereas HCC is seen in older children and adolescents. The presentation in both hepatoblastoma and HCC is similar, with most patients presenting with abdominal distension and a right upper quadrant mass. Additional features, particularly for HCC, include abdominal pain, nausea, weight loss, anorexia and jaundice. Features of underlying chronic liver disease may be present with HCC.

Diagnosis

The liver mass may be seen on ultrasound examination of the abdomen and **CT scan (if available)**. The diagnosis should be confirmed by biopsy. *Alpha-fetoprotein levels are elevated* in nearly all cases of hepatoblastoma and in about 65% of cases of HCC. *In these patients, the alpha-fetoprotein level may be used as a tumour marker to monitor progress.* A chest X-ray should be taken to look for evidence of lung metastases.

Treatment and prognosis

Surgical excision is the definitive treatment for both tumours. *Hepatoblastoma is a chemosensitive tumour, and pre-operative chemotherapy significantly improves the prognosis, facilitating surgical excision and the control of distant metastases. The most active agents are doxorubicin and cisplatin. Cisplatin monotherapy along with surgery is recommended for localised and non-metastatic tumours.* The prognosis for patients with these tumours is around 50%, although the surgery is difficult and carries significant risks.

The overall prognosis for HCC is very poor. This disease is much less responsive to chemotherapy than hepatoblastoma, and unfortunately these tumours are often multi-centric or extensively invasive, making resection possible in less than 30% of patients. Of these cases, only one-third survive long term.

Soft-tissue sarcomas

These tumours arise from undifferentiated embryonic tissue. The most common of these is rhabdomyosarcoma, a tumour of striated muscle. Rhabdomyosarcomas can arise anywhere where there is such striated muscle or embryonic remnants thereof, but the most common sites include the orbit, head and neck (including the nasopharynx), the genito-urinary tract in both boys and girls, and the extremities. Two main histological types are recognised, namely the more common embryonal type, and the less common alveolar type, which generally carries a much poorer prognosis.

Presentation

Most rhabdomyosarcomas present as diffuse masses, but orbital lesions generally present with proptosis and diplopia, and nasopharyngeal lesions often present with nasal obstruction, epistaxis and pain. At least 25% of sarcomas will have metastases at diagnosis, most commonly to the lungs and lymph nodes.

Diagnosis

Histological confirmation is required by biopsy or excision of the primary tumour. Initial radical surgery should not be performed. Primary tumours should be defined by **CT scan (if available)** (this is particularly important for head and neck and orbital tumours), although other techniques such as tomography and ultrasound examination may be useful. For head and neck lesions, lumbar puncture with careful CSF examination is required. Parameningeal tumours are those in which CSF invasion is demonstrated or possible due to the proximity of the tumour to the meninges based on **CT scanning (if available)**. Metastatic surveillance includes chest X-ray, abdominal ultrasound examination **or CT scanning (if available)**, and bilateral bone-marrow aspiration.

Treatment

In view of the high rate of local and distal dissemination, chemotherapy is required for all patients. The VAC regimen (vincristine, actinomycin D and cyclophosphamide, four to nine courses), is most commonly used. In more recently devised regimens, ifosfamide has replaced cyclophosphamide (IVA ifosfamide, actinomycin D and vincristine), although ifosfamide carries a far greater risk of side effects, including haemorrhagic cystitis and nephropathy. Unless the tumour can be completely excised, local therapy should generally be performed after cytoreductive chemotherapy (e.g. after three to six courses). Surgery is the usual local therapy for sites such as the extremities and genito-urinary system. For head and neck tumours, surgical excision of the primary tumour is usually extremely difficult, and **radiotherapy should be considered**.

Radiotherapy is the treatment of choice following chemotherapy for orbital tumours.

For parameningeal tumours, whole CNS radiotherapy and intrathecal methotrexate is advised.

Prognosis

For completely resected tumours, the prognosis is good, with at least 70% survival. For those with regional disease the prognosis is less good, with about 40–50% survival. Survival is particularly poor for patients with metastatic disease (less than 20%) and for parameningeal tumours, so careful consideration is needed before embarking on a curative treatment for these categories. Alveolar histology confers a significantly worse prognosis for all stages and sites.

Kaposi's sarcoma

This tumour has become a major healthcare problem in areas affected by the HIV pandemic. Younger children tend to present with disseminated suppurative lymphadenopathy and conjunctival disease, whereas in older children, skin nodules predominate.

Treatment

Radiotherapy may control locally aggressive tumours. Kaposi's sarcoma may also respond to chemotherapy, including agents such as vincristine, actinomycin D and DTIC.

Bone sarcomas

About 50% of all sarcomas occur in the bone, the predominant types being osteosarcoma and Ewing's sarcoma.

Presentation

A bone sarcoma usually presents as a painful mass which may be hot and tender, mimicking osteomyelitis. Around 95% of osteosarcomas arise in long bones, and about 50% occur in the upper tibia or lower femur. Around 50% of Ewing's sarcomas occur in long bones, usually in the shaft, with the remainder occurring in the pelvis, shoulder, skull and vertebrae. About 20% of patients with Ewing's sarcoma and 10–20% of those with osteosarcoma have metastatic disease at diagnosis.

Diagnosis

The diagnosis is suggested on plain X-ray with osteosarcoma showing bony expansion with osteoblastic and/or lytic activity. Ewing's sarcoma generally appears as an ill-defined lytic lesion. Diagnosis is confirmed with biopsy, preferably using an open technique under direct vision. Chest X-ray or *CT of the chest (if available)* is used to detect lung metastases, the lung being the most common metastatic site for both tumours.

Treatment and prognosis for Ewing's sarcoma
Chemotherapy using vincristine, actinomycin D, Adriamycin and cyclophosphamide should be given to control both local and metastatic disease. Local therapy with wide surgical excision should be performed. **If this is not possible, high-dose radiotherapy (e.g. 45–50 Gy) should be given**, although for long bone sites amputation may be more appropriate.

The overall prognosis is around 40%, but depends on the site and the adequacy of local tumour control. The prognosis for patients with metastatic disease is very poor.

Treatment and prognosis for osteosarcoma
Amputation of the long bone containing the primary tumour only gives a cure rate of about 20%. *Chemotherapy either before or after local therapy has increased survival to around 50% for non-metastatic patients. Six courses of cisplatinum and doxorubicin (three pre- and three post-surgery) may be feasible in many resource-limited countries. The current American and European protocols use a combination of cisplatinum, doxorubicin and high-dose methotrexate.*

Local control is either with amputation or (if available) with tumour resection and **endoprosthetic bone replacement or rotation plasty**.

Germ-cell tumours (GCTs)
Around 3% of tumours in children are GCTs, which are seen mainly in infants and adolescents. They include benign (mature and immature teratoma) and malignant (e.g. yolk sac tumour, germinoma) subtypes.

Presentation
In infancy, the usual presentation is a pelvic or sacrococcygeal mass often noticed after birth (or sometimes prior to birth on antenatal scans). In adolescents, GCTs present either as an enlarged mass in the gonads (testicular enlargement or a pelvic mass arising from the ovary) or in the mediastinum with signs of airway or superior vena cava obstruction.

Diagnosis
Initial assessment is by X-ray and CT (if available) for mediastinal masses, and ultrasound examination for abdominal and pelvic masses. Assessment of serum alpha-fetoprotein and β-human chorionic gonadotrophin levels can assist in diagnosis and monitoring of the disease.

Treatment and prognosis
For mature and immature teratoma as well as malignant GCTs Stage I, surgery alone can be sufficient, with a survival of more than 90%. For more advanced malignant GCTs, four to six cycles of platinum-compound-based chemotherapy in addition to surgery can achieve a survival of around 70%.

Palliative chemotherapy and radiotherapy
As stated above, if curative treatment is not possible or has failed, the focus must then be on providing palliative care,

particularly symptom control, including adequate pain relief (*see* Section 1.15 and Section 1.16). Occasionally, palliative chemotherapy may be appropriate, such as the use of steroids with or without vincristine in relapse or incurable acute lymphoblastic leukaemia and lymphomas. Steroids are also used in the control of symptoms such as headache due to certain brain tumours. Palliative radiotherapy may be useful for treating bone pain caused by tumour infiltration (e.g. in neuroblastoma) and by bone tumours themselves, and may be helpful in controlling symptoms caused by compression of nerves (including the spinal cord) or other vital organs.

Conclusion
Although in many resource-limited countries the curative treatment of children with cancer may not be achievable currently, children will present with often distressing symptoms, which we must strive to alleviate and palliate. As infections in particular become more controllable in resource-limited settings, cancer starts to emerge as a major cause of morbidity and mortality. Some allocation of resources becomes inevitable, and as paediatric oncology requires a multidisciplinary approach, thinking about and acting on the problems faced by children with cancer can lead to improvement of care for all children in hospital.

Organisations working to advance paediatric oncology around the world
World Child Cancer (www.worldchildcancer.org): currently working in Mexico, Colombia, Cameroon, Ghana, Malawi, Mozambique, Bangladesh, the Philippines and the Pacific Islands.

International Confederation of Child Cancer Parent Organisations (ICCCPO) (http://icccpo.org/index.cfm): **an international network of parent support groups and survivor networks that provide psychosocial care for children and their families.**

Maternal Childhealth Advocacy International – Cameroon (www.mcai.org.uk).

St Jude Children's Research Hospital based in the USA (www.stjude.org): a paediatric treatment and research facility. It develops advanced cures for and means of prevention of paediatric cancer through research and treatment. It is involved worldwide in supporting projects through its International Outreach programme, including twinning. It includes the following:

- Cure4kids (www.cure4kids.org): a free online education and collaboration resource dedicated to supporting the care of children with cancer and other catastrophic diseases worldwide.
- Pond4kids (www.pond4kids.org): provides a free database collecting epidemiological data and including a cancer registry.

International Society of Pediatric Oncology (SIOP) (Société Internationale d'Oncologie Pédiatrique) (www.siop-online.org): this organisation has a special focus on paediatric oncology in developing countries (PODC). Some of the relevant working groups include the following:

- twinning, collaboration and support
- graduated-intensity treatment guidelines
- providing advice and support to low-income countries on the most appropriate protocols to use based on the resources available, including financial resources,

training, supportive care, monitoring and investigations, and infection control

- abandonment of treatment
- palliative care
- essential drugs.

International Network for Cancer Treatment and Research (INCTR) (www.inctr.org): this organisation is dedicated to helping to build capacity for cancer research and treatment in developing countries, and it focuses on palliative care, cancer registration, research, training, nursing and pathology services.

Union for International Cancer Control (UICC) World Cancer Congress (www.uicc.org): this organisation focuses

on raising awareness, education, and developing a global network of influence.

Franco-African Pediatric Oncology Group (GFAOP) (www.gfaop.org): this runs projects for children with cancer in Africa, including a recent Wilms' tumour protocol trial.

Further reading

Pinkerton R, Plowman PN and Pieters R (eds) (2004) *Paediatric Oncology*, 3rd edn. London: Hodder Arnold.

Pizzo PA and Poplack DG (eds) (2010) *Principles and Practice of Pediatric Oncology*, 6th edn. Philadelphia, PA: Lippincott Williams & Wilkins.

Steven MCG, Caron HN and Biondi A (eds) (2012) *Cancer in Children: clinical management*, 6th edn. Oxford: Oxford University Press.

5.15 Eye disorders

> **BOX 5.15.1 Minimum standards**
> - Vitamin A.
> - Ocular antibiotics.
> - Fluorescein.
> - Ocular steroids.
> - Aciclovir.
> - Occlusive pads.
> - Glasses and other visual aids.

Introduction

Two of the most important eye disorders in children in resource-limited countries are vitamin A deficiency (xerophthalmia) and trachoma. Both of these can be prevented by appropriate action in the community, which is cheap and very effective for both disorders.

Eye examination and diagnosis: basic equipment

- Vision-testing chart. Show only one letter at a time and get the child to match the letter on a chart (*see* Figure 5.15.1).
- A bright torch light which can give a focused beam of light.
- An ophthalmoscope:
  - The ophthalmoscope is mainly used for examination of the ocular fundus (i.e. the retina, choroid and optic nerve).
  - It can also be used for examination of the ocular media (i.e. the cornea, lens, and aqueous and vitreous humour). Dial a small positive lens (about +2 or +3) in the ophthalmoscope, and hold it about 20 cm from the patient's eye. In the healthy eye with a dilated pupil, there will be a clear red glow of light reflected from the retina, called the red reflex, and any opacity in the cornea, lens or aqueous or vitreous

humour will appear as a black shadow against this red reflex.
  - The ophthalmoscope can also be used to act like a magnifying lens to examine in detail the conjunctiva, sclera, iris, etc. To do this a very strong positive lens (about +20) is dialled in the ophthalmoscope, which is then held very close to the patient's eye.

An ultra-low-cost ophthalmoscope, otoscope and loupe which is solar powered is now available (www.arclightscope.com).

- Mydriatic drops:
  - **Cyclopentolate 1%, or cyclopentolate 0.5%** in children less than 6 months old. **Atropine 0.5%**

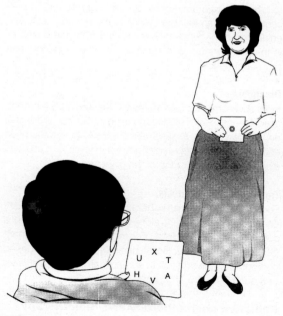

FIGURE 5.15.1 Eye testing.

ointment is very long-acting. It can be given to parents to put into the eyes for 2 days prior to a clinic appointment, especially if an initial attempt at refraction and fundus examination has been unsuccessful because of the child becoming distressed when drops were used in the clinic.

- Local anaesthetic drops:
  - **Proxymetacaine 0.5% is ideal for children because it stings less than other topical anaesthetic drops. Tetracaine 0.5% or 1%** is an alternative which is less quickly degraded when not stored in the refrigerator.
- Sterile **fluorescein** paper strips.
- Binocular telescopic magnifying glasses (loupes) are very useful but not essential. Some magnification will be achieved by using a strong pair of reading glasses (+3.00–4.00 DS) perched as far down your nose as possible.
- More sophisticated equipment, such as a tonometer for measuring intra-ocular pressure, a slit lamp and a binocular indirect ophthalmoscope, may only be available in a specialist clinic. However, if available, they greatly add to the diagnosis and treatment that can be offered.

Gaining the confidence and trust of the child is the most important step in a successful eye examination, which should not be painful or unpleasant, except possibly unavoidably when drops are put in the child's eye. If the child finds it hard to cooperate, examine the parents' or older siblings' eyes first to gain the child's confidence. A general anaesthetic may sometimes be required in small children where a serious eye problem (e.g. retinoblastoma) is suspected.

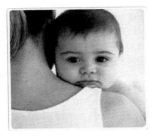

FIGURE 5.15.2 Position in which to examine the eye of a young child.

Three ways of examining the eyes of young children

Examining the eyes of babies and young children is often difficult. Patience and encouragement are required to gain the confidence of the child. If it is still difficult to get a good view, the following techniques may be helpful:

1 Let the parent cuddle the child as he or she faces backwards over the parent's shoulder (see Figure 5.15.2), especially if the parent's anxiety and sense of obligation to restrain the child is adding to the child's fears. You may then be able to attract the child's interest in participating in the examination from this secure position.

2 In the case of infants, wrap the baby in a sheet or blanket, with their head on the examiner's lap, and their body on their mother's lap (see Figure 5.15.3). Gently hold open their lids with the fingers and thumb of one hand. The other hand is then free to instil any eye drops, or hold a torch or condensing lens. This is probably the best way

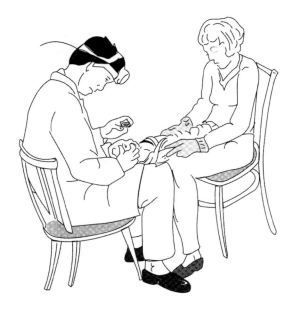

FIGURE 5.15.3 Supine posture for eye examination.

to get a satisfactory view of the eye, but it also provokes the greatest resentment from the baby.

3 If it is difficult to get drops into the child's eye, try lying the child flat on their back, create a puddle of drops at the inner canthus, and wait while the child is held facing upwards (see Figure 5.15.4). The child will eventually open their eye, and the medication in the puddle of drops at the inner canthus will then go into the eye.

4 In difficult cases, where a serious eye condition is suspected, it may be necessary to instil a drop of local anaesthetic, and use a speculum to hold open the eyelids. However, this should only be done by an experienced professional in controlled circumstances, and must not be attempted in the face of determined resistance from any but the smallest child.

Presenting symptoms of eye disease

These include the following:
- red, sore, irritable or discharging eyes
- impairment or loss of vision
- squint.

Red, sore, irritable or discharging eyes

- A sticky discharge with no redness, normal cornea and apparently normal vision in a child up to the age of 18 months (and occasionally older) is commonly caused by a blocked tear duct. Teach the mother to express the lacrimal sac with firm pressure to the side of the nose at the inner canthus.
- Bilateral sore red irritable eyes are usually caused by conjunctivitis. If the symptom is **unilateral** the usual cause is an ulcer or injury to the cornea or iritis. Evert the upper eyelid to inspect the upper tarsal conjunctiva. Apply fluorescein stain to the cornea to diagnose an ulcer or identify a foreign body. The green fluorescein dye will stain the ulcer. A foreign body, especially if lodged under the upper lid, may be associated with staining of the cornea.

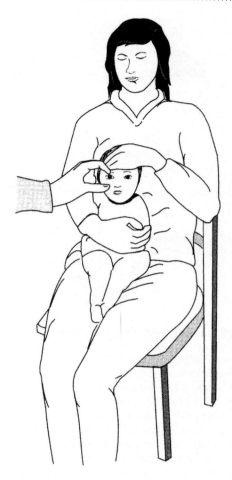

FIGURE 5.15.4 Seated posture for eye examination.

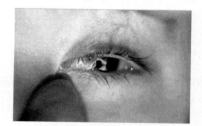

FIGURE 5.15.5 Expressing the lacrimal duct. © www.medscape.com

Conjunctivitis

- **Acute** bacterial conjunctivitis causes a mucopurulent discharge from the conjunctiva and is usually self-limiting, resolving after a few days. Give topical antibiotics as drops or ointment to speed recovery.
- Acute bacterial conjunctivitis is **dangerous in neonates** when caused by sexually transmitted disease. The cornea in a neonate is at much greater risk, and neonates produce less tears to wash away bacteria. **Treatment is urgent.**
- The WHO-recommended treatment for severe neonatal conjunctivitis is a single IM injection of either **ceftriaxone** 50 mg/kg (maximum 125 mg) or **kanamycin** 25 mg/kg (maximum 75 mg) and hourly **tetracycline ointment** or **chloramphenicol drops or ointment**.

- In presumed gonococcal infection, empirical treatment for possible co-infection with chlamydia – that is, ceftriaxone **and** erythromycin to prevent chlamydial pneumonia in the baby – should be strongly considered.

In addition, we recommend diagnosis and treatment of the mother for uro-genital disease due to gonococcus and/or chlamydia in order to prevent salpingitis.

- **Acute viral conjunctivitis** is a self-limiting disease that usually lasts for a week or so. Tear secretions are watery rather than mucopurulent. There is no specific treatment, but it is customary to give antibiotic drops.
- **Vernal conjunctivitis** is a chronic allergic conjunctivitis which is very common and causes recurrent severe itching of the eyes. Affected children are usually atopic (i.e. suffer from asthma and eczema). In addition to itchy eyes, there may be redness, watering, lid swelling and a mucus discharge. Typically there are papillae of the conjunctiva under the upper lid. In some cases these can be massive in size and may be associated with corneal ulceration in the upper third of the cornea. There may be nodular swelling and opacity at the corneo-scleral junction (i.e. the limbus). Anti-inflammatory drops such as cromoglycate relieve the symptoms, but in severe cases use topical steroids (e.g. hydrocortisone 1%, betamethasone 0.1%, or dexamethasone 0.1% eye drops). However, prolonged use of topical steroids has a high risk of causing steroid-induced glaucoma.

Trachoma
See Section 6.1.M.

Corneal ulcers

- Corneal ulcers are usually **unilateral**. There is usually pain and photophobia. Staining the eye with fluorescein will show the outline of the ulcer.
- **Herpes simplex** ulcers are typically branched and irregular. Treat by applying **aciclovir ointment 3%** every 2 hours until the epithelium has healed.
- **Bacterial corneal ulcers** are more serious and can rapidly progress to destroy the cornea and the eye. They must be treated as an emergency. If possible, first perform a Gram stain and microscopy of tissue scraped with great care from the edge of the ulcer with a scalpel blade. This will often give helpful information about the cause of the ulcer and so make the treatment more specific. Antibiotic drops should be given hourly or 2-hourly for 48 hours and then four times a day. The choice of antibiotic depends on the availability and also the results of the Gram stain. Ofloxacin (0.3%) or ciprofloxacin (0.3%) both have a good spectrum of activity against Gram-positive and Gram-negative bacteria. **In most circumstances one of these is the first choice.** Concentrated locally made antibiotic drops are very helpful if pre-prepared drops are not available. These can be made up by diluting antibiotic powder for injection in 5 mL of sterile water or 0.9% saline. These home-made eye drops should only be used for 48 hours, and should then be discarded. The following are the recommended strengths: gentamicin 15 mg/mL or amikacin 50 mg/mL for Gram-negative organisms; cefuroxime, ceftazidime or cefazolin 50 mg/mL for Gram-positive organisms. If a Gram stain is not possible, two types of drops can be given alternately every hour. Chloramphenicol (0.5%

drops and 1% ointment) is a cheap and readily available alternative if none of the above are available.

- **Fungal corneal ulcers** are very common in hot humid climates. The branching filaments of the fungus can be identified on a Gram stain. The treatment is unfortunately very difficult because topical antifungal drugs are hard to obtain and the response to treatment is slow. Natamycin is sometimes available as an eye ointment. Econazole, clotrimazole and ketoconazole are all available as skin creams, and it may be necessary to use either these or systemic antifungal agents in difficult cases.

Iritis

Iritis is a less common cause of acute red eye. The pupil is constricted and irregular and there are often deposits known as keratic precipitates on the posterior surface of the cornea. Give intensive topical steroids hourly (prednisolone, betamethasone or dexamethasone drops) and keep the pupil dilated with mydriatics (atropine 0.5–1% twice daily).

Vitamin A deficiency (xerophthalmia)

Xerophthalmia usually only affects malnourished children (*see* Section 5.10.A on vitamin A deficiency).

- In the early stages, the conjunctiva appears dry and wrinkled, but this is not easy to detect.
- As the disease progresses, the cornea also appears dry and then shows signs of corneal ulceration. Ulcers may progress very rapidly to destroy the entire cornea. Eventually the whole eye shrinks or the child may be left with a dense corneal scar.
- In communities where vitamin A deficiency is common, older children are frequently found with corneal scars dating from early childhood. In most cases malnutrition is a chronic problem, and the disease is precipitated by an acute infective illness, which is nearly always measles. Xerophthalmia and measles are particularly important because these ulcers are very frequently bilateral, whereas most other causes of corneal ulceration and scarring usually only affect one eye.

There are three other factors which may precipitate corneal destruction in xerophthalmia:

- **Herpes simplex:** severe and often bilateral herpes simplex ulcers may develop.
- **Traditional eye medicines:** application of toxic substances may cause damage and chemical burns to the conjunctiva and cornea.
- **Exposure:** sick and malnourished children may lie with their eyes open and exposed, so the cornea is not protected by the eyelid.

Management

- Apply topical antibiotics and ensure adequate closure of the eyelids. Give **local aciclovir** if **herpes simplex** is suspected. Give **topical steroids** (hydrocortisone 1% or betamethasone 0.1% eye drops or ointment) if a clear history of toxic traditional eye medication is obtained.
- Give vitamin A capsules (200 000 IU/day in children over 1 year of age, 100 000 IU/day for those aged 6–12 months, and 50 000/day for those under 6 months, for 2 days, then another dose in 2 weeks). Systemic antibiotics and rehydration may also be indicated.

The child who cannot see or who cannot see well

If only one eye is affected, the child and their family may not be aware of the problem. However, a child with poor vision in one eye only will often develop a squint in that eye (see below).

Cornea

Bilateral corneal scarring that is severe enough to cause serious visual impairment is most commonly a consequence of xerophthalmia and measles (both of which are preventable, by giving vitamin A and immunisation). Careful refraction may improve the sight. An optical iridectomy or a corneal graft may also help.

Cataract

Cataract is the most common congenital ocular abnormality. It may be present at birth, or may develop in early childhood. It may be complete, presenting as a dense white opacity in the pupil, or be incomplete and less obvious. There will be a normal pupillary light reflex, so that the pupil constricts when a light is shone into the eye. In other causes of a white appearance of the pupil, including retinoblastoma, the reaction of the pupil to a light shone in the affected eye is usually lost.

Congenital cataracts require **early expert surgical treatment**, otherwise the child will develop nystagmus, which will prevent the development of good vision.

Congenital glaucoma

Congenital glaucoma usually presents with photophobia, a hazy cornea and often enlargement of the eye called buphthalmos. Urgent specialist surgery is required to control intra-ocular pressure and save what sight is available, otherwise the child will become irreversibly blind.

Retinal diseases

- **Retinopathy of prematurity** is the commonest cause of acquired retinal disease. It is associated with excessive oxygen given to premature babies (*see* Section 3.4). It is now particularly common in middle-income countries, such as Latin America, Eastern Europe, the Middle East and Asia. In countries with highly developed intensive neonatal care services it is uncommon, and in resource-limited countries most very premature babies do not survive.
- **Retinitis pigmentosa** is the most common congenital disorder of the retina. It affects the peripheral retina and causes night blindness.
- **Vitamin A deficiency** also causes night blindness by affecting rod photoreceptors in the peripheral retina.
- **Retinoblastoma** is important because **it is one of the few eye diseases that can be fatal in a child if not properly treated.** The tumour can present in one eye or in both eyes as a white mass in the pupil, a squint, a painful inflamed eye or a mass in the orbit. If the eye is removed before the tumour has spread, the child's life may be saved.

Optic nerve

Optic nerve hypoplasia or optic atrophy may be congenital. It may also be acquired following meningitis, or rarely following an infection such as typhoid or measles. There is no effective treatment.

Cortical blindness

Cortical blindness occurs following severe brain insults such as meningitis or cerebral malaria. The pupillary light reflex is normal, but the child cannot see. In some cases the vision gradually improves with time.

Management of blindness

- In the majority of cases, management is with rehabilitation and education rather than medical treatment.
- Cataracts and glaucoma in particular must be recognised and diagnosed early to preserve and save as much sight as possible.
- Most blind children have some sight and should have an opportunity to use low-cost visual aids. Simple aids, manufactured locally, may enable children to read and so transform their opportunities for education. These aids may consists of a strongly positive lens worn as spectacles or used as a stand magnifier.

Squint

Squint, or misalignment of the eyes (also known as strabismus), is common in children. When assessing a child for squint, consider the following:

- **Does the child really have a squint?** Look at the corneal light reflexes. If the reflection of light is in the same position in each eye, there is no squint, but if one is asymmetrical then that eye is squinting.
- **Does the squint alternate?** Cover the non-squinting

eye. If the squinting eye moves to look at the light or object being held, and if the child can use either eye to fixate, then the squint alternates. This means that the vision is fairly good in each eye, and the treatment of the squint is purely cosmetic.

- **If the squint does not alternate, is there any disease in the squinting eye?** Test the pupillary light reflex and then dilate the pupils with mydriatic eye drops. Look for diseases such as cataract, retinal scar and in particular retinoblastoma. Refer the child for treatment if you find cataract or an abnormality in the retina. Treatment for retinoblastoma is urgent enucleation.
- **Is there a refractive error, such as hypermetropia (long sight) or myopia (short sight)?** This requires refraction tests.
- **Is the squinting eye amblyopic (i.e. is there poor vision in the squinting eye)?** At first, squints cause double vision (diplopia), which the child finds confusing. As time passes, the visual acuity in the squinting eye becomes permanently suppressed. The treatment for amblyopia is to force the child to use the squinting eye by wearing an occlusive patch over the healthy eye for about 1 hour a day for several weeks.

Amblyopia only develops in young children, and it can only be treated in children under 5 years of age. Surgery may be required, but should not be considered until eye disease and refractive errors have been excluded and amblyopia has been treated.

5.16 Neurological disorders

5.16.A Coma

> **BOX 5.16.1 Minimum standards**
> - **ABC** and high-dependency care.
> - Clinical chemistry.
> - Haematology, including blood film for malaria.
> - Toxicology, chest X-ray, cultures and lumbar puncture.
> - Neuroimaging: CT and MRI (if available).

Introduction

Coma is a state of unresponsiveness, in which the child is unable to be aroused by external stimuli (physical, verbal or sensory) or inner needs. It results from a process either diffusely affecting the cerebral hemispheres or directly impairing the function of the reticular activating system in the brainstem.

It may be caused by:
- systemic disorders (e.g. metabolic encephalopathies)
- intracranial diseases which are either diffuse or focal.

Primary assessment and resuscitation

Coma is a medical emergency that requires immediate assessment and detection of reversible causes. Initial quick resuscitative measures are paramount, before undertaking a full clinical assessment of the child.

History

A detailed history should be taken from the parent or carer, with a focus on the following:
- possible cause of coma
- onset and progression of unconsciousness
- extent of injury
- signs of deterioration or recovery
- past medical history.

Examination

Clinical examination is directed towards identifying signs suggesting the following:

- cause or causes
- extent of injury
- level of consciousness.

A general examination should be undertaken guided by the history and presumptive cause of coma. Identify immediate reversible causes of coma, such as hypoglycaemia, hyperglycaemia, trauma and seizures, and treat them accordingly (*see* Table 5.16.A.1). Look for rashes (e.g. purpura of meningococcaemia), tick bites, signs of trauma, evidence of ingestion of drugs or chemicals, and evidence of organ failure.

TABLE 5.16.A.1 Causes of coma

Trauma	**Head injury** (consider child abuse)
Seizure	Overt **seizures**, status epilepticus, subclinical seizures, post-ictal state
Infections	**Bacterial (meningitis):** *Streptococcus pneumoniae, Haemophilus influenzae, Neisseria meningitidis,* streptococci (group B), *Pseudomonas* species, tuberculosis Consider cerebral abscess
	Viruses: herpes simplex, Japanese B virus (JBV), herpes zoster
	Acute spirochaetaemia: syphilis, Lyme disease, leptospirosis
	Parasitic: malaria, rickettsial
	Fungal: *Cryptococcus neoformans*
Metabolic	**Hypoglycaemia:** Excess insulin or metabolic disorders
	Hyperglycaemia: Diabetic ketoacidosis
	Hypoxaemia
	Electrolyte imbalance: hyponatraemia or hypernatraemia
	Severe dehydration
	Severe malnutrition
	Organ failure: Liver failure, renal failure, Addison's disease, respiratory failure
	Drugs: Opiates, salicylates, organophosphates, benzodiazepines, thiazines, aluminium in patients undergoing dialysis, barbiturates, antidepressants
	Other: Porphyrias, Reye's syndrome
Poisoning	Alcohol, recreational drugs, accidental/deliberate poisoning
Tumours	**Primary:** medulloblastoma, astrocytoma
	Secondary: leukaemias, sarcomas
Vascular	Haemorrhage (subdural/subarachnoid), hypertension, hypotension, thrombosis, aortic stenosis, cardiac asystole, vacuities and collagen vascular syndromes
Shock syndromes	Sepsis, trauma, burns, peritonitis

Causes of coma

The following features found on examination may be indicative of specific causes.

- **Pulse:** bradycardia may indicate raised intracranial pressure (RICP) or reflect the effects of poisons or drug overdose.
- **Blood pressure:** hypertension may indicate hypertensive encephalopathy or signs of RICP; hypotension occurs in shock.
- **Temperature:** this may indicate sepsis.
- **Respiratory pattern:** this may be irregular due to brainstem lesion or RICP, rapid due to acidosis or aspirin ingestion, or slow due to opiate ingestion.
- **Pupil size and reactivity:** pupil may be small due to opiate ingestion, or large due to amphetamine ingestion or RICP; pupils may be unequal and/or unreactive due to RICP.
- **Skin rashes:** these may be due to infections (e.g. meningococcal septicaemia, dengue fever).
- **Breath odour:** this may be caused by diabetic ketoacidosis, alcohol ingestion, or inborn errors of metabolism.
- **Hepatomegaly:** this may indicate Reye's syndrome or other metabolic disorders.
- **Fundi:** Papilloedema may indicate RICP; dilated veins may indicate RICP; retinal haemorrhages may indicate trauma or malaria; and exudates, retinal whitening and orange coloration of vessels may indicate other signs of malaria retinopathy
- **Posture/oculocephalic reflexes** (*see* Figure 5.16.A.2): these are abnormal in RICP.

Neurological examination

The purpose of the neurological examination is not only to identify features of raised intracranial pressure (including herniation syndromes), focal deficits (e.g. space-occupying lesions) and lateralising signs (hemiplegic syndromes), but also to establish a baseline for comparison on subsequent evaluations. Examination may also help to provide prognostic information.

Level of consciousness

Many methods exist for establishing the level of consciousness. Two that are commonly used are the AVPU system, and coma scales.

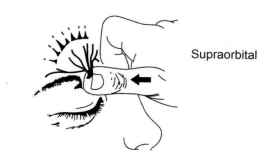

Supraorbital

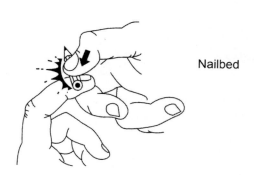

Nailbed

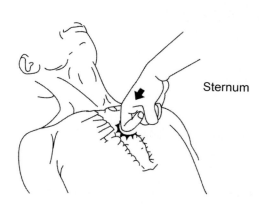

Sternum

FIGURE 5.16.A.1 Sites for the application of a painful stimulus to elicit a response.

AVPU system

A = Alert
V = Response to Voice command
P = Response to Pain
U = Unresponsive

In this test:

- 'A' means that the patient is awake, alert and interacting with the environment.
- 'V' means that the patient appears to be asleep, but when spoken to opens their eyes.
- 'P' indicates that there is no response to a voice. but a painful stimulus will produce some response (e.g. a withdrawal).
- 'U' indicates that the patient is completely unresponsive to any stimulus.

Figure 5.16.A.1 shows sites for the application of a painful stimulus in order to elicit a response.

TABLE 5.16.A.2 Glasgow Coma Scale

Activity	Best response	Score
Eye opening	Spontaneous	4
	To verbal stimuli	3
	To pain	2
	None	1
Verbal	Orientated	5
	Confused	4
	Inappropriate words	3
	Incomprehensible sounds	2
	None to pain	1
Motor	Follows commands	6
	Localises pain	5
	Withdraws in response to pain	4
	Abnormal flexion in response to pain (decorticate)	3
	Abnormal extension in response to pain (decerebrate)	2
	No response to pain	1

TABLE 5.16.A.3 Adelaide Coma Scale

Activity	Best response	Score
Eye opening	Eyes open spontaneously	4
	To request	3
	To pain	2
	No response to pain	1
Verbal	Orientated, alert	5
	Recognisable and relevant words but less than usual, spontaneous cry	4
	Cries only to pain	3
	Moans only to pain	2
	No response to pain	1
Motor	Obeys commands	6
	Localises painful stimulus	5
	Withdrawal from pain	4
	Abnormal flexion to pain (decorticate)	3
	Abnormal extension to pain (decerebrate)	2
	No response to pain	1

Coma scales

These have been devised to measure the depth of coma and improve agreement between clinicians. Coma scales can also be used to monitor progression or regression of the depth of coma. Although many different versions exist, the most widely used ones are the paediatric modification of the Glasgow Coma Scale (for children between the ages of 4 years and 15 years) and the Adelaide Coma Scale (for children under 4 years of age).

Pupillary reactions

Use a bright torch and from the side shine the light on the cornea of each eye in turn. Observe for pupillary size (constricted or dilated) and the reaction to light (normal, sluggish or non-reactive). While doing this test consider the effect of drugs used in treatment (e.g. benzodiazepines).

Ocular movements
- Eyelid response.
- Corneal response.

Oculocephalic reflexes (doll's head manoeuvre)

In the normal state while turning the head sharply to one side, the eyes move to the opposite side. In the abnormal state the eyes only partly deviate or remain fixed (*see* Figure 5.16.A.2).

Before performing this test it is important to check that there is no cervical injury.

Oculo-vestibular or caloric response

Tilt the head forward at 30 degrees, and instil ice cold water in the ear. In the normal state the eyes turn to the side of the stimulus (*see* Figure 5.16.A.2). This manoeuvre tests brainstem function.

Before doing this test it is important to ascertain that the tympanic membrane is intact and there is no wax in the external meatus.

Motor function and activity

Observe for tremors, abnormal movements and tone. The presence of hypertonia or hypotonia indicates a neuro-muscular problem. Exaggerated deep tendon reflexes and clonus may indicate an upper motor neuron type lesion, whereas their absence may indicate a lower motor neuron type problem.

Abnormal postures in an unconscious patient (e.g. decerebrate or decorticate rigidity) may indicate brain damage at cerebral or cortical level (*see* Figure 5.16.A.3).

Respiratory pattern

Abnormal variations in breathing pattern may be difficult to identify in children. The following may be sought for:
- **irregular:** consider seizures
- **Cheyne–Stokes:** raised intracranial pressure, cardiac failure
- **Kussmaul breathing:** acidosis, central neurogenic hyperventilation, midbrain injury, tumour or stroke

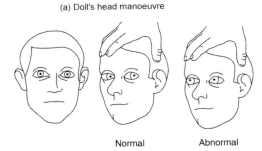

(a) Doll's head manoeuvre

Normal   Abnormal

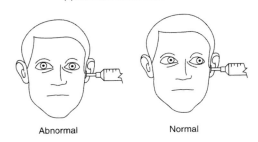

(b) Ice-water caloric response

Abnormal   Normal

FIGURE 5.16.A.2 Oculocephalic reflex (doll's head manoeuvre) and oculo-vestibular response (ice-water caloric response).

- **apneustic (periodic) breathing:** pontine damage, central herniation.

Signs and symptoms of raised intracranial pressure
- Preceding history of headache.
- Recurrent vomiting.
- Sixth (abducens nerve) cranial nerve palsy.
- Sluggish or no pupillary reaction.
- Dilated retinal veins with reduced pulsations.
- Papilloedema.
- Subhyaloid retinal haemorrhages.
- Bradycardia.
- Raised blood pressure.
- Irregular respiration.

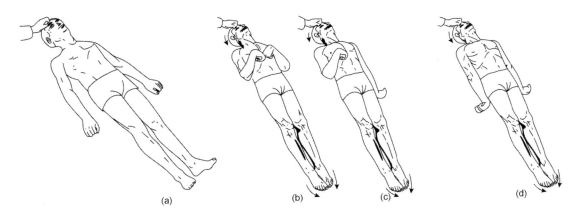

(a)   (b)   (c)   (d)

FIGURE 5.16.A.3 Abnormal postures elicited in an unconscious patient by a painful stimulus. (a) No response. (b) Decorticate. (c) Mixed decorticate/decerebrate. (d) Decerebrate.

Investigations

These are guided by the presumptive clinical diagnosis. Essential tests may include the following:

- **Clinical chemistry** for blood glucose, electrolytes, creatinine, urea, blood gases and liver function tests (including clotting profile).
- **Blood film** for malarial parasites.
- **Haematological parameters** such as full blood count and peripheral blood film. Toxicological tests for salicylates, organophosphates, opiates, alcohol and paracetamol.
- **Blood cultures.**
- **Lumbar puncture** if there is a high index of suspicion of central nervous system infection. This should be delayed if there are features suggestive of raised intracranial pressure, the child is too sick, there is infection at the puncture site, there is a bleeding tendency or there is rash of meningococcal septicaemia. The child should be given antibiotics to cover the possibility of bacterial meningitis, and lumbar puncture should be deferred until a later date.
- **Chest X-ray** if there is suspicion of tuberculosis or severe pneumonia.

If facilities are available, consider the following:

- **Computerised tomography (CT) scan** or preferably **magnetic resonance imaging (MRI) scan.** These are particularly useful for detecting space-occupying lesions and traumatic injury. Contrast dye should be given if an infection or a tumour is suspected.
- Plasma ammonia level and plasma and CSF lactate levels.
- Urine and plasma for organic and amino acids.

Other investigations (if available)

These will depend on the cause of the coma, and include the following:

- **Hormonal assays:** thyroid hormones, cortisol, ketosteroids (adrenal insufficiency).
- **Electroencephalography (EEG):** this may be helpful in detecting seizures or encephalitis. It may also be useful in establishing the prognosis.
- **Evoked potential responses:** these may help to detect brainstem lesions.
- **Neuroimaging:** magnetic resonance angiography or MRI or CT scan.

Differential diagnosis

A simple way to establish a cause would be to determine whether it is primarily intra- or extracranial. Intracranial conditions may be subdivided into those with or without focal signs. Extracranial causes include encephalopathies arising from metabolic derangements or exogenous toxins. The common causes are listed in Table 5.16.A.1.

Management

The prognosis depends on the aetiology, age of the patient, and level of consciousness at presentation. The presumptive cause of coma guides the treatment and the initial response to appropriate interventions.

See subsequent subsections and disease-specific sections (e.g. meningitis (Section 5.16.B), malaria (Section 6.3.A.d), tuberculosis (Section 6.1.N)). Consider the following interventions for general coma management.

Immediate general management: overview – see relevant sections for detail

ABC support of vital functions (*see* Section 1.11)

- **Support respiration** if respiratory effort is not adequate to maintain the desired oxygen saturation and/or carbon dioxide excretion.
- **Support circulation** to maintain adequate cerebral perfusion (aim to keep systolic blood pressure at normal values for age, and avoid hypotension).
- Assess for and treat **hypoglycaemia** (*see* Section 5.8.B)
- **Maintain normoglycaemic state:** be cautious about administering insulin to hyperglycaemic patients, as hyperglycaemia may be stress induced.
- **Assess and maintain electrolyte balance:** avoid hyponatremia: use Ringer-lactate or Hartmann's solution, both with added glucose (50 mL of 50% glucose in 500 mL of crystalloid gives a 5% solution, 100 mL gives a 10% solution). If possible keep serum sodium levels in the normal range (135–145 mmol/litre).
- **Treat seizures** if present and give prophylactic anticonvulsants if the child has repeated seizures (*see* Section 5.16.E and 5.16.D).
- Treat for meningitis if this is an acute illness (*see* Section 5.16.B).
- Treat for cerebral malaria if history and test confirm (*see* Section 6.3.A.d).
- Insert a nasogastric tube to **aspirate the stomach contents.** Perform gastric lavage in circumstances such as drug or chemical ingestion.
- Assess for and treat hypoglycaemia (*see* Section 5.8.B)
- **Regulate the body temperature** (avoid hyperthermia, i.e. temperature > 37.5°C).
- Undertake appropriate **medical management of raised intracranial pressure**.
- **Support ventilation** (maintain a **pCO_2** of 3.5–5.0 kPa).
- **Reduce raised intracranial pressure** by using the following:
  - **Mannitol:** 250–500 mg/kg, i.e. 1.25–2.5 mL/kg of 20% IV over 15 minutes; repeat as required based on response and clinical signs (maximum total dose 2 grams/kg).
  - **Hypertonic saline:** 3 mL/kg of 3% sodium chloride as required, to a maximum increase of plasma sodium level of 10 mmol/litre.
- **Dexamethasone** (for life threatening cerebral oedema surrounding a space-occupying lesion):
  - Child under 35 kg; 20 mg initially then 4 mg 3 hourly for 3 days, then 4 mg every 6 hours for 1 day, then 2 mg every 6 hours for 4 days then decrease by 1 mg daily.
  - Child over 35 kg; 25 mg initially, then 4 mg 2 hourly for 3 days, then 4 mg 4 hourly for 1 day, then 4 mg 6 hourly for 4 days then decrease by 2 mg daily.
- **Catheterisation** for bladder care and urine-output monitoring.
- Plan for continued **regular clinical assessment**, mainly nursing observations of pulse, respiration, blood pressure and level of consciousness.

Intermediate general management

- Prevent the child from falling out of the bed.
- Nutritional support: give enteral nutrients to prevent malnutrition during periods of unconsciousness.
- Skin care: prevent bed sores by turning the patient.
- Use eye padding to avoid xerophthalmia.

- Family counselling, support and consent in the case of invasive procedures.
- Chest physiotherapy is needed to avoid hypostatic pneumonia.
- Restrict fluids to 80% of maintenance if evidence of water retention is seen.
- Prevent deep vein thrombosis by physiotherapy and/or use of anti-embolism stockings.
- Maintain oral and dental hygiene.
- To avoid infection, provide appropriate care for central and peripheral venous or arterial access by maintaining sterility when handling the sites.
- Be alert for hospital-acquired infection.

Long-term management

Provide rehabilitation, family education and support for disabilities that may arise. Seizures need to be looked for and treated.

Cerebral malaria (see Section 6.3.A.d)

In endemic areas, malaria is by far the commonest cause of coma. The majority of children affected are in the second year of life. Onset of coma is dramatic: the child may be well in the morning and comatose by the evening. The fatality rate is high even after prompt administration of antimalarial drugs. Neurological sequelae (i.e. hemiplegia, spasticity, blindness, deafness) may occur.

5.16.B Bacterial meningitis

> **BOX 5.16.B.1 Minimum standards**
> - Lumbar puncture.
> - Early parenteral antibiotics.
> - Antituberculous drugs (if indicated).
> - Dexamethasone (if indicated).
> - Anticonvulsants.
> - Monitoring of vital signs, fluid balance, blood glucose and electrolytes.
> - Immunisation and/or prophylaxis for contacts.
> - Follow-up for neurological sequelae.

The incidence of bacterial meningitis is about ten times higher in resource-limited than in well-resourced countries, and the outcome is worse. Mortality is reported to be 12–44% in resource-limited countries, and less than 5% in well-resourced countries. In the former, sequelae are under-reported and frequent (20%), including significant neurological impairment and hearing loss.

Pathogens that cause meningitis

- Worldwide, the commonest pathogens are *Streptococcus pneumoniae*, *Haemophilus influenzae* and *Neisseria meningitidis*. **Local incidence varies, and in many countries has been altered by vaccine availability.**
- Neonatal meningitis is most commonly caused by group B streptococcus (*Streptococcus agalactiae*) and *E. coli*. Other coliforms and streptococci, as well as *Neisseria meningitidis* and *Listeria monocytogenes*, may also occur. *Listeria monocytogenes* and Group B streptococci cause both early and late neonatal infections, and may have a better prognosis than infections caused by coliforms. Neonatal meningitis has a poorer prognosis than most community-acquired meningitis of later childhood.

Diagnosis of meningitis

Clinical

- **In infants and children:** fever, neck stiffness, bulging fontanelle (in infants), vomiting, headache, altered consciousness and possibly convulsions. In meningococcal meningitis there may be a maculopapular or petechial rash.
- **In neonates:** signs are more subtle and non-specific and include poor feeding, hyper- or hypothermia, convulsions, apnoea, irritability and a bulging fontanelle.

Laboratory

- Contraindications to lumbar puncture include evidence of raised intracranial pressure (especially coma or focal neurological signs), the child being too sick to tolerate a flexed position, infection at the puncture site, bleeding tendency (blood clotting or platelet disorder), or a widespread petechial rash suggesting meningococcal disease. In these situations, antibiotics should be started and lumbar puncture delayed until it is safe to undertake.
- Gram stain of CSF may identify bacteria in about two-thirds of cases, and provides a guide to choice of antibiotic therapy in the absence of culture facilities.
- Other laboratory tests of use include blood culture and polymerase chain reaction (PCR) of CSF, and for general management, full blood count, serum electrolytes and glucose levels, and urine specific gravity. In malarial areas, undertake a blood smear and treat appropriately. Both meningitis and malaria may coexist in a patient and be difficult to distinguish from each other.

Other pathogens

Consider tuberculous meningitis in children who do not respond to the initial antibiotics, particularly if two or more of the following are present: history more than 7 days, HIV known or suspected, patient remains unconscious, CSF has a moderately high white blood cell count (typically > 300–500/mL, mostly lymphocytes), elevated protein levels (0.8–4 grams/litre) and low glucose levels (< 1.5 mmol/litre), Chest X-ray suggests tuberculosis, optic atrophy, focal neurological deficit or extrapyramidal movements (*see* Section 6.1.N).

Children with HIV are more prone to meningitis and septicaemia caused by *Streptococcus pneumoniae* and *Salmonella* species, and relapse is more frequent. Non-typhoidal *Salmonella* (NTS) meningitis is common in post-malarial anaemia and malnutrition, and requires lengthy antibiotic treatment (at least 1 month).

Fungal infections (e.g. *Cryptococcus neoformans*),

TABLE 5.16.B.1 Bacterial meningitis: typical findings in cerebrospinal fluid

Condition	White cell count (×10⁹/L)	Cell differential	Protein (g/litre)	Glucose (mmol/litre)
Normal	0.5 < 22 in full term, < 30 in premature neonates	PMN ≤ 2 but < 15 in neonate	< 0.5	Two-thirds blood glucose
Acute bacterial meningitis*	100 to > 300 000	Mostly PMN. Monocytes in *Listeria* infection	> 1.0	< 2.5
Tuberculous meningitis	50–500 sometimes higher	Lymphocytes early but also PMN	> 1.0	< 2.5, Usually 0
Herpes encephalitis	usually < 500	Mostly lymphocytes PMN early in the disease	> 0.5	Normal
Cerebral abscess	10–200	PMN or lymphocytes	> 1.0	Normal
Traumatic tap	WBC and RBC	RBC/WBC =500/1	Increases by 0.001 g/L per 1000 RBC	

*Bacterial meningitis can occur without a pleocytosis. Partial treatment will alter these findings. PMN, polymorphonuclear granulocytosis; WBC, white blood cell count; RBC, red blood cell count.

mostly in children with HIV, often cause severe headache without neck stiffness. Lumbar puncture may improve symptoms.

Therapy

Antibiotic choices depend upon activity against the infecting organism, CSF penetration, cost and availability of the antibiotic, route of administration, and local patterns of antibiotic resistance (see Tables 5.16.B.2, 5.16.B.3 and 5.16.B.4). If national guidelines are available they should be followed. The degree of diagnostic certainty is also important, especially in the case of meningitis with minimal rash, as treatment should be given for all the common causes of bacterial meningitis according to the child's age group.

It is important to know the antimicrobial sensitivities in the local area. Antimicrobial resistance has emerged among the three major bacterial pathogens that cause meningitis outside the neonatal period. In the meningococcus, intermediate penicillin resistance may occur and chloramphenicol resistance is emerging. *Haemophilus influenzae* infections are also frequently beta-lactamase resistant, and chloramphenicol resistance has been described. Third-generation cephalosporins are therefore the drugs of choice for both organisms, although if they are precluded on the basis of cost, chloramphenicol (plus penicillin or ampicillin) is an alternative. Pneumococci resistant to penicillin and to chloramphenicol are widespread in Asia and some parts of Africa, and third-generation cephalosporins are again the drugs of choice. However, pneumococcal resistance to third-generation cephalosporins may occur. Treatment of these strains requires the addition of vancomycin or rifampicin to therapy with third-generation cephalosporins.

Third-generation cephalosporins (ceftriaxone or cefotaxime) may be necessary first-choice antibiotics in some areas. In neonates, ceftazidime, which is also active against *Pseudomonas* infections, may be the most suitable drug.

The antibiotic regimen should be rationalised once culture and sensitivity results for the infecting organism become available.

During confirmed epidemics of meningococcal meningitis and where there are other signs such as petechial rash, lumbar punctures are unnecessary. If resources are very limited, oily chloramphenicol (100 mg/kg IM) as a single

dose of up to 3 grams can be curative. If the oily dose is too large for one buttock, divide it into two doses. Alternatively, single-dose IM ceftriaxone, 100 mg/kg up to 4 grams, may be recommended.

Duration of therapy

Neonates require 14–21 days of treatment. In infants and children, a 10-day course is usually adequate for pneumococcal and *Haemophilus* infections, and a 7-day course for meningococcal infections. Seven days of ceftriaxone treatment is usually sufficient. Where antibiotic availability is very limited, some authors have used 5- to 7-day courses of ceftriaxone for uncomplicated meningococcal, pneumococcal or *Haemophilus* meningitis in infants and children.

Corticosteroids

Dexamethasone may reduce the incidence of neurological sequelae and deafness in bacterial meningitis, **although studies in resource-limited countries have been inconclusive. The usually recommended dose of dexamethasone is 0.15 mg/kg four times daily for 4 days (or if this is not available, prednisolone 2 mg/ kg per day for 4 days).** The first dose should be given concurrently with, or a maximum of 4 hours after, first antibiotic administration.

There is **no** evidence that corticosteroids are helpful in bacterial meningitis where there is delay in presentation and antibiotics have already been given some hours earlier. Steroids are generally not indicated in meningococcal disease.

Do not use steroids in the newborn or in children younger than 3 months, or in patients with suspected cerebral malaria or viral encephalitis.

Nursing and ongoing care
Monitoring

- Careful observation is essential.
- Raised ICP and shock are the most severe complications. Early recognition and treatment are essential.
- Daily weights and urine specific gravity aid the assessment of fluid requirement.
- Temperature, pulse, blood pressure, capillary refill time (normal value is less than 3 seconds), respiratory rate

and effort, conscious level and pupillary responses should be monitored frequently after admission (4- to 6-hourly), particularly in patients with meningococcal disease (see Section 6.1.G). Pulse oximetry is valuable (if available) for monitoring oxygenation and for identifying early evidence of respiratory compromise.

- A critical care pathway is an ideal way of incorporating observations, treatment and laboratory findings on one chart. Doses and treatments can be standardised and incorporated on the chart.

- Ideally, if available, monitor electrolytes (sodium, potassium, calcium and magnesium, urea and/or creatinine) and replacement of fluid deficits (hyponatraemia due to excessive IV administration of hypo-osmolar solutions is common, and can predispose to seizures). Monitoring of full blood count and coagulation screen should be undertaken regularly if these are initially abnormal.

Supportive care
Fluids

Maintenance fluids should be given once any shock or dehydration has been corrected, initially by the IV route but later by nasogastric tube or orally. The degree of dehydration may be underestimated, and deep breathing may be a sign of acidosis. Low serum sodium levels often occur in meningitis. Avoid over-hydration by maintaining careful fluid balance, and in particular avoid IV fluids with low sodium levels such as 5% glucose. Use Hartmann's solution with added glucose (5–10%) or a similar proprietary fluid. If electrolytes are being measured, maintain serum Na^+ in the high normal range and above 135 mmol/litre.

Fluid balance

Urine output should be monitored, particularly in the unconscious child. Weighing nappies can be useful in the infant or young child. Catheterisation, unless undertaken in an aseptic way, can lead to urinary tract infection and is unwise if resources are limited.

Cerebral support

Seizures must be controlled with anticonvulsants, but there are no data to support routine use of prophylactic anticonvulsants (see Section 5.16.D and Section 5.16.A on seizures and coma).

If there is a high **fever** (> 39°C), apply temperature reduction methods, including paracetamol.

Blood glucose levels must be monitored every 4 hours, particularly in the infant and young child. Hypoglycaemia must be considered in any child with seizures or altered consciousness and corrected as follows: give 2–5 mL/kg of 10% glucose IV and recheck blood glucose levels 30 minutes later. If they remain low (less than 2.5 mmol/litre), repeat the IV glucose dose (5 mL/kg) and ensure that glucose is included in any infusion.

Gastric and airway protection

A **nasogastric tube** may be helpful in unconscious children or in those who are vomiting, in order to protect the airway. A small amount of milk (1 mL/kg/hour) passed down this nasogastric tube may prevent gastric erosions. Gastric protection may also be provided by using drugs such as ranitidine or omeprazole (if available).

Nutritional support

A **nasogastric tube** should be inserted if the child is unable to feed orally after 24 hours. Continue expressed breast milk if the child is breastfed, or give milk feeds 15 mL/kg every 3 hours.

Bedside care

Turn an unconscious child 2-hourly, keeping them dry, and prevent overheating. Insert a nasogastric tube if there is persistent vomiting.

Include the mother or family members in progress reports, and make them part of the caring team.

Complications

- Convulsions with or without hypoglycaemia (see Sections 5.16.D and E for management of convulsions).

- If fever does not settle within 48 hours and if the child's condition deteriorates or is not improving, repeat lumbar puncture and review the CSF findings, and consider drug resistance and tuberculous meningitis.

- If the fontanelle is patent, monitor the head circumference daily to detect hydrocephalus. Consider a head ultrasound scan to look for ventriculitis, ventricular dilatation, subdural effusion or brain abscess. In older children, computed tomography or magnetic resonance imaging may be helpful for assessing the size and position of any intracranial lesion (if available and if intervention is possible).

- Aspiration pneumonia may occur in the unconscious child.

- Hydrocephalus, deafness, visual loss, epilepsy and neurological deficits may develop and be evident either early in disease or at follow-up. Around 20% of cases worldwide will develop serious sequelae.

Follow-up

- Undertake hearing tests in all children, and neurological assessments and head circumference measurements (in infants) on discharge from hospital and at post-discharge visits 1 month and 6 months after recovery. In the absence of effective treatment, a deaf child will require training in lip-reading and sign language, and they and their family will need significant support.

- New sequelae are unlikely to develop after discharge, but may have been missed.

- Physiotherapy may be required if neurological sequelae have resulted in contractures.

Immunisation to prevent meningitis

Highly effective protein-conjugated polysaccharide vaccines are available against *Haemophilus influenzae* and several serogroups of *Streptococcus pneumoniae* and *Neisseria meningitidis*. They are effective in young infants as well as in older children and adults. If they are unavailable, plain polysaccharide vaccines against *Neisseria meningitidis* and *Streptococcus pneumoniae* may be provided. Vaccine availability may be limited in low-income countries.

TABLE 5.16.B.2 Antibiotic choices by age group for immediate treatment and where the infecting organism is not known

Age group	Probable pathogen	Antibiotics of choice	Alternative antibiotics
Neonates	Gram-negative bacteria Group B streptococci *Listeria* *Neisseria meningitidis* *Streptococcus pneumoniae* *Haemophilus influenzae*	Ampicillin **plus** third-generation cephalosporin: cefotaxime/ceftriaxone	Penicillin (but use ampicillin if *Listeria* is suspected) **plus** gentamicin or ceftazidime
1 month to 5 years	*Neisseria meningitidis* *Streptococcus pneumoniae* *Haemophilus influenzae*	Third-generation cephalosporin: cefotaxime/ceftriaxone Add vancomycin or rifampicin if there is *S. pneumoniae* resistance	Chloramphenicol **plus** ampicillin Add vancomycin or rifampicin if there is *S. pneumoniae* resistance
Children over 5 years	*Neisseria meningitidis* *Streptococcus pneumoniae*	Third-generation cephalosporin: cefotaxime/ceftriaxone Add vancomycin or rifampicin if there is *S. pneumoniae* resistance	Chloramphenicol **plus** ampicillin Add vancomycin or rifampicin if there is *S. pneumoniae* resistance

For all age groups, if there is no improvement after the third day, look for evidence of cerebral abscess or subdural effusions, where relevant. These would manifest as continuing fever, localising neurological signs or decreased consciousness. Ultrasound or CT (if available) would be helpful. Seek neurosurgical advice (if available). Repeat the lumbar puncture, looking for evidence of improvement such as a reduced white cell count or increased CSF glucose levels. Add in a third antibiotic. Consider other sites of infection, such as cellulitis, pneumonia with empyema, arthritis or osteomyelitis.

Give all antibiotics parenterally (IV or IM) for at least 3 days. Chloramphenicol can then be given orally if the child is significantly improved.

The IM route may be used if the IV route cannot be accessed. High oral doses of chloramphenicol can be used if there is no alternative, but are not recommended for infants under 3 months of age.

TABLE 5.16.B.3 Antibiotic therapy in bacterial meningitis where the infecting organism is known

Organism	Antibiotics of choice	Alternative antibiotics	Duration
Haemophilus influenzae	Ceftriaxone/cefotaxime	Ampicillin **plus** chloramphenicol*	10–14 days
Streptococcus pneumoniae†	Ceftriaxone/cefotaxime	Ampicillin/benzylpenicillin **plus** chloramphenicol*	10–14 days
Neisseria meningitidis	Ceftriaxone/cefotaxime	Benzylpenicillin **plus** chloramphenicol*	7 days
Gram-negative bacilli (including *E. coli*)	Ceftriaxone/cefotaxime with or without gentamicin	Ampicillin **plus** gentamicin or chloramphenicol*	At least 21 days‡
Salmonella enteritidis	Ceftriaxone/cefotaxime **plus** IV ciprofloxacin (if available)	Meropenem or chloramphenicol* **plus** ampicillin (may be incomplete cover and excess mortality compared with cephalosporins)	At least 21 days‡
Listeria monocytogenes	Ampicillin **plus** gentamicin		10–14 days
Group B streptococcus	Benzylpenicillin **plus** gentamicin or ceftriaxone/cefotaxime		10–14 days
Staphylococcus species	Flucloxacillin **plus** gentamicin	Flucloxacillin **plus** chloramphenicol*	10–14 days

* Chloramphenicol should be used with caution in children under 3 months of age. Monitoring of serum levels is advisable in this group.

† *Streptococcus pneumoniae* infections that are resistant to penicillins and cephalosporins are increasingly prevalent. If resistance is suspected, add either rifampicin or vancomycin (see doses below).

‡ Gram-negative infections are difficult to treat and have a high rate of sequelae. A repeat lumbar pucture to ensure response to antibiotics may be indicated if the clinical picture is not improving.

The choice of antibiotic depends on local antibiotic resistance patterns, national guidelines and drug availability.

Give all antibiotics parenterally for at least 3 days.

Once culture and sensitivity results are available, empirical antibiotics should be changed accordingly.

Do not delay antibiotic therapy if cephalosporins are unavailable; use the next most appropriate antibiotic combination.

Bacterial meningitis: prophylaxis for contacts
Neisseria meningitidis

Give rifampicin to all household contacts for 2 days as follows: adults, 600 mg twice daily; children aged 1 month to 12 years, 10 mg/kg twice daily; neonates, 5 mg/kg twice daily (*see* Section 6.1.G for alternative antibiotics and vaccination regimes).

In many countries, rifampicin is protected from use in any disease other than TB. In this case consider giving ciprofloxacin orally as a single dose as follows: adults, 500 mg; children aged 5–12 years, 250 mg; children aged 1 month to 5 years, 125 mg.

Haemophilus influenzae

Give rifampicin to all non-vaccinated household contacts for 4 days at the doses stated above.

TABLE 5.16.B.4 Bacterial meningitis: antibiotic doses

Antibiotic	Route	Dose
Ampicillin	IV	100 mg/kg/4–6 hourly (max. single dose 2 g every 4 hours)
Benzylpenicillin	IV	50 mg/kg/4 hourly (max. single dose 2.4 g)
Cefotaxime	IV	50 mg/kg/6 hourly (max. daily dose 12 g)
Ceftriaxone	IV or IM	80 mg/kg/24 hours once daily* (max. single dose 4 g) large doses preferably IV
Chloramphenicol	IV	25 mg/kg 6 hourly† (after loading dose of 50 mg/kg)
	Oral	25 mg/kg 6 hourly†
	IM	An oily preparation of chloramphenicol is available and is usually used in a single dose of 50–100 mg/kg with a maximum dose of 3 g. The dose may be repeated after 24 hours. It is recommended only if more suitable alternatives are unavailable
Flucloxacillin or cloxacillin	IV	50 mg/kg 6 hourly (max. dose 8 g/day)
Gentamicin	IV or IM	1 month–12 years 2.5 mg/kg 8 hourly‡ (*see* Section 3.4 for neonatal doses)
Ciprofloxacin	IV	10 mg/kg 8 hourly (10 mg/kg/12 hourly in the neonate)
Meropenem	IV	1 month to 12 years body weight < 50 kg; 40 mg/kg 8 hourly; body weight > 50 kg; 2 g every 8 hours (maximum single dose 2 g) by slow IV injection over 5 minutes
		12–18 years 2 g every 8 hours
Vancomycin	IV	15 mg/kg loading dose and then 10 mg/kg 6 hourly‡ (total daily dose should not exceed 2 g)

* Ideally, 80 mg/kg 12-hourly should be given for the first two doses, followed by 80 mg/kg/24 hours.

† Although not recommended in children under 3 months old or in malnourished children, the evidence for this is slight.

‡ Monitoring of drug levels is strongly advised if at all possible, with adjustment of doses.

For doses in the neonatal period, *see* Section 3.4

5.16.C Encephalitis

BOX 5.16.C.1 Minimum standards
- ABCD and intensive care.
- Lumbar puncture, basic clinical chemistry and haematology.
- Temperature control.
- Anticonvulsants.
- Antiviral and antibiotic drugs.

Introduction

Encephalopathy refers to a clinical syndrome of reduced consciousness for which there may be a variety of causes. Encephalitis is an inflammatory process involving primarily the brain parenchyma, but sometimes also the meninges (meningoencephalitis) or spinal cord (encephalomyelitis). Primary encephalitis refers to cases in which the causative agent invades and replicates within the nervous system, whereas in post-infectious encephalitis the clinical manifestations appear to be caused by an immunological response to the agent. In practice it can be difficult to differentiate between the two entities. This subsection focuses on primary infectious encephalitis.

Aetiology

- In many instances no specific aetiological agent can be identified.
- Geographical location and seasonal variation influence the frequency of infection with specific organisms.
- Viruses are the responsible pathogen in the majority of cases (*see* Table 5.16.C.1).
- Arboviruses are an important cause of encephalitis worldwide, but the major contributor within the arbovirus group, the Japanese encephalitis virus (JEV), is limited to Asia and the Pacific Rim.
- Enteroviruses are a common seasonal cause of encephalitis in Europe and the USA. In the last decade there have been periodic large outbreaks of enterovirus 71 infections in Asia, and the overall incidence of enterovirus 71 is increasing in this region.

TABLE 5.16.C.1 Causes of viral encephalitis according to geographical region

America	Europe and the Middle East	Africa	Asia	Australasia
• West Nile Virus • La Crosse • St Louis • Dengue • Rabies	• Tick-borne encephalitis • West Nile virus • Rabies	• West Nile virus • Rift Valley fever virus • Congo-Crimean haemorrhagic fever • Dengue • Rabies	• Enterovirus 71 • Japanese encephalitis • West Nile virus • Dengue • Murray Valley encephalitis • Rabies • Nipah	• Murray Valley Encephalitis • Japanese Encephalitis
• Sporadic causes	• Herpes simplex 1 and 2 • Varicella zoster virus • Epstein–Barr virus • Cytomegalovirus • Human herpes virus 6 and 7 • Coxsackieviruses • Echoviruses • Enteroviruses 70 and 71 • Parechovirus • Poliovirus • Measles • Mumps • Rubella			

TABLE 5.16.C.2 Suggested investigations in children with acute encephalitis, with reference to differential diagnosis

Investigation	Relevance
Blood glucose levels	Hypoglycaemia (common in infants and children with severe infections and poor oral intake/vomiting)
	Hyperglycaemia (diabetes)
	Metabolic encephalopathies, inborn errors of metabolism
Full blood count, blood film	Cerebral malaria (in endemic regions, returning travellers, etc.)
Urea and electrolytes	Hyponatraemia, syndrome of inappropriate secretion of antidiuretic hormone
Liver function tests	Reye's syndrome, metabolic encephalopathies
	Liver failure
Arterial blood gas	Metabolic encephalopathies
	To assess severity, particularly in individuals with brainstem compromise
Ammonia	Reye's syndrome, metabolic encephalopathies
Blood culture and Widal test	Typhoid and other septicaemias may have encephalopathic features
Acute and convalescent serology	To include locally relevant pathogens (e.g. Japanese encephalitis serology in Asia) and those suggested by history and examination (e.g. measles, mumps, varicella, HSV, *Mycoplasma*, *Legionella*)
Toxicology	Heavy metals, pesticides
Erythrocyte sedimentation rate	Collagen vascular disorders
Autoantibodies	Collagen vascular disorders
Cerebrospinal fluid (CSF) • Examination and culture • CSF PCR	Bacterial meningitis
	Tuberculous meningitis
	Intracranial haemorrhage
	HSV
	Enterovirus 71
Electroencephalography (EEG)	Status epilepticus
Neuroimaging (with contrast enhancement)	Space-occupying lesion (malignancy, brain abscess)
	Tuberculous meningitis
	Intracranial haemorrhage

• Herpes simplex type 1 (HSV-1) causes sporadic encephalitis worldwide.

• The common childhood viral infections such as measles, mumps, rubella and chickenpox (varicella zoster virus, VZV) may all involve the nervous system.

• Spirochaetal infections including syphilis, leptospirosis and Lyme disease are a well-recognised cause of meningoencephalitis. Other organisms such as *Brucella* are occasionally implicated. *Mycoplasma pneumoniae* is an important and treatable cause. Neurological involvement may occur in chlamydial and rickettsial infections, and both fungi (e.g. *Cryptococcus*) and parasites (e.g. *Angiostrongylus cantonensis*) may cause meningoencephalitis.

- Immunocompromised individuals are at particular risk of developing parasitic and fungal infections.
- Encephalitis has been noted to occur following a wide variety of immunisations. Fortunately, improvements in vaccine technology in recent years have meant that such complications are now rare.

Clinical features

Presentation

The following clinical manifestations commonly occur, whatever the aetiological agent:

- An acute systemic illness with fever, headache, nausea and vomiting.
- Generalised seizures, less commonly focal.
- Behavioural or personality changes.
- Deteriorating conscious level, confusion and drowsiness, lapsing into coma.
- Neck stiffness is common but not invariable.
- Signs of involvement of any part of the nervous system may be present (e.g. hemiparesis, ataxia, myelitis, movement disorder, brainstem abnormalities).
- A rash may point to a specific diagnosis (e.g. measles, VZV, enteroviruses).
- Presentation may be subtle and/or subacute in immunocompromised individuals.
- Signs of raised intracranial pressure (ICP) may be present. The possible contribution of raised ICP to the

clinical picture should always be considered, as this may be amenable to treatment.

Severity ranges from a mild illness with fever, a single brief seizure and confusion lasting for 2–3 days, to a more prolonged illness with a fluctuating level of consciousness and evolution of neurological signs over several weeks. Occasionally the course may be fulminating, with death occurring within a few days.

Diagnosis

The following investigations (*see* Table 5.16.C.2) should be considered in all cases but may be constrained by lack of resources. Efforts should be directed towards identifying those diseases that are treatable, common locally, or indicated by specific details in the history.

CSF examination and culture provide valuable diagnostic information, but if the child shows evidence of raised ICP, has signs suggestive of a space-occupying lesion or has cardiovascular compromise, lumbar puncture may be contraindicated. Lumbar puncture should be deferred until considered clinically safe, and antimicrobial therapy should be prescribed empirically, directed towards the common pathogens and antibiotic sensitivity patterns in the region.

Typical findings in the CSF in viral encephalitis are documented in Table 5.16.C.3, together with characteristic features on EEG and neuroimaging. In general it is possible to differentiate between viral and bacterial CNS infections on the basis of the CSF picture. If there is doubt, however, empirical antibiotic therapy should be given pending CSF culture results (*see* Section 5.16.B). Alternatively, if the child is stable, the lumbar puncture should be repeated after 24–48 hours while observing the clinical condition closely.

TABLE 5.16.C.3 Typical findings in viral encephalitis

Investigation	Findings
CSF microscopy and biochemistry	<ul><li>Rarely may be normal</li><li>Usually lymphocyte-predominant pleocytosis (from a few to several thousand white blood cells/mm³)</li><li>In early disease, polymorphonuclear cells may predominate</li><li>Mildly elevated or normal protein levels</li><li>Normal CSF/plasma glucose ratio</li><li>Absence of microorganisms on Gram stain</li><li>Eosinophilia suggests parasitic infection</li><li>India-ink stain: cryptococcus</li><li>Normal CSF opening pressure ($< 25\,cmH_2O$)</li></ul>
Electroencephalography (EEG)	<ul><li>Virtually always abnormal</li><li>Diffuse slow waves; occasionally unilateral patterns may suggest particular causative agents, such as HSV (see below) or subacute sclerosing panencephalitis</li></ul>
Neuroimaging: CT or MRI	<ul><li>May be normal</li><li>Cerebral oedema is common</li><li>Features may suggest particular causative agents (e.g. HSV, Japanese encephalitis virus)</li></ul>

Management

In the majority of cases no specific treatment is available, and management is primarily supportive.

- Provide bed rest, and analgesia for headaches. Care is needed with sedation, as a deterioration in conscious level may be obscured and/or respiratory depression may occur.
- Antipyretics may be used to alleviate distress, but are no longer recommended solely to reduce the temperature.
- Ensure adequate oxygenation ($SaO_2 > 94\%$).
- Regularly monitor electrolytes and review fluid balance.

Fluid restriction may not be appropriate if the cardiac output is low. Aim to keep the serum sodium level (and other electrolytes) within the normal range. Consider the possible causes of hyponatraemia (e.g. vomiting/gastrointestinal losses, excessive hypotonic intravenous fluids, over-hydration, syndrome of inappropriate secretion of antidiuretic hormone) and act accordingly.

- Critically ill children, particularly those with evidence of brainstem involvement or raised ICP, should be managed in an intensive-care unit if possible. Assisted ventilation and cardiovascular support should be instituted early if there is evidence of compromise. Children should be nursed with the head in the midline and tilted 20 degrees up. If they are ventilated, normocapnia should be maintained.

- Control of seizures (see Section 5.16.D and E). Caution is required when using anticonvulsant drugs with the potential to cause respiratory depression. EEG monitoring may reveal subclinical seizure activity.
- Intermittent use of mannitol (250–500 mg/kg per dose, which may be repeated after 1 hour) or hypertonic saline may be helpful if there is evidence of raised intracranial pressure (ICP), but remember that electrolyte and fluid balance monitoring are critical (hypernatraemia is as dangerous as hyponatraemia). ICP monitoring should only be undertaken in centres that are experienced in this technique.
- If there are pointers in the history, examination and/or preliminary investigations that suggest a specific diagnosis such as HSV, *Mycoplasma* or Lyme disease, the relevant treatment should be given (see below).
- If bacterial or tuberculous meningitis cannot be excluded, and the child is severely ill, consider providing cover with appropriate drugs until these diagnoses can be definitively ruled out (see Section 5.16.B and Section 6.1.N). A second lumbar puncture performed 24–48 hours after admission may aid this decision (provided that raised ICP is not present).

Long-term prognosis

The illness may be prolonged, and survivors may be left with significant neurological sequelae. Physiotherapy and rehabilitation should be commenced once the acute stage of the illness is over and the child is stable. Some children remain in hospital for many months, and relatives require considerable support to cope with the often devastating effects on the family. A number of children without overt neurological sequelae are left with subtle problems, including visual and hearing impairments, learning difficulties and behavioural problems. Long-term follow-up is needed to detect and manage these problems.

Features of specific viral infections that cause encephalitis

Enterovirus 71

- There have been recurrent outbreaks in Asia since the 1990s, and a rising prevalence in the region.
- Children under 5 years of age are most commonly affected.
- These infections can be associated with hand, foot and mouth disease (HFMD) (with vesicular lesions on the hands, feet or mouth) or herpangina (mouth ulcers)
- Neurological involvement includes aseptic meningitis, acute flaccid paralysis, Guillain–Barré-type illness and brainstem encephalitis (cranial nerve involvement, myoclonic jerks and autonomic disturbance). The onset of neurological problems is commonly within the first 3 days of illness.
- Diagnosis is primarily clinical, but viral culture on throat, rectal or vesicle swabs provides supportive evidence. If available, PCR is advisable to identify the specific serotype of enterovirus.
- Children affected with brainstem encephalitis are at risk of cardiopulmonary complications such as shock,

pulmonary oedema and/or haemorrhage. They should be managed in a paediatric intensive care unit if possible.

- Polyclonal IgG (2 grams/kg in 24 hours) may be given when there is neurological involvement, although there is no direct evidence to support this therapy at present. There are potential adverse effects, such as anaphylaxis, and IVIG should only be administered with cardiac monitoring facilities.
- High-level supportive care is necessary for patients with cardiopulmonary compromise, but there is a high case fatality and morbidity in this group.

Japanese encephalitis virus

- This is the most common cause of encephalitis worldwide. There are an estimated 50 000 cases and 15 000 deaths each year.
- It is currently limited to Asia and the Pacific Rim, but there is evidence that previously non-endemic regions such as Tibet have cases.
- The virus is transmitted by *Culex* mosquitoes, with an enzootic cycle involving pigs and birds.
- Most infections are asymptomatic (200–300 asymptomatic cases for every case of encephalitis).
- Extrapyramidal and brainstem involvement is common in patients with encephalitis. Patients may have Parkinsonian features acutely, with some later developing choreoathetoid movement disorders. Gradual improvement over several months is usual in survivors.
- Myelitis may occur, usually accompanied by some encephalitic features. The prognosis for recovery from myelitis is poor.
- Diagnosis rests on IgM/IgG capture ELISA in serum and CSF. Viral isolation is difficult, as the viraemia is short-lived.
- Thalamic, basal ganglia and brainstem lesions are often apparent on CT or MRI imaging (if available).
- There are no specific features on EEG.
- Treatment is supportive only, but effective vaccines are available.
- The prognosis is poor. Up to 30% of patients with encephalitis die in the acute stage. Neurological sequelae are common in survivors, but do tend to improve with time.

Herpes simplex virus

- This causes sporadic encephalitis worldwide.
- Encephalitis is more frequently a manifestation of recurrent than primary infection. There is no correlation between the presence of herpetic skin lesions and the diagnosis of HSV encephalitis.
- Seizures (both focal and generalised) are a prominent feature.
- Personality changes, temporal lobe phenomena, and dysphasia are also common.
- CSF findings:
  - Lymphocytic pleocytosis: < 50 to 2000/mm^3.
  - Red blood cells are present in CSF in more than 80% of cases, reflecting haemorrhagic necrosis.
  - Protein levels are usually moderately elevated, but may reach very high levels as the disease progresses (3–5 grams/litre).
  - Up to 25% of cases may have a relatively low CSF glucose concentration.

— Occasionally the CSF is entirely normal in early disease.

- Diagnosis is by polymerase chain reaction (PCR) or serology on CSF. Viral isolation is difficult.
- If the initial CSF PCR is negative but there are ongoing clinical features suggestive of HSV infection (e.g. deteriorating level of consciousness, focal seizures), a repeat lumbar puncture more than 72 hours after the onset of neurology is advisable. Early CSF for PCR may be falsely negative.
- EEG may show a typical pattern of multifocal periodic lateralising episodic discharges (PLEDs) on a slow background, often with a temporal lobe focus.
- CT and MRI (if available) may show lesions (often haemorrhagic) in the temporal lobes. In early disease, scans may be normal.
- **Treatment is with high-dose IV aciclovir for 21 days as an infusion over one hour** (neonate to 3 months 20 mg/kg; 3 months–12 years 500 mg/m^2 (*see* Section 9 for chart on surface area); 12–18 years 10 mg/kg. All doses given 8 hourly: in older child use ideal weight for height if obese).
- Treatment may be stopped if the patient is diagnosed with a clear alternative cause of the encephalitis.
- In those with a definitive diagnosis, it is advisable to have a negative CSF PCR at the end of the treatment course.
- Early diagnosis and treatment improve the outcome significantly. HSV is a possibility in all patients with encephalitis, although in areas of the world where other pathologies such as enterovirus 71 encephalitis are endemic, HSV is responsible for only a very small minority of the total number of cases. **If resources permit, start aciclovir (at the dosage stated above) in all cases without a definitive diagnosis and continue until HSV has been excluded, or an alternative diagnosis has been reached.**
- Mortality can still be up to 20%, with around 15% of cases left with severe sequelae. Relapses occur occasionally, but these are less likely to occur if treatment is continued for 21 days.

Varicella zoster virus (VZV)
- VZV infection usually only results in mild encephalitis, with acute cerebellar ataxia as the main feature. Seizures and coma are rare, and the prognosis is good.

Measles (*see* Section 6.2.E)
- Acute encephalitis may occur 6–8 days after the onset of the rash, and may be severe, with up to 10% mortality and frequent sequelae.
- Delayed chronic encephalitis may also occur in the form of subacute sclerosing panencephalitis (SSPE), presenting with cognitive deterioration and myoclonic jerks. In such cases the EEG shows stereotypic polyphasic complexes on a background of excess slow activity.

Rabies (*see* Section 6.2.H)
- Saliva (plus virus) from an infected mammal enters via a bite, skin abrasion, or rarely through intact skin or mucous membranes.
- The incubation period varies from a few days to many months. A history of animal bite may not be elicited at the time of presentation.
- There is an initial prodrome of fever and malaise lasting

a few days, followed by a second phase of excitement, hyperacusis, hydrophobia and pharyngeal spasms.
- Lastly, a paralytic phase occurs (rarely this may be the only manifestation).
- Death is inevitable once neurological signs are apparent.
- Effective prevention is available with the human diploid cell vaccine, and should be combined with passive immunisation if exposure has occurred.

Other organisms
Mycoplasma
- Neurological involvement occurs in up to 7% of infections.
- Both direct invasion of CNS and immune-mediated disease occur.
- Aseptic meningitis, transverse myelitis and Guillain–Barré syndrome are the most common manifestations.
- Diagnosis is by complement fixation titres (if available).
- If the diagnosis is suspected, treat intravenously or enterally if tolerated, with erythromycin, 12.5 mg/kg/dose 6-hourly for 10 days. However, this is not effective for the immune-mediated disease.

Cryptococcus
- This can cause acute fulminant meningoencephalitis in immunocompromised children.
- It may present more subtly in an immunocompetent child.
- Consider when there is prolonged headache, fever, vomiting and focal neurology.
- It it important to have a baseline CSF opening pressure (provided that there are no contraindications).
- There may be normal CSF biochemistry and cell count.
- Diagnosis is based on India ink smear or CSF culture or rapid antigen assay in CSF or serum.
- Start with a 2-week induction treatment phase of an IV infusion over 4–6 hours of amphotericin 250 micrograms/kg once daily increasing as tolerated to 1.5 mg/kg once daily (after a test dose of 100 micrograms/kg to be included in the first calculated dose) plus flucytosine 25 mg/kg/every 6 hours, or fluconazole 6–12 mg/kg/day up to a maximum of 800 mg/day.
- Children with HIV may require higher doses of amphotericin (up to 5 mg/kg/day)
- Amphotericin therapy requires pre-hydration and close supervision for toxicity, including hepatic and renal function tests, electrolyte monitoring and regular full blood counts.
- In settings where amphotericin is not available, fluconazole 12 mg/kg/day up to 1200 mg/day with or without flucytosine 100 mg/kg/day **or** fluconazole 12 mg/kg/day up to 1200 mg/day alone may be used.
- Initial treatment should be followed by an 8-week consolidation phase using fluconazole 6–12 mg/kg/day, up to a maximum of 400–800 mg/day.
- For the maintenance treatment phase, fluconazole 6 mg/kg/day up to a maximum of 200 mg/day is used.
- Raised intracranial pressure may develop during treatment, and prompt recognition is important. If identified, repeated therapeutic lumbar punctures can be helpful in controlling headache and limiting the development of ventricular dilatation, blindness and cranial nerve palsies.
- In HIV-infected individuals, consider antiretroviral therapy

once antifungal treatment is established, but there is a risk of immune reconstitution syndrome.

Human angiostrongylus

- This is predominantly found in the Pacific Islands and Asia, where it is the most common cause of eosinophilic meningoencephalitis.
- The main mode of infection is via consumption of raw snails or other molluscs, freshwater prawns, frogs and contaminated vegetables.
- The hands may become contaminated with larvae that are then directly carried to the mouth by small children.
- Presentation is commonly with acute severe headache, low-grade fever, cranial nerve involvement, visual disturbances, paraesthesia or hyperaesthesia, and raised intracranial pressure.
- Peripheral blood eosinophilia may be very marked.
- Eosinophils are also seen in the CSF. Organisms may

invade both the meninges and the brain parenchyma, especially involving the posterior fossa.

- Diagnosis is primarily clinical, relying on a history of likely ingestion of contaminated food, with typical clinical findings and an eosinophilic CSF picture. Serological tests are available, but may be normal in the early stages, and are also difficult to interpret because there is great cross-reactivity with other parasites.
- MRI (if available) may show multiple micronodular enhancing lesions.
- In many cases the symptoms spontaneously resolve within several weeks (mean period of 20 days).
- It is rarely fatal, and sequelae are usually minimal. A minority of patients have persistent paraesthesia and weakness associated with chronic infection.
- Provide analgesia for headache: consider giving a 2-week course of albendazole and prednisolone orally, but the evidence for treatment regimes in children is lacking, and most cases resolve with time.

5.16.D Epilepsy

> **BOX 5.16.D.1 Minimum standards**
> - Anticonvulsants: phenobarbitone, phenytoin, sodium valproate, carbamazepine, ethosuximide.
> - Temperature control.
> - Prednisolone.
> - EEG and neuroimaging with CT and MRI (if available).

Introduction

Epilepsy is a symptom caused by a central nervous system (CNS) disorder, and is usually defined as the occurrence of two unprovoked seizures. In over 70% of cases a cause cannot be identified (idiopathic epilepsy), although genetic causes may be important, as there is often a family history. Most children with epilepsy live in disadvantaged communities where the incidence rates are estimated to be twice those in western countries, and where more than 70% of affected individuals are untreated.

The impact of epilepsy on children and families is wide-ranging. To reduce disability, management is best shared with other healthcare workers who can visit the family closer to home, such as community doctors, and healthcare or disability workers.

Confirming the diagnosis of epilepsy

There is no justification for a trial of anti-epileptic drugs if the diagnosis is unclear. The diagnosis of epilepsy is purely a clinical one, and is usually based on a good history or eyewitness account or ideally a video (often taken with a mobile phone) of an event.

Important features of the seizures include the following:
- timing and duration
- provocation factors
- the early phase of the attack; look for localising features
- movements
- sensory symptoms

- level of responsiveness
- nature of offset.

In early childhood, breath-holding attacks, reflex anoxic seizures and febrile syncope may be commonly mistaken for epileptic seizures. Syncope, hypoglycaemia and non-epileptic attacks such as extensor spasms also enter the differential diagnosis.

Role of investigations

The history and sometimes the examination will usually indicate the cause. Children can be managed without the need for an electroencephalogram (EEG) or neuroimaging. EEG and neuroimaging (preferably an MRI scan, but sometimes a CT scan may be informative) should be reserved for intractable cases or those with neurological signs suggesting a space-occupying lesion. Such problems, and the imaging needed to identify them, will usually require the support of a specialised neurosurgical centre, at least one of which should exist in every country.

Prognostic features of epilepsy

When a syndrome cannot be identified precisely, the features in Table 5.16.D.2 can serve as a guide to the prognosis.

Once the diagnosis and prognosis have been assessed, draw up a problem list as follows:
- What effect does the epilepsy have on the development of the child?
- Are learning or motor problems present?
- Is the child attending school and getting opportunities to play with other children?
- Are there any behavioural problems?

Selecting appropriate anti-epilepsy drugs

Phenobarbitone, phenytoin, carbamazepine and sodium valproate should be available.

Convulsive status epilepticus (see Section 5.16.E).

TABLE 5.16.D.1 Clinical classification: most common syndromes of epilepsy in children

Syndrome	Features	Treatment
Generalised		
Tonic or tonic–clonic (grand mal)	Loss of consciousness Stiffening, convulsive movements Incontinence Post-ictal drowsiness, headache	Phenobarbitone Phenytoin Sodium valproate Carbamazepine
Absences	Vacant stare, with decrease in awareness, responsiveness and memory Precipitated by hyperventilation	Ethosuximide (may not be affordable) Sodium valproate **Avoid** carbamazepine and phenytoin
Myoclonic	Head nodding or jerks of limbs	Ethosuximide (may not be affordable) Sodium valproate **Avoid** carbamazepine and phenytoin
Infantile spasms	Sudden flexion of head, trunk and limbs; sometimes extensor spasms Associated with hypsarrhythmia on the EEG and developmental delay	Steroids (these require careful monitoring; **avoid** using them if this is not feasible) Sodium valproate
Lennox–Gastaut syndrome	Multiple seizure types: tonic (especially night), atonic, absences, generalised tonic–clonic. Associated with slow spike and wave on EEG and developmental delay	Sodium valproate Carbamazepine Phenytoin Combinations of the above
Secondary generalised seizures	Seizures starting as partial, and developing (sometimes rapidly) into generalised tonic–clonic seizures	Carbamazepine Sodium valproate Phenytoin Phenobarbitone
Partial		
Simple	Convulsive movements involving the eyes, face and parts of limbs. May have sensory symptoms	Carbamazepine Sodium valproate
Complex	Aura of abdominal discomfort, vacant stare, loss of contact with surroundings, lip smacking, chewing, swallowing, facial flush, hallucinations Post-ictal tiredness and headaches May produce apnoea	Carbamazepine Sodium valproate Phenobarbitone
Benign epilepsy of childhood with Rolandic spikes	Most common, usually starts at 3–10 years of age Predominantly simple partial seizures involving oropharyngeal muscles (gurgling), face or limbs, mostly during sleep Characteristic EEG, normal intelligence	Often do not need treatment Carbamazepine Sodium valproate Phenobarbitone

TABLE 5.16.D.2 Prognosis in epilepsy

Good outcome	Adverse outcome
Single seizure type	Multiple seizure types
No additional impairment	Additional neurological impairment (especially cognitive)
Late age of onset (for the syndrome)	Early age of onset (for the syndrome)
Provoked by illness, stress, flashing lights	Unprovoked
Short seizures	Status epilepticus
Low frequency of seizures	High frequency of seizures
Good initial response to anti-epileptic drugs	Poor initial response to anti-epileptic drugs, requiring polytherapy

How to start treatment

- Monotherapy is the aim, to reduce the side effects and interactions.
- Try to avoid using drugs that impair development (e.g. phenobarbitone, except in infancy).
- If possible, always prescribe the same brand, as there may be pharmacodynamic differences.
- Always start in low doses to minimise side effects and increase the likelihood of compliance.
- Remember to warn the child and their family about any likely side effects, especially if they are temporary, such as drowsiness.
- Increase the drug dose gradually (every 2–4 weeks) until the seizures stop or are significantly reduced, or side effects become significant (*see* Table 5.16.D.3).

How to monitor treatment

- Case notes should record the diagnosis, problem list, dates and types of seizures, indication for treatment, past treatment with response and side effects of treatment, and information that has been given to the child and their parents or carers.

- Hand out medical cards to be kept as a seizure diary, reminder of prescription and clinic dates. Graphic symbols can be used for the illiterate.
- Regularly review the child to check on their progress. Review them more often if seizure control has not been achieved, or if are side effects or drug changes.

When to change treatment

- Consider changing treatment if side effects are troublesome.
- Introduce the second anti-epileptic drug in the normal way, first checking for possible drug interactions. Once established, begin to withdraw the first anti-epileptic gradually. If seizure control is not achieved with monotherapy, seek a specialist referral.

When and how to stop treatment

In children with a good prognosis, 12–24 months of freedom from seizures is associated with a 70% risk of continuing seizure remission. Withdrawal must be a gradual and closely monitored process. If seizures recur after a decrease in drug dose, they usually remit once the last decrease has been reversed. The withdrawal period depends on the drug (e.g. phenobarbitone over 4–6 months, carbamazepine over 2–3 months).

Whom to refer

This depends upon local facilities. One-third of patients will be intractable to treatment with first-line anti-epileptic drugs. Some of them may not have epilepsy, and others may have syndromes with a poor prognosis. They will require specialist assessment and treatment advice. Epilepsy may also be a part of complex developmental disorders involving the CNS, and these children may also benefit from specialist input.

TABLE 5.16.D.3 Doses of common anti-epileptic drugs

Drug	Usual dose	Side effects and toxicity
Carbamazepine	1 month–12 years initially 5 mg/kg at night or 2.5 mg/kg twice daily increasing to 5 mg/kg three times a day Maximum dose 20 mg/kg per day 12–18 years Initially 100–200 mg 1–2 times daily increasing to 200–400 mg two or three times daily. Maximum up to 1.8 g daily	Ataxia, diplopia, aplastic anaemia (bruising, mouth ulcers)
Phenobarbitone	One month to 12 years initial dose 1.5 mg/kg twice daily increasing to 2.5–4 mg/kg/day once or twice daily 12–18 years 60–180 mg once daily	Drowsiness, agitation, rashes, developmental impairment
Phenytoin	1 month–12 years initial dose 1.5–2.5 mg/kg twice daily then increasing to 2.5–5 mg/kg twice daily 12–18 years initial dose 75–150 mg twice daily increasing to 150–200 mg twice daily (maximum 300 mg twice daily)	Gum hypertrophy, hirsutism, acne, ataxia, diplopia, nystagmus, neuropathy, choreoathetosis, encephalopathy, lymphoma, megaloblastic anaemia
Sodium valproate	1 month–12 years initial dose 5–7.5 mg/kg twice daily increasing to 12.5–15 mg/kg twice daily 12–18 years initial dose 300 mg twice daily increasing to 0.5–1 g twice daily	Nausea, epigastric pain, alopecia, weight gain, tremor, hepatitis, pancreatitis, encephalopathy

Social issues
Promoting social integration
Children need to participate as fully as possible in the normal activities of their peers, at school, at play, in the home and preparing for employment. Community workers should be involved in the wider management, and parents' fears and anxieties discussed.

Supporting parents
Parents often tend to overprotect their children who have epilepsy, and may lack confidence in dealing with seizures. In many societies epilepsy carries a stigma. Opportunities to discuss first aid, behaviour and other concerns are vital, and can be provided by healthcare workers or parent groups.

First-aid advice
The general theme to be emphasised is that children with epilepsy should be encouraged to live as full and normal a life as possible. There are very few absolute restrictions, but these include climbing trees or riding bikes or motorcycles. Children should be accompanied when swimming or when

near to hazards such as stoves and fires. During a convulsion, place the child in the recovery position, protect them from hard or sharp objects in the vicinity, and cushion their head. Do not put anything in their mouth or try to restrain their limbs. Let them recover by themselves. They may need to rest or sleep, but keep them under observation because they may start convulsing again. As a rough guide, a convulsion that does not stop spontaneously within about 10 minutes is likely to continue for longer, and may need intervention with anti-epileptic drugs given IV, rectally or bucally. The use of rectal diazepam at home by parents and carers is described later in this subsection.

Febrile seizures

A febrile seizure is a seizure that occurs in children aged between 6 months and 7 years with febrile illness not caused by an intracranial disease. The commonest age of onset is 14–18 months. Febrile seizures are common, occur in 2–5% of all these children, and account for about one-third of all childhood seizures.

Clinical presentation

Febrile seizures are usually brief, generalised, clonic or tonic–clonic convulsions lasting less than 10 minutes with minimal post-ictal confusion or weakness. About 20% of febrile seizures are complex (i.e. focal), or last longer than 15 minutes, or occur more often than once in 24 hours. Complex febrile seizures may suggest an underlying central nervous system cause and are associated with a poorer outcome (cognitive impairment or epilepsy).

Febrile seizures occur while the child has a recognisable infection, most commonly an upper airway infection or a viral illness such as gastroenteritis. Other causes include pneumonia, urinary tract infections and after vaccinations. Shigellosis, roseola infantum and malaria have an unusually high incidence of seizures. Most children have a core temperature of 38–41°C, but it may occur at the onset of the febrile illness, and the child may have a normal temperature at the time of seizure.

An increased frequency of febrile seizures occurs in the children of parents and siblings who have had febrile seizures, and siblings with epilepsy.

Identify the cause

Check blood glucose levels (by finger-prick test if available), take a careful history and examine the patient thoroughly, especially with regard to alertness and ability to play, looking for common and serious sites of infection. Where relevant, look at rapid test or film for malaria parasites, and full blood count. Consider urinalysis, lumbar puncture, cultures of blood, urine, pharyngeal swab and cerebrospinal fluid, and relevant X-rays in children whose history and examination offer clues to serious infection. A lumbar puncture is mandatory if meningitis is thought to be a possibility (unless there is evidence of raised intracranial pressure, when IV antibiotics should be given until meningitis can be excluded; *see* Section 5.16.A and Section 5.16.B).

Differential diagnosis

Exclude the following:
- meningitis
- encephalitis
- acute encephalopathies of metabolic or toxic origin
- cerebral malaria
- electrolyte disorders
- hypoglycaemia
- anoxia
- trauma
- haemorrhage
- tumour.

Other entities that can be confused with febrile seizures include the following:

- febrile delirium (in which the patient is speaking but not making sense)
- febrile rigors (in which the patient is shaking with a fine tremor).

Treatment

No treatment is necessary in simple self-limiting febrile seizures provoked by a minor febrile illness. Advice to parents should consist of the following:

- Reassurance that the condition is almost always benign and that the large majority of children stop having seizures after 5 or 6 years of age, while many have only one seizure.
- Practical demonstration of the recovery position for use if a further seizure occurs (*see* Section 5.16.E).
- Advice to seek medical help if a further seizure occurs, both in case it is prolonged (less than 5% of cases, but see below) and, importantly, so that the source of the provoking infection can be identified.

Sequelae

- About one-third of children with febrile seizures will have another febrile seizure.
- Around 3% will have at least one afebrile seizure.
- Around 2% may develop epilepsy (recurrent afebrile seizures).
- Approximately 65% of children with simple febrile seizures will have had no further seizures by 7 years of age.
- Recurrent seizures tend to re-occur, particularly in children aged less than 1 year at the onset of the febrile convulsions or those with a positive family history.

Risk of later epilepsy

The risk factors for the development of epilepsy are as follows:
- complex febrile seizures
- previous abnormal neurological function
- multiple febrile seizures
- family history of epilepsy
- age less than 1 year at the first seizure.

Long-term care: home treatment

- Rectal diazepam for parents to administer if there are prolonged seizures (2.5 mg for children under 1 year, 5 mg for those aged 1–3 years, 10 mg for those aged over 3 years). **The parents must also be taught what to do if their child stops breathing (i.e. they should be equipped with a bag and mask and shown how to use it).**
- Oral or rectal paracetamol to prevent or treat febrile seizures.
- Advice to parents as described above.

5.16.E Convulsive status epilepticus

BOX 5.16.E Minimum standards
- ■ **ABC** and high-dependency care.
- ■ Anticonvulsants:
  - — lorazepam
  - — phenobarbitone
  - — phenytoin
  - — paraldehyde
  - — diazepam
  - — midazolam
  - — thiopentone.
- ■ Temperature control.
- ■ Mannitol.
- ■ Dexamethasone.

Introduction

Convulsive status epilepticus (CSE) is a life-threatening condition in which the brain is in a state of prolonged electrical discharge. It is defined as a generalised convulsion lasting for more than 30 minutes, or recurrent convulsions which occur very frequently over a 30-minute period, where the patient does not regain consciousness between seizures.

The duration of the convulsion is highly relevant, as the longer the duration of the episode, the more difficult it becomes to control it. Convulsions that persist for longer than 10 minutes are much less likely to stop spontaneously. Therefore it is usual practice to institute anticonvulsive treatment when the episode has lasted for 5 minutes or more.

Common causes of convulsions in children

These include the following:
- fever with a predisposition to febrile convulsions (usually between the ages of 6 months and 6 years)
- meningitis
- epilepsy
- hypoxia
- metabolic abnormalities
- abrupt withdrawal of anti-seizure medication, especially phenobarbitone
- an acute cerebral event or injury (e.g. haemorrhage, trauma)
- ingestion of medication.

Tonic–clonic status occurs in approximately 5% of patients with epilepsy. Up to 5% of children with febrile seizures will present with status epilepticus. The mortality rate of status epilepticus can be high (up to 20% in adults), especially if treatment is not initiated quickly. However, with optimal management and adherence to a structured and standardised management plan, the mortality in children is much lower and patients can survive with minimal or no brain damage.

Evaluation and immediate management of status epilepticus

During a seizure:
- Turn the child on their side.
- **Adopt an ABC approach. It is vital to ensure satisfactory**

respiration and circulation and to exclude or treat hypo-glycaemia before giving anti-epileptic drugs.
- Ensure that the airway is patent and that there is adequate respiratory effort and circulatory volume. Institute corrective measures immediately if these are required.
- If available, administer oxygen via a mask.
- Check glucose levels and treat if they are low (< 2.5 mmol/litre or 45 mg/dL). If in doubt or unable to check the levels, it is safer to treat as if hypoglycaemia is present and give 10% dextrose IV 2–5 mL/kg as an initial bolus and, if safe to do so, follow this with an infusion containing a glucose-containing fluid to avoid the risk of rebound hypoglycaemia.
- If the seizure has lasted more than 5 minutes (or if the duration is not known), prepare for anticonvulsant treatment. Short recurrent seizures lasting less than 5 minutes should also be treated (see Figure 5.16.E.1).
- **A self-inflating bag with non-return valve (e.g. Ambubag) and a suitably sized face mask must be available in case excessive respiratory depression is caused by benzodiazepines** (see Section 1.12).
- Treat the fever (if present) with exposure, tepid sponging and rectal paracetamol (40 mg/kg loading dose, 20 mg/kg if less than 3 months of age).

Drugs
Lorazepam (intravenous or intra-osseous route)

Lorazepam is a benzodiazepine with a fast onset of action and a longer duration of effect (12ldren zures lasting with diazepam (which is less than 1 hour). It produces less respiratory depression than other benzodiazepines, and is less likely to require additional anticonvulsants to stop the seizure. However, absorption from the rectal route is poor. Lorazepam is not available in every country, but is no more expensive than diazepam.

Dose: 50–100 micrograms/kg/dose by IV or intra-osseous route (the dose can be repeated after 10 minutes if necessary).

Midazolam (buccal application)

Midazolam is an effective fast-acting anticonvulsant that has an onset of action within minutes but has a shorter lasting effect (15–20 minutes). Most children do not convulse again once the seizure has been terminated.

Buccal midazolam is twice as effective as rectal diazepam, but both drugs produce the same degree of respiratory depression. This occurs only in about 5% of patients, is short-lived, and is usually easily managed with bag-valve-mask ventilatory support.

Midazolam can be given by the buccal or IV route. However, the ready-made buccal midazolam may not be available in some countries. In such situations the standard IV preparation can be used instead via the buccal route. Simply draw the required dose in a syringe using a needle so as to filter off any glass fragments, and after removing the needle apply the drug on the buccal mucosa between the lower lip and the gum.

Dose:

- 500 micrograms/kg/dose (maximum 10 mg) with buccal application (the dose may be repeated).

Diazepam

Diazepam is an effective, commonly used, readily available and fast-acting anticonvulsant with similar characteristics to midazolam. It is widely used, but may now be superseded by the more effective lorazepam or buccal midazolam where the latter is available. The rectal dose is well absorbed.

Dose:

- 500 micrograms/kg/dose rectally
- 200–300 micrograms/kg/dose by the IV or intra-osseous route (the dose may be repeated).

Lorazepam (intranasal route)

This has been found to be safer than IM paraldehyde, and is also less expensive and easier to access. It is directly instilled into one nostril, with the patient in a supine position, drop by drop over 30–60 seconds.

Dose: 50–100 micrograms/kg/dose intranasally.

Paraldehyde

Paraldehyde is an effective and cheap anticonvulsant with a sustained level of effect and a good safety profile. However, it may be difficult to find in some countries. Paraldehyde takes 10–15 minutes to start to take effect, and its action is sustained for 2–4 hours.

It is generally given by the rectal route after mixing the required dose with an equal amount of any edible oil (e.g. olive oil). This mixture is then quickly pushed up the rectum using a simple feeding tube attached to a syringe. **Do not leave paraldehyde standing in a plastic syringe for longer than a few minutes, as the drug dissolves plastic.** The IM route can also be used, but is very painful and can lead to abscess formation, so is better avoided. Paraldehyde causes little respiratory depression, but should not be used in patients with liver disease.

Dose: 0.4 mL/kg rectally (0.4 grams/kg).

Phenytoin

Phenytoin is a readily available anticonvulsant that can give very good results with little effect on respiration. It has a peak action within 1 hour, and a long half-life. Its action is therefore more sustained than that of diazepam.

It is administered as an IV infusion mixed with 0.9% sodium chloride solution made up to a concentration of 10 mg/mL, given over a 20-minute period. Phenytoin can cause dysrhythmias and hypotension (especially if given rapidly), so it is important to monitor the electrocardiogram (ECG) and blood pressure if these are available. In addition, local irritation, phlebitis and dizziness may accompany IV administration.

If the child is known to be on oral phenytoin it is better to either avoid using phenytoin (use phenobarbitone instead) or use a lower loading dose (i.e. 10 mg/kg).

Dose: 20 mg/kg IV infusion given over 20 minutes (only use normal (0.9%) saline for dilution).

Phenobarbitone

Phenobarbitone is a time-tested anticonvulsant and readily available in many countries; the parenteral preparation is on the WHO essential drug list. It can be used to good effect in all age groups, and causes little respiratory depression.

It is given by the IV route as a slow injection over 5–15 minutes, and can also be given by the IM route, although the absorption is variable. It has a sustained effect that lasts over 12–24 hours.

There is now evidence to suggest that phenytoin and phenobarbitone may have some synergistic effect when used sequentially. It is thought that one primes the brain in readiness for the other, thus producing a beneficial effect. However, there is controversy about which drug should be used first.

Dose: 20 mg/kg IV infusion over 5–10 minutes.

Thiopental

Thiopental (thiopentone) sodium is a drug better used by experienced staff who are familiar with it (usually anaesthetists: see Section 1.24) and who are capable of intubating difficult cases. It is a general anaesthetic agent with no analgesic properties but with marked cardiorespiratory effects. It is usually given after paralysis and intubation in induction of anaesthesia. Other anti-epileptic medication must be continued. The child should not remain paralysed, as continued seizure activity cannot otherwise be monitored. A paediatric neurologist should continue to give clinical advice and support.

General measures once seizures are controlled

- **Maintain a normoglycaemic state** using 5% glucose-containing solutions (10% in young infants). Often children may show a hyperglycaemic pattern following seizures as a stress-induced response. This does not require correction with insulin.
- **Normal maintenance fluid volume** can be given to avoid hypoglycaemia and to maintain electrolyte balance. However, evidence of raised intracranial pressure or increased antidiuretic hormone secretion should necessitate fluid restriction.
- **Assess and maintain electrolyte balance**, maintaining serum sodium levels within the normal range (135–145 mmol/litre). Avoid hyponatraemia by using Ringer-lactate or Hartmann's solution.
- **Aspirate the stomach contents** by inserting a gastric tube, and perform gastric lavage or give charcoal (1 gram per year of the child's age) if appropriate for specific drug ingestion.
- **Regulate the temperature**, ensuring that temperatures above 37.5°C are avoided.
- **Treat raised intracranial pressure**, if clinically present (see Section 5.16.K), as follows:
  - Support ventilation (maintain a pCO_2 of 4.5–5.5 kPa).
  - Maintain a 20-degree head-up position.
  - Give 20% mannitol, 250–500 mg/kg (1.25–2.5 mL/kg) IV over 15 minutes. This may be repeated on a 2-hourly basis as required.
  - Alternatively, hypertonic saline can be used (2.7% or 3% at a dose of 3 mL/kg). This may not be associated with a 'rebound' rise in pressure or induce a diuresis like mannitol but rather augments plasma volume.
  - Give dexamethasone, 500 micrograms/kg twice daily (for oedema surrounding a space-occupying lesion).
- **Catheterise the bladder**, as distension may aggravate raised intracranial pressure.
- **Frequent reassessment of ABC** is mandatory, as

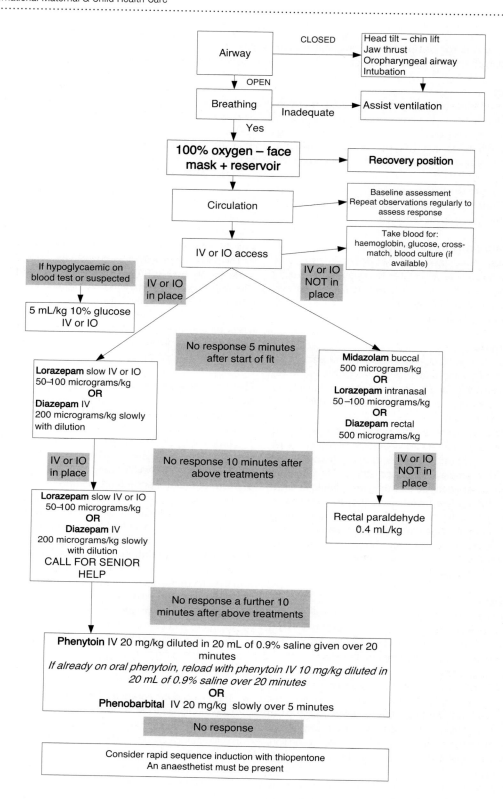

FIGURE 5.16.E.1 Algorithm for the treatment of status epilepticus in children.

therapy may cause depression of ventilation or hypotension, especially if benzodiazepines or barbiturates have been used.

- If available, a standard EEG can be done to establish cessation of electrical seizure activity.

- **Identify and treat the underlying cause** of the convulsion.
- Following seizure control there are several regimes for continued drug control of the convulsions, but they are beyond the scope of this text.

5.16.F Neuropathies

Introduction

Neuropathies are diseases that affect the anterior horn cells and/or the peripheral nerves.

Anterior horn cell disease

The most common neuropathies are:
- poliomyelitis (*see* Section 6.2.G)
  - spinal muscular atrophy.

Spinal muscular atrophy

This is a motor neuron disease of the spinal cord and brainstem, inherited as an autosomal-recessive disorder and associated with deletions of the survival motor neuron (SMN) and neuronal apoptosis inhibitory protein (NAIP) genes. It is the second commonest autosomal-recessive disorder after cystic fibrosis.

Clinical features

These children have delayed motor development but normal social, language and intellectual development. They are floppy and weak. The weakness is proximal more than distal, and affects the lower limbs more than the upper ones. The children are areflexic, and fasciculation of the tongue is diagnostic (observed with the tongue at rest in the mouth). There are three clinical subtypes based on severity.

- **Severe infantile type:** These infants never sit, crawl or walk. The onset is before or soon after birth. They have severe intercostal and bulbar weakness but the diaphragm is spared. Most die from respiratory failure before their second birthday.
- **Intermediate type:** These infants can sit but are unable to walk. They may or may not have respiratory and bulbar weakness, and this factor determines their prognosis. If it is absent, these children can survive into adulthood.
- **Mild type** (also known as Kugelberg–Welander type). The onset is later and these children can walk, but they do so late and with difficulty. Respiratory and bulbar weakness is not usually present. A coarse tremor of the hands is frequently seen in this and the intermediate form. This is a useful sign for distinguishing this type from muscular dystrophy, with which it is often confused (*see* Table 5.16.F.1).

Diagnosis

Since the discovery of the gene defect, muscle biopsy is rarely needed. Deletion of the *SMN* gene is found in almost all cases of spinal muscular atrophy of all three types. It can be detected rapidly by the polymerase chain reaction (PCR). Blood (2–5 mL in an EDTA tube), or DNA extracted from it, can be sent by post to a laboratory that will perform the test and confirm the diagnosis within a few days.

TABLE 5.16.F.1 Comparison of spinal muscular atrophy (mild type) and Duchenne muscular dystrophy

Feature	Spinal muscular atrophy	Duchenne muscular dystrophy
Motor milestones	Delayed	Normal or delayed
Hypotonia	+++	+/–
Pseudohypertrophy	+/–	+++
Hand tremor	+++	–
Tongue fasciculation	+	–
IQ	Normal	Normal or low
ECG	Baseline tremor	R- and Q-wave changes
Creatine kinase	Normal or slightly raised ($\times$ 2)	Very high ($\times$ 100)
EMG	Chronic denervation	Myopathic
Muscle biopsy	Denervation	Dystrophic

Management

Management is supportive. The most important complication in the intermediate form is the development of scoliosis. This can be delayed by getting the child to stand with support of lightweight callipers for as long as possible. If the child is confined to a wheelchair, a brace may be needed to control the scoliosis. Surgery (fusion of the spine) may be necessary. Children with symptoms of nocturnal hypoventilation (disturbed sleep, headaches, daytime drowsiness and poor concentration) may benefit from assisted non-invasive night-time ventilation with a nasal mask (*see* Section 8.2).

Peripheral neuropathy

The two commonest causes of peripheral neuropathy in children are Guillain–Barré syndrome (*see* Section 5.16.G) and hereditary motor and sensory neuropathy.

Hereditary motor and sensory neuropathy

This is the commonest chronic peripheral neuropathy in children. It is progressive, and there are several types, but the commonest is type I (peroneal muscular atrophy). It is dominantly inherited, and most children are asymptomatic until late childhood, when unsteady clumsy gait with frequent falls develops. There is weakness and wasting of the muscles of the anterior compartment of the leg. The parents are often asymptomatic. The diagnosis is confirmed by the finding of very low motor conduction velocities in both the child and one of the parents, indicating demyelination. Type II is similar, but rare, and shows axonal rather than demyelinating changes in nerve conduction studies. There are no treatments for these diseases other than special boots and ankle orthoses to stabilise the ankle.

Other peripheral neuropathies

These include leukodystrophies (where peripheral nerve demyelination occurs as part of CNS demyelination), toxic neuropathy (due to glue or benzene sniffing, lead, or drugs) and diphtheria (see Section 6.1.C).

5.16.G Guillain–Barré syndrome

BOX 5.16.G Minimum standards
- ABC resuscitation and emergency care.
- Lumbar puncture.

Introduction

This is the commonest peripheral neuropathy seen in childhood. It is a demyelinating neuropathy induced by an autoimmune process that is precipitated by a preceding viral or other infection. It has a peak incidence at around 8 to 9 years of age in well-resourced countries and 3 to 4 years of age in resource-limited ones, possibly due to overcrowding. Rarely, an acute axonal form occurs, especially in some countries, such as China.

Clinical features

The onset is usually acute. There is often a history of a preceding upper respiratory or gastrointestinal tract infection and insidious sensory symptoms (e.g. muscle tenderness, occasionally an unsteady gait, and frequent falls). The weakness starts in the lower limbs and ascends to affect the trunk, upper limbs, and the respiratory (intercostal and diaphragm), bulbar and facial muscles. It is usually symmetrical and affects both proximal and distal muscles, and may take 10–30 days to reach its maximum. Cranial nerve involvement often precedes respiratory difficulties. Reflexes are frequently absent. Sensory loss is minimal and of the 'glove-and-stocking' distribution. Ophthalmoplegia, papilloedema and bladder involvement rarely occur. Autonomic dysfunction occurs in many children, resulting in hypertension, hypotension and cardiac arrhythmias. In some patients the paralysis occurs rapidly with quadriplegia and respiratory paralysis within 2–5 days.

Chronic inflammatory demyelinating polyradiculoneuropathy

The disease may evolve into chronic inflammatory demyelinating polyradiculoneuropathy. This disease is similar to Guillain–Barré syndrome, consists of progressive or relapsing motor and sensory dysfunction, and lasts at least 2 months, with hyporeflexia of all four limbs. The importance of identifying this condition is that it responds to steroids (prednisolone 2 mg/kg/day).

Diagnosis

The diagnosis is confirmed by an abnormal nerve conduction stimulation, but a high CSF protein level and almost normal cell count are very suggestive. These findings are usually present after the first week of onset. Other causes of acute flaccid paralysis such as poliomyelitis in endemic countries need to be considered (see Table 5.16.G.1).

Management

Supportive care is the cornerstone of successful management of the acute patient. Of greatest concern is respiratory failure due to paralysis of the diaphragm (the muscle that is most important for breathing). **Intubation** may be needed if there is evidence of impending respiratory failure. The following steps in management should be taken:

- Admit the child to hospital to monitor for impending respiratory and bulbar paralysis and autonomic dysfunction.
- Measure the respiratory rate, heart rate and blood pressure, perform pulse oximetry and if possible measure vital capacity (or peak flow), and check airway protection frequently. Blood gas analysis may be helpful.
- If the vital capacity is less than 50% of normal for age **and/or there is significant respiratory failure with hypoxaemia and hypercapnia**, ventilate the child if possible.
- If bulbar and respiratory paralysis occurs, airway protection, tube feeding and ventilatory support will be necessary. Airway protection can be achieved by intubation or tracheostomy.
- Plasma exchange (also called plasmapheresis) and high-dose immunoglobulin therapy may lessen the severity of the illness and accelerate recovery in some patients, but are not widely available. These two treatments are equally effective, and a combination of the two is not significantly better than either alone. However, immunoglobulin is easier to administer.
- Children who require ventilation can be given high-dose human immune globulin if available (0.4 grams/kg IV over 6 hours daily for 5 days). This can be repeated if there is no response, if deterioration occurs or if there is a relapse.

Prognosis

Recovery is usually complete within 4–6 months in most children, but may take up to 2 years. About 5% of children will have minor motor sequelae, and around 2–3% will die from respiratory failure or autonomic dysfunction. Poor prognostic factors include onset of weakness within 8 days of preceding infection, rapid progression, cranial nerve involvement and a CSF protein level of > 800 mg/litre in the first week of the disease. The prognosis is generally better in children than in adults.

TABLE 5.16.G.1 Other causes and features of acute flaccid paralysis

Cause	Features
Spinal cord	
Poliomyelitis	Preceding fever, headache and meningeal irritation, asymmetrical weakness, CSF pleocytosis
Enterovirus: Japanese B encephalitis	Similar to poliomyelitis
Trauma	History and evidence of trauma
Myelitis	Paraplegia, segmental sensory loss
	Bladder and bowel sphincter disturbance
Epidural abscess	Fever, vertebral tenderness
Neuropathies	
Guillain–Barré syndrome	Symmetrical, areflexia, ascending weakness
Diphtheria	Preceding history of diphtheric pharyngitis, cardiac involvement, deep sensation impaired
Botulism	Bulbar symptoms before onset of weakness, ophthalmoplegia
Tick paralysis	Rapid progressive paralysis, no sensory loss,
	normal CSF protein levels
	Resolves quickly once tick has been removed
Metabolic	
Acute intermittent porphyria	Family history, other symptoms
Hereditary tyrosinaemia	
Muscle	
Myasthenia gravis (rare but treatable)	Fluctuating weakness that is worsened by activity and better after rest
	Tensilon test is positive
Acute viral myositis	Tender muscles, limp, fever, elevated muscle enzymes (creatine phosphokinase or aldolase)
Other causes	
Organophosphate poisoning	History of exposure, excessive salivation, twitching of muscles, meiosis, tachycardia

5.16.H Muscular dystrophy

BOX 5.16.H.1 Minimum standards
- Creatine kinase measurement.
- Prevention of scoliosis and contractures.
- Prednisolone.

Introduction

The muscular dystrophies are a group of inherited disorders that cause progressive muscle weakness and share a common pathological process of muscle fibre degeneration and fibrosis.

Duchenne muscular dystrophy

This is the most common muscular dystrophy, caused by deficiency of dystrophin, a structural protein found on the inner side of the sarcolemmal membrane. The deficiency is caused by deletions or point mutations of the dystrophin gene, which is located on the short arm of chromosome Xp21.

Clinical features

Duchenne muscular dystrophy is X-linked; it affects boys and is transmitted by females. Affected infants are normal in the first 2 years but will have very high serum creatine kinase levels. They usually present between 2 and 5 years of age with delayed walking, frequent falls, and difficulty in climbing stairs and in getting up from the floor. The weakness affects proximal more than distal muscles, and the pelvic girdle more than the shoulder girdle. The facial muscles are unaffected. Prominent calves and thighs are characteristic. With time, these children walk on their toes with marked lumbar lordosis and a waddling gait. The arm reflexes are lost early but ankle jerks are preserved. Once confined to a wheelchair, they rapidly develop contractures of the knees, hips and ankles and scoliosis. Intellectual impairment may occur or develop in some patients, often related to the onset of respiratory failure. The ECG shows dominant R waves in right-sided leads, deep Q waves in left-sided leads, and inverted T waves in most patients.

Diagnosis

The serum creatine kinase activity is very high (100 times normal). The electromyogram (EMG) is myopathic, and muscle biopsy shows dystrophic changes and absent dystrophin. Deletions in the dystrophin gene can be identified by the polymerase chain reaction (PCR) in DNA extracted from blood in 60–80% of patients.

Management

There is no effective drug treatment. A course of oral prednisolone (0.75 mg/kg/day) for 3–6 months can produce a small but significant improvement in muscle strength, but has many side effects, and these must be weighed against the slight benefit. Night splints to keep the ankles at 90 degrees may delay shortening of the tendo-achilles. When walking is becoming difficult, the fitting of lightweight callipers and intensive physiotherapy may keep the child ambulant for a few more years. Once the child is wheelchair-bound, a rigid seat and adequate postural support of the spine may prevent scoliosis.

Prognosis

The weakness is progressive, and by 10–12 years of age a wheelchair will be needed. Later, as respiratory muscle weakness develops, nocturnal hypoventilation may cause disturbed sleep and morning headaches (due to hypoventilation and carbon dioxide retention). Assisted non-invasive ventilation (using a nasal mask) at night will improve the child's quality of life (see Section 8.2). Death occurs in the twenties from respiratory or cardiac failure.

Genetic counselling

An elevated creatine kinase activity (on three separate occasions) in female relatives indicates carrier status. Some will also have an abnormal muscle biopsy, with some fibres showing normal and others absent dystrophin. Normal creatine kinase and muscle biopsy does not exclude the carrier state. Prenatal diagnosis is possible in some but not all families, but requires specialised molecular genetic techniques.

Becker muscular dystrophy

This is a milder variant of Duchenne muscular dystrophy, and is rare. Onset is between 5 and 10 years of age, and ambulation is maintained beyond 15 years and often into adulthood. This disorder is caused by partial deficiency of dystrophin.

Limb girdle muscular dystrophies

These are rare and vary in severity. A severe form is prevalent in North Africa. It has a clinical picture similar to Duchenne muscular dystrophy, but affects boys and girls and has more prominent involvement of the shoulder girdle muscles, with winging of the scapulae. It is associated with deficiency of one of the sarcoglycans, a group of sarcolemmal proteins intimately linked to dystrophin. This can be demonstrated in muscle biopsy specimens. The intelligence remains normal and the heart is unaffected. Genetic tests for diagnosis are available in specialised laboratories.

Congenital muscular dystrophy

Infants with congenital muscular dystrophy are born floppy and weak and have contractures. They have delayed motor milestones, and most are unable to walk. They develop a characteristic long thin expressionless face with an open mouth. There is no ophthalmoplegia. There are several subgroups, some with eye or brain abnormalities and demyelination. Merosin is deficient in one subgroup. Inheritance is autosomal recessive and the gene defect is known for most of them. The creatine kinase may be elevated or normal, and the diagnosis is made by muscle biopsy or genetic testing. Management is supportive. Congenital muscular dystrophy must be distinguished from other causes of hypotonia (i.e. other congenital myopathies, infantile spinal muscular atrophy and organic acidaemias).

5.16.I Breath-holding episodes

> **BOX 5.16.I.1 Minimum standards**
> - Haemoglobin measurement.
> - Oxygenation measurement.

Introduction

Breath-holding episodes occur in about 4% of children under the age of 5 years. They typically start between the ages of 6–18 months, and usually cease before the age of 5 years. They are infrequent, usually occurring less than once a month, but occasionally occur more often. There are two types of episodes, which are differentiated by the presence of **cyanosis** or **pallor**. The underlying mechanism of the two types is different.

Type of episodes
Cyanotic breath-holding episodes

These are provoked by anger, frustration, fright or pain. The infant cries vigorously, holds their breath in expiration, goes blue, loses consciousness and becomes limp. Rarely this is followed by a brief stiffening of the body. The infant then starts breathing again and the attack ends. These attacks may be due to cerebral ischaemia from a sudden rise in intrathoracic pressure that impedes venous return. Intrapulmonary right–left shunting also plays a part.

Pallid asystolic spells

These are less common than the cyanotic type (about 20% of all cases), and may occur in the context of a minor illness. The attack is provoked by pain, usually from a mild injury on the head. The child cries, loses consciousness, develops marked pallor and goes stiff. Occasionally the child loses consciousness immediately after the injury without crying. A few clonic jerks (reflex anoxic seizures) may occur. These pallid spells are caused by vagal asystole, and can be induced by pressure on the eyeballs (oculo-cardiac reflex), although it is not necessary to elicit this reflex, and if thought to be important, this should only be done under controlled conditions with EEG and ECG monitoring. **There is also a risk of damaging the eyeballs when pressing on them.**

Diagnosis

The diagnosis is based on a careful history of the sequence of events. These attacks are frequently confused with epilepsy. In epilepsy, the cyanosis occurs after the tonic–clonic phase of the seizure. In breath-holding spells cyanosis occurs before but, more importantly, the diagnosis rests on the fact that the attacks are always precipitated by an appropriate stimulus. An EEG is not necessary except when the diagnosis is in doubt and epilepsy is suspected. **An ECG must be done in pallid asystolic spells to exclude long QT interval syndromes. Always exclude anaemia, which is a well-documented cause of breath-holding episodes. Also exclude chronic hypoxaemia, which is also a cause from unrecognised cardiac or respiratory disease.**

Prognosis

These attacks are frightening for the parents, but are harmless. They eventually cease with time, and if there is no underlying pathology they do not have any long-term effects. There is no risk of subsequent epilepsy. Some infants with the pallid type go on to develop faints in later childhood.

Management

The parents need to be given an explanation of these attacks and reassured about their harmless nature. There is no effective drug and no need for drug treatment. Treat anaemia and hypoxaemia if these are present.

5.16.J Migraine

BOX 5.16.J.1 Minimum standards
- Paracetamol and ibuprofen.
- Anti-emetics.
- Propranolol, clonidine and pizotifen.

Introduction

Migraine is a common cause of recurrent headaches in children. Its prevalence increases with age. It may be preceded by a history of recurrent abdominal pain and vomiting at a younger age (abdominal migraine, cyclical vomiting). The headache is typically throbbing in nature, temporal or frontal in location, more often bilateral than unilateral (in contrast to adult migraine), and commonly associated with nausea, vomiting, pallor and sometimes photophobia. It usually lasts for 1–3 hours, but sometimes persists for 24 hours, and it is relieved by sleep. Migraine is precipitated by stress (e.g. school examinations, family pressure, unrealistic expectations) and sometimes by hunger, fatigue, lack of sleep, exposure to sun, and some foods (e.g. chocolates, Coca-Cola, caffeinated drinks, nuts, cheese). A positive family history of migraine, especially on the maternal side, is found in over 90% of patients, and the diagnosis of migraine must be questioned in the absence of such a history. Between the attacks the child is well.

Classification of migraine

Migraine is classified into three types.
- **Common migraine:** There is no aura in this type. It is the commonest form in children, accounting for over 80% of children with migraine.
- **Classical migraine:** An aura precedes the headache, which is rare in children (about 10%). Visual aura include hemianopia (loss of half of the visual field), scotoma (small areas of visual loss), fortification spectra (brilliant white zigzag lines), blurred vision and flashes of lights. Occasionally sensory auras occur, consisting of paraesthesia round the mouth and numbness of the hands and feet.
- **Complicated migraine:** Rarely neurological signs occur during the headache and persist for varying periods after it. Ophthalmoplegic migraine (third cranial nerve palsy) is rare, and must be distinguished from a berry aneurysm or other space-occupying lesion compressing the third cranial nerve.
  - **Hemiplegic migraine** is the occurrence of hemisyndrome (weakness or numbness down one side of the body) with the headache. Recurrent attacks of hemiplegic migraine are rare in children, but occasionally, starting in infancy, a child may have alternating hemiplegia as a manifestation of migraine.
  - **Basilar migraine** results from vasoconstriction of the basilar and posterior cerebral arteries. Symptoms include vertigo, tinnitus, diplopia, blurred vision, ataxia and occipital headaches. There is complete recovery after the attack. Minor head trauma may precipitate basilar migraine.

Management

A careful history and examination is essential to confirm the diagnosis of migraine. Investigations are rarely needed. Explanation of the attacks and the relatively benign nature and good prognosis will reassure the parents and the child, and by itself will lead to a reduction in frequency and severity of the headaches in over 50% of these children. Where possible, precipitating factors need to be identified and eliminated or reduced. In particular, dietary factors such as chocolate, Coca-Cola, caffeinated drinks and cheese should be avoided.

Acute attack

Rest and sleep in a quiet darkened room is usually preferred by patients. A simple analgesic alone or in combination with a non-steroidal anti-inflammatory agent is often all that is required, and if given at the onset will abort or reduce the severity of the headaches. Paracetamol (20 mg/kg per dose, repeated every 6 hours as necessary) and ibuprofen (5 mg/kg per dose) are useful agents.

If nausea and vomiting are troublesome, an anti-emetic may be prescribed, such as metoclopramide. Aged 5–9 years 2.5 mg and 9–18 years 5 mg three times daily orally or 100–150 microgram/kg slowly (over 2 minutes) by IV injection (maximum 1 mg). Children weighing over 60 kg can have metoclopramide orally 10 mg three times daily

Prochlorperazine is also useful, 200 micrograms/

kg (maximum 12.5 mg) orally IM or IV immediately, then 100 micrograms/kg per dose 6- to 8-hourly, orally or rectally. Prochlorperazine is not licensed for use in children who weigh less than 10 kg. Extrapyramidal side effects may occur.

The triptans (sumatriptan, zolmitriptan and rizatriptan) are serotonin-receptor agonists and are highly effective for the acute attack, but their use in children under 12 years of age awaits further evaluation. The dose of sumatriptan for adults is 50–100 mg orally as soon as possible after onset. It must not be used for basilar or hemiplegic migraine.

Prophylactic treatment

If the headaches are frequent (at least three to five per month) and troublesome, continuous prophylaxis is required, usually for a period of 1 year. If the headaches recur, the course of treatment is repeated. The drug of choice for children is propranolol, but pizotifen and clonidine have both been tried in children, with varying degrees of success.

- Propranolol is a beta-blocker, and can be given to children over 2 years of age (the dose for children aged 2–12 years is 200–500 micrograms/kg three times daily orally; for children over 12 years it is 20–40 mg two to three times daily). **Propranolol must not be given to children with asthma or diabetes, and it may cause depression.**
- Clonidine can be given at a dose of 2 micrograms/kg every 8 hours (maximum dose 200 micrograms/day).
- Pizotifen is given for children aged 5–10 years at an initial dose of 500 micrograms, increasing to 1 mg at night or 500 micrograms 8-hourly. For children aged 10–12 years give 1 mg at night or 500 micrograms 8-hourly. For children aged 12–18 years give 1.5 mg at night, increasing to 1.5 mg 8-hourly. It may cause weight gain.

Prognosis of migraine

The prognosis is generally good. About 50% of children with migraine will undergo spontaneous prolonged remission after the age of 10 years. In most children the headaches are infrequent and rarely interfere with schooling or daily activities. In some the headaches are frequent and troublesome, and these will require prophylactic treatment.

5.16.K Neurosurgical disorders

BOX 5.16.K.1 Minimum standards
- Maternal folic acid before and during pregnancy.
- Dexamethasone and mannitol.
- High-dependency care.
- Antibiotics.
- Anticonvulsants.
- Shunts.
- Regional/national centre (with CT and MRI scanning facility).

Introduction

Every country needs at least one hospital equipped to manage children with neurosurgical problems. The central and essential component of accurate assessment of the most frequently encountered intracranial neurosurgical emergencies is the prompt identification of the presence of raised intracranial pressure (ICP). Once this is recognised and controlled, the precise diagnosis of the site and cause can await sophisticated neuroimaging by ultrasound examination, computed tomography (CT) or magnetic resonance imaging (MRI).

Raised intracranial pressure

The signs and symptoms are different for pre-speech and younger infants compared with older children.

Babies and children under 2 years

The signs and symptoms are as follows:
- abnormally rapid head growth
- separation of cranial sutures
- bulging of the anterior fontanelle (note that the anterior fontanelle usually closes by 18 months of age)
- dilatation of scalp veins

- irritability
- vomiting
- loss of truncal tone
- fluctuating level of responsiveness
- irregular rate and rhythm of breathing, usually with slowing of the respiratory rate
- irregular heart rate, usually with bradycardia, but occasionally with tachycardia
- decerebrate attacks.

It is important to note that features may be non-specific (as in irritability and vomiting), that there may be marked fluctuations in the younger child's condition from minute to minute and from hour to hour, and that frank unconsciousness occurs relatively late, often being preceded by apnoea. Decerebrate attacks can be mistaken for epileptic seizures; in the former, the child extends all four limbs and trunk, whereas in the latter, flexion of the upper limbs is more usual and there are clear tonic–clonic phases.

Older children

The signs and symptoms are as follows:
- headaches
- vomiting
- loss of postural control of the trunk
- **failing vision**
- diplopia
- **neck pain and extension**
- **decerebrate attacks**
- irregular rate and rhythm of breathing, usually with **slowing of the respiratory rate**
- irregular heart rate, usually with bradycardia, but occasionally with tachycardia, and mounting hypertension with widening pulse pressure
- **diminishing level of consciousness.**

The most urgent features are failing vision, neck pain and extension, decerebrate attacks, diminishing level of consciousness and cardiorespiratory failure, as they all indicate incipient terminal events. Failing visual acuity is also urgent, as it indicates severe papilloedema and a danger of permanent visual loss. The absence of papilloedema does not exclude raised intracranial pressure; its presence does indicate that there is a risk of permanent visual loss.

Accurate cerebral localisation on a clinical basis is difficult in children and virtually impossible in babies and young children, but the following can be fairly dependable features of a supra-tentorial mass lesion:

- dysphasia
- visual field defects
- epileptic seizures.

Unilateral pupillary dilatation indicates a mass ipsilateral to the dilated pupil, or on the side of the pupil that dilated first in the case of bilateral pupillary dilatation.

Management

Although the definitive solution is removal of the causative lesion, this will often have to await the availability of imaging by computed tomography and transfer to a neurosurgical facility. The emergency relief of raised intracranial pressure can be achieved by one or more of the following medical measures:

- dexamethasone by slow IV injection (500 micrograms/kg immediately and then 100 micrograms/kg every 6 hours)
- 20% mannitol by IV infusion (250–500 mg/kg and repeated as required based on response and clinical signs; maximum total dose 2 grams/kg infusion over 20 minutes).
- alternatively, hypertonic saline can be used (2.7% or 3% at a dose of 3 mL/kg). This may not be associated with a rebound rise in pressure as may occur with mannitol and does not induce a diuresis like mannitol but rather augments plasma volume.
- intubation and artificial ventilation to $PaCO_2$ of about 4 kPa (if available).

In an extreme emergency, and faced with a rapidly deteriorating child with no immediate prospects of evacuation for neuroimaging and specialist neurosurgical care, the following measures can be employed if there is no history of head injury.

Babies

Trans-fontanelle needle tapping of the subdural space is undertaken, and if there is no subdural effusion, the needle is then advanced into the cerebral ventricle in the hope of finding and relieving hydrocephalus.

Infants and children

Right frontal burr-hole and ventricular drainage is undertaken (see below).

If there is a history of head injury, the procedure for 'blind' burr-holes is followed (see below).

Head injuries (*see* Section 7.3.C).

Intracranial abscesses

Spontaneous extradural, subdural or intracerebral abscesses most commonly arise in children as a complication of an acute, or very occasionally chronic, episode of infection in the paranasal sinuses or middle ear. The cardinal clinical features are as follows:

- raised intracranial pressure
- signs of focal neurological disturbance, including epileptic seizures
  - systemic signs of sepsis; these may be absent.

The diagnosis can be confirmed by CT scan with IV contrast enhancement (if available).

- Evacuation of pus is important both to relieve raised intracranial pressure and mass effect, and to provide material for accurate microbiological diagnosis. Intracerebral abscesses can often be drained satisfactorily by burr-hole aspiration, which may have to be repeated. Extradural and subdural collections will usually require a major craniotomy.
- Raised intracranial pressure will usually be very severe, and may require the use of mannitol.
- Pending microbiological diagnosis, or in the absence of such support, the most useful antibiotics are a combination of cefuroxime (IV 60 mg/kg 6-hourly for 3 days, then 25 mg/kg 6-hourly) and metronidazole (7.5 mg/kg by IV infusion over 20 minutes every 8 hours) for a minimum of 3 weeks. A further 6 weeks of an appropriate oral antibiotic, such as amoxicillin, is usually necessary.
- Amoxicillin route: oral:
  - Dose: 1 month to 18 years of age, 40 mg/kg daily in 3 divided doses maximum dose 1.5 g daily in 3 divided doses.
- An ENT surgeon may need to drain fronto-ethmoid sinuses or mastoids to prevent recurrence.

Hydrocephalus

Hydrocephalus can be diagnosed by trans-fontanelle ultrasound in infants with an open anterior fontanelle, and by CT (if available) in older infants and children. CT will also demonstrate the likely cause.

- The emergency relief of hydrocephalus, or suspected hydrocephalus, is by trans-fontanelle needle drainage in babies, or by burr-hole drainage and insertion of an external ventricular drain in older children.
- The best site for burr-hole drainage is on the right coronal suture in the mid-orbital line. The landmarks for trans-fontanelle puncture are the same as for subdural puncture (see above), but the needle is angled more steeply. Most babies will tolerate venting of up to 50 mL of CSF. Following withdrawal of the needle, the skin puncture is closed with a suture to prevent external leakage of CSF.
- It is important to have the CSF examined by a microbiology laboratory, remembering that sub-acute, partially treated, 'neglected' pyogenic meningitis and tuberculous meningitis can present with hydrocephalus.
- Definitive treatment may involve removal of the obstructing lesion in the case of a tumour or other mass, or establishment of a permanent CSF diversion by inserting an implanted ventriculo-peritoneal shunt.
- Shunt blockage is common and must be diagnosed quickly. The symptoms of shunt blockage are essentially those of raised intracranial pressure, and require urgent attention if death or disability is to be avoided. **The most reliable eye sign is loss of upward gaze.** Blockages

usually affect the ventricular end of the catheter rather than the peritoneal end. Many children develop abdominal distension after shunting. This is due to the unusual load of CSF. In the absence of vomiting and constipation, it should be treated conservatively.

- Shunt infections can present acutely with features of cerebral irritation, fever and seizures if there is major ventriculitis occurring within a few days of insertion; however, this is relatively rare. **The only method that is guaranteed to eliminate shunt infection is removal of all components, including any loose or retained fragments from earlier procedures, interval external drainage, appropriate antibiotics and shunt reinsertion through fresh incisions. As with all serious infections, success is dependent upon accurate microbiological diagnosis.** The most frequently encountered organisms are *Staphylococcus epidermidis* and *Staphylococcus aureus*. The most useful antibiotic is vancomycin by IV injection children 1 month to 18 years 15 mg/kg every 8 hours to a maximum daily dose of 2 grams. The duration of treatment depends on how rapidly the CSF becomes sterile, but a minimum of 7 days is recommended.

Myelomeningocoele

Myelomeningocoele is the commonest major congenital malformation compatible with survival. Its incidence has been progressively falling for 20 years. Although there are regional variations, the overall frequency is 0.7–0.8 per 1000 live births. The objective of management in the immediate postnatal period is the prevention of infection of the central nervous system. This is achieved by early closure of the lesion.

- The level of the open lesion is noted and an assessment made of the sensorimotor level, the state of the sphincters, any orthopaedic deformity, and the presence of major hydrocephalus, as evidenced by signs of raised intracranial pressure (see above).

- **The ideal is to achieve closure within 24 hours of birth. The majority of lesions have adequate skin in the wall of the sac, as long as this is not unnecessarily sacrificed by a wide incision. The technique employed involves mobilisation of the neural placode, watertight dural repair and closure of the skin.** While awaiting closure, the lesion should be protected with a dressing of moist sterile 0.9% saline, which must be replaced every few hours to prevent desiccation.

- Most babies will require surgical treatment for hydrocephalus in the first few weeks of postnatal life.

In children who are paralysed and without urinary or bowel control, the commitment is a lifelong one, and this is a challenge to families and healthcare systems. Before offering treatment to these children, it is important that their future prognosis and quality of life is discussed with the parents.

The aim should be to prevent as many as possible of these anomalies by adequate maternal nutrition prior to conception and during pregnancy.

Folic acid taken prior to conception and for the first trimester of pregnancy abolishes 75% of cases of myelomeningocoele and anencephaly.

See Section 5.10.A.

5.17 Orthopaedic problems

BOX 5.17.1 Minimum standards
- Antibiotics.
- X-rays.
- Erythrocyte sedimentation rate (ESR) and C-reactive protein (CRP).
- Antituberculous drugs.
- Orthopaedic procedures.

Introduction

Injuries are by no means the only paediatric orthopaedic problems in resource-limited countries. There is a great burden of orthopaedic infective conditions which, if treated suboptimally, can lead to considerable handicap. Furthermore, there is the same spectrum of non-infective conditions as is seen in well-resourced countries which, due to the limited resources available in under-resourced healthcare systems, represents a considerable diagnostic and therapeutic challenge.

Infections

Paediatric musculoskeletal infections are a common presentation in resource-limited countries. Morbidity and mortality can be prevented by prompt diagnosis, antibiotics and surgery where indicated. Infection should be suspected in any child presenting with pain or swelling in the limbs, spine or pelvis.

Pyomyositis
- Pus is present within skeletal muscle, most commonly in the thigh and gluteal regions.
- It is caused by bacterial infection of muscle, in nearly 70% of cases due to *Staphylococcus aureus*.
- It is common in the tropics, but exceedingly rare in the developed world.
- There may be a history of previous injection or trauma to the site.
- Signs include general malaise, swinging fever, decreased range of motion, fluctuant swelling in the later stages, and tenderness.

Treatment

If diagnosed early (which is unusual), pyomyositis may respond to antibiotic therapy (flucloxacillin), but most cases will require incision and drainage of the abscess under general anaesthesia.

At operation

- Incise along the long axis of the tender/swollen area.
- **Mark this area prior to giving anaesthesia.**
- Drain all pus.
- Irrigate thoroughly.
- Insert a wick to maintain drainage and prevent recurrence of the abscess.

Post-operative care

- Give analgesia.
- Give a 5-day course of antibiotics.
- Change the dressings daily.
- Evaluate for signs of recurrence and other foci of infection.

Osteomyelitis

This is infection within bone. It is common in resource-limited countries, and has a number of different manifestations:

- acute haematogenous osteomyelitis
- neonatal osteomyelitis
- subacute haematogenous osteomyelitis
- chronic osteomyelitis.

Acute haematogenous osteomyelitis
Pathogenesis

- The causes are unknown.
- Infection starts in metaphyseal venous sinusoids.
- There is thrombosis of the vessels.
- Pus develops in the medullary cavity, leading to a build-up of pressure.
- If untreated, pus bursts through the cortex and spreads under the periosteum, rendering bone ischaemic (see **chronic** osteomyelitis below).
- In infants and children the pathogen is almost always *Staphylococcus aureus* (for neonates, see below). The exception is in sickle-cell disease, where *Salmonella paratyphi* is common. In this situation, use cefotaxime or ciprofloxacin.

Diagnosis

- Any child with fever and unexplained bone pain.
  - High index of suspicion.
  - Around 50% of cases will have a history of recent infection.
  - The child refuses to move the affected limb.

Investigations

- In resource-limited countries, **clinical examination is the mainstay of diagnosis**.
- White blood cell count is unreliable.
- Erythrocyte sedimentation rate is raised in 90% of cases.
- Blood culture is positive in 40–50% of cases.
- Plain X-rays: bony changes take 7–14 days.
- Aspiration and Gram stain; look for acid-fast bacilli.
- Bone scan (if available).

Treatment

- Prior to the formation of pus in the medullary cavity, antibiotics alone may suffice.
- Due to the predominance of *Staphylococcus aureus* as the causative organism, the initial antibiotic should be flucloxacillin while culture results are awaited (50 mg/kg IV or orally (maximum individual dose 2 grams) 6-hourly for 3 weeks).
- Once an abscess has formed this should be drained surgically.

Operative treatment

- Undertake incision, drilling and drainage of the osteomyelitic abscess.
- Mark the area of maximal swelling and tenderness prior to anaesthesia.
- Make a longitudinal incision.
- Dissect on to and incise the periosteum.
- Drill the cortex of the bone. If there is no pus at one site, drill further holes proximally and/or distally until pus is obtained.
- Copious irrigation is needed.
- Leave the wound open, and apply a dry or antiseptic dressing.
- Monitor post-operatively for recurrence and other foci of infection, and leave the wound to granulate.

Neonatal osteomyelitis

There are several features unique to neonatal osteomyelitis.

- In the neonate, metaphyseal vessels communicate with epiphyseal ones, thus permitting the spread of infection into the epiphysis and ultimately into the joint. Therefore acute haematogenous osteomyelitis and septic arthritis may occur together. This can lead to complete lysis of areas such as the femoral head and neck and the proximal humerus, or premature physeal arrest.
- As the immune system of the neonate is immature, there may be a less marked inflammatory response to infection, with an absence of fever, raised white blood cell count or erythrocyte sedimentation rate.
- Multiple foci of infection are more common.
- A wider spectrum of infecting organisms is found (not only *Staphylococcus aureus* but also group B streptococci and Gram-negative coliforms).
- Antibiotic treatment consists of gentamicin plus flucloxacillin.

Subacute haematogenous osteomyelitis

This differs in presentation from acute haematogenous osteomyelitis in the following ways:

- It often has an insidious onset.
- The clinical signs are less marked.
- Investigations may be inconclusive or equivocal.
- The location is usually metaphyseal, with plain X-rays showing a solitary lytic lesion (abscess) with a sclerotic margin.
- The differential diagnosis includes a neoplasm.

The usual **causative organism** is, as for acute haematogenous osteomyelitis, *Staphylococcus aureus.*

Treatment consists of surgical curettage of the lesion followed by antibiotic therapy.

Chronic osteomyelitis

If acute osteomyelitis goes untreated, the pressure due to the intramedullary pus eventually increases until it bursts through the cortical bone into the subperiosteal space. If still undecompressed, the pus spreads proximally and distally, stripping the periosteum and thus rendering this cortical bone ischaemic (having been deprived of both intramedullary and periosteal blood supply).

The avascular cortical bone therefore dies and becomes a focus of chronic infection called a 'sequestrum'. Simultaneously, a periosteal reaction occurs under the stripped periosteum, resulting in the laying down of new bone or 'involucrum'.

The appearance on plain X-ray is characteristic, with sclerotic sequestrum separated (by the abscess cavity) from an irregular and enveloping involucrum.

Chronic osteomyelitis is difficult to treat even with optimal resources. Some guidelines on its management are as follows:

- If an osteomyelitic abscess is beginning to point, or there are signs of an underlying abscess, this should be incised and drained.
- In weight-bearing bones there should be no attempt at removal of sequestrum until the overlying involucrum is mature. This maintains the potential for weight bearing and ambulation.
- Periods of immobilisation should be minimised in order to retain ranges of motion and function of nearby joints.
- Sequestrum that begins to point through the skin can be removed or excised.
- In many cases the clinical picture that results is one of intermittent flare-ups of infection which can be treated by incision and drainage of abscesses, excision of sequestrate, and antibiotic (flucloxacillin) suppression of infection as required.
- Curative treatment is often elusive even in specialised centres, and a degree of morbidity is unfortunately inevitable.

Septic arthritis

Septic arthritis is infection of a synovial joint.

Features

- It is more common in males than in females.
- The peak incidence is at around 2 years of age.
- The first symptom may be a reluctance to use the limb.
- There is a swollen tender warm joint with a restricted range of motion.
- There is commonly fever (38–40°C).
- The patient is usually **systemically unwell**.

Diagnosis

- The mainstay of diagnosis is **clinical examination**.
- The white blood cell count is raised in 30–60% of cases.
- Elevation of the erythrocyte sedimentation rate is more sensitive (except in the neonate).

Plain X-rays are often normal until there is evidence of bone destruction at 7–14 days. Common pathogens include *Staphylococcus aureus*, *Haemophilus influenzae*, group A and B streptococci, pneumococci and Gram-negative coliforms (in neonates).

Aspiration of the joint is the definitive test.

Treatment

- Antibiotic therapy should not begin until after joint aspiration and blood cultures have been taken.
- Start with flucloxacillin (infants and children) or flucloxacillin and gentamicin (neonates).
- Some studies have shown that a combination of **aspiration** and antibiotic therapy is sufficient treatment, but this must be followed by close monitoring to ensure improvement.
- If the child fails to improve, surgical washout and drainage is required either via open arthrotomy or by arthroscopic means (but only if a skilled operator and equipment are available).

Post-operative care

- Continue antibiotic therapy, and monitor for recurrence.
- Early mobilisation of the affected joint is needed to prevent stiffness.
- If treated early, the prognosis for functional recovery is good. However, if presenting late there may already have been destruction of the articular surface.
- Be alert for coexisting osteomyelitis, which is present in around 15% of cases of septic arthritis.

Tuberculosis

Tuberculosis as an entity is covered in detail in Section 6.1.N, but it is important to remember the potential orthopaedic manifestations.

- It can cause both osteomyelitis and septic arthritis.
- In both cases the signs are less marked than in their non-mycobacterial forms, and the history is usually more chronic.
- It may be associated with systemic manifestations of tuberculous disease (respiratory and renal).
- Spinal tuberculosis (Pott's disease) can be the cause of both paraplegia and scoliotic deformity.
- Treatment consists of surgical drainage and curettage of abscess cavities combined with antituberculous chemotherapy. For chronic disease and joint destruction, spinal stabilisation and joint arthrodeses may be indicated.

Non-infective conditions

The non-infective paediatric orthopaedic conditions described below can be extremely difficult to treat in resource-limited settings. First, without any form of population screening procedure in place or comprehensive primary healthcare provision, many cases will present late. Secondly, the advanced diagnostic modalities (ultrasound and arthrography) that are needed to direct treatment may not be available. Finally, where surgery is indicated, the operative techniques often need highly specialist training and/or specialised resources such as internal fixation and perioperative fluoroscopy, which are unlikely to be available in most resource-limited countries.

Fortunately, the conditions described are rare, typically occurring at a rate of less than 0.1%. They thus present far less commonly than the orthopaedic paediatric infections, and cause a lesser burden of handicap overall.

Developmental dysplasia of the hip

Formerly known as 'congenital dislocation of the hip', this complex condition has now been renamed 'developmental dysplasia' in recognition of its variable characteristics, such as the fact that it is not always present at birth, nor does it always feature hip dislocation.

- Reported initial (neonatal) rates range from 3 to 17 per 1000 live births, but the rate of established dislocation is much lower, at around 1 per 1000.
- The aetiology is multifactorial; increased rates are seen in female children, firstborns, breech position and oligohydramnios, and there is undoubtedly a genetic influence (increased rates are associated with a positive family history and affected siblings).
- Early detection depends upon neonatal screening, which is often not available in resource-limited countries.
- If screening is to be carried out, it should involve Barlow and Ortolani tests for newborns followed by subsequent re-examination and ultrasonography of suspected cases at 1 month of age.
- Plain X-rays are of limited use before 6 months of age.

Treatment

As mentioned above, treatment of this condition in resource-limited settings is extremely difficult.

- Up to 6 months of age, gentle closed reduction can be undertaken, and then maintained in a Pavlik harness.
- If a Pavlik harness is unavailable, a plaster spica, maintaining the hips in flexion and abduction, will achieve the same objective.
- In children over 6 months of age, closed reduction can still be attempted, but is increasingly less likely to be successful due to the interposed joint capsule preventing stable concentric reduction.
- If closed reduction fails, open reduction can be attempted if surgical skills allow and infection is avoided.
- Later presentation with proximal femoral and acetabular abnormalities may require complex secondary reconstructive procedures, but these can only be undertaken in specialist hospitals by a specialist surgeon.

The reality of developmental dysplasia of the hip in resource-limited countries is that cases will often not present until after the age of 18 months, when the child has failed to walk or has an obviously abnormal gait. By this time bony changes may have occurred, the only treatment then being complex secondary procedures, the skills and resources for which are usually unavailable in a resource-limited setting.

Congenital talipes equinovarus

More than two-thirds of cases of talipes equinovarus occur in developing countries. Most children receive either no treatment or substandard care. This results in physical disability that is entirely preventable.

There are three classes of talipes equinovarus (clubfoot):

- **Postural:** this arises from intrauterine positioning, and resolves fully with passive stretching within a few weeks of birth. Parents can be trained to do this.
- **Congenital:** this arises in an otherwise normal child, and has varying degrees of severity. It occurs in 1 in 1000 live births, and is bilateral in 30–40% of cases.
- **Syndromic:** this is associated with other syndromes, such as arthrogryposis, is often severe and is refractive to treatment.

Treatment

- The goal of talipes treatment is to obtain a functional plantigrade stable foot by the time the child begins to walk (i.e. before 1 year of age).
- If it is recognised in the neonatal period, gentle daily parental manipulation may be successful, or alternatively manipulation and taping by qualified healthcare professionals (e.g. a physiotherapist). Ponseti management has gained popularity as it does not require surgery and is easily learned (www.global-help.org/publications/books/help_cfponseti.pdf).
- For cases that fail to resolve in the first 6–12 weeks, serial manipulation and plaster casting is indicated, with cast changes every 2–4 weeks.
- If the deformity still fails to resolve, there may be a place for limited percutaneous soft tissue releases (Achilles tendon or plantar fascia) at the age of 3–9 months. These techniques are relatively easily learned, have low morbidity, and are user-friendly in resource-limited settings. They should be combined with manipulation and casting.
- For the case that still fails to resolve, more extensive surgery, such as a postero-medial release, is required. The timing of this surgery is usually between 6 months and 1 year of age. Although specialist training is required to learn this operation, it can be relatively easily assimilated by the non-orthopaedic surgeon and, being only a soft tissue release, does not require any 'high-tech' surgical resources.
- Unfortunately, as with developmental dysplasia of the hip, children with this condition in resource-limited countries commonly present late (over 18 months of age), when the deformity is fixed and secondary bony changes have occurred. Correction at this stage requires a combination of bony and soft tissue surgery which can really only be undertaken by an orthopaedic specialist surgeon.
- In the adolescent child with fixed chronic deformity, the procedure of choice may be an arthrodesis (fusion) combined with correction of deformity performed at skeletal maturity.

Perthes disease (Legg–Calve–Perthes disease)

Perthes disease is a disease of uncertain aetiology involving a process of fragmentation and repair of the femoral head, possibly due to underlying idiopathic osteonecrosis.

- It usually occurs in susceptible children between 4 and 8 years of age, but can occur in children as young as 2 years or as old as 12 years.
- It is five times more common in boys, 10% of cases are bilateral, and it is associated with hyperactivity.
- It presents with a limping or waddling gait with groin, thigh or knee pain.
- X-rays show varying degrees and stages of fragmentation and repair of the femoral head.
- The prognosis depends on the degree of fragmentation and the potential for repair and remodelling prior to epiphyseal closure. A good prognosis is therefore associated with early onset and male gender (as the epiphyses close later).

Treatment

- In the majority of cases no specific treatment is indicated. The femoral head will repair and remodel satisfactorily, and the eventual outcome will be good. Bed rest, activity restriction and abduction braces have no proven impact on the natural history of the disease.

- In the small proportion of cases that may benefit from surgery, the issue is **containment**. A very deformed femoral head may not sit or move properly in the acetabulum, and thus leads to secondary arthrosis. A proportion of these cases may benefit from varus osteotomies of the proximal femur or pelvic osteotomies. Assessment for these procedures requires arthrography at the very least, and the procedures themselves are very much the preserve of the orthopaedic specialist surgeon in a specialist hospital.

Slipped upper femoral epiphysis

Slipped upper femoral epiphysis (SUFE) (also known as slipped capital femoral epiphysis, SCFE) is a disease in which the epiphysis becomes posteriorly displaced on the femoral neck.

- The prevalence is 1–10 per 100 000, and is higher in black populations.
- It is twice as common in boys as in girls, the at-risk age group being 10–17 years for boys, and 8–15 years for girls. Most affected children are obese, and in 40% of cases there is bilateral hip involvement.
- The aetiology is unknown, but is possibly endocrine related.
- The onset may be abrupt or gradual. Sudden slips present with severe pain and inability to walk; chronic slips present with pain often referred to the knees, a slight limp, and limited internal rotation of the hip.
- Plain antero-posterior and lateral X-rays are the most important diagnostic investigations. Severity can be classified according to the degree of epiphyseal displacement. Greater than 30% displacement can result in premature osteoarthrosis.

Treatment

- The goal of treatment for SUFE is to stabilise the slippage and to promote premature fusion of the epiphysis if possible.
- Ideal treatment is fixation *in situ* with a single cannulated screw. Given the posterior position of slippage, the point of entry of the screw needs to be anterior on the femoral neck. This procedure needs to be done under fluoroscopic or X-ray control in a specialist hospital.
- Where internal fixation or peri-operative imaging is not available, an alternative would be spica cast immobilisation. However, this is often logistically difficult, and the physis may still be open even after cast removal.
- For the most severe degrees of slippage, in the hands of a specialist surgeon, reduction and fixation of the slip or femoral neck realignment osteotomies may be indicated.
- The commonest complications of operative treatment for SUFE are chondrolysis and osteonecrosis of the femoral head due to vascular compromise.

Genu varum and genu valgum

Varying degrees of bowed knees and knock-knee are common in the paediatric population. Most of these are merely variants of the normal physiological knee-angle development appropriate to the child's age. Very few will require any form of intervention.

- Normal development: Babies are born with a varus knee angle that reduces with growth to become neutral at 18 months to 2 years of age. Thereafter the knee becomes increasingly valgus, reaching a peak at 5–7 years, after which the angle gradually declines to the 5–9 degrees of valgus seen in most adults.
- **Blount's disease** is a developmental condition that affects the proximal tibial physis and results in progressive varus deformity.
- Treatment of degrees of genu valgum and genu varum depends upon the age of the child and the severity of the condition. Bracing is of no proven benefit. Various corrective osteotomies are possible, but these should be restricted to those cases with functional handicap, and are certainly not indicated merely on cosmetic grounds.

Scoliosis

Scoliosis is deformity of the spine characterised by lateral curvature and rotation.

- The commonest cause of paediatric scoliosis in resource-limited countries is probably tuberculosis (Pott's disease). X-ray appearances can be strongly suggestive of this diagnosis, and then antituberculous chemotherapy is commenced.
- The scoliotic deformity is described as idiopathic where there is no known aetiology. Contrary to popular belief, most idiopathic scoliosis is only of cosmetic significance; only the most severe cases will have any degree of cardiorespiratory compromise.
- Scoliotic bracing is expensive, has compliance problems and is unlikely to be available in resource-limited countries. If available it may have a role in slowing the progression of curves which are between 20 and 40 degrees.
- Curves that are under 40 degrees at the time of skeletal maturity are unlikely to progress further.
- Surgical correction requires a specialised hospital and a skilled fully trained surgeon and support staff.

5.18 Skin disorders

Section 5.18

BOX 5.18.1 Minimum standards
- Anti-scabies treatment.
- Antibacterial treatment.
- Antifungal treatment.
- Topical steroids.
- Emollients.
- Antiviral treatment.

Introduction

In resource-limited countries, skin disease is dominated by bacterial infections such as impetigo and parasitic conditions such as scabies and pediculosis. It is often poorly managed, and may incur a significant economic cost to families through use of ineffective remedies. It is important to recognise whether cases reflect individual or community problems; treatment of single cases of scabies will have little impact if there is widespread infection in the community.

Scabies

Scabies is a parasitic infection caused by the mite, *Sarcoptes scabiei*, which spreads from person to person, usually by direct contact. The adult female burrows a tunnel into the stratum corneum or outer skin layer, producing eggs which hatch into larvae within 3–4 days.

'Outbreaks' in communities may follow a cyclical pattern, with peaks of incidence occurring every 4–7 years. Infection in adults usually reflects overcrowding in households and transmission through contact with infected individuals, including infants.

Clinical presentation

The main sites of infection include fingers, wrists, elbows, ankles, genitals and buttocks; the face and head may be affected in babies, but these sites are seldom involved in older children. Important clues include the following:
- itching in several members of the same household
- lesions in characteristic sites, particularly the lateral borders of the fingers
- papules, pustules and sinuous tracks or burrows (5–10 mm).

In onchocerciasis (*see* Section 6.3.C.g), itching is also common but lesions are seldom found on the fingers.

Diagnosis

Remove mites from their burrows with a sterile needle and examine them under low power of the microscope.

Complications

Secondary bacterial (streptococcal) infection is common (see below). In severely immunocompromised individuals (e.g. those with AIDS) a crusted form of scabies, without severe itching but with large numbers of mites, may occur.

Treatment

The cheapest treatment options are sulphur based. However, they are slow to take effect, and require daily applications for 7–14 days. Permethrin is the most rapidly active but also the most expensive option.

All potentially affected areas are treated, including the soles of the feet and, in babies, the scalp.

Failure of anti-scabetic agents often occurs because there is no place where individuals can apply these treatments in privacy. Treat all members of the household, including those without itching.

Clothes should be cleaned or changed after the first treatment. Resistance to gamma-benzene hexachloride occurs. Ivermectin (oral) is highly effective for crusted scabies, but is not suitable for children under 5 years (single dose of 150 micrograms/kg). No food should be taken for 2 hours before or after the dose.

Community-based treatments, although ideal, are seldom practised as they are difficult and, although individually cheap, comparatively costly to apply to large numbers.

TABLE 5.18.1 Topical treatment of scabies

Anti-scabies preparation	Treatment	Side effects
Sulphur	Given as a 5–10% application in white soft paraffin or as soap. Treat for 1–2 weeks	Local irritation
25% Benzyl benzoate emulsion	Initial application, followed by a second one 2–3 days later	Local itching, eczema
5% Permethrin cream	One application (another is often necessary)	Minimal itching
0.5% Malathion lotion	One or two applications	Itching
1% Gamma-benzene hexachloride lotion	One to four applications	Use with caution in children; seizures have been recorded
1% Crotamiton cream	1–2 weeks of treatment	Not very effective, although it can reduce itching

Impetigo

The term **pyoderma** is used to describe a range of superficial bacterial infections that include impetigo, folliculitis, abscesses (furunculosis) or secondary bacterial infection (e.g. of scabies). Impetigo is a form of pyogenic infection that involves the epidermis and is caused by Group A streptococci or *Staphylococcus aureus*. It is not possible to separate the two infections clinically.

Ecthyma occurs when impetigo penetrates deeper, to affect the dermis and cause ulceration.

Clinical presentation

Impetigo presents with oozing and yellowish crusted plaques, often on exposed sites such as the face. These plaques may be multiple, and form blisters, in which case *Staphylococcus aureus* is the usual cause. This may be transmitted to other parts of the body and to other children. Secondary infection of scabies may occur; papules become pustular and there may be surrounding impetiginised crusts on scabetic burrows.

Boils (furuncles) are also common, and are always caused by *Staphylococcus aureus*. Lesions are large tender fluctuant masses with surrounding inflammation. They may occur in other members of the same household.

Complications

A serious complication of streptococcal impetigo or pyoderma is glomerulonephritis, which follows infection by nephritogenic strains. In tropical environments, post-streptococcal glomerulonephritis more often follows skin infection rather than throat infection.

Management

Impetigo is transmissible, and treatment should include other contacts with lesions. Cover both *Staphylococcus aureus* and streptococci, unless laboratory facilities for culture are available. A topical agent may be used, but for widespread lesions oral treatment is usual (*see* Table 5.18.2). The choice of medication is influenced by cost, extent of disease and type of lesions.

Most *Staphylococcus aureus* strains, even in remote communities, are resistant to both penicillin and tetracycline. Most topical azole antifungal agents (e.g. clotrimazole, miconazole), apart from ketoconazole, have activity against Gram-positive bacteria. Boils are best managed by incision and drainage.

TABLE 5.18.2 Treatment of impetigo

Agent	Route	Use	Cost
Cloxacillin, flucloxacillin	Oral: 12.5–25 mg/kg four times a day	For widespread and severe impetigo. Rapid effect, with clearance in 3–5 days	Expensive
Mupirocin	Topical	For localised infections. Rapid effect, with clearance in 3–7 days	Moderate
Fucidin	Topical	As for mupirocin	Moderate
Clioquinol	Topical	Slow to take effect (7–14 days). May stain skin; irritant	Cheap
Potassium permanganate (alternatives are chlorhexidine and povidone iodine)	Topical	Simple to use, stains skin. Slow to take effect (7–14 days)	Cheap

Tropical ulcer (tropical phagedenic ulcer)

Tropical ulcer mainly occurs in children and teenagers, but is seldom seen in developed countries. It is patchily distributed in endemic foci throughout Africa, India and the West Pacific. It is associated with humid regions or areas subject to local flooding.

Tropical ulcer is considered to result from synergistic bacterial infection, of which one anaerobic organism is usually *Fusobacterium ulcerans*. Other bacteria present in lesions include spiral bacteria and Gram-negative bacteria. *F. ulcerans* has also been isolated from mud and stagnant water in the vicinity of cases.

The initial lesion is a soft papule with surrounding hyper-pigmentation overlying an area of skin necrosis. This develops over at least 1 week, and when the overlying skin sloughs a regular and deep ulcer, 3–10 cm in diameter, is revealed.

Complications

With proper care and regular irrigation or cleansing of lesions the area will heal. About 5–10% of lesions may progress to chronic ulceration, and in some cases secondary squamous carcinoma or more serious infection (e.g. underlying osteomyelitis) may develop.

Management

The objective of treatment is to allow rapid healing without secondary infection.

Regimen

- Dilute antiseptic (e.g. potassium permanganate solution), or 0.9% saline for cleansing the ulcer and surrounding skin.
- Daily dressings.
- A single IM dose of benzyl penicillin (50 mg/kg) or oral metronidazole (7.5 mg/kg every 8 hours for 5 days). The former is particularly important in areas where yaws is also endemic, as it will cover both conditions.
- If healing is delayed, local pinch grafting may be necessary.

Cutaneous leishmaniasis (*see* Section 6.3.A.c).

Superficial fungal infections

Common childhood fungal infections are scalp ringworm or tinea capitis and oropharyngeal candidiasis.

Tinea infections are caused by dermatophyte fungi, which are adapted to survive on the outer layer of the skin, the stratum corneum, or structures such as hair or nails derived from it. Dermatophyte infections are caused by one of three genera of fungi, *Trichophyton*, *Microsporum* and *Epidermophyton*, which are acquired by spread from soil, animal or human sources (geophilic, zoophilic or anthropophilic infections, respectively). By convention they are referred to by the term tinea followed by the appropriate Latin word for the site affected – for example, tinea pedis (feet), tinea corporis (body) or tinea capitis (scalp).

Tinea capitis is often endemic in rural or urban areas of resource-limited countries and inner-city areas of industrialised countries. Prevalence rates may reach over 20% in some communities.

The main signs of infection are as follows:

- scaling
- hair loss: this may be diffuse or in localised patches; scalp hairs in affected areas may break at scalp level or a few millimetres above the skin
- itching: this is variable.

The key to the diagnosis is the presence of broken hairs. Confirmation is by culture of scrapings taken from the scalp surface with a sterilised scalpel or sterile scalp brushes. The presence of infection can also be verified by microscopy of hair samples.

Complications

- Kerion is a severe pustular reaction on the scalp, which accompanies a strong immune response to ringworm infection.
- Favus is a widespread crusting form.
- Secondary infection with bacteria may occur, usually where there are crusts overlying the surface of inflamed lesions.

Management

Culture of fungus can distinguish whether infection is from a human or animal source, i.e. zoophilic species (*Microsporum canis*, from cats and dogs; *Trichophyton verrucosum*, from cattle) or anthropophilic species (*Trichophyton violaceum*, *T. tonsurans*, *T. soudanense* or *Microsporum audouinii*).

The presence of infections in close contacts (e.g. schoolmates or family) may signal child-to-child spread and alert schools to other infected children. In resource-limited countries, mass treatments have a low priority because of health resources and because cases usually self-heal.

Children with severe symptoms (e.g. kerions, favus or widespread hair loss) should be treated.

- Whitfield's ointment or imidazole antifungal agents (e.g. clotrimazole) are generally ineffective in scalp ringworm.
- The treatment of choice is griseofulvin, which is available in oral tablet or solution form, 10 mg/kg once daily (after food) and up to 20 mg/kg in refractory infections. Single-dose treatments with a 1-gram immediate dose, sometimes repeated after 1 month, have been successful for mass treatment of infected classes in school.
- Terbinafine child 10–20 kg 62.5 mg; child 20–40 kg 125 mg; child > 40 kg 250 mg all once daily for 4 weeks in tinea capitis is an alternative.
- If possible, a topical treatment such as an imidazole cream (clotrimazole) two or three times daily, ketoconazole shampoo or selenium sulphide shampoo should be given to prevent spread to others. Occasionally, kerions may require topical or oral steroids, but these are not part of their initial treatment.

Eczema (atopic dermatitis)

Eczema is a specific inflammatory disease involving the epidermis and dermis. In childhood the commonest form of eczema is atopic dermatitis. The latter is uncommon in rural areas of resource-limited countries, and appears to be associated with urban environments and increased affluence.

Clinical presentation

Severe itching and a scaling rash affect the skin flexures (e.g. the elbows, behind the knees, the neck). Scratching may be very severe, and sufficient to disturb sleep.

Management principles

- **Moisturise the skin with emollients.** Thicker more greasy preparations such as white soft paraffin or a 50:50 mixture of white soft paraffin and liquid paraffin are preferred to creams, as they provide longer-lasting effects.
- **Treat inflammatory lesions with topical corticosteroids** (once or twice daily). Weaker-strength preparations (1% hydrocortisone) are best, although it may be necessary to use medium to strong topical steroids in some cases (never use the latter on the face). Use corticosteroids only intermittently, relying on emollients for long-term management.
- **Treat complications.** These are secondary bacterial infections, usually *Staphylococcus aureus* and acute herpes simplex (eczema herpeticum): apply aciclovir cream five times a day for 5–10 days (until healed) or aciclovir orally if severe, 20 mg/kg four times a day for 5–7 days, and contact dermatitis which may include allergy to topical medicaments such as lanolin and corticosteroids. An oral antibiotic (e.g. cloxacillin or flucloxacillin 12.5–25 mg/kg four times a day) in acute flare-up of eczema may produce a good response.

Atopic eczema ranges from a mild skin rash to a severe condition that can dominate family life and may cause major family stress. Food allergy is a rare cause, and skin testing for precipitating factors is usually not helpful. In industrialised countries there are patient organisations (e.g. the National Eczema Society in the UK) which provide support and advice to patients and their families.

Hypopigmentation and hyperpigmentation disorders

These are often secondary to other inflammatory processes which should be treated. There are no effective, cheap or easily administered treatments for the pigmentary changes themselves. The common fungal disease, pityriasis versicolor, may present with hypopigmented patches on the trunk which coalesce; however, these are scaly. Treatment with topical antifungal azole creams (e.g. clotrimazole, miconazole) is effective.

Further reading

Regular updates on the management of skin disease in resource-limited environments are available in the *Community Dermatology Journal*, which can be accessed without charge on www.ifd.org

WHO (1997) *Drugs used in skin diseases.* http://apps.who.int/medicinedocs/en/d/Jh2918e

5.19 Surgical disorders

BOX 5.19.1 Minimum standards
- ■ Surgeon experienced in working with children's disorders.
- ■ Anaesthetist experienced in children's anaesthesia.
- ■ Equipped theatre with appropriately sized instruments where relevant.
- ■ Pain relief.
- ■ Fluid management.
- ■ Ultrasound.
- ■ Radiography.
- ■ Blood transfusion
- ■ Cytology.
- ■ Chest drain insertion.

Introduction

Children's surgery is a specialist subject. There are some emergency operations that may have to be performed by a competent general surgeon, such as appendectomy and surgery for a strangulated inguinal hernia, but most of the operations that are needed on very young children and infants require specialist knowledge and experience. Children's surgery is therefore likely to be a tertiary-level referral service.

Indirect inguinal hernia

This is the protrusion of the abdominal viscus into a peritoneal sac (the processus vaginalis) in the inguinal canal. The contents of the sac are usually intestines, but may be omentum, Meckel's diverticulum, or ovary and Fallopian tube in females.
- Around 50% of cases are seen in the first year of life, mostly before 6 months of age.
- Patent processus vaginalis (not a hernia) is present in 80% of boys at birth, in 40% at 2 years, and in 20% of adult men.
- A bulge in the groin, which sometimes extends to the scrotum, and which appears when the child cries or strains but disappears when he relaxes, is certainly a hernia. Hernias are seldom symptomatic except when they are very large or are incarcerated or strangulated. On physical examination, cough or crying impulse is the most important sign. A soft bulge that is reducible on digital pressure is also a diagnostic feature. Hernia in neonates may be transilluminant, so it is not a very reliable test to differentiate with hydrocoele.

Needle aspiration is contraindicated in any inguinal swelling because of the risk of perforating the intestines.

Differential diagnosis
This should include the following:
- **Lymphadenopathy:** firm, immobile, non-reducible, and no cough impulse.

- **Hydrocoele:** can reach the upper pole of the swelling, transilluminant, no cough impulse is present.
- **Hydrocoele of the cord:** separate from testes, non-reducible, no cough impulse, upper limit is reachable, moves on pulling on the same-sided testis.
- **Undescended testis:** scrotum empty and hypoplastic, cough impulse, may be reducible.
- **Femoral and direct inguinal hernias:** rare, but should be kept in mind.

Treatment
All inguinal hernias should be promptly repaired unless there is another medical condition that makes the anaesthetic risks prohibitive. Premature infants with hernia should not be discharged without a repair of the hernia, as the risk of incarceration is high. An anaesthetist with paediatric anaesthesia experience is required, as anaesthesia-related risks are higher in children. Post-operative apnoea may occur in premature babies and at times may require ventilatory support. If these facilities are not available, the baby should be referred to higher centres or the surgery deferred until the risks associated with anaesthesia are low.

There are reasons for avoiding delay, especially in infants.
- Spontaneous disappearance of inguinal hernia does not occur.
- The risk of incarceration is greater in infants.
- Operation is technically more difficult and the risk of injury to the vas and testicular vessels is greater in long-standing and incarcerated hernia.
- Increasing age does not affect the risk of anaesthesia so long as an experienced anaesthetist is available.

A herniotomy is performed through an incision in the lowermost transverse inguinal skin crease. The sac is identified and transfixed. Herniorrhaphy is not required, as the cause is a patent processus vaginalis. Bilateral exploration and repair are indicated in patients with bilateral hernias, but routine contralateral prophylactic exploration is no longer recommended.

Incarcerated hernia

This occurs when the intestine becomes stuck at the internal inguinal ring. If it is prolonged, the blood supply may also become compromised, causing strangulation. There is a sudden increase in the size of the hernia with severe pain and symptoms of bowel obstruction (vomiting and abdominal distension). On examination a hard tender fixed mass in the groin is palpable, with increased bowel sounds on auscultation. It may be confused with the torsion of testis, acute inguinal lymphadenitis and tense infected hydrocoele.

Treatment
This includes the following:

- adequate sedation and administration of analgesics to calm the baby
- cold fomentation (to reduce the oedema)
- the application of gentle pressure to reduce the hernial contents (however, signs of peritonitis are a contraindication).

After reduction of the hernia, the child should be admitted to the hospital and checked hourly to ensure that there is no damage to the intestine or testis, and to reduce a recurrent incarceration promptly if it occurs.

Herniotomy is performed after 48 hours to allow tissue oedema to subside.

Hydrocoele

This is accumulation of fluid in the scrotum; there is communication via a patent processus vaginalis (PPV) with the peritoneal cavity. Rarely hydrocoele is secondary to epididymo-orchitis, tumour and torsion of the testis.

- It is usually asymptomatic.
- The testis is not palpable separately, and the upper pole of the swelling is reachable, reduces on lying down and is transilluminant (hernia in a neonate may also be transilluminant).
- No cough impulse is present.

Differential diagnosis

Hydrocoele should be differentiated from **inguinal hernia**, and underlying pathology such as **tumours** and **torsion of testis** should not be missed. In older children, **spermatocoele** and **varicocoele** are non-transilluminant, have a worm-like feeling on palpation, and are separate from the testes.

Surgical treatment

This is rarely indicated. More than 90% of hydrocoeles will spontaneously disappear. **Surgery is indicated if it has not disappeared by the age of 2 years**, and for hydrocoeles that are larger and symptomatic. Herniotomy or PPV ligation, as performed for inguinal hernia, is the procedure of choice.

Undescended testis (cryptoorchidism)

An undescended testis is one that cannot be made to reach the bottom of the scrotum. It is the second most common problem in paediatric surgery after indirect inguinal hernia, and should be distinguished from the more common **retractile testis**.

The incidence of undescended testis is 2.7–3% at birth in full-term infants, decreasing to 1.5% after 1 year of age, and thereafter the incidence remains the same. It is more common in premature infants, approaching 100% at a gestational age of 32 weeks or less.

- An **ectopic testis** is one that has strayed from the inguinal canal, usually to the thigh, perineum, base of the penis, or femoral or abdominal region.
- An **ascending testis** is one that is in the scrotum at birth, but the spermatic cord fails to elongate at the same rate as body growth, so the testis becomes progressively higher in the inguinal canal during childhood.

An **impalpable testis** is quite uncommon (less than 10%),

and **agenesis** is rare (20% of all impalpable testes). A fully descended but grossly hypoplastic testis may be impalpable and only identified by exploration. Normal descent of testes occurs around the seventh month of fetal life when the gubernaculum swells and shortens, drawing the testis through the inguinal canal into the scrotum. Failure of descent may occur because of hormonal failure (inadequate gonadotrophins and testosterone), a dysgenetic testis, or an anatomical abnormality such as an abnormal or malplaced gubernaculum, obstruction of the inguinal canal or scrotum, or a short vas or vessels.

Sequelae of non-descent

- The higher temperature of the extrascrotal testis causes testicular dysplasia with interstitial fibrosis and poor development of seminiferous tubules, thus hampering spermatogenesis. Testosterone production is unaffected by position. Thus a male with bilateral undescended testes will develop secondary sexual characteristics, but will be sterile.
- Due to dysplasia, there is an increased risk of malignancy (10- to 20-fold higher). The risk of malignant degeneration is not altered greatly by orchidopexy, but a position where it is palpable helps early diagnosis and gives a better prognosis. Malignancy usually develops in the second or third decade of life.
- A testis in the inguinal region is more prone to direct trauma and torsion.

Examination

An unhurried examination with warm hands and environment greatly helps in picking up a testis in an abnormal position. A hypoplastic scrotum may suggest that it has never housed a testis. In older children, squatting may coax the testis into the normal position, thus differentiating a retractile testis. Always look for an associated hernia. The position and size of the testis should be noted. If it is impalpable, ectopic locations of the testis should be examined. For a testis that cannot be felt at all, an ultrasound examination may be helpful. Bilateral non-palpable testes may require laparoscopic examination and hormonal profiles in a higher centre.

Treatment

The histological changes in the testes occur as early as 6 months of postnatal life, and therefore a child who has an undescended testis should be operated at the earliest time possible to prevent such changes.

The best time for orchidopexy is about 1 year of age, and preferably before the child's second birthday.

- The hernial sac should be dissected from the cord structures and a high ligation done.
- The testis is placed in an extra-dartos pouch in the scrotum after an adequate dissection and mobilisation of the vas and vessels. Retroperitoneal dissection and careful snipping off of lateral peritoneal bands will give an adequate length to the cord.
- In about 50% of cases of impalpable testis a useful testis can be brought down, and in the remaining 50% there is either no testis present (testicular agenesis or intrauterine torsion-vanishing testis), or there is a useless and potentially neoplastic testis, which is removed.
- For an abdominal testis, laparoscopy is useful for identifying and confirming the position of the testis and

simultaneously permitting the ligation of spermatic vessels (Fowler–Stephen's stage I operation). Later the testis can be brought into the scrotum after dividing the artery, the testicular blood supply being supported by the artery to the vas.

- For psychological reasons, if orchidectomy has been undertaken, prosthetic replacement should be performed later on.
- In bilateral undescended testes, especially with hypospadias, an intersex disorder should be suspected and the child should be further investigated.

Prognosis
There is a 2% recurrence rate, 2–5% incidence of atrophy, 70–80% fertility after unilateral orchidopexy, and 40% fertility after bilateral orchidopexy.

Phimosis
Phimosis is defined as excessive tightness of the foreskin, preventing retraction behind the glans. It occurs in 1–2% of males. The foreskin normally cannot be retracted in infants, and non-retractability of the foreskin is not pathological until the age of 3 years. Forced retraction may cause phimosis by producing tears in the foreskin, which heals with scarring and contraction. If there is pooling of urine and repeated attacks of balanoposthitis, simple dilatation of the foreskin can be done and the mother given advice about local hygiene.

After the age of 3 years, the foreskin becomes naturally retractile. Explain to the mother that daily retraction and cleansing of the glans will prevent recurrence of the phimosis. At the same time it is of utmost importance to emphasise the importance of reducing the prepuce over the glans to avoid paraphimosis, which is an inability to bring the foreskin into its natural position because it is trapped in the sulcus at the base of the glans.

Circumcision for phimosis is only indicated where the prepucial skin is scarred and fibrotic due to balanitis xerotica obliterans.

Hypospadias
This is a condition where the urethra opens on the ventral aspect of the penis at a point proximal to the normal site. When it opens on the dorsal aspect (termed 'epispadias') there is usually associated exstrophy of the bladder.

- Hypospadias is one of the commonest congenital anomalies of the male genitals, occurring in 1 in 300 male births. There are various degrees of severity depending on how far back the urethral meatus lies. It may be associated with undescended testes, and in severe cases there is a possibility of an intersex problem.
- Ventral curvature of the shaft of the penis is called a 'chordee'. It is due to fibrosis of the urethral plate, shortened skin, or fibrosis of the corpora cavernosa. The prepuce is deficient ventrally, and an unsightly dorsal hood of redundant skin is present.
- Congenital short urethra is a deformity where there is ventral curvature of the shaft of the penis without hypospadias.

The disabilities of hypospadias are cosmesis of the penis, a stream that is deflected downwards or splashes, and in severe hypospadias, boys have to void in a sitting position (like females). Uncorrected chordee interferes with intercourse, and there is infertility in severe hypospadias (penoscrotal and perineal), as semen is not directed into the vagina.

Treatment
Hypospadias should be corrected before school age so that the child does not feel ostracised in society. In severe cases of hypospadias, intersex disorders and associated urological abnormalities such as pelvic-ureteric junction obstruction or renal agenesis should be ruled out.

Principles of surgery
These are as follows:

- correction of chordee to straighten the penis (orthoplasty)
- movement of the urinary meatus to its normal position on the tip of the penis (urethroplasty)
- correction of the deformity of the glans to give it a conical shape (glansplasty).

No infant with hypospadias should be circumcised, as the prepuce is essential for the repair. Repair can be undertaken as a one-time or staged procedure. It depends on the degree of chordee and the severity of the hypospadias.

Bladder stones
In resource-limited countries, bladder stones are quite common due to the prevalence of malnutrition. The stones are composed of ammonium acid urate and oxalate, and are seen in lower socio-economic groups. Such stones are usually related to a high dietary intake of rice or wheat and low intake of milk and animal protein (see Section 5.10.B).

Children present with increased frequency of urine and strangury or haematuria (the child usually holds the penis and rubs it with the finger and cries during micturition). Children may present with an episode of retention of urine if the bladder stone becomes impacted at the bladder neck or in the urethra.

During rectal examination, a stone may be palpable on bimanual palpation. A plain abdominal X-ray may reveal calcified stones. Abdominal ultrasonography will detect non-calcified stones.

Treatment
Open stone surgery is the modality of choice. Endoscopic removal can be performed in some children if the necessary equipment and expertise are available.

If there is no infection, two-layered closure of the bladder is sufficient, requiring no catheter or suprapubic drainage. Once the stones have been removed, recurrence is rare.

Cervical swellings
The neck is one of the commonest sites of cystic and solid swellings during childhood. Lesions are either developmental anomalies arising from the remnants of branchial arches, thyroglossal tract, jugular lymphatics or the skin, or acquired as in diseases of the salivary gland, lymph nodes or thyroid gland.

- Lymphangiomas (cystic hygroma).
- Branchial cysts/fistulae.
- Thyroglossal cyst.

- Ectopic thyroid/thyroid swellings.
- Epidermal cyst.
- Swelling of salivary glands.
- Haemangiomas.
- Lymph-node swellings.

Lymphadenopathy

Enlargement of the lymph nodes may result from acute or chronic infection and from primary or secondary neoplasia.

- Infection is the commonest cause of lymph node enlargement in childhood, secondary to scalp and skin infections, including lice.
- Tuberculosis is the most important pathogen in resource-limited countries.
- In many cases the lymph nodes are reacting to an upper respiratory tract infection or an ear infection. This is known as **non-specific reactive hyperplasia**, and is much more common. Thus not every enlarged lymph node needs a surgical biopsy.
- Primary tumours of the lymph nodes include lymphoma and leukaemia.

Enlargement of a lymph node by more than 1 cm is significant, and a persistent node more than 3 cm in diameter requires fine-needle aspiration cytology or surgical biopsy.

A careful history with regard to repeated upper respiratory tract infections, boils on the scalp or drainage area, and ear discharge, should be taken. A positive family history of tuberculosis is an important feature of tubercular lymphadenitis. A history of the pattern of fever, loss of weight and appetite, and the presence of night sweats are important features when making a differential diagnosis.

On careful physical examination, all sites of lymph nodes (cervical, axillary, inguinal and abdominal) should be examined. The size, number, consistency, tenderness, and presence or absence of fluctuations should be noted. On abdominal examination, liver, spleen and mesenteric lymph nodes should be palpated. The drainage area of the lymph nodes should be examined for boils, furuncles, injury or neoplastic swelling. The tonsils should be inspected for enlargement and suppuration.

- In **acute lymphadenitis**, the affected nodes are enlarged, painful and tender, restricting movement of local areas of the body. Fever and leukocytosis are common. Untreated infections may resolve spontaneously, progress to suppuration and abscess formation, or become chronic.
- In **tubercular lymphadenitis**, lymph nodes are enlarged and painless, and become matted together and fixed to adjacent structures. Caseation leads to the formation of 'cold' abscesses, which lack the local and systemic signs of acute inflammation (fever, tenderness and erythema). When a cold abscess ruptures through the deep fascia (a 'collar-stud abscess') the skin becomes red and thin, takes on a blue tinge and then gives way to establish an indolent tubercular sinus. On aspiration, straw-coloured fluid is present, in contrast to the thick pus that is usually present in an acute abscess. Confirmation depends on culture of the organisms or visualisation of acid-fast bacilli on microscopy.
- In **primary neoplasia (e.g. leukaemia)** the nodes are painless, rubbery in consistency and discrete. Liver and spleen enlargement may or may not be present.

Systemic features of low-grade fever, night sweats, or loss of weight and appetite point towards the diagnosis.

- **Secondary enlargement of the lymph nodes** due to neoplasia is rare in childhood.
- **Primary cancers** are soft-tissue sarcomas and very rare. The nodes are large, firm to hard in consistency, and fixed to underlying structures.

Investigations

- Full blood count.
- The erythrocyte sedimentation rate is usually raised in chronic infection and neoplasms. Leukocytosis is seen in acute lymphadenitis and abscess formation. Leukaemia will usually be diagnosed by the appearance of leukaemic cells in peripheral blood.
- Mantoux test. To diagnose tuberculosis, start with 1 in 10 000 and then 1 in 1000. A strongly positive test is a pointer towards the diagnosis; if the test is negative, it does not rule out the disease (especially in the presence of HIV infection).
- X-ray of the chest.
- To identify there is the pulmonary lesion of primary complex or the hilar lymphadenopathy seen in cases of tuberculosis. Mediastinal widening is seen in patients with lymphomas.
- Fine-needle aspiration cytology (FNAC) is helpful if there are persistent lymph nodes that do not decrease in size after a 1-week course of antibiotics and another week of observation. Lymphomas cannot be definitely diagnosed on FNAC, and a surgical biopsy is mandatory.

Treatment
Acute lymphadenitis

- Antibiotics are prescribed. Penicillin is usually appropriate, as most infections occur outside the hospital setting. Oral or IV preparations may be used. If improvement has not occurred within 48 hours, a broad-spectrum antibiotic such as an oral or IV cephalosporin may be started.
- Anti-inflammatory medication (to relieve the pain and reduce the swelling).
- Hot fomentation (to relieve the pain and reduce the swelling).

Fluctuation, or other local signs of abscess formation, indicate the need for **incision and drainage of pus**, which is best performed under general anaesthesia. All of the loculi are broken and necrotic material is curetted out. **Always visualise and remember the important structures nearby.** A sample should be sent for microscopy (including Ziehl–Neelsen staining), culture and sensitivity, and appropriate antibiotics prescribed. The precipitating cause of acute lymphadenitis should also be treated.

Tubercular lymphadenitis

Antitubercular treatment leads to resolution (a full course of 9 months should be undertaken, with four drugs for 2 months and two drugs for the next 7 months; see Section 6.1.N).

Cold abscesses require drainage, and repeated aspirations may be preferable to avoid sinus formation, pending diagnosis and initiation of treatment.

Lymphomas and leukaemias

After diagnosis, further investigations will be required to stage the disease and its treatment (*see* Section 5.14).

Cystic hygroma

This is a hamartoma of the jugular lymph sac which presents in infancy and is more common in boys than in girls. It produces a major neck swelling and is diagnosed by inspection. The swelling is usually found as a unilateral, fluctuant, transilluminant swelling centred on the carotid triangle. The cysts are of varying sizes and contain clear fluid. A haemangiomatous element may be present in the swelling, giving it a reddish tinge instead of a light blue colour. Cysts may enlarge suddenly due to viral or bacterial infection or haemorrhage. If the cyst compresses airways and vessels, it may cause stridor, respiratory distress and superior vena caval syndrome. Initially these lesions can be treated by aspiration and intralesional injection of bleomycin (a less expensive anti-cancer drug), at a dose of 300–600 micrograms/kg; these procedures can be repeated every 2–6 weeks, producing excellent results in the majority of cases. Surgical excision is difficult, and removal should be attempted without sacrificing important structures, in some cases in conjunction with sclerotherapy.

Branchial cysts, sinuses and fistulae

Sinuses and fistulae most commonly arise from the second branchial cleft, and occasionally from the first or third one. They present as a small discharging sinus on the skin overlying the lower third of the sternomastoid muscle. Parents often notice a drop of clear fluid coming from a very small opening. Sinuses and fistulae usually present in early childhood, and may sometimes be complicated by infection and abscess formation. Treatment consists of surgical excision of the whole tract up to the pyriform fossa to prevent recurrence. Methylene blue is injected or a nylon thread guided in the fistula to delineate it during surgical dissection for appropriate excision.

Thyroglossal cyst

The descent of the thyroid gland from the floor of the fetal mouth leaves a tract from the foramen caecum of the tongue to the thyroid isthmus. A cyst lined by respiratory epithelium may arise anywhere along the tract, but is usually subhyoid (75%). The swelling is in the midline and moves with swallowing and also with protrusion of the tongue. An infected cyst may be mistaken for acute bacterial lymphadenitis, or an ectopic thyroid may cause a similar swelling.

The thyroglossal cyst and the entire tract along with the central portion of hyoid bone should be excised to minimise the risk of recurrence (Sistrunk's operation).

Epidermoid cyst

Inclusion dermoid cysts arise from ectodermal cells that become detached during fetal growth. They are often in the midline or along lines of embryonic fusion. They contain sebaceous cheesy material surrounded by squamous epithelium. They enlarge slowly and should be removed completely; the capsule should not be breached to prevent recurrence.

Haemangiomas

These are the most common tumours of infancy and the most common congenital anomalies. They are present in around 1–3% of all newborn infants. This figure increases to 10% by 1 year of age. Haemangiomas can be capillary or cavernous, although both types may be present.

The natural history of capillary haemangiomas is as follows:

- They initially present shortly after birth as a pale pink or bright red spot or patch on the skin.
- There is subsequently rapid growth in infancy for 3–6 months, followed by a static phase.
- At 18–24 months the lesion starts to involute. Around 50% will involute by 5 years and 90% by 7 years. Rarely the lesion persists and requires excision.

A cavernous haemangioma has a deeper component in subcutaneous tissues or muscles, and is less likely to regress completely.

Management

Management of these lesions consists of an accurate diagnosis and careful observation. Parents need reassurance when the lesion is growing rapidly. Problems of ulceration, bleeding and (rarely) infection occur secondary to minor trauma. These are best treated non-operatively.

- Surgical excision is indicated when there is functional or gross cosmetic disability (e.g. a haemangioma on the eyelid), or a vital organ is threatened.
- Steroids may be used to induce involution in large haemangiomas (prednisolone 1–2 mg/kg/day for 2–4 weeks; the dose is tapered off before stopping the therapy). These can be repeated in cycles, with a gap of 4–6 weeks. Intra-lesional steroids can be used to induce regression in the size of haemangiomas in and around the eye.

Obstructive jaundice in infancy

This is most commonly caused by extrahepatic biliary atresia, choledochal cyst or inspissated bile syndrome.

- The most difficult differential diagnosis is neonatal hepatitis.
- If jaundice in the newborn persists, the stools are never yellow or green, and the urine is brown, a conjugated bilirubin level should be measured and urobilinogen and bilirubin looked for in the urine.
- Ultrasound may help in diagnosis. Strongly suspected cases need referral for radioactive scan and further management.

Empyema thoracis (*see* Section 5.3.B)

This is defined as an accumulation of pus in the pleural space. In most children this results from an infected pleural effusion associated with ongoing uncontrolled pulmonary sepsis or pneumonia. An infection of the pleural space is unlikely when there is a healthy underlying lung that is completely expanded. Empyemas and effusions may be diffuse and involve the entire pleural space, or they may be intralobar, diaphragmatic or paramediastinal.

Before the advent of antibiotic therapy, *Pneumococcus* and *Streptococcus* species were the organisms most frequently associated with empyema. Currently

Staphylococcus aureus is the most common organism. In resource-limited countries, *Mycobacterium tuberculosis* is an important cause.

Other reasons for empyema include extension of lung abscess, trauma and extension of subphrenic abscess.

An empyema usually presents with pleuritic chest pain and a heavy sensation on the involved side. The child is febrile, tachypnoeic, tachycardic and may have a cough that is productive (purulent sputum).

Examination

On examination there is reduced respiratory excursion, pain and dullness on percussion. A friction rub or distant to absent breath sounds may be heard on auscultation of the involved side.

- Chest X-rays in the antero-posterior and lateral views are necessary for the accurate localisation of the empyema. The underlying lung may show consolidation or evidence of infection by tubercular organisms. There may be evidence of a mediastinal shift to the opposite side. The presence of pneumatocoeles indicates staphylococcal infection.
- An ultrasound scan may help to distinguish fluid from consolidation in a patient with complete opacification. It is also helpful for localising a loculated empyema that may be drained. It is essential for evaluating the condition of the underlying lung in order to decide whether to proceed with decortication or pneumonectomy.

Management

Treatment depends on the cause, whether the condition is acute or chronic, the state of the underlying lung, the presence of a bronchopleural fistula, the ability to obliterate the space, and the patient's clinical condition and nutritional status.

- Fluid from the effusion should be aspirated (by thoracocentesis) under ultrasound control after giving local anaesthesia (*see* Section 5.3.B).
- If the fluid is serosanguinous, thoracocentesis and appropriate antibiotics (benzylpenicillin and flucloxacillin) given by the IV route until the temperature settles (change the antibiotics according to sensitivity), and then orally, for a total period of 6 weeks, can be a definitive treatment.
- If the fluid is thick and purulent, a tube thoracostomy is indicated. An intercostal tube should be placed in a dependent position to encourage the pleural space to drain completely. Simultaneously, physiotherapy should be instituted to expand the lung and obliterate the space (*see* Section 8.3 for placement of chest drains).
- If loculated and undrained pockets are present and the lung is not expanding on tube thoracostomy, an open surgical procedure (decortication) will be required, but adequate time should be given to non-operative treatment. If the underlying lung is badly damaged, and will not expand on vigorous physiotherapy, pneumonectomy is indicated.
- In tubercular empyema, a 6- to 8-week course of antitubercular treatment (*see* Section 6.1.N) is essential for optimum results. Surgical therapy should be withheld, except for emergency drainage, until the tubercular disease in the lung has regressed or stabilised, as shown on the serial chest X-rays.

Urinary tract infection (UTI) due to surgical causes

Recurrent UTI requires investigation to exclude the following structural and functional abnormalities:

- vesico-ureteric reflux (*see* Section 5.6.B)
- posterior urethral valves
- neurogenic bladder (*see* Section 4.2.D)
- urethral strictures
- bladder stones (see above)
- diverticulum of the bladder and urethra
- voiding dysfunction.

Umbilical pathology
Umbilical hernia

- This is a defect in the umbilical ring, which generally closes at birth, leading to protrusion of a loop of bowel or omentum through it. Some degree of herniation is seen in 20% of newborn babies, and still more in premature babies or when there is any increase in intra-abdominal pressure (e.g. due to ascites or VP shunt).
- Swelling appears on crying and straining, and decreases when the child is calm.
- It can be reduced with an audible gurgle.

Most umbilical hernias close spontaneously in the first 12 months of life, but they may take up to 3 years. Strangulation and incarceration are virtually unknown; therefore it is safe to wait. **Strapping with coin application is contraindicated**, as it leads to maceration of skin and infection, without any real advantage of inducing closure.

Surgical indications are a large hernia that has not closed by 3 years of age or an incarceration.

Umbilical discharge

- **Purulent discharge** is seen in umbilical sepsis. **Neonatal tetanus** is a serious condition in which mortality is very high (*see* Section 3.4) (cow dung application, as practised in rural India, is one cause). Portal thrombosis may occur secondary to it and manifest later as portal hypertension. Appropriate antibiotics (benzylpenicillin) should be instituted at the earliest possible stage, and local hygiene maintained.
- **Mucus/serous discharge** is seen in umbilical polyps and **granulomas**. Silver nitrate application will enable these to epithelialise. If these persist, excision will be required. Umbilical fistula may be present and require exploration and excision.
- **Urinary discharge** is seen with a patent urachus in association with a lower urinary tract obstruction. It is quite rare. Surgical treatment involves excision of the urachal remnant after investigation and relief of any underlying outlet obstruction.
- **Faecal discharge** is seen with a patent vitello-intestinal duct. This is a persistence of the connection between the yolk sac and the midgut, which normally disappears at about the sixth week of gestation. All remnants need to be excised, which may necessitate a laparotomy to search for any discontinuous segments of the tract.

Appendicitis

Appendicitis is the most common abdominal surgical emergency. Although diagnosis and treatment have improved, appendicitis continues to cause significant morbidity, and is still (although rarely) a cause of death. However, abdominal pain unrelated to appendicitis is also common, and in many cases a few hours of active observation are recommended before proceeding to surgery.

Appendicitis results from luminal obstruction following infection or impaction by a faecolith. Inflammation of the appendix does not inevitably lead to perforation, as spontaneous resolution may occur.

Clinical presentation

- Presentation is very variable.
- Pain is invariably present and nearly always the first symptom. Early visceral pain is non-specific in the epigastric or umbilical region, and **only later does pain become localised over the appendix**, most typically at McBurney's point. Pain with a pelvic appendix is often delayed in onset because the inflamed appendix does not contact the peritoneum until rupture occurs and infection spreads. Pain of a retrocaecal appendix may be in the flank or back.
- Anorexia, nausea and vomiting typically follow the onset of pain within a few hours.
- Diarrhoea occurs more frequently in children than in adults, and can result in misdiagnosis. It may indicate a pelvic abscess.
- The child with acute appendicitis lies in bed with minimal movement. There may be fever and tachycardia.
- The patient may be asymptomatic before perforation occurs, and symptoms may be present for longer than 48 hours without perforation. In general, however, the longer the duration of symptoms, the greater the risk of perforation.

Examination

Examination of the chest to rule out a lower respiratory tract infection is essential.

The single most important aspect of evaluation is serial examination undertaken by the same person. This decreases the number of unnecessary operations. Analgesia should not be withheld as was previously advised.

Investigation

There may be an increase in the white blood cell count, but this is unreliable.

Ultrasonography is an effective diagnostic aid, with a sensitivity of about 85% and a specificity of about 90%. Demonstration of a non-compressible appendix that is 7 mm or larger in antero-posterior diameter is the primary criterion.

Management

- The initial management involves IV fluids and adequate analgesia.
- In a patient who presents with peritonitis, adequate fluid resuscitation (see Section 5.5.B) must be performed before surgery is undertaken.
- For early non-ruptured appendicitis, peri-operative antibiotics (cefuroxime and metronidazole) should be given.
- For perforated appendicitis after appendicectomy, saline irrigation of the peritoneal cavity with the patient in the head-high position is advisable in an attempt to remove as much infected material as possible. Intravenous antibiotics should be given for at least 5 days:

— Cefuroxime (50 mg/kg 8- to 12-hourly) plus metronidazole (7.5 mg/kg 8-hourly IV over 20 minutes)
OR
— Ampicillin IV (25–50 mg/kg 8-hourly; maximum 4 grams/day) plus gentamicin (7 mg/kg once daily) plus metronidazole (7.5 mg/kg 8-hourly).

- If the initial presentation is with an appendicular mass, conservative treatment with IV antibiotics is given until the symptoms subside, with a plan for an interval appendicectomy.

Complications

Complications following appendicectomy include wound infection, abscess formation (local, subphrenic or pelvic) and paralytic ileus. A late complication may be an adhesive bowel obstruction.

Pyloric stenosis

This is a classical cause of gastric outlet obstruction in infants. It has a prevalence rate of about 1.5 to 4 in 1000 live births among white populations, but is less common in Africans and Asians. It is more common in males than in females, with a ratio of between 2:1 and 5:1. There appears to be an increased risk to firstborn infants with a positive family history.

Cause

No definite cause has been established. Pathologically there is marked muscle hypertrophy, primarily involving the circular layer, which produces partial or complete luminal obstruction.

Presentation

Pyloric stenosis typically presents at 2–8 weeks of age, with a peak occurrence at 3–5 weeks. The **vomiting is projectile and non-bilious**. Occasionally there is coffee-ground vomiting due to gastritis or oesophagitis. The child remains hungry after vomiting, and is otherwise not ill looking or febrile. Around 2–5% of infants have jaundice associated with indirect hyperbilirubinaemia. Non-bilious projectile vomiting, visible gastric peristalsis in the left upper abdomen, and in those presenting late a hypochloraemic hypokalaemic metabolic alkalosis are the cardinal features of pyloric stenosis.

Diagnosis

A definite diagnosis can be made in 75% of infants with pyloric stenosis by careful physical examination of the upper abdomen. **An absolute prerequisite for this is a calm and cooperative child, a warm environment, good light and patience.** With the patient in the supine position, in the mother's left arm and sucking on the left breast, and the surgeon sitting on the left side of the patient, the left hand is used to feel the classically described 'olive' to the right of the rectus muscle, often palpated against the spinal column. Visible gastric peristalsis is often noticed.

Investigations

- Ultrasonography is the most commonly used imaging technique for diagnosis. A positive finding is a pyloric canal length of 16 mm or more and a pyloric muscle thickness of 4 mm or more. A diameter of more than 14 mm is also considered abnormal.

- Blood investigations in an advanced situation may show the typical hypochloraemic hypokalaemic metabolic alkalosis.

Management

- It is most important to prepare the patient appropriately and adequately for anaesthesia and surgery.
- Intravenous fluid resuscitation with 5% glucose in 0.9% saline with 20–40 mEq/litre of potassium chloride is the optimal fluid.
- Urine output and serum electrolytes should be monitored.
- The stomach should be aspirated before the operation.
- Ramstedt's pyloromyotomy performed through a right upper quadrant or supraumbilical incision is curative, and is associated with a low morbidity.
- The majority of these patients can be started on feeds about 6 hours after surgery.
- Those who present with haematemesis from gastritis may benefit from delay of feeding for an additional 6–12 hours after surgery.
- Vomiting in the early post-operative period is thought to be secondary to discordant gastric peristalsis or atony.

Intussusception

This is the telescoping of a portion of the intestine into the lumen of an immediately adjoining part. Typically it occurs in a well-nourished child aged 4–12 months. The male:female ratio is 3:2, and it is more common in Caucasians.

The pathogenesis of intussusception is unclear. It usually originates in the ileum close to the ileocaecal junction and proceeds into the ascending colon. In 2–8% of cases there is a specific lead point such as a Meckel's diverticulum, polyp or duplication cyst. Adenoviral infection resulting in lymphoid hyperplasia may act as a lead point.

Clinical presentation

- The infant is suddenly disturbed by what appears to be violent abdominal pain. The pain is colicky, intermittent and severe. With spasms the infant draws up the knees to the abdomen, screams, becomes pale and may sweat, and vomiting occurs soon afterwards. The infant may pass a normal stool, appears to recover immediately, and may resume normal eating habits, until stricken by another bout of colicky abdominal pain. The vomiting is initially reflex, but with a delayed diagnosis becomes secondary to intestinal obstruction and is often bile-stained.
- Classically, the infant passes stool that resembles redcurrant jelly. Many parents describe this as the presenting symptom, and consequently it is often treated as bacillary dysentery initially.
- **The triad of pain, vomiting and blood per rectum is present in only one-third of patients.** One in 10 infants with intussusception will have diarrhoea before signs and symptoms attributable to intussusception become obvious. This is often a cause for delay in diagnosis.
- Pallor, persistent apathy and dehydration are common signs.
- Abdominal examination reveals emptiness in the right lower quadrant and a **sausage-shaped mass in the right hypochondrium**, extending along the line of the transverse colon. **The mass is not always easy to palpate, and its absence does not rule out an intussusception.**
- Fever and leukocytosis are common, and tachycardia results from episodes of colic and hypovolaemia from dehydration.

Investigations

- Abdominal X-ray may show a soft tissue mass across the central abdomen with dilated loops of bowel.
- **Ultrasonography has become the standard non-invasive diagnostic test, and is very reliable. Doughnut (target or concentric ring) and pseudo-kidney sign suggest a diagnosis of intussusception.**

Management

The most important aspect of treatment is adequate resuscitation prior to intervention. This involves establishing reliable IV access, collecting blood for baseline investigations and for cross-matching, passing a nasogastric tube for decompression, and giving IV fluids and analgesia. Some patients may require one or more boluses of 10–20 mL/kg of albumin or Ringer-lactate solution when first seen.

Broad-spectrum IV antibiotics such as a combination of cefuroxime (25–50 mg/kg 8-hourly, depending on the degree of infection) and metronidazole (7.5 mg/kg 8-hourly IV over 20 minutes) are started, and the urine output is monitored.

Management is initially non-surgical (i.e. with the use of air or barium enema). Sedation should be used for the procedure.

- **A surgeon and theatre should be ready when the radiologist attempts reduction. If perforation occurs, surgery should be performed immediately.**
- **An absolute contraindication to rectal reduction is evidence of peritonitis, indicating the presence of a gangrenous intestine.**

If hydrostatic reduction fails and if the patient is stable, a repeat reduction may be attempted. Once the intussusception reduces, the child should be observed overnight with careful monitoring of fluid and electrolytes.

If reduction fails, the child is taken for surgery, where by gentle manipulation (pushing and not pulling) the intussusception can be reduced. The appendix may be removed, recorded and the parents informed. If a pathological lead point is found, a resection anastomosis is performed. If the bowel is not viable, it is resected and a primary anastomosis is performed. Feeds are started the day after the operation and increased gradually.

Intravenous antibiotics should be given for at least 48 hours, and longer (for 7 days) if peritonitis is present.

The interval between the onset of symptoms and institution of treatment is of paramount importance, and mortality can be reduced if the condition is recognised and treated early.

Intestinal obstruction

This is the most common condition requiring emergency surgery in infants and children. Most causes result from complications of congenital anomalies or from inflammatory conditions that affect the bowel.

Causes

- **Extrinsic causes:** incarcerated hernia and vascular bands, intussusception, anomalies of rotation (volvulus and Ladd's bands, paraduodenal and paracaecal hernias), post-operative adhesions.
- **Intrinsic causes:** inspissation of bowel contents (meconium ileus, distal intestinal obstruction syndrome in patients with cystic fibrosis), roundworm obstruction.
- **Peristaltic dysfunction:** Hirschsprung's disease.
- **Inflammatory lesions:** tuberculosis, Crohn's disease.

Symptoms and signs

Patients present with cramping abdominal pain with anorexia, nausea and vomiting, which progresses to become bile-stained. Abdominal distension occurs, with the degree being directly related to the site of obstruction in the gastrointestinal tract, such that the distension is greater the more distal the obstruction.

On examination, the patient may have tachycardia and signs of dehydration. Tenderness and hyperactive bowel sounds are present on abdominal examination.

Chest and abdominal films are taken to confirm the diagnosis of obstruction and rule out the presence of free air.

Treatment

- The goal of treatment is to relieve obstruction before ischaemic bowel injury occurs.
- Intravenous access is established and blood collected for baseline investigations, including a full blood count, urea, creatinine and electrolytes, and cross-matching.
  - Intravenous fluids (Ringer-lactate or Hartmann's solution with 10% glucose) are started according to the guidelines of 4 mL/kg/hour for the first 10 kg, 2 mL/kg/hour for the next 10 kg, and 1 mL/kg/hour for the next 10 kg.
  - For example, a child weighing 22 kg would need 40 + 20 + 2 = 62 mL/hour.
- Some patients may need one or more IV boluses (10–20 mL/kg) with Ringer-lactate or Hartmann's solution or albumin at the start of resuscitation.
- A nasogastric tube is passed for decompression.
- Give broad-spectrum IV antibiotics such as:
  - cefuroxime 50 mg/kg 8-hourly or 12-hourly in the neonate, and metronidazole 7.5 mg/kg 8-hourly IV **or**
  - benzylpenicillin 50 mg/kg 6-hourly plus gentamicin 7 mg/kg once daily plus metronidazole 7.5 mg/kg 8-hourly.
- Once the patient is adequately resuscitated and fluid and electrolyte imbalances have been corrected, laparotomy is performed and the cause treated. Transfer to a facility where paediatric surgical and anaesthetic skills are available should be undertaken if the patient's condition will tolerate this. Otherwise, or in the absence of such a facility in the country, surgery should be performed.
- At all times adequate analgesia should be given (*see* Section 1.15).

Hirschsprung's disease

This is characterised by an absence of ganglion cells in the affected intestine. The incidence is about 1 in 4400–7000 live births; the male:female ratio is about 4:1, and in long segment disease it approaches 1:1. The longer the segment of aganglionosis, the higher is the familial incidence.

Associated conditions

These include Down's syndrome (4–16%), Waardenburg syndrome, multiple endocrine neoplasia 2A and Von Recklinghausen's disease. A higher incidence of enterocolitis has been noted in patients with Hirschsprung's disease and Down's syndrome.

Presentation

The usual presentation is with delay of passage of meconium beyond 48 hours after birth. (Around 95% of full-term infants pass meconium within 24 hours after birth, and the remainder pass it within 48 hours.) The child then has episodes of constipation, abdominal distension, vomiting and poor feeding, and fails to thrive. They may also present with a history of constipation with explosive diarrhoea, the latter indicating the development of enterocolitis.

Differential diagnosis

Hirschsprung's disease should be considered in the differential diagnosis of any child who has constipation dating back to the newborn period. However, childhood constipation related to dietary and habitual problems needs to be carefully ruled out in order to avoid unnecessary X-rays and biopsies.

Examination

On examination the child has a distended abdomen, and after a rectal examination there is often explosive passage of flatus and faeces.

- A plain X-ray of the abdomen may show dilated bowel loops with paucity of air in the location of the rectum. Barium enema may show the characteristic coning, although a simple colonic dilatation can occur in any chronic constipation.
- Rectal biopsy remains the gold standard for diagnosis. It should be performed at least 2 cm above the anal valves, as the normal anus has a paucity or absence of ganglion cells at the level of the internal sphincter. Although suction rectal biopsy with acetylcholinesterase staining has become the accepted standard for diagnosis in most centres, a full-thickness rectal biopsy under general anaesthesia is equally useful if such facilities are not available.

Treatment

Enterocolitis remains the major cause of morbidity, and has a mortality rate of around 6–30%. It manifests clinically as explosive diarrhoea, abdominal distension and fever. The pathophysiology is not fully understood. The diagnosis is made on clinical grounds, and treatment is conservative, consisting of IV fluids and rectal washouts to decompress the colon.

Surgery

The surgical treatment of Hirschsprung's disease has evolved from a three-stage procedure (initial colostomy with multiple seromuscular biopsies, pull-through of the ganglionic colon as the second stage, and closure of colostomy as the third stage) through a two-stage procedure (colostomy at the transition zone initially, and pull-through as a second stage) to a one-stage procedure without a colostomy. The essential prerequisite for a primary pull-through is adequate preparation with colonic washouts.

Perforative peritonitis

The causes of perforation include amoebiasis, typhoid, tuberculosis, roundworm perforation and Hirschsprung's disease (*see* Section 6).

Management starts with an adequate history and clinical examination, followed by chest and abdominal X-rays. Adequate resuscitation should be carried out as outlined in the section on intestinal obstruction. After this a laparotomy is performed and the cause treated. Treatment includes fluid resuscitation if necessary, and antibiotics (either a third-generation cephalosporin or an aminoglycoside plus metronidazole).

Further reading

Coran AG, Caldamone A, Adzick NS *et al.* (2012) *Paediatric Surgery*, 7th edn. St Louis, MO: Mosby Year-Book.

Holcomb III GW and Murphy JP (2012) *Ashcraft's Pediatric Surgery*, 5th edn. Philadelphia, PA: Saunders.

Spitz L and Coran AG (2007) *Rob & Smith's Operative Surgery. Pediatric Surgery*, 6th edn. London: Chapman & Hall.

Section 6

Infections in children

6.1 Bacterial infections

6.1.A Botulism

BOX 6.1.A.1 Minimal standards
- Consider the diagnosis.
- Ideally give specific anti-toxin.
- Wound care when appropriate including antibiotics.
- High dependency care.

Introduction

Botulism intoxication is a rare, potentially fatal (5–10%) paralytic illness caused by botulinum toxin. The disease is caused by ingestion of the anaerobic *Clostridium botulinum* bacterium, which produces toxin in the intestinal tract or secretes the toxin directly into a wound. Person-to-person transmission of botulism does not occur.

Botulism can be prevented by killing the spores by pressure cooking or autoclaving at 121°C (250°F) for 3 minutes or providing conditions that prevent the spores from growing. Food-borne botulism results from contaminated foodstuffs in which *C. botulinum* spores have been allowed to germinate in anaerobic conditions. This typically occurs in home-canned food substances which have been inadequately heated and in fermented uncooked dishes. Given that multiple people often consume food from the same source, it is common for more than a single person to be affected simultaneously. Symptoms usually appear 12–36 hours after eating, but can also appear within 6 hours to 10 days.

Wound botulism results from the contamination of a wound with the bacteria, which then secrete the toxin into the bloodstream. Wounds may not be obviously or grossly infected but are usually deep and contain avascular areas.

The toxin, which is absorbed from the bowel or wound into the blood stream, causes paralysis by blocking the release of acetylcholine at the neuromuscular junction.

Signs and symptoms

Muscle weakness starts in the muscles supplied by the cranial nerves controlling eye movements, the facial muscles and the muscles controlling chewing and swallowing. Double vision, drooping of both eyelids, loss of facial expression and swallowing problems may occur, as well as difficulty with talking. The weakness then spreads to the arms (starting in the shoulders and proceeding to the forearms) and legs (again from the thighs down to the feet) (a symmetric descending flaccid paralysis in a proximal to distal pattern).

Severe botulism leads to reduced power in the muscles of respiration. There may be hypoventilation and difficulty coughing which when severe can lead to respiratory failure, coma from hypoxaemia and carbon dioxide retention and eventually death if untreated. Infants may present with prolonged apnoeic episodes.

Botulism can also cause disruptions to the autonomic nervous system. This is experienced as a dry mouth and throat (due to decreased production of saliva), postural hypotension (decreased blood pressure on standing, with resultant light-headedness and fainting), and eventually constipation (due to decreased bowel peristalsis). Some of the toxins (B and E) also precipitate nausea and vomiting.

The classic triad described is bulbar palsy and descending paralysis, lack of fever, and full consciousness.

Differential diagnosis

Botulism differs from other flaccid paralyses in that it always manifests initially with prominent cranial paralysis and its invariable descending progression, in its symmetry, and in its absence of sensory nerve damage.

In children the differential diagnosis is as follows:
- Guillain–Barré syndrome
- tick paralysis
- poisoning
- poliomyelitis
- psychiatric illness.

In infants it is as follows:
- meningitis
- electrolyte–mineral imbalance
- Reye's syndrome
- rare congenital abnormalities.

Infant botulism

Infants, especially those under 6 months of age, are susceptible to botulism. Infant botulism results from the ingestion of the *C. botulinum* spores, and subsequent colonisation of the small intestine. The composition of the intestinal microflora (normal flora) in infancy is insufficient to competitively inhibit the growth of *C. botulinum* and levels of bile acids (which normally inhibit clostridial growth) are lower than later in life. Ingestion of honey is a recognised source of botulism in infants.
- Typical symptoms of infant botulism include diminished suckling and crying ability (difficulty or poor feeding and an altered cry).
- Neck weakness progressing to generalised floppiness with a complete descending flaccid paralysis.
- Constipation. Although constipation is usually the first symptom of infant botulism, it is commonly overlooked.

Honey is the only known dietary reservoir of *C. botulinum* spores linked to infant botulism. For this reason honey should not be fed to infants under 1 year of age. Other cases of infant and paediatric botulism are acquired from spores in the soil.

Complications

Botulism is very dangerous when affecting the respiratory system leading not only to respiratory failure, but also impaired clearing of secretions leading to pneumonia.

Laboratory confirmation is undertaken by demonstrating the presence of toxin in serum, stool, or food, or by culturing *C. botulinum* from stool, a wound or food.

However, laboratory testing may take hours or days. Initial diagnosis and appropriate treatment depend on clinical diagnosis through a thorough history and physical examination.

Diagnosis

Diagnosis is likely in resource-limited settings to be made on clinical grounds.

Consider diagnosing botulism if the patient's history and physical examination suggest botulism. However, other diseases such as Guillain–Barré syndrome, poliomyelitis and poisoning can appear similar to botulism, and special tests (when available) may be needed to exclude these other conditions. The presence of more than one affected family member is strongly suggestive of botulism.

A definite diagnosis can be made if botulinum toxin is identified in the food, wound or stool. Botulinum toxin can be detected by a variety of techniques, including enzyme-linked immunosorbent assays (ELISAs), electrochemiluminescent (ECL) tests and mouse inoculation or feeding trials.

Treatment

Botulinum antitoxin (if available) should be administered as soon as possible. Antitoxin does not reverse paralysis, but arrests its progression.

Before administration of antitoxin, skin testing should be performed for sensitivity to serum or antitoxin.

After skin testing, and ensuring that treatment for potential anaphylaxis is immediately available (adrenaline, IV fluids and bag-valve-mask), administration of one vial of antitoxin IV is recommended. There is no need to re-administer the antitoxin since the circulating antitoxins have a half-life of 5–8 days.

Close monitoring of respiratory function (including SpO$_2$ monitoring) is essential to detect respiratory failure. Physiotherapy to encourage deep breathing exercises may help to prevent retained secretions and pneumonia. When required, and available, artificial ventilation may be needed often for 2–8 weeks' duration in severe cases.

The treatment of children, pregnant women or immunocompromised patients with botulism does not differ from the above approach.

Antibiotics are required to remove the bacteria in cases of wound botulism. Oral (or intravenous) metronidazole (30 mg/kg per day, given at 6-hourly intervals; maximum 4 grams/day) is effective in decreasing the number of vegetative forms of *C. botulinum* and is the antimicrobial agent of choice. Penicillin V orally 25 mg/kg 6-hourly is an alternative treatment. Therapy for 10–14 days is recommended.

Other antibiotics may be required to treat secondary chest infections.

Remember that the child is fully conscious and can feel pain. Good nursing care is essential.

If a deep wound is thought to be responsible it should be treated to remove dead tissue and the source of the toxin-producing bacteria.

Each case of food-borne botulism is a potential public health emergency and it is important to identify the source of the outbreak and ensure that all persons who have been exposed to the toxin have been identified, and that no contaminated food remains.

6.1.B Buruli ulcer

BOX 6.1.B.1 Minimum standards
- WHO global public health initiative.
- Antibiotics: rifampicin, streptomycin and clarithromycin.
- Surgery.
- Dry reagent-based polymerase chain reaction (PCR) assay.

Introduction

Buruli ulcer is a highly destructive ulcerating condition caused by *Mycobacterium ulcerans*, which ranks third among mycobacterial infections affecting immunocompetent humans.

Any part of the body may be affected, particularly areas exposed to minor trauma. Management is a combination of medical treatment to eradicate the infective agent and surgical to excise the infected tissue.

Background and epidemiology

The disease occurs in several parts of Africa, Papua New Guinea, the Americas, South East Asia, China and Australia. The organism is found in soil or stagnant water and predominantly affects children in whom infection usually occurs following a minor penetrating injury.

Intercurrent helminthic infections may also predispose to ulceration. HIV infection, and other immunodeficiency states, can exacerbate Buruli ulcer and lead to severe complications.

Clinical features

A non-ulcerative lesion usually precedes ulceration. Four non-ulcerative presentations are recognised:
- **papule:** painless, may be itchy, non-tender intradermal lesion
- **nodule:** painless firm lesion 1–2 cm diameter in the subcutaneous tissue, usually attached to the skin

- **plaque:** painless well-demarcated elevated dry indurated lesion > 2 cm in diameter
- **oedematous:** diffuse extensive non-pitting swelling, ill-defined margin, firm, usually painful, with or without colour change over affected skin.

Subsequently an ulcer forms with central necrosis and often spreads very rapidly in all directions.

Characteristic features

- Ulcer is usually painless (hence delay in healthcare-seeking behaviour).
- Edge of ulcer is deeply undermined.
- Satellite ulcers often communicate with the original ulcer by subcutaneous tunnels.
- Skin between adjacent ulcers is often unattached to the underlying tissues.
- The extent of damage is always greater than it appears from the surface.
- Regional adenitis and systemic symptoms are unusual (and if present suggest primary or secondary bacterial infection).
- Erosion of underlying tissue may involve nerves, blood vessels and bone (in up to 15% of cases).

Complications

These include the following:
- tetanus
- osteomyelitis
- scarring
- ankylosis
- contractures.

Around 25% of patients develop long-term complications that may include amputation or loss of sight.

Differential diagnosis

- **Papule:** granuloma annulare, herpes, insect bites, leishmaniasis, acne, pityriasis, psoriasis.
- **Nodule:** boil, cyst, leishmaniasis, lipoma, lymphadenitis, mycosis, onchocerciasis.
- **Plaque:** cellulitis, haematoma, insect bites, leishmaniasis, leprosy, mycosis, psoriasis.
- **Oedema:** actinomycosis, cellulitis, elephantiasis, necrotising fasciitis, onchocerciasis, osteomyelitis.
- **Ulcer:** cutaneous diphtheria, guinea worm, leishmaniasis, necrotising fasciitis, neurogenic ulcer, tropical ulcer, tuberculosis, sickle-cell disease, squamous-cell carcinoma, syphilis, venous ulcer, cutaneous amoebiasis, yaws.

Investigations

- Slough from ulcer usually contains numerous acid-fast bacilli on Ziehl–Neelsen stain (sensitivity 40%).
- Culture unhelpful (sensitivity 20–60%, time consuming (8 weeks), expensive, frequently gives false-positive results).
- Biopsy and histopathology (sensitivity is 90%).
- Polymerase chain reaction (PCR) is increasingly used in diagnosis (it is rapid, only taking 2 days, and has a sensitivity of more than 95%). Recently, a highly sensitive dry reagent-based PCR assay has been developed that is better suited for use in most endemic countries.

Management

The current recommendation is for combined medical and surgical management.

1 **Small early lesion (e.g. nodules, papules, plaques, ulcers < 5 cm in diameter):** for papules and nodules, if immediate excision and suturing is possible, start antibiotics at least 24 hours before surgery and continue for 4 weeks. Otherwise, treat all lesions in this category with antibiotics for 8 weeks.
2 **Non-ulcerative and ulcerative plaque and oedematous form: large ulcerative lesions (> 5 cm in diameter): lesions in the head and neck region, particularly the face:** treat with antibiotics for at least 4 weeks, then surgery (if necessary), followed by another 4 weeks of antibiotics.
3 **Disseminated/mixed forms (e.g. osteitis, osteomyelitis, joint involvement):** treat with antibiotics for at least 1 week before surgery and continue for a total of 8 weeks.

Necrotic ulcers should be excised with care to remove all affected tissue by extending the margin into healthy tissue. Excision is followed by primary closure or split-skin grafting. Reconstructive surgery and physiotherapy may be required for patients with contractures and other permanent disabilities and disfigurements.

Antibiotics

Antibiotic combination treatment, by reducing ulcer size, makes larger ulcers more amenable to surgery and grafting.

Africa

Oral rifampicin (10 mg/kg) once daily plus intramuscular streptomycin (15 mg/kg) once daily for 8 weeks.

Overall treatment success rate 96% when used in conjunction with surgery depending on size of ulcer at presentation.

Note: for treatment of early (less than 6 months' duration) ulcers of limited size (< 10 cm), 4 weeks of streptomycin and rifampicin followed by 4 weeks of rifampicin and clarithromycin is as effective as 8 weeks of streptomycin and rifampicin.

Australia

Oral rifampicin plus one other oral antibiotic (either clarithromycin or ciprofloxacin) for 3 months:

1 when histology of resection margins shows either necrosis or acid-fast bacilli or granulomata, **or**
2 when initial lesion was large enough to require grafting, **or**
3 for complex recurrent disease.

Amikacin (IV) is recommended where surgical resection is necessarily incomplete.

Recommended antibiotics and doses for children are as follows:
- Rifampicin 10–20 mg/kg/day up to maximum 600 mg daily.
- Clarithromycin 15–30 mg/kg/day in two divided doses if under 12 years, up to a maximum of 500 mg twice daily if over 12 years.
- Ciprofloxacin 20 mg/kg/day in two divided doses, up to a maximum of 500–750 mg twice daily.

Prevention and public health aspects

Long trousers and other mechanical barriers.

BCG offers some protection.

The *Global Buruli Ulcer Initiative*, launched by the WHO in 1998, advocates the following:

- health education and staff training in the communities most affected
- development of educational materials adapted to the needs of the countries
- community-based surveillance system to increase early

detection and referral for treatment in collaboration with diseases such as leprosy and Guinea worm

- assessment of local health services and resources currently available for the diagnosis and treatment of Buruli ulcer in endemic areas
- strengthening of the capacity of health systems in endemic areas by upgrading surgical facilities and improving laboratories
- rehabilitation of those already deformed by the disease.

6.1.C Diphtheria

> **BOX 6.1.C.1 Minimum standards**
> - ABC (especially airway protection).
> - Immunisation and prophylaxis of contacts.
> - Early parenteral antibiotics.
> - Dexamethasone.
> - Early antitoxin.
> - Bed rest, close observation and ECG monitoring.
> - Intubation/tracheostomy.

Introduction

In countries with adequate coverage of immunisation (over 70%), diphtheria is now uncommon. Epidemics still occur associated with a fall in level of immunisation, as happened in the mid-1980s and early 1990s in Russia and Ukraine and other republics of the former USSR. The disease affects all ages.

Epidemiology

- When levels of immunisation are low, children are the

major group affected. Young infants are protected by maternal antibody.

- With improvement in immunisation rates, affected age groups shift to older children and adults. Boosters at school entry and school leaving are essential to provide adequate herd immunity.
- Mass movement of people, for example refugees or army personnel, are important sources of spread in epidemics.
- It is more common in autumn and winter.
- In tropical countries, skin infection by *Corynebacterium diphtheriae* provides a reservoir that results in natural immunity of the carrier and subclinical spread within the community.

Pathogenesis

C. diphtheriae invades the upper respiratory tract. The incubation period is 2–4 days.

TABLE 6.1.C.1 Clinical features of diphtheria

Site	Comments
Pharynx + + +	Affected in over 90% of cases
Tonsil ±	Yellow/white to grey/black (if haemorrhagic) thick membrane which extends beyond the tonsils and covers the adjacent pharyngeal wall. Bleeds when separated from underlying tissue. Pharyngeal membrane may extend to nares, palate or larynx. There may be distortion of soft palate, tonsils, etc. If confined to tonsils, little toxaemia
Nasal ±	Serosanguinous discharge, sore nose and lip
	Little toxaemia Highly infectious
Neck	Enlarged, tender cervical nodes, 'bull neck'
Skin 0– +	Any type of lesion (e.g. bites, impetigo) may be infected. May progress to ulcer with punched-out sharp edges. Important reservoir for transmission and natural immunisation. May result in respiratory colonisation
Other sites	Conjunctiva, ear and vulva
Levels of toxaemia 0, ±,+ +, + + +	Low-grade fever (rarely > 38.9°C)
	Weak, rapid pulse, limp, apathetic, restless
	Rarely haemorrhagic diathesis

- Diphtheria toxin causes necrosis and exudation in local tissue which results in formation of the 'membrane'. An attempt at removal of the membrane causes bleeding.
- Toxin is distributed by blood and lymphatic system resulting in toxaemia, and causing cardiac and neurological complications.

- Non-toxin-producing *C. diphtheriae* may cause focal disease but not cardiac and neurological complications. Vaccination does not protect against this organism.

TABLE 6.1.C.2 Complications of diphtheria

Complication	Weeks	Comments
Toxaemia	1	Related to extent of membrane and amount of toxin absorbed. May result in cardiovascular (CVS) collapse in first 10 days. Disseminated intravascular coagulation. Survivors of severe toxaemia usually have further CVS and neurological complications
Myocarditis	2–3 Range 1–6	Onset related to severity of toxaemia Soft first heart sound, apical systolic murmur ECG: conduction abnormalities, ST-T wave changes. **Echocardiogram:** left ventricular dilation, reduced contractility, hypertrophied left ventricle, sometimes pericardial fluid Biochemistry: **blood myoglobin levels elevated, elevated lactate dehydrogenase, elevated creatine phosphokinase** Mortality: high in early onset, severe carditis
Palatal paralysis	1	Probably due to local absorption of toxin: 'fluids come down nose' Resolves in a few days
Visual accommodation	4–5	Blurring of vision, sometimes strabismus
Bulbar, heart, respiratory and limb nerves	6–8	Bilateral, resolve completely if patient survives

Clinical features

Symptoms are initially due to disease of upper respiratory tract and associated toxaemia. Later symptoms relate to the level of toxin absorbed into the circulation. Cases with small membranes and low toxaemia recover spontaneously and most remain subclinical.

Diagnosis

- Unless all children with upper respiratory symptoms, including croup, have an appropriate examination, diphtheria will be missed.
- A portion of membrane or a swab taken from beneath it should be sent for Gram stain and culture. The laboratory should be informed of suspected diagnosis so that appropriate culture medium is used.

Management

See also Section 5.1.

The aim is to neutralise toxin released into blood by the bacillus and to kill the bacteria.

- Admit to isolation (on ICU if possible) cared for by staff who are fully immunised.
- Be prepared for intubation/tracheostomy, especially if laryngeal diphtheria is suspected.
- Dexamethasone (150 microgram/kg twice daily IV or orally) should be given in cases of moderate to severe airway obstruction and when there is swelling of the neck until airway obstruction resolves.
- Take great care when examining the throat or taking a sample of the membrane as it may precipitate complete airway obstruction.
- Give intravenous or nasogastric maintenance fluids if the child cannot drink.
- Give benzylpenicillin 50 mg/kg 4-hourly IV. Change to procaine benzylpenicillin 25 000–50 000 units/kg IM once daily (must not be given IV) when toxic symptoms have subsided or where toxicity is slight or, if the child can drink, to penicillin V 12.5 mg/kg 6-hourly. Erythromycin 40–50 mg/kg per day in four divided doses (maximum 2 grams/day) IV, and orally when child can swallow, is an alternative. Antibiotics should be given for 7–10 days.
- **Antitoxin must be given as soon as possible** (after the test dose). The dose is dependent on the severity of the disease rather than the site of the membrane, although the two usually coincide:
  - Nasal and tonsillar (mild disease): 20 000 units IM.
  - Laryngeal with symptoms (moderately severe): 40 000 units IM or IV.
  - Nasopharyngeal (moderately severe): 60 000–100 000 units IV depending on severity and combined sites/delayed diagnosis (malignant disease), also 60 000–100 000 units IV.
  - In practice, give 60 000 units to all cases with visible membrane and neck swelling.

Commercially available antitoxin is extremely expensive but highly purified. Some countries (e.g. Vietnam) make their own antitoxin but it is much **less purified** than the Aventis Pasteur vaccine for example, and **cannot be given intravenously**.

Test dose and desensitisation
See also *Section 5.1.B on anaphylaxis.*

- As antitoxin is from horse serum, a test dose with 0.1 mL of 1 in 1000 dilution in saline is given intradermally.
  - Positive reaction is 10 mm erythema occurring within 20 minutes.
  - If there is no reaction, give full-dose IV/IM as appropriate.
- Have adrenaline 1 in 1000 and syringe available to give IM if anaphylaxis occurs (10 micrograms/kg).
- Desensitisation: (if test dose is positive) give graduated doses of increased strength every 20 minutes commencing with:
  - 0.1 mL of 1 in 20 dilution in saline subcutaneously followed by 1 in 10 dilution
  - then 0.1 mL of undiluted subcutaneously, then 0.3 mL and 0.5 mL IM
  - then 0.1 mL undiluted IV.

Additional treatment

- Give oxygen if cyanosed or $SaO_2 < 94\%$. Use nasal cannulae or a face mask held close to the child's face by the mother. **Do not use nasal or nasopharyngeal catheters** as these can precipitate complete airway obstruction. Be aware that giving oxygen does **not** compensate for hypoventilation which, if severe, will require intubation and cricothyroidotomy or tracheostomy (see Section 8.2). Note that intubation may dislodge the membrane, causing complete airway obstruction.
- Bed rest and observation for 2–3 weeks at least, depending on severity.
- Regular monitoring of cardiac function. Serial ECGs two or three times per week through the critical period from admission until towards the end of the second week of illness. Rhythm disturbances, particularly atrioventricular block sometimes going on to complete heart block are not uncommon, and are often the earliest evidence of cardiac involvement.
- With severe cardiac involvement (which often follows from severe local disease) the children develops a low-output state and may die from cardiac failure or arrhythmias. Poor urine output and rising creatinine are early indicators of poor prognosis and should be monitored, together with serum potassium which should be kept in the normal range (see Section 9.A). Strict bed rest is essential for all children until the critical period for cardiac complications has passed (minimum of 2 weeks from onset).
  - Captopril at the earliest sign of any cardiac involvement may be helpful (100 micrograms/kg once daily as a test dose with the child supine and monitoring blood pressure carefully, followed by 100–200 micrograms/kg 8-hourly).
  - Prednisolone 1.5 mg/kg/day for 2 weeks may be of value in reducing the incidence of myocarditis.
- Nasogastric feeds if palatal or bulbar paralysis occurs. Bulbar problems rarely become evident until several weeks later, so even if children come through the phase of upper airway obstruction and survive the cardiac problems, they should remain in close contact with the hospital for at least 6 weeks.
- Immunise on discharge.

Prevention

- Maintaining immunity at all age levels in the community is important. Additional immunisation at school entry and leaving (see Section 1.17).
- Give immunised household contacts a booster of toxoid.
- Give all unimmunised contacts one dose of IM benzathine benzylpenicillin (600 000 units for children under 5 years and 1.2 million units for those over 5 years). This drug must not be given IV. Immunise and check daily for signs of diphtheria.

6.1.D Leprosy

> **BOX 6.1.D.1 Minimum standards**
> - Public health measures.
> - Clinical awareness.
> - Multi-drug treatment (MDT) with rifampicin, dapsone and clofazimine.
> - Protective footwear.
> - Support and counselling.
> - Reconstructive surgery.

Introduction

A campaign to eliminate leprosy below a prevalence of 1 in 10 000 greatly reduced total numbers, but new cases, especially in India and Brazil, are still being detected in worryingly large numbers. It remains the prototype of a disfiguring skin disease. It is caused by *Mycobacterium leprae*, an organism that invokes an immunological response in the skin and especially focusing on superficial cutaneous nerves, resulting in anaesthesia and paralysis of hand, foot and facial muscles. There is a range of disease from an effective immune response with few surviving bacteria termed paucibacillary leprosy, to a poor immune response with very large numbers of bacteria termed multibacillary leprosy. Unfortunately, the present public health picture of leprosy is that the majority of new cases are multibacillary and the percentage of children affected is greater than before. The incubation period is very long (up to 8–10 years) and disability is often present by the time it is diagnosed.

In countries where the prevalence is low, leprosy may be forgotten and those trained to recognise it disbanded. The expectation is that general health services will oversee the patient as he or she moves from an anxious family to a traditional health practitioner to a health centre. The latter will be overwhelmed by common skin disease such as impetigo, cutaneous fungus disease and scabies, and current policy is to train all health workers in health centres to manage these correctly and thereby increase the likelihood of detection and better management of rarer diseases such as leprosy. Conditions not diagnosed or not responding should be guided through an effective referral system to greater expertise.

The global registered prevalence of leprosy at the beginning of 2009 stood at 213 036 cases, while the number of new cases detected during 2008 was 249 007. The number of new cases detected globally has fallen by 9126 (a 4% decrease) during 2008 compared with 2007.

Pockets of high endemicity still remain in some areas of Angola, Brazil, Central African Republic, Democratic Republic of Congo, India, Madagascar, Mozambique, Nepal, and the United Republic of Tanzania.

Diagnosis

At one end of the clinical spectrum of leprosy is an early single lesion with very few bacilli which may resolve spontaneously and certainly responds well and quickly to antibiotics. It is hypopigmented, flat and insensitive to light touch, pinprick and hot and cold.

The spectrum passes through an increasing number of such lesions that are unlikely to resolve spontaneously, and increasingly, over a period of years, infiltration and swelling which is often nodular, from asymmetry to symmetry, to greater numbers of bacilli, to eventual widespread infiltration of the skin. The bacteria are shed into the environment from the nose and wounds.

Early diagnosis requires a full examination of all the skin, tests of any suspicious lesion for numbness, and a biopsy of infiltrated lesions, especially nodules, the presence of a granuloma alerting to the need for bacterial stains.

Cutaneous nerves, ulnar, radial, posterior cervical, lateral popliteal and muscular cutaneous on the dorsum of the foot must be palpated for thickening. Early signs include flexion of the fourth and fifth finger, dropped foot, and reduction in blinking.

Differential diagnosis

Vitiligo is totally de-pigmented, whiter than leprosy and usually symmetrical. There is no sensory loss. It is long lasting.

Pityriasis alba is very common, mild, dry eczema, usually symmetrical on both cheeks and the extensor surface of both limbs. It varies over days or weeks and responds to moisturising ointments or hydrocortisone.

Pityriasis versicolor is a common infection of the skin from *Malassezia furfur* producing depigmentation and fine scaling especially of the upper trunk. The organism and the slight inflammation it causes accounts for a dull red to brown discolouration of white skin. Pigmented skin loses pigment due to exfoliation. It responds to selenium sulphide shampoo, Whitfields (benzoic acid and salicylic acid) ointment or ketoconazole, plus sun exposure for rapid re-pigmentation.

Post-inflammatory depigmentation is preceded by undisputed injury such as a burn, chickenpox, fungal infection or psoriasis. There may be loss of normal skin texture as in a scar.

Reactions

Reactions are immunological responses to *Mycobacterium leprae* or its antigen. There are two types.

Erythema nodosum-like with multiple tender, symmetrical red lumps anywhere in the skin due to immune complexes and accompanied by fever and malaise. It often responds to rest and non-steroidal anti-inflammatory drugs but persistent reactions will need oral steroids. There is usually a history of prior diagnosis of leprosy.

The other type of reaction is focused on a previous plaque or infected nerve. There is redness, swelling and tenderness. It is destructive of nerves. An early prescription of an initially high dose of prednisolone is necessary (1 mg/kg/day). Complete withdrawal of steroids should only occur after several weeks if nerve destruction is to be avoided

Treatment

Multidrug therapy cures leprosy. Multidrug therapy should be given under supervision by experts able to provide full advice on the preventive management of disability, who may confirm the diseases by skin smears or biopsies and can manage reactions. Standard drug therapy is available free from government programmes for the elimination of leprosy. WHO guidelines for multidrug therapy include a single dose for a single lesion, or two drugs for lesions which contain more than one bacteria. A daily regimen for 1 year of three drugs is necessary for more widespread multibacillary disease. Lepromatous leprosy is subject to reaction even after 1 year of therapy and patients must be educated to return for diagnosis and appropriate therapy promptly. Relapse after completion of therapy is uncommon but well documented.

WHO-recommended treatment for paucibacillary leprosy in children (10–14 years)

Once a month: On day 1, two capsules of rifampicin (300 mg + 150 mg) plus one tablet of dapsone (50 mg).

Once a day: On days 2–28, one tablet of dapsone (50 mg).

Full course: six blister packs over 6 months.

For children younger than 10 years, the dose must be adjusted according to body weight.

WHO recommended treatment for multibacillary leprosy in children (10–14 years)

Once a month: On day 1, two capsules of rifampicin (300 mg + 150 mg) plus three capsules of clofazimine (50 mg × 3) plus one tablet of dapsone (50 mg).

Once a day: On days 2–28, one capsule of clofazimine every other day (50 mg), plus one tablet of dapsone (50 mg) daily.

Full course: 12 blister packs over 12 months.

For children younger than 10 years, the dose must be adjusted according to body weight.

Children may be more troubled by the haemolytic side effect of dapsone, and are less tolerant to rifampicin. New drug regimens include ofloxacin, minocycline and clarithromycin. Several experimental and clinical studies have demonstrated that these drugs either alone or in combination with other anti-leprosy drugs have significant bactericidal activity. Patients presenting with single skin lesion paucibacillary leprosy can be treated with only one dose containing rifampicin 20 mg/kg, ofloxacin 15 mg/kg and minocycline 100 mg (only for children over 12 years).

Multibacillary leprosy patients who do not accept clofazimine can be treated with this combination given monthly for 24 months.

There is still a fear of the stigma of leprosy. The emphasis of therapy is that it is a cure and rapidly renders the patient non-infectious.

Support and counselling is necessary for the patient along with education for family and community, or else the cured patient may still not be acceptable to either family or community.

6.1.E Leptospirosis

BOX 6.1.E.1 **Minimum standards**
- Recognition and treatment of shock.
- Antibiotics: amoxicillin, penicillin (parenteral for severe disease), doxycycline.
- Public health measures.

Introduction

Leptospirosis is a zoonotic disease caused by *Leptospira* species with a worldwide distribution. It is endemic in the tropics and its incidence in these countries appears to be increasing. The possible reasons include an increase in the rat population and seasonal flooding. Transmission to humans is from infected animal urine. The onset is usually abrupt. It is an acute febrile disease with varied manifestations characterised by vasculitis. The severity of disease ranges from asymptomatic or subclinical to self-limited systemic illness (approximately 90% of patients) to life-threatening illness with jaundice, renal failure, and hemorrhagic pneumonitis. The clinical course is usually biphasic and with multisystemic involvement. The initial (septicaemic) phase lasts 4–7 days, the second (immune) phase 4–30 days. It can be lethal in the acute period, and is similar to diseases such as dengue, malaria, hepatitis and viral illnesses.

Risk factors for infection include occupational exposure (farmers, ranchers, abattoir workers, veterinarians, loggers, sewer workers, rice field workers, laboratory workers), recreational activities (fresh water swimming, canoeing, trail biking), household exposure (pet dogs, domesticated livestock, rainwater catchment systems, and infestation by infected rodents), and skin lesions (contact with wild rodents).

History and examination

- **Enquire about** headache, fever, abdominal pain, breathing difficulties and cough, diuresis, bleeding, diarrhoea or vomiting.
- **Assess** vital signs (blood pressure, pulse, respiratory rate), 'alarm signs', blood film for malaria parasite. Consider dengue fever.
- **Watch out for** 'alarm signs' of leptospirosis: abdominal pain, respiratory distress, jaundice, bleeding and oliguria.

Clinical manifestations

Leptospirosis is associated with a variable clinical course. The disease may manifest as a subclinical illness followed by seroconversion, a self-limited systemic infection, or a severe, potentially fatal illness accompanied by multiorgan failure. Physical examination is often unrevealing. An important but frequently overlooked sign is **conjunctival suffusion**.

Below are common clinical manifestations:

- **General symptoms:** headache, myalgia, vomiting and anorexia, arthralgia, macular rash.
- **Central nervous system:** CSF pleocytosis and elevated protein, meningism, neurological symptoms.
- **Renal system:** pyuria, haematuria, proteinuria, oliguria/anuria, dysuria, back pain.
- **Gastrointestinal system:** abdominal pain, diarrhoea, constipation, abnormal liver function tests, hepatomegaly, jaundice, gastrointestinal bleeding.
- **Respiratory system:** cough, pharyngitis, otitis media, chest pain, pneumonitis, pulmonary oedema and haemoptysis.
- **Cardiac system:** arrhythmias, conduction and other ECG abnormalities.
- **Haematology:** blood clotting disorder, petechiae, bruises, epistaxis, thrombocytopenia, lymphadenopathy, splenomegaly.
- **Eyes:** conjunctival bleeding, photophobia, retro-orbital pain, uveitis, papilloedema.

Classification

- **Mild disease:** headache, fever, myalgia, no evidence of bleeding.
- **Moderate disease:** headache, fever, myalgia, abdominal pain and jaundice.
- **Severe disease:** Weil's disease or icterohaemorrhagic fever: shock, abdominal pain, respiratory failure, pulmonary haemorrhage, acute renal failure, altered consciousness and bleeding.

Diagnosis

1 **Clinical:** Features that are significantly associated with leptospirosis include:
   - conjunctival suffusion
   - haemorrhage
   - abdominal pain
   - hepatosplenomegaly
   - oedema.
2 **Laboratory:**
   - **Cultures:** blood culture in initial phase and urine in the second phase. Blood (50% yield) and CSF specimens are positive during the first 10 days of the illness. Urine cultures become positive during the second week of the illness.
   - **Serology:** Serological tests (microscopic agglutination test (MAT), macroscopic agglutination test, indirect haemagglutination, and enzyme linked immunosorbant assay – ELISA) are most often used for confirmation.
     - The gold standard is considered to be the MAT. However, this test is cumbersome which requires live organisms, considerable expertise, and is performed only by reference laboratories. MAT is most specific when a fourfold or greater rise in titre is detected between acute and convalescent serum specimens. However, a single titre of > 1:800 is strong evidence of current or recent infection with leptospira.
     - Rapid diagnosis with specific IgM (ELISA) can be made by two commercially available rapid tests, the microplate IgM ELISA and an IgM dot-ELISA dipstick test. If one of these assays is positive, sera for MAT can be sent to a reference laboratory.
     - **Newer tests:** Polymerase chain reaction (PCR), not widely available, but shows considerable promise for a quick, accurate diagnosis.

- **Routine labs:** white blood cell (WBC) counts may range between 3000 and 26 000/microlitre; thrombocytopenia, raised serum bilirubin, hyponatremia, proteinuria, pyuria, microscopic haematuria, elevated creatine kinase and minimal to moderate elevations of hepatic transaminases may be seen.
3 **X-rays:** chest radiographs may show small nodular densities, confluent consolidation or a ground-glass appearance.

Differential diagnosis

Malaria, dengue fever, scrub typhus, acute viral illnesses including influenza, other rickettsial disease, typhoid fever and rare causes such as ehrlichiosis and hantavirus infections.

Complications

These include renal failure, uveitis, haemorrhage, acute respiratory distress syndrome, myocarditis and rhabdomyolysis. Vasculitis with necrosis of extremities may be seen in severe cases. Severe leptospirosis may require ICU admission. Multi-organ failure in 75% and mortality in over 50% of these patients may be seen.

Management

The majority of *Leptospira* infections are self-limiting. Many antibiotics have antileptospiral activity, and if the illness is severe and the diagnosis is recognised, antibiotic therapy should be given.

Mild disease:

- Discharge home with advice about hydration and 'alarm signs'.
- Antibiotics:
  - Children under 10 years of age: amoxicillin 15 mg/kg three times daily for 7 days or, if allergic, erythromycin 10–15 mg/kg/day three times daily for 7 days.
  - Children over 10 years: doxycycline 100 mg twice daily for 7 days.

Moderate disease:

- Observe for 48 hours, monitor vital signs 4-hourly.

- If abdominal pain and respiratory distress settle, discharge.
- Antibiotics: benzylpenicillin 25–50 mg/kg IV 6-hourly for 3 days, then change to oral penicillin. Amoxicillin is an alternative.

Severe disease:

- Give oxygen as required, IV fluids (*see* Section 5.5), and pass a nasogastric tube.
- Keep an accurate fluid-balance chart.
- Pulmonary haemorrhage may require assisted ventilation with PEEP.
- Pulmonary oedema: treat with fluid restriction, oxygen and diuretics.
- Management of disseminated intravascular coagulation, renal failure and myocarditis.
- Antibiotics: Intravenous therapy with benzylpenicillin (250 000 to 400 000 units/kg/day in four to six divided doses; maximum dose 6 million units daily: note 600 mg = 1 million units), or doxycycline (4 mg/kg/day in two equally divided doses; maximum dose 200 mg daily), or ceftriaxone (80–100 mg/kg once daily; maximum dose 4 grams daily), or cefotaxime (150–200 mg/kg/day in three to four equally divided doses; maximum dose 12 grams daily). Doxycycline should be avoided in children less than 8 years of age.
- For children less than 8 years of age with severe penicillin allergy, therapy with oral azithromycin (10 mg/kg once on day 1, maximum dose 500 mg/day, followed by 5 mg/kg/day once daily on subsequent days, maximum dose 250 mg/day) or oral clarithromycin (15 mg/kg/day divided into two equal doses, maximum dose 1 gram/day) may be given.
- The duration of treatment is usually 5–7 days.

Prevention

Vaccination of domestic animals against leptospirosis provides substantial protection. The major control measure is to avoid potential sources of infection such as stagnant water, water derived from run-off from animal farms, rodent control, and protection of food from animal contamination.

Currently no vaccine is available for human immunisation, but doxycycline prophylaxis during period of exposure has been shown to be protective.

6.1.F Lyme disease

BOX 6.1.F.1 Minimum standards
Antibiotics: doxycycline, amoxicillin and ceftriaxone.

Introduction

This disease is caused by the bacterium *Borrelia*. *Borrelia burgdorferi* is the main cause in North America, whereas *Borrelia afzelii* and *Borrelia garinii* cause most European cases. The prevalence of Lyme disease in sub-Saharan Africa is presently unknown, but cases have been reported. The abundance of hosts and tick vectors would support the presence of this infection in Africa where it is probably grossly under-diagnosed.

Transmission

Lyme disease is transmitted to humans from a natural reservoir among rodents by ticks that feed on both rodents and other animals, such as deer.

Tick bites often go unnoticed because of the small size of the tick in its nymphal stage, as well as tick secretions that prevent the host from feeling any itch or pain from the bite. However, transmission is quite rare, with only about 1% of recognised tick bites resulting in Lyme disease. This may be because an infected tick must be attached for at least a day for transmission to occur.

Days to weeks following the tick bite, the spirochetes spread via the bloodstream to joints, heart, nervous system, and distant skin sites, where their presence gives rise to the variety of symptoms of disseminated disease.

If untreated, the bacteria may persist in the body for months or even years, despite the production of antibodies against *Borrelia* by the immune system.

Diagnosis

Lyme disease is diagnosed clinically based on symptoms, objective physical findings (such as erythema migrans (EM), facial palsy or arthritis) or a history of possible exposure to infected ticks, as well as serological blood tests. The EM rash is not always a bull's-eye (see below) (i.e. it can be red all the way across). When making a diagnosis of Lyme disease, healthcare providers should consider other diseases that may cause similar illness. Not all patients infected with Lyme disease will develop the characteristic bull's-eye rash, and many may not recall a tick bite.

Signs and symptoms

Many of the symptoms are not specific to Lyme disease.

The incubation period from tick bite to the onset of symptoms is usually 1–2 weeks, but can be much shorter (days), or much longer (months).

Early localised infection

The classic sign of early local infection with Lyme disease is a circular, outwardly expanding rash called erythema chronicum migrans (also erythema migrans or EM), which occurs at the site of the tick bite 3–30 days after the bite. The rash is red, and may be warm, but is generally painless. Classically, the innermost portion remains dark red and becomes thicker and firmer; the outer edge remains red; and the portion in between clears, giving the appearance of a bull's-eye. EM is thought to occur in about 80% of infected patients. Patients can also experience flu-like symptoms, such as headache, muscle soreness, fever, and malaise. Lyme disease can progress to later stages even in patients who do not develop a rash.

Early disseminated infection

Within days to weeks after the onset of local infection, the *Borrelia* bacteria begin to spread through the bloodstream. EM may develop at sites across the body that bear no relation to the original tick bite. Other discrete symptoms include migrating pain in muscles, joints, and tendons, and heart palpitations and dizziness.

Various acute neurological problems appear in 10–15% of untreated patients. These include facial palsy, arthritis and meningitis. Radiculoneuritis causes shooting pains that may interfere with sleep, as well as abnormal skin sensations. Mild encephalitis may lead to memory loss, sleep disturbances, or mood changes.

The disease may also have cardiac manifestations including cardiac arrhythmias.

Late disseminated infection

After several months, untreated or inadequately treated patients may go on to develop severe and chronic symptoms that affect many parts of the body, including the brain, nerves, eyes, joints and heart. Many disabling symptoms can occur.

Chronic encephalomyelitis, which may be progressive, can involve cognitive impairment, weakness in the legs, awkward gait, facial palsy, bladder problems, vertigo, and back pain. In rare cases untreated Lyme disease may cause frank psychosis, which has been misdiagnosed as schizophrenia or bipolar disorder. Panic attacks and anxiety can occur; there may also be delusional behaviour, including somatoform delusions, sometimes accompanied by a depersonalisation or derealisation syndrome, where the patients begin to feel detached from themselves or from reality.

Lyme arthritis usually affects the knees.

Treatment

In most cases, the infection and its symptoms are eliminated by antibiotics, especially if the illness is treated early. Delayed or inadequate treatment can lead to the more serious symptoms, which can be disabling and difficult to treat.

The antibiotics of choice for early infections are given orally for 10–28 days:

1 In children over 8 years: doxycycline, 4 mg/kg/day in two divided doses (maximum of 100 mg per dose).
2 In younger children (less than 8 years): amoxicillin 50 mg/kg/day in three divided doses. Doxycycline should not be given in pregnancy, instead use amoxicillin 250–500 mg three times daily for pregnant girls. If early infection is severe, ceftriaxone 50 mg/kg IV/IM once daily can be given at any age.

Late-diagnosed chronic Lyme disease is treated with oral or intravenous antibiotics for a minimum of 4 weeks, frequently ceftriaxone 50–75 mg/kg once a day IV.

6.1.G Meningococcal disease

BOX 6.1.G.1 Minimum standards
- Early parenteral antibiotics.
- Treatment of shock.
- Neurological assessment and cerebral protection.
- Frequent reassessment of clinical status.
- Electrolyte monitoring and replacement.
- Replacement of platelets, clotting factors and red cells.
- Follow public health procedures.

Introduction

Meningococcal disease is caused by *Neisseria meningitidis*, a Gram-negative diplococcus which is a commensal of the human nasopharynx. Endemic meningococcal disease primarily affects children under 5 years old. Some areas, in particular the meningitis belt in sub-Saharan Africa, suffer from epidemics of meningococcal disease. Temperate climates usually experience an increase in disease during winter months, whereas in sub-Saharan Africa, conditions during the dry season cause a sharp rise in incidence.

Predominant disease-causing organisms are sero-groups A, B and C and W135, with other serogroups generally only causing infection in specific patient groups (e.g. complement deficiency and the immunocompromised). Serogroup A is associated with epidemic disease in the meningitis belt of Africa, Middle East and southern Mediterranean regions, and less commonly in other developing countries. Serogroups B and C are largely responsible for endemic disease in temperate countries, although serogroup C is now less common in countries where the serogroup C vaccine has been widely introduced.

TABLE 6.1.G.1 Signs and symptoms of meningococcal meningitis and septicaemia

Meningococcal meningitis	Meningococcal septicaemia
Symptoms	*Symptoms*
Fever	Fever
Headache	Petechial/purpuric rash
Nausea and vomiting	Shivering/rigors
Rash	Malaise and lethargy/confusion
Drowsiness or irritability	Headache
Neck and back pain, and stiffness	Nausea and vomiting
Convulsions	Limb and joint pain
Signs	Absence of neck stiffness
Fever	Collapse
Non-blanching rash	*Signs*
Neck stiffness/positive Kernig's sign/opisthotonus	Fever
Decreased conscious level	Petechial/purpuric rash
Infants	Shock:
Signs of meningitis may be non-specific with neck stiffness frequently absent.	Tachycardia
	Low pulse volume
	Cool peripheries
Bulging fontanelle may be present.	Capillary refill time > 3 seconds
Suspect meningitis in any febrile infant, especially where there is marked irritability, vomiting and poor feeding	Hypotension (late sign)
	Urine output reduced (< 1 mL/kg/hour)
	Tachypnoea
Both meningitis and septicaemia can coexist in the same child.	Hypoxaemia
	Decreased conscious level

Clinical features

In general, meningococcal disease presents either as **meningitis** or as **meningococcal septicaemia**, although many patients present with a mixed picture. In developed countries, the majority of cases may present with septicaemia and frequently with shock, whereas in African serogroup A epidemics, meningitis is the commonest presentation.

Meningococcal disease should be suspected in any patient who presents with a non-blanching (petechial or purpuric) rash. However, 13% of cases may present with a maculopapular rash and 7% may have no rash. Severity of rash does not correlate with severity of disease.

Life-threatening features of meningococcal disease

- **Shock:** particularly uncompensated shock (hypotension and tachycardia). Shock causes the majority of deaths due to meningococcal disease and is a medical emergency.
- **Raised intracranial pressure:**
  - Decreased conscious level (Glasgow Coma Scale score or Modified Children's Coma Score < 8 or deteriorating).
  - Focal neurological abnormalities, especially false localising signs (e.g. pupillary dilatation).
  - Abnormal postures (decorticate or decerebrate).
  - Convulsions.
  - Rising blood pressure with falling pulse rate.

CSF features consistent with meningococcal meningitis

- Turbid or purulent (may be clear or blood stained), white blood cell count > 500 cells/mm^3 (< 3 cells/mm^3 in normal CSF).
- Protein usually > 0.8 grams/litre (< 0.6 grams/litre in normal CSF).
- Glucose reduced compared with blood glucose concentration.
- Gram-negative diplococci (intra- or extracellular) in 72% of previously untreated cases.

When not to perform a lumbar puncture

Lumbar puncture may precipitate coning if there is significantly raised intracranial pressure. In septicaemia, lumbar puncture is unlikely to be helpful and may cause rapid deterioration in an unstable child.

Contraindications to lumbar puncture: suspected critically raised intracranial pressure

- Glasgow Coma Scale score/Modified Children's Coma Score < 8 (or if child is unresponsive to pain).
- Focal neurological signs, including pupillary abnormalities.
- Unexplained hypertension/bradycardia.
- Shock (see below).
- Significant clotting disorder or low platelet count (50 × 10^9/litre) is present.

Management of meningococcal disease

See Section 5.16.B for a discussion of isolated meningococcal meningitis.

Principles

In suspected cases, give an injection of benzylpenicillin before transfer of child to hospital. Recommended doses of benzylpenicillin by age group are as follows:

- < 1 year: 300 mg
- 1–10 years: 600 mg
- > 10 years: 1.2 grams.

On admission, early antimicrobial therapy should be given, such as benzylpenicillin with chloramphenicol (for dose and alternatives, *see* Table 6.1.G.3). Ideally this should be given intravenously, but if this is not possible it can be given intramuscularly.

Close monitoring and aggressive supportive therapy

TABLE 6.1.G.2 Investigations in meningococcal disease

Investigations		Comment
Microbiology	Lumbar puncture†	For Gram stain and culture
		(remember contraindications for performing lumbar puncture)
	Throat swab	Culture*
	Blood culture	Gold standard diagnostic test for septicaemia, positive in 30% or more of previously untreated cases
Special microbiology: advanced methods	Meningococcal serology: CSF or blood. Meningococcal PCR	Acute and convalescent blood samples required
Haematology	Full blood count	Low haemoglobin
		In early septicaemia or in lone meningitis usually high neutrophil count. Low white cell count with neutropenia in severe septicaemia. Low platelet count ($< 50 \times 10^9$/litre) in disseminated intravascular coagulation
	Coagulation screen	Prolonged PT, KCTT and TT
		Raised fibrin degradation products
Biochemistry	Urea, creatinine, electrolytes including calcium, magnesium, phosphate	Hypokalaemia
		Hypocalcaemia
		Hypophosphataemia
		Metabolic acidosis
		Raised urea and creatinine (if severe, suspect pre-renal failure)

* Meningococci should be cultured on Mueller–Hinton or chocolate agar to identify and serogroup with antibiotic sensitivities.

† Where laboratory facilities are scarce, diagnosis of meningitis is made on CSF alone: appearance, cell count, glucose sticks, Albustix.

are needed if features of shock or raised intracranial pressure develop.

Never delay antimicrobial therapy if facilities are not available for immediate lumbar puncture or blood culture.

The most appropriate available antibiotic should be used. In general, intravenous benzylpenicillin with intravenous chloramphenicol are the drugs of choice where meningococcal disease is the most likely diagnosis. Where the diagnosis is uncertain, or where there is a high prevalence of penicillin resistant meningococci, broad-spectrum antibiotics should be used (see Table 6.1.G.3), ideally including a third-generation cephalosporin.

Do not delay administration if cefotaxime or ceftriaxone are unavailable (use benzylpenicillin, ampicillin or chloramphenicol instead for the initial dose).

The risk of transmission disappears after 24–48 hours of antibiotic therapy. Isolation is not essential, but staff should maintain good hygienic practice and wear masks and gloves during invasive procedures such as intubation, airway and mouth care, and line insertion.

Parenteral antibiotic treatment should be given for 7–14 days if the diagnosis of meningococcal disease is certain. Once culture and sensitivity results are available, treatment should be modified appropriately.

TABLE 6.1.G.3 Antibiotic doses in meningococcal disease

Antibiotic	Route	Dose and frequency
Ampicillin	IV	400 mg/kg/24 hours in four divided doses (maximum single dose 3 grams)
Benzylpenicillin	IV	300 mg/kg/24 hours in six divided doses (maximum single dose 2.4 grams)
Cefotaxime	IV	200 mg/kg/24 hours in four divided doses (maximum single dose 4 grams)
Ceftriaxone	IV/IM	80 mg/kg/24 hours once daily (maximum single dose 4 grams)
Chloramphenicol	IV	100 mg/kg/24 hours in four divided doses*
	Oral	100 mg/kg/24 hours in four divided doses†

* Chloramphenicol should be used with caution in infants less than 3 months of age. Monitoring of serum levels is recommended, and lower doses with wider dosage intervals may be required.

† Oral chloramphenicol is usually used only following 3–4 days of parenteral antibiotics. Although not recommended for children less than 3 months of age or in malnourished children, the evidence for harmful effects is slight.

Important notes

- Early recognition of life-threatening disease (shock and raised intracranial pressure) is vitally important. There is a very high risk of death if patients are not resuscitated aggressively at presentation.
- Assess airway patency, breathing and circulation (ABC) and examine for signs of shock and raised intracranial pressure (see above). Management regimens differ for different presentations: shock; raised intracranial pressure; meningitis uncomplicated by either shock or raised intracranial pressure.
- Many children present with a mixed picture and may require treatment of shock as well as management of neurological complications.

- Meningococcal disease is often progressive and patients may continue to deteriorate after antibiotic and supportive therapy have been initiated. All suspected cases should be closely monitored for cardiovascular and neurological deterioration for at least 24 hours.
- Management of children with severe shock or raised intracranial pressure who do not respond fully to initial resuscitation is complex. Every effort should be made to admit these patients to an appropriate intensive-care facility.

Shock

This is a medical emergency (*see also* Section 5.5.A and 5.5.C)

- Assess **ABC** and give high-flow oxygen.
- Check blood glucose levels (e.g. using BM Stix).
- Obtain intravenous or intra-osseous access.
- Take blood for culture, full blood count, grouping and cross-matching, coagulation screen, and urea and electrolytes.
- Commence appropriate intravenous antibiotics.
- Do not perform a lumbar puncture.
- Commence fluid resuscitation immediately using 20 mL/kg of crystalloid or colloid given as fast as possible. Reassess and use further fluid boluses of 20 mL/kg if signs of shock persist. Use either Ringer-lactate or Hartmann's solution (or 0.9% saline if neither of these are available) or other non-glucose-containing crystalloid or a colloid such as 4.5% human serum albumin.
- Blood products such as packed cells, plasma and platelets may be required. Arrange for supplies if available.
- Patients who remain shocked after 40 mL/kg colloid/crystalloid will probably benefit from inotropic support (e.g. dopamine 10–20 micrograms/kg/minute IV by peripheral intravenous cannula).
- Shocked patients are at significant risk of developing pulmonary oedema as fluid therapy increases. Ideal therapy is mechanical ventilation for patients who require more than 40 mL/kg fluids.
  - In resource-limited countries, where facilities for mechanical ventilation are unavailable, further fluid boluses should be undertaken cautiously with repeated boluses of 5–10 mL/kg of crystalloid, colloid or blood products as appropriate.
  - If pulmonary oedema develops (with tachypnoea, hypoxia, cough and fine crackles, raised jugular venous pressure and hepatomegaly) further fluid administration should be withheld until the patient stabilises. Inotropic support, as described above, may be of benefit.
- Full neurological and cardiovascular assessment with regular (at least hourly) assessment of: pupillary responses, conscious level, pulse, blood pressure, capillary refill time, respiratory rate and effort, pulse oximetry (if available) and temperature.
- Regular (ideally 4-hourly initially) monitoring of electrolytes (sodium, potassium, **calcium and magnesium, phosphate**, urea and/or creatinine) and glucose and replacement of deficits.
- **Blood gases should be undertaken to detect metabolic acidosis from shock or respiratory acidosis due to ventilatory insufficiency.**

- Severe metabolic acidosis (pH < 7.0), which does not respond to fluid therapy, may require cautious sodium bicarbonate correction (1 mEq/kg slowly IV).
- Regular blood gas monitoring is essential for ventilated patients.
- Monitor full blood count and coagulation regularly if initially abnormal.
  - Blood or packed cell transfusion should aim to maintain haemoglobin levels around 7–10 g/dL in the early phases of shock.
  - Platelets and coagulation factors (usually fresh frozen plasma and cryoprecipitate) should be replaced as required in order to control bleeding.
- Hydration will usually be via the intravenous route, but nasogastric feeding is appropriate if tolerated.
  - Urine output should be monitored (by an indwelling catheter if the conscious level is depressed). Insert a nasogastric tube for gastric drainage if there is persistent vomiting or if the conscious level is decreased.

Suspected raised intracranial pressure

This is a medical emergency.

Actions

- Assess ABCD, give high-flow oxygen (10 litres/minute), and obtain intravenous or intra-osseous access.
- Treat shock (see above), if present.
  - Exercise caution with fluid therapy as there is a conflict of need between raised intracranial pressure (RICP) and shock. The former requires less fluid, and the latter needs more.
- Do not perform a lumbar puncture.
- Give mannitol 250–500 mg/kg IV (this should be repeated if signs of raised intracranial pressure persist, up to a maximum total dose of 2 grams/kg or if available a serum osmolality up to 325 mOsm/litre).
  - Hypertonic saline may be used as an alternative (e.g. 3% saline 3 mL/kg).
  - If mannitol or 3% saline is unavailable, give furosemide 1 mg/kg IV.

If signs of raised intracranial pressure persist, ideal management would include:

- Rapid sequence induction of anaesthesia and intubation for both airway protection (if Glasgow Coma Scale score is < 8 and/or the child is unresponsive to painful stimuli) and stabilisation of PCO_2.
- Mechanical ventilation with optimal sedation and maintenance of PCO_2 within the normal range (ideally 4.5–5.5 kPa).

Other useful techniques include the following:

- Place the patient supine in a 30-degree head-up position.
- Avoid placing a central venous catheter in the internal jugular vein.
- Give antipyretics to maintain normal temperature.
- Undertake a full neurological and cardiovascular assessment with regular (at least hourly) assessment of: pupillary responses, conscious level, pulse, blood pressure, capillary refill time, respiratory rate and effort, pulse oximetry (if available) and temperature.
- Monitor electrolytes, gases, clotting and full blood count as recommended for shock.

Prognosis

- Even with optimal intensive care, around 5–10% of patients with meningococcal septicaemia will die. Where intensive care is unavailable this may rise to more than 40%.
  - Mortality of other causes of acute meningitis is generally much lower (around 2%).
- The most frequent complication of meningitis is hearing impairment or deafness, which may affect up to 10% of survivors.
- Survivors of septicaemia may require skin grafting of necrotic lesions and amputation of necrotic digits or limbs.
- In general, most survivors make a virtually complete recovery, although subtle neurological abnormalities (e.g. behavioural and developmental problems, mild motor abnormalities) are not uncommon.

Prevention of meningococcal disease
Education

Increasing awareness of primary healthcare workers and general public about the presenting symptoms of meningococcal disease and emphasising the need for early presentation and treatment may have a major impact on mortality and morbidity.

Prophylaxis of contacts

Transmission is via droplet spread to close contacts. Around 4–25% of people are colonised at any one time, but outbreaks of disease are not generally related to colonisation rate. Household contacts of a case may be at 800 times increased risk of disease compared with the general population.

Chemoprophylaxis is used to prevent secondary cases by eliminating nasal carriage. Administer as soon as possible (within 48 hours after presentation of the index case).

Follow local public health guidelines when determining who should receive antibiotic prophylaxis. In general, only immediate family (or those sharing accommodation) and kissing contacts should be treated. Healthcare workers should receive prophylaxis only where they have experienced extensive contact with the patient's respiratory secretions (e.g. during intubation).

Drugs for prophylaxis

Give rifampicin for 2 days for all household contacts:

- adults: 600 mg twice daily
- children aged 1 month to 12 years: 10 mg/kg twice daily
- neonates: 5 mg/kg twice daily.

In many countries rifampicin is protected from use for any disease other than TB. In this case consider giving ciprofloxacin orally as a single dose: adults, 500 mg; children aged 5–12 years, 250 mg; children aged 1 month to 5 years, 125 mg.

Vaccination

Where the index case has proven serogroup A or C disease, consideration should be given to vaccinating close contacts with appropriate polysaccharide or polysaccharide conjugate vaccine.

During larger outbreaks or epidemics, wider-scale prophylaxis is occasionally used, but should only be carried out under guidance of local/national public health authorities. Public education regarding presenting symptoms of meningococcal disease and emphasising the need for early presentation may be more beneficial than wide-scale distribution of antibiotics.

Vaccines based on the **capsular** polysaccharide of serogroups A and C (±Y and W-135) have been available for several years, and have been used for vaccination of contacts (as above) and for protection of travellers to endemic areas. They are unable to reliably induce immunity in infants and young children as their duration of protection is short.

They are not generally used for population vaccination campaigns except in epidemic situations.

Conjugated polysaccharide vaccines for serogroups A, C, Y and W-135 are now available and offer the possibility of inducing long term immunity in all age groups.

A vaccine against serogroup B has recently received a license.

Where widespread epidemics of meningococcal disease occur (e.g. in the meningitis belt in sub-Saharan Africa), mass vaccination campaigns have proved useful in reducing attack rate. Such campaigns are administered by local public health authorities.

6.1.H Pertussis

BOX 6.1.H.1 Minimum standards
- Immunisation.
- Erythromycin.
- Oxygen.
- Close monitoring for apnoea and hypoxaemia.

Introduction

Infection with the organism *Bordetella pertussis* (a Gram-negative bacillus) causes a clinical syndrome commonly referred to as 'whooping cough'. The illness classically has three stages.

- Stage 1: **Catarrhal stage** (1–2 weeks). The symptoms are those of an upper respiratory infection.

- Stage 2: **Paroxysmal stage** (2–4 weeks). The child has severe episodes of coughing – usually up to 10 coughs without drawing breath, and then a sharp inspiration or 'whoop'. The prolonged coughing (often with vomiting) may lead to poor feeding, with weight loss and sometimes rectal prolapse. Other complications such as subconjunctival haemorrhages and ulceration of the frenulum may develop.

- Stage 3: **Convalescent stage** (1–2 weeks). The episodes of coughing subside. Occasionally the child may continue to cough for months.

Pertussis should be prevented by universal infant immunisation. In some countries, immunisation is also given to the mother during pregnancy (28 to 38 weeks gestation) to prevent pertussis in infancy.

Effects on the young infant

Infants may become infected with pertussis before they have been immunised, or if immunisation is not available (or the parents have refused it). Young infants with pertussis have a different and serious clinical picture that includes the following:

- apnoea with hypoxaemia
- bradycardia
- seizures
- cough and poor feeding.

Diagnosis

The laboratory facilities needed to diagnose pertussis are not available in many hospitals. **Culture from a pernasal swab should be undertaken on Bordet–Gengou medium.** An absolute lymphocytosis (with a typical clinical picture) is highly suggestive (the total lymphocyte count may be over 30×10^9/litre).

Treatment

The following groups of children should be admitted to hospital

- infants under 6 months of age
- children with complications such as pneumonia, convulsions, dehydration or severe under-nutrition
- those with apnoea or cyanosis.

Supportive treatment

- Maintain nutrition and hydration.
- Give oxygen according to the criteria for acute lower respiratory infection (ALRI) (*see* Section 5.3.A).

- Give gentle suction of secretions (avoid triggering coughing).
- Low-dose continuous oxygen (0.5–1.0 litre/minute) via nasal cannulae may reduce apnoeic episodes in infants. Do not use nasopharyngeal cannulae, which can provoke coughing spasms.
- Do not give cough suppressants, sedatives or antihistamines.
- Encourage breastfeeding. If the infant cannot drink, pass a nasogastric tube.
- If there is severe respiratory distress, consider intravenous maintenance fluids to avoid aspiration, but avoid malnutrition.
- In some infants, the frequency of apnoeic episodes is high and requires ventilatory support.

Specific treatment

- Treat pneumonia that is complicating pertussis, according to the ALRI protocol in Section 5.3.A.
- Give DTP vaccine to any unimmunised siblings (*see* Section 1.17).
- Treat convulsions (*see* Section 5.16.E).
- Erythromycin will eradicate pertussis from the nasopharynx but has little effect on the severity or duration of clinical symptoms unless it is started very early in the disease. The oral dose of erythromycin is 12.5 mg/kg 6 hourly for neonates for 7 days and 125 mg 6 hourly for age 1 month to 2 years for 7 days. Azithromycin (10 mg/kg once daily) may also be given, and the course is shorter (3 days) but is not recommended under 6 months of age. Prophylaxis of other infants in the family is of no proven benefit, and has side effects.

6.1.I Relapsing fevers

> **BOX 6.1.I.1 Minimum standards**
> - Public health measures to kill lice.
> - Antibiotics: erythromycin, ceftriaxone.
> - Close observation for the Jarisch–Herxheimer reaction.

Epidemiology

Epidemic or louse-borne relapsing fever (LBRF), caused by *Borrelia recurrentis*, is transmitted by the human body louse (*Pediculus humanus*) (and occasionally the head louse (*P. capitis*) or, possibly, the crab louse (*Phthirus pubis*)), which becomes infected following a blood meal and remains infected for life. Humans are the reservoir host. The louse is crushed when the host scratches. *Borrelia* enters the new host via abrasions and mucous membranes. Bloodborne and congenital infections may also occur. Currently only endemic in Ethiopia, LBRF occurs in epidemics in situations of poor hygiene and overcrowding.

Endemic or tick-borne relapsing fever (TBRF) occurs in widespread endemic foci: central, eastern and southern Africa (*Borrelia duttonii*); north-western Africa and the Iberian peninsula (*B. hispanica*); central Asia and parts of the Middle East, India and China (*B. persica*); and various

regions of the Americas (*B. hermsii*, *B. turicatae*, *B. venezuelensis*). Animal reservoirs include wild rodents, lizards, toads, owls, pigs and chickens. Transmission to humans occurs following the bite of an infected argasid (soft) tick of the genus *Ornithodorus* via tick saliva or coxal fluid. Human congenital infections may also occur. TBRF is a common and under-diagnosed cause of fever in many parts of Africa.

Pathology

Borreliae multiply in blood by simple fission. They have a predisposition for reticulo-endothelial system and CNS, causing widespread vascular endothelial damage and platelet sequestration in the bone marrow. Clinical severity tends to correlate with the level of spirochaetaemia and relapses result from antigenic variation.

Clinical features

- Incubation period usually 4 to 8 days (range 2–15 days).
- TBRF usually clinically milder, but may be associated with up to 11 relapses.
- LBRF more severe, and rarely gives rise to more than three relapses.

- Typical features include sudden-onset high fever, headache, confusion, meningism, myalgia, arthralgia, nausea, vomiting, dysphagia, dyspnoea and cough (which may be productive of sputum containing *Borrelia*).
- Hepatomegaly is common (associated with jaundice in 50% of patients with LBRF, and in less than 10% of those with TBRF). Splenomegaly is common and splenic rupture may occur.
- Petechiae, erythematous rashes, conjunctival injection and haemorrhages are more common in LBRF.
- Complications include myocarditis, pneumonia, nephritis, parotitis, arthritis, neuropathies, meningoencephalitis, meningitis, acute ophthalmitis and iritis.
- The case fatality rate (CFR) may reach 70% in epidemics of LBRF, and is lower in children than in adults.
- CFR is usually less than 10% in untreated cases of TBRF, but tends to be higher in children and pregnant women.

Differential diagnosis

Malaria, typhus, typhoid, meningococcal septicaemia/meningitis, dengue, hepatitis, leptospirosis, yellow fever, other viral haemorrhagic fevers.

Diagnosis

- Giemsa- or Field-stained blood films reveal spirochaetes.
- *Borrelia* is also visible on unstained blood films using dark-field or phase-contrast microscopy.
- Centrifuge anticoagulated whole blood to concentrate spirochaetes above the buffy coat.
- The acridine orange-coated quantitative buffy coat (QBC) technique is also useful.
- Polymerase chain reaction (PCR) assays are now available for diagnosis and speciation.
- Serology is unreliable.
- Examination of the vector may be useful.

Treatment

- A single dose of antibiotic is effective in about 95% of cases of LBRF, and in up to 80% of cases with TBRF.
- Single-dose treatment is recommended in LBRF epidemics.
- TBRF relapses are less likely with a 5- to 10-day course of treatment.

Effective antibiotics include tetracycline, doxycycline, penicillin, erythromycin, chloramphenicol and ciprofloxacin. Choice will depend on the patient's age, contraindications and drug availability.

Ceftriaxone is recommended for patients presenting with meningitis or encephalitis.

In epidemics of LBRF, treatment of close contacts may also be recommended.

Usual dosage recommendations:

- LBRF: a single dose of one of the following:
  - doxycycline, 100 mg (non-pregnant adults)
  - tetracycline, 500 mg (non-pregnant adults)
  - erythromycin, 500 mg in adults and children over 5 years
  - erythromycin, 250 mg in children up to 5 years.
- TBRF: a 5-day course of one of the following:
  - doxycycline, 100 mg twice daily (non-pregnant adults)
  - erythromycin, 2 grams divided into two to four doses daily (adults)
  - erythromycin, 50 mg/kg divided into two to four doses daily (children).

Complications

A Jarisch–Herxheimer reaction (JHR) may occur in up to 80–90% of patients treated for LBRF, and in up to 50% of those treated for TBRF. This may be fatal in around 5% of cases.

- The reaction usually commences within 2 hours of the first dose of antibiotic.
- Symptoms include rigors, restlessness and anxiety, then a sharp rise in temperature, tachycardia and initial rise blood pressure, followed by marked vasodilation and sweating, which may result in collapse and shock.
- All patients must be closely monitored for a JHR. Intravenous fluids may be required to maintain blood pressure.
- Steroids are of no benefit.

Prevention and control

LBRF: improve hygiene, reduce crowding, delouse (DDT, permethrin or malathion powder to skin and clothing), heat treat/destroy clothing. Antibiotic prophylaxis may be recommended in high-risk situations.

TBRF: avoid tick habitats.

6.1.J Sexually transmitted diseases

> **BOX 6.1.J.1 Minimum standards**
> - Health education programmes.
> - Child protection in cases of abuse.
> - Antibacterial drugs.
> - Antiviral drugs.
> - Podophyllin/trichloroacetic acid.

Introduction

Anogenital infections in childhood are most commonly acquired through sexual contact or abuse, but may also arise as a result of close personal contact within the family or on the playground, and some systemic infections may be transmitted by sexual means without being considered venereal illnesses.

The diagnosis of sexually transmitted disease is considered in the following circumstances:

- a history of recent sexual abuse
- the isolation of sexually transmitted organisms in cases without obvious trauma leading to a diagnosis of chronic sexual abuse
- specific syndromes and diseases usually transmitted by the sexual route in adults
- congenital syphilis or perinatally acquired chlamydia

or gonorrhoea transmitted from the mother *in utero* or postnatally (*see* Section 3.4)

- HIV infection not acquired perinatally, through transfusion or another known mechanism.

There are more than 20 different infections that may be spread by the sexual route. These range from the classic sexually transmitted diseases (e.g. syphilis, gonorrhoea), through conditions that are mainly sexually transmitted (e.g. genital herpes, human papillomavirus), to those infections that can also be transmitted by sexual means (e.g. hepatitis B and C).

Sexual abuse
Children known to have been abused recently
Sexually abused children are at risk of acquiring an infection from the perpetrator. In relation to the high frequency of sexual abuse, the typical sexually acquired infections are fairly rare, but the risk depends on a number of epidemiological factors.

The diagnosis of potential infection of a child presenting with sexual abuse includes an active microbiological search by culture of vulval, perineal or anal swabs. Bacterial infections such as gonorrhoea, syphilis or chlamydia are usually manifested soon after the assault, with the development of local ulcers and infected vaginal or vulval discharge.

The sexually transmitted viral diseases such as herpesvirus type 2 can also become evident soon after the incident, but diseases with a longer latency period such as human papillomavirus are more difficult to link directly to the episode of sexual abuse.

The management of the child potentially infected after sexual abuse consists of the following:

- management of the sexual abuse (*see* Section 7.6)
- local management of injuries, including tetanus toxoid if applicable
- bacteriological swabs
- serological tests for syphilis, hepatitis B and HIV, repeated 6 weeks later
- prophylactic broad-spectrum antibiotics: ceftriaxone 50 mg/kg IM as a single dose (maximum dose 4 grams) plus erythromycin 20–40 mg/kg/day in three divided doses for 7 days
- post-exposure hepatitis B vaccination if not previously vaccinated; follow-up doses at 1–2 and 4–6 months after the first dose
- assessment of the risk of HIV transmission and prophylaxis if indicated.

Children are at higher risk because episodes of assault are often multiple and mucosal trauma is likely.

Factors that should be assessed include the following:
- assailant's HIV status or likelihood of having HIV
- time elapsed since incident (< 72 hours)
- exposure characteristics
- possible benefits and risks associated with post-exposure prophylaxis (PEP).

PEP is generally well tolerated in children. The choice of antiretroviral drugs will depend on local availability and policy. An example is a combination of zidovudine, lamivudine and lopinavir/ritonavir. Follow-up and appropriate treatment of identified infection (see below) should be undertaken.

The presence of a sexually transmissible infection in a child alerting to the possibility of sexual abuse
This group of children presents with symptoms and signs suggestive of genital, urinary or lower intestinal infection. In children aged around 2–10 years, the finding of genital, anal or pharyngeal infection with *Neisseria gonorrhoeae*, *Treponema pallidum* or *Chlamydia trachomatis* should prompt a search for evidence of sexual abuse. However, herpesvirus type 2, *Trichomonas vaginalis*, *Mycoplasma* species and bacterial vaginosis are not so commonly acquired as a result of sexually transmitted infection in this age group. Although human papillomavirus types 6, 11, 16 and 18 are also usually transmitted by sexual means and may present with condylomata, a long latency in the onset of clinical signs means that these may have been transmitted from mother to child during birth, and close domestic contact other than sexual abuse has also been shown in such cases.

Specific syndromes or diseases usually associated with sexual transmission in adolescent children
These conditions occur particularly in sexually active adolescents. In view of the rampant spread of HIV infection, the approach to the management of sexually transmitted diseases in children and adolescents must include the following aspects:

- Treatment of the symptoms and causes in a typical syndromic approach to STDs, as described below.
- Identification of those without symptoms. There is a recognised risk of co-infection, and as both syphilis and HIV may be asymptomatic, serological tests for syphilis (VDRL or RPR) and HIV (ELISA) should be offered with appropriate counselling in all patients.
- Prevention of new infection by education about safe sex practices and condom use.
- Motivation to engage in health-seeking behaviour.

Genital ulcers and lymphadenitis
The infections presenting with genital ulcers with or without inguinal adenopathy and bubos are most often acquired as a result of voluntary or involuntary sexual activity, but may occur as a result of non-sexual inoculation through close domestic or play contact or indirect transmission. The patient should be carefully examined to determine the site, number, size and appearance of the ulcers, the type of exudate, the presence of associated pain, erythema and swelling, or of draining lymphadenopathy.

Regional epidemiological factors determine the relative frequency and likelihood of genital herpes (herpesvirus type 2), syphilis, chancroid, lymphogranuloma venereum or granuloma inguinale.

Genital herpes
This causes painful vesicular or shallow ulcerative lesions on the genitals. Grouped or single lesions occur on a thin erythematous base but with generally uninflamed intervening epithelium. These regress spontaneously but may recur. Oral aciclovir 200 mg five times daily for 5 days does not

prevent future recurrences, but if started early, will reduce the intensity and duration of symptoms. Locally, anaesthetic and antiseptic creams help to relieve symptoms.

Chancre of primary syphilis

This is a painless ulcer with a serous exudate which is highly infectious. The diagnosis can be made by direct dark-field examination or immunofluorescent antibody stains. At this stage, serological tests for syphilis are usually still negative. The treatment in children over 12 years consists of benzathine benzylpenicillin, 50 000 U/kg IM as a single dose (50 000 U = 37.5 mg). Benzathine benzylpenicillin must not be given IV.

Chancroid

This is caused by *Haemophilus ducreyi*. Painful papulovesicles or ulcers on the genitals are associated with suppurative inguinal adenopathy. In the absence of adenopathy, the condition has to be differentiated from herpes or syphilis, the latter of which is usually painless. In treatment of children over 12 years of age, the following are satisfactory: azithromycin 1 gram orally as a single dose, ceftriaxone 250 mg IM as a single dose, or erythromycin base 500 mg orally four times daily for 7 days.

Lymphogranuloma venereum

Patients with lymphogranuloma venereum (LGV) commonly present with unilateral tender inguinal and/or femoral lymphadenopathy. Genital ulcers are usually less obvious and have often disappeared by the time of presentation. LGV is caused by *Chlamydia trachomatis.* Treatment for children over 12 years of age is with doxycycline 100 mg orally twice daily or erythromycin 500 mg orally four times daily, and should be continued for 21 days.

Granuloma inguinale

Klebsiella granulomatis is the cause of this ulcerative disease. The lesions are painless and slowly progressive. Subcutaneous granulomas often occur on the genitals and perineum, but regional lymphadenopathy is absent. Treatment is with doxycycline or erythromycin, as for LGV. Alternatively azithromycin, ciprofloxacin or trimethoprim-sulfamethoxazole can be used.

Urethritis and vulvovaginitis

These patients present typically with a discharge from urethra or vagina. The character of the discharge may be non-specific or it may have typical features allowing a presumptive diagnosis concerning its aetiology. Together with the discharge, there may be other features such as itching, discomfort or dysuria. There may be inflammatory erythema and swelling of the tissues. Where pruritus is a major symptom, *Trichomonas* or *Candida albicans* should be suspected. The appearance of the discharge may be typically white cheesy in *Candida*, or creamy-purulent and frothy in *Trichomonas* infection, but often is fairly non-specific.

The organisms responsible for this mode of presentation include *Neisseria gonorrhoeae, Chlamydia trachomatis, Trichomonas, Candida* species, *Gardnerella vaginalis* and *Ureaplasma* species. In the syndromic approach to the management of patients with surface epithelial infection, broad-spectrum treatment aimed at gonorrhoea, *Chlamydia* and *Trichomonas* or *Candida* is given at the same time as

bacterial swabs are taken for culture. Where laboratory resources are scarce, bacteriological investigations may be reserved for those not responding appropriately to the first course of therapy.

Recommended treatment for children over 12 years of age includes ceftriaxone 250 mg IM as a single dose, or cefixime 400 mg orally in a single dose, against *Neisseria gonorrhoeae*. Azithromycin, 1 gram orally as a single dose, or doxycycline 100 mg orally twice daily for 7 days (alternatively, erythromycin 40–50 mg/kg/day given as 4 divided doses 6 hourly for 14 days for children under 12 years) should be added for *Chlamydia*. If *Trichomonas* or bacterial vaginosis due to *Gardnerella vaginalis* is identified or strongly suspected, metronidazole is added as 15–30 mg/kg/day in three divided doses for 7 days. *Candida* infection can be treated with a short course (3 days) of topical azoles such as clotrimazole, miconazole or butoconazole cream. An alternative is treatment with local nystatin (100 000 U/mL three to four times daily), but this is less effective.

Acute balanoposthitis

Inflammation of the glans and prepuce can have a large number of infectious and also non-infectious causes. In the usual case, there is erythema and swelling of the glans and prepuce together with local exudate. Most such cases are not due to sexually transmitted infection, but are caused by beta-haemolytic streptococci, *Staphylococcus aureus* or *Candida albicans*. These may arise secondary to local trauma including ritual circumcision. Allergic contact dermatitis and rarer causes such as psoriasis or pemphigus should also be considered. Sexually transmitted organisms include *Chlamydia, Gardnerella vaginalis, Trichomonas, Candida albicans*, syphilis, herpes virus and papillomavirus. If 'milking' along the length of the urethra produces a purulent discharge, STDs are also more likely.

Accordingly, the evaluation of a boy presenting with balanoposthitis includes examination for the presence of urethral discharge and a urine dipstick. A swab should be sent for microbiological confirmation. A suggested treatment for children over 12 years is azithromycin 1 gram orally in one dose, or erythromycin 40–50 mg/kg per day in four divided doses for 14 days, plus metronidazole 15–30 mg/kg per day in three divided doses for 7 days. In the presence of urethral discharge, treatment should also include antibiotic cover for gonorrhoea.

Genital warts

Condylomata acuminata are fleshy, soft, pedunculated or flat warty lesions that may sometimes have quite a narrow base. They occur singly or in clusters. In sexually active adolescent boys, they may occur on the shaft or corona of the penis, and in girls on the genital mucosal surface both inside and outside the vagina. Perineal cutaneous condylomata are not always acquired sexually. Human papillomavirus (HPV) types 6 and 11 cause these warts. Apart from the visible wart, the infection may be quite asymptomatic, particularly where lesions occur intravaginally. They must be differentiated from the flat papular condylomata lata of syphilis, skin tags and molluscum contagiosum.

Local treatment is satisfactory in most instances, although recurrences occur. Trichloroacetic acid or 10–25% podophyllin may be applied to external lesions, taking care not to involve normal skin. Other precautions to avoid the development of complications include limiting the application to less than 0.5 mL of podophyllin and an area of over 10 cm^2 of warts per session. The preparation should be washed off 1–4 hours after application to reduce local irritation. The process can be repeated in 7 days. Other treatment modalities include cryotherapy, surgical excision, curettage or electrocautery. An alternative is not to treat, and to await possible spontaneous resolution.

The association with genital dysplasia and carcinoma should be remembered, and therefore Pap smears and regular follow-up are indicated in girls with human papillomavirus infection.

Two HPV vaccines are now available. They offer protection against HPV types that cause a large percentage of carcinomas as well as genital warts.

Pelvic inflammatory disease (PID) and epididymitis

The deep infections of the upper female genital tract present with features of infection, such as fever and leucocytosis, together with lower abdominal pain and a vaginal discharge. There may be signs of pelvic peritonitis or a tender mass on vaginal or rectal examination. Epididymitis in males presents typically with unilateral pain, swelling and tenderness of the testis, together with urethral discharge. This can be distinguished from testicular torsion by means of an ultrasound examination. In sexually active adolescents, these infections are most often caused by *Neisseria gonorrhoeae* or *Chlamydia trachomatis*. Such patients may be very ill and require hospitalisation including possible surgical drainage. General supportive therapy is given as required. The antibiotic therapy aims at the above two organisms and outpatient treatment typically includes a third-generation cephalosporin like ceftriaxone plus doxycycline. Metronidazole may be added to treat bacterial vaginosis which frequently accompanies PID.

In severe cases, or where there is no response to the above treatment within 72 hours, intravenous broad-spectrum antibiotics including an aminoglycoside and clindamycin should be given.

6.1.K Streptococcal disease

BOX 6.1.K.1 Minimum standards
- Antibiotics: penicillin and erythromycin.
- For resistant pneumococci: cefotaxime/ceftriaxone, vancomycin.
- Pneumococcal vaccine post-splenectomy and in sickle-cell disease.

Introduction

Streptococci are Gram-positive bacteria, of which the most important are:
- Group A streptococcus
- Group B streptococcus
- *Streptococcus pneumonia*.

Group A streptococci (GAS) *Streptococcus pyogenes*

This is a common commensal in the throat. It causes many diseases, as described below.

Head and neck
- Acute pharyngitis, retropharyngeal abscess and otitis media (*see* Section 5.1.C).
- Tonsillitis: GAS likely if exudate, tender anterior cervical lymph nodes, fever, no cough. Penicillin V for 10 days is the treatment of choice, but amoxicillin may be better tolerated in liquid form. GAS is always sensitive to penicillin. In penicillin allergy use a macrolide (although there is resistance to this group of antibiotics).
- Sinusitis: follows otitis media: coryza, postnasal drip, headache, fever.
- Brain abscess: this is a rare complication resulting from direct extension of an ear or sinus infection, or from haematogenous spread (*see* Section 5.16.K).

Skin and soft tissue
- Impetigo: purulent, yellow-crusted skin lesions (*see* Section 5.18).
- Pyoderma: papule becomes vesicular then pustular with a thick crust and surrounding erythema.
- Erysipelas: erythematous warm painful skin lesions with raised borders associated with fever.
- Cellulitis: local pain, tenderness, swelling and erythema associated with fever.

Skin infections are commonly co-infected with *Staphylococcus aureus*, which should be treated with flucloxacillin. Treat invasive disease with IV flucloxacillin, benzylpenicillin and clindamycin.

Necrotising fasciitis
- Pain disproportionate to physical findings: erythema may be absent or rapidly progress to purple with haemorrhagic fluid-filled blisters or bullae. Fever, malaise, myalgia, diarrhoea, anorexia. Spread through fascial planes requires early surgical exploration and resection. Give intravenous immunoglobulin (IVIG) (if available).

Myositis
- CT or MRI (if available) is useful for diagnosis.

Scarlet fever
- This presents with tonsillitis and a characteristic rash, circumoral pallor and strawberry tongue. Rash starts with generalised blanching erythema which is punctate (i.e. like sandpaper) and palpable, followed by desquamation.

Pneumonia
- Invasive GAS can rapidly progress to necrotising pneumonia with empyema (*see* Section 5.3.B).

Septicaemia
- Risk factors include burns and chickenpox. The main symptoms are fever, tachycardia, tachypnoea and hypotension.

Mediastinitis
- Rare but serious, frequent fatalities as often diagnosed late.

Toxic shock syndrome
- Systemic shock with multi-organ failure. Give IVIG (if available) (*see* Section 5.5.C).

Rheumatic fever
Acute rheumatic fever
- **Major criteria:** carditis, Sydenham chorea, polyarthritis, erythema marginatum, subcutaneous nodules.
- **Minor criteria:** fever, arthralgia, raised ESR or CRP, prolonged PR interval on ECG.

Two major or one major and two minor criteria with evidence of preceding GAS throat infection confirm a diagnosis of rheumatic fever (*see* Section 5.13).
   Rheumatic heart disease results in chronic valvular damage, predominantly of the mitral valve.

Glomerulonephritis
- Acute renal failure with haematuria and proteinuria days after streptococcal pharyngitis (*see* Section 5.6.A).

Group B streptococci (GBS)
Streptococcus agalactiae
This species colonises 15–45% of healthy women and can cause severe infections in the puerperium and in the neonate.
   Postpartum infection (*see* Section 2.5.G).

Neonatal infection
- Early onset (first week of life) (*see* Section 3.4) associated risk factors: prematurity, prolonged rupture of membranes, maternal intrapartum fever, chorioamnionitis, maternal UTI, previous baby with GBS disease.

- Late onset (1 week to 3 months of age) causes sepsis and meningitis: not prevented by peripartum antibiotics.

Empirical IV treatment with ampicillin and gentamicin for 5 days. Then, once GBS is confirmed, treat sepsis with benzyl penicillin for 7 days if meningitis is excluded by lumbar puncture. If meningitis is not excluded, treat for 14 days.

Maternal
- Septic abortion, puerperal sepsis, urinary tract infection.

Streptococcus pneumoniae
Gram-positive diplococcus (lancet shaped). At least 85 pathogenic serotypes are known. Types 1, 3, 4, 6, 7, 8, 9, 12, 14, 18, 19 and 23 are the most virulent.
- Common infections include pneumonia, meningitis, peritonitis, otitis media, sinusitis, arthritis and conjunctivitis.
- Pneumococcal infections are more common in children with defective splenic function (e.g. sickle-cell anaemia, splenectomy); also nephrotic syndrome, chronic renal failure, diabetes mellitus, malabsorption, heart failure, skull fracture, neurosurgery and those with congenital or acquired immunodeficiency such as agammaglobulinaemia, and HIV infection.
- Patients with white blood cell counts of more than 15×10^9/litre are likely to have bacteraemia.
- Culture of *Streptococcus pneumoniae* from the respiratory tract is not useful because many people are asymptomatic carriers.

Treatment
- In the last two decades, resistance of *S. pneumoniae* to antibiotics such as penicillin and chloramphenicol has emerged.
- In many countries, up to 5–40% of isolates may be resistant to penicillin G.
- If resistance to chloramphenicol or penicillin is suspected, give either cefotaxime or ceftriaxone. If resistance to these two drugs is considered, add vancomycin to ceftriaxone or cefotaxime. If results of sensitivity confirm susceptibility to penicillin G, ceftriaxone or cefotaxime should be given and vancomycin should be stopped.

TABLE 6.1.K.1 Antibiotic doses for streptococcal disease

Disease	Antibiotic	Dose and route	Dose interval	Duration/comments
Otitis media	Amoxicillin (oral)	12.5 mg/kg orally	8 hours	5–7 days
	Amoxicillin – clavulanic acid	12.5 mg/kg orally	8 hours	5–7 days
	Cefaclor	12.5 mg/kg orally	8 hours	5–7 days
	Erythromycin	12.5 mg/kg orally	6 hours	5–10 days
Sinusitis	As for otitis media	As for otitis media	As for otitis media	As for otitis media
Meningitis	Penicillin G	50 mg/kg IV	4–6 hours	10–14 days for all antibiotics below
	Chloramphenicol	Load 50 mg/kg IV, then 25 mg/kg	6 hours	
	Cefotaxime	50 mg IV	6–8 hours	Maximum single dose 4 grams
	Ceftriaxone	100 mg IV	24 hours	Maximum single dose 4 grams/day
	Vancomycin	Load 15 mg/kg IV then 10 mg/kg IV	6 hours	Total daily dose not more than 2 grams Drug levels needed
	Meropenem	10–20 mg/kg slow IV injection over 5 minutes	8 hours	Maximum single dose 2 grams

Pneumococcal vaccine

- Give pneumococcal conjugated vaccine (e.g. Prevenar 13), two doses starting at 2 months of age, with 2 months between doses, with a reinforcing dose at 12–13 months, or if over 1 year old give a single dose.
- At-risk groups (see above) should have conjugate vaccine (any age) followed by polysaccharide vaccine (23 serotypes) over 2 years of age with a repeat dose every 5 years.

Chemoprophylaxis

- Daily oral penicillin V (125 mg twice daily for children

under 5 years, 250 mg twice daily for older children) is recommended for children at risk (see above).

Other groups of streptococci (C, D, E, F, G, H, K, L, M, N, O and V)

- These cause diseases such as infective endocarditis, urinary tract infection and pneumonia. Susceptibility to penicillin is variable, and treatment with an aminoglycoside (e.g. gentamicin) and penicillin G or ampicillin is recommended.

TABLE 6.1.K.2 Streptococci and related conditions

Streptococci	Group Lancefield	Reaction (Haemolytic)	Disease caused
S. pyogenes (GAS)	A	J	Tonsillitis, pyoderma, impetigo, scarlet fever (subsequent rheumatic fever, acute glomerulonephritis)
			Necrotising fasciitis, toxic shock syndrome
S. agalactiae (GBS)	B	J	Neonatal sepsis/meningitis
S. equisimilis (GCS)	C	J	Endocarditis, pneumonia, cellulitis, septicaemia
S. faecalis (GDS)	D	J or none	Normal gut flora. May cause peritonitis, urinary tract infection, endocarditis and septicaemia
S. viridians	–	I	Mouth commensal. May cause endocarditis, dental caries
S. pneumoniae	–	–	Pneumonia, meningitis, otitis media, sinusitis

6.1.L Tetanus

BOX 6.1.L.1 Minimum standards
- Immunisation and prevention.
- ABC, especially airway protection.
- Anti-tetanus immunoglobulin and tetanus toxoid.
- Wound care.
- Diazepam, magnesium sulphate and phenobarbitone for acute spasms.
- Morphine.
- Early IV penicillin and/or metronidazole.
- Close observational care in a high-dependency area.

Introduction

Generalised tetanus (lockjaw) is a neurological disease manifesting as trismus and severe muscular spasms. It is caused by a neurotoxin produced by the anaerobic bacterium *Clostridium tetani* in a contaminated wound. The different forms of tetanus include the following:

- **Neonatal tetanus** is a form of generalised tetanus occurring in newborn infants lacking protective passive immunity because their mothers are not immune.
- **Localised tetanus** manifests as local muscle spasms in areas contiguous to a wound.
- **Cephalic tetanus** is a dysfunction of cranial nerves associated with infected wounds on the head and neck. Both of the latter conditions may precede generalised tetanus.

Tetanus continues to cause thousands of deaths per year worldwide (*see* Figure 6.1.L.1). The World Health

Organization estimates that 59 000 newborns worldwide died in 2008 as a result of neonatal tetanus.

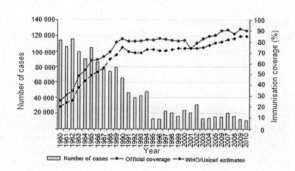

FIGURE 6.1.L.1 Total tetanus global annual reported cases and coverage, 1980–2010. Source: WHO/IVB Database, 2011.

For infection to occur, two conditions must be met:
1. a wound with a degree of necrosis
2. a wound contaminated with material containing *Clostridium tetani* (a Gram-positive obligate anaerobe widely distributed in the environment).

The umbilical stump is a common site of entry for neonatal tetanus, which carries up to 60–80% mortality. Ear piercing in neonates is also a common cause (e.g. in Vietnam). In up to 30% of infected children no wound can be found. Cases of tetanus in older children follow small puncture wounds, accidents and trauma in the partial or unvaccinated child.

Pathogenesis

Once the *C. tetani* spore is inoculated into necrotic tissue with a low oxygen concentration it changes into a vegetative form, which elaborates the powerful toxin, tetanospasmin, which ascends peripheral nerves to the spinal cord where it binds to cerebral gangliosides and impairs inhibitory synapses. This causes muscle rigidity, spasm and autonomic overactivity.

Clinical presentation

A previously well neonate presents at 3–20 days with irritability, decreased sucking, trismus, muscle spasms or convulsions. An older child presents following a minor injury or bite. Some infections follow chronic otitis media.

The clinical presentation depends upon the distance the injury is from the spinal cord. The incubation period ranges from 3 to 21 days. The shorter the incubation period and the time from onset of symptoms to the first spasm, the worse the outcome.

More than 90% of patients develop trismus ('locked jaw') due to the short pathway of the fifth cranial nerve. As the disease progresses, spasm of muscle groups supplied by other cranial nerves occurs, including the seventh cranial nerve, resulting in facial muscle rigidity and risus sardonicus. Spasm of the pharyngeal muscles may result in dysphagia, and spasm of the laryngeal muscles may result in asphyxia. The **generalised muscle spasms are extremely painful**, and may be prolonged, giving rise to opisthotonus. The sympathetic system can be affected, causing lability of temperature, blood pressure and cardiac function.

Early signs will be helpful in making the diagnosis. The mother may complain of an abnormal cry ('baby cannot cry well'), because she has noticed that trismus prevents the mouth from opening. This happens before suckling is affected. If one is uncertain, a slight touch stimulus may initiate spasm or rigidity. History of the birth (usually at home) and of how the cord was cut is informative, although not particularly discriminating. Contamination at birth (e.g. being born on to the floor with or without cord cutting with an unsterile instrument) is more likely to result in tetanus than for example contamination following a circumcision, but either could be responsible.

The diagnosis of tetanus is made clinically by excluding other causes of tetanic spasms, such as hypocalcaemic tetany, phenothiazine reaction, strychnine poisoning, and hysteria in the older child.

Management of established tetanus

The approach to treatment given in this subsection is appropriate for both neonatal and childhood tetanus.

The aims of management are as follows:
- neutralising existing toxin and preventing its further production
- control of spasms
- prevention of complications
- providing adequate nutrition.

On admission

- Secure and maintain the airway, and ensure adequacy of ventilation.
- Insert an intravenous line. IV infusions, even slow IV administration of drugs, may not be possible, because of lack of a suitable IV giving set (even as simple as a burette type) equipment or skilled time. However, an IV cannula should be left *in situ* for drug and antibiotic administration.
- **IM injections must be avoided at all costs, as they will provoke spasms.**
- If the baby or child is in **acute spasm**, this should be terminated by giving **diazepam by bolus IV infusion over 15 minutes (dose 300 micrograms/kg) or rectally (400 micrograms/kg)**. Ensure that for intravenous infusion, diazepam is diluted to 100 micrograms/mL and that extravasation does not occur (very irritant).
- Also give an IV loading dose of 25–40 mg/kg of magnesium sulphate over 20–30 minutes (maximum loading dose is 2 grams).
- **Always have a bag-mask available in case the patient stops breathing as a result of the diazepam and/or magnesium.**
- When the patient is stable, a nasogastric tube, ideally passed by an anaesthetist, will allow fluids, food and drugs to be given with minimal disturbance. Feeds need to be given frequently (ideally hourly) and in small amounts due to reduced gut motility. **In the neonate, regular breast milk feeds via a nasogastric tube are essential.**
- Any obvious wound should be debrided and cleansed, especially if extensive necrosis is present, and previously ill-advised sutures should be removed. In neonatal tetanus, wide excision of the umbilical stump is not indicated.
- Finally, the disease itself does not induce immunity, so after recovery tetanus vaccine must be given for future prevention.

Antibiotics

- Oral (or intravenous) metronidazole (30 mg/kg per day, given in divided doses at 6-hourly intervals; maximum dose 400 mg) is effective in decreasing the number of vegetative forms of *C. tetani* and is the antimicrobial agent of choice.
- IV benzylpenicillin 100–200 mg/kg/day, given in divided doses at 4- to 6-hourly intervals; (75 mg/kg/day in the neonate in 3 divided doses) for the first 48 hours then oral penicillin V 25 mg/kg 6 hourly is an alternative treatment. Therapy for 10–14 days is recommended. Oral therapy can be given after the initial period.

Associated septicaemia is not uncommon in the neonate, and additional broader-spectrum antibiotics will often be required (*see* Section 3.4 for treatment of neonatal sepsis). Hospital-acquired infections are also common, especially pneumonia, and should be appropriately treated.

Neutralisation of toxin

Antitetanus human immunoglobulin (HTIG) is the preparation of choice for neutralising unbound tetanospasmin. It is given by intravenous infusion over 30 minutes at a dose of **5000–10 000 units immediately on admission.** Adverse reactions are rare. **Local instillation is of no benefit.**

For neutralisation of the toxin, HTIG is not available in most countries where it is needed. An equine immunoglobulin may be available and is used (500–1000 units/kg IM; maximum dose 20 000 units). There is a risk of anaphylaxis (*see* Section 5.1.B for management), so adrenaline must be immediately available if equine immunoglobulin is given. Immune globulin intravenous (IGIV) contains antibodies to tetanus and can be considered for treatment in a dose of 200–400 mg/kg if HTIG is not available.

Management of spasms and hypertonicity

- Spasms can usually be controlled by slow IV injection of diazepam, 200 micrograms/kg followed by IV 25–40 mg/kg of magnesium sulphate over 20–30 minutes (maximum loading dose 2 grams).
- Subsequently give IV diazepam (200 micrograms/kg every 4–6 hours) and magnesium sulphate (10–20 mg/kg 2- to 4-hourly IV).
- Stop diazepam if magnesium alone controls the spasms.
- Reduce the dose of diazepam if apnoeic episodes occur.
- **Always have a bag-mask available in case the patient stops breathing as a result of the diazepam and/or magnesium.**
- Give paracetamol 25 mg/kg 6-hourly for pain (20 mg/kg in the neonate). If this is insufficient, the WHO pain ladder approach should be adopted. Oral or IV morphine may be needed (*see* Section 1.15).

Alternative antispasmodic or sedative drugs

- Phenobarbitone (15 mg/kg in one or two divided doses) as a loading dose then 5 mg/kg given once daily can be used for breakthrough spasms.

Ventilation and prevention of complications

Hospitals in regions with a high prevalence of neonatal tetanus may not have appropriate facilities for ventilation, or even for emergency intubation of neonates; bag-and-mask ventilation, when apnoeic attacks occur, may be the only alternative.

Many patients have major problems with pharyngeal spasms/upper airway obstruction and are sometimes best managed with a tracheostomy and pharmacological control of the spasms (sometimes the tracheostomy may need to be undertaken as an emergency procedure). Up to a third of those who need a tracheostomy do not require ventilation.

- Intubation can be very difficult because of pharyngeal/laryngeal spasm, and often a mini-tracheostomy without prior intubation may be appropriate, provided experts for the procedure and anaesthesia are present.
- Infusions of morphine are essential to minimise suffering due to severe pain. Under no circumstances should paralysing drugs be given to children who are intubated and ventilated without infusions of morphine.

Neonates rarely receive ventilation. Also, few places where tetanus occurs will have appropriate ventilators, or staff who are skilled in intubation and ventilation of children. An alternative way to support breathing is by bag-and-mask ventilation as often as necessary for the apnoeas that occur secondary to bouts of spasms and/or the drugs given to treat the spasms.

Good nursing and frequent monitoring, with particular attention to gentle suction under direct vision of secretions from the airway, maintenance of adequate hydration, temperature, mouth hygiene, turning of the patient to avoid orthostatic pneumonia and bed sores, will reduce complications.

- The child should be nursed in a quiet environment with low-level lighting. Sudden loud noises should be avoided.
- It will be helpful to involve the mother in management to call the staff if the baby goes into spasm or stops breathing. She can also be taught to feed the baby by tube (including checking position by suction of the tube before each feed) and taught minimal handling techniques. She could also count minor spasms, although she may not be able to chart them.
- Invasive procedures should be kept to a minimum and preceded by appropriate analgesia. There must be **continuous** observation by experienced personnel.
- In a high-dependency care unit, cardiac function should ideally be monitored by ECG to detect toxin-induced arrhythmias and autonomic instability.

TABLE 6.1.L.1 Guide to tetanus prophylaxis in routine wound management in children

History of absorbed tetanus toxoid (doses)	Clean, minor wounds		All other wounds[a]	
	Td or Tdap[b]	HTIG[c]	Td or Tdap[b]	HTIG[c]
Less than 3 or unknown	Yes	No	Yes	Yes
3 or more[d]	No[e]	No	No[f]	No

Td = adult-type diphtheria and tetanus toxoid vaccine, Tdap = booster tetanus toxoid, reduced diphtheria toxoid and acellular pertussis, HTIG = human tetanus immune globulin.

[a] Such as, but not limited to, wounds contaminated with dirt, faeces, soil and saliva, as well as puncture wounds, avulsions, and wounds resulting from missiles, crushing, burns and frostbite.

[b] Tdap is preferred to Td vaccine for adolescents who never have received Tdap vaccine. Td is preferred to tetanus toxoid (TT) vaccine for adolescents who have received Tdap vaccine previously, or when Tdap vaccine is not available.

[c] Immune globulin intravenous should be used when HTIG is not available.

[d] If only three doses of fluid toxoid have been received, a fourth dose of toxoid, preferably an adsorbed toxoid, should be given. Although licensed, fluid tetanus toxoid rarely is used.

[e] Yes, if 10 years or more have elapsed since the last tetanus-containing vaccine dose.

[f] Yes, if 5 years or more have elapsed since the last tetanus-containing vaccine dose. More frequent boosters are not needed, and can accentuate adverse effects.

- High-dependency care of severe cases of tetanus may be necessary for up to 3–4 weeks.

It is important to realise that the child/baby has unimpaired consciousness and is aware of what is taking place. Prescribe regular and frequent analgesia, as antispasmodics alone do not prevent the suffering resulting from painful spasms or painful procedures. The spasms are also very frightening and distressing for the parents.

Rigidity will take longer to resolve than the spasms.

Monitoring
Only absolutely essential blood tests should be performed, to avoid precipitating spasms.

- Glucose, urea and electrolytes.
- A chart of the occurrence of spasms can be helpful.
- Cardiac monitoring.
- Pulse oximetry.
- Fluid input/output.
- Calorific intake.

Prognosis
The prognosis for neonatal tetanus is poor, especially with a short incubation period (< 7 days) or with rapid evolution of symptoms. Pyrexia, tachycardia and frequent spasms (> 20 spasms in 24 hours) also indicates a poor prognosis. Quality of nursing care and the **availability of high-dependency care facilities greatly affect the outcome, and where these facilities are available mortality may be as low as 20%.**

In children who survive neonatal tetanus, motor difficulties may be permanently present. Older children may have muscle weakness and atrophy, and difficulties with speech, balance and memory.

Prevention
Every child should receive tetanus vaccine according to the expanded programme of immunisation (EPI). All pregnant women should receive two doses antenatally, as this will protect the baby for the first 4–6 months of age.

Tetanus toxoid should be given, combined with diphtheria and pertussis, to infants according to national schedules. Note that both HIV infection and placental malaria reduce the transplacental transfer of anti-tetanus antibodies *in utero*. Sterile handling of the umbilical cords by midwives or appropriately trained traditional birth attendants should also reduce the incidence of neonatal tetanus. Sterilisation of hospital supplies will prevent the rare instances of tetanus that may occur in a hospital from contaminated sutures, instruments or plaster casts.

A booster tetanus toxoid vaccine with or without tetanus immune globulin (TIG) in the management of wounds depends on the nature of the wound and the history of immunisation with tetanus toxoid (*see* Table 6.1.L.1).

Further reading
World Health Organization (2014) *Immunisation Surveillance, Assessment and Monitoring.*
www.who.int/immunization_monitoring/diseases/tetanus/en/

6.1.M Trachoma

> **BOX 6.1.M.1 Minimum standards**
> - Bilamellar tarsal rotation.
> - Oral azithromycin.
> - Ocular tetracycline.
> - The WHO SAFE strategy: Surgery for trichiasis, Antibiotics to clear infection, and Facial cleanliness and Environmental improvement.

Introduction
Trachoma is the most common infectious cause of blindness worldwide. It is caused by *Chlamydia trachomatis*, certain serotypes of which preferentially infect the conjunctival epithelium. The organism is transmitted from person to person by direct contact, fomites (objects capable of carrying infectious organisms), and eye-seeking flies. Disease clusters in families; the greatest risk factor for infection is sharing a bedroom with an active case. Repeated episodes of infection over many years cause an accumulation of scar tissue in the tarsal plate and tarsal conjunctivae of the upper lids. Contraction of the scar may produce trichiasis and/or entropion, and the resulting corneal abrasion by in-turned lashes leads to corneal scarring. This eventually causes blindness. In paediatric practice in endemic areas, active trachoma is seen frequently. Blinding complications may start to appear in the second and third decades of life.

Clinical features
These are best presented using the framework of the WHO simplified clinical grading system. Examination for trachoma involves inspection of the lashes and cornea, followed by eversion of the upper eyelids to examine the tarsal conjunctivae (*see* Figure 6.1.M.1). A ×2.5 magnifying loupe and torch (or daylight) should be used. These tools are sufficient to determine the presence or absence of signs that are considered in this grading scheme. Each eye is graded separately.

Trachomatous inflammation – follicular (TF): the presence of five or more follicles at least 0.5 mm in diameter in the central part of the upper tarsal conjunctiva. Follicles appear as white or yellow-grey semitransparent patches or swellings beneath the conjunctiva. Fewer than five follicles, or follicles at the nasal or temporal margin, may be normal.

Trachomatous inflammation – intense (TI): pronounced inflammatory thickening of the upper tarsal conjunctiva obscuring more than half of the normal deep tarsal blood vessels.

TF and TI are both forms of 'active trachoma'; they are associated with infection with *Chlamydia trachomatis*, although **not all infected individuals exhibit these signs, and not all individuals with these signs are infected.** Patients with active trachoma may be asymptomatic or complain of irritable red eyes or a whitish discharge.

Trachomatous scarring (TS): the presence of easily visible scars in the tarsal conjunctiva. Scars appear as white bands, lines, or sheets. TS is the result of repeated cycles of inflammation and resolution over many years and itself is virtually asymptomatic, although scarring of eyelid glands may produce symptoms of dry eye.

Trachomatous trichiasis (TT): at least one eyelash rubs on the eyeball, or there is evidence of recent removal of in-turned eyelashes. TT is intensely irritating to the sufferer, and they may choose to pull out their eyelashes in an attempt to reduce the discomfort. There may be discharge from superadded bacterial infection of the abraded cornea. Except in hyperendemic areas, it is unusual to observe TT in children.

Corneal opacity (CO): easily visible corneal opacity over the pupil, so dense that at least part of the pupil margin is blurred when viewed through the opacity. Such corneal opacities cause significant visual impairment.

It is important to remember that these grades are not mutually exclusive. A patient with active trachoma (TF and/or TI) may also show signs of the late complications of the disease.

There are other signs of trachoma that are not included in the simplified grading scheme:

- Papillae are often visible in individuals with active trachoma, but are not specific for trachoma. These are small elevations of the conjunctival surface that give the conjunctiva a velvety appearance. They are more easily seen using a slit lamp.
- Fibrovascular connective tissue may grow inwards from the limbus to invade the anterior layers of the superior cornea in response to infection. The ingrowth is known as pannus. The new blood vessels may persist after resolution of infection.
- Sometimes follicles are found under the bulbar conjunctiva at the limbus as well as deep to the tarsal conjunctiva. Scarring of limbal follicles may subsequently leave small depressions known as Herbert's pits.

Treatment

For active trachoma (TF and/or TI), antibiotics are required. Topical tetracycline eye ointment 1% is effective when applied to both eyes twice daily for 6 weeks. A single dose of oral azithromycin (20 mg/kg, up to a maximum dose of 1 gram) is just as effective, is better tolerated than topical tetracycline, and can be directly observed, so is associated with higher compliance rates.

Trichiasis or entropion requires surgical management to restore the margin of the eyelid to its normal position, so that contact between the lashes and globe is interrupted. Bilamellar tarsal rotation is the procedure currently recommended by the World Health Organization; it is performed under local anaesthetic and can be undertaken at the village level by trained ophthalmic nurses or ophthalmic assistants.

Corneal opacity can theoretically be managed by corneal graft. Unfortunately, few endemic countries have the resources to establish a transplant programme, and because of new vessel growth from the limbus and abnormalities of the tear film in the trachomatous eye, the risk of graft rejection or failure is very high.

The identification of signs of trachoma in an individual should prompt screening of other members of that individual's community. Antibiotic treatment of individuals presenting

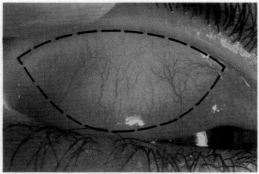

a *Normal tarsal conjunctiva (×2 magnification). The dotted line shows the area to be examined.*

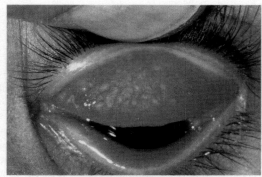

b *Trachomatous inflammation – follicular (TF).*

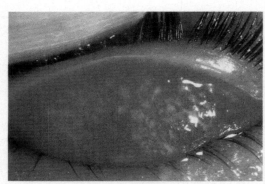

c *Trachomatous inflammation – follicular and intense (TF + TI).*

FIGURE 6.1.M.1 (a) Normal tarsal conjunctiva (×2 magnification). The dotted line shows the area to be examined. (b) Trachomatous inflammation – follicular (TF). (c) Trachomatous inflammation – follicular and intense (TF + TI).

to healthcare facilities is unlikely to have any impact on the incidence of blindness from trachoma in the communities from which those individuals come. Comprehensive community-based management of trachoma is necessary wherever the prevalence of disease is high.

Prevention

Blindness from trachoma is preventable. The acronym SAFE has been adopted by the WHO and partners to encapsulate the recommended approach to controlling trachoma. It comprises Surgery for trichiasis, Antibiotics to clear infection, and Facial cleanliness and Environmental improvement (provision of water and acceptable means for disposal of human faeces) to reduce transmission. Surgery should be offered to all individuals with trichiasis. The 'A', 'F' and 'E' components should be implemented district-wide

wherever the prevalence of TF in 1- to 9-year-olds is 10% or higher. The WHO plans to use the 'SAFE' strategy to achieve the elimination of trachoma as a public health problem by the year 2020.

6.1.N Tuberculosis

BOX 6.1.N.1 Minimum standards
- All children with suspected TB should be tested for human immunodeficiency virus (HIV).
- All children with HIV should have a chest X-ray to look for TB.
- Children who cannot expectorate spontaneously should have induced sputum or gastric aspirate.
- Specimens should be sent for both microscopy for acid-fast bacilli and TB culture or Xpert MTB/RIF test.
- Drug-resistant TB needs expert supervision.
- Tracing, screening and prophylaxis of contacts.

Introduction

The global incidence of tuberculosis (TB) has been falling since 2002. However, in 2009 there were still almost 10 million children who were orphans as a result of parental deaths caused by TB. About 13% of TB cases occur among people living with HIV. India and China accounted for 40% of notified cases and Africa accounted for another 24%. Treatment for smear-positive pulmonary TB was 87% in 2009.

Major factors in the global increase in tuberculosis since the mid-1980s include the HIV pandemic, migration of people from countries with a high prevalence of tuberculosis to industrialised countries (particularly refugees), poverty, overcrowding and failure of investment in tuberculosis control programmes. Multi-drug resistance is a major concern.

Epidemiology
- In low-income countries, the risk of developing infection is up to 2.5% per annum.
- The age group at highest risk of developing disease is 0–5 years, with risk up to 30–40% (especially under 1 year) and at puberty.
- Spread is by untreated smear-positive adults who may infect up to 10–15 people per year.
- Children are generally non-infectious, except for older children and adolescents with cavitary TB.
- Children with untreated tuberculosis contribute to the pool of adults with reactivated disease.
- The WHO estimates that TB in children contributes to 1.3 million annual cases (or 15%) in low-income countries and 450 000 deaths worldwide.

Factors that predispose tuberculosis-infected children to develop systemic disease
- Age under 5 years, and especially under 1 year.
- Household contact with smear-positive disease.
- Malnutrition.
- Tuberculosis infection in previous 2 years.
- Immunosuppression, especially HIV infection.

Tuberculin skin test
- The tuberculin skin test (TST), also called the Mantoux test, is useful for screening contacts. The TST is less useful for diagnosing active TB because a negative result does not exclude TB. If TB is clinically suspected, efforts should be made to collect diagnostic specimens, exclude other causes, and then treat if TB is the most likely diagnosis (do not treat as a diagnostic test).
- Use either 5 TU of tuberculin (PPD-S) or the 2 TU of tuberculin (PPD RT2 3).
- Inject tuberculin (PPD-S) **intradermally** into the upper third of the flexor surface of the forearm with a 1-mL syringe and a short bevel gauge 25–27 needle producing a wheal of at least 5 mm. Read the transverse diameter of induration at 48–72 hours. Regard induration of 0–5 mm as negative, 6–9 mm as indeterminate, and likely to be associated with environmental mycobacteria, and 10 mm or more as indicative of infection with *Mycobacteria tuberculosis*, except in the child who has had BCG in the previous few years, when induration of 15 mm is required.
- In resource-limited countries where BCG is given at birth, most children will have a negative tuberculin test by 10 years of age, and thus an induration of 10 mm in children this age or older may be regarded as supportive of *M. tuberculosis* infection.
- Negative or reduced response to tuberculin occurs in malnutrition, immunosuppression associated with HIV or other immunodeficiency states, recent viral or some bacterial diseases such as pertussis, overwhelming tuberculosis and non-respiratory tuberculosis. Thus with these conditions an induration of 6–9 mm may be indicative of tuberculosis.
- Remember that a negative tuberculin does not exclude tuberculosis, and additional work-up may be warranted in any suspected child.
- Tuberculin skin test interpretation must be undertaken bearing in mind the age, epidemiology and underlying illness, if any.

Serology

Antibody tests are inconsistent and imprecise. They do not improve outcomes for patients and should not be used. The WHO recently gave guidelines recommending against the use of serology tests for TB. It is the first negative recommendation to be made by the WHO, describing it as 'inaccurate and useless', after 'overwhelming' evidence that suggested it produced an 'unacceptable level' of false-positive or false-negative results.

Pathogenesis

- Inhalation of the tubercle bacillus into an alveolus establishes the primary (Ghon) focus. In the 4- to 8-week period before the cell-mediated immune (CMI) response develops, there is spread to regional lymph nodes, and small numbers of bacilli disseminate throughout the body in the lympho-haematogenous system.
- Certain organs favour survival of tubercle bacilli, including regional nodes, epiphyseal lines of bones, cerebral cortex, renal parenchyma and apical regions of the lungs (Simon focus).
- Establishment of an adequate CMI response (which coincides with the appearance of sensitisation to tuberculin) in most cases results in control or eradication of proliferating tubercle bacilli at these sites.
- The primary focus is seldom detected on chest X-ray; enlarged hilar/paratracheal nodes or parenchymal complications are the usual evidence of the primary complex.
- **Primary tuberculosis of the lung** is usually a manifestation of lympho-bronchial disease, with local compression or erosion of the bronchi. **Extrathoracic disease** is due to local spread of disease at metastatic sites (e.g. lymph nodes, brain, bone, kidney and abdomen).
- Dissemination of large numbers of tubercle bacilli may result in acute miliary disease or, less commonly, a chronic disseminated (cryptic) tuberculosis.
- Erythema nodosum and phlyctenular conjunctivitis are hypersensitivity reactions which may occur during primary tuberculosis.
- The risk of developing symptomatic disease following primary tuberculosis is highest (around 50%) in the first 1 to 2 years after infection and the rest in the individual's lifetime.

Tuberculosis in adolescence

This may result from reactivation of a primary infection, exogenous infection, or both. There is a strong hypersensitivity reaction in the lungs with local infiltration and often cavity formation. Pulmonary lymph node enlargement and extra-thoracic dissemination is uncommon.

Clinical features

In well-resourced countries, the majority of children with respiratory tuberculosis are asymptomatic and are picked up through contact tracing and will generally have early primary disease. In resource-limited countries, only children with symptomatic disease present, and they are therefore only 'the tip of the iceberg'.

The following are some of the key features of tuberculosis in children:

- Fever, cough, anorexia, weight loss, wheezing, night sweats and malaise are common.
- Extrapulmonary disease may involve other tissues and organs, such as the central nervous system, lymph nodes and gastrointestinal tract.
- Findings can include lung findings (dull resonance) or involvement of other organs in extrapulmonary tuberculosis, such as hepatosplenomegaly, lymphadenopathy, mass, etc. (see Table 6.1.N.1).

HIV and tuberculosis

Children living with HIV who have poor weight gain, fever or current cough, or contact history with a TB case, may have

TABLE 6.1.N.1 Typical features of common forms of extrapulmonary TB in children

Type of extrapulmonary TB	Key clinical findings
TB lymphadenitis (most common)	Enlargement and swelling of lymph nodes
Pleural/pericardial TB	Cough and shortness of breath
TB meningitis	Headache, vomiting, fever, neck stiffness, seizures, confusion and coma
Miliary TB	Very sick, respiratory distress, hepatosplenomegaly, diffuse lymphadenopathy
Gastrointestinal TB	Abdominal pain, diarrhoea, mass or ascites
Spinal TB	Backache with or without loss of function in lower limbs
TB arthritis	Pain and swelling of joints (usually monoarthritis)

TB and should be evaluated for TB and other conditions. If the evaluation shows no TB, children should be offered isoniazid preventive therapy (IPT) regardless of their age.

Children living with HIV who do not have poor weight gain, fever or current cough are unlikely to have active TB. Children living with HIV who are more than 12 months of age and who are unlikely to have active TB on symptom-based screening and have no contact with a TB case should receive 6 months of IPT (10 mg/kg/day, maximum 300 mg/day) as part of a comprehensive package of HIV prevention and care services.

With regard to children living with HIV who are less than 12 months of age, only those who have contact with a TB case and who are evaluated for TB (using investigations) should receive 6 months of IPT if the evaluation shows no TB disease. All children living with HIV after successful completion of treatment for TB disease should receive isoniazid for an additional 6 months.

- Features of tuberculosis in children with perinatally acquired HIV infection are not well defined.
- Many HIV-infected infants probably succumb to bacterial infections and *Pneumocystis jirovecii* pneumonia before contracting tuberculous infection.
- In older children, there is difficulty in diagnosis due to the following reasons:
  - The tuberculin reaction is positive in only 20% of cases.
  - There is confusion with HIV-related respiratory disorders, including lymphocytic interstitial pneumonitis (LIP), superimposed viral/bacterial infections, chronic interstitial pneumonitis, Kaposi's sarcoma and bronchiectasis.
  - There is often a lack of facilities for culturing *M. tuberculosis*.
- Atypical clinical and radiological features of TB are much more common in children with HIV with more severe and complicated disease.
- HIV/tuberculosis co-infected children are more likely to develop disseminated tuberculosis and meningitis, have cavitary pulmonary disease and may have a poor response to treatment and a higher mortality if not started on ART.

- Because of the difficulty in confirming tuberculosis in symptomatic HIV-infected children, many children probably receive unnecessary tuberculous chemotherapy.
- Finger clubbing may be seen in chronic tuberculosis, and is common in HIV-related pulmonary disorders.
- Standard 6-month chemotherapy is given in uncomplicated pulmonary tuberculosis.

Respiratory tuberculosis
- Most respiratory tuberculosis results from complications of lympho-bronchial disease and includes segmental lesions, consolidation, collapse and obstructive emphysema.
- In young children, small cavities may develop during the course of primary (especially progressive) tuberculosis, but they are classically seen in the adolescent period.
- Large pleural effusions usually occur in older children and adolescents.
- Radiological features of pulmonary tuberculosis may be atypical in HIV infection, other immunosuppressed states and/or malnutrition.

Pericarditis
Tuberculosis should be considered in all cases of pericarditis. *M. tuberculosis* may be cultured from a pericardial tap in over 50% of the cases.

Lymph node disease
- This may result from a focus in the upper lung fields or from haematogenous spread.
- Diagnosis may be made by biopsy or fine-needle aspiration.
- Swelling and softening of nodes may continue for months after treatment has been completed.
- In well-resourced countries, environmental mycobacteria are now a far commoner cause of chronic granulomatous disease of cervical lymph nodes than tuberculosis in indigenous young children.

Miliary tuberculosis
- This is commonest in young children and in those who are immunosuppressed, usually occurring within 3–12 months of primary infection.
- Chest X-ray (except in the early stages) will demonstrate a 'snowstorm' or miliary appearance.
- Meningitis is a common complication. Therefore a lumbar puncture should be performed in all cases.
- The WHO advises 9–12 months of anti-TB chemotherapy.

Meningitis
- This is commonest in children under 5 years, and often occurs within 6 months of infection.
- The onset is usually insidious and the diagnosis is often delayed. Late diagnosis is invariably complicated by neurological dysfunction or death.
- Prolonged fever, irritability, headache, vomiting, mental status changes, visual symptoms, focal neurological deficits or cranial nerve palsies, and seizure are some of the common presentations in children with tuberculous meningitis.
- CSF: cell count is usually less than 500/mm^3 and mainly lymphocytic, but polymorpho-neutrophils may be prominent early on, which may cause confusion with partially treated bacterial meningitis. Protein levels are usually

raised (0.8–4 grams/litre) and glucose levels are low. However, on admission CSF values may be within normal limits and lumbar puncture must be repeated if there is any doubt.
- **Brain imaging, such as CT or MRI (if available)**, should be undertaken at diagnosis and at 3–4 months, and at any time when there is neurological deterioration, to detect complications such as hydrocephalus and tuberculomata.

Management
- A four-drug regimen in the upper range of drug doses is recommended for 2 months, followed by a two-drug regimen for 10 months in uncomplicated tuberculosis meningitis. It consists of the following four drugs given for first 2 months:
  - H: isoniazid 20 mg/kg once daily orally, or by IM or slow IV injection; (maximum 300 mg daily) **plus**
  - R: rifampicin 15–20 mg/kg once daily orally or by IV infusion over 2–3 hours; (maximum 600 mg daily) **plus**
  - Z; pyrazinamide 40 mg/kg once daily orally; (maximum 2 grams daily) **plus**
  - E: ethambutol 20 mg/kg once daily orally (maximum 1.5 grams daily).

Thereafter, isoniazid **plus** rifampicin alone are continued for 10 months. The WHO also now advises 12 months of therapy, although shorter regimens have been shown to be adequate in some studies.

Corticosteroids must be given in all cases with initiation of therapy. Dexamethasone 0.6 mg/kg/day in two divided doses or prednisolone 2–4 mg/kg/day is given for 4 weeks and tapered over 2 weeks for a total duration of 6 weeks.

A ventriculo-peritoneal shunt may be required for obstructive hydrocephalus (if available).

Bone and joints
- These are frequently missed in the early stages because of a low index of suspicion.
- The spine is affected in 50% of the cases, followed by knee, hip and ankle. The most serious complication is spinal compression.
- The diagnosis is made by histology, Ziehl–Neelsen (ZN) stain and mycobacterial culture of tissue that may be positive, and **if in doubt specimens should be sent for polymerase chain reaction (PCR)**.
- **The WHO advises the standard 12 months of anti-TB chemotherapy, similar to that for TB meningitis.**

Abdominal tuberculosis
- This may present with ascites, abdominal nodes or masses, or diarrhoea with or without abdominal pain, or as gastrointestinal obstruction.
- The diagnosis is usually made on bacteriological examination of ascitic fluid or a biopsy.
- The standard three- to four-drug regimen is used for therapy for a total of 6–9 months in uncomplicated cases.
- Ultrasound and **CT or MRI (if available) may be required in evaluation and to detect any complications**.

Perinatal tuberculosis
- Congenital tuberculosis is rare but should always be

considered in sick neonates or infants, especially in areas where HIV/tuberculosis co-infection is common.

- If a mother has completed tuberculosis chemotherapy during pregnancy or has inactive disease, her infant should be given BCG at birth.
- If she has active disease or is still requiring treatment, the infant should be given isoniazid 10 mg/kg once daily for 3–6 months.
- Once the mother and infant are both on appropriate treatment, the infant may breastfeed unless the mother has multi-drug-resistant TB. A tuberculin test and chest X-ray is then performed on the infant. If they are negative, BCG is given; if it is positive, full investigations for tuberculosis are undertaken. If no evidence of disease is detected, isoniazid is continued for another 3–4 months. If tuberculosis is suspected, full treatment with 4 drugs is given at standard doses (see Table 6.1.N.2 and Table 6.1.N.3 on management).

Danger signs for TB
- Suspicion of tuberculous meningitis.
- Extensive pulmonary or miliary TB.
- TB in an infant or a child with HIV.
- Symptoms and signs such as seizures, coma, severe respiratory distress, gastrointestinal obstruction or severe malnutrition.

Diagnosis of TB

Diagnosis depends on eliciting key points that may increase the yield of TB cases. A high index of suspicion in a child who has prolonged or unexplained illness should warrant investigation for TB. Sputum or gastric aspirate for acid-fast bacilli (AFB) stain and culture should always be attempted.

Standard methods for diagnosis are the tuberculin test and a chest X-ray. Even in resource-limited countries, every effort should be made to obtain a diagnostic specimen from gastric aspiration or sputum induction (see below). In poor communities the tuberculin test is often negative (or unavailable) and the chest X-ray might not be available, easy to interpret or have films of good enough quality. Many children are often over-diagnosed, especially in areas with high HIV prevalence.

TB infection is diagnosed using the tuberculin skin test. It is considered positive if there is Mantoux induration of ≥ 10 mm in children who have not received BCG vaccination or ≥ 15 mm in children who have received BCG recently. Interferon-gamma release assays (IGRA) detect latent and active infection but cannot differentiate between the two. They may be positive in some cases of HIV infection and malnutrition when the tuberculin test is negative, but in these circumstances there is also a higher rate of false-negative IGRA results. However, they are currently too expensive for resource-limited countries, and their routine use is not advised by the WHO.

Key features suggestive of pulmonary TB
Three or more of the following should strongly suggest a diagnosis of TB:
- chronic symptoms suggestive of TB (prolonged fever, cough, night sweats weight loss)
- physical signs suggestive of TB (chronic lymphadenopathy, abdominal mass, gibbus or monoarthritis)
- a positive tuberculin skin test (induration > 10 mm)
- chest X-ray suggestive of TB (hilar adenopathy, cavitation, pleural effusion, infiltrate; see below for pictures).

Investigations
- Tuberculin test > 10 mm or > 5 mm in malnutrition or HIV.
- Chest X-ray: lymphadenopathy, collapse/consolidation with or without persistent opacity, cavitation, miliary appearance.
- Histology: lymph node or other tissue biopsy.
- Smear/culture: gastric aspirate, induced sputum, nasopharyngeal aspirate, laryngeal swab, bronchoscopy or body fluids.
- Ultrasound: chest, abdomen, lymph nodes, pericardium and brain.
- **CT or MRI (if available).**
- HIV antibody tests (if relevant).

Except in adolescents with cavitary disease, most tuberculosis in children is paucibacillary (low number of mycobacteria). Young children cannot expectorate.

Tuberculosis may be evident on chest X-ray, especially in older children.
- Gastric aspiration should be undertaken in the early morning while the child is lying down. Ziehl–Neelsen (ZN) staining of gastric aspirate is positive in only about 10% of children with advanced pulmonary tuberculosis, and culture is positive, under optimal conditions, in only 30–50% of cases.
- Alternative methods are sputum induction using nebulised 3% hypertonic saline, nasopharyngeal aspiration and laryngeal swabs. None of these has a sensitivity of more than 25–30%. Sputum induction requires a nebuliser and appropriate equipment, and must be undertaken in a room with adequate ventilation.
- **The polymerase chain reaction (PCR) on histological specimens may be useful if the ZN stain is negative.** In CSF it has similar sensitivity (around 50%) to culture. It is reserved for special cases where an urgent diagnosis is required.
- Young children, especially those who are sick, malnourished or deteriorating, or where tuberculous meningitis is suspected, should be considered for treatment even though investigations are inconclusive. In other cases with pulmonary disease where the diagnosis is not clear, a course of appropriate antibiotics should be given for 7–10 days and the chest X-ray repeated after 2 weeks or so. If there is no improvement or deterioration, a full course of anti-tuberculosis chemotherapy may be given and progress carefully monitored to document the response. If the tuberculin test is negative initially it should be repeated after 3 months, when the patient's immune system has normalised, and it may become reactive at that time.
- Increase in weight (measured daily or weekly) and loss of fever (measured twice daily) indicate a response to treatment. If treatment is given for suspected rather than proven tuberculosis, and no resolution or improvement in symptoms occurs within 4 weeks, this suggests that tuberculosis is unlikely. However, the course should still be completed and an alternative diagnosis sought, such as drug-resistant tuberculosis, fungal infection or malignancy.

Xpert MTB/RIF test

The Xpert MTB/RIF is a test for rapid diagnosis of TB and drug-resistant TB. It is a TB-specific automated, cartridge-based nucleic amplification assay, and it detects *Mycobacterium tuberculosis*, as well as mutations conferring resistance to rifampicin, directly from sputum in an assay that provides results within 100 minutes.

Results from field demonstration studies found that a single Xpert MTB/RIF test can detect TB in 99% of patients with smear-positive pulmonary TB and more than 80% of patients with smear-negative pulmonary TB. The co-existence of HIV does not significantly affect the performance of Xpert MTB/RIF.

Furthermore, Xpert MTB/RIF can detect rifampicin resistance with 95.1% sensitivity and exclude resistance with 98.4% specificity. The WHO endorsed the Xpert MTB/RIF assay in December 2010. It should be used as the initial test in individuals with suspected multi-drug-resistant TB (MDR-TB) or HIV/TB. It may be used as a follow-on test to microscopy where MDR-TB and/or HIV is of lesser concern, especially in smear-negative specimens. It is effective in children where sputum may need to be obtained by induction via nasopharyngeal aspirate after salbutamol and then saline nebuliser.

Management of TB in children

With the exception of CNS and osteo-articular disease (see below), both pulmonary and extra-pulmonary tuberculosis may be treated with standard 6-month chemotherapy. The standard treatment regimen for all patients with drug-susceptible, uncomplicated TB is made up of an intensive phase lasting 2 months and a continuation phase lasting 4 months. During the intensive phase 4 drugs (isoniazid, rifampicin, pyrazinamide, and ethambutol) are used to rapidly kill the tubercle bacilli. Infectious patients become less infectious within approximately 10–14 days of starting treatment and symptoms abate. In the continuation phase, 2 drugs (isoniazid, rifampicin) are used, over a period of 4 months.

For non-HIV-infected children with a low risk of isoniazid resistance, ethambutol can be omitted. Ethambutol should not be given in a dose higher than 20 mg/kg/day to children under 5 years, as they may be unable to report visual disturbance associated with optic neuritis.

TABLE 6.1.N.2 Regimens for treatment of uncomplicated susceptible pulmonary tuberculosis

Regimen	Total duration
Standard daily	
Isoniazid, rifampicin, pyrazinamide ethambutol* for 2 months, then isoniazid, rifampicin for 4 months†	6 months
Intermittent three times weekly	
Isoniazid, rifampicin, pyrazinamide, ethambutol for 2 months, then isoniazid, rifampicin three times weekly for 4 months	6 months

* In HIV-uninfected children with a low risk of isoniazid resistance, ethambutol can be omitted.

† For central nervous system and osteo-articular disease, the continuation phase should be 10 months (total duration 12 months).

Thiacetazone is no longer used as a first-line drug. Thiacetazone may cause severe reactions in HIV-infected patients.

Presently DOTS (directly observed treatment, short course) is not generally practised for children, as it is assumed that parents will supervise treatment, but where DOTS is practised in the community it may be appropriate to include children.

During the continuation phase of treatment, thrice-weekly regimens can be considered for children known to be HIV-uninfected and living in an area of low HIV prevalence and settings with well-established directly-observed therapy (DOT). However, our advice is that in low resource settings, all children with TB should be treated with daily regimes (for dosage *see* Table 6.1.N.4).

For central nervous system and osteo-articular disease, the continuation phase should be 10 months (total duration 12 months).

Adverse reactions to tuberculosis chemotherapy are uncommon and if they occur it is usually within 6–8 weeks of starting treatment. Liver transaminases may increase two- to threefold during treatment with isoniazid and rifampicin, but drug therapy may be continued if there is no jaundice or symptoms of liver toxicity (e.g. nausea, vomiting, malaise or liver tenderness). Viral hepatitis (especially hepatitis A) should be considered if jaundice occurs. Adjunct treatment with corticosteroids in meningitis is indicated at initiation of therapy (see above) and may enhance resolution of disease in lympho-bronchial disease, pericarditis, pleural effusion and severe miliary disease with alveolar capillary block. Prednisolone 1.5–2.0 mg/kg/day is given for 2–3 weeks and then tailed off over 2 weeks (see treatment of meningitis).

Follow-up

All children who are started on anti-tuberculous therapy must be followed closely, preferably every month. Clinical, radiologic and mycobacteriologic improvement and adverse effects of drugs must be monitored. In children, weight gain and resolution of signs and symptoms are indicators of a good response to treatment. Routine laboratory tests such as liver function tests and X-rays are rarely needed in children. Those children with severe disease, poor response,

TABLE 6.1.N.3 Summary of treatment of pulmonary or peripheral lymph node TB

Area of low HIV prevalence with low levels of isoniazid resistance and child HIV-negative	*2-month intensive phase* Isoniazid Rifampicin Pyrazinamide *4-month continuation phase* Isoniazid Rifampicin
Area of high HIV prevalence or high levels of isoniazid resistance or extensive pulmonary disease	*2-month intensive phase* Isoniazid Rifampicin Pyrazinamide Ethambutol *4-month continuation phase* Isoniazid Rifampicin

TABLE 6.1.N.4 Daily dosage schedule for anti-tuberculous drugs and side effects

Drug	Children: once daily dose	Adolescents under 50 kg: once daily dose	Adolescents over 50 kg: once daily dose	Side effects
Isoniazid daily	10 mg/kg range 7–15 mg/kg Maximum 300 mg 15–20 mg/kg for meningitis	5 mg/kg Maximum 300 mg	5 mg/kg Maximum 300 mg	Hepatic enzyme elevation, hepatitis, peripheral neuropathy, hypersensitivity
Rifampicin	15 mg/kg range 10–20 mg/kg Maximum 600 mg 15–20 mg/kg in meningitis	10 mg/kg Maximum 600 mg	10 mg/kg Maximum 600 mg	Orange discoloration of urine and secretions (and contact lenses), nausea, vomiting, hepatitis, febrile reactions, thrombocytopenia
Pyrazinamide	35 mg/kg range 30–40 mg/kg 40 mg/kg in meningitis	25 mg/kg Maximum 1.5 gram	25 mg/kg Maximum 2.0 gram	Hepatotoxicity, hyperuricaemia, gastrointestinal upset, arthralgia, skin rash
Ethambutol	20 mg/kg range 15–25 mg/kg 20 mg/kg in meningitis	15 mg/kg Maximum 2.5 grams	15 mg/kg Maximum 2.5 grams	Optic neuritis, skin rash

Higher range of isoniazid applies to young children. Use mean dosage and round up rather than round down when prescribing except when prescribing ethambutol.

TABLE 6.1.N.5 Three times weekly dosage schedule for anti-tuberculous drugs (from the WHO)

Drug	Children: three times weekly dose given once daily	Adolescents under 50 kg: three times weekly dose given once daily	Adolescents over 50 kg: three times weekly dose given once daily
Isoniazid	20–40 mg/kg Maximum 900 mg	10 mg/kg Maximum 900 mg	10 mg/kg Maximum 900 mg
Rifampicin	10–20 mg/kg Maximum 600 mg	10–20 mg/kg Maximum 600 mg	10 mg/kg Maximum 600 mg
Pyrazinamide	50–70 mg/kg Maximum 3 gram	35 mg/kg Maximum 3 gram	35 mg/kg Maximum 2.5 gram
Ethambutol	25–30 mg/ kg	25–30 mg/kg	25–35 mg/kg

unusual presentations or suspected resistant TB must be referred to an expert.

Multi-drug-resistant TB (MDR-TB) and extreme-drug-resistant TB (XDR-TB)

Rapid drug susceptibility testing of isoniazid and rifampicin should be done at the time of diagnosis (if available). After treatment is started for MDR-TB, further sputum (induced or gastric aspirate) should be obtained monthly to ensure successful treatment. An expert in the management of paediatric TB must be involved in choosing the optimal regimen for a child with drug-resistant TB.

Fluoroquinolones may be used in treatment of MDR-TB in children. Theoretical concerns about cartilage damage from early trials in young dogs have not been evident in children, and these are far outweighed by the benefits in treatment of TB. Later-generation fluoroquinolones (see below) are more effective than earlier ones. Four second-line anti-tuberculous drugs should be used and the intensive phase should include ethionamide or prothionamide, pyrazinamide, a parenteral agent, and cycloserine (or para-aminosalicylic acid (PAS) if cycloserine cannot be used).

The intensive phase should be at least 8 months and the total duration at least 20 months if there was no previous MDR-TB treatment. The continuation phase is usually given as the same oral drugs while stopping the injectable drugs. In children with HIV and MDR-TB, antiretrovirals should be started as soon as possible following initiation of anti-tuberculous therapy, irrespective of CD4 count. The preferred regimen is zidovudine, lamivudine and efavirenz, but if already on antiretrovirals, continue the same regimen. Co-trimoxazole should be added for pneumocystis prophylaxis.

Treatment should be ambulatory rather than in hospital as much as possible.

Groups of second-line anti-tuberculosis agents
Second-line parenteral agent (injectable anti-tuberculosis drugs)
- Kanamycin (Km), 15–30 mg/kg/day (maximum 1000 mg).
- Capreomycin (Cm), 15–30 mg/kg/day (maximum 1000 mg).
- Streptomycin (S) 15–20 mg/kg/day (maximum 1.0 gram).

Fluoroquinolones
- Levofloxacin (Lfx), 15–25 mg/kg/day (maximum 1000 mg).
- Moxifloxacin (Mfx), 7.5–10 mg/kg/day (maximum 400 mg).
- Ofloxacin (Ofx), 15–20 mg/kg/day (maximum 800 mg).

Oral bacteriostatic second-line anti-tuberculosis drugs
- Ethionamide (Eto), 15–20 mg/kg/day (maximum 1000 mg).
- Cycloserine (Cs), 10–20 mg/kg/day (maximum 1000 mg).

TABLE 6.1.N.6 Recommended anti-tuberculous drugs according to resistance pattern of TB culture from list above

Resistance pattern	Change to:
Pan-susceptible	Category 1 (HREZ) (Isoniazid: H Rifampicin: R Ethambutol: E Pyrazinamide: Z)
H (with or without Streptomycin (S))	R − E − Z (6–9 months)
Polyresistant but not MDR	Continue the empirical second-line regimen. Consult with a specialist. Patient may require a combination of first- and second-line drugs
HR HRE	Z − S − Lfx − Eto − Cs − PAS
HREZ	S − Lfx − Eto − Cs − PAS
HRS HRES HREZS	Km − Lfx − Eto − Cs − PAS
Resistance to any second-line drug	Continue the empirical second-line regimen. Consult with a specialist

- Terizidone (Trd), 10–20 mg/kg/day (maximum 1000 mg).
- p-aminosalicylic acid (PAS), 150 mg/kg/day (maximum 8 grams (PASER)).

Prevention of TB

- Diagnosis and treatment of 'smear-positive' tuberculosis in adults combined with contact tracing is the key to prevention of childhood tuberculosis.
- Tuberculin-positive children with normal chest X-rays should be given prophylaxis, either isoniazid (10 mg/kg/day, maximum dose 300 microgram) alone for 6 months or in low-incidence countries, isoniazid and rifampicin for 3 months. The age limit for prophylactic therapy depends on national policy, for example, under 5 years in low-income countries as per WHO recommendations.
- HIV-infected infants and children exposed to tuberculosis infection but without active disease should

receive isoniazid prophylaxis as described above. The WHO advises that HIV-infected children over 1 year old who are unlikely to have tuberculosis, even in the absence of exposure to tuberculosis, should receive a routine course of isoniazid for 6 months. There must be facilities for investigation of tuberculosis and regular follow-up. However, a recent double-blind, randomised, placebo-controlled trial (*see* Further reading below) of pre-exposure isoniazid prophylaxis against tuberculosis showed that this does not work for primary prophylaxis. It did not improve tuberculosis-disease-free survival among HIV-infected children or tuberculosis-infection-free survival among HIV-uninfected children immunised with BCG vaccine.

- Neonatal BCG may reduce the risk of tuberculosis meningitis and disseminated disease by 60–80%, especially in children under 5 years of age. However, it has a limited efficacy against pulmonary disease. Because of the increased risk of disseminated BCG infection in HIV-infected infants, the WHO advises that all infants **known to be HIV-infected** should **not** receive BCG. However, this has practical implications in resource-limited countries where PCR is not usually available to detect HIV infection in infants under 18 months of age.

Further reading

World Health Organization (2012) *Global Tuberculosis Control*.

World Health Organization (2009) *Treatment of Tuberculosis*, 4th edn.

World Health Organization (2010) *Rapid Advice: Treatment of tuberculosis in children*.

World Health Organization (2010) *Antiretroviral Therapy for HIV Infection in Infants and Children: towards universal access*.

World Health Organization (2011) *Guidelines for the Programmatic Management of Drug-Resistant Tuberculosis*.

World Health Organization (2008) *Management of MDR-TB: a field guide*.

World Health Organization (2011) *Guidelines for intensified tuberculosis case-finding and isoniazid preventive therapy for people living with HIV in resource-constrained settings*.

World Health Organization (2014) *Guidance for National Tuberculosis Programmes on the management of Tuberculosis in Children, Second edition*. www.who.int/tb/publications/childtb_guidelines/en/

Madhi SA, Nachman S, Violari A *et al.* (2011) Primary isoniazid prophylaxis against tuberculosis in HIV-exposed children. *New England Journal of Medicine*, **365**, 21–31.

British National Formulary for Children (BNFC) 2014–15.

Donald PR, Shoeman JF, Van Zyl LE *et al.* Intensive short course chemotherapy in the management of tuberculous meningitis. *Int J Tuberc Lung Dis.* 1998; **2**: 704–11.

6.1.O Typhoid or paratyphoid

BOX 6.1.0.1 Minimum standards
- Blood culture and full blood count.
- Antibiotics: chloramphenicol, amoxicillin, ceftriaxone, ciprofloxacin.
- Public health measures.
- Sanitation, hygiene and preventive vaccines.

Typhoid

Epidemiology

Despite major advances in public health and hygiene in much of the developed world, typhoid fever continues to plague many resource-limited countries. Although accurate community-based figures are unavailable, it is estimated that over 30 million cases occur annually, with the vast majority of cases in Asia leading to an estimated 200 000 deaths. Population-based incidence rates are estimated at 500–1000 cases per 100 000 population in endemic areas. However, there is a paucity of information from Africa, and preliminary data indicate that the burden in Africa, in urban settings, may also not be far behind that of Asia.

In recent years, typhoid fever has been notable for the emergence of drug resistance. The first cases of chloramphenicol-resistant typhoid emerged in the early 1970s, followed by the emergence of multi-drug-resistant (MDR) typhoid in the mid-1980s. This organism is resistant to ampicillin, chloramphenicol and trimethoprim-sulphamethoxazole (co-trimoxazole)). Over the last few years, however, the development of quinolone and third-generation cephalosporin resistance in *Salmonella typhi* from various parts of Asia has raised the extremely worrying prospect of a 'super-resistant' variant of typhoid in addition.

In contrast to classic descriptions of milder disease, because of increasing drug resistance in *Salmonella paratyphi*, paratyphoid fever is now of comparable severity and virulence to typhoid fever. Both types of illness will therefore be described.

TABLE 6.1.0.1 Common clinical features of typhoid fever in childhood (Karachi, Pakistan)

High-grade fever	95%
Coated tongue	76%
Anorexia	70%
Vomiting	39%
Hepatomegaly	37%
Diarrhoea	36%
Toxicity	29%
Abdominal pain	21%
Pallor	20%
Splenomegaly	17%
Constipation	7%
Headache	4%
Jaundice	2%
Obtundation (reduced alertness)	2%
Ileus	1%
Intestinal perforation	0.5%

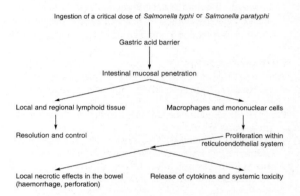

FIGURE 6.1.0.1 The pathogenesis of typhoid.

Pathogenesis

The disease is spread by the ingestion of a Gram-negative flagellar organism, *Salmonella enterica* serovar Typhi (*S. typhi*). A larger infecting dose leads to a shorter incubation period and a more severe infection.

The organism crosses the intestinal mucosal barrier after attachment to the microvilli by an intricate mechanism involving membrane ruffling, actin rearrangement and internalisation in an intracellular vacuole. Once inside the intestinal cells, *S. typhi* bacteria find their way into the circulation and reside within the macrophages of the reticulo-endothelial system.

The clinical syndrome is produced by the release of pro-inflammatory cytokines (the interleukins IL-6 and IL-13 and tumour necrosis factor-α, TNF-α) from the infected cells, leading to fever, rigors, inanition (the exhausted condition that results from lack of food and water) and anorexia. Local effects such as intestinal haemorrhage and perforation are comparatively rare in childhood, as there is relative lymphoid hyperplasia of the intestinal wall. However, malnourished children, especially adolescents, may be at greater risk of these complications.

Clinical features

The classic stepladder rise of fever is relatively rare in childhood. Much of the presentation of typhoid fever in

various geographical locations and populations is modified by coexisting morbidities and early administration of antibiotics. In malaria-endemic areas and in parts of the world where schistosomiasis is common, the presentation of typhoid may also be atypical. Data in Table 6.1.0.1 from a consecutive series of 2000 cases show the common clinical features of typhoid in endemic areas.

Although data from South America and parts of Africa suggest that typhoid may present as a mild illness in young children, this may vary in different parts of the world. There is emerging evidence from South Asia from both community and health facility settings that the presentation of typhoid may be more dramatic in children under 5 years of age, with comparatively higher rates of complications and hospitalisation. Diarrhoea, toxicity and complications such as disseminated intravascular complications are also more common in infancy, with higher case-fatality rates. However, some of the other features of typhoid fever seen in adults, such as relative bradycardia, are rare, and rose spots may only be visible at an early stage of the illness in fair-skinned children.

It must also be recognised that MDR typhoid appears to be a more severe clinical illness with higher rates of toxicity, complications and case-fatality rates. This appears to be a consistent finding and potentially related to the increased virulence of MDR *S. typhi* as well as higher rates of bacteraemia. In endemic areas, therefore, it may be prudent to treat all severely ill toxic children, especially those requiring hospitalisation, with second-line antibiotics.

Acute perforation of the intestine with haemorrhage and peritonitis can occur. This presents with severe abdominal pain, vomiting, abdominal tenderness, severe pallor and shock. An abscess may form together with enlargement of the liver and spleen. Management of peritonitis is described in Section 5.19.

Diagnosis of typhoid

The sensitivity of blood cultures in diagnosing typhoid fever in many parts of the developing world is limited, as microbiological facilities may be basic, and widespread antibiotic prescribing may render bacteriological confirmation difficult. Although bone marrow and **duodenal fluid cultures** may increase the likelihood of bacteriological confirmation of typhoid, these are difficult to obtain and they are invasive.

The serological diagnosis of typhoid is also fraught with problems, as a single Widal test may be positive in only 50% of cases in endemic areas, and serial tests may be required in cases presenting in the first week of illness. **Newer serological tests such as a dot-ELISA, co-agglutination and the Tubex® are promising**, but are comparatively expensive, may not be effective in primary care settings and have yet to find widespread acceptability.

The mainstay of diagnosis of typhoid in endemic areas therefore remains clinical. **Thus any high-grade fever of more than 72 hours' duration associated with any of the above-mentioned features, especially with no localising upper respiratory signs or meningitis or malaria, must be suspected as typhoid and managed accordingly.** While leucopenia (white blood cell count $< 4 \times 10^9$/litre) with a left shift in neutrophils may be seen in a third of children, young infants may also commonly present with a leucocytosis.

Typhoid treatment

Making an early diagnosis of typhoid fever and instituting appropriate supportive measures and specific antibiotic therapy is the key to the appropriate management of typhoid fever. The following are the important principles of management:

- Adequate rest, hydration and attention to correction of fluid-electrolyte imbalance.
- Antipyretic therapy (paracetamol) as required if fever is > 39°C.
- A soft, easily digestible diet should be continued unless the child has abdominal distension or ileus.
- Regular monitoring for clinical recovery and potential complications.
- Antibiotic therapy: the right choice, dosage and duration are critical to curing typhoid with minimal complications. Traditional therapy with either chloramphenicol or amoxicillin is associated with relapse rates of 5–15% and 4–8%, respectively.
- **If drug resistance is not locally a problem**, start with oral chloramphenicol and/or oral amoxicillin/ampicillin (initially intravenous if vomiting).
- **If drug resistance is prevalent**, use cefixime or ceftriaxone or ciprofloxacin (associated with higher cure rates).

Although epidemics are usually associated with a single dominant clone of *S. typhi*, in endemic situations there may be several coexistent strains of *S. typhi*, and a clinical judgement may need to be made when instituting antibiotic therapy before culture results become available. This is particularly important as delay in the institution of appropriate second-line antibiotic therapy in resistant cases of typhoid leads to a significant increase in morbidity and mortality. Despite the availability of newer orally administrable drugs such as quinolones and third-generation cephalosporins, blanket administration of these agents to all cases of suspected typhoid is expensive and will only lead to the rapid development of further resistance.

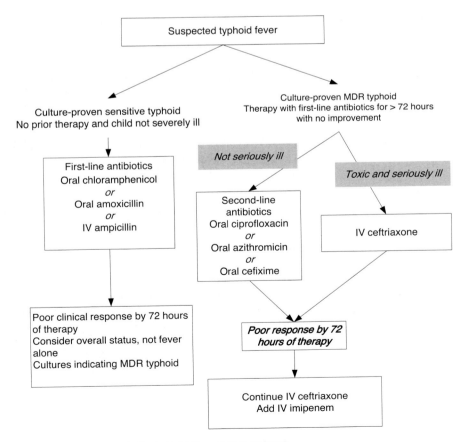

FIGURE 6.1.0.2 Algorithm for the treatment of typhoid. MDR, multi-drug-resistant.

Given the recent evidence that MDR typhoid is a more severe clinical illness from the outset, the algorithm in Figure 6.1.O.2 may be acceptable for selection of antibiotics and management of typhoid.

Table 6.1.O.2 shows the main antibiotics that can be employed for the treatment of both sensitive and MDR infections with *S. typhi*.

Corticosteroids

In severely ill and toxic children with typhoid requiring hospitalisation, past studies have shown that **dexamethasone IV** (0.5–1 mg/kg/day 8-hourly for up to six doses) **may be life-saving in some contexts**. However, **avoid using steroids in ambulatory settings**, as they mask abdominal complications and peritonitis.

Preventive measures for typhoid

The continued presence of typhoid in much of the developing world is an indication of the poor state of public health and sanitation. It is important therefore to be aware of the important risk factors for developing typhoid, in order to institute preventive measures during outbreaks.

There is some epidemiological evidence that prior usage of antibiotics is associated with an increased risk of subsequent development of typhoid. The precise reasons for this are unclear, but may be related to alterations in intestinal flora, increasing the predisposition to colonisation and infection with pathogenic strains of *S. typhi*. Thus controlling indiscriminate use of antibiotics may not only reduce the emergence of drug-resistant strains, but also reduce the risk of development of typhoid.

Of the major risk factors for outbreaks of typhoid, contamination of water supplies with sewage is the most important. Therefore during outbreaks a combination of central chlorination and domestic water purification is important. In endemic situations, consumption of street foods, especially ice cream and cut fruit, has been recognised as an important risk factor. The human-to-human spread by chronic carriers is also important, and attempts should therefore be made to target food handlers and high-risk groups for *S. typhi* carriage screening. There is an urgent need to define the extent of carriage among food handlers in areas of high burden.

Of the available vaccines against typhoid, the classic heat-inactivated whole-cell vaccine is associated with an unacceptably high rate of side effects and is no longer in use. There are two newer vaccines which offer protection in older school-age children, but these are not recommended for use in children under 2 years of age:

- The Vi polysaccharide (Vi-CPS) vaccine can be administered in two doses at any stage, and has a 60–70% protective efficacy for at least 5 years. Recent large-scale demonstration projects in South Asia indicate that the Vi-CPS vaccine has considerable potential for use in school-age populations. The protective efficacy in children under 5 years of age has varied between studies.
- The oral attenuated ty-21a vaccine has also been evaluated and found to be comparably effective. However, it is generally available in capsule form and therefore difficult to administer to young children, especially those of preschool age.

Given the high rates and morbidity of typhoid in young children, there is a clear need for the development of a Vi-conjugate vaccine, which could be potentially employed within the Extended Programme of Immunisation vaccination schedule. Studies in Vietnam confirm the protective efficacy of such candidate vaccines, and several candidates are in an advanced stage of clinical development.

TABLE 6.1.0.2 Antibiotics in *S. typhi* infections

Drug	Route	Dose (frequency)	Duration (days)
Chloramphenicol	Oral	60–75 mg/kg/day (6-hourly)	14 days
Ampicillin/amoxicillin	IV/oral	100 mg/kg/day (6- to 8-hourly)	14 days
Ciprofloxacin	Oral/IV	20–30 mg/kg/day (12-hourly)	7–10 days
Gatifloxacin	Oral	10 mg/kg/day (once daily)	7 days
Ceftriaxone	IV/IM	65–100 mg/kg/day (once daily)	7–14 days
Cefixime	Oral	8 mg/kg/day (12-hourly)	14 days
Azithromycin	Oral	10–20 mg/kg/day (once daily)	5–7 days

Non-typhoidal salmonella infections

These infections usually give rise to a self-limiting gastroenteritis. This is manifested as diarrhoea with abdominal cramping pains, nausea and vomiting. There is usually a fever and there may be blood and mucus in the stools (*see* Section 5.12.A for treatment of this level of infection). A reactive polyarticular arthritis may develop 2 weeks after the diarrhoea.

Occasionally, particularly in the neonate and in the immunosuppressed, the malnourished, or children with sickle-cell disease, these infections can become very serious by spreading to the following sites: meninges (meningitis), bones (osteomyelitis) and joints (septic arthritis), lungs (pneumonia and empyema) and soft tissues (giving abscesses). This is a particular problem in children with HIV infection.

Treatment for metastatic infections should be urgently given by intravenous or intramuscular injection. Initial treatment should ideally be with the broad-spectrum antibiotics cefotaxime or ceftriaxone, and if later sensitivity tests become available the organisms may be sensitive to amoxicillin (usually resistant now), co-trimoxazole and ciprofloxacin. Chloramphenicol may be effective in the absence of the above.

Drug dosage schedules

- Cefotaxime:
  - Neonates less than 7 days old: 50 mg/kg every 12 hours.
  - Neonates over 7 days old: 50 mg/kg every 8 hours.
  - Infants and children: 50 mg/kg every 6 hours.
- Ceftriaxone: All ages 50 mg/kg once daily. In very severe

infections 80–100 mg/kg once daily may be given (maximum dose 4 grams/day).

- Co-trimoxazole: 18 mg/kg by IV infusion 12-hourly. In very severe infections, 27 mg/kg co-trimoxazole IV 12-hourly (maximum dose 1.44 gram).
- Ciprofloxacin: 10–15 mg/kg twice daily by IV infusion.

6.1.P Rickettsial diseases

> **BOX 6.1.P.1 Minimum standards**
> - Supportive care and hydration.
> - Early treatment with doxycycline or chloramphenicol.
> - Public health measures and vector control.

Introduction

Rickettsial diseases are caused by obligate intracellular Gram-negative coccobacillary forms that multiply within eukaryotic cells. They take on a characteristic red colour when stained by the Giemsa or Gimenez stain.

- Illnesses are restricted by geography to places where both the natural animal host and its insect vector are present, and the vector has contact with humans.
- These diseases affect all ages, including children.

Aetiology and types

Rickettsial illnesses can be divided into the following biogroups:

1. **Spotted fever biogroup:**
   - Rocky Mountain spotted fever (RMSF), caused by *Rickettsia rickettsia*.
   - Rickettsial pox, caused by *Rickettsia akari*.
   - Boutonneuse fever (i.e. Kenya tick-bite fever, African tick typhus, Indian tick typhus, etc.).
2. **Typhus group:**
   - The causative organisms (*Rickettsia prowazekii* and *Rickettsia typhi*) are similar to those of epidemic typhus.
   - Examples include Brill–Zinsser disease (i.e. relapsing louse-borne typhus) and murine (endemic or flea-borne) typhus.
3. **Scrub typhus biogroup (Tsutsugamushi disease):**
   - These are a heterogeneous group of organisms that differ strikingly from rickettsial species and have a single taxonomic name, *Orientia tsutsugamushi* (*see* Section 6.1.Q).
4. **Other rickettsioses and closely related illnesses:**
   - New or re-emerging rickettsioses have been described, including tick-borne lymphadenopathy (TIBOLA) and *Dermacentor*-borne-necrosis-eschar-lymphadenopathy (DEBONEL).
   - *Ehrlichia* organisms (the cause of human monocytic ehrlichiosis and *Ehrlichia ewingii* infection), *Anaplasma phagocytophilum* (the cause of human granulocytic anaplasmosis), and *Bartonella* species (the cause of catscratch disease, relapsing fever and trench fever) are organisms related to the rickettsiae.
   - Q fever is a disease caused by *Coxiella burnetii*, which has recently been removed from the Rickettsiales.

Clinical presentation

There are so many clinical similarities among the diseases caused by rickettsiae that certain clinical and epidemiological features should suggest their presence:

1. Most of these infections are spread through ticks, mites, fleas or lice.
2. All rickettsial infections cause fever, headache and intense myalgias.
3. All rickettsial infections are arthropod-borne, so exposure to ticks or mites is an important clue to their early diagnosis.
4. Rash and/or a localised eschar occur in most patients.
   - Illnesses are generally characterised by fever, rash and malaise. They are often misdiagnosed as measles, meningococcaemia, typhoid or rheumatic fever, or investigated as pyrexia of unknown origin.
   - Disease is caused by a vasculitis of small blood vessels, which on the skin is seen as a petechial or haemorrhagic rash. The vasculitis may affect many organ systems, and explains the wide range of symptoms seen.
   - There are features specific to individual rickettsia, including meningoencephalitis (in Rocky Mountain spotted fever), myocarditis and cough (in Q fever) or lymphadenopathy and hepatosplenomegaly (in scrub typhus).
   - An eschar at the site of the infecting bite is helpful in the diagnosis of tick-borne and mite-borne rickettsial infections, and is recognised as a necrotic black papule.
   - The severity of illness varies with the organism, and the age of the patient. For example, in Rocky Mountain spotted fever, the untreated acute illness has a case fatality rate of 20%, with two-thirds of cases occurring in children under 15 years of age. In contrast, louse-borne typhus may only cause mild symptoms in children, with deaths occurring mainly in adults.
   - Other manifestations may occur, such as gastrointestinal, conjunctival, hepatic and pulmonary manifestations, that are more common in some illnesses than in others.

Differential diagnosis

Depending on local diseases, the combination of clinical manifestations, laboratory data and geographical areas, other causes to consider include the following:

- malaria
- measles
- typhoid

- dengue haemorrhagic fever
- Kawasaki disease
- leptospirosis
- meningococcal infections
- rubella
- group A streptococcal infection
- syphilis
- toxic shock syndrome
- vasculitis and thrombophlebitis.

Diagnosis

Confirmation of diagnosis of rickettsial infections is usually clinical, with the following methods used for confirmation as appropriate:

1 **Isolation:**
   - Rickettsiae can be isolated following inoculation into animals, such as guinea pigs in special reference laboratories.

2 **Serology:**
   - Serological detection of convalescent antibodies is the mainstay of diagnosis of rickettsial infection. The following serologic tests can be used:
     — the Weil–Felix (WF) agglutination test; **this is not used for rickettsial pox, Q fever or ehrlichiosis, for which specific diagnostic serological tests are available**
     — microimmunofluorescent (MIF) antibody test
     — enzyme-linked immunosorbent assay (ELISA)
     — Western blot immunoassay.

   The WF test is neither specific nor sensitive, and is not helpful. None of these methods are normally useful in the initial clinical management of patients with acute illness. A modification of the ELISA test has been developed to serologically confirm the specific species of rickettsiae.

3 **Immunologic detection of rickettsiae in tissue:**
   - Biopsies of skin rash, an eschar, or other tissues can be useful but are rarely performed, as these require specialised laboratories.

4 **PCR amplification of rickettsial DNA:**
   - PCR amplification, especially by the new 'suicide PCR' primers from rickettsial genes from blood, skin biopsy samples and other tissues can be performed in reference laboratories for detection of rickettsial DNA. It has estimated sensitivity and specificity of 68% and 100%, respectively.

5 **Routine blood examinations:**
   - These are unhelpful but are required to rule out other diseases, such as malaria, typhoid, dengue haemorrhagic fever and leptospirosis.

Treatment

- Treatment should not await serological diagnosis, as this is often delayed.
- In children over 8 years of age, give tetracyclines, particularly doxycycline (2.2 mg/kg twice daily up to a maximum of 100 mg twice daily). The use of these drugs is not advised in children under 8 years of age because of dental staining. Under 8 years give co-trimoxazole 24 mg/kg twice daily for 2 weeks.
- Oral chloramphenicol (25 mg/kg four times daily up to a maximum of 3 grams/day) is also effective.
- For scrub typhus (see Section 6.1.Q), rifampicin and azithromycin have been used successfully in areas where the rickettsia is resistant to conventional treatment.
- Treatment should be for 7–14 days.
- Fluoroquinolones (e.g. ciprofloxacin) may be effective and are being evaluated.
- Supportive care for complications affecting the cardiac, renal and pulmonary systems may be necessary in patients with severe disease.

Control

- Insect vector control is important for human louse-borne typhus, which occurs in cold mountainous areas where people live close together, or in internally displaced or refugee populations. In these situations, delousing of individuals with insecticides prevents and controls epidemic typhus.
- For scrub typhus, mite bites can be prevented by using topical insect repellents.
- A vaccine is also available for Rocky Mountain spotted fever.

Health education

This may include the following:
- community education on the risks of living in very close proximity to animals
- the need for regular re-facing of mud walls and floors
- for human louse-borne typhus, the importance of washing and sunning clothes and bedding.

TABLE 6.1.P Some major rickettsia and their distribution

Disease	Agent	Vector	Reservoir	Distribution
Rocky Mountain spotted fever	*R. rickettsii*	Ticks	Rodents, dogs, rabbits	USA, South America, Canada
Rickettsial pox	*R. akari*	Mite	Mouse	Worldwide
Louse-borne typhus	*R. prowazekii*	Lice	Human	Worldwide
Murine typhus	*R. typhi*	Flea	Mouse (urban)	Worldwide
Scrub typhus	*Orientia tsutsugamushi*	Mite	Rodents	Australia, India, SE Asia
Q fever	*Coxiella burnetii*	None	Cattle, goats	Worldwide

6.1.Q Scrub typhus

BOX 6.1.Q.1 **Minimum standards**
- Serology.
- Chest X-ray.
- Doxycycline and tetracycline.

Epidemiology

- Geographical distribution: Asia, Australia and Pacific Islands.
- Agent: *Orientia tsutsugamushi* (Rickettsia tsutsugamushi).
- Hosts: Rodents are reservoir hosts, and humans are accidental hosts. The most commonly affected age group is 5–14 years, and the disease is more common in boys.
- Vector: Larva of trombiculid mite. Mites live on jungle grass and become infectious by biting and sucking tissue fluid of infected rodent or by transovarian transmission to the next generation of mites.

Clinical manifestations

- Incubation period is 5–18 days.
- Abrupt onset of fever, severe headache, myalgia, cough, suffused conjunctivae, dark red papular or maculopapular rash (5–7 days after fever) on the trunk, arms and thighs.
- Eschar (19–28% in children, 46–82% in adults) may be seen at the site of the mite bite, especially in the perineum, axilla or trouser-belt region. Eschar is a firmly adherent black scab, 3–6 mm in diameter, with a raised red margin.
- There is regional or generalised lymphadenopathy, hepatomegaly and sometimes a maculopapular rash. Moderate leucocytosis may be seen, and occasionally thrombocytopenia.
- **In severe cases**, complications include meningoencephalitis, myocarditis, pneumonitis, respiratory distress syndrome or (rarely) renal failure.
- **In non-severe cases**, fever subsides within 2 weeks. Indigenous people in endemic areas usually have mild illness without rash or eschar.

Diagnosis

- Diagnosis is based on clinical manifestations, geographical distribution and history of contact with jungle-grass exposure in the bush.
- Confirmation is by serology or polymerase chain reaction (PCR). Weil–Felix test titres of 1:160 (or a fourfold rise after 2–4 weeks) occur in only 50% of cases. **More sensitive serological tests are the indirect immunoperoxidase test and the indirect immunofluorescent tests. For individuals living in endemic areas the positive titre is ≥ 1:400 or a fourfold rise in acute and convalescent sera. The positive titre indicating infection may be lower in non-endogenous children. PCR on the eschar material is more sensitive than on the blood.**

- Routine blood examinations are unhelpful, but are required to rule out other diseases such as dengue haemorrhagic fever, malaria and leptospirosis.
- Blood culture to exclude septicaemia (e.g. typhoid).
- Chest X-ray is indicated if there is cough and dyspnoea to detect pneumonitis, pleural effusion or respiratory distress syndrome.
- Perform lumbar puncture if there is meningism or severe headache to rule out other causes of CNS infection. CSF commonly shows a picture of aseptic meningitis.
- A fall in body temperature usually occurs within 24–48 hours after treatment.

Management

- The drug of choice is doxycycline orally 2.2 mg/kg initially followed by 2.2 mg/kg 12 hours later, then 1.1 mg/kg every 12 hours until the patient is afebrile for 2–3 days, **or** continue treatment for 5–7 days.
- Alternative drugs are tetracycline 250 mg orally four times a day for 7 days (in children over 8 years) or chloramphenicol 15–25 mg/kg orally four times a day for 7 days, depending on severity.
- In a few cases, fever returns 5–7 days later. If this happens, repeat the dose of antibiotic.
- Tetracycline should not be given to oliguric patients. Doxycycline is safe in renal impairment.
- Rifampicin and azithromycin have been used successfully in areas where the rickettsia is resistant to conventional treatment.
- In severe cases, the risk of dying outweighs the risk of tooth discoloration from doxycycline or tetracycline.
- **Remember that antimicrobial agents only suppress infection. Cure depends on host immunity.**
- Treatment should not be withheld pending laboratory confirmation for a clinically suspected infection.

6.1.R Yaws

BOX 6.1.R.1 **Minimum standards**
- Azithromycin.
- Benzathine penicillin.

Introduction

Yaws is caused by the bacterium *Treponema pallidum* subspecies *pertenue*. It is closely related to the bacterium that causes syphilis, but this disease is not sexually transmitted. Yaws mainly affects children in rural tropical areas, such as the Caribbean Islands, Latin America, West Africa, India, and South-East Asia. Yaws is transmitted by direct contact with the skin sores of infected people.

Symptoms

About 2–4 weeks after infection, the child develops a sore called a 'mother yaw' where bacteria entered the skin. The sore is reddish and looks like a berry. It is usually painless but does cause itching.

These sores may last for months. More sores may appear shortly before or after the mother yaw heals as the person scratches or spreads the bacteria from the mother yaw to uninfected skin. Eventually the skin sores heal.

Some patients develop destructive ulcerations of the nasopharynx, palate and nose (termed gangosa), painful skeletal deformities, especially in the legs (termed saber shins), and other soft-tissue changes (gummas, inflammatory cell infiltration). In the advanced stage, sores on the skin and bones can lead to severe disfigurement and disability.

Signs and tests

A sample from a skin sore is examined using a dark-field microscope. There is no blood test for yaws. However, the blood test for syphilis is usually positive in children with yaws, because the bacteria that cause these two conditions are closely related.

Treatment

Recently a single dose of oral azithromycin (30 mg/kg) has been shown to be as effective as a single IM injection of benzathine benzylpenicillin 50 000 units/kg (37.5 mg/kg) with less risk of a dangerous anaphylactic response and the need for needles. If the child vomits within 30 minutes of the oral dose of azithromicin, a repeat dose should be given. Benzathine benzylpenicillin must not be given IV.

Anyone who lives in the same house with someone who is infected should be examined for yaws and treated if they are infected. Skin lesions may take several months to heal. By its late stage, yaws may have already caused damage to the skin and bones. It may not be fully reversible, even with treatment for the infection.

6.1.S Other bacterial infections

> **BOX 6.1.S.1 Minimum standard**
> - Anthrax: ciprofloxacin, doxycycline, rifampicin, vancomycin, gentamicin, chloramphenicol, penicillin, amoxicillin, imipenem, meropenem and clindamycin.
> - Brucellosis: co-trimoxazole.
> - *Chlamydia*: erythromycin.
> - *Haemophilus influenzae*: amoxicillin, Hib vaccine.
> - Plague: streptomycin, tetracycline, chloramphenicol.
> - *Staphylococcus*: cloxacillin, flucloxacillin, sodium fusidate.

Anthrax

This is an infection from animals caused by *Bacillus anthracis*.

Cutaneous

Major features:
- surrounded by extensive oedema
- painless and non-tender (although may be pruritic or accompanied by a tingling sensation).

Minor features:
- development of black eschar
- progresses over 2–6 days through papular, vesicular and ulcerated stages before eschar appears
- most commonly affects the hands, forearms, face and neck
- discharge of serous fluid
- local erythema and induration
- local lymphadenopathy
- associated with systemic malaise including headache, chills and sore throat, but afebrile.

Take initial diagnostic tests:
Swab from lesion for stain and culture.
Blood cultures (prior to antimicrobial use, if possible).

Start antibiotic treatment to cover *B. anthracis.*

Ciprofloxacin orally is given under 8 years of age. In children older than 8 years doxycycline can be given. Either drug is combined with one or two other antibiotics (such as amoxicillin, benzylpenicillin, or chloramphenicol). When the condition improves and the sensitivity of the *Bacillus anthracis* strain is known, treatment may be switched to a single antibiotic. Treatment should continue for 60 days because germination may be delayed.

Features of inhalation anthrax
- Rapid onset of severe unexplained febrile illness (fever, chills, fatigue, non-productive cough).
- Rapid onset of severe sepsis not due to a predisposing illness.
- Abrupt onset of respiratory failure and the presence of widened mediastinum or pleural effusions on chest X-ray.
- Nausea.
- Sweats (often drenching).
- Confusion or altered mental status.
- Vomiting.
- Pallor or cyanosis.
- Dyspnoea.
- Tachycardia.
- Abdominal pain.
- Pleuritic chest pain.
- Sore throat.

Take initial diagnostic tests:
- Chest X-ray: **mediastinal widening**, pleural effusion, pulmonary infiltrate.
- Full blood count: to look for raised haemocrit, raised white cell count, especially neutrophilia.
- Liver function tests: to look for high transaminase activity.
- CT of chest (if available) if high suspicion and normal chest X-ray.

- Blood culture.

Start antibiotic treatment to cover *B. anthracis*.

Give ciprofloxacin intravenously in combination with one or two other antibiotics (agents with *in-vitro* activity include rifampicin, vancomycin, gentamicin, chloramphenicol, penicillin, amoxicillin, imipenem, meropenem and clindamycin) until sensitivity testing is available. Treatment should continue for 60 days because germination may be delayed.

It is important to notify public health authorities if such an infection is identified.

Brucellosis

This is an infection from animals caused by *Brucella* species, usually through infected milk. It causes a chronic illness with fever, pain and swelling of the joints, and anaemia.

Treatment is with co-trimoxazole for 4 weeks: give 18–24 mg co-trimoxazole/kg twice daily.

- **Or** give paediatric liquid 240 mg/5 mL (200 mg sulfamethoxazole plus 40 mg trimethoprim):
  - Age 6 weeks to 6 months: 2.5 mL twice daily.
  - Age 6 months to 6 years: 5 mL twice daily.
  - Age 6–12 years: 10 mL twice daily.

Campylobacter infection

This causes acute gastroenteritis with **considerable abdominal pain**, fever and bloody diarrhoea (*see* Section 5.12.A). Most children recover without treatment with antibiotics, although erythromycin and ciprofloxacin are both effective.

Chlamydia infections

Chlamydia trachomatis causes trachoma (*see* Section 6.1.M), infections of the genital tract (*see* Section 6.1.J), and conjunctivitis in the newborn which is less severe than that due to the gonococcus (*see* Section 3.4).

Chlamydia pneumoniae produces a chronic pneumonitis in the infant. It is important not to forget this cause of acute respiratory infection, which responds well to erythromycin.

Haemophilus influenzae infections

Haemophilus influenzae causes serious infections in infants and young children, including:

- pneumonia (*see* Section 5.3.A)
- middle ear infections (*see* Section 5.1.C)
- acute epiglottitis (*see* Section 5.1.A)
- meningitis (*see* Section 5.16.B).

Infections can be prevented by an extremely effective conjugate vaccine. **Every country should attempt to immunise their infants against this cause of many serious illnesses, deaths and handicap.**

Plague

Yersinia pestis is transmitted to children by the fleas of infected rats. It occurs in epidemics.

It presents with an acute fever and painful tender large swollen lymph nodes (buboes). It can cause pneumonia and septicaemia.

Prompt treatment on suspicion is essential.

- Streptomycin is the treatment of choice for severe cases (15 mg/kg IM daily, maximum dose 1 gram) for 7 days.
- Tetracycline (in children over 8 years, 250–500 mg 6-hourly) and chloramphenicol (15–25 mg/kg 6-hourly) are alternative drugs, which are also given for 7 days.

Shigellosis

- This causes an acute gastroenteritis, which particularly affects the large bowel. There is blood and mucus in the diarrhoea.
- There is often a high fever.
- Shigellosis may cause seizures.
- There may be tenesmus (a continuous feeling of wanting to defecate).
- Septicaemia may occur.

See Section 5.12.A for advice on treatment.

Staphylococcal infections

The most common presentation is with a pus-forming skin infection (impetigo) (*see* Section 5.18).

However, this bacterium can be transported in the blood to other parts of the body, where it produces serious infections:

- Pneumonia is particularly dangerous (*see* Section 5.3.A).
- Osteomyelitis is also dangerous and difficult to diagnose (*see* Section 5.17).
- Pyomyositis can occur.
- Occasionally staphylococcal infections cause mastoiditis (*see* Section 5.1.C) and laryngotracheitis (*see* Section 5.1.A).

The two groups of antibiotics most effective against this organism are flucloxacillin or cloxacillin and sodium fusidate (fucidin).

Treatment with sodium fusidate/fusidic acid

Use in combination with another antistaphylococcal agent if possible, to avoid the development of resistance.

Oral route

Absorption is not as good as with the IV route, but the oral route should be used when possible. Doses as fusidic acid:

Neonate to 1 year	15 mg/kg	3 times daily
1 year to 5 years	250 mg	3 times daily
5 years to 12 years	500 mg	3 times daily
12 years to 18 years	750 mg	3 times daily

The suspension usually contains 250 mg of fusidic acid in 5 mL.

Intravenous infusion

Give 6–7 mg/kg of sodium fusidate 8-hourly (for children over 50 kg in weight, give 500 mg IV 8-hourly).

The dose may be doubled in severe infections.

Dilute in 5% glucose to a concentration of 1 mg/mL, and give slowly over at least 6 hours.

See Section 5.12.A for further information on *Campylobacter* and cholera infections.

6.2 Viral infections

6.2.A Chickenpox

BOX 6.2.A.1 Minimum standards
- Antipyretics and antipruritus treatment (e.g. chlorpheniramine/promethazine).
- Antibiotics for secondary infection.
- Aciclovir in immunosuppressed, neonates and other at-risk groups.
- VZIG IM (if available) for immunocompromised patients.
- Live attenuated varicella vaccine (for susceptible groups when in remission).

Introduction

Chickenpox is caused by varicella zoster virus (VZV), a member of the herpesvirus family. It is spread by direct contact, droplet or airborne transmission, and is very contagious.

Chickenpox manifests as a generalised pruritic vesicular rash typically consisting of crops of lesions in varying stages of development and resolution (crusting), mild fever, and other systemic symptoms. Varicella tends to be more severe in adolescents and adults than in young children.

The peak age for infection is 5 to 9 years. In immunocompetent children it is usually a mild disease, and lifelong immunity follows an infection.

Groups at increased risk include those with immunodeficiency (mainly those with HIV infection), those on chemotherapy or long-term steroids (defined as those who within the previous 3 months received prednisolone, or its equivalent, at a daily dose of 2 mg/kg/day or more than 40 mg/day for at least 1 week or 1 mg/kg/day for 1 month), and neonates whose mothers have had chickenpox just before or just after the birth. Patients on lower doses of steroids plus another immunosuppressant drug and patients with an additional medical problem (e.g. nephrotic syndrome) should be included, plus those on salicylate therapy or with chronic lung or skin problems, including eczema. Acyclovir should be used in these groups.

Children with chickenpox are at increased risk of developing Reye's syndrome if given aspirin and other non-steroidal anti-inflammatory drugs.

Clinical presentation

- The incubation period is 14–21 days. There is low-grade fever and headache, followed by the rash, which is mostly on the trunk and face. The rash develops into successive small single oval vesicles with an erythematous base which break within 2 days to develop into scabs and heal. It is very itchy, and scratching may result in secondary bacterial infection and scar formation.
- The course of the disease is about 1 week. Children are infectious from 1 or 2 days before the rash appears until 1 or 2 days after all of the lesions have formed scabs.
- Complications include septicaemia, bronchopneumonia, hepatitis, thrombocytopenia, purpura, pericarditis, myocarditis, endocarditis, arthritis, myositis, glomerulonephritis, ascending mediastinitis and post-infectious encephalitis, especially with cerebellar involvement. Any fever or other symptom occurring within a few days of apparently resolving chickenpox must be taken seriously.
- Guillain–Barré syndrome, facial nerve palsy, transverse myelitis, hypothalamic involvement, optic neuritis and transient loss of vision have been reported.
- Intrauterine infection, especially in the first two trimesters, may result in a congenital varicella syndrome (i.e intrauterine growth retardation, scarred skin, limb atrophy, mental retardation, CNS and eye complications). Only 1–2% of infants with intrauterine exposure develop complications.
- In mothers, chickenpox but not shingles, occurring between 5 days before and 2 days after delivery, may result in a **severe infection in the neonate**. This is probably due to lack of formation of VZV IgG antibodies that would have crossed the placenta and would be protective for the newborn baby. The infant should be treated as soon as possible with **varicella-zoster immunoglobulin** (if available) and with **IV aciclovir** as well if infection manifests (see below and Section 2.8.1).

Management

- Keep the child clean, and cut and clean under their nails to discourage scratching and prevent secondary skin infection.
- Baking soda baths or calamine lotion may relieve the itching.
- Antihistamines, such as chlorpheniramine 1 mg twice daily (1 month to 2 years of age), 1 mg three to six times a day; maximum 6 mg daily (2–6 years), 2 mg three to four times a day; maximum 12 mg daily (6–12 years), or 4 mg three to six times a day; maximum 24 mg daily (over 12 years) may reduce scratching.
- Give paracetamol for fever.
- Appropriate antibiotics should be given for secondary bacterial infection, which is mostly due to *Staphylococcus aureus* or *Streptococcus pyogenes*.
- Aciclovir IV 10 mg/kg 8-hourly or 250 mg/m² 8-hourly for 7–10 days is recommended for immunocompromised children who develop chickenpox. Oral aciclovir (20 mg/kg four times a day) is given for HIV-infected patients whose **CD4+ counts** are relatively normal. It should

be considered for HIV-infected children with a CD4+ T-lymphocyte percentage of 15% or greater.

- If available, IM varicella-zoster immunoglobulin (VZIG) should be given at the following doses: birth to 5 years, 250 mg (one vial); 6–10 years, 500 mg (two vials); 10–15 years, 750 mg (three vials) and 15–18 years, 1 gram. This may modify the disease if given shortly (not more than 4 days) after exposure. Indications include immunocompromised children, such as HIV-infected pregnant women and premature infants born at less than 28 weeks' gestation, who have had intimate contact (face to face) with chickenpox or herpes zoster. Neonates whose mothers develop varicella between 7 days before and 28 days after delivery are offered VZIG 250 mg as a single IM injection.
- If VZIG is not available, oral or IV aciclovir (at the above doses) may be given.
- In addition to standard precautions, airborne and contact precautions are recommended for patients with varicella for a minimum of 5 days after the onset of rash and until all lesions are crusted, which in immunocompromised patients can be 1 week or longer.

Prevention

- Live attenuated varicella vaccine (monovalent varicella vaccine or measles, mumps, rubella, varicella: MMRV) given as two subcutaneous or intramuscular injections confers over 95% protection against severe disease. Both have been licensed for use in healthy children from 12 months to 12 years of age. Children in this age group should receive two 0.5-mL doses of varicella vaccine administered subcutaneously, separated by at least 3 months.
- Susceptible children aged 13 years or older without immunocompromise should receive two 0.5-mL doses of varicella vaccine separated by at least 28 days.
- Patients in whom vaccine is contraindicated include those who are immunocompromised children and those receiving aspirin.
- Patients who are receiving immunosuppressive treatment (including steroid therapy) are generally immunised when in complete remission. The total lymphocyte count should be $> 1.2 \times 10^9$/litre and there should be no other evidence of a lack of cellular immune competence.
- The vaccine should not be given within 3 months of VZIG.

6.2.B Dengue

BOX 6.2.B.1 Minimum standards

- ■ Airway, Breathing and Circulation assessment and management.
- ■ Recognition and treatment of shock.
- ■ Blood transfusion and replacement of clotting factors and platelets.
- ■ High-dependency/intensive care.
- ■ Vector control.

Introduction

Dengue infection is caused by an RNA virus of the Flaviviridae family. The disease first appeared in an epidemic in the Philippines in 1957, subsequently in Thailand, and then in other South-East Asian countries. It is now an important health threat in most Asian and South American countries, with an estimated 50–100 million dengue infections worldwide every year and a fatality rate of about 2.5% in hospitalised cases, although this could be reduced by earlier detection and access to good medical care.

Epidemics occur every year during the rainy season, and the mosquitoes *Aedes aegypti* and *Aedes albopictus* are the main vectors.

The dengue virus comprises four serotypes (type 1, 2, 3 and 4) which cause lifelong specific antibody responses. Unusually, a second infection with a different serotype of the virus puts the sufferer at greater risk of more severe illness.

Dengue hemorrhagic fever or severe dengue is the

TABLE 6.2.B.1 Increasing signs of severity in dengue

Dengue: diagnosis	Warning signs of severity	Severe dengue
Probable dengue	*Require close observation and medical care*	*Any of the following:*
Live in or travel to dengue endemic area	Persistent vomiting	Severe plasma leakage showing as shock or respiratory distress
	Clinical fluid accumulation	
Fever and two of the following:	Mucosal bleed	Severe bleeding as evaluated by clinicians
Nausea, vomiting	Lethargy, restlessness	
Rash	Liver enlargement > 2 cm	
Aches and pains	Laboratory: increase in haematocrit concurrent with rapid decrease in platelet count	Severe organ involvement:
Tourniquet test positive		• liver (AST, ALT ≥ 1000)
and either		• CNS: impaired consciousness
Supportive serology	Abdominal pain and tenderness	• heart and other organ failure
or		
Occurrence at the same location and time as other confirmed dengue cases		

AST, aspartate aminotransferase; ALT, alanine aminotransferase; CNS, central nervous system.

severe clinical illness, and involves plasma leakage, significant bleeding and shock with a significant fatality rate, especially where intensive-care facilities are lacking. There are no available vaccines for dengue and no specific antiviral treatment. Treatment is supportive. Control is currently by control of the vectors.

Diagnosis

In 2009, the WHO classification of dengue infection was revised to simplify diagnosis and management. Table 6.2.B.1 shows the warning signs that severe dengue may develop.

This new WHO guideline classifies the infection either as dengue or as severe dengue. The old definition of (non-severe) dengue is the same as that of dengue fever (A90 according to the ICD code) and severe dengue means dengue hemorrhagic fever (A91 according to the ICD code).

The alternative differential diagnosis of acute febrile illness with non-specific symptoms is as follows:

- septicaemia
- scrub typhus
- viral infection

- enteric fever
- leptospirosis.

Pathogenesis of severe dengue or dengue haemorrhagic fever (DHF)

Infection with one dengue serotype gives specific lifelong antibody with only partial protection against other serotypes. Therefore, unusually, severe dengue or DHF occurs predominantly in patients with second infections who have a different serotype in their second infection from their first (previous dengue fever). Antibody-dependent enhancement, immune enhancement and T-cell (T8) proliferation and apoptosis are important in the development of disease.

Hypotheses for severe dengue or DHF include the following:

- Non-neutralising antibodies to dengue virus enhance viral uptake and replication in target cells (monocytes).
- Enhanced viral replication in the presence of T-cell apoptosis, resulting in large antigen load in the face of massive T-cell activation, releasing cytokines that lead to tissue damage and vascular leakage.

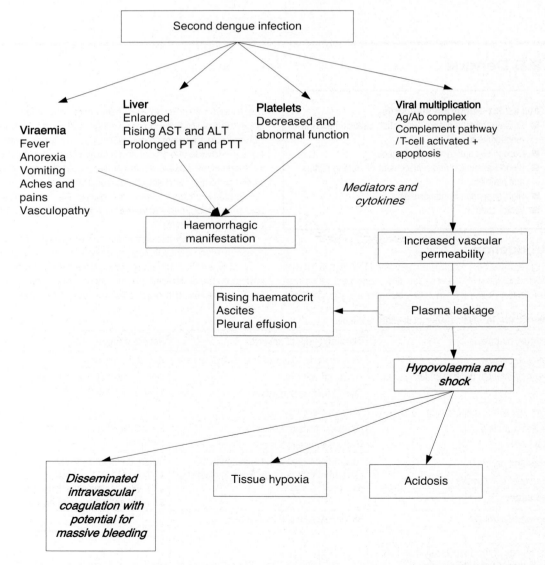

FIGURE 6.2.B.1 Pathophysiology of severe dengue or dengue haemorrhagic fever. AST, aspartate aminotransferase; ALT, alanine aminotransferase; PT, prothrombin time; PTT, partial thromboplastin time.

TABLE 6.2.B.2 Clinical course of severe dengue or DHF

Phase	Symptoms	Signs	Laboratory test
1. Febrile phase duration 3–5 days (days 1–5)	High continuous fever (39–40°C), headache, anorexia, nausea, vomiting, myalgia, arthralgia, epigastric discomfort, right upper quadrant pain, fine rubelliform maculopapular rash, mucosal bleeding	Facial flushing, injected conjunctivae Tourniquet test positive (*see* Figure 6.2.B.2), tenderness at right upper quadrant, hepatomegaly, lymphadenopathy, dry lips and mucosa	Not significant
2. Haemorrhagic shock or toxic phase duration 1–2 days (days 4–6)	Fever declines, abdominal pain especially in the right upper quadrant, bleeding in skin and mucosa (nose, gums, gastrointestinal tract) About 30% of cases will develop shock (irritability, restlessness, severe abdominal pain, sweating) Shock is less common when IV fluids have been given early	Right upper quadrant tenderness, hepatomegaly, tourniquet test positive, bleeding of mucosa, signs of dehydration (dry lips and mucosa, dark yellowish urine) Cold clammy skin (prolonged capillary refill time > 2 seconds) Thready pulse, tachycardia, narrow pulse pressure (≤ 20 mmHg, e.g. 90/70, 100/80)	Blood count: rising haematocrit, decreased platelet count (< 100 × 10⁹/litre), leucopenia Abnormal liver function test (albumin, liver enzyme: AST, ALT), renal function, calcium, electrolyte, blood gas in severe dengue with intractable and prolonged shock
3. Convalescence phase Duration 2–3 days	No fever or low-grade biphasic fever Increased appetite Diuresis	Convalescence rash on extremities with itching Widespread petechial rash with scattered round pale areas Sinus bradycardia	Stable haematocrit (or slowly increasing is a good clinical sign due to diuresis in some cases) Rising platelet count

Dengue or dengue fever (non-severe dengue) has only phases 1 and 3.

- Antibodies against dengue virus bind to complement pathway, releasing mediators that lead to vascular leakage as well.

Figure 6.2.B.1 shows a proposed pathophysiological pathway for severe dengue.

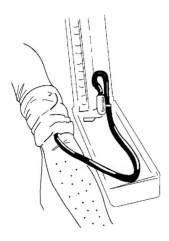

FIGURE 6.2.B.2 Tourniquet test showing petechiae.

Tourniquet test:
1 Apply an appropriate blood pressure cuff (it should be two-thirds of upper arm length)
2 Inflate to the level of mean arterial pressure (systolic plus diastolic blood pressure, divided by 2) for 5 minutes.
3 Positive test: petechiae > 10/square inch after removing the cuff for 2 minutes or longer.

Management of dengue and severe dengue (dengue haemorrhagic fever, DHF)

The aim of management of dengue and severe dengue is supportive, aiming to maintain adequate intravascular volume to prevent shock and to use blood and blood products to combat severe bleeding.

Management of severe dengue with shock and respiratory distress

Initial management of shock
1 Give high-flow oxygen with a mask with reservoir or nasal cannulae.
2 Give a bolus of Ringer-lactate or Hartmann's or 0.9% saline solution (20 mL/kg).
3 If the child shows improvement, give 10 mL/kg of Ringer-lactate or Hartmann's solution or 0.9% saline with 5% dextrose over 1 hour (add 50 mL of 50% dextrose to each 500-mL bag).
4 Reduce IV fluids (Ringer-lactate or Hartmann's solution or 0.9% saline plus 5% dextrose) to 7 mL/kg/hour for 6 hours if vital signs improve.
5 Check vital signs every 15 minutes until stable, then every hour for 4 hours, then every 2–4 hours.
6 Check haematocrit every 4 hours.
7 If vital signs are stable, haematocrit declines to 36–40% and no warning signs appear, then reduce IV fluid to 5 mL/kg/hour for 6 hours followed by maintenance fluids (2–3 mL/kg/hour).
8 Stop IV fluid when the child drinks more than half of the required intake or there is a diuresis.

TABLE 6.2.B.3 Management of dengue and severe dengue without shock

Day of illness	Assessment	Management
Days 1–3 (febrile phase)	**Monitor** temperature, blood pressure and pulse rate at least every 4–6 hours **Do** tourniquet test **Look for** signs of dehydration (dry lips and mucosae, low urine output) **Look for** warning signs (*see* Table 6.2.B.1)	1 Tepid sponge, paracetamol (do not give salicylate or other non-steroidal anti-inflammatory drugs, as they may cause bleeding, acidosis, hepatotoxicity and Reye's syndrome) 2 Give ORS/fruit juice/water frequently and in small amounts 3 If the child is vomiting, try domperidone 0.2 mg/kg 6- to 8-hourly 4 Admit if the child has signs of dehydration, gastrointestinal bleeding or cannot drink 5 Give IV fluid: 5% dextrose in Ringer-lactate or Hartmann's or 0.9% saline 1–3 mL/kg/hour depending on oral intake and haematocrit
Days 4–6 (toxic phase)	**Monitor** vital signs every 2–4 hours **Do:** • tourniquet test if previously negative • complete blood count (CBC) • serial haematocrit every 4 hours • palpate liver • record intake and output **Look for** warning signs (*see* Table 6.2.B.1)	1 Admit if the child has signs of dehydration or warning signs 2 Give IV fluid: 5% dextrose in Ringer-lactate or Hartmann's or 0.9% saline = maintenance + 3–5% deficit depends on haematocrit (maintain latter at 36–43 vol%) 3 If haematocrit is rising above 44% (or above 5% of previous value) increase rate of IV fluid to 6–7 mL/kg/hour (or 7% deficit) to prevent shock 4 If haematocrit is still high (> 45%), change IV fluid to low dose of colloid, e.g. Dextran 40 (maintenance + 3% deficit) or 2–4 mL/kg/hour (maximum dose of 30/kg/day) 5 Decrease IV fluid when vital signs are stable, haematocrit declines and urine is clear 6 Stop IV fluid when the child can drink more than half of normal or there is a diuresis

Haematocrit of normal child is usually 35–36%, so if a child has haematocrit > 42% this means that it has risen to 20% or more above normal level.

Shock that does not improve with the first 20 mL/kg bolus of Ringer-lactate or Hartmann's or 0.9% saline solution

1 Continue high-flow oxygen.
2 Give a bolus of Dextran 40 (especially if the haematocrit is very high (> 50%) or the child has a puffy face or distended abdomen), 10 mL/kg over 15–30 minutes.
3 If the haematocrit is < 42% or has decreased by more than 5% consider careful transfusion of packed red cells, 5–10 mL/kg over 30 minutes to 1 hour.
4 If the child improves, revert to Ringer-lactate or Hartmann's solution or 0.9% saline plus 5% dextrose, 5–7 mL/kg/hour for 6 hours and follow management in steps (7) and (8) above, 5 mL/kg/hour for 6 hours.
5 Check vital signs every 15 minutes until the child is stable, then every hour.
6 Check haematocrit every 4 hours and aim to maintain it at 40–45%.
7 Measure fluid intake and output every 4–8 hours.

Shock that does not improve with Dextran 40 bolus

1 Consider giving 4.2% sodium bicarbonate, 1–2 mL/kg IV slowly over 10 minutes.
2 Continue giving Dextran 40 at 7 mL/kg/hour.
3 Consider using an inotropic drug, such as dopamine or dobutamine 5–15 micrograms/kg/minute, if the child is still shocked or not improving.
4 Consider transfusion with packed red cells if the child is shocked with haematocrit < 42% or haematocrit declines by more than 5% of previous value.

Intractable shock with respiratory distress

1 Continue high-flow oxygen.

2 If calculated total intake is maximum (≥ 7 mL/kg/hour), haematocrit is > 40%, and shock has been present for > 24 hours, try furosemide 200–500 microgram/kg IV or 5–10 mg per dose for most children > 1 year of age.
3 If total intake is maximum (≥ 7 mL/kg/hour), haematocrit is > 40% and duration since first shock is < 24 hours **consider giving sodium bicarbonate, give inotropic drugs and consider positive pressure ventilation with PEEP** (if available).
4 Drain pleural effusion if it is interfering with ventilation (and if high pressure settings are needed on the ventilator); diagnose from chest X-ray or ultrasound.
5 Monitor electrolytes, calcium, albumin, renal function, blood gas and blood clotting according to clinical severity.

Blood and blood components should be given only in cases of suspected or severe bleeding or intractable shock.

Fluid management
Plasma expanders
Colloid solutions to expand the intravascular volume:
• Dextran 40 (osmolarity = 600 mOsmol/litre), maximum 30 mL/kg/day
• 6% hydroxyethyl starch (osmolarity = 308 mOsmol/litre)
• 4.5% albumin in severe hypoalbuminaemia with moderate to massive effusion/ascites and respiratory distress.

Blood products to combat bleeding:
• fresh frozen plasma (FFP), 10 mL/kg/dose
• packed red cells (PRC), 5–10 mL/kg/dose
• platelet transfusion, 0.2 units/kg/dose.

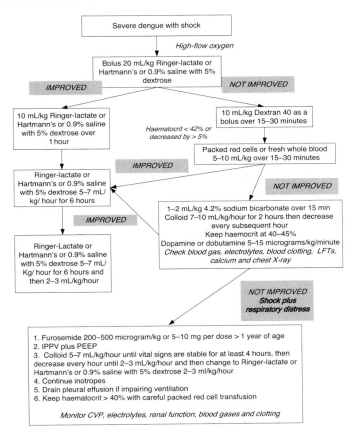

FIGURE 6.2.B.3 Management of severe dengue with shock. LFTs, liver function tests; IPPV, intermittent positive pressure ventilation; PEEP, positive end-expiratory pressure; CVP, central venous pressure.

Crystalloids

Normal maintenance fluids are 5% dextrose in Ringer-lactate or Hartmann's or 0.9% saline solution, about 2–3 mL/kg/hour or:

Up to 10 kg	= 100 mL/kg/day
From 11–20 kg	= 100 mL/kg/day × 10 kg for the first 10 kg, PLUS 50 mL/kg/day × body weight in kg above 10 kg
> 20 kg	= 1500 mL PLUS 20 mL/kg/day × body weight in kg > 20 kg

Example: body weight of 14 kg = 1000 mL + (4 × 50) = 1200 mL.

Example body weight of 30 kg = 1500 mL + (10 × 20) = 1700 mL.

In an obese child, use ideal body weight to calculate IV fluids. For example, for an obese 7-year-old girl with body weight 40 kg, IV fluids should be calculated from her age multiplied by 2 plus 8 (7 × 2 + 8 = 22 kg).

In practice, based on the above we can calculate IV fluids easily and rapidly as follows:

- 5 mL/kg/hour is equal to a 5% deficit if body weight < 40 kg
- 4 mL/kg/hour is equal to a 5% deficit if body weight > 40 kg

The maximum fluid that should be given in 24 hours (maximum fluid = resuscitation [20 mL/kg] + 10% deficit + maintenance) is 7 mL/kg/hour.

Inotropic drugs

- Dopamine will increase renal blood flow: dose is 5–15 micrograms/kg/minute.
- Dobutamine is usually used in patients with poor peripheral circulation: dose is 5–15 micrograms/kg/minute.

Severe dengue with organ involvement

Vital organs are not primarily involved in severe dengue, but are affected secondarily to plasma leakage, shock, haemorrhage and hypoxia. Notably, hepatic dysfunction and renal failure may occur especially in cases with prolonged shock.

Central nervous system involvement may be manifested by convulsions, spasticity and/or change in consciousness. Some cases have reported dengue virus in cerebrospinal fluid as in encephalitis.

Prevention and control

There is no vaccine to protect against dengue. Development of a vaccine against dengue infection has been challenging, although there has been recent progress.

At present, the only method for controlling or preventing the transmission of dengue virus is to combat vector mosquitoes by preventing them from accessing egg-laying habitats. This is achieved by environmental management and modification, with community participation and active monitoring.

6.2.C Acute hepatitis

BOX 6.2.C.1 Minimum standards
- Liver function tests.
- International normalised ratio (INR) or prothrombin time.
- Blood glucose measurement.
- Vitamin K.
- Immunisation against hepatitis B: population vaccination.

Introduction
- Acute hepatitis results in liver dysfunction of duration less than 6 months.
- Transaminases (AST and ALT) are abnormal, but patients are not necessarily jaundiced.
- Acute hepatitis may be cholestatic, and may be complicated by acute liver failure as described in Section 5.7.A.
- Hepatitis A is common and usually self-limiting, but other important diseases may occur at the same time or appear similar and be overlooked (*see* Table 6.2.C.1).

TABLE 6.2.C.1 Causes of acute hepatitis-like presentation

Aetiological group	Examples	Possible cholestasis
Viral	Hepatitis A virus, hepatitis B virus, hepatitis C virus, hepatitis E virus, delta superinfection, cytomegalovirus, Epstein–Barr virus, herpes simplex, parvovirus, measles, mumps, varicella, rubella, adenovirus, ECHO, coxsackie, flaviviruses (e.g. yellow fever, dengue, Lassa, Ebola, Rift Valley fever).	Hepatitis A virus, hepatitis B virus, hepatitis E virus
Bacterial/fungal	*Salmonella*, *Leptospira*, any septicaemia	Not usually
Protozoal + parasitic	*See* Section 6.3.A.d and 6.3.C	Not usually
Drugs and toxins	*See* Section 7.4	Drug cholestasis
Shock	Cardiac arrest, post surgery, heat stroke, radiation	Occurs 7–10 days after injury
Immune	Autoimmune, lupus, Kawasaki disease	Autoimmune, lupus, Kawasaki disease
Infiltrative	Leukaemias, haemophagocytic syndromes, Hodgkin's disease	Leukaemias, Hodgkin's disease
Metabolic	Urea cycle disorders	Usually not
	Wilson's disease	Yes

Management of acute hepatitis
- Exclude hepatitis A with HAV IgM and attempt diagnosis with tests (if available).
- Monitor hepatic synthetic function for liver failure using prothrombin time or INR, having given IV vitamin K.
- Monitor for complications, including hypoglycaemia, encephalopathy, bone-marrow aplasia, secondary sepsis and pancreatitis (*see* Section 5.7.A).
- Treat complications when possible.
- Give vitamin K, 300 micrograms/kg.
- Give anti-emetics if there is severe nausea and vomiting.
- Give intravenous fluids **only if oral or nasogastric rehydration is not possible**.
- *See* Section 5.7.A for the management of acute liver failure if this develops.
- If available, immunise all family contacts for HAV and HBB (HAV A, two doses 2 weeks apart; HAV B, three doses, the first being given immediately, the second 1 month later, and the third 3–6 months later).

Hepatitis A
- Hepatitis A (HAV) is a picornavirus spread by the faecal–oral route.
- The incubation period from infection to raised transaminases is 10–20 days.
- Before jaundice is seen there may be anorexia, nausea, vomiting, fever and liver tenderness.

- Jaundice is related to age, with more than 90% of children under 2 years being asymptomatic, and only 76% of teenagers jaundiced.
- A minority of cholestatic cases have a relapsing course, and 0.1–0.2% develop acute liver failure. The prognosis for almost all is excellent with symptomatic treatment.
- Chronic liver disease does not develop, but occasional patients have a transient nodular regenerative phase with evidence of portal hypertension lasting up to 1 year. Aplastic anaemia is a rare complication.
- HAV vaccine is highly efficacious and without side effects.

Hepatitis B
Acute hepatitis B (see also section on chronic hepatitis)
- This is spread by blood and body fluid products, vertical transmission from mother to baby, and sexual contact. The risk of all such spread is much greater than for HIV infection.
- The incubation period is 60–90 days, but rarely up to 7 months.
- The risk of acute liver failure is less than 1%, and the risk of chronic liver disease depends on the patient's age: it is approximately 90% at birth, 25% in childhood and less than 10% in adults.
- Hepatitis B vaccine is usually given by three injections over 6 months, but an accelerated course can be given

over 21 days, and post-exposure vaccination is usually given in combination with immunoglobulin in a different site. All healthcare workers should be immunised against HBV and their immunity status checked.

Hepatitis C
- The mechanisms of spread are the same as for hepatitis B, but vertical spread is rare (around 4%).
- The incubation period is 2–26 weeks, followed by acute hepatitis that is almost always asymptomatic.
- Chronic hepatitis ensues in 30–90% of cases.
- Symptomatic liver disease is almost never seen in childhood.
- Treatment with a combination of pegylated interferon and ribavirin is becoming progressively more successful (if available).

Hepatitis E
- Spread is by the faecal–oral route and is endemic in Southern Europe, the Middle East and Asia.

- It is rare in children, and the highest rate in adolescents is 3%.
- A relapsing course is seen.
- The prognosis is usually good, but mortality is recognised in pregnant women.

Epstein–Barr virus (EBV)
- EBV infection is accompanied by hepatosplenomegaly and hepatitis.
- The prognosis is usually good, but rare cases are complicated by lymphoproliferative disease or haemophagocytic syndrome in immune-deficient individuals.

Cytomegalovirus (CMV)
- Spread is the same as for EBV and hepatitis, but symptoms are usually only seen in the newborn and immunocompromised.

Parvovirus B19
- This infection can be accompanied by acute liver failure and aplastic anaemia.

6.2.D Human immunodeficiency virus (HIV) infection

BOX 6.2.D.1 Minimum standards
- Preventive campaigns.
- Antenatal HIV screening.
- Antenatal and postnatal antiretroviral (ARV) drugs.
- Paediatric HIV testing.
- Antiretroviral drugs (triple drug regimes for all), including those to prevent vertical transmission guaranteed.
- Health system strengthening to provide a capacity to treat all with ARV and give supportive treatment.
- Correction of nutritional deficiencies.
- Antibacterial drugs, including anti-TB and antifungal drugs.
- Analgesia and palliative care.
- Counselling and family support.

Introduction

The human immunodeficiency virus (HIV) epidemic has spread to all corners of the world, affecting millions of infants, children and adults. It is the most common cause of acquired immune deficiency in children. The timely and early diagnosis of neonates, infants and children with HIV is vital. However, the healthcare system of resource-limited countries has its own strengths and limitations. Pitfalls in accurate testing, poor access to health, and high financial costs are a few of the many factors that hamper efforts to limit the spread of diseases such as HIV. In addition, the management of HIV is complex and intricate. Many factors, including proper assessment and indication, counselling, availability and choice of antiretroviral drugs, toxicity, monitoring, financial burden, and social and psychosocial support have to be addressed for HIV care to be successful. Education, evaluation, building expertise, establishing HIV referral centres with diagnostic testing (including virological testing), ensuring availability of antiretroviral drugs,

monitoring and follow-up are some of the key elements necessary for programmes to have adequate impact.

Epidemiology
- There are two major strains of the human immunodeficiency virus: HIV1 and HIV2. HIV1 is the more pathogenic, and is responsible for the global epidemic. HIV2 is largely confined to West Africa. This subsection reflects current management of HIV1, but the principles apply to both strains.
- Infection with HIV leads to progressive destruction of the cellular immune system, ultimately resulting in an acquired immune deficiency syndrome (AIDS) in the vast majority of infected individuals.
- HIV/AIDS is now one of the leading causes of death in children.
- Mother-to-child transmission results in approximately 1000 children becoming infected with HIV each day worldwide. There were 2.5 million children under 15 years old living with HIV in 2009.
- Around 97% of the world's new HIV infections occur in people living in low- and middle-income countries. About 92% of children living with HIV are from sub-Saharan Africa.
- The number of new infections fell from a peak in the late 1990s, but has now plateaued at a high incidence of 2.6 million new infections per year, just below the maximum level reached previously.
- Deaths from AIDS have decreased by 19% between 2004 and 2009 with increasing access to antiretroviral therapy.
- Around 95% of the world's HIV-infected children have been from resource-limited countries. About 90% have been from sub-Saharan Africa, but the prevalence elsewhere is rising, particularly in India, South-East Asia, and countries of the former Soviet Union.

- More than 90% of children acquire HIV perinatally (vertically) from their mothers. The rest are infected through transfusion of infected blood products or via unsterilised needles (extent unknown but probably small), or via sexual transmission among adolescents, or in younger children through child sexual abuse.
- In non-breastfed infants, vertical transmission occurs mainly around the time of delivery, with transmission rates in resource-limited countries ranging from 17% to 24%. Breastfeeding roughly doubles the risk of transmission. In breastfed cohorts from resource-limited countries the rates of transmission are 25–45%.
- Management ideally begins before birth, with counselling and voluntary testing of HIV-infected women during pregnancy, and institution of measures to reduce transmission. In almost all countries, antiretroviral therapy for mothers and infants, elective (pre-labour) Caesarean section and avoidance of breastfeeding have reduced transmission rates to less than 2%.
- Without prenatal counselling and screening, as is frequently the case in resource-limited countries, management begins only when the child becomes symptomatic, with subsequent identification of the HIV infection in the mother.
- Treatment may not be successful if presentation is at an advanced stage of immunosuppression.
- In all societies, even those with a high prevalence, HIV is a potentially stigmatising condition, and the mother or both parents may be reluctant to undergo testing. Confidentiality is essential.
- Counselling must be confidential, requires time and should be undertaken by trained staff.
- Even if a child born to an infected mother is uninfected, he or she will inevitably be affected. Between 14.4 and 18.8 million children were estimated to have lost one or both parents to AIDS in 2010 (UNAIDS data). These children may be abandoned by relatives, ostracised by the community, poorly educated and highly vulnerable. Many support themselves and surviving siblings by commercial sex work, and may acquire HIV infection as a result.

Natural history data

- Before the advent of **highly active antiretroviral therapy (HAART)**, infant mortality doubled and mortality in children aged 1–5 years increased from 8 to 20 per 1000 in Harare between 1990 and 1996.
- However, even in resource-limited countries, some children may be symptom-free into the second decade of life. There is no upper age limit at which it is appropriate to test for HIV if the mother does not have a negative test after the child's birth.
- Data from large long-term prospective perinatally recruited cohort studies are limited in resource-limited countries.
- Growth failure, generalised lymphadenopathy, hepatosplenomegaly, persistent diarrhoea, pulmonary infections, chronic cough and recurrent fevers are the most frequent clinical manifestations.
- The most common causes of death are pneumonia, diarrhoea and malnutrition. Post-mortem studies from the Cote d'Ivoire and clinical studies in Malawi and South Africa showed that *Pneumocystis jiroveci* pneumonia (PCP) is a frequent cause of death in children under 15 months of age.
- Malignancy is a relatively rare AIDS-defining illness in children, compared with HIV-infected adults. However, substantial increases in Kaposi's sarcoma in children have been reported from East and Central Africa. Co-infection with the human herpes virus (HHV8) is a crucial aetiological factor. Kaposi's sarcoma typically presents with large non-tender firm mobile lymph nodes in the head and neck region, and there may be skin lesions and pulmonary disorders. Median survival in one series was only 3 months.

Diagnostic issues

Confirming a diagnosis of HIV infection in young children can be difficult in resource-limited settings.

Early infant diagnosis of HIV: exposed infants should be tested at 6 weeks or as soon as possible thereafter. Infant blood samples are sent as dried blood spots to a laboratory that has the required equipment for HIV PCR testing. This laboratory may be close by, but could also be far from the site. The results then need to be sent back to sites and returned to caregivers in a timely manner. Finally, infants who have tested positive must be started on ART.

In areas of high HIV prevalence, WHO *Integrated Management of the Child* recommends that, when

TABLE 6.2.D.1 Signs and symptoms for use in endemic areas with limited access to diagnostic laboratories

Signs or illness specific to HIV infection	Signs or illness uncommon in HIV-negative children	Signs common in both HIV-positive and ill non-HIV-infected children
Pneumocystis pneumonia	Molluscum contagiosum with multiple lesions	Persistent diarrhoea (> 14 days)
Oesophageal candidiasis	Oral thrush (especially after the neonatal period) without antibiotic treatment and lasting > 1 month or recurrent	Failure to thrive
Herpes zoster	Generalised pruritic dermatitis	Persistent cough > 1 month
Lymphoid interstitial pneumonia	Recurrent severe infections (three or more per year)	Generalised lymphadenopathy
Kaposi's sarcoma	Persistent and/or recurrent fever lasting > 1 week	Hepatosplenomegaly
Chronic parotid enlargement	Neurological dysfunction (progressive neurological impairment, delayed development, intellectual impairment, hypertonia)	Chronic otitis media
Recto-vaginal fistula (rare)	Failure to thrive in a fully breastfed infant < 6 months of age	Moderate or severe malnutrition

assessing sick children aged 2 months to 5 years, health-care workers ask about a history of pneumonia, persistent diarrhoea, ear discharge or very low weight, and look for oral thrush, parotid enlargement and generalised persistent lymphadenopathy. If there are two or more of the above, HIV infection should be suspected and an HIV antibody test performed.

Clinical diagnosis

- The symptoms and signs are often non-specific. The most recent modified WHO clinical case definition for paediatric AIDS is a useful tool for epidemiological surveillance, but lacks sensitivity and has a low positive predictive value (PPV). It is therefore not useful for confirming a diagnosis of HIV infection in an individual child.
- The presence of oral candidiasis does not distinguish HIV-infected from HIV-uninfected children. However, failure of oral candidiasis to respond to treatment or rapid relapse is a highly specific sign of HIV infection. After the neonatal period, the presence of oral thrush without antibiotic treatment, or lasting over 30 days despite treatment, or recurring, or extending beyond the tongue, is highly suggestive of HIV infection. Also typical is extension to the back of the throat, which indicates oesophageal candidiasis.
- Chronic parotitis, the presence of unilateral or bilateral parotid swelling (just in front of the ear) for 14 or more days, with or without associated pain or fever or shingles, is highly suggestive of HIV infection.
- Shingles is unusual in healthy children. Herpes zoster ophthalmicus (i.e. shingles around one eye) is said to have greater than 95% PPV for HIV infection in African children.
- Geographical variation in patterns of disease must be recognised. *Penicillium marneffei* infection, an opportunistic fungal disease that presents with nodular skin lesions, is an AIDS-defining illness that has been reported in South-East Asia. Giant molluscum contagiosum has been a presenting sign in children in Eastern Europe.
- None of these clinical features is a sensitive marker of HIV infection in childhood populations, in that a minority of HIV-infected children manifest them.

There are many clinical signs or conditions that are quite specific to HIV infection, which should be strongly suspected if these conditions are present (*see* Table 6.2.D.1). Some of these features are listed below.

1 Signs or conditions that are very specific to HIV-infected children:
- Pneumocystis pneumonia (PCP).
- Oesophageal candidiasis.
- Lymphoid interstitial pneumonia (LIP).
- Kaposi's sarcoma.

2 Signs that may indicate possible HIV infection:
- **Recurrent infection:** three or more severe episodes of a bacterial infection (e.g. pneumonia, meningitis, sepsis, cellulitis) in the past 12 months.
- **Oral thrush:** after the neonatal period, the presence of oral thrush in the absence of antibiotic treatment, or lasting over 30 days despite treatment, or recurring, or extending beyond the tongue.
- **Chronic parotitis:** the presence of unilateral or bilateral parotid swelling for 14 or more days.

- **Generalised lymphadenopathy:** the presence of enlarged lymph nodes in two or more non-inguinal regions without any apparent underlying cause.
- **Hepatomegaly** with no apparent cause.
- **Persistent and/or recurrent fever.**
- **Neurological dysfunction:** progressive neurological impairment, microcephaly, developmental delay, hypertonia, encephalopathy.
- **Herpes zoster.**
- **HIV dermatitis:** typical skin rashes include erythematous papular rashes, extensive fungal infections of the skin, scalp and nails, and extensive molluscum contagiosum.
- **Chronic suppurative lung disease.**

3 Signs that are common in HIV-infected and non-HIV-infected children:
- Chronic otitis media.
- Persistent diarrhoea.
- Moderate or severe malnutrition.

Counselling and testing

If there are reasons to suspect HIV infection, and the child's HIV status is not known, the family should be offered diagnostic testing for HIV.

Counselling used to be more complex when there was no treatment available. There is now no question that it is in the child's best interest to be tested so that treatment can be given to prolong life if they are HIV-positive. The lessons of obtaining informed consent still apply, just as with any other important investigation. If the mother has not already been tested, a positive result in a child is most likely to mean that the mother is infected, too. However, if the mother is not present when the child presents, the onus of responsibility of the paediatrician is to the child, and testing should not be delayed.

The additional consideration with testing for HIV is the stigma associated with the diagnosis. When HIV meant inevitable death, there was enormous fear of the diagnosis. The potentially better prognosis has been hard to accept when so many present too late. Stigma is also associated with the fact that it is a sexually transmitted disease. This raises issues of where the infection was acquired and contact tracing. The fear of domestic violence and social ostracisation sometimes creates reluctance to allow children to be tested.

The process of counselling starts with always ensuring that the test is done with consent. The person giving consent should be the carer at the time when the test is indicated. If the child is of an age at which they can be responsible for taking their own medicines, they can give their own consent for testing. There are no surrogate tests for HIV, such as lymphocyte counts; the appropriate test according to what is available should always be done. If there is delay in getting a result it may be necessary to start appropriate treatment – for example, for suspected PCP pneumonia with IV co-trimoxazole.

If there is refusal to allow testing, the test cannot be carried out. If the test is positive, the family need to have confidence in the healthcare professionals to ensure adherence to treatment. Counselling requires time, and must be done by trained staff. If staff at the first referral level have not been trained, assistance should be sought from other sources, such as local community AIDS support organisations. A time limit should be set to prevent repeated procrastination and the risk of death from opportunistic infection.

HIV counselling should take account of the child as part of a family. This should include the psychological implications of HIV infection for the child, mother, father and other family members. Counselling should stress that, although cure is currently not possible, there is much that can be done to improve the quality and duration of the child's life. Antiretroviral treatment (ART) is available and greatly improves survival and the quality of life of the child and the parents. Counselling should make it clear that the hospital staff want to help, and that the mother should not be frightened of going to a health centre or hospital early in an illness, even if this is only to ask questions.

HIV is talked about much more openly now than was the case at the start of the epidemic, and testing is seen as an expected part of routine healthcare. The request for testing should not be built up as a major event, but included as part of the diagnostic work-up along with malaria, TB and other investigations.

As mentioned above, counselling requires time, and must be done by trained staff.

Indications for HIV counselling
HIV counselling is indicated in the following situations.

Child with unknown HIV status presenting with clinical signs of HIV infection and/or risk factors (e.g. a mother or sibling with HIV/AIDS)
- Make time for the counselling session.
- Take advice from local people experienced in offering testing, so that any advice given is consistent with what the mother will receive from professional counsellors at a later stage.
- Where available, arrange an HIV test, according to national guidelines, to confirm the clinical diagnosis, alert the mother to HIV-related problems, and discuss prevention of future mother-to-child transmission.

Note the following:
1 If HIV testing is not available, discuss the presumptive diagnosis of HIV infection in the light of the existing signs and symptoms and risk factors.
2 In countries with generalised HIV epidemics, routine healthcare provider-initiated testing and counselling (PITC) is recommended for all children seen in paediatric health services (World Health Organization, 2007).

Child known to be HIV-infected but responding poorly to treatment, or needing further investigations
Discuss the following:
- the parents' understanding of HIV infection
- management of current problems
- the role of ART and adherence to regular drug administration
- the need to refer to a higher level, if necessary
- support from community-based groups (if available).

Child known to be HIV-infected who has responded well to treatment and is to be discharged (or referred to a community-based care programme)
Discuss the following:
- the reason for referral to a community-based care programme, if appropriate
- follow-up care

- risk factors for future illness
- immunisation and HIV
- adherence and ART treatment support.

Laboratory diagnosis
The definitive diagnosis of HIV requires laboratory confirmatory testing. The HIV antibody test is commonly used as a screening test. However, in the neonatal and infantile period, the antibody test is not recommended. This is because the maternal HIV antibodies readily cross the placenta and persist in the neonate for up to 18 months. Also, all screening tests should be confirmed by a second test. The following are some of the tests used for laboratory diagnosis of HIV in children:
- Antibody tests:
  - HIV IgG antibody tests.
  - Rapid Test.
- Virological tests:
  - HIV DNA polymerase chain reaction (PCR).
  - HIV RNA PCR.
  - HIV culture.
- P24 antigen assay:
  - Direct.
  - Acid hydrolysis.

DNA-based assays are the most reliable for diagnosis, and are recommended for diagnosis in infants. However, the cost and availability of tests may be an issue in resource-limited countries. The simplest laboratory test is an HIV antibody test, usually done by enzyme-linked immunosorbent assay (ELISA). However, even this may not be affordable or available in many settings.

The WHO recommends the use of a presumptive clinical diagnosis of severe HIV disease in the **absence** of virologic testing **if**:
- an infant's HIV exposure is confirmed by antibody testing **and** if either:
  - clinical stage 3 or 4 or AIDS-indicator condition(s) are present **or**
  - the child has two or more of the following: oral thrush, severe pneumonia, severe sepsis.

A **presumptive** diagnosis of AIDS can also be made in an antibody-positive infant **if** CD4 percentages are below 20% **or** other factors are present, including recent HIV-related maternal death or advanced HIV disease in the mother.

Infants acquire maternal HIV IgG transplacentally, and this can be detected by ELISA up to 18 months of age. Thus antibody tests cannot reliably distinguish infected from uninfected children until they are 18 months old. Additional diagnostic challenges arise if the child is still breastfeeding or has been breastfed. Although HIV infection cannot be ruled out until 18 months for some children, many children will have lost HIV antibodies between 9 and 18 months of age. The importance of this is that a rapid antibody test can be done if the mother is unwilling or unavailable to be tested herself. If the antibody test is negative and the child has not been breastfed in the last 6 weeks, there is then no need for further testing unless there is ongoing exposure (e.g. through breastfeeding). If the antibody is positive, this does not mean that the child is infected, but if other signs of immune deficiency are present it may warrant empirical treatment according to WHO guidelines if PCR testing is not available.

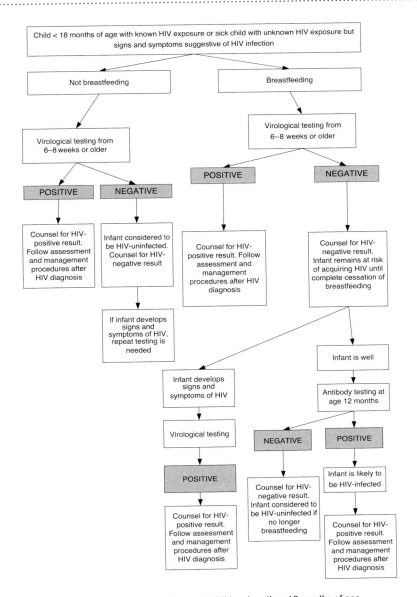

FIGURE 6.2.D.1 Algorithm for diagnosing HIV infection in infants and children less than 18 months of age.

Many children born to HIV-infected mothers may die before this age, and a diagnosis of HIV infection may be presumptive, dependent on signs and symptoms. Thus, based on age, the clinical, serological and virological tests and status of breastfeeding will determine the diagnosis of a child undergoing evaluation (see Table 6.2.D.2).

TABLE 6.2.D.2 Proposed methods for diagnosing HIV in children (born to mothers identified as HIV-positive or with unknown HIV status) in resource-limited settings* (see Figure 6.2.D.1)

Diagnostic method	Age of child		
	< 12 months	12–18 months	> 18 months
Clinical staging	Yes	Yes	Yes
Serological (antibody)	May be helpful[†]	Yes[‡]	Yes
Virological	Yes	Yes, if serology is positive	No, serology is definitive

*If the child is breastfeeding, a negative diagnostic test, either serological or virological, would have to be repeated 6 weeks after cessation of all breastfeeding.

[†] A positive antibody test in a child under 12 months of age defines the exposure status of the child and may be helpful when the mother's HIV status is unknown.

[‡] By the age of 12 months, HIV antibody-positive testing can be considered indicative of probable HIV infection, and should be confirmed by a second antibody test after 18 months.

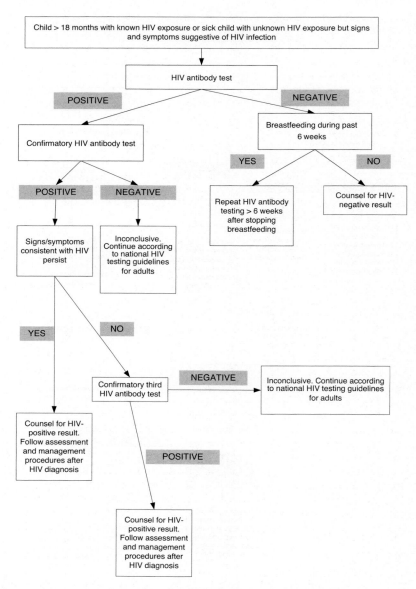

FIGURE 6.2.D.2 Algorithm for diagnosing HIV infection in infants and children aged 18 months or older.

Algorithms for diagnosis are shown in Figures 6.2.D.1 and 6.2.D.2.

Notes to Figure 6.2.D.1.

1 If HIV exposure is not certain, consider testing the mother first before doing a virological test on the child. If the mother tests negative for HIV, explore other risk factors for HIV transmission.

2 In infants and children under 18 months of age considered to be HIV-uninfected who develop signs or symptoms suggestive of HIV, virological testing should be performed.

3 If virological testing is not available, antibody testing can be performed. By the age of 12 months most uninfected children will have lost maternal antibody, and positive antibody testing at this time usually indicates HIV infection in the child (96% specificity). In infants younger than 12 months where antibody testing is still positive, a presumptive clinical diagnosis of severe HIV disease may need to be made, as it is not possible to reliably establish HIV infection with antibody testing before the

age of 12 months (i.e. specificity at age 9–12 months is 74–96%). In this situation, confirmation of the presumptive clinical diagnosis of HIV infection by virological testing should be sought as soon as possible.

4 Antibody testing can be performed at the age of 12 months (see above).

5 Where the infant is being considered to be HIV-infected based upon a positive antibody test performed at 12 months of age or older, the result should be confirmed by virological testing (in children less than 18 months of age) or by antibody testing (once they are over 18 months of age).

Notes to Figure 6.2.D.2.

1 A definitive diagnosis of HIV infection in children aged ≥ 18 months can be made with antibody testing. HIV testing procedures for children aged ≥ 18 months follow the national HIV testing guidelines for adults. Virological testing can be used to diagnose HIV infection at any age.

2 One positive HIV antibody test (rapid test or ELISA) should be confirmed by a second HIV antibody test

(rapid test or ELISA) using an assay that relies on a different antigen or has different operating characteristics. In low-HIV-prevalence settings, a third confirmatory test may be required.

3 Children who are breastfed have an ongoing risk of acquiring HIV infection. Therefore HIV infection can be excluded only after stopping breastfeeding for more than 6 weeks.

HIV antibody test (ELISA or rapid tests)

Rapid tests are widely available and are safe, effective, sensitive and reliable for diagnosing HIV infection in children above the age of 18 months. For those under 18 months, HIV antibody tests are a sensitive reliable way to exclude HIV infection in non-breastfeeding children. For those children under 18 months, confirm all positive HIV antibody tests by virological tests as soon as possible (see below). Where this is not possible, repeat antibody testing at 18 months.

Rapid HIV tests can be used to exclude HIV infection in a child presenting with malnutrition or other serious clinical events in areas with high HIV prevalence.

To confirm the diagnosis, it is necessary to use assays that detect the virus itself or viral components. Such tests include **antigen detection tests, viral culture, amplification techniques and HIV-specific IgA tests**.

Virological testing

Virological testing for HIV-specific RNA or DNA is the most reliable method of diagnosing HIV infection in children under 18 months of age. This requires sending a blood sample to a specialised laboratory that can perform this test, and these are becoming increasingly available in large centres in many countries. It is relatively inexpensive, easy to standardise, and can be done using dried blood spots. In infants and children undergoing virological testing, the following assays (and respective specimen types) are potentially available:

- HIV DNA on whole blood specimens or dried blood spots (DBS)
- HIV RNA on plasma or DBS
- ultrasensitive p24 antigen (Up24 Ag) on plasma or DBS.

The new ultrasensitive p24 assay is as accurate as PCR virology, significantly less expensive, and less resource demanding when used to diagnose HIV. It is particularly valuable in infants under 12 months old.

A test at birth will only detect *in-utero* infection, whereas most infection occurs at delivery. Infected infants can suffer life-threatening infections in the first weeks of life. Where there is a high risk of infection (e.g. a mother who seroconverts in pregnancy, has a low CD4 count or other genital lesions and has had no antiretrovirals), testing should be done at 2 weeks of age. Where the risk is low (e.g. a mother who has been on HAART throughout pregnancy), the test can be delayed until 6 weeks of age. At the first DTP immunisation of all infants, the maternal HIV status should be checked from records or rapid testing. If it is positive or unavailable, the child should be tested. All HIV-exposed infants should have HIV virological testing at 4–6 weeks of age or at the earliest opportunity thereafter.

If the child has had zidovudine (ZDV) prophylaxis during and after delivery, virological testing is not recommended until 4–8 weeks after delivery, as ZDV interferes with the reliability of the test.

One virological test that is positive at 4–8 weeks is sufficient to diagnose infection in a young infant. If the young infant is still breastfeeding, and the DNA virological test is negative, it needs to be repeated 6 weeks after the complete cessation of breastfeeding to confirm that the child is not HIV infected.

Infants with signs or symptoms suggestive of HIV infection must undergo HIV serological testing and, if this is positive, virological testing. In breastfeeding infants or children it is strongly recommended that breastfeeding is not discontinued in order to perform any kind of diagnostic HIV test. In sick infants in whom HIV infection is being considered as an underlying cause of symptoms and signs, and virological testing is not available, HIV serological testing and the use of a clinical algorithm for presumptive clinical diagnosis of HIV infection are strongly recommended.

In infants with an initial positive virological test result, it is strongly recommended that ART be started without delay and, at the same time, a second specimen be collected to confirm the initial positive virological test result. **Do not delay ART. In infected infants, immediate initiation of ART saves lives, and commencement of ART should not be delayed while waiting for the results of the confirmatory test. Results from the CHER trial suggest initiation of ART before 12 weeks of age results in a 75% reduction in early mortality.**

(Cotton MF, Violari A, Otwombe K, *et al.* (2013) Early time-limited antiretroviral therapy versus deferred therapy in South African infants infected with HIV: results from children with HIV early antiretroviral (CHER) randomised trial. *Lancet* 382: 1555–63.)

Test results from virological testing in infants should be returned to the clinic and the child and their mother or carer as soon as possible, but at the very latest within 4 weeks of specimen collection. Positive test results should be fast-tracked to the mother–baby pair as soon as possible to enable prompt initiation of ART.

All infants with unknown or uncertain HIV exposure who are being seen in healthcare facilities at or around the time of birth or at the first postnatal visit (usually 4–6 weeks), or at another child health visit, should have their HIV exposure status ascertained.

Clinically well, HIV-exposed infants should undergo HIV serological testing at around 9 months of age (or at the time of the last immunisation visit). Those who have positive serological assays at 9 months should have a virological test to identify whether they need ART.

Recently the WHO Technical Reference Group for Paediatric HIV/ART and Care made the following key recommendations with regard to when and how to test for HIV in children:

1 Infants known to have been exposed to HIV should have a virological test (HIV nucleic acid test) at 4–6 weeks of age, or at the earliest opportunity for infants seen after 4–6 weeks.

2 Urgent HIV testing is recommended for any infant presenting to healthcare facilities with signs, symptoms or medical conditions that could indicate HIV.

3 All infants should have their HIV exposure status established at their first contact with the healthcare system, ideally before 6 weeks of age.

4 Infants under 6 weeks of age, of unknown HIV exposure status and in settings where local or national antenatal HIV seroprevalence is greater than 1%, should be offered maternal or infant HIV antibody testing and counselling in order to establish their exposure status.

Other laboratory tests

- **A low CD4 count or CD4:CD8** ratio suggests HIV infection, but requires specialised equipment. **A low total lymphocyte count** is a much less expensive though less specific surrogate marker of HIV infection and immunosuppression.
- HIV infection can also cause anaemia or thrombocytopaenia. It is appropriate to test for HIV in children who present with low platelet counts.
- Lack of thymic shadow on chest X-ray is a feature of advanced disease, but is clearly not specific, as the thymus tends to shrink in volume in response to a variety of acute infections in childhood.

Assessment of HIV-infected and HIV-exposed children

Any child with an illness compatible with HIV infection should be properly evaluated irrespective of HIV exposure. This includes neonates, infants and children with perinatal exposure, and those with specific signs and symptoms suggestive of HIV infection, chronic or unexplained illness, or known exposure during childhood. Figure 6.2.D.3 shows a useful algorithm that can be used by paediatricians and other clinical care providers for the initial evaluation and management of children with known exposure to HIV, or sick children with symptoms suggestive of HIV infection but unknown history of exposure.

Notes to Figure 6.2.D.3.

1. An expert in the management of children with HIV should be consulted wherever this is feasible.
2. If HIV is suspected, compassionate counselling before HIV testing should be arranged.
3. Maternal advanced HIV disease and low CD4 are risk factors for HIV transmission.
4. Successful treatment with ART in mothers reduces the risk of transmission.
5. PMTCT using ZDV monotherapy alone, ZDV plus NVP single dose, and NVP single dose alone is associated

---

Left-hand flow chart:

Child with known HIV exposure

↓

Assess the likelihood of acquiring HIV infection by asking for the following history:
- Mother's history: maternal HIV disease status, mother alive or dead, ART or prophylaxis for MTCT, mode of delivery, breastfeeding
- Father's history: HIV status, father alive or dead, travel/employment away from home, etc.
- Blood transfusion: source of blood and was it tested

↓

- Perform history and physical examination for child who has symptoms and/or signs of HIV infection
- Look for opportunistic infections
- Undertake appropriate investigation and treatment for opportunistic infection

↓

Identify needs for ART for prevention of MTCT and CTX to prevent PCP

↓

Perform HIV diagnostic testing
Methods depend on child's age

Right-hand flow chart:

Ill child with unknown HIV exposure but with suspected HIV infection

↓

Identify whether there are HIV risk factors in the family, possible MTCT, blood transfusion, injecting drug use, history of migrant work, or high number of sexual contacts

↓

Perform history and physical examination
Child has signs and symptoms of HIV infection including opportunistic infections
Appropriate investigations/treatment for opportunistic infections

↓

- Perform HIV diagnosis testing if there are risk factors and/or signs or symptoms consistent with HIV infection or HIV-related opportunistic infections
- Diagnostic methods used depend on child's age
- In cases where maternal HIV status cannot be confirmed and virological testing is not available to diagnose HIV infection in a child younger than 18 months, HIV antibody test should be performed to confirm HIV exposure via MTCT

FIGURE 6.2.D.3 Initial assessment of a child with known HIV exposure or a sick child with unknown HIV exposure but with suspected HIV infection. MTCT, mother-to-child transmission; ART, antiretroviral therapy; PCP, pneumocystis pneumonia.

with transmission rates of approximately 5–10%, 3–5% and 10–20%, respectively.

6 An infant remains at risk of acquiring HIV for as long as he or she is breastfed.

Perinatally acquired HIV infection

HIV1 transmission occurs more frequently than that of HIV2. It occurs in late pregnancy, during delivery and through breastfeeding, and transmission is more likely if any of the following factors are present:

- advanced maternal HIV disease
- premature labour
- prolonged rupture of membranes
- contact with maternal blood
- in the first twin
- maternal genital infection.

Prevention of mother-to-child transmission (PMTCT) of HIV and infant feeding in the context of HIV

HIV transmission may occur during pregnancy, labour and delivery, or through breastfeeding. The best way to prevent transmission is to prevent sexually acquired HIV infection, especially in pregnant women, and to prevent unintended pregnancies in HIV-positive women. If an HIV-infected woman becomes pregnant, she should be provided with services including antiretroviral drugs, safe obstetric practices, and infant feeding counselling and support (*see* Section 2.8.C).

The key recommendations of the 2010 WHO guidance on ARV drugs for treatment of pregnant women and prevention of HIV in infants are as follows:

Women who are immunocompromised

As early as possible, provide ART for all HIV-positive pregnant women both to benefit the health of the mother and to prevent HIV transmission to her child during pregnancy and breastfeeding.

Start lifelong ART for all pregnant women with severe or advanced clinical disease (stage 3 or 4), or with a CD4 count of ≤ 350 cells/mm^3, regardless of symptoms. HIV-positive pregnant women in need of treatment for their own health (i.e. as soon as the eligibility criteria are met) should start ART irrespective of gestational age, and should continue with it throughout pregnancy, delivery, during breastfeeding and thereafter.

The recommended first-line regimens for pregnant women are as follows:

- AZT + 3TC + NVP **or**
- AZT + 3TC + EFV **or**
- TDF + 3TC (or FTC) + NVP **or**
- TDF + 3TC (or FTC) + EFV.

The infant is given NVP or AZT starting as soon as possible after birth (aim for less than 6 hours postpartum) and continued for 4–6 weeks.

Women who are not immunocompromised

Antiretroviral (ARV) prophylaxis is indicated for HIV-positive pregnant women with relatively strong immune systems who do not need ART for their own health. This would reduce the risk of HIV transmission from mother to child. There are two options, both of which should start early in pregnancy, at 14 weeks or as soon as possible thereafter.

The two options provide a significant reduction in MTCT with equal efficacy in this group of women who are not eligible for ART.

Option A: Twice daily AZT for the mother during pregnancy; if the mother has less than 4 weeks of AZT, give single-dose nevirapine during labour, and AZT and lamivudine during labour and for 7 days postpartum. Give the infant prophylaxis with either AZT or NVP for 6 weeks after birth if he or she is not breastfeeding. If the infant is breastfeeding, daily NVP infant prophylaxis should be continued for 1 week after the end of the breastfeeding period.

or

Option B: a three-drug prophylactic regimen for the mother, taken during pregnancy and throughout the breastfeeding period, as well as infant prophylaxis for 6 weeks after birth, whether or not the infant is breastfeeding.

Option B+: all pregnant and breastfeeding women infected with HIV should initiate ART as lifelong treatment.

Breastfeeding

The global availability of ART means that there is enough evidence for the WHO to recommend breastfeeding for mothers with HIV.

Even with ART there is still a small risk of HIV transmission, particularly if there is any interruption to treatment, either in supply or absorption (due to diarrhoea or vomiting). HIV can be transmitted through breast milk at any point during lactation, so the rate of infection in breastfed infants increases with duration of breastfeeding.

In many countries, public health services where there is poor access to clean drinking water and alternatives to breastfeeding have not been able to adequately support and provide safe replacement feeding. HIV-positive mothers have faced the dilemma of whether to give their babies all the benefits of breastfeeding but expose them to the risk of HIV infection, or avoid all breastfeeding and increase the risk of their baby's death from diarrhoea and malnutrition.

The effectiveness of ART in reducing transmission through breastfeeding has resulted in two major changes in 2012 from previous guidelines:

1 National health authorities should decide whether health services will principally counsel and support HIV-positive mothers to either:

- breastfeed and receive ARV interventions **or**
- avoid all breastfeeding, as the strategy that is most likely to give infants the greatest chance of HIV-free survival.

2 In settings where national authorities recommend that HIV-positive mothers should breastfeed, and provide ARVs to prevent transmission, mothers should exclusively breastfeed their infants for the first 6 months of life, introducing appropriate complementary foods thereafter, and should continue breastfeeding for the first 12 months of life.

Mothers who are known to be HIV infected and who decide to stop breastfeeding at any time should stop gradually over 1 month. Stopping breastfeeding abruptly is not advisable (World Health Organization, 2010).

These new guidelines have great potential to improve the mother's own health and to reduce the mother-to-child HIV transmission risk to 5% or lower in a breastfeeding population in the absence of any interventions and with continued breastfeeding. With ART the WHO is aiming for complete prevention of mother-to-child transmission worldwide by 2015.

Where a decision has been made to continue breast-feeding because the child is already infected, infant feeding options should be discussed for future pregnancies. This should be carried out by a trained and experienced counsellor.

If a child is known to be HIV-infected and is being breastfed, encourage the mother to continue breastfeeding if living in a resource-limited country, as there is usually a high risk of gastroenteritis in such regions.

If the mother is known to be HIV-positive and the child's HIV status is unknown, the mother should be counselled about the benefits of breastfeeding as well as the risk of HIV transmission through breastfeeding. If replacement feeding is acceptable, feasible, affordable, sustainable and safe, avoidance of further breastfeeding is recommended. Otherwise, exclusive breastfeeding should be practised if the child is less than 6 months of age, and breastfeeding should be discontinued as soon as these conditions are in place.

Infants born to HIV-positive mothers who have escaped perinatal infection have a lower risk of acquiring HIV if they are not breastfed. However, their risk of death may be increased if they are not breastfed in situations where there is no regular access to nutritionally adequate, safely prepared breast milk substitutes, and there is a high risk of gastroenteritis.

Counselling should be provided by a trained and experienced counsellor. Take advice from local people experienced in counselling so that any advice given is consistent with what the mother will receive from professional counsellors at a later stage.

If the mother decides to use breast milk substitutes, counsel her about their correct use and demonstrate their safe preparation.

Management of the child with a suspected or proven HIV infection

- The aim of treatment should be to maintain the best possible quality of life for the child for as long as possible, without bankrupting the family. This disease affects the whole family, and the child must be treated in the context of the needs of all of the family.
- Currently there are far more questions than evidence-based answers; published data on many management issues in the context of resource-limited countries are not available.
- Much can be achieved with compassionate supportive care, by applying existing guidelines (such as Integrated Management of Childhood Illness algorithms) with an awareness of the need for early diagnosis and intervention in the HIV-infected child.
- Diagnosis of infections such as tuberculosis, lower respiratory infections, bacteraemia (particularly with non-typhoid salmonellae, staphylococci or streptococci) and opportunistic infections can be difficult, and often relies on empirical trials of therapy.

A low threshold for antibiotic use is appropriate, but may exacerbate diarrhoea and candidiasis, and may only be effective if given IV or IM, in the presence of diarrhoea and malabsorption.

Most infections in HIV-positive children are caused by the same pathogens as in HIV-negative children, although they may be more frequent, more severe and occur repeatedly. There is recent evidence that *Staphylococcus aureus* may be more invasive in children with HIV.

Clinical staging of HIV infection

In a child with diagnosed or highly suspected HIV infection, a clinical staging system helps to identify the degree of damage to the immune system and to plan treatment and care options. The stages determine the likely prognosis of HIV, and are a guide as to when to start, stop or substitute ARV therapy in HIV-infected children.

The clinical stages identify a progressive sequence from least to most severe, such that the higher the clinical stage the poorer the prognosis. For classification purposes, once a stage 3 clinical condition has occurred, the child's prognosis will probably remain that of stage 3, and will not improve to that of stage 2, even with resolution of the original condition, or the appearance of a new stage 2 clinical event. ART with good adherence dramatically improves the prognosis.

The clinical staging events can also be used to identify the response to ARV treatment if there is no easy or affordable access to viral load or CD4 testing.

TABLE 6.2.D.3 WHO paediatric clinical staging system for use in children under 13 years with confirmed laboratory evidence of HIV infection (HIV antibody where age is > 18 months, DNA or RNA virological testing where age is < 18 months)

Stage 1	• Asymptomatic • Persistent generalised lymphadenopathy (PGL)
Stage 2	• Unexplained persistent hepatosplenomegaly • Papular pruritic eruptions • Fungal nail infections • Lineal gingival erythema (LGE) • Extensive wart virus infection • Extensive molluscum infection (> 5% of body area) • Recurrent oral ulcerations (two or more episodes in 6 months) • Parotid enlargement • Herpes zoster • Recurrent or chronic upper respiratory tract infections (otitis media, otorrhoea, sinusitis, two or more episodes in any 6-month period)
Stage 3	• Unexplained moderate malnutrition not responding to standard therapy • Unexplained persistent diarrhoea (for > 14 days) • Unexplained persistent fever (intermittent or constant, for > 1 month) • Oral candidiasis (outside the neonatal period) • Oral hairy leukoplakia • Pulmonary tuberculosis[1] • Severe recurrent presumed bacterial pneumonia (two or more episodes in 6 months) • Acute necrotising ulcerative gingivitis or periodontitis • Lymphoid interstitial pneumonia (LIP) • Unexplained anaemia (< 8 grams/dL), neutropenia (< 500/mm³) or thrombocytopenia (< 30 000/mm³) for > 1 month

(continued)

Stage 4	• Unexplained severe wasting or severe malnutrition not responding to standard therapy • Pneumocystis pneumonia • Recurrent severe presumed bacterial infections (two or more episodes within 1 year, e.g. empyema, pyomyositis, bone or joint infection, or meningitis, but excluding pneumonia) • Chronic orolabial or cutaneous herpes simplex infection (for > 1 month) • Disseminated or extrapulmonary tuberculosis • Kaposi's sarcoma • Oesophageal candidiasis • Symptomatic HIV seropositive infant < 18 months of age with two or more of the following: oral thrush, with or without severe pneumonia, with or without failure to thrive, with or without severe sepsis[2] • CMV retinitis • CNS toxoplasmosis • Any disseminated endemic mycosis, including cryptococcal meningitis (e.g. extrapulmonary cryptococcosis, histoplasmosis, coccidiomycosis, penicilliosis) • Cryptosporidiosis or isosporiasis (with diarrhoea for > 1 month) • Cytomegalovirus infection (onset at age > 1 month in an organ other than liver, spleen or lymph nodes) • Disseminated mycobacterial disease other than tuberculous • Candida of trachea, bronchi or lungs • Acquired HIV-related recto-vesical fistula • Cerebral or B-cell non-Hodgkin's lymphoma • Progressive multifocal leukoencephalopathy (PML) • HIV encephalopathy • HIV-related cardiomyopathy • HIV-related nephropathy

[1] TB may occur at any CD4 count, and CD4% should be considered where available.

[2] Presumptive diagnosis of stage 4 disease in seropositive children under 18 months of age requires confirmation with HIV virological tests, or with HIV antibody test if over 18 months of age.

Antiretroviral therapy (ART)

Antiretroviral (ARV) drugs are becoming more widely available, and have revolutionised the care of children with HIV/AIDS. ARV drugs are not a cure for HIV, but they have dramatically reduced mortality and morbidity, and improved the quality and length of life. The WHO recommends that in resource-limited settings, HIV-infected adults and children should start ARV therapy based upon clinical or immunological criteria, and using simplified standardised treatment guidelines.

Resistance to single or dual agents is quick to emerge, so **single-drug regimens are contraindicated**. Indeed **at least three drugs are the recommended minimum standard for all settings**. Although new ARV drugs are coming on to the market, frequently these are not available for use in children, due to lack of suitable formulations or dosage data, or their high costs.

As children with HIV are often part of a household that includes an adult with HIV, ideally access to treatment and ARV drugs needs to be ensured for other family members, and where possible similar drug regimens should be used. Fixed-dose combinations are increasingly available, and are preferred as they promote and support treatment adherence, as well as reducing the cost of treatment. Existing tablets often cannot be divided into lower dosages for children (under 10 kg), so syrups or solutions and suspensions are needed.

The underlying principles of ART and the choice of first-line ART in children are largely the same as for adults. However, it is also important to consider the following:
• availability of a suitable formulation that can be taken in appropriate doses
• simplicity of the dosage schedule
• taste/palatability and thus compliance in young children
• the ART regimen that the parent(s) or carers are or will be taking.

Suitable formulations for children are not available for some ARVs (particularly the protease inhibitor class of drugs).

Antiretroviral drugs

Antiretroviral drugs fall into three main classes, namely nucleoside analogue reverse transcriptase inhibitors (NRTIs), non-nucleoside reverse transcriptase inhibitors (NNRTIs), and protease inhibitors (PIs) (see Table 6.2.D.4).

Triple therapy is the standard of care.

The WHO currently recommends that first-line regimens should be based upon two nucleoside analogue reverse transcriptase inhibitors (NRTIs) plus one non-nucleoside drug (NNRTI). The use of triple NRTI as first-line therapy is currently considered a secondary alternative because of recent research findings in adults. Protease inhibitors are usually recommended as part of second-line regimens in most resource-limited settings.

Efavirenz (EFV) is the NNRTI of choice in children who are on rifampicin, if treatment needs to start before antituberculous therapy is completed.

For drug dosages and regimens, see Appendix 4.

Calculation of drug dosages

Drug doses are given per kg for some drugs and per m² surface area of the child for others. A table giving the equivalent weights of various surface area values is provided in Section 9 of this textbook, to aid dosage calculation. In general, children metabolise PI and NNRTI drugs faster than adults, and require higher than adult equivalent doses to achieve appropriate drug levels. Drug doses have to be increased as the child grows, otherwise there is a risk of under-dosage and development of resistance.

Formulations

Liquid formulations may not be readily available, are more expensive, and may have a reduced shelf-life. As the child gets older, the amount of syrup that needs to be taken becomes quite considerable. Therefore, in patients over 10 kg in weight, it is preferable to give parts of scored tablets or combination preparations (see Appendix 4).

TABLE 6.2.D.4 Classes of antiretroviral drugs recommended for use in children in resource-limited settings

Nucleoside analogue reverse transcriptase inhibitors (NRTIs)		
Zidovudine	ZDV/AZT	180–240 mg/m^2 twice daily
Lamivudine	3TC	4 mg/kg twice daily up to a maximum of 150 mg twice daily
Stavudine	d4T	1 mg/kg twice daily up to 30 mg twice daily
Didanosine	ddl	90–120 mg/m^2/dose twice daily
Abacavir	ABC	8 mg/kg/dose given twice daily up to 300 mg twice daily
Non-nucleoside reverse transcriptase inhibitors (NNRTIs)		
Nevirapine	NVP	160–200 mg/m^2 up to a maximum of 200 mg twice daily
Efavirenz	EFV	15 mg/kg/day up to 600 mg once daily
Etravirine	ETV	200 mg twice daily for adolescents
Protease inhibitors (PIs)		
Lopinavir/ ritonavir	LPV/r	230–350 mg/m^2 twice daily
Darunavir	DRV	10–20 mg/kg twice daily
Atazanavir	ATV	7 mg/kg once daily
Ritonavir	RTV	Given as a 'booster' with another PI
Integrase inhibitors		
Raltegravir	RAL	400 mg twice daily for adolescents

First-line ART for children under 3 years of age

An LPV/r-based regimen should be used as first-line ART for all children infected with HIV who are under 3 years (36 months) of age, regardless of NNRTI exposure. If LPV/r is not feasible, treatment should be initiated with an NVP-based regimen.

Where viral load monitoring is available, consideration can be given to substituting LPV/r with an NNRTI after virological suppression is sustained.

For infants and children under 3 years of age who are infected with HIV, ABC + 3TC + AZT is recommended as an option for children who develop TB while on an ART regimen containing NVP or LPV/r. Once TB therapy has been completed, this regimen should be stopped and the initial regimen should be restarted.

For infants and children under 3 years of age who are infected with HIV, the NRTI backbone for an ART regimen should be ABC + 3TC or AZT + 3TC (this is a strong recommendation but with low-quality evidence).

First-line ART for children aged 3 years or older (including adolescents)

For children aged 3 years or older (including adolescents) who are infected with HIV, EFV is the preferred NNRTI for first-line treatment, and NVP is the alternative.

For children aged 3–9 years (and adolescents weighing less than 35 kg) who are infected with HIV, the NRTI backbone for an ART regimen should be one of the following, in order of preference:
- ABC + 3TC
- AZT or TDF + 3TC (or FTC).

For adolescents who are infected with HIV (10–19 years old, weighing 35 kg or more), the NRTI backbone for an ART regimen should align with that of adults and be one of the following, in order of preference:
- TDF + 3TC (or FTC)
- AZT + 3TC
- ABC + 3TC.

When to start ART

About 20% of HIV-infected infants in developing countries progress to AIDS or death by 12 months of age (with a substantial contribution from PCP infections in infants under 6 months of age who are not receiving co-trimoxazole treatment).

ART should be initiated in all children infected with HIV below 5 years of age, regardless of WHO clinical stage or CD4 count, that is:
- Infants diagnosed in the first year of life.
- Children infected with HIV when aged 1–4 years.

ART should be initiated in all children infected with HIV aged 5 years or older with a CD4 cell count of less than 500 cells/mm^3, regardless of WHO clinical stage, that is:
- CD4 count less than 350 cells/mm^3.
- CD4 count between 350 and 500 cells/mm^3.

ART should be initiated in all children infected with HIV with severe or advanced symptomatic disease (WHO clinical stage 3 or 4) regardless of age and CD4 count.

ART should be initiated in any child younger than 18 months who has been given a presumptive clinical diagnosis of HIV infection.

Infants and children with specific conditions

- For children or adolescents with severe anaemia (< 7.5 g/dL) or severe neutropenia (< 0.5/mm^3), avoid AZT.
- For adolescents over 12 years of age with hepatitis B, the preferred regimen is tenofovir (TDF) + emtricitabine (FTC) or 3TC + NNRTI.

Side effects of antiretroviral therapy and monitoring

The response to antiretroviral treatment and the side effects of treatment both need to be monitored. Where CD4 cell count or viral load monitoring is available, this should be done every 3 to 6 months and can provide information on the success or failure of the response to treatment, and therefore guide changes to treatment. Where this is not possible, clinical parameters, including clinical staging events, need to be used (see Table 6.1.D.3).

Monitoring the response after ARV initiation

- After ARV initiation or a change in ARVs see the child at 2 and 4 weeks after the start or change.
- All children should be seen if there are any problems that concern the caregiver, or inter-current illness.

Long-term follow-up

- A clinician should see the child at least every 3 months.
- A non-clinician (ideally the provider of ARV medication, such as a pharmacist, who would assess adherence and provide adherence counselling) should see the child monthly.
- The child should be seen more frequently, preferably by a clinician, if clinically unstable.

Monitoring the response (*see* Appendix 1)

At entry into care and at initiation of ART, and then at regular intervals and as required by symptoms, monitor the following:

- weight and height (monthly)
- neurodevelopment (monthly)
- adherence (monthly)
- CD4 (%) if available (then every 3 to 6 months)
- viral load if available (every 3 to 6 months)
- baseline haemoglobin or haematocrit (if on ZDV/AZT), full chemistry (renal function, liver enzymes, especially ALT for liver toxicity) and lipids (if available)
- symptom-related determination: haemoglobin or haematocrit or full blood count, ALT.

General long-term side effects of antiretroviral therapy include lipodystrophy. The specific side effects of individual antiretroviral drugs are summarised in Appendix 5.

When to change treatment

Drugs need to be substituted for others when there is:

- treatment-limiting toxicity, such as:
  - Stevens–Johnson syndrome (SJS)
  - severe liver toxicity
  - severe haematological findings
- drug interaction (e.g. tuberculosis treatment with rifampicin interfering with NVP or PI)
- potential lack of adherence by the patient if they cannot tolerate the regimen.

TABLE 6.2.D.8 Clinical and CD4 definition of ARV treatment failure in children (after 6 months or more of ARV)

Clinical criteria	CD4 criteria
Lack of or decline in growth among children with an initial growth response to ARV	Return of CD4% if aged < 6 years (% or count if aged ≥ 6 years) to pre-therapy baseline or below, without other cause
Loss of neurodevelopmental milestones or onset of encephalopathy	≥ 50% fall from peak CD4% if aged < 6 years (% or count if aged ≥ 6 years), without other aetiology
New or recurrent WHO clinical Stage 4 conditions	

First-line regimen treatment failure; when to switch regimens

1 A switch to a second-line regimen is recommended when:
   - clinical failure is recognised **and/or**
   - immunological failure is recognised **and/or**
   - virological failure is recognised.
2 Clinical failure is defined as the appearance or reappearance of WHO clinical stage 3 or stage 4 events after at least 24 weeks on ART in a treatment-adherent child. It is important to exclude TB as a cause of clinical failure, especially when there is poor growth.

3 Immunological failure is defined as developing or returning to the following age-related immunological thresholds after at least 24 weeks on ART, in a treatment-adherent child:
   - CD4 count of < 200 cells/mm³ or CD4+% < 10% for a child between 2 and 4 years of age
   - CD4 count of < 100 cells/mm³ for a child aged 5 years or older.

4 Virological failure is defined as a persistent viral load above 5000 RNA copies/mL, after at least 24 weeks on ART, in a treatment-adherent child.

Principles

Virological failure is due to resistance mutations acquired either at the time of infection or as a result of poor adherence. Even a resistance test before starting treatment (not widely available) will not always show archived mutations (not in the majority of the virus tested). Acquired resistance is more likely if there is initial improvement (ideally documented virologically). A history of missed doses is usually not given readily, but it is essential that support to ensure 100% adherence is put in place before second-line treatment is started.

In the absence of routine CD4 or viral load assays, judgements should be made about treatment failure based on:

- clinical progression
- CD4 decline as defined in Table 6.2.D.8.

Generally, patients should have received 6 months or more of ARV therapy, and adherence problems must be ruled out where possible before considering treatment failure and switching ARV regimens.

If an apparent deterioration is due to the immune reconstitution inflammatory syndrome (IRIS), this is not a reason for switching therapy. IRIS usually starts within weeks or the first few months after starting ART in children who have very low CD4 counts (< 15%). The most common initiator is TB which has been latent, but the symptoms of other opportunistic infections can develop as the immune recovery enables a response. Treatment is of the infection, and ART should be continued.

Immune reconstitution inflammatory syndrome (IRIS)

It is important to differentiate IRIS clinically from treatment failure, because the symptoms may be similar. IRIS can be confused with several other clinical events that are also observed in children with advanced HIV disease, such as opportunistic infections, ARV-related toxicity, or HIV disease clinical progression.

What is IRIS?

IRIS is an exaggerated immune response to antigens or organisms. The related organisms could be mycobacteria (e.g. *Mycobacterium tuberculosis*, non-tuberculosis mycobacteria), viruses (e.g. herpes zoster, herpes simplex) or fungi (e.g. *Cryptococcus neoformans*).

Who is at risk of developing IRIS?

It usually occurs in a child with low baseline CD4 or WHO clinical stage 3 or 4 before initiation of ART. The incidence rate of IRIS could be as high as 15–25%.

When does IRIS develop?

It usually occurs during the first 6 months after initiation of ART, although it commonly manifests during the first month. During the initial period of ART, antiretroviral drugs cause a rapid decline in HIV viral load and a rapid rise in CD4, so a brisk immune response to antigen is developed.

What are the common manifestations of IRIS?

There are two types of IRIS:

- 'Worsening type': clinical worsening of a previously treated opportunistic infection. For example:
  - worsening of respiratory symptoms and/or chest X-ray finding in a child with previously treated pulmonary tuberculosis
  - severe headache in a child with previously treated cryptococcal meningitis.
- 'Unmasking type': unmasking of a previously subclinical infection with exaggerated inflammatory response. For example:
  - suppurative lymphadenitis from *Mycobacterium* infection
  - development of an abscess at the BCG vaccination site.

How should IRIS be managed?

- ARVs should be continued.
- For the 'unmasking type', the appropriate anti-infective agents are needed.
- In most cases, the symptoms of IRIS resolve after a few weeks. However, some reactions can be severe or life-threatening, requiring a short course of steroid treatment (e.g. IRIS from pulmonary tuberculosis with acute respiratory distress syndrome (ARDS), IRIS from *M. avium* complex infection with high-grade fever and severe abdominal pain, IRIS from cryptococcal meningitis with a severe increase in intracranial pressure).

Second-line treatment regimens in the event of treatment failure

After failure of a first-line NNRTI-based regimen, a boosted PI plus two NRTIs are recommended for second-line ART. LPV/r is the preferred boosted PI.

After failure of a first-line LPV/r-based regimen, children younger than 3 years should remain on their first-line regimen, and measures to improve adherence should be undertaken.

After failure of a first-line LPV/r-based regimen, children aged 3 years or older should be switched to a second-line regimen containing an NNRTI plus two NRTIs. EFV is the preferred NNRTI.

After failure of a first-line regimen of ABC or TDF + 3TC (or FTC), the preferred NRTI backbone option for second-line ART is AZT + 3TC.

After failure of a first-line regimen containing AZT or d4T + 3TC (or FTC), the preferred NRTI backbone option for second-line ART is ABC or TDF + 3TC (or FTC).

Third-line ART

Third-line regimens should include new drugs with minimal risk of cross-resistance to previously used regimens, such as integrase inhibitors and second-generation NNRTIs and PIs.

Patients on a failing second-line regimen with no new ARV options should continue with a tolerated regimen.

Strategies that balance the benefits and risks for children need to be explored when second-line treatment fails.

- For older children and adolescents who have more therapeutic options available to them, constructing third-line ARV regimens with novel drugs used to treat adults, such as ETV, DRV and RAL, may be possible.
- Children on a second-line regimen that is failing with no new ARV drug options should continue with a tolerated regimen. If ART is stopped, opportunistic infections still need to be prevented, symptoms relieved and pain managed.

Nutritional care and failure to thrive (*see* Appendix 3)

Nutrition is a long-term concern in all HIV-infected children. Stunting frequently develops within the first 12 months, although most children maintain normal weight-for-height ratios. Close monitoring of growth, and early protein/calorie, vitamin A and other micronutrient supplementation need to be evaluated.

- Regular vitamin A as per WHO guidelines.
- Supplementary feeding if possible (aim for 150 kcal/kg/day).
- Exclude or treat *Candida*.
- Exclude or treat enteric infection.
- Consider zinc deficiency (*see* Section 5.10.A).
- Consider fever.
- Consider depression.
- Consider pain.

Clinical management

1. HIV-infected children should be assessed routinely for nutritional status, including weight and height, at scheduled visits, particularly after the initiation of ART.
2. HIV-infected children on or off ART who are symptomatic, who have conditions requiring increased energy (e.g. TB, chronic lung disease, chronic oral infections, malignancies) or who have weight loss or evidence of poor growth, should be provided with 25–30% additional energy.
3. HIV-infected children who are severely malnourished should be managed as per the guidelines for uninfected children and provided with 50–100% additional energy.
4. HIV-infected children should receive one recommended daily allowance of micronutrients daily. If this cannot be ensured through the diet, or there is evidence of deficiency, supplementation should be given.
5. HIV-infected infants and children should receive high-dose vitamin A supplementation every 6 months between 6 and 59 months of age, as per the guidelines for uninfected children (*see* Section 5.10.A).
6. HIV-infected children who have diarrhoea should receive zinc supplementation as part of management, as per the guidelines for uninfected children.

7 For infants and young children who are known to be HIV infected, mothers are strongly encouraged to exclusively breastfeed for 6 months and to continue breastfeeding as per recommendations for the general population (i.e. up to 2 years of age and beyond).

Respiratory disorders in children with HIV infection

Symptoms include cough, shortness of breath, fever, sweats and cyanosis.

The aetiology of acute respiratory infections is similar to that of community-acquired infections in immunocompetent children (*Mycobacterium tuberculosis*, *Pneumococcus*, *Haemophilus influenzae*, *Staphylococcus aureus*, *Mycoplasma pneumonia*) (*see* Section 5.3.A and Section 6.1.N). However, children with HIV may require more prolonged courses of treatment.

Studies on the aetiology of pneumonia among HIV-infected children in resource-limited countries have identified *Streptococcus pneumoniae*, *Staphylococcus aureus*, *Haemophilus influenzae* and *Klebsiella* species as the major bacterial pathogens in HIV-infected children. HIV-negative children are affected by the same pathogens, although at lower rates. The post-mortem studies showed similar results, except that *H. influenzae* was slightly less prominent. *M. tuberculosis* was prevalent regardless of HIV status, reflecting its significance in resource-limited countries. From the limited data available, **RSV** and **parainfluenza** appear to be the most prevalent viral causes of pneumonia.

In cases of failed treatment, consider using a second-line antibiotic.

Treatment of recurrent infections is the same, regardless of the number of recurrences.

Specific HIV-related causes of infection and illness

Pneumocystis jiroveci (formerly carinii) pneumonia (PCP)

- PCP should be suspected and anti-pneumocystis therapy considered in any HIV-positive infant with severe pneumonia.
- Severe generalised pneumonia usually includes ventilation/perfusion mismatch and severe hypoxaemia.
- High fever is uncommon compared with bacterial pneumonia.

PCP is most likely to develop in a child whose HIV infection occurred in the previous 12 months (the peak time is 4–6 months), or over 12 months if they have a low CD4 count and are not on co-trimoxazole prophylaxis. There is an absent or low-grade fever, non-productive cough and difficulty breathing. Signs include severe respiratory distress (tachypnoea, chest indrawing), which is disproportionate to findings on auscultation (usually normal breath sounds or only a few crackles). If an oxygen saturation monitor is available, check at rest and, if normal, again after exercise. The latter may show hypoxia or, if there is a severe infection, cyanosis.

There may be a history of a poor response to 48 hours of first-line antibiotics, and elevated levels of lactate dehydrogenase.

PCP is often the first clinical indicator of HIV infection, and is a WHO clinical stage 4 criterion.

Clinical and radiological signs are not diagnostic. However, a clear chest or diffuse chest signs on auscultation are typical with PCP infection, as is the presence of diffuse infiltrates and areas of hyperinflation rather than focal signs on a chest X ray.

Induced sputum and nasopharyngeal aspiration are useful for obtaining sputum for examination. Nasopharyngeal aspirate has a low sensitivity with conventional staining techniques, and requires **PCR**. Induced sputum techniques greatly increase the diagnostic yield. Beware the risk of infection being transmitted to operators, especially of multiple drug-resistant tuberculosis, for example. **Bronchoalveolar lavage** may provide a diagnosis if adequate resources are available.

Treatment of PCP

Severe disease (severe respiratory distress, severe hypoxia): treat with co-trimoxazole 60–90 mg/kg IV 12-hourly for a minimum of 7 days, followed by oral drugs in the same doses for another 2 weeks (IV if there is severe nausea). In addition, give high-dose dexamethasone for the first 5 days (150 micrograms/kg/dose 6-hourly for 4 days) or prednisolone 0.5 mg/kg 12-hourly for 5 days, then 0.25 mg/kg 12-hourly for 5 days, then 0.25 mg/kg daily for 5 days. The response usually occurs after more than 5–7 days of appropriate high-dose therapy.

Less severe disease: treat with oral co-trimoxazole 30 mg/kg 6-hourly for 21 days (trimethoprim (TMP) 5 mg/kg; sulfamethoxazole (SMX) 25 mg/kg).

If the child has a severe drug reaction, change to pentamidine (4 mg/kg once a day by IV infusion) for 3 weeks, or trimethoprim 5 mg/kg/dose orally 6-hourly and dapsone 100 mg/kg once a day for 21 days.

Continue co-trimoxazole prophylaxis (see below) on recovery, and ensure that ART is being given.

Co-trimoxazole prophylaxis

Co-trimoxazole prophylaxis has been shown to be very effective in HIV-infected infants and children in reducing mortality and the likelihood of PCP as a cause of severe pneumonia. PCP is now unusual in countries where prophylaxis is routine.

Co-trimoxazole also protects against common bacterial infections, toxoplasmosis and malaria.

Who should be given co-trimoxazole?

- All HIV-exposed children (children born to HIV-infected mothers) from 4–6 weeks of age, whether or not they are part of a prevention of mother-to-child transmission (PMTCT) programme.
- Any child under 5 years old identified as HIV-infected, regardless of CD4 count.
- Any child over 5 years old with a CD4 count of less than 25%.
- Any child with a history of PCP.

See Appendix 2 for management.

For how long should co-trimoxazole be given?

- HIV-exposed children: for the first year, or until HIV infection has been definitively ruled out and the mother is no longer breastfeeding.

- HIV-infected children:
  - Indefinitely where ARV treatment is not yet available.
  - Where ARV treatment is being given, co-trimoxazole may only be stopped once clinical or immunological indicators confirm restoration of the immune system for 6 months or more (also see below). On the basis of current evidence it is not yet clear whether co-trimoxazole continues to provide protection after immune restoration is achieved.
  - If there is a history of PCP pneumonia, continue indefinitely.

Under what circumstances should co-trimoxazole be discontinued?

- If severe cutaneous reactions such as Stevens–Johnson syndrome occur with co-trimoxazole or other sulpha drugs, or if there is renal and/or hepatic insufficiency or severe haematological toxicity (severe anaemia or pancytopenia). It is contraindicated in children with glucose-6-phosphate dehydrogenase (G6PD) deficiency.
- **In an HIV-exposed child**, only after HIV infection has confidently been excluded:
  - For a non-breastfeeding child under 18 months of age, this is by negative DNA or RNA virological HIV testing.
  - For a breastfed HIV-exposed child under 18 months of age, negative virological testing is only reliable if performed 6 weeks after cessation of breastfeeding.
  - For a breastfed HIV-exposed child over 18 months of age, negative HIV antibody testing 6 weeks after stopping breastfeeding.
- **In an HIV-infected child:**
  - If the child is on ARV therapy, co-trimoxazole can be stopped only when evidence of immune restoration has been obtained. Continuing co-trimoxazole may continue to provide benefit even after the child has clinically improved.
  - If ARV therapy is not available, co-trimoxazole should not be discontinued.

What doses of co-trimoxazole should be used?

- Recommended dosages of 6–8 mg/kg TMP once daily should be used.
  - For children under 6 months of age, give 2.5 mL of suspension (40/200 mg in 5 mL) or 1 paediatric tablet (or ¼ adult tablet, 20 mg TMP/100 mg SMX: tablets can be crushed).
  - For children aged 6 months to 5 years, give 5 mL of suspension or 2 paediatric tablets (or ½ adult tablet).
  - For children aged 6–14 years, give 10 mL of suspension or 1 adult tablet.
  - For children over 14 years, give 2 adult tablets.
- Use weight-band dosages rather than body-surface-area doses.
- If the child is allergic to co-trimoxazole, dapsone is the best alternative. Give dapsone after 4 weeks of age in an oral dose of 2 mg/kg/24 hours once daily.
- If the patient is G6PD-positive, consider giving pentamidine or atovaquone.

What follow-up is required?

Co-trimoxazole prophylaxis should be a routine part of the care of HIV-infected children, and must be assessed for tolerance and adherence at all regular clinic visits or follow-up visits by healthcare workers and/or other members of the multidisciplinary care team. It is suggested that initial clinic follow-up in children takes place monthly, and then every 3 months if co-trimoxazole is well tolerated.

Lymphocytic interstitial pneumonitis (LIP)

LIP is a non-infectious pulmonary disorder caused by white cell infiltration into alveolae. It is most common in children over 2 years old, and is a clinical stage criterion which is an indication for starting ART.

LIP is common in children (it occurs in at least 40% of children with perinatal HIV), but rare in adults (it occurs in about 3% of adults with HIV). Various studies in Africa have documented a 30–40% prevalence of LIP in HIV-infected children, and up to 60% prevalence in those with chronic lung disease. LIP is often mistaken for pulmonary TB (miliary) because of the chronic cough and the miliary-like pattern on chest X-ray.

Pathogenesis: Possible explanations for LIP include a co-infection of the lungs by HIV and Epstein–Barr virus (EBV), leading to immune stimulation with lymphoid infiltration and chronic inflammation.

The child is often asymptomatic in the early stages, but may later have a mild persistent cough, with or without difficulty in breathing, bilateral parotid swelling, persistent generalised lymphadenopathy, poor growth, hepatomegaly and other signs of heart failure (tender hepatomegaly, bilateral pitting pedal oedema, loud second heart sound and finger clubbing). Chest auscultation may be normal, or there may be widespread crackles. It may produce severe ventilatory perfusion mismatch with hypoxaemia, but may be asymptomatic.

There is an increased risk of lower respiratory tract infection, including bronchiectasis. It is also associated with parotid, adenoid and tonsillar enlargement (and may produce sleep-related upper airway obstruction; see Section 5.1.D).

LIP may be mistaken for miliary TB, but the child is systematically too well.

Suspect LIP if the chest X-ray shows a bilateral reticulo-nodular interstitial pattern that is prominent in the lower lobes, nodules less than 5 mm in diameter, a single patchy alveolar opacity, hyperinflation or isolated bullae. It must be distinguished from pulmonary tuberculosis and bilateral

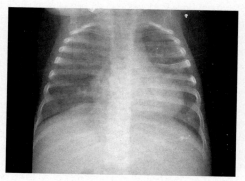

FIGURE 6.2.D.4 Chest X ray showing lymphocytic interstitial pneumonia (LIP): typical is hilar lymphadenopathy and lacelike infiltrates.

hilar adenopathy (see Figure 6.2.D.4). Chest X-ray diffuse infiltrations and hilar lymphadenopathy persisting for more than 2 months despite antibiotic treatment are also a clue.

X-ray appearances are often more severe than the clinical features.

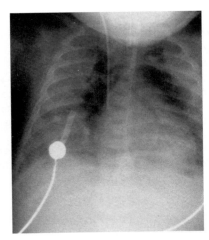

FIGURE 6.2.D.5 Pneumocystis jiroveci pneumonia (PCP): typical is a ground glass appearance.

Treatment of LIP

- Give oxygen therapy during episodes of hypoxia.
- Give a trial of antibiotic treatment for bacterial pneumonia before starting treatment with prednisolone.
- Start treatment with steroids only if there are chest X-ray findings suggesting lymphocytic interstitial pneumonitis, plus any of the following signs:
  - fast or difficult breathing
  - cyanosis
  - pulse oximetry reading of oxygen saturation < 90% (normal value is > 93%).
- Bronchodilators (e.g. salbutamol) are of benefit where wheezing is a problem. For moderate symptoms give oral prednisone, 1–2 mg/kg daily for 3 days, and for more severe symptoms for up to 4 weeks. Then slowly decrease the dose over 2–4 weeks depending on the treatment response. If there is no response by 4 months, slowly taper the dose to stop over a further 2 months.
- Only start steroid treatment if it is possible to complete the full treatment course (which may take several months depending on the resolution of signs of hypoxia), as partial treatment is not effective and could be harmful. Beware of reactivation of TB.

Tuberculosis (see also Section 6.1.N)

In a child with suspected or proven HIV infection, it is important always to consider the co-diagnosis of tuberculosis, a diagnosis which is often difficult. Early in HIV infection, when immunity is not impaired, the signs of tuberculosis are similar to those in a child without HIV infection. Pulmonary tuberculosis is still the commonest form of tuberculosis, even in HIV-infected children. As HIV infection progresses and immunity declines, dissemination of tuberculosis becomes more common. Tuberculous meningitis, miliary tuberculosis and widespread tuberculous lymphadenopathy occur.

All children with HIV should be screened for TB.

Avoid, if practicable, children with HIV being in contact with a TB-infected person.

Isoniazid preventive therapy (IPT)

1. All HIV-infected infants and children who are exposed to TB through household contacts, but show no evidence of active disease, should begin isoniazid preventive therapy (IPT).
2. Children who have either poor weight gain, fever, cough or a contact with TB should be evaluated for active TB. If TB is excluded, give IPT.
3. Children living with HIV (over 12 months of age, and including those previously treated for TB), who are not likely to have active TB, and who are not known to be exposed to TB, should receive 6 months of IPT as part of a comprehensive package of HIV care.
4. Infants living with HIV, who have been exposed to TB but are evaluated as not having active TB, should receive IPT as part of a comprehensive package of HIV care.
5. The recommended dose of isoniazid (INH) for preventive therapy in HIV co-infection is 10 mg/kg daily for 6 months (maximum 300 mg/day).
6. See the child monthly and give a 1-month supply of isoniazid at each visit.

Investigations

A tuberculin skin test (TST, Mantoux) is unreliable in HIV and should not be used. Since a definitive diagnosis of TB in children is difficult, there could be clinical features that are very suggestive of TB, leading to a high index of suspicion. In such cases a negative TST should not prevent you from starting anti-TB treatment. Furthermore, several people develop TB infection when they come into contact with the TB pathogens, but they do not go on to develop signs and symptoms of TB disease, because their immune systems control the infection. When the immune systems break down, such individuals develop signs and symptoms suggestive of TB disease. A TST can be positive in either state, and without signs and symptoms would be suggestive of TB infection and not TB disease.

Chest X-ray: this may be normal, or it may show non-specific infiltrates, hilar or paratracheal lymphadenopathy, persistent opacities after an antibiotic trial, or a miliary pattern.

Microscopy (alcohol and acid-fast bacilli, AAFB), Ziehl–Neelsen (ZN) stain) **and culture:** this is the most important investigation. Sputum which may need to be induced by saline nebuliser (in an isolation room with staff wearing a fine-particle (FP3) mask), and gastric aspirate (if the child is coughing, take this in the early morning before they have had anything to eat or drink). Collect at least three specimens.

Treatment of infants and children diagnosed with TB and HIV

Treat TB in HIV-infected children with the same anti-TB drug regimen as for non-HIV-infected children with TB.

Thiacetazone is associated with a high risk of severe, and sometimes fatal, skin reactions in HIV-infected children, and must not be given. These reactions can start with itching, but progress to severe reactions.

Recommended ART regimens for children who need TB treatment

Recommended regimens for children and adolescents initiating ART while on TB treatment

Younger than 3 years

Two NRTIs + NVP, ensuring that the dose is 200 mg/m^2

or

Triple NRTI (AZT + 3TC + ABC).

3 years or older
Two NRTIs + EFV

or

Triple NRTI (AZT + 3TC + ABC).

Recommended regimens for children and infants initiating TB treatment while receiving ART
Child on standard NNRTI-based regimen (two NRTIs + EFV or NVP)

Younger than 3 years
Continue NVP, ensuring that the dose is 200 mg/m^2

or

Triple NRTI (AZT + 3TC + ABC).

3 years or older
If the child is receiving EFV, continue the same regimen. If the child is receiving NVP, substitute with EFV

or

Triple NRTI (AZT + 3TC + ABC).

- TB should be treated with standard regimes, the emphasis being on achieving high adherence rates. The development of multi-drug-resistant TB is a very real threat if compliance is poor. Directly observed therapy (DOT) may be the best approach.
- Any child with active TB disease and HIV infection should begin TB treatment immediately, and start ART as soon as tolerated in the first 8 weeks of TB therapy, irrespective of CD4 count and clinical stage.
- For all HIV-infected children, anti-TB therapy should be started immediately upon the diagnosis of TB, and ART should continue.

Bronchiectasis
Suspect bronchiectasis if there is a persistent cough productive of copious sputum (in vomit in young children) or haemoptysis associated with fever, anorexia and failure to thrive. There may be clubbing and localised coarse crackles on auscultation. Obtain a chest X-ray and sputum for Gram stain and culture as well as AAFB; differential diagnoses include TB and LIP. Treatment consists of physiotherapy with postural drainage, bronchodilators and antibiotics. Intravenous amoxicillin (50 mg/kg 6-hourly) and gentamicin (7.5 mg/kg daily) may be required for 2 weeks.

Cytomegalovirus (CMV)
CMV can present with pneumonia with fever, dry cough, respiratory distress and hypoxia. CMV also causes oesophagitis and gastroenteritis presenting with nausea, difficulty swallowing, diarrhoea and vomiting. CMV retinitis is often asymptomatic or may cause blurred vision, strabismus and ultimately blindness. The fundi show white perivascular infiltrates and haemorrhages, reduced acuity and field defects.

A chest X-ray may show diffuse interstitial infiltrates. Oesophageal endoscopy may show linear, localised or punctate ulcers. Biopsies show typical inclusion cells.

Treatment is with ganciclovir 6 mg/kg 12-hourly for 14 days.

Other lung infections
Other opportunistic lung infections that may occur include *Pseudomonas aeruginosa*, *Chlamydia*, *Mycoplasma*, *Cryptococcus neoformans*, *Aspergillus*, cytomegalovirus, *Histoplasma*, *Coccidioides*, *Legionella* and *Nocardia*.

Gastrointestinal disorders
Oral and oesophageal problems
Oral candidiasis

This is the most common form of fungal infection and the most common orofacial manifestation encountered in HIV-infected children. It progresses to involve the oesophagus in 20% of cases, and denotes significantly impaired T-cell function.

It presents as white plaques on mucosa that are difficult to remove, loss of taste, pain on swallowing, reluctance to eat, increased salivation and crying during feeds.

Treatment for oral candida
- Nystatin 100 000 IU/mL oral suspension, 1–2 mL four to six times a day for 7 days **or**
- Local gentian violet 0.5% aqueous solution twice daily for 7 days (dissolve one teaspoonful (5 mL) of crystals in 1 litre of water, filter off the residue, and use within 7 days) **or**
- Clotrimazole 1%, miconazole 2% gel, or amphotericin B suspension/lozenges three times daily **or**
- Fluconazole 3–6 mg/kg on the first day, then 3 mg/kg (maximum 100 mg) daily for 1–2 weeks. If there is rare resistance to fluconazole, give ketoconazole oral tablets, 3.3–6.6 mg daily.

Oesophageal candidiasis
Oesophageal candidiasis is a stage 4 clinical feature indicating profound immune impairment (advanced HIV disease). The only clinical symptom may be reluctance to feed. It presents as difficulty or pain while vomiting or swallowing, reluctance to take food, excessive salivation, or crying during feeding. The condition may occur with or without evidence of oral candida. If oral candida is not found, give a trial of treatment with fluconazole (3–6 mg/kg once a day). Exclude other causes of painful swallowing (e.g. cytomegalovirus, herpes simplex, lymphoma and, rarely, Kaposi's sarcoma), if necessary by referral to a larger hospital where appropriate testing is possible.

Treatment for oesophageal candidiasis
- Give oral fluconazole, 3–6 mg/kg once a day for 7 days, except if the child has active liver disease.
- Give amphotericin B, 0.5–1 mg/kg/dose once a day) by IV infusion for 10–14 days to children with liver disease and in cases where there is a lack of response to oral therapy, inability to tolerate oral medications, or the risk of disseminated candidiasis (e.g. in a child with leukopenia).

Viral oesophagitis
Herpes simplex virus (HSV)

Herpes simplex virus (HSV) infection may either be primary (herpetic gingivostomatitis) or secondary (herpes labialis). The prevalence of oral HSV infection ranges from 10% to 35% in adults and children with HIV infection. The presence of HSV infection for more than 1 month constitutes an AIDS-defining condition.

Clinical appearance

HSV infection appears as a crop of vesicles, usually localised on the keratinised mucosa (hard palate, gingiva) and/or the vermillion borders of the lips and perioral skin. The vesicles rupture and form irregular painful ulcers. They may interfere with mastication and swallowing, resulting in decreased oral intake and dehydration.

Systemic therapy with antiviral agents is recommended. The treatment is more effective if it is instituted in the prodromal stage of infection. Treat with aciclovir 20–40 mg/kg orally or IV four times daily for 7 days (maximum single dose is 800 mg).

Cytomegalovirus (CMV) infection: treat with ganciclovir IV 5 mg/kg every 12 hours for 14–21 days.

Reflux oesophagitis may also be present. Treat with antacids and/or an H_2-antagonist, such as ranitidine 2 mg/kg twice daily (*see* Section 5.12.E).

Idiopathic aphthous ulcers: if possible these need to be differentiated from HSV **by viral culture**. Pay attention to oral hygiene. Thalidomide is useful if they are severe.

Severe periodontal and gingival disease (cancrum oris)

Periodontal (gum) disease is common among HIV-infected patients. It is characterised by bleeding gums, bad breath, pain or discomfort, mobile teeth, and sometimes sores. Its reported prevalence ranges widely, from 0% to 50%. If left untreated, HIV-associated periodontal disease may progress to life-threatening infections, such as Ludwig's angina and noma (cancrum oris).

Noma is a gangrenous condition that primarily affects children. It is a multifactorial disease. The most important risk factors are poverty, chronic malnutrition, poor oral hygiene and severe immunosuppression. Although it is considered to be a preventable disease, noma has a case-fatality rate of 70–90% if left untreated.

- Treat with benzylpenicillin 50 mg/kg 4-hourly or amoxicillin 40–60 mg/kg IV 8-hourly. Change to oral antibiotics once the child is able to swallow (usually after 24–48 hours).
- Provide materials for and education on dental hygiene.

Rarely, **malignancy** (Kaposi's sarcoma or non-Hodgkin's lymphoma) or oral hairy leukoplakia (white lacy markings on the sides of the tongue associated with Epstein–Barr virus infection; no treatment required) occur. Visceral Kaposi's sarcoma may present with persistent diarrhoea, intestinal obstruction and abdominal pain.

Persistent diarrhoea (see Section 5.12.B)

Case management should start with management of dehydration with oral rehydration solution. Dysentery (loose stools with blood) should be managed in the same way as for non-HIV-infected children (e.g. for *Shigella* infection). Concur with the local prevalence of treatable infections. Giardiasis, cryptosporidiosis, microsporidiosis, *Shigella*, *Salmonella*, *Campylobacter*, enteropathogenic *E. coli* and *Yersinia* may each contribute to gastrointestinal dysfunction. HIV itself may cause an enteropathy, and in highly immunosuppressed children, atypical mycobacterial infection and protozoa such as *Blastocystis hominis* may cause diarrhoea. Even with sophisticated microbiology, no pathogen may be found, and malabsorption due to lactase deficiency and other brush-border defects should be considered. All antiretroviral drugs (except AZT) can cause diarrhoea, particularly ritonavir.

Chronic or recurrent diarrhoea

Normal endemic pathogens may be responsible, such as rotavirus, *Giardia lamblia*, *Campylobacter jejuni* (see Section 5.12.A and Section 5.12.B), salmonellae (typhoid and non-typhoid), *E. coli*, *Shigella*, *Entamoeba histolytica* and *Strongyloides stercoralis*.

Investigations

- Fresh stool microscopy and culture: *Giardia*, *Entamoeba*.
- Ova and cysts: helminths.
- ZN stain: cryptosporidia, cyclospora.
- pH and reducing substances: lactose intolerance.
- CD4 count < 50: CMV, mycobacterium avium intracellulare
- CD4 count < 100: cryptosporidium, microsporidiosis.

Look for signs of vitamin deficiencies:

- Vitamin A: night blindness, dry eyes, Bitot's spots (on conjunctivae).
- Vitamin D: rickets (wide wrist, double malleoli, bow legs, rachitic rosary, Harrison's sulcus).
- Vitamin E: dry rough skin.
- Vitamin K: ecchymosis, purpura.

Opportunistic infections such as those listed below may be responsible:

- Bacterial: atypical mycobacterial infections, such as *Mycobacterium avium* complex (MAC) (see below).
- Protozoa and parasites: cryptosporidia, microsporidia, *Isospora belli*. Treat with azithromycin 10 mg/kg once daily.
- Viral: cytomegalovirus, herpes simplex virus.
- Fungal: histoplasmosis, coccidiomycosis, *Candida*. If severe, treat with fluconazole 3 mg/kg once daily.

Diarrhoea may be secondary to antibiotics, either by direct effects or through *Clostridium difficile*. Stop antibiotics as soon as possible. Give live yoghurt with or without oral vancomycin.

If lactose intolerance is present, give lactose-free feeds.

Treat dysentery with ciprofloxacin 15 mg/kg 12-hourly for 3 days, or ceftriaxone 50 mg/kg once a day for 2–5 days, plus metronidazole 7.5 mg/kg 8-hourly for 7 days.

Nutritional management includes calorie replacement, which may need to be nasogastric, but always encourage eating. Ensure that additional food is not just recommended but actually given. Vitamin A, multivitamins and zinc (10–20 mg once a day for 10–14 days) supplementation may be of benefit (*see* Section 5.10.A).

Prevention: Use hygienic practices during food preparation, always use clean water, avoid bird and animal faeces, avoid swimming in fresh water, and avoid reptiles (salmonellae).

Abdominal pain

This is most frequently related to infections, but occasionally is caused by tumours (non-Hodgkin's lymphoma and Kaposi's sarcoma).

Malabsorption

HIV can be directly associated with an enteropathy. Lactase deficiency and other brush-border defects can also be responsible. Consider trial of a lactose-free diet.

Central nervous system disorders

A myriad of HIV-related CNS diseases have been described. Primary CNS infection by HIV is quite common, as it is a neurotropic virus. Various abnormalities of the central nervous system (CNS) and peripheral nervous system (PNS) are associated with HIV and AIDS. These abnormalities may be attributable to the following causes: HIV infection, complications related to immunosuppression, neurotoxic effects of antiretroviral treatments, and other systemic complications of HIV that affect brain function.

Neurological disorders in people with HIV infection include peripheral neuropathies (nerve disorders that affect the limbs or feet and hands), myelopathy (disorders of the spinal cord), focal cerebral mass lesions (brain tumours such as CNS lymphoma), CNS complications of opportunistic infections, vascular (blood vessel) abnormalities, seizures and encephalopathies. Developmental delays and regression are also important CNS-related problems in HIV-infected children.

The neurological manifestations of HIV infection include the following:
- progressive or static encephalopathy
- seizures
- strokes
- HIV myopathy
- HIV myelopathy
- peripheral neuropathy
- psychiatric manifestations
- sleep problems.

The effect of HIV on the brain ranges from severe effects, found in more than 50% of patients dying of AIDS at postmortem, to the much more common and milder effects on the developing brain in children, which result in mild learning difficulties. It is particularly important to recognise this so that appropriate support can be given (e.g. reminding the patient to take ART).

TABLE 6.2.D.10 Comparison of features of major CNS mass lesions in HIV

Clinical			Neuroimaging (if available)		
Disease	Timing	Fever	Number of lesions	Type of lesions	Location of lesions
Cerebral toxoplasmosis	Acute onset of symptom	Common	Multiple	Enhancing spherical rings; mass effect	Basal ganglia
Primary CNS lymphoma	Insidious onset of symptom	Usually absent	One or few	Irregular shape, weakly enhancing, mass effect	Periventricular, peri-ependymal, corpus callosum
Tuberculoma	Insidious onset of symptom	Common	One or few	Discrete lesions, significant surrounding oedema, mass effect	Supratentorial in adults, infratentorial in children (at the base of the brain near the cerebellum)
Cryptococcoma cryptococcal meningitis	Acute onset of symptom	Common	Variable	Mass lesions, dilated perivascular spaces, oedema	Basal ganglia

Care of HIV-infected children with CNS involvement requires a thorough evaluation and stepwise therapy according to the underlying aetiology. A multidisciplinary approach is usually needed for appropriate care.

Specific neurological problems
HIV encephalopathy
- Rapid onset or chronic and relapsing forms.
- Hypertonic (spastic) diplegia and expressive language delay.
- Acquired microcephaly with developmental regression (loss of skills).
- White-matter disease predominates. It does not cause seizures, and therefore seizures need to be fully investigated for another pathology.

Encephalitis
Toxoplasma gondii
- Prevention: avoid cats and cat faeces:
  - avoid raw uncooked or partially cooked food
  - can be acquired congenitally.
- Diagnosis: CT/MRI of the brain, and serology (if available).
- Treat with co-trimoxazole 60 mg/kg orally (IV if there is severe nausea) 12-hourly for 2 weeks.
- Then give lifelong prophylaxis: sulfadiazine 85–120 mg/kg/day in two doses, pyrimethamine 1 mg/kg/day (maximum 25 mg) and folinic acid 5 mg every 3 days.

JC virus (papovavirus)
The JC virus is associated with progressive multifocal leukoencephalopathy, a disease characterised by altered mental status, limb weakness, or both. Patients may also exhibit personality changes with frequent emotional outbursts. There is no treatment for this illness, but strong antiretroviral medications (if available) can sometimes improve the symptoms.

Fungal lesion
This is rare.

Diffuse CMV encephalitis
Treat with ganciclovir 5 mg/kg orally or IV 12-hourly for 14–21 days.

Malaria
See Section 6.3.A.d.

Meningitis
Bacterial meningitis
This has the usual spectrum of pathogens, such as

TABLE 6.2.D.11 Neurological manifestations of paediatric HIV infection

Abnormality	Clinical findings	Diagnostic studies (if available)
Focal cerebral mass lesions	Headache, nausea/vomiting, motor deficits (usually asymmetrical), discoordination, visual changes, altered mental status	CT/MRI: enhancing lesions Lumbar puncture: CSF may reveal abnormal cytology or Epstein–Barr virus via PCR Brain biopsy: sometimes needed to confirm diagnoses
Myelopathy	Gait disturbances, lower-extremity weakness/spasticity incontinence, sensory abnormalities, abnormal lower-extremity reflexes	CT/MRI on mass lesions seen; nerve-root thickening may be present CSF: polymorphonuclear pleocytosis
Myopathy	Muscle weakness, muscle soreness, weight loss	EMG: irritative myopathy Muscle biopsy: inflammation, degeneration
Opportunistic infections	Headache, nausea/vomiting, fever, seizures, altered mental status, malaise	CT/MRI: multiple enhancing lesions (toxoplasmosis), periventricular and meningeal abnormalities (CMV)
Peripheral neuropathy	*Distal symmetrical neuropathy* • Distal numbness/pain • Paraesthesias • Stocking/glove sensory loss • Decreased ankle reflexes	*Distal symmetrical neuropathy* EMG: distal axonopathy
	Inflammatory demyelinating polyneuropathy • Progressive weakness • Paraesthesias • Areflexia • Mild sensory loss	*Inflammatory demyelinating polyneuropathy* EMG: demyelination
	Progressive polyradiculopathy • Lower-extremity weakness • Paraesthesias • Urinary incontinence and retention • Diminished reflexes	*Progressive polyradiculopathy* EMG: polyradiculopathy Serum: increased creatine kinase
Progressive encephalopathy	Fine and gross motor deficits (usually symmetrical), abnormal tone, neurodevelopmental delay, microcephaly, altered mental status	CT/MRI: brain atrophy, white-matter abnormalities
Seizures	Focal or generalised seizures, post-ictal stare (fatigue and confusion following seizure)	EEG: abnormal patterns CT/MRI and CSF studies: mass lesions may be seen via imaging, and CSF may be positive for pathogens and abnormal cells if aetiology is infectious or neoplastic Lumbar puncture: may reveal infection
Strokes (cerebrovascular accidents)	Rapid onset of focal neurological signs, seizures, altered mental status	CT/MRI: extent of bleeding seen (in ischaemic strokes, CT may not show changes during the first 2–1 hours): contributing factors such as CNS neoplasms may be identified Lumbar puncture: with subarachnoid haemorrhages, blood will be present in the CSF

Pneumococcus, *Haemophilus influenzae*, *Meningococcus* and *Mycobacterium TB*. (*see* Section 5.16.B).

Viral meningitis
See Section 5.16.C.

Cryptococcosis and other fungi
- Prevention: avoid bird faeces.
- Clinical features: chronic onset, headache (common), fever, meningism (usually but not always present), and there may be a change in mental state.
- Diagnosis: based on staining of CSF sample with Indian ink.
- Treatment:
  – Fluconazole 6–12 mg/kg orally or, if there is severe nausea, IV once daily for 14 days. There is a high relapse rate, therefore give prophylactic fluconazole 3–6 mg/kg/day **or** amphotericin IV 0.5–1.5 mg/kg/day for 14 days followed by oral fluconazole for 8 weeks.

Syphilis
Treat with benzylpenicillin IV 50 mg/kg every 6 hours for 48 hours, then oral penicillin 25 mg/kg 6-hourly for 3 weeks (20% of cases may have a systemic febrile response to penicillin).

Tuberculosis
See Section 6.1.N.

Cerebral abscess
Acute bacterial or tuberculosis.

TABLE 6.2.D.12 Care guidelines for children with neurological manifestations of paediatric HIV infection

Abnormality	Care guidelines
Focal cerebral mass lesions	• Assess for signs of increased intracranial pressure, fever, focal neurological signs and behavioural changes • Administer chemotherapy or antibiotics as needed • Provide support to family and education regarding specific medications needed by patients
Myelopathy	• Assess for pain, muscle weakness, lower-extremity weakness, incontinence and spasticity • Administer HAART to reverse immune suppression • Administer muscle relaxants as needed • Provide physical therapy for weakened muscles and to maintain range of motion • Teach exercises to the family so that they can help the patient at home
Myopathy	• Assess for pain, muscle weakness and range of motion • Consider discontinuing medications that may be contributing to the condition • Administer corticosteroids and pain medications as needed • Provide physical therapy for weakened muscles and to maintain range of motion • Teach exercises to the family so that they can help the patient at home

Opportunistic infections	• Assess for signs of increased intracranial pressure, fever, focal neurological signs and behavioural changes
	• Administer appropriate medication based on the suspected or confirmed pathogen:
	   — toxoplasmosis: pyrimethamine, sulfadiazine, clindamycin
	   — cryptococcosis: fluconazole, flucytosine, amphotericin B
	   — herpes simplex: aciclovir
	   — cytomegalovirus: ganciclovir, foscarnet

Peripheral neuropathy	• Assess for numbness, paraesthesias, pain and weakness • Administer analgesics, tricyclic antidepressants, anticonvulsants and steroids as needed • Provide support to the family and education regarding progression of symptoms
Progressive encephalopathy	• Assess for progressive motor dysfunction, and failure to reach or loss of age-appropriate milestones • Administer antiretroviral medications and muscle relaxants as needed • Assist with ambulation and activities of daily living • Provide information to the family regarding progression of symptoms
Seizures	• Assess for seizure activity • Protect the patient from injury during seizure activity • Monitor respiratory status: suction airway and administer oxygen as needed • Administer anticonvulsant medications as needed • Provide support to the family during seizures • Educate the patient and the family about long-term use of anticonvulsant medications and seizure precautions (e.g. patients with seizures should never swim alone or climb to high places from which they could fall during a seizure)
Strokes	• Intensive care, including neurosurgical intervention, is often needed immediately after a stroke occurs • Look for contributing factors, such as low platelet levels, which may be correctable • Assess for seizures • Assist with ambulation and activities of daily living • Provide physical therapy as needed • Provide support and education to the family regarding the long-term prognosis

Skin disorders

Cutaneous lesions are often the first manifestation of HIV noted by patients and healthcare professionals. These can be due to infectious or non-infectious causes. Viral, bacterial and fungal infections have been very frequently reported in HIV-infected children. These usually tend to be more severe and resistant to therapy. Common skin diseases may present with unusual skin lesions such as Norwegian scabies and disseminated, confluent and large lesions of molluscum contagiosum (see Table 6.2.D.13).

Seroconversion rash

Maculopapular erythematous rash (very rarely observed in infants).

Viral infections
Varicella

• Chickenpox: can be very severe (affecting the lungs and brain) or even fatal.

• Herpes zoster: can involve single or multiple dermatomes and may affect the eyes.

Treat with:

1 IV aciclovir (poorly absorbed by the oral route):
  • Age < 3 months: 10 mg/kg 8-hourly.
  • Age > 3 months: 20 mg/kg 8-hourly.
2 Valacyclovir is the prodrug of aciclovir, and achieves better blood levels orally and is an alternative to IV aciclovir (if available).
3 VZIG within 96 hours of contact (if available).

HSV 1 and 2

Infection appears as a crop of localised vesicles. It may affect the lips, mouth and anogenital areas (rare in children unless sexually abused). The vesicles rupture and form irregular painful ulcers. They may interfere with mastication and swallowing, resulting in decreased oral intake and dehydration.

TABLE 6.2.D.13 Common infectious and non-infectious skin lesions in paediatric HIV

Infectious disorders and lesions	Non-infectious disorders and lesions
Viral infections • Herpes simplex, herpes zoster • Molluscum contagiosum • CMV • Warts Fungal infections • Candida • Tinea onychomycosis Bacterial infections • Impetigo • Scabies	Seborrhoeic dermatitis, atopic dermatitis, general dermatitis Nutritional deficiency Eczema Psoriasis Drug eruptions Vasculitis Alopecia

- May be recurrent and severe.
- Treat with oral aciclovir, 20 mg/kg four times daily for 5–7 days (maximum single dose 800 mg).

Molluscum contagiosum

Umbilicated papular lesions. Treat with ARVs (no other measures are effective). If neglected, giant lesions can result which require surgical excision.

Measles

- Prevent by immunisation (see below and Section 6.2.E).
- May not have a rash.
- Giant-cell pneumonitis may occur.
- Treat with Vitamin A and human immunoglobulin (if available).

Viral warts

These can be persistent and severe. Topical treatment is ineffective (*see* molluscum contagiosum above), and ARVs are the only effective treatment.

Bacterial infections

Impetigo and furunculitis due to *Staphylococcus aureus* are common. Treat with (flu)cloxacillin, 12.5–25 mg/kg four times daily orally, or a first-generation cephalosporin such as cephradine.

Fungal infection

Fungal infection is common and involves the feet, hands and groin. Treat with topical imidazole (e.g. miconazole 2% twice daily until healed) or terbinafine cream. If severe, widespread or for nail infections, use itraconazole or terbinafine. Treatment will be needed for 4–6 weeks.

Antifungal drugs commonly used in paediatric patients include the following:

- **Itraconazole:** children aged 1–12 years: course ('pulse') of 5 mg/kg (maximum 200 mg) daily for 7 days, with subsequent courses repeated after 21-day intervals; fingernails need two courses, and toenails need three courses. For children aged 12–18 years: either 200 mg once daily for 3 months or course ('pulse') of 200 mg twice daily for 7 days, with subsequent courses repeated after 21-day intervals; fingernails need two courses, and toenails need three courses.
- **Terbinafine:** children aged over 1 year: body weight 10–20 kg, 62.5 mg once daily; body weight 20–40 kg, 125 mg once daily; body weight over 40 kg, 250 mg once daily, for 6 weeks to 3 months.
- **Fluconazole:** 6 mg/kg weekly.
- **Griseofulvin:** 20–25 mg/kg/day (microsize formulation) or 10–15 mg/kg/day (ultramicrosize formulation) for 6–12 weeks.

Seborrhoeic dermatitis and pityriasis versicolor

Seborrhoeic dermatitis occurs in up to 85% of adults and children with HIV infection. It may be an early sign of HIV. It is caused by the yeast *Malassezia furfur.*

It is characterised by thick yellow hypopigmented scaly macules occurring on the scalp but also on the face or in the diaper (nappy) area. Older children may also have involvement of the nasolabial folds, the skin behind the ears, and the eyebrows.

Treatment consists of selenium-based or ketoconazole shampoo, topical coal tar or antifungal creams, aqueous cream, UVB light therapy or salicylic acid. To decrease inflammation, 1% hydrocortisone cream can be applied to the affected area (except for the face) three times per day. Parents should be instructed to use 1% hydrocortisone cream sparingly in the diaper area.

If the condition is severe, give oral fluconazole 3 mg/kg once daily.

Non-specific pruritic papular rash

This is a common and severe problem in children with HIV infection. In a previously untested child it should be an indication for HIV testing. In a child who is known to have HIV, the CD4 count should be checked and ARV started if appropriate.

Treatment

- Bathe in a skin antiseptic wash (e.g. dilute chlorhexidine solution).
- Antihistamines: give chlorpheniramine:
  - Age < 1 year: 1 mg twice daily.
  - Age 1–5 years: 1–2 mg three times daily.
  - Age 6–12 years: 2–4 mg three times daily.
  - Age > 12 years: 4 mg three times daily.
- Aqueous cream and calamine lotion may be of benefit.

Drug side effects

Drug eruptions can occur in patients who are receiving treatment for HIV infection. These can be severe (e.g. erythema multiforme, Stevens–Johnson syndrome, toxic epidermal necrolysis).

Drug side effects are most common with co-trimoxazole, sulfadiazine, anti-tuberculous drugs (e.g. thiacetazone, which is contraindicated in HIV infection), penicillin, cephalosporins and dapsone.

Drug eruptions usually appear as pink to erythematous papules that run together and create a blotchy appearance, but may include elevated patches (hives), mucous membrane ulceration, scaling and light sensitivity.

NRTIs (nevirapine and efavirenz) have been associated with pruritic maculopapular eruptions. Most eruptions are mild, and the medication can be continued with eventual spontaneous resolution of the eruption.

To promote comfort, the patient can be given oral antihistamine such as diphenhydramine hydrochloride 1 mg/kg every 6 hours. In more severe cases, the eruptions resolve when the medication is discontinued.

Most drug eruptions are mild and resolve after the causative medication is discontinued.

Infestations

Sarcoptes scabiei (*see* Section 5.18) may present as in children without HIV infection. It is characterised by pruritic papular lesions that most commonly occur in the webs of the fingers and toes, the folds of the wrist, the antecubital area and the axilla. Infants may also have lesions on the palms and soles of the feet. Scrapings observed under a microscope may reveal the mite, eggs or faeces.

Treatment consists of an application of topical benzyl benzoate lotion, 25%, which is left on the skin to dry and repeated the next day. HIV-infected patients with advanced disease can experience a variant of scabies called Norwegian scabies. This type of scabies is characterised by generalised scaling and enlarged crusted plaques. After a patient is treated for scabies, the family should be advised to wash all clothing and bedclothes in hot water and iron them to kill any mites that may be living in the cloth.

Malignancy

Consider Kaposi's sarcoma in children presenting with nodular skin lesions, diffuse lymphadenopathy and lesions on the palate and conjunctiva with peri-orbital bruising. The diagnosis is usually clinical, but can be confirmed by a needle biopsy of skin lesions or a lymph node biopsy. Suspect Kaposi's sarcoma also in children with persistent diarrhoea, weight loss, intestinal obstruction, abdominal pain or a large pleural effusion. Consider referral to a larger hospital for management.

Eye involvement (*see* Section 5.15)

- Malignancy (e.g. non-Hodgkin's lymphoma, Kaposi's sarcoma).
- HIV retinopathy: this is a microangiopathy with soft exudates. It is asymptomatic and does not require treatment. It needs to be differentiated from tuberculosis.
- Cytomegalovirus retinitis: this is the most common cause of visual loss in HIV. Treat with ganciclovir 5 mg/kg IV or orally 12-hourly for 14–21 days.
- Herpes zoster: this may produce corneal ulceration and retinal necrosis.
- Toxoplasmosis: this usually causes CNS disease and reactivation disease, and may cause visual problems or blindness. Treatment includes pyrimethamine, 1–2 mg/kg/day orally for 2 days, then 1 mg/kg/day orally for 2 months, then 1 mg/kg/day orally for 3 days a week (maximum 50 mg). Secondary prophylaxis may also be given to prevent reactivation.

Prophylaxis for any opportunistic infections consists of the following:
- **Primary prophylaxis:** giving medication to prevent infection that has not yet occurred.
- **Secondary prophylaxis:** giving medication to prevent recurrence of an infection after an episode.

Prophylaxis can often be stopped after sustained immune reconstitution secondary to ART, but not in all cases.

Mycobacterium avium complex (MAC)

- This produces a systemic infection with fever, chronic diarrhoea, abdominal pain, chronic malabsorption, generalised lymphadenopathy and obstructive jaundice (from lymph node enlargement around the porta hepatis).
- Treat with clarithromycin 7.5 mg/kg twice daily IV or orally **or** azithromycin 10 mg/kg once daily **and** ciprofloxacin and rifabutin.
- Consider prophylaxis with the above drugs if **CD4 cell counts are persistently < 50/mm³ despite antiretroviral therapy, as the risk of MAC is high.** The opportunistic infection guidelines recommend that all HIV-infected individuals with CD4 counts of < 50 cells/mm³ should have primary prophylaxis against disseminated MAC initiated. Prior to initiating prophylaxis, patients should be evaluated for active MAC infection by clinical assessment.

Fever of unknown origin

- HIV infection itself can cause fever.
- In an endemic area, always treat for malaria (ideally after a blood film). Malaria has not usually been reported to be more severe in HIV-infected children in terms of parasite density or response to treatment. The main interaction between the two diseases has been the acquisition of HIV by children through blood transfusion for malaria-associated anaemia.
- Have a low threshold for diagnosing septicaemia and meningitis and giving powerful empirical antibiotics if severe sepsis is suspected.
- Consider tuberculosis and non-Hodgkin's lymphoma.

Immunisation

Early immunisations can help HIV-infected children who are more likely to acquire diseases that are preventable by immunisation because of their compromised immune system. Appropriate immunisations vary according to geographical location.

Routine immunisations appear to be generally safe for children with HIV infection without fever. Although immune responses may be suboptimal in some HIV-infected children, because of the severe nature of infections and associated mortality, routine immunisation of all children with HIV exposure or confirmed HIV infection is recommended with few exceptions.

Immunisations should generally follow the Expanded Programme on Immunisation (EPI) scheme. The current EPI schedule includes DTP, OPV, hepatitis B, *Haemophilus influenzae* type B vaccine (Hib) and measles vaccine. The difference in HIV-infected children is an extra dose of measles vaccine to be given at the age of 6 months. **BCG and yellow fever vaccines should not be given to HIV-symptomatic children.**

In HIV-endemic areas, BCG is routinely administered postnatally. This should be given even to infants of mothers known to be HIV-infected, as the damage to the immune system generally occurs after the onset of viraemia (i.e. after the first 6 weeks of life). There is no evidence of frequent dissemination occurring after neonatal administration of BCG, although BCG-osis is not an easy diagnosis to establish, and there may be unrecognised cases.

Because most HIV-positive children have an effective immune response in the first year of life, EPI should be started as early as possible after the recommended age of vaccination.

There are theoretical risks associated with giving live oral polio vaccine, particularly to other immunocompromised members of the household. However, cases of vaccine-associated paralytic illness are rare, and oral poliomyelitis vaccine (OPV) continues to be recommended.

Live attenuated measles vaccine is recommended by the WHO for children in resource-limited countries, where the risks from wild-type measles virus are high. Responses to the vaccine tend to be lower in HIV-infected children with more advanced disease. The WHO recommends giving an extra dose of measles vaccine at 6 months, as well as the standard dose at 9 months, to HIV-infected children. It is important to be aware of measles in the differential diagnosis of any child with fever or pneumonia and HIV, as a typical morbilliform rash and standard symptoms may not be present.

Other non-EPI vaccines are encouraged and recommended, especially in children whose immune systems have recovered. These more expensive but strongly recommended vaccines include MMR, pneumococcal conjugate vaccine, hepatitis A, typhoid and varicella vaccines. Diseases caused by these organisms have a greater propensity to cause severe life-threatening infections in HIV-infected children.

Terminal care of children dying from HIV infection

See also Section 1.16.

Despite the increased availability and effectiveness of ARVs, death is still a possible outcome of HIV/AIDS. Each year, millions of children lose one or both parents to AIDS. Although relatives often go to heroic lengths to provide orphans with food, shelter and housing, often the children's psychosocial needs are overlooked, and these young people are not given full recognition or support after their loss. This is usually due to the belief that children are too young to understand what is happening or are better off not dwelling on their loss. Consequently, they are not properly supported in their time of mourning.

Local groups for the support of families with HIV infection are essential, and ideally should be funded by local government.

Give end-of-life (terminal) care if:
- the child has had a progressively worsening illness
- everything possible has been done to treat the presenting illness.

Keep up to date on how to contact local community-based home care programmes and HIV/AIDS counselling groups. Find out whether the carers are receiving support from these groups. If not, discuss the family's attitude towards these groups and the possibility of linking the family with them.

Pain control for children with HIV
See Section 1.15.

Need for referral
Often the facilities or expertise that are needed will not be available at the health centre or hospital to which a child with suspected or confirmed HIV has come for treatment. If the child is not suffering from a life-threatening condition that requires urgent treatment, and referral can be arranged, it is advisable to refer the child to a paediatric infectious disease specialist or HIV treatment centre for the following:
- HIV testing with pre- and post-test counselling
- further investigations to confirm the diagnosis
- evaluation of immunological status and the need to initiate ART
- management of complicated HIV-related conditions and infections
- evaluation of possible treatment failure
- second-line treatment if there has been little or no response to treatment
- HIV medication-related toxicities
- HIV-related expert counselling.

Summary

- The major practical focus should be on prevention of childhood HIV infection. This means implementing effective strategies for reduction of mother-to-infant transmission, such as prenatal screening of mothers and administration of ARV drugs for mother and baby.
- Unfortunately, establishing the infrastructure that is required to implement effective interventions is lagging far behind the scientific advances in this field. Surmounting the sense of hopelessness among health-care professionals who are dealing with overwhelming numbers of patients without resources is a critical issue. This may come in part from research that identifies practical interventions which improve the quality of life for HIV-infected children and their families.
- Limiting the use of blood transfusions and ensuring that the blood supply is safe, and preventing sexual transmission among adolescents, are vital public health issues.
- Positive education is required to encourage testing in the knowledge that there is now accessible safe treatment to keep children alive so that they can have a full healthy life.
- The key to successful treatment is 100% adherence. Do not start outpatient treatment until the child's carer and ideally all the family have expressed a commitment to treatment. Choose ART regimens which are simple, and ensure that there is no problem with swallowing.
- Predict growth for dosing so that the child is never under-dosed.
- Frequent review is necessary to re-emphasise the importance of adherence and education of young people.
- It is essential that resource-limited countries are permitted by multinational drug companies to develop low-cost and effective forms of HAART, without being limited by international patent regulations.
- Without question, health system strengthening is essential if the advent of ARVs for all is to be adequately managed.

This is a very optimistic time in the field of paediatric HIV, with the potential to aim for eradication of mother-to-child transmission, and to provide successful treatment.

Appendix 1

TABLE 6.2.D.14 Monitoring children on ART

Item	Before or at ART initiation	Month (M) 1	M 2	M 3	M4	M5	M 6	Every 2–3 months	Symptom-directed
Clinical evaluation: history and physical examination (including neurodevelopment)	X	X	X	X	X	X	X	X	X
Weight and height	X	X	X	X	X	X	X	X	
Calculation of ART dose[1]	X	X	X	X	X	X	X	X	
Concomitant medications[2]	X	X	X	X	X	X	X	X	
Check ART adherence[3]		X	X	X	X	X	X	X	
Haemoglobin and white blood cell count[4]	X								X
Full chemistry[5]									X
CD4% or count[6]	X							X*	X
HIV viral load measurement[7]									X

* If signs of clinical progression of disease are seen, the CD4 count should be done earlier.
- The child should be seen again within 1 week of starting ART to resolve any problems.
- If the child has missed a visit, attempts should be made to call or visit the child's home.
- In addition to these suggested appointments, caregivers should be encouraged to bring the child in if he or she is sick, especially during the first few months of ART when the child may experience ART side effects and intolerance.

[1] Children may show rapid weight and height gain after ART, in addition to expected normal growth. Therefore the ART dose should be recalculated at every visit. Under-dosing of ART can lead to the development of resistance.

[2] Concomitant drugs should be asked for at every visit to ensure that the child is on appropriate CTX dosing (if indicated) and is not taking drugs that have potential interactions with ART.

[3] ART adherence can be assessed by asking questions about missed doses and the times when the child takes ART. Performing a pill count is time consuming, but may give a more accurate indication of adherence, if done correctly.

[4] Haemoglobin (Hb) and white blood cell count (WBC) monitoring may be considered in children on ZDV at 1, 2 and 3 months.

[5] Full chemistry includes but is not restricted to liver enzymes, renal function, glucose, lipids, amylase, lipase and serum electrolytes. Monitoring depends on symptoms and regimens. Regular liver enzyme monitoring during the first 3 months of treatment may be considered for certain children using nevirapine-based regimens, in particular for adolescent girls with a CD4 count of > 250 cells/mm^3, and for infants and children who are co-infected with hepatitis B or hepatitis C virus, or other hepatic disease.

[6] TLC is not suitable for monitoring of therapy; therefore it cannot be a substitute for CD4. If CD4 is not available, clinical monitoring alone is used.

[7] At present, viral load measurement is not recommended for decision making about the initiation or regular monitoring of ART in resource-limited settings. Tests for assessment of HIV RNA viral load can also be used to diagnose HIV infection, and to assess discordant clinical and CD4 findings in children in whom ART is suspected of failing.

Appendix 2
Treatment of PCP infection

TABLE 6.2.D.15 Starting co-trimoxazole (CTX) prophylaxis for *Pneumocystis jiroveci* pneumonia (PCP)

HIV-exposed infants and children	Confirmed HIV-infected infants and children		
	Under 1 year	1–5 years	6 years or older
CTX prophylaxis is universally indicated, starting at 4–6 weeks after birth, and maintained until cessation of risk of HIV transmission and exclusion of HIV infection	CTX prophylaxis is indicated regardless of CD4 percentage or clinical status	WHO stages 2, 3 and 4 regardless of CD4 percentage **or** Any WHO stage and CD4 < 25%	Any WHO clinical stage and CD4 < 350 cells/mm^3 **or** WHO stage 3 or 4 and any CD4 level

Patient information: It needs to be explained to patients that although CTX does not cure HIV, regular dosing is essential for protection of children from infections that are more common or more likely to occur in HIV infection. CTX does not replace the need for antiretroviral therapy.

TABLE 6.2.D.16 Dosing for PCP: once-daily CTX dosing

Weight	Suspension: 40 mg TMP + 200 mg SMX/5 mL	Tablets (SS): 80 mg TMP/400 mg SMX	Tablets (DS): 160 mg TMP/800 mg SMX
1–4 kg	2.5 mL	–	–
5–8 kg	5 mL	½ tablet	–
9–16 kg	10 mL	1 tablet	½ tab
17–50 kg	20 mL	2 tablets	1 tablet
> 50 kg	20 mL	2 tablets	1 tablet

Appendix 3
Summary of nutritional recommendations and support for HIV-infected children

- Regular growth monitoring.
- Safe infant feeding advice (the emphasis is on an **exclusive** infant feeding option). Substitute feeds if they are acceptable, affordable, feasible, sustainable and safe, otherwise exclusive breastfeeding, and early weaning. Avoid all mixed feeding.
- Dietary counselling for asymptomatic children to increase energy intake by 10% compared with HIV-uninfected children.
- Dietary counselling for symptomatic children to increase energy intake by 20–30% compared with HIV-uninfected children.
- Counselling on the importance of a balanced diet, including affordable choices from all food groups (micronutrient requirement of 1 RDA for age).
- Counselling on high-energy affordable food options for children with growth failure.
- Counselling on the use of clean water and hygienic food preparation.
- Vitamin A supplementation to prevent vitamin A deficiency in children aged 6 to 59 months with dosing schedule as follows:
  - Children aged 6–11 months: 100 000 IU (30 mg) once every 6 months.
  - Children aged 12–59 months: 200 000 IU (60 mg) once every 6 months.
- Zinc supplementation during diarrhoeal episodes: 10 mg once daily for 10 days in children older than 6 months if weight is ≤ 10 kg, and 20 mg if weight is > 10 kg.
- Assessment and management for underlying HIV-associated illnesses.
- Assessment for need to initiate ART.
- Referral to outreach service providers for food assistance, if needed.

Appendix 4

TABLE 6.2.D.17 Formulations and dosages of ART drugs for children

Name of drug	Formulation	Age	Age (weight), dose and dose frequency	Other comments
Nucleoside analogue reverse transcriptase inhibitors (NRTIs)				
Zidovudine (ZDV) AZT	Syrup: 10 mg/mL Capsules: 100 mg, 250 mg Tablet: 300 mg	All ages	< 4 weeks: 4 mg/kg/dose twice daily 4 weeks to 13 years: 180–240 mg/m²/dose twice daily Maximum dose: ≥ 13 years: 300 mg/dose twice daily	Large volume of syrup is not well tolerated in older children, Syrup needs to be stored in glass jars and is light sensitive Can give with food Doses of 600 mg/m²/dose per day required for HIV encephalopathy Capsule can be opened and its contents dispersed, or tablet crushed and its contents mixed with a small amount of water or food and immediately taken (solution is stable at room temperature) Do not use with d4T (antagonistic antiretroviral effect)
Lamivudine (3TC)	Oral solution: 10 mg/mL Tablet: 150 mg	All ages	< 30 days: 2 mg/kg/dose twice daily ≥ 30 days or < 60 kg: 4 mg/kg/dose twice daily Maximum dose: > 60 kg: 150 mg/dose twice daily	Well tolerated Can give with food Store solution at room temperature (use within 1 month of opening) Tablet can be crushed and its contents mixed with a small amount of water or food and immediately taken
Fixed-dose combination of ZDV plus 3TC	No liquid formulation available Tablet: 300 mg ZDV plus 150 mg 3TC	Adolescents and adults	Maximum dose: > 13 years old or weight > 60 kg: 1 tablet per dose twice daily (should not be given if weight is < 30 kg)	Ideally, tablet should not be split Tablet can be crushed and its contents mixed with a small amount of water or food and immediately taken At weights of < 30 kg, ZDV and 3TC cannot be dosed accurately in tablet form
Stavudine (d4T)	Oral solution: 1 mg/mL Capsules: 15 mg, 20 mg, 30 mg, 40 mg	All ages	< 30 kg: 1 mg/kg/dose twice daily 30–60 kg: 30 mg/dose twice daily Maximum dose: > 60 kg: 40 mg/dose twice daily	Large volume of solution Keep solution refrigerated; it is stable for 30 days, but must be shaken well. It needs to be stored in glass bottles Capsules can be opened and their contents mixed with a small amount of food or water (stable in solution for 24 hours if kept refrigerated) Do not use with ZDV (antagonistic antiretroviral effect)
Didanosine (ddI, dideoxyinosine)	Oral suspension paediatric powder/water: 10 mg/mL (In many countries needs to be made up with additional antacid) Chewable tablets: 25 mg, 50 mg, 100 mg, 150 mg, 200 mg Enteric-coated beadlets in capsules: 125 mg, 200 mg, 250 mg, 400 mg	All ages	< 3 months: 50 mg/m²/dose twice daily 3 months to < 13 years: 90–120 mg/m²/dose twice daily or 240 mg/m²/dose once daily Maximum dose: ≥ 13 years or > 60 kg: 200 mg/dose twice daily or 400 mg once daily	Keep suspension refrigerated; it is stable for 30 days, but must be shaken well Administer on an empty stomach, at least 30 minutes before or 2 hours after eating If tablets are dispersed in water, at least 2 appropriate-strength tablets should be dissolved for adequate buffering Enteric-coated beadlets in capsules can be opened and sprinkled on a small amount of food

(continued)

Name of drug	Formulation	Age	Age (weight), dose and dose frequency	Other comments
Abacavir (ABC)	Oral solution: 20 mg/mL Tablet: 300 mg	Over 3 months	< 16 years or < 37.5 kg: 8 mg/kg/dose twice daily Maximum dose: > 16 years or ≥ 37.5 kg: 300 mg/dose twice daily	Can give with food Tablet can be crushed and its contents mixed with a small amount of water or food and immediately ingested **Warn parents about hypersensitivity reaction** ABC should be stopped permanently if a hypersensitivity reaction occurs

Non-nucleoside reverse transcriptase inhibitors (NNRTIs)

Name of drug	Formulation	Age	Age (weight), dose and dose frequency	Other comments
Nevirapine (NVP)	Oral suspension: 10 mg/mL Tablet: 200 mg	All ages	15–30 days: 5 mg/kg/dose once daily for 2 weeks, then 120 mg/m²/dose twice daily for 2 weeks, then 200 mg/m²/dose twice daily > 30 days to 13 years: 120 mg/m²/dose once daily for 2 weeks, then 120–200 mg/m²/dose twice daily Maximum dose: > 13 yrs: 200 mg/dose once daily for first 2 weeks, then 200 mg/dose twice daily	If rifampicin co-administration, avoid use Store suspension at room temperature, but it must be shaken well Can give with food Tablets are scored and can be divided into two equal halves to give a 100 mg dose; can be crushed and combined with a small amount of water or food and immediately administered Warn parents about rash Do not dose escalate if rash occurs (if mild or moderate rash, hold drug; when rash has cleared, restart dosing from beginning of dose escalation; if severe rash, discontinue drug)
Efavirenz (EFV)	Syrup: 30 mg/mL (note that syrup requires higher doses than capsules; see dosing chart) Capsules: 50 mg, 100 mg, 200 mg	Only for children over 3 years of age or who weigh > 10 kg	Capsule (liquid) dose: 10–15 kg: 200 mg (270 mg = 9 mL) once daily 15–19 kg: 250 mg (300 mg = 10 mL) once daily 20–24 kg: 300 mg (360 mg = 12 mL) once daily 25–32 kg: 350 mg (450 mg = 15 mL) once daily 33–39 kg: 400 mg (510 mg = 17 mL) once daily Maximum dose: ≥ 40 kg: 600 mg once daily	Capsules may be opened and added to food, but have a very peppery taste; however, can mix with sweet foods or jam to disguise taste Can give with food (but avoid giving after high-fat meals which increase absorption by 50%) Best given at bedtime, especially in the first 2 weeks, to reduce CNS side effects
Etravirine	100 mg, 200 mg dispersible tablets	Child over 6 years	16–20 kg, 100 mg twice a day, 21–25 kg, 125 mg twice a day 26–30 kg, 150 mg twice a day > 30 kg, 200 mg twice a day	AUC decreased by 50% if taken on an empty stomach

Protease inhibitors (PIs)

Name of drug	Formulation	Age	Age (weight), dose and dose frequency	Other comments
Nelfinavir (NFV)	Powder for oral suspension (mix with liquid): 200 mg per level teaspoon (50 mg per 1.25 mL scoop): 5 mL Tablet: 250 mg (tablets can be halved; can be crushed and added to food or dissolved in water)	All ages However, extensive pharmacokinetic variability in infants, with requirement for very high doses in infants under 1 year	< 1 year: 50 mg/kg/dose three times daily or 75 mg/kg/dose twice daily ≥ 1 year to < 13 years: 55–65 mg/kg/dose twice daily Maximum dose: ≥ 13 years: 1250 mg/dose twice daily	Powder is sweet, faintly bitter, but gritty and hard to dissolve; must be reconstituted immediately prior to administration in water, milk, formula, pudding, etc.; do not use acidic food or juice (which increase the bitter taste); solution is stable for 6 hours Because of difficulties with use of powder, the use of crushed tablets is preferred (even for infants) if the appropriate dose can be given

(continued)

Name of drug	Formulation	Age	Age (weight), dose and dose frequency	Other comments
Nelfinavir (NFV) (*cont.*)				Powder and tablets can be stored at room temperature Take with food Drug interactions (less than with ritonavir-containing protease inhibitors)
Lopinavir/ ritonavir (LPV/r)	Oral solution: 80 mg/ mL lopinavir plus 20 mg/mL ritonavir Note that oral solution contains 42% alcohol Capsules: 133.3 mg lopinavir plus 33.3 mg ritonavir	6 months or older	> 6 months to 13 years: 225 mg/m² LPV and 57.5 mg/ m² ritonavir twice daily, or weight-based dosing as follows: 7–15 kg: 12 mg/kg LPV and 3 mg/kg ritonavir twice daily 16–40 kg: 10 mg/kg lopinavir and 5 mg/kg ritonavir twice daily Maximum dose: > 40 kg: 400 mg LPV and 100 mg ritonavir (3 capsules or 5 mL) twice daily	Preferably oral solution and capsules should be refrigerated; however, they can be stored at room temperature up to 25°C (77°F) for 2 months; at temperatures > 25°C (77°F) the drug degrades more rapidly Liquid formulation has low volume but bitter taste Capsules are large Capsules should **not** be crushed or opened, but must be swallowed whole Should be taken with food
Saquinavir/r	Soft gel capsule: 200 mg Hard gel capsule: 200 mg, 500 mg	> 25 kg	Approved dosing in adults: SQV 1000 mg and RTV 100 mg twice daily There are no data for children For children who weigh > 25 kg, the approved adult dosing can be used If possible, monitoring of SQV level is recommended	Capsules are large Capsules should **not** be crushed or opened, but must be swallowed whole Should be taken with food
Darunavir plus Ritonavir (RTV)	75 mg (white), 150 mg (white), 400 mg (light orange), 600 mg (orange)		**PI experienced, 3–6 years:** 10–11 kg: 200 mg twice a day + RTV 32 mg twice a day 11–12 kg: 220 mg twice daily + RTV 32 mg twice a day 12–13 kg: 240 mg twice a day + RTV 40 mg twice a day 13–14 kg: 260 mg twice a day + RTV 40 mg twice a day 14–15 kg: 280 mg twice a day + RTV 48 mg twice a day **6 years:** 15–30 kg: 375 mg twice a day + RTV 50 mg twice a day 31–40 kg: 450 mg twice a day + RTV 60 mg twice a day. > 40 kg: 600 mg twice a day + RTV 100 mg twice a day	DRV and RTV levels reduce in combination

Integrase inhibitor

Raltegravir	400 mg tablets (pink)	> 6 years	> 25 kg: 400 mg twice a day	With or without food Avoid indigestion remedies

Appendix 5

TABLE 6.2.D.18 Side effects of ARVs

Drug		Side effects	Comments
Nucleoside analogue reverse transcriptase inhibitors (NRTIs)			
Lamivudine	3TC	Headache, nausea, abdominal pain, diarrhoea, fatigue, pancreatitis	Well tolerated, can be crushed
Stavudine	d4T	Headache, abdominal pain, neuropathy, pancreatitis, lactic acidosis, hepatitis, lipodystrophy	Large volume of suspension, capsules can be opened
Zidovudine	AZT	Headache, anaemia, neutropenia, nausea, hepatitis, neuropathy, nail pigmentation	Do not use with d4T (antagonistic ARV effect)
Abacavir	ABC	Hypersensitivity reaction, with fever, mucositis and rash; this is rare, but if it occurs stop the drug	Tablets can be crushed
Didanosine	ddI	Peripheral neuropathy, diarrhoea, nausea, abdominal pain, lipodystrophy. Lactic acidosis and pancreatitis (especially with d4T)	On empty stomach, give with antacid
Non-nucleoside reverse transcriptase inhibitors (NNRTIs)			
Efavirenz	EFV	Vivid dreams, sleepiness, rash, mood changes, hypercholesterolaemia	Take at night, avoid taking with fatty food
Nevirapine	NVP	Rash (Stevens–Johnson syndrome), liver toxicity (check liver function tests at 2, 4 and 8 weeks)	When given with rifampicin, increase NVP dose by 30% or avoid use
Protease inhibitors (PIs)			
Lopinavir/ritonavir*	LPV/r	Diarrhoea, nausea, vomiting, headache	Liquid: bitter taste. Take with food
	NFV	Diarrhoea, vomiting, rash	Take within 2 hours of food
	SQV	Diarrhoea, abdominal discomfort	
Darunavir	DRV	Rash, nausea, diarrhoea, headache	
Atazanavir	ATV	Rash, nausea, jaundice, headache	Avoid antacids
Ritonavir*	RTV	Rash, nausea, diarrhoea, peri-oral paraesthesia, flushing, hepatitis	Liquid: bitter taste
Integrase inhibitor			
Raltegravir		Nausea, dizziness, insomnia, rash, pancreatitis, elevated ALT, AST, GGT	Avoid indigestion remedies

*Requires cold storage and cold chain for transport.

TABLE 6.2.D.19 Number of tablets of child-friendly solid formulations for twice daily dosage (morning and evening)

Drug	Strength of paediatric tablet (mg)	Children aged ≥ 6 weeks										Strength of adult tablet (mg)	Number of tablets by weight-band	
		Number of tablets by weight-band morning and evening												
		3–5.9 kg		6–9.9 kg		10–13.9 kg		14–19.9 kg		20–24.9 kg			25–34.9 kg	
		am	pm	am	pm	am	pm	am	pm	am	pm		am	pm
Single drugs														
AZT	60	1	1	1.5	1.5	2	2	2.5	2.5	3	3	300	1	1
ABC	60	1	1	1.5	1.5	2	2	2.5	2.5	3	3	300	1	1
NVP	50	1	1	1.5	1.5	2	2	2.5	2.5	3	3	200	1	1
DdI	25	2[a]	2[a]	3	2	3	3	4	3	4	4	25	5	5
Combinations														
AZT/3TC	60/30	1	1	1.5	1.5	2	2	2.5	2.5	3	3	300/150	1	1
AZT/3TC/NVP	60/30/50	1	1	1.5	1.5	2	2	2.5	2.5	3	3	300/150/200	1	1
ABC/AZT/3TC	60/60/30	1	1	1.5	1.5	2	2	2.5	2.5	3	3	300/300/150	1	1
ABC/3TC	60/30	1	1	1.5	1.5	2	2	2.5	2.5	3	3	[b]		
d4T/3TC	6/30	1	1	1.5	1.5	2	2	2.5	2.5	3	3	30/150	1	1
d4T/3TC/NVP	6/30/50	1	1	1.5	1.5	2	2	2.5	2.5	3	3	30/150/200	1	1
LPWr[c]	100/25	NR	NR	NR	NR	2	1	2	2	2	2	100/25	3	3

[a] This dose of DdI is only approximate for children aged 3 months or older and weighing between 6 kg and 6.9 kg.

[b] See ABC/3TC FDC dosing table.

[c] Higher doses of LPWr may be required when co-administered with enzyme-inducing drugs such as NVP, EFV, fos-amprenavir (FPV) and rifampicin.

TABLE 6.2.D.20 Number of tablets or capsules of child-friendly solid formulations for once-daily dosage

Drug	Strength of tablet or capsule (mg)	Number of tablets or capsules by weight-band once daily					Strength of tablet/capsule (mg)	Number of tablets or capsules by weight-band once daily
		3–5.9 kg	6–9.9 kg	10–13.9 kg	14–19.9 kg	20–24.9 kg		25–34.9 kg
		Once daily	Once daily	Once daily	Once daily	Once daily		Once daily
Single drugs								
EFV[a]	200 mg	NR	NR	1	1.5	1.5	200	2
DdI[b]	125 mg or 200 mg EC	NR	NR	1 (125 mg)	1 (200 mg)	2 (125 mg)	125 mg EC	2

[a] EFV is not recommended for children under 3 years and weighing less than 10 kg.

[b] DdI EC is not recommended for children weighing less than 10 kg.

NR, not recommended; EC, enteric coated.

Further reading

World Health Organization (2010) *Antiretroviral Therapy for HIV Infection in Infants and Children: towards universal access.* http://whqlibdoc.who.int/publications/2010/9789241599801_eng.pdf

6.2.E Measles

BOX 6.2.E.1 Minimum standards

- Immunisation.
- Vitamin A.
- Oral rehydration solution and nutritional provision.
- Antibiotics for secondary infection.
- Oxygen.
- Nebulised adrenaline and corticosteroids for croup.
- Eye pads.
- Public health measures.

Introduction

Measles is an acute viral disease characterised by fever, cough, coryza, conjunctivitis, an erythematous maculopapular rash, and typical oral lesions (Koplik's spots). It is caused by an RNA virus, a member of the genus *Morbillivirus* in the Paramyxoviridae family. Humans are the only natural hosts. It is transmitted by direct contact with infectious droplets or, less commonly, by airborne spread. It has a high incidence in winter. Measles is one of the most highly communicable of all infectious diseases.

Measles occurs worldwide, and is a significant cause of morbidity and mortality worldwide. It is the fifth most common cause of death in children under 5 years of age. There has been a 78% reduction in measles mortality worldwide in recent years, largely as a result of immunisation, from 733 000 deaths in 2000 to 164 000 in 2008, and a reduction in the total number of cases from 39.9 to 20 million.

Epidemiology

- Measles is transmitted by droplet spread of virus in nasopharyngeal secretions. It is most infectious before the appearance of rash, and for at least 7 days after the onset of the first symptoms. The incubation period is 10–12 days. Quarantine can be lifted 2 days after the fever subsides.
- Epidemic cycles of infection in urban areas may occur every 2 years. In isolated communities, all age groups are affected. In resource-limited countries, the population peak incidence is at 1–2 years, with a mortality of 1–5%, although during epidemics it may rise to 30%. Mortality is low in the well nourished. Children who acquire infection in overcrowded conditions tend to have more severe disease, probably due to a larger infecting dose of the virus.
- Pneumonia and upper airway obstruction account for about 75% of measles deaths. Measles is more severe in HIV-infected children.
- In resource-limited countries, measles commonly occurs in previously vaccinated children. This is partly explained by a persistent maternal antibody at 9 months of age when vaccine is usually given, and also a relatively poor efficacy of the vaccine and waning immunity.
- It rarely occurs in infants under 3 months of age because of maternal immunity transferred *in utero*.

Clinical features

Prodromal period (3–5 days): acute coryza-like illness with high-grade fever, cough and conjunctivitis. Febrile seizures may occur. Koplik's spots (tiny bluish-white specks on a red base on the buccal mucosa of the cheeks, resembling grains of salt) appear by days 2–4.

A maculopapular rash commences on day 4 on the face and neck, behind the ears and along the hairline, and spreads to become generalised and reaches the feet after 3 more days). Fades after 5–6 days in order of appearance, developing a brownish colour and often becoming scaly. If severe, there may be petechiae and ecchymoses. The rash is due to infiltration of lymphocytes into areas of virus replication in skin.

Persistence of fever beyond day 3 of the rash is usually due to complications (see below).

Diagnosis

This is mostly clinical (diagnosis is based on the specific pattern of rash, history of contact with a measles patient, and Koplik's spots). Serology, viral culture or PCR may be used to confirm it.

Laboratory findings

Leukopenia and thrombocytopenia may be observed during measles infection. Chest radiography may demonstrate interstitial pneumonitis.

Complications

Recovery following acute measles may be delayed for weeks or months due to failure to thrive, recurrent infections, persistent pneumonia and diarrhoea.

Pneumonia (*see* Section 5.3.A)
- Bacterial pneumonia usually occurs during convalescence and after several days of an afebrile period. It is the most frequent cause of death with an incidence of 10–25% of hospitalised cases in developing countries.
- Viral pneumonia occurs during the acute phase of measles, and may progress to giant-cell pneumonia in the immunosuppressed (e.g. leukaemia, HIV).
- Mediastinal emphysema occurs in 1 in 300 measles cases, and may lead to subcutaneous emphysema.

Diarrhoea

Incidence 20–40%. May become persistent and frequently precipitates malnutrition (*see* Section 5.12.A).

Tracheobronchitis

This presents as croup. Laryngeal tissue sometimes becomes necrotic, which may lead to laryngeal obstruction (*see* Section 5.1.A).

Otitis media

This is common, especially in infants. Mastoiditis may develop. It is an important cause of chronic otitis media and hearing impairment (*see* Section 5.1.C).

Stomatitis

There is mucosal inflammation and ulceration with bleeding gums and secondary *Candida albicans* and herpes simplex infections. Stomatitis causes difficulty in eating and worsens malnutrition. Cancrum oris (noma) may develop.

Xerophthalmia

Vitamin A deficiency may combine with measles to pre-cipitate xerophthalmia and blindness (*see* Section 5.10.A).

Malnutrition

Malnutrition secondary to measles results from anorexia and poor nutrition following infection. Mortality is high (> 15%) (*see* Section 5.10.B).

Tuberculosis

Tuberculosis, including tuberculous meningitis, may first be noticed in the post-measles period (*see* Section 6.1.N).

Encephalitis

- **Acute allergic encephalitis:** this is a demyelinating disorder and the most common CNS complication of measles. Onset is often in the second week as exan-thema is clearing. It occurs in one or two per 1000 cases of measles, and can be fatal. Virus is not found in the brain.
- **Acute measles inclusion-body encephalitis:** this results from direct invasion of brain cells by virus (which may be isolated from CSF). There is a more rapid onset if there is immunosuppression or malignancy.
- **Subacute sclerosing panencephalitis (SSPE):** there is a long latent period (several years) between infec-tion and the onset of symptoms. Commonly, measles occurred at an early age. SSPE is characterised by lethargy, psychological changes, myoclonic jerks and mental deterioration, eventually leading to death. Virus has been isolated from brain biopsy specimens.
- Atypical measles may have prolonged fever and present with pneumonia or rarely encephalitis. Rash may or may not appear. Prolonged fever for 2–3 weeks with diarrhoea may simulate enteric fever.

Differential diagnosis

- Other exanthema and drug reactions.
- Koplik's spots are the most helpful diagnostic feature in the prodromal period.

Case assessment and classification

Cases may be classified into:
- uncomplicated measles
- severe measles requiring treatment or urgent referral.

TABLE 6.2.E.1 Clinical features of severe disease

Symptom	Complication
Cough, tachypnoea or indrawing	Pneumonia
Stridor when quiet	Croup, necrotising tracheitis
Severe diarrhoea	Dehydration
Recent severe weight loss	Malnutrition
Corneal damage or Bitot spots	Blindness
Ear discharge	Otitis media, deafness
Lethargy, convulsions	Encephalitis
Inability to drink or eat	Dehydration, malnutrition
Blood in the stools	Dysentery, haemorrhagic measles
Severe stomatitis	Cancrum oris

Danger signs

These include the following:
- breathing difficulty
- cyanosis
- bleeding
- corneal/mouth ulcers
- coma/lethargy
- seizures
- inability to eat or drink.

Management
Mild measles

- Give small frequent feeds. Infants should continue breastfeeding. Extra energy should be provided by adding vegetable oil or sugar to cereals (1 teaspoon of each). Follow-up nutritional support is needed.
- Give paracetamol for temperature > 39°C. Saline drops for blocked nose.
- Maintain oral hygiene by rinsing the mouth several times daily. Apply 1% gentian violet to mouth sores. Treat oral thrush with nystatin drops.
- If mouth ulcers are secondarily infected, give an antibiotic (penicillin or metronidazole orally for 5 days).
- If the mouth is too sore to feed or drink, a nasogastric tube may be required.
- Maintain ocular hygiene for purulent conjunctivitis, with daily washings with sterile 0.9% saline or boiled water (using cotton-wool swabs) and the application of tetracycline eye ointment three times daily. **Never use topical steroids.** Consider using protective eye pads.
- **Vitamin A treatment** of children with measles in devel-oping countries has been associated with decreased morbidity and mortality rates. The dose is 100 000 IU as a capsule (in children under 1 year old) or 200 000 IU (in those over 1 year old). **Give a second capsule the next day.**
- Give oral rehydration solution (ORS) for diarrhoea.
- Give an oral antibiotic (co-trimoxazole, amoxicillin, ampi-cillin) if there is a clear indication of lower respiratory tract infection (*see* Section 5.3.A).
- Admit the child to hospital if they show signs or symp-toms of severe measles.

Severe measles

Admit the child to hospital and isolate them. Airborne trans-mission precautions are indicated for 4 days after the onset of rash in otherwise healthy children, and for the duration of illness in immunocompromised patients.

In addition to the care for mild measles described above:
- Give parenteral antibiotics for pneumonia or septicaemia (e.g. benzylpenicillin or ceftriaxone/cefotaxime if avail-able). Give (flu)cloxacillin plus gentamicin or cefuroxime (if available) if *Staphylococcus aureus* is suspected. If stridor associated with fever is present use ceftriaxone/cefotaxime (if available) or chloramphenicol. Rapidly spreading pulmonary tuberculosis may be difficult to distinguish from a progressive pyogenic pneumonia.
- Give oxygen as required to keep $SpO_2 \geq 94\%$.
- Croup: nebulised adrenaline, 1 mL adrenaline (1 in 1000) mixed with 1 mL of saline every 2 hours, **careful observation** (*see* Section 5.1.A, which also describes the use of oral steroids or nebulised budesonide, either of which can be life-saving in this situation).
- Diarrhoea: give oral rehydration and appropriate

antibiotic if the child passes bloody stools. Persistent diarrhoea requires nutritional support.

- Otitis media: give antibiotics and maintain regular aural hygiene. Screen for hearing impairment during follow-up.
- Xerophthalmia: use protective eye pads, and give vitamin A capsules (see above).
- Malnutrition: treat according to management guidelines (see Section 5.10.B).
- Encephalopathy: follow the management guidelines for coma and convulsions (see Section 5.16.A and Section 5.16.E).

Prevention and follow-up

- Give 'normal immunoglobulin' (if available) for susceptible immunocompromised contacts of measles cases or those under 1 year old. It is given intramuscularly to

prevent or modify measles in a susceptible child within 6 days of exposure. The usual recommended dose is 0.25 mL/kg given intramuscularly; immunocompromised children (e.g. those with HIV) should receive 0.5 mL/kg intramuscularly (the maximum dose is 15 mL).

- Improve vaccination coverage (see Section 1.17).
- Give a follow-up vitamin A dose (after 2 weeks) if the child is malnourished or has an eye disorder.
- Measles control by immunisation is one of the most important public health interventions in reducing child mortality. If a child with measles is admitted, immunise all other unimmunised children under 6 months of age in the hospital, with a follow-up second dose in all aged 6–9 months as soon after 9 months as possible. A second dose is given at 12–15 months of age.

6.2.F Mumps

BOX 6.2.F.1 Minimum standards
Measles, mumps, rubella (MMR) vaccination two-dose schedule.

Introduction

Mumps is a systemic disease characterised by swelling of one or more of the salivary glands, usually the parotid glands. It is caused by a virus of the paramyxovirus family (which also includes measles and parainfluenza). The virus is spread by airborne droplets through the respiratory tract, mouth and possibly the conjunctivae and urine, and is present in saliva, CSF, blood and urine. Other viruses and bacteria (cytomegalovirus, parainfluenza virus types 1 and 3, influenza A virus, coxsackieviruses and other enteroviruses, human immunodeficiency virus (HIV), *Staphylococcus aureus* and non-tuberculous *Mycobacterium*) may also cause parotitis.

Clinical presentation

- The incubation period is 14–24 days. Onset is with painful swelling of parotid glands, fever, general malaise, and occasionally headache. Parotid swelling may be unilateral at first, followed a couple of days later by swelling of the opposite parotid gland, with pain on opening the dry mouth.
- Mild meningoencephalitis is common and usually neither serious nor recognised clinically. There may be nausea and vomiting, and abdominal pain.
- Orchitis presents with fever and tender oedematous swelling of the testis. In 10–20% of cases the second testicle may be affected. However, infertility is rare.
- Differential diagnosis of parotitis includes cervical

adenitis, pyogenic parotitis, recurrent parotitis, tumours of the parotid and tooth infections.

- Mumps orchitis can mimic hernias, tumours, haematomas, epididymo-orchitis and testicular torsion.

Complications

Complications include oophoritis, mastitis, pancreatitis, nephritis, myocarditis, thyroiditis, labyrinthine disturbance, painful swelling of the lacrimal glands, optic neuritis, uveokeratitis, rapid loss of vision, arthritis, jaundice, pneumonia and thrombocytopenia. Transient or permanent unilateral nerve deafness has been reported. Infection during pregnancy very rarely causes disease of the fetus (e.g. aqueductal stenosis, hydrocephalus).

Management

Symptomatic treatment includes analgesics, fluids, and scrotal support for orchitis. Antibiotics are usually not warranted for the uncomplicated disease, but each complication should be treated on its own merits with antibiotics (in the case of pneumonia or wherever a secondary bacterial infection is suspected), or with appropriate local treatment and monitoring. The value of corticosteroids for orchitis is not established.

Prevention

Measles, mumps, rubella (MMR) immunisation is routine in well-resourced countries, and has reduced mumps by over 90%. The recommended two-dose vaccine schedule has an effectiveness of approximately 90% (range 88–95%).

6.2.G Poliomyelitis

BOX 6.2.G.1 Minimum standards
- Immunisation.
- ABC, including airway protection if there is bulbar palsy.
- Public health measures.
- Bed rest and physiotherapy.
- Nutritional support and hydration.
- Nasogastric feeding and airway protection if there is bulbar palsy.

Introduction

Poliomyelitis is caused by polioviruses type 1, 2 and 3, which are ingested and then multiply in the tonsils and Peyer's patches of the gut. In most cases, infection is contained at this point and the child is asymptomatic.

Due to both vertical and mass vaccination campaigns, the number of reported cases has fallen by 90% since 1988. Wild poliovirus is now mainly found in Afghanistan and a few countries in sub-Saharan Africa.

Severity
Minor illness
This is associated with viraemia and non-specific symptoms, such as nausea, vomiting, abdominal pain and sore throat.

Major illness
Non-paralytic poliomyelitis
This occurs in a minority of symptomatic children. Incubation period is 10–14 days and symptoms include: fever, headache and two to five days later, signs of meningeal irritation with severe pain and stiffness of neck, back and limbs.

Paralytic poliomyelitis
- Paralysis occurs within the first 2 days of major illness.
- It can affect any muscles, but particularly large ones and those of the lower limbs.
- Asymmetrical paralysis, flaccid muscles and absent tendon reflexes are characteristic. There is intact sensation. Paralysis is maximal within 3–5 days of onset, and rarely extends once the temperature has settled.
- In **bulbar form**, the involvement of cranial nerve nuclei and vital centres in the brainstem results in paralysis of the facial, pharyngeal, laryngeal and tongue muscles, causing swallowing difficulties, aspiration and respiratory failure.
- Hypertension may occur, as well as transient bladder paralysis.

Diagnosis
CSF initially shows neutrophil predominance, but after 5–7 days is mainly lymphocytic. CSF protein levels are normal or slightly elevated. CSF glucose levels are normal. Virus can be isolated from throat and stool for up to 3 months after onset. The differential diagnosis includes other causes of acute flaccid paralysis (*see* Section 5.16.F).

Prognosis
- This depends on the extent of paralysis and the quality of care during the acute phase.
- Early identification of and intervention for respiratory and bulbar paralysis will reduce mortality to 5–10%.
- With appropriate physiotherapy, improvement in the function of paralysed muscles can occur for up to 18 months.
- Factors that adversely affect outcome include intramuscular injections, muscle fatigue, corticosteroid therapy and immunocompromised states. Removal of tonsils or teeth during the incubation period increases the risk of bulbar paralysis.

Management
Acute phase
- Absolute bed rest is mandatory. Avoid intramuscular injections and exercise.
- Analgesics should be given for severe pain. Keep paralysed muscles in a neutral position to prevent contractures.
- Gentle passive exercises and warm compresses should be used to help to relieve pain. Active exercises are introduced a few days after the temperature has settled.
- Respiratory paralysis requires ventilatory support (if available) (*see* Sections 1.25 and 8.3).
- Bulbar paralysis requires nasogastric tube feeding and, to protect the airway, may require tracheostomy.

Convalescent phase
- Aim to improve motor function, prevent deformities and generally reintegrate the child into society.
- Encourage active participation by the parents in the rehabilitation process. The educational and emotional needs of the child must not be neglected. The services of an orthopaedic surgeon and an orthoptist may be required.
- *See* Sections 4.2.C, 4.2.D and 4.2.E for further information on the long-term care of children with a disability.

Prevention
See Section 1.17 on immunisation.

6.2.H Rabies management and prevention after animal bites

> **BOX 6.2.H.1 Minimum standards**
> - Palliative care, including morphine.
> - Wound care.
> - Rabies vaccine.
> - Rabies immunoglobulin.

Rabies encephalitis

Furious and paralytic (dumb) forms of human rabies can occur. Furious rabies is characterised by agitation, hyper-excitability and hydrophobia, which is due to spasms of the inspiratory muscles, accompanied by an inexplicable feeling of terror. Spasms occur on attempting to drink water or from a draught of air. Flaccid paralysis without hydrophobia occurs in some patients, but this paralytic rabies is rarely recognised. It is likely to be misdiagnosed as another encephalitis or cerebral malaria. Once symptoms of encephalitis have begun there is no treatment. The disease is always fatal in Asia, Africa and Europe. A very few patients have survived infection after contact with bats in the Americas. North and South American bat rabies viruses appear to be less pathogenic.

Management

The treatment of established rabies is palliative. Sedatives (e.g. diazepam, midazolam) and strong analgesics (e.g. morphine) may be given parenterally to control symptoms and relieve anxiety. An IV infusion assuages the feeling of thirst. Relatives and staff should wear gloves when handling the child, their vomitus or their saliva. Close attendants are at risk of exposure to the virus, but there is no documented case of transmission of rabies to a carer. However, if anti-rabies vaccine is available it should be offered to them, but rabies immunoglobulin (RIG) is not needed.

Rabies prophylaxis

Dog bites are the usual cause of rabies in humans, but cats, foxes, bats, jackals, wolves, mongooses and domestic mammals may also transmit the infection.

Estimating the risk of exposure to rabies

1. Is there a bite wound with broken skin? Have mucous membranes or an existing skin lesion been contaminated by virus in the animal's saliva? Intact skin is a barrier against the virus.
2. How did the animal behave? An unprovoked attack by a frantic dog is a high risk, but so is contact with a paralysed animal, or an unusually tame wild mammal.
3. Is rabies known to occur in the biting animal species?
4. Regularly vaccinated animals are unlikely to be rabid, but vaccinated dogs or cats can transmit the infection.
5. Try to have the animal's brain examined for rabies. If this is not possible, the animal may be kept under safe observation, but post-exposure treatment must not be delayed. If the animal is still healthy after 10 days, vaccine treatment of the patient can be stopped.

Post-exposure treatment

Table 6.2.H.1 lists the criteria for initiating treatment. All

three parts of post-exposure therapy are always **urgent**. The aim is to chemically kill or neutralise the rabies virus at the wound site before it can enter a nerve ending and travel to the brain. Neutralising antibody is provided by local injection of rabies immunoglobulin, or it may be present already in previously vaccinated individuals.

1. Wound care: this is important for all bites, irrespective of the rabies risk.
2. Rabies vaccine (active immunisation).
3. Rabies immunoglobulin (RIG) is passive immunisation which provides antibody locally for the first week, until the vaccine-induced antibody appears.

Wound care

- Scrub and flush the lesion repeatedly and energetically with **soap or detergent and water.** Remove any foreign material. Local analgesia may be necessary.
- Apply povidone iodine (or 70% ethyl alcohol, but this is painful).
- Do not suture the wound, or at least delay suturing.
- Give tetanus immunisation if appropriate.
- Treat bacterial infection of wounds with an oral antibiotic, such as amoxicillin/clavulinic acid or tetracycline.

Rabies vaccine

Active immunisation with vaccine should be given whenever there is a risk from contact with a suspect rabid animal. Rabies vaccines are suitable for people of all ages, including pregnant women.

Vaccines accredited by the WHO include the following:

- Purified chick embryo cell vaccine (PCEC) (Rabipur®, RabAvert®) (1.0 mL/ampoule).
- Purified vero cell vaccine (PVRV) (Verorab®) (0.5 mL/ampoule).
- Purified duck embryo vaccine (PDEV) (Vaxirab®) (1.0 mL/ampoule).
- Human diploid cell vaccine (HDCV) by Sanofi (1.0 mL/ampoule).

These vaccines are interchangeable, so a change may be made to a different vaccine during a course of treatment.

The side effects of these vaccines are mild local or non-specific generalised symptoms. Transient maculopapular or urticarial rashes are occasionally seen.

Other vaccines

1. Tissue culture rabies vaccines not listed above should be used according to the manufacturer's instructions.
2. Vaccines of nervous tissue origin (e.g. Semple vaccine and suckling mouse brain vaccine) should only be used if no other vaccine is available.

Three post-exposure regimens (see Table 6.2.H.2)

Standard five-dose intramuscular (IM) 'Essen' regimen

- Days 0, 3, 7, 14 and 28: Inject one IM dose (1 mL or 0.5 mL) into the deltoid or antero-lateral thigh in small children. Do not inject into the gluteal region.

Economical four-site intradermal (ID) regimen

The intradermal dose is **0.1 mL per site for vaccines containing 0.5 mL/ampoule** (e.g. Verorab®), and **0.2 mL per site for vaccines containing 1 mL/ampoule** (e.g. Rabipur®).

- Day 0: draw up a whole ampoule of vaccine into a 1-mL (Mantoux-type) syringe. Give intradermal injections at four sites (deltoid, and either thigh or suprascapular areas) using all of the vaccine.
- Day 7: give an intradermal dose (**0.1 mL or 0.2 mL**) at two sites (deltoid areas).
- Day 28: give one intradermal dose.

Practical points

- Intradermal injections should raise a **papule** as with BCG vaccine.
- Inject using strict aseptic precautions. If ampoules are shared, use a new **sterile needle and syringe** for each patient. If there is difficulty in injecting 0.2 mL intradermally, withdraw the needle and inject the remainder at an adjacent site.
- **Do not waste vaccine.** Ampoules shared between patients must be stored at 5°C and used on the same day.
- If few patients are treated, on day 0 ask the patient to bring their relatives and friends for pre-exposure vaccine on day 7.
- If vaccine is very scarce or unaffordable, and 1-mL vaccines (e.g. Rabipur®) are used, half the dose (i.e. 0.1 mL per intradermal site) may be used.
- The timing of the final dose can be varied for economy. A clinic could assign 1 or 2 days a week for intradermal rabies vaccination for the day 28 doses and pre-exposure immunisation (see below).
- This is the **most economical** rabies post-exposure regimen both for the healthcare provider and for the patient.
- This regimen is as immunogenic as IM vaccination, and may become the treatment of choice in Asia and Africa.

Economical two-site ID regimen

The **intradermal dose is 0.1 mL per site for vaccines containing 0.5 mL/ampoule** (e.g. Verorab®). The equivalent dose is **0.2 mL for vaccines containing 1 mL** (e.g. Rabipur®), but half the dose (i.e. 0.1 mL per site) is used.

- Days 0, 3, 7 and 28: give an intradermal dose at two sites (deltoids).

The same precautions for intradermal use as described above apply. This regimen is less economical if few patients are being treated. It has mainly been used in large clinics.

Rabies immunoglobulin (RIG)

- Passive immunisation with RIG is recommended to accompany vaccine following contact with suspected rabid animals where the skin has been broken or mucous membranes have been contaminated (*see* Table 6.2.H.2).
- It is vital for bites with a high risk of infection (on the head, neck or hands) or for multiple bites.
- If supplies are limited, ensure that the high-risk, severely exposed patients have access to RIG.
- If RIG is not available immediately, it should be given up to 7 days after the first dose of vaccine. After that it is no longer needed.

- RIG is not required if a course of vaccine has been completed previously.

Dosage: equine RIG (40 IU/kg) or human RIG (20 IU/kg) is infiltrated into and around the wound on day 0. If this is not anatomically possible (e.g. on a finger), inject any remainder IM, at a site remote from the vaccine site, but not into the gluteal region.

- Skin tests are **not** useful for predicting anaphylactoid reactions to equine RIG, and should not be used.
- In very rare cases there may be **anaphylaxis**.

Anaphylaxis treatment (see also Section 5.1.B)

Adrenaline (epinephrine) intramuscular treatment is essential.

Dosage:

- Age < 6 years: 150 micrograms or 0.15 mL of 1:1000 (1 mg/mL).
- Age 6–12 years: 300 micrograms or 0.3 mL of 1:1000.
- Age > 12 years: 500 micrograms or 0.5 mL of 1:1000.

The dose can be repeated at 5-minute intervals if necessary.

In addition, if available give the following:

Chlorpheniramine maleate IM or by slow IV injection

Dosage:

- Age 6 months to 6 years: 2.5 mg.
- Age 6–12 years: 5 mg.
- Age > 12 years: 10 mg.

Hydrocortisone sodium succinate by slow IV injection or IM

Dosage:

- Age 1–5 years: 50 mg.
- Age 6–12 years: 100 mg.
- Age > 12 years: 200 mg.

Post-exposure treatment for previously vaccinated adults

Thorough wound care and vaccine treatment are always **urgent** following possible exposure to a rabid animal. Patients who have previously had a complete pre-exposure (three doses) or post-exposure course of vaccine only require a short booster course, and RIG is not necessary.

Two post-exposure booster regimens (see Table 6.2.H.2)

Standard two-dose IM regimen

- Days 0 and 3: inject one IM vaccine dose.

Economical single-day four-site ID regimen

- Day 0: Give 0.1 mL intradermal injections at four sites (deltoids, and either thigh or suprascapular areas).
- The intradermal dose is 0.1 mL, which is sufficient for vaccines of any volume. For Verorab® (0.5 mL/ampoule) a whole ampoule is used.
- For 1 mL vaccines, the total dose is half an ampoule. **Do not waste vaccine.** Ampoules may be shared between patients or used as pre-exposure prophylaxis for relatives, hospital staff, etc. on the same day. **See above for precautions when sharing ampoules.** If the ampoule cannot be shared, give the whole 1 mL to the patient at four sites, as for the primary four-site intradermal regimen described above.

Pre-exposure treatment

Pre-exposure vaccination is the best means of rabies prophylaxis. No one who has had pre-exposure treatment and a post-exposure booster injection is known to have died of rabies.

Indications for pre-exposure rabies prophylaxis

People working with dogs, bats or other wild mammals should be immunised. Anyone in an area where dog rabies is enzootic is at risk of infection, especially children. Ideally, rabies should be included as part of the routine Expanded Programme on Immunisation (EPI). Pre-exposure vaccine should be given whenever it is affordable to residents of dog rabies areas, and should be strongly encouraged if RIG may not be available locally.

Pre-exposure three-dose regimen (see Table 6.2.H.2)

Days 0, 7 and 28: Inject one dose of a vaccine IM (1 ampoule) or intradermally (0.1 mL). Variation in timing does not matter. The final dose may be given from day 21 to months later, but aim for a total of three doses. Having had one or two doses is still an advantage if the individual is exposed to rabies in the future, especially if RIG may not be available.

- Patients on chloroquine, steroids or other immunosuppressive drugs should have IM not intradermal injections for pre-exposure treatment.
- Patients who have been vaccinated should keep a record of their immunisations.
- Routine booster doses are only recommended for people at high occupational risk of exposure.
- If contact with a rabid animal occurs, **post-exposure booster vaccine treatment is still required**.

Summary

- The only treatment for rabies encephalitis is palliative care.
- Rabies can be prevented by education about the

TABLE 6.2.H.1 Recommended criteria for post-exposure treatment

Type of exposure	Criteria	Action
No exposure*	Touching animals, or being licked on intact skin	No treatment
Minor exposure, WHO Category II	Nibbling (tooth contact) with uncovered skin, or minor scratches or abrasions without bleeding	Start vaccine immediately
Major exposure, WHO Category III	Single or multiple bites or scratches that break the skin, or licking on broken skin, or licking or saliva on mucosae, or physical contact with bats	Immediate rabies immunoglobulin and vaccine
Severe exposure, WHO Category III	Bites on the head, neck or hands, or multiple bites	Immediate rabies immunoglobulin is mandatory with vaccine

For all cases:
- Stop treatment if the dog or cat remains healthy for 10 days.
- Stop treatment if the animal's brain is shown to be negative for rabies by appropriate investigation.

*The confusing term 'WHO Category I' should be avoided, as misunderstanding leads to unnecessary treatment.

dangers of animal contact, the need for vaccination of pets, first-aid cleaning of wounds with soap, and the need to attend a clinic for vaccine.
- Pre-exposure vaccination should be encouraged, especially for children and if RIG is not available locally.
- Post-exposure prophylaxis is urgent.
- If rabies vaccine is unaffordable or in short supply use robust economical ID regimens that are suitable for use globally.

This scheme is a modification of WHO recommendations.

TABLE 6.2.H.2 Selected standard intramuscular and economical intradermal rabies vaccine regimens

Vaccine regimen and route	Days of injection (number of sites injected denoted by superscript number)					Visits to clinic	Total vaccine used (ampoules)
Pre-exposure:							
IM	0		7		28	3	3
ID 0.1 mL‡	0		7		28	3	< 1–3
Post-exposure (+ RIG day 0):							
IM five-dose	0	3	7	14	28	5	5
ID four-site†	0^4		7^2		28	3	< 2–3
Post-exposure booster if previous vaccine course:							
IM	0	3				2	2
ID*	0^4					1	1 (or < 1)*

IM, intramuscular; ID, intradermal.

* 0.1 mL/site, whole ampoule used for 0.5 mL vaccines. For 1 mL ampoules share between two, or alternatively use the whole dose to avoid wastage.

† Intradermal doses are 0.1 mL/site for PVRV vaccine (0.5 mL/ampoule) or the equivalent dose, 0.2 mL/site of injection, for PCECV vaccine (1.0 mL/ampoule).

‡ Intradermal doses are all 0.1 mL/site of injection.

6.2.I Viral haemorrhagic fevers

BOX 6.2.I.1 Minimum standards
- ■ ABCD.
- ■ Management of shock.
- ■ Blood transfusion and clotting factors.
- ■ Isolation and infection control.
- ■ Public health measures.

Introduction

Viral haemorrhagic fevers (VHFs) are a group of severe infections caused by viruses that normally affect animals. Human infection is characterised by high fever and, in a proportion of cases, haemorrhage. Animal hosts such as rodents are usually asymptomatic and are often infected with virus from birth, excreting it in urine or body fluids throughout life.

In primary cases, transmission to humans occurs by a variety of routes, such as food contaminated with urine (e.g. Lassa, Junin, Machupo and Hantaan fevers) via arthropod vectors such as ticks (e.g. Crimean-Congo and Omsk fevers) or mosquitoes (e.g. Rift Valley fever). The hosts for Ebola and Marburg haemorrhagic fevers are not yet known.

Humans with disease are usually highly infectious. Most VHFs cause severe disease with a high mortality, especially following human-to-human spread (secondary cases). Some (e.g. Lassa fever) may also cause asymptomatic or mild illness.

Symptomatic disease is commonly mistaken for other febrile illnesses, typically malaria, typhoid fever or *Shigella* dysentery, which fail to respond to treatment. Individual VHFs are geographically restricted in distribution. As with all geographical illnesses, clinicians only need to know of those present in the local area. VHFs are fortunately rare.

Lassa fever

- Distribution: West Africa (Nigeria, Sierra Leone, Liberia and Guinea).
- Host: Mastomys rat (habitat is rural).
- Transmission:
  - **Primary:** mainly from contact with host (rat) urine. Food may be contaminated.
  - **Secondary:** transmission from patient to carer, or to hospital and laboratory staff is common, particularly from haemorrhagic cases. Maternal illness is particularly severe, with a high risk of vertical transmission to the baby (which is invariably fatal).

Prevalence

This disease is relatively common. Most primary human infections are not severe, and many are subclinical. Childhood seroprevalence in Sierra Leone can be as high as 20% in some rural villages. Outbreaks may occur in displaced communities or when humans enter host habitat.

Clinical features

- High fever (>39°C) with cough and vomiting in 65% of hospital cases.
- Abdominal pain and diarrhoea are common (around 35% of cases).

- In children, wheeze and pleural effusions are more frequent than in adults.
- Sore throat and pharyngeal ulcers occur less frequently in children than in adults, but are highly suggestive of Lassa fever.
- In children, oedema (especially of the face) and overt bleeding are seen in 10% of cases, and in a febrile child from an appropriate area should suggest Lassa fever.
- At the epicentre of the transmission area, Lassa fever is a common cause of a febrile child with convulsions.

Diagnosis of Lassa fever
Clinical case diagnosis
- An unexplained febrile illness compatible with Lassa fever, in a child from an area of known transmission, with no response of either fever or illness to an anti-malarial drug plus a broad-spectrum antibiotic (e.g. chloramphenicol).
  - Note that malaria parasitaemia in an area of endemic malaria transmission is not sufficient to exclude other causes of fever (e.g. VHF) as the cause of a febrile illness, as many adults and older children may have coincidental asymptomatic malaria parasitaemia as the cause of a febrile illness.

Supportive indirect laboratory tests
- Raised liver transaminases (AST/SGOT) (in adults this reflects a poorer prognosis).
- Low initial white blood cell counts, but often a normal platelet count.

Confirmation of diagnosis
- **Positive specific IgM serology** (on admission only 50% of cases are positive).
- **Rising IgG titres** to Lassa on acute and convalescent serum.
- Isolation of virus: this is rarely appropriate and, **due to the high risks of laboratory infection, samples should not be taken without senior expert advice**.
  - Samples must be marked as high infection risk, ideally with standard yellow hazard tape, and sent in two sealed plastic bags. Samples should only be taken if laboratory staff are aware of the potential risks, and are able to take the necessary precautions to handle such specimens safely. The laboratory should be informed that the specimen has been sent.

Management
- Appropriate symptomatic management of fever, distress and pain.
- Fluid and nutritional requirements.
- Supportive care includes oxygen (if hypoxic) and initial IV volume replacement if the patient is hypovolaemic (see Section 5.5).
- Blood transfusion may be required for a falling PCV or haemorrhage. Fresh-frozen plasma (FFP) may not be of benefit, as inhibitors of clotting factors may cause bleeding.
- **Early ribavirin can improve the prognosis in severe disease, but is very expensive.**

Infection control
See below and Section 1.2.

Ebola

- Distribution: Central Africa (Sudan, Democratic Republic of the Congo, Gabon, Cote d'Ivoire, Uganda) and West Africa (Guinea, Liberia and Sierra Leone).
- Host: the main animal reservoir is unknown.
- Transmission:
  - **Primary:** infection occurs mainly in adults trekking in tropical Central African forests. Transmission from primates to humans has been recorded.
  - **Secondary:** patients with advanced disease are viraemic and highly infectious. Once in a human host, transmission to carers, hospital and laboratory staff is frequent (30% of doctors developed Ebola during an outbreak in Kikwit, Democratic Republic of the Congo). However, once effective infection control measures have been implemented, secondary cases are rare.

The disease is invariably severe, with a high death rate, but only 20% of cases in the Democratic Republic of the Congo outbreak were under 15 years of age. Children are at low risk in the community, and boys have half the incidence of girls, possibly because they are less involved in the care of sick adults.

Invariably, in children, there is a history of contact with a primary case, and an outbreak of an illness that could be Ebola is present in the hospital and/or community. Post-mortem transmission does occur, possibly through skin contact.

Prevalence

Prevalence is low: the disease occurs sporadically in well-localised outbreaks.

Clinical disease (data for adults)

- Fever is invariably present, and diarrhoea occurs in 85% of cases. This is bloody in 20% of cases, and can be confused with *Shigella* dysentery.
- Vomiting and abdominal pain are common (75% of cases).
- Headaches, myalgia or arthralgias are reported in 50% of cases.
- Sore throat occurs in 50% of cases, and is a distinguishing feature, as is conjunctival injection (45%).
- A maculopapular rash, although poorly visible on black African skin, is common.
- Cough occurs in 10% of cases.
- Bleeding is seen in 40% of cases, and is usually either gastrointestinal, oral, at injection sites or as skin petechiae. This is a major diagnostic sign.
- Hospital mortality is around 80%. Recovery starts 2 weeks into the illness.

Diagnosis of Ebola
Clinical diagnosis

- **Suspected clinical case (during epidemic):** any febrile illness associated with haemorrhage. No contact history is required.
- **Probable case (during epidemic):** a febrile illness occurring within 3 weeks of contact with a case of Ebola

or

a febrile illness in which three or more of the above clinical features are present.

- **Possible clinical case (non-epidemic):** an unexplained severe febrile illness, particularly with haemorrhage, in an area of Ebola transmission, with no response to an antimalarial drug plus a broad-spectrum antibiotic (e.g. chloramphenicol).

Indirect laboratory tests supportive of diagnosis
- Raised liver transaminases (AST/SGOT).
- Low or normal initial white blood cell count.

Confirmation of diagnosis

Early serological tests were difficult to interpret, but newer specific IgM ELISAs may allow diagnosis of acute cases on a single positive test. However, IgM is not always positive at presentation.

- **Specific IgG (by ELISA) rises too slowly to be used as a test of acute infection, but may be useful in epidemiological surveys.**
- **Isolation of the virus is not appropriate outside a specialised laboratory.**
- **A post-mortem skin biopsy (in formalin at room temperature) is not infectious, and can allow a diagnosis to be made using immunohistochemistry.**

Samples need to be marked as **high infection risk**, ideally with standard yellow hazard tape, and sent in two sealed plastic bags. Samples should only be taken where laboratory staff are aware of the potential risks and can take the necessary precautions to handle such specimens safely. The laboratory should be informed that the specimen has been sent.

Infection control
See below and Section 1.2.

Notification

Consider formal identification of a possible outbreak of Ebola if there is a new illness of high mortality in adults in a recognised area of transmission, particularly if hospital-acquired secondary cases have occurred.

Management
- Apart from supportive care, particularly with regard to adequate fluid and nutritional intake, there are no specific treatments that modify the course of the illness.
- Antimalarial and antibiotic therapy should be given routinely, directed at treating possible alternative diagnoses (e.g. shigellosis, typhoid).

Infection control of VHFs

At increased risk are laboratory staff, midwives, and those staff and family members who are handling body fluids and excreta. High-risk patient groups are those with active haemorrhage, those who are confused and agitated, and pregnant mothers.

Barrier nursing
- Secondary spread is usually by contact with blood, urine-infected secretions, used needles or stool, but

some viruses (e.g. Ebola) have also been found on patients' skin.

- There is little clinical evidence of respiratory aerosol spread for the VHFs, although virus may be present in the nose and oropharynx.
- Surgical and obstetric procedures carry a particularly high risk of infection for staff.
- **Transmission is substantially reduced by strict adherence to barrier nursing, disinfection of excreta, and clear labelling of 'at risk' specimens.**
  - **Only essential samples should be taken.**
  - The laboratory should be aware of and prepared to receive specimens.
  - Family contact should be restricted to the minimum required for care.
  - Soap and water should be available for hand washing before and after patient contact.
  - **For all carers, including family members, careful barrier nursing with gloves and plastic aprons is mandatory, and stocks of these must be readily to hand.**
  - Hospital staff and carers are advised to wear double gloves, plastic aprons, gowns (with boots), a head covering, HEPA-type face masks and goggles or eye shields. However, in a tropical setting these can only be tolerated for a few hours at a time, so arrange work to account for this.
  - If outer gloves are not changed between patients, gloved hands should be washed in 1:100 bleach.
  - Appropriate disposal of excreta and clinical waste is essential, so incinerate burnable clinical waste daily, and flush excreta down a dedicated toilet, having added 1:10 household bleach (0.5% chlorine) first.

(a) Disinfect bedpans and urine bottles with 1:10 bleach.
(b) Disinfect beds and equipment with 1:100 bleach.
(c) Disinfect the dead with 1:10 bleach before burying in a sealed plastic bag.

Consider using seropositive staff to nurse these patients. The identification and involvement of these staff has been successful in some outbreaks. They must follow the ward infection control measures. Remember that convalescent patients may continue to excrete virus for many months (in both Lassa and Ebola).

Fear among staff and the community needs to be addressed openly, and staff and carers must be educated about the role of barrier nursing measures, and the risks involved if these are not implemented.

Careful attention should be paid where local culture and customs (e.g. burial rites, 'widow cleansing', care of the sick, etc.) cause 'high-risk' activity. Education and participation of community leaders is important to ensure safe practice.

Which patients should be isolated?
Isolation of all patients who are likely to have a VHF on admission

- The different categories of **clinical diagnostic probability** are based on fever, contact history, haemorrhagic and non-haemorrhagic clinical signs, initial laboratory tests and geography. These categories are as follows:

  - suspected clinical VHF
  - probable VHF
  - illness probably not a VHF.
- Distinguishing signs (e.g. conjunctivitis in Ebola) are particularly helpful for categorising cases.

Isolation of suspected and probable cases on presentation to hospital

- Isolation should ideally be in single rooms, but an identified separate communal ward for probable and confirmed cases is often all that is available.
  - This should have an adjoining toilet, for safe waste disposal.
  - There should be a separate adjoining area for changing into and storing isolation clothing.
  - Supplies of gloves, gowns, etc. need to be readily available.
  - Hand-washing facilities are mandatory.
- The area should be marked as 'access restricted' to only those trained in VHF isolation precautions, and attention should be paid to screening windows.

Written infection control measures should be clearly displayed on the ward.

Differential diagnosis of VHFs

- The important differential diagnoses are, depending on geography, falciparum malaria, typhoid, meningococcaemia, *Shigella* or non-specific bloody dysentery, severe sepsis, leptospirosis, plague, yellow fever and dengue.
- It is crucial to exclude other treatable disease in patients presenting with symptoms suggestive of a VHF, and to initiate therapy directed at these.
- All patients should therefore receive a broad-spectrum antibiotic (e.g. chloramphenicol), and in some areas an antimalarial drug.
- In an endemic area, or during a known outbreak, the clinical diagnosis of a VHF is relatively straightforward. Difficulty arises when sporadic or new cases occur.
- A history of contact with a case in the previous 3 weeks and a history of recent travel to a transmission area should be sought. As no VHF has an incubation period longer than 3 weeks, travellers or contacts of known or suspected cases who are well after this period are unlikely to be infected.

Further reading
The following very practical resources are for those who require additional VHF control information.

Medicins Sans Frontieres 2014 on the Ebola epidemic in West Africa www.msf.org.uk/ebola

WHO fact sheet on Ebola 2014 www.who.int/mediacentre/factsheets/fs103/en/

World Health Organization Global Alert and Response on the Ebola epidemic 2014. www.who.int/csr/disease/ebola/en/

World Health Organization (1997) *WHO Recommended Guidelines for Epidemic Preparedness and Response: Ebola Haemorrhagic Fever (EHF).* www.fas.org/nuke/intro/bw/whoemcdis977E.pdf

6.2.J Yellow fever

> **BOX 6.2.J.1 Minimum standards**
> - Immunisation.
> - Intensive supportive care.
> - Blood transfusion.
> - Vector control.
> - Internationally notifiable.

Introduction

Yellow fever is a flavivirus infection spread by the bite of *Aedes* and other mosquitoes.

Epidemiology

- Yellow fever is currently confined to tropical Africa and parts of South America, especially around the Amazon basin. It does not occur in Asia.
- A reservoir of infection exists in jungle primates, and mosquitoes which bite the animals in the tree canopy.
- Three transmission cycles are recognised:
  - sylvatic (jungle), in which a reservoir is maintained among jungle primates by mosquitoes, with humans being infected incidentally
  - intermediate (savannah), the commonest cycle occurring in Africa, in which semi-domestic mosquitoes may cause small epidemics in rural villages
  - urban, in which infected humans introduce infection to urban areas, where the day-biting *Aedes aegypti* flourishes and may cause major epidemics in unvaccinated populations.

Pathophysiology

Symptoms are due to toxic effects on the liver, kidneys and sometimes other organs, such as the heart and brain. Asymptomatic infections may also occur.

Clinical features

- The incubation period is 3–6 days.
- Many patients have an initial febrile illness, with chills and muscle pains, from which they recover.
- Others, after an illness of about 5 days, have a brief period of apparent improvement followed by deterioration and the following complications:
  - vomiting: first bilious and then black ('coffee grounds')
  - jaundice, liver failure and hypoglycaemia
  - bleeding of the gums, nose and stomach
  - proteinuria, oliguria and renal failure
  - delirium and coma.

- Mortality among complicated cases is 20–50%.

Laboratory diagnosis

- Leukopenia, thrombocytopenia, initial haemoconcentration and then haemodilution.
- Raised transaminases and bilirubin levels.
- Abnormal clotting.
- Proteinuria and impaired renal function.
- Rapid detection methods for yellow fever virus include PCR and antigen detection.
- The serum IgM-ELISA assay is 95% sensitive if performed within 7–10 days of clinical onset.
- **A probable case is defined as positive IgM-ELISA taken within days 3–10** of symptoms.
- A confirmed case is defined as a clinically compatible case plus a fourfold rise in antibody titre in a patient with no history of recent yellow fever vaccination and having excluded cross-reactivity with other flaviviruses.
- Post-mortem liver biopsy specimens show mid-zone necrosis of hepatic lobules, often with eosinophilic Councilman bodies. Antigen may also be detected in tissue.

Management

- **Universal cross-infection precautions**, careful nursing and symptom control.
- Nurse suspected patients under permethrin-treated bed nets, as blood may remain infective for mosquitoes up to 5 days after onset.
- Supportive management, fluids, blood transfusion, fresh-frozen plasma, inotropes, dialysis, and ventilation if required.
- No specific antiviral treatment is available. Caution in prescribing and beware risk of bleeding, hepatic and renal impairment. H2-receptor antagonists may reduce risk of gastric bleeding.
- **Suspected cases of yellow fever must be notified within 24 hours** to national public health authorities, which in turn notify the WHO.

Prevention

- Elimination of the breeding sites of *Aedes aegypti* mosquitoes around human dwellings.
- Immunisation of the local population with live attenuated 17D yellow fever vaccine. Immunisation becomes effective after 10 days. Vaccine may be given to children aged 6 months or older unless there are specific contraindications (e.g. if they are immunocompromised).

6.3 Other parasitic infections

6.3.A Systemic protozoal infections

6.3.A.a African trypanosomiasis

BOX 6.3.A.A.1 Minimum standards
- Hydration, nutritional support, and treatment of intercurrent infections.
- Confirm the diagnosis, including lumbar puncture for clinical staging.
- Pentamidine, suramin, melarsoprol, eflornithine and nifurtimox.
- Prednisolone.
- Public health measures and vector control.

Introduction

Gambian trypanosomiasis, caused by *Trypanosoma brucei gambiense*, is a slowly progressive disease of West and Central Africa. Rhodesian trypanosomiasis, caused by *T. b. rhodesiense*, is a subacute infection found in East and Southern Africa. Trypanosomiasis of wild and domestic animals is often caused by other 'subspecies' of *T. brucei* which are indistinguishable morphologically from those that cause human infection.

Transmission
- By the bite of infected tsetse flies (*Glossina*).
- Riverine tsetse (*Glossina palpalis* group) are responsible for transmission of *T. b. gambiense*, chiefly from a human reservoir. Infection may be endemic or epidemic.
- Savannah tsetse flies (*Glossina morsitans* group) are mainly responsible for sporadic transmission of *T. b. rhodesiense* from animals to humans.
- Congenital transmission is also well recognised.

Clinical features

A painful bite lesion (the trypanosomal chancre) may form at the site of the infected bite and last for up to 3 weeks. Among indigenous people in endemic areas, this is more commonly seen in *T. b. rhodesiense* (19%) than in *T. b. gambiense* infections. However, a chancre may be seen in 25–40% of early presentations of *T. b. gambiense* among expatriates. Clinical staging is essential for planning treatment, and depends on evidence of CNS involvement based on lumbar puncture findings.

Haemolymphatic stage 1
- Symptoms of fever and malaise that last for about a week are associated with waves of parasitaemia.

Lymph nodes (especially those at the back of the neck in Gambian disease) become enlarged.
- There may be short-lived oedematous swellings of the face or limbs, and sometimes a patchy circular erythematous rash or skin itching.
- Early symptoms are often milder in Gambian disease, and this stage may last for months to years.
- In Rhodesian disease, patients are usually more ill with tachycardia, high fever, hepatosplenomegaly, myocarditis, anaemia and sometimes jaundice.

Meningo-encephalitic stage 2
- Severe headache and altered behaviour are often seen.
- Patients may become apathetic, depressed or frankly psychotic.
- Sleep is disturbed, so that patients are often awake during the night and sleep by day; eventually deep coma results.
- Ataxia and cerebellar signs are frequent.
- Delayed response to pain after deep pressure, the appearance of primitive reflexes and altered tendon reflexes may be seen.
- Death often results from intercurrent infection.

Diagnosis
- In *T. b. rhodesiense* infections, trypanosomes can usually be observed in thick blood films. These are also useful for *T. b. gambiense* infections, but may be negative during periods of low parasitaemia.
- More sensitive methods of examining the blood include microhaematocrit centrifugation, use of the quantitative buffy coat (QBC) technique, and the mini-anion exchange column method.
- When there are enlarged lymph nodes, particularly posterior cervical nodes in *T. b. gambiense* infections (Winterbottom's sign), microscopy of a node aspirate may demonstrate trypanosomes.
- **Serological methods: The card agglutination test for trypanosomiasis (CATT) is useful only for population screening for *T. b. gambiense* infections. Positive results need to be confirmed by the finding of parasites. Other serological tests exist that may be useful for screening suspected cases of *T. b. gambiense*, but are rarely available in resource-limited settings. Seropositives require parasitological confirmation. Negative serology does not exclude the diagnosis. Always search for**

parasites. No serological screening tests are currently available for *T. b. rhodesiense*.

- Treatment depends on evaluation of the stage of infection, so lumbar puncture is essential. Criteria for stage 2 disease in a previously untreated patient include either the presence of trypanosomes in the CSF, or a raised CSF lymphocyte count (> 5 cells/mm³) in the absence of another cause. CSF protein levels are usually raised. CSF IgM (if available) may be useful as an early marker of CNS invasion.

Treatment

Drug resistance is becoming more widespread. Check local resistance patterns and treatment recommendations.

The drugs used for treatment are toxic. They should only be started after a parasitological diagnosis has been confirmed and, particularly in stage 2 *T. b. gambiense* disease, after the patient's general condition has been improved by attention to hydration, nutrition and intercurrent infections.

T. b. gambiense stage 1

- Give pentamidine isethionate 4 mg/kg IM daily for 7–10 days.
- Children should be given a meal or a sweet drink 1 hour prior to treatment (to reduce the risk of hypoglycaemia), and must lie down for an hour after an injection and have careful checks of pulse and blood pressure (there is a **risk of severe hypotension**).
- **Side effects:** hypoglycaemia (may occur up to 7 days after treatment), arrhythmias, bone-marrow suppression, electrolyte disturbances (low K⁺, Ca²⁺, Mg²⁺). Monitoring is recommended if possible.

T. b. gambiense stage 2

- **Recommended treatment is nifurtimox–eflornithine combination treatment (NECT).**
- Give nifurtimox 5 mg/kg orally three times daily for 10 days plus eflornithine 200 mg/kg every 12 hours by IV infusion (over 2 hours) for 7 days.
- Second choice, if nifurtimox is not available and the patient is under 12 years of age, is to give eflornithine 150 mg/kg every 6 hours by IV infusion (over 2 hours) for 14 days. If the patient is over 12 years of age, give eflornithine 100 mg/kg every 6 hours by IV infusion (over 2 hours) for 14 days.
- There is a risk of infection and phlebitis at the IV site. Care is needed with regard to sterile procedures and securing the IV line. Change the IV site every 2 days.
- Side effects include **CNS abnormalities (due to nifurtimox), convulsions**, and bone-marrow suppression (due to eflornithine).
- **Relapse after NECT or eflornithine:** Give **melarsoprol,** 2.2 mg/kg/day slowly IV for 10 days. **Encephalopathy occurs in up to 15% of patients treated with melarsoprol, and is associated with a 50% case-fatality rate.** Co-administration of prednisolone reduces the risk of encephalopathy to less than 5%. Prior to the first dose of melarsoprol, start prednisolone orally 1 mg/kg (maximum 40 mg/day) daily for 10 days, then taper and stop over 3 days.

- **Side effects include encephalopathy, peripheral neuropathy, skin reactions including Stevens–Johnson syndrome, and phlebitis.** Note that melarsoprol IV is very painful, particularly if extravasation occurs, and may cause tissue necrosis.

T. b. rhodesiense stage 1

- **Suramin:** initial test dose of 4–5 mg/kg slowly IV over 5 minutes on day 1, then 20 mg/kg slowly IV on days 3, 10, 17, 24 and 31. Maximum single dose 1 g/injection.
- The initial test dose is to reduce the risk of idiosyncratic anaphylactic reactions to suramin. Have IM adrenaline available (*see* Section 5.1.B).
- Test the urine for albumin before each dose, and modify the regime if more than a trace of protein is seen.
- This regime may also be used for **stage 1** *T. b. gambiense* if pentamidine is unavailable.
- **Side effects include hypersensitivity, nephrotoxicity** (monitor urine albumin levels before each dose, and modify the regime if more than a trace of protein is seen) and peripheral neuropathy.

T. b. rhodesiense stage 2

- **Melarsoprol:** 3.6 mg/kg slowly IV for 3 or 4 days repeated three or four cycles with an interval of 7–10 days between treatment series.
- **Prednisolone:** 1 mg/kg (maximum 40 mg/day) orally daily throughout the course of melarsoprol, then gradually taper and stop. Note that the recommendation for use in *T. b. rhodesiense* stage 2 is largely based on evidence for use in *T. b. gambiense* stage 2.
- Side effects: see previous notes.

Follow-up

- **Notify all cases** so that effective surveillance and public health action is taken.
- All patients should have follow-up lumbar puncture for 2 years (*T. b. gambiense*, lumbar puncture 6-monthly; *T. b. rhodesiense*, 3-monthly for 1 year and then 6-monthly).
  If initially stage 1 but at follow-up:
  (i) CSF 6–19 white blood cells/mm³: repeat lumbar puncture in 1–2 months.
  (ii) CSF ≥ 20 white blood cells/mm³: treat as stage 2.

  If initially stage 2, CSF white cell count trend at follow-up is more important than the actual value.
- Drug resistance is increasing – if suspected seek expert advice.

6.3.A.b American trypanosomiasis (Chagas disease)

BOX 6.3.A.B.1 Minimum standards
- Bed nets.
- Vector control.
- Benznidazole.
- Nifurtimox.

Introduction

American trypanosomiasis is potentially life-threatening and is caused by the protozoan parasite, *Trypanosoma cruzi*.

An estimated 10 million people are infected worldwide, mostly in Latin America, where it is endemic. In 2008 it killed more than 10 000 people. It is increasingly being detected in the USA, Canada, many European and some Western Pacific countries.

In Latin America, *T. cruzi* is mainly transmitted by the infected faeces of blood-sucking triatomine bugs. These bugs typically live in the cracks of poorly constructed homes in rural or suburban areas. They become active at night when they feed on human blood by biting an exposed area of skin such as the face, where the bug defecates close to the bite. The parasites enter the body when the person instinctively smears the bug faeces into the bite, the eyes, the mouth, or any break in the skin.

T. cruzi can also be transmitted in the following ways:
- via food contaminated with the parasite through, for example, contact with triatomine bug faeces
- by blood transfusions from infected donors
- by transmission from an infected mother to her newborn during pregnancy or childbirth.

Clinical management

Signs and symptoms

The disease presents in two phases. The initial acute phase lasts for about 2 months after infection. During the acute phase, a high number of parasites circulate in the blood. In most cases, symptoms are absent or mild, but can include fever, headache, enlarged lymph glands, pallor, muscle pain, difficulty in breathing, swelling and abdominal or chest pain. In less than 50% of people bitten by a triatomine bug, the characteristic first visible signs can be a skin lesion or a purplish swelling of the lids of one eye.

During the chronic phase, the parasites congregate in the heart and digestive tract. Up to 30% of patients suffer from cardiac disorders, and up to 10% suffer from digestive (typically enlargement of the oesophagus or colon), neurological or mixed pathology. The infection can lead to sudden death or heart failure caused by progressive destruction of the heart muscle.

Treatment

Benznidazole and nifurtimox are both almost 100% effective in curing the disease if given soon after infection. However, the efficacy of both diminishes the longer a person has been infected. Treatment is also indicated for those in whom the infection has been reactivated (e.g. due to immunosuppression), for infants with congenital infection, and for patients during the early chronic phase. The potential benefits of medication in preventing or delaying the disease should be weighed against the long duration of treatment (up to 2 months) and possible adverse reactions (occurring in up to 40% of treated patients).

Benznidazole and nifurtimox should not be taken by pregnant women or by people with kidney or liver failure. Nifurtimox is also contraindicated in people with a history of neurological or psychiatric disorders. In addition, specific treatment for cardiac or digestive manifestations may be required.

Benznidazole 100 mg tablets

Acute or early chronic phase:
- Full term newborn infant give 5 mg/kg daily in 3 divided doses increasing after 3 days to 10 mg/kg daily if no leukopenia or thrombocytopenia occurs. Treat for 60 days.
- Infant or child, 40 kg body weight give 7.5 mg/kg daily in 2–3 divided doses for 60 days.
- Child > 40 kg give 5 mg/kg daily in 2–3 divided doses for 60 days.

Chronic phase:
Infant or child 5 mg/kg daily in 2–3 divided doses for 60 days.

Nifurtimox Tablets 30, 120 and 250 mg

Acute or early chronic phase:given after meals
- Neonate, infant or child < 40 kg give15–20 mg/kg daily in 3 divided doses for 60 days
- Child > 40 kg 12.5–15 mg/kg daily in 3 divided doses for 60 days

Chronic phase:
Infant or child 8–10 mg/kg daily in 3 divided doses for 60 days.

Vector control and prevention

There is no vaccine for Chagas disease. Vector control is the most effective method of preventing this disease in Latin America. Blood screening is necessary to prevent infection through transfusion.

The WHO recommends:
- insecticide spraying of houses and surrounding areas
- house improvements to prevent vector infestation
- personal preventive measures such as bed nets
- good hygiene practices in food preparation, transportation, storage and consumption
- screening of blood donors
- screening of newborns from infected mothers, and of siblings of infected children to provide early diagnosis and treatment.

6.3.A.c Leishmaniasis

BOX 6.3.A.C Minimum standards
■ Public health measures and vector control.

Leishmaniasis: visceral
■ Bone-marrow, splenic and lymph-node aspirate.
■ Pentavalent antimonials.
■ Amphotericin B.
■ Paromomycin.

Leishmaniasis: cutaneous and mucocutaneous
■ Pentavalent antimonials.
■ Topical 15% aminosidine plus 12% methyl benzethonium.
■ Ketoconazole.

Introduction

Leishmaniasis is caused by *Leishmania*, a protozoon whose reservoir is in animals, including rodents and dogs, and in some areas (e.g. India) in humans. The vector is the female sandfly.

There are three main clinical types of disease:
● cutaneous (CL)
● mucocutaneous (MCL)
● visceral leishmaniasis (VL) or kala-azar.

Parasite and life cycle

● About 21 of the 30 or more species of *Leishmania* infect humans. They are morphologically similar and can only be differentiated by isoenzyme analysis which identifies the zymodeme in the cultured parasite.
● In animals and humans, *Leishmania* lives in macrophages in the reticulo-endothelial system in the form of amastigotes (Leishman–Donovan bodies). When taken up by the biting sandfly it transforms into a promastigote, which has a flagellum.
● There are two main genera of sandfly responsible for transmission, *Phlebotomus* in the Old World and *Lutzomyia* in the New World (Central and South America). Sandflies breed in organic material in dark moist sites, such as cracks in masonry, termite hills, or leaves on the forest floor. The female obtains her blood meal at night by feeding on animals, and also on humans if they are living or working in the vicinity.

Epidemiology

The Old World comprises Africa, Asia and Europe (collectively known as Afro-Eurasia), plus the surrounding islands. It is used in the context of, and contrast with, the 'New World' (i.e. the Americas and sometimes Oceania). Old world CL and VL are found in the Mediterranean basin, the Middle East, the Sudan, Ethiopia, Kenya, Afghanistan, the Indian subcontinent, and southern regions of the former Soviet Union, and China. Where HIV infection and VL coexist, there are major problems in the treatment of VL. Drug resistance in VL is a serious concern in India and the Sudan. Bihar State has 90% of VL in India and 45% of world cases.

In the New World, CL and MCL are the main forms of infection. VL occurs mainly in North-East Brazil.

Currently, leishmaniasis occurs in four continents and is considered to be endemic in 88 countries, 72 of which are resource-limited:
● 90% of all visceral leishmaniasis cases occur in Bangladesh, Brazil, India, Nepal and Sudan
● 90% of mucocutaneous leishmaniasis cases occur in Bolivia, Brazil and Peru
● 90% of cutaneous leishmaniasis cases occur in Afghanistan, Brazil, Iran, Peru, Saudi Arabia and Syria.

Leishmaniasis is a disease of poverty associated with malnutrition, displacement, poor housing and migration of non-immune people to endemic areas. It is linked with deforestation and urbanisation.

Immunology

● A strong cell-mediated immune (CMI) response is required for control of and recovery from disease. Polyclonal stimulation of B cells results in high levels of IgG.
● Subclinical infection is common. CL usually heals spontaneously, but untreated MCL will progress, and VL will result in death. Development of VL indicates that the host's CMI is unable to control the infection, and if untreated, progressive immunosuppression will develop.
● Death is usually due to a secondary infection (e.g. respiratory tract or gut infection).

Cutaneous and mucocutaneous leishmaniasis

Cutaneous leishmaniasis

The species responsible are *L. tropica, L. major, L. aethiopica* in the Old World, and *L. mexicana* and *L. amazonensis* in the New World. Single or multiple nodules develop on exposed areas, especially the face or extremities, and usually ulcerate. Most heal spontaneously within months to a year or so, leaving scars.

Mucutaneous leishmaniasis

The species responsible is *L. braziliensis*. A nodule develops initially, as in CL, but at about the time of healing, metastatic lesions occur on mucosal surfaces, such as the nasal mucosa and oropharynx. If these are left untreated, progressive destruction of local tissue occurs.

Diagnosis

● Slit skin smear or aspiration should be undertaken from the raised margin of the lesion (not the base of the ulcer). Material is spread on a slide, dried, fixed in methanol and stained with Giemsa or Leishman.
● If a biopsy is undertaken (e.g. in MCL), impression smears should be done before fixing.
● If available, the specimen should be cultured.

Management

Most CL lesions are self-limiting. Treatment is indicated for multiple, large and disfiguring lesions and all MCL. Clean the lesion, and give antibiotics if necessary.

Standard treatment for CL and MCL is with pentavalent antimonials (Sb): **sodium stibogluconate** (Pentostam, 100 mg Sb/mL) or **meglumine antimoniate** (Glucantime, 85 mg Sb/mL). **It is essential to remember that the doses of these two drugs are different, because they contain different concentrations of antimony (Sb).** Give 20 mg Sb/kg/day IV or IM in a single dose for 20–28 days depending on the species of *Leishmania* (e.g. MCL requires 28 days or more). The IV infusion is stopped if coughing or substernal pain occurs. Urinary excretion of Sb is rapid (its half-life is 2 hours), although slow accumulation occurs.

For *L. major*, weekly or twice weekly intra-lesional injections of Sb (which are painful) may be administered (1 mL/lesion at four sites per ulcer) to adolescents or adults, using a 1-mL syringe and a fine (24-gauge) needle, for 4–8 weeks. A topical ointment containing 15% aminosidine and 12% methylbenzethonium chloride applied twice daily for 10–20 days may be tried. Efficacy is variable, but it may be combined with intra-lesional Sb injections.

Oral fluconazole, 3 mg/kg once daily (maximum 100 mg) for up to 6 weeks, may be effective, but there is a **danger of liver dysfunction**.

In areas where there is antimonial resistance, pentamidine (IM 2 mg/kg every second day for seven injections), amphotericin B and oral miltefosine may be required (see management of VL below).

All three of these drugs have potentially serious side effects.

Visceral leishmaniasis (kala azar)

Epidemics occur in situations of famine, complex emergencies and mass movements of populations. It has a high fatality rate if untreated. It is estimated that there are 360 000 new cases every year globally, of which more than 60% occur in Northern India (Bihar).

The species responsible are *L. donovani* and *L. infantum* in the Old World, and *L. chagasi* in the New World.

- The major presenting features include the triad of prolonged fever, anaemia and moderate to marked splenomegaly. In the early stages the child is often only mildly unwell and may have a reasonable appetite. In a minority of cases, the onset may be acute, with a high temperature, toxaemia and mild splenomegaly.
- Pancytopenia is the main laboratory finding.

Diagnosis

- In children, the diagnosis is usually confirmed by demonstrating amastigotes on bone-marrow aspirate.
- Splenic aspirates have a higher sensitivity, and this procedure is safe in skilled hands so long as the platelet count is above 40 × 10⁹/litre and coagulation is normal.
- Repeat bone-marrow or splenic aspiration to monitor progress if required.
- If there is lymphadenopathy, diagnosis may be attempted by fine-needle aspiration.
- **Serological antibody tests such as ELISA have a high sensitivity, and are particularly helpful if a parasitological diagnosis cannot be obtained.**
- If a microscopic diagnosis cannot be made, **the polymerase chain reaction (PCR) should be undertaken. The value of the PCR is being evaluated**.

Differential diagnosis

- Differential diagnosis of marked hepatosplenomegaly, anaemia and pancytopenia includes hyper-reactive splenomegaly (tropical splenomegaly) syndrome and schistosomiasis, as well as myeloid leukaemia and myelofibrosis.
- In acute-onset disease, malaria, disseminated tuberculosis, typhoid, brucellosis, African trypanosomiasis, relapsing fever and leukaemia should be considered.
- **HIV infection greatly increases the risk of visceral leishmaniasis, and thus co-infection is common.**

TABLE 6.3.A.C.1 Clinical features of visceral leishmaniasis

Incubation period: 2–4 months (weeks to two years)
Fever: intermittent at first
Anaemia: bone-marrow depression, hypersplenism
Splenomegaly: progressive enlargement
Hepatomegaly
Weight loss
Epistaxis: haemorrhage from other sites may occur in advanced disease
Diarrhoea: invasion of gut by amastigotes, secondary infection
Cough
Oedema: hypoalbuminaemia
Hair and skin signs of malnutrition in chronic forms
Lymphadenopathy: in some African countries

TABLE 6.3.A.C.2 Clinical pathology of visceral leishmaniasis

Haemoglobin: low; normochromic, normocytic film
White blood cells: low, 2–3 × 10⁹/litre Eosinophils low
Platelets: low, < 100 × 10⁹/litre
Reticulocytes: low
Serum albumin: low
Serum globulin: elevated
Liver transaminases and serum bilirubin: normal

Management of visceral leishmaniasis

Consider HIV co-infection and secondary disorders such as malaria, respiratory and gut infections, and tuberculosis. Blood transfusion for anaemia is seldom required, as the child has usually adapted to the low haemoglobin level. Give haematinics and vitamin supplements during nutritional rehabilitation and convalescence.

Liposomal amphotericin B used to be expensive, but following a campaign the WHO has brought about a 90% reduction in price, and consequently this is now the treatment of choice.

The alternative treatment is with antimoniates (Sb), for which again the WHO has obtained a substantial reduction in cost. Meglumine antimoniate and sodium stibogluconate are available. The duration of Sb treatment is usually 4 weeks, but prolonged treatment (up to 6 weeks) may be necessary in resistant cases (*see* Table 6.3.A.c.3).

For relapse, a second course can be given after a few weeks. Serious toxicity is rare in children, but if a prolonged course of high dosage is required, or toxicity is suspected, liver function tests and an ECG looking for conduction disorders should be undertaken. Serious toxicity may require dimercaprol to chelate and remove the antimony.

In areas where there is resistance to Sb, such as Bihar state in India, and the Sudan, alternative drugs are required as follows: amphotericin B by slow infusion; paromomycin (aminoglycoside, identical to aminosidine); or oral miltefosine. Combinations of drugs (e.g. paromomycin and Sb) may be more effective. In patients with HIV/VL co-infection, management is difficult because of frequent relapse when treatment is stopped. HAART combined with maintenance anti-leishmanial therapy is important.

TABLE 6.3.A.C.3 Drugs used in the treatment of visceral leishmaniasis

Drug	Doses	Contraindications and cautions	Side effects
Liposomal amphotericin B	4 mg/kg IV over 30–60 minutes once daily by IV infusion on days 1, 2, 3, 5 and 10	An initial test dose of 100 micrograms/kg (maximum 1 mg) is infused over 15 minutes. Observe for 1 hour to ensure that anaphylaxis does not occur, then proceed	May produce hypotension, fever, vomiting, headache, and muscle and joint pain. Less commonly, chest pain, hypoxia, severe abdominal pain, flushing, urticaria, and flank or leg pain
Sodium stibogluconate (100 mg Sb/mL) or meglumine antimoniate (81 mg Sb/mL)	20 mg/kg (minimum 200 mg) IV infusion or deep IM injection over over 5–10 minutes once daily for 28 days Prolonged treatment for 6 weeks in resistant cases	Pre-existing severe cardiac, liver, renal, pancreatic or haematological abnormalities Not to be given during pregnancy Filter solution through 5-micron filter immediately before infusion	Vomiting, abdominal pain, myalgia and arthralgia, headache, metallic taste. Rarely sudden death with prolonged QT interval; therefore monitor ECG and stop infusion if QT exceeds 0.5 seconds
Conventional amphotericin B	Slow IV infusion, 1 mg/kg every second day for 15 days, or daily for 20 days. (daily dose must never exceed 1.5 mg/kg)	An initial test dose of 100 micrograms/kg (maximum 1 mg) is infused over 15 minutes. Observe for 1 hour to ensure that anaphylaxis does not occur, then proceed	May produce hypotension, fever, vomiting, headache, and muscle and joint pain
Paromomycin	Daily IV or IM injections 16–20 mg/kg/day for 21 days	Do not give at the same time as gentamicin or other aminoglycosides. Avoid if there is renal impairment	Vomiting, diarrhoea, abdominal pain, fever and ototoxicity
Miltefosine	2.5 mg/kg/day orally for 28 days	Not in pregnancy	Nausea and vomiting

A limited stock of the above drugs is kept by the WHO in Geneva for rapid response to an epidemic.

A study looking at the effectiveness of a single-dose treatment (by IV infusion) using liposomal amphotericin B is currently in progress in India.

Follow-up and prognosis

Symptomatic improvement usually occurs within a few days, and a haematological response occurs within 2 weeks. Splenomegaly slowly regresses, but may take a year or more to resolve. Prolonged follow-up (at least 1 year) is necessary to detect relapse. Relapse is treated with a repeat prolonged course of antimonials (up to 8 weeks). Unresponsiveness will require alternative drugs such as liposomal amphotericin B (if available), aminosidine, standard amphotericin B or pentamidine. Trials of miltefosine are in progress.

Prevention and control

Prevention is similar to that of malaria, and includes insect repellents and the use of fine-mesh bed nets impregnated with permethrin. Control includes spraying of sandfly resting sites and human dwellings, destruction of animal reservoirs and treatment of cases.

Further reading

Murray HW, Berman JD, Davies CR et al. (2005) Advances in leishmaniasis. Lancet, **366**, 1561–77.
World Health Organization (2014) Leishmaniasis. www.who.int/leishmaniasis/en/

6.3.A.d Malaria

BOX 6.3.A.D.1 Minimum standards for an effective malaria control programme

1 Prevention:
- Impregnated bed nets (ITNs), preferably long-lasting insecticidal nets (LLINs).
- Where appropriate, intermittent preventive treatment in infants (IPTi) and seasonal malaria chemoprevention (SMC) for older children.
- Other methods of vector control, such as indoor residual spraying (IRS), personal protection (e.g. mosquito coils, impregnated clothing, repellents, etc.).

2 A well-informed population to improve early care seeking and adherence to treatment and preventive regimes.

3 Good case management:
- Early accurate diagnosis: all patients should have a biological test before treatment:
  - Quality-assured thick blood film and/or rapid diagnostic test (RDT).
  - Haemoglobin measurement to detect and treat malaria anaemia (e.g. using a haemocue machine).
  - In severe disease, facilities to measure blood glucose levels and provide safe blood transfusion.
- Effective treatment:
  - Treatment for simple malaria.
    - » Artemisinin combination therapy (ACT) (following the national protocol for recommended ACT).
  - Treatment for severe disease.
    - » IV or IM artesunate (IM artemether, rectal artesunate, or IV or IM quinine if artesunate is not available).
  - Pre-referral treatment.
    - » Rectal artesunate (if artesunate is not available, rectal quinine) or if injections are safe IV or IM artesunate or IM artemether, or IM quinine.

4 Accessible, acceptable and affordable care:
- Consider training community health workers in remote areas to diagnose and treat malaria.
- Make treatment free for pregnant girls and children under five.
- Set up a good referral system from community and first-level health facilities to facilities with means to treat severe cases, including transport and facilities to access resources to pay for treatment if needed.

BOX 6.3.A.D.2 Minimum standards for hospital treatment of severe malaria

- A triage system.
- RDTs and microscopy for initial diagnosis, plus laboratory facilities to determine levels of parasitaemia.
- Antimalarial drugs for IV, IM and oral treatment.
- Oxygen.
- Antibiotics and anticonvulsants.
- Safe blood transfusion services.
- Nasogastric feeding.
- Good nursing care (monitoring of vital signs and fluid balance, nasogastric feeding).

Malaria is estimated to cause at least 650 000 deaths each year, mostly among African children.

- Unlike anywhere else in the world, children aged 6–24 months in Africa are most at risk of the worst forms of malaria. Every 30 seconds an African child dies of malaria.

There are five *Plasmodium* species known to be infective to humans, namely *Plasmodium falciparum*, *P. vivax*, *P. ovale*, *P. malariae* and *P. knowlesi*.

P. falciparum causes severe disease and is the most prevalent form in sub-Saharan Africa (most sub-Saharan Africans are protected against *P. vivax* due to lacking a protein in their red blood cells (the Duffy antigen)). *P. falciparum* differs from the other species in that infected erythrocytes adhere to capillary epithelium, thus disappearing from the circulation and evading destruction by the spleen.

P. vivax and *P. ovale* can cause recurrent malaria attacks due to the formation of a dormant form existing as hypnozoites in the liver, which are periodically released into the blood. Drugs to eliminate the hypnozoites from the liver are limited (primaquine).

P. malariae can cause long-term problems, including kidney failure, and *P. knowlesi* is a newly emerging form which has caused severe disease in Asia (Papua New Guinea and Thailand).

Life cycle

The infected *Anopheles* female mosquito injects sporozoites into the bloodstream of an individual. Sporozoites circulate for less than 30 minutes before being phagocytosed or entering liver parenchymal cells. The blood and liver phase prior to re-entry into the circulation is called the pre-erythrocytic phase, and it varies in length according to the species. At the end of this phase, merozoites invade the red blood cells and begin the erythrocytic phase. Parasites rapidly multiply within the red blood cells, which finally burst, releasing more merozoites into the bloodstream to invade further red blood cells.

Periodic bouts of fever are associated with the release of the merozoites. After some time, sexual forms of the parasites (gametocytes) are formed which are then ingested by a female mosquito to complete the cycle in humans. In the mosquito stomach, the gametocytes merge and eventually form sporozoites which migrate to the salivary

Introduction

Malaria is an extremely important public health burden in Africa, disproportionately affecting the youngest and most vulnerable. Children under 5 years and pregnant women, especially in the first pregnancy, suffer from severe forms of the disease. In Asia, the disease is more common in men and older children.

- Nearly 80% of the world's malaria burden is in Africa.

glands, where they are injected into the bloodstream by the mosquito as it takes a blood meal to support its own reproductive effort.

In two species (*P. vivax* and *P. ovale*) some hepatic-stage parasites remain within the liver cells with the formation of the dormant phase, called hypnozoites. For various reasons (perhaps including waning immunity), at a later date the dormant phases activate and reseed blood. This leads to manifestations of malaria not from a new infection but from the latent exo-erythrocytic phase.

P. falciparum differs from the other species in that infected erythrocytes adhere to capillary epithelium, thus disappearing from the circulation and evading destruction by the spleen.

P. falciparum is the most likely species to cause life-threatening disease, and is a major cause of mortality in children.

Plasmodium falciparum

Clinical features

- Typical symptoms include high-grade fever alternating with cold spells, rigors, chills and sweating. There are usually associated myalgias and arthralgias.
- However, features in children under 5 years of age may be non-specific, with fever, vomiting, diarrhoea and abdominal pain being the main symptoms.
- In older immune individuals the only symptoms may be fever with headache and joint pains.
- All fevers in children from a malaria-endemic area are therefore due to malaria until proven otherwise.

Diagnosis
Microscopy

- Blood smear for malaria remains the gold standard: a thick film for diagnosis, and a thin film to confirm the type of malarial parasite. Typically species-specific ring forms inside red blood cells are seen, but there may also be gametocytes.
- The level of parasitaemia is usually scored as 1–5+. If the malarial smear is 3+ or more, there is a high level parasitaemia. In areas where parasitic density is measured the smear is reported as parasites/mm^3.
- Malaria microscopy in district hospitals can be of very poor quality. A quality assurance programme should be in place that includes the following:
  - a properly trained and regularly updated microscopist
  - adequate time to look at slides, particularly for low-level parasitaemia
  - the correct stains and good-quality slides
  - a binocular microscope that is properly serviced and maintained
  - a system of internal and preferably external cross-checking of a sample of slides, especially the low parasitaemias and negative slides.
  - If possible examination requires a reliable electricity supply or good lighting near a window in the day time. Many modern microscopes have an inbuilt LED light.

Rapid diagnostic tests

Antigen-capture test kits use a rapid simple dipstick test from a finger-prick blood sample to give a result in 10–20 minutes. RDTs should be used in circumstances where microscope facilities and/or diagnostic expertise are limited.

There are two main forms of rapid test.

Histidine-rich protein 2 (HRP2) tests

These only detect *P. falciparum*. HRP2 tests have a sensitivity of 97–100% (i.e. there are very few false-negative results). These tests can lack specificity (which may be as low as 59% in some studies), so there can be a high frequency of false-positive results, especially in a high transmission zone where malaria infection is frequent (children can have as many as six attacks a year). HRP2 remains in the bloodstream for at least 2 weeks after all viable parasites have been killed, and often for considerably longer (6–8 weeks), so patients returning with fever within 4 weeks after treatment cannot be diagnosed using an HRP2-based RDT. However, a presumptive diagnosis that fever equals malaria has an even lower specificity.

HRP2 tests are very heat stable, but are sensitive to humidity. They have a shelf-life of 2 years, and their use can be taught to healthcare workers, even at village level, in a few hours. They are especially suitable for use in sub-Saharan Africa, where other species of malaria are rare.

Parasite lactate dehydrogenase (pLDH) tests

The parasite lactate dehydrogenase (pLDH) antigen is produced by all four *Plasmodium* species. The pLDH-based tests detect the antigen using a panel of monoclonal antibodies. They can have high sensitivity for *P. falciparum*, and are more specific than HRP2. They return to negative in 3–14 days (the majority do so within 7 days).

Some pLDH tests are able to differentiate between *P. falciparum* and other *Plasmodium* species, and between viable and non-viable parasites, thereby enabling their use for monitoring therapy and for detecting new infections within 2 weeks of successful treatment.

The tests currently on the market are available in two forms. The first has a pan-pLDH antibody that can detect any species of malaria. When positive, it produces a single test line. The second produces two test lines, a pan-specific line and a line that detects *P. falciparum*. In theory, there are monoclonal antibodies that can individually detect all of the different species, but these have not yet been validated.

pLDH tests are not as heat stable as HRP2 tests. Although pLDH has a high sensitivity for *P. falciparum*, its sensitivity for *P. vivax* appears to be less satisfactory if the patient has a low parasitaemia. pLDH tests are more expensive than HRP2 tests, and are not therefore recommended in sub-Saharan Africa, where 97% of infections are due to *P. falciparum*.

Advantages of RDTs over microscopy

- The result is available within 15–20 minutes and one person can set up a new test every 1 or 2 minutes. In contrast, there are more steps involved in microscopy (i.e. slide preparation, drying, staining, and drying stained slides), and a negative slide requires 6 minutes of reading time (a microscopy report can be delayed up to an hour from collecting the blood).
- Training takes 2 hours with minimally educated workers.
- Many more tests can be done in one clinic or outreach session.

A quality control/quality assurance system for RDTs should be in place at the level of importation where the Compliance with last Malarial Treatment (CMT) is based, and at project level after transportation, to ensure that tests remain in good condition (lot testing). Monitoring of the conditions to which the tests are subjected during transportation may account for problems with their function at project level.

Field teams need to monitor the performance of healthcare staff regularly to ensure that tests are performed properly.

Other diagnostic tests that should be available in malaria programmes

- Haemacue to determine haemoglobin levels.
- Tests to deliver safe transfusion: two instant HIV tests, syphilis, hepatitis B and hepatitis C screen.
- Tests for G6PD deficiency if primaquine is to be used for radical treatment to eliminate hypnozoites and/or gametocytes of *P. falciparum*.
- Polymerase chain reaction (PCR) tests. These can be used to detect very low levels of parasitaemia. Work is progressing to develop a bedside PCR detection machine. PCRs are very important in elimination scenarios to detect very low parasitaemias, and in drug efficacy studies.

Case definitions of malaria

Suspected malaria: a patient with a fever or history of fever in the last 48 hours who lives in or has come from a malaria-endemic area.

Uncomplicated (simple malaria): a patient with a fever or history of fever in the last 48 hours who has a positive biological test and no symptoms of severe disease.

Complicated malaria: a patient with the signs and symptoms of simple malaria who is unable to take oral drugs.

Non-severe malaria may be associated with a variety of other symptoms, including cough, vomiting, diarrhoea, abdominal pain, myalgia, headache, sweating and rigors.

Severe malaria

A patient with one or more of the following signs or symptoms, with biologically confirmed *P. falciparum* infection (and occasionally *P. vivax*) and parasitaemia:

- prostration (inability to sit, or to drink or breastfeed)
- impaired consciousness (cerebral malaria)
- respiratory distress
- multiple convulsions
- circulatory collapse
- severe anaemia (haemoglobin concentration < 5 grams/ dL or haematocrit of < 15%) may be the presenting symptom, especially in children and pregnant women, and can rapidly lead to death.

Other conditions that may be associated with severe malaria

Hyperparasitaemia may be associated with severe malaria, but is not pathognomonic of severe disease in itself. It has been associated with a higher risk of mortality and needs to be rigorously treated, preferably in the first instance with parenteral medications. If there are no other signs of severity, the patient may not need hospital admission.

Hypoglycaemia often causes unconsciousness or death if not detected and treated rigorously. It is especially dangerous in children, malnourished patients and pregnant women, and is exacerbated by quinine treatment.

Pulmonary oedema is a grave and often fatal complication of malaria. It can occur spontaneously (particularly during pregnancy), but it is often a result of fluid overload during treatment.

Metabolic (lactic) acidosis: see section on severe malaria below.

Abnormal bleeding is associated with thrombocytopaenia, and leads to bleeding of gums and epistaxis, and sometimes more severe internal bleeding.

Jaundice is more common in adults than in children. Mild jaundice only reflects haemolysis, whereas very high bilirubin levels suggest hepatic dysfunction.

Haemoglobinuria is common, but its more extreme form, blackwater fever, is rare. It is associated with quinine therapy.

Oliguria/anuria can be a sign of renal dysfunction, but make sure that the patient is adequately rehydrated before commencing therapy for renal failure. **Fluid balance charts should be instituted and monitored closely for all patients with severe malaria.**

Uncomplicated/simple malaria

There is a fever and a positive blood smear. There is no evidence of altered consciousness, hypoglycaemia, severe anaemia, jaundice or respiratory difficulties.

Management
Management of children who have always lived in an endemic area

- There is no need to admit the child to hospital (unless they are under 4 months of age or less than 5 kg in weight, or pregnant).
- A diagnostic test should be done before treatment (microscopy if available and quality assured, or an RDT). This will confirm malaria and also ensure that patients who do not have malaria receive appropriate treatment. **Note that malaria is frequently accompanied by other serious infections, such as pneumonia.** Signs of bacterial or viral infections should be looked for and treated appropriately even if the malaria diagnostic test is positive.
- Give first-line antimalarial treatment (ACTs) as recommended in local national guidelines.
- Ensure that tablets or syrup are swallowed and not vomited.
- Give the first dose under direct observation and advise the carer on how to administer the drug to young children by dissolving tablets in breast milk or syrup and giving this slowly with a syringe.
- If the child vomits within the first 30 minutes, repeat the full dose. If they vomit after 1 hour give a half dose. Advise the carer to return if further doses are vomited. Remember to advise the carer to give the dose with food if artemether/lumefantrine is used, to improve absorption of the lipophilic lumefantrine.
- Encourage oral fluid intake and continued feeding with light nutritious foods plus catch-up meals when the child recovers. Measures to lower the body temperature may be necessary (tepid sponging and paracetamol).
- Test for iron deficiency, and if the patient is pale and anaemic (based on palmar and conjunctival examination and/or haemoglobin test), give haematinics (iron

and folic acid, **but** if sulfadoxine-pyrimethamine has been used for malaria treatment, do not give folic acid for 2 weeks).

Management of children visiting or returning from an endemic area for the first time

Hospital admission for management of *P. falciparum* is always advisable.

Treat with an ACT

The WHO recommends the use of **fixed-dose combinations (FDCs)** if available, or pre-packaged drugs if FDCs are not available. **The WHO discourages the use of monotherapies, to reduce the risk of resistance developing.** In particular, the use of artesunate monotherapy, which is commonly available on the private market, is strongly discouraged.

ACTs recommended by the WHO

- Artesunate/amodiaquine (AS/AQ FDC).
- Artesunate + mefloquine (AS+MQ or AS/MQ FDC).
- Artesunate + sulphadoxine/pyrimethamine (AS + SP).
- Artemether + lumefantrine (AM/LM FDC).
- DHA/piperaquine (Duo-Cotecxin, Eurartesim) FDC.
- Artesunate/pyronaridine (Pyramax) FDC.

Non-ACTS

- Malarone (atovaquone/proguanil) FDC: this is very expensive and usually only used where there is artemisinin resistance, or for prophylaxis in western travellers.
- Quinine tablets in IV, IM and rectal forms: for true treatment failures.
- Chloroquine: only for non-*P. falciparum* malaria.
- Primaquine and its derivatives (tafenoquine): for radical treatment of *P. vivax* (and *P. falciparum* in elimination areas).

Paediatric formulations

- AS/AQ infant dose is dispersible, and suitable for children who weigh 4.5–8 kg.
- Paediatric Coartem® (AM/LM) is dispersible and available as cherry-flavoured tablets for children who weigh 5–25 kg.
- Artequin (Mepha) FDC AS/MQ is available as mango-flavoured pellets/granules that can be swallowed directly without water. It is not WHO prequalified.
- AS/MG FDC produced in Brazil for Drugs for Neglected Diseases (DNDi).

Drugs frequently available but not WHO prequalified

- ASMQ Artequin (also in paediatric granules).
- Artemisinin/piperaquine (Artequick).
- Artemisinin and naphthoquine.

Drugs in development

- Artemisone (partner drug not yet decided).
- Synthetic AS called OZ (Sanofi Aventis).
- Semi-synthetic artemisinin (One World Health).

Advice for carers

Discuss preventive efforts with carers (e.g. bed net at night, ideally impregnated with insecticide). Give LLIN if possible.

Tell the mother to return after 2 days if fever persists, and earlier if the child deteriorates.

If the child is repeatedly vomiting and the area is remote and admission to hospital difficult, give rectal artesunate until the vomiting settles. Then give a full 3-day course of ACT.

Management of severe malaria
Severe malaria is a complex multi-system disease that constitutes a medical emergency.

Mortality approaches 100% without treatment, and death often occurs within the first few hours. Prompt initiation of antimalarial treatment in peripheral healthcare facilities and comprehensive management in hospital are necessary to prevent deaths.

Neurological sequelae of cerebral malaria affect about 10% of African children who survive cerebral malaria. These sequelae are severe and permanent in up to 19000 children annually, and include spastic paresis and epilepsy.

Care should be provided within 15 minutes of arrival at a healthcare facility. Triage systems should be in place in health centres and hospitals to pick up severely ill patients, referral should be rapid, and emergency facilities must be instituted in hospitals, with a high standard of medical and nursing care available 24 hours a day.

Any seriously ill or unconscious patient in a malaria-endemic area must be tested for malaria by RDT (remember that parasites may not be present in the peripheral blood of a patient with cerebral malaria). Malaria should be assumed in any child with severe anaemia, convulsions, hyperpyrexia and/or hypoglycaemia either in hospital or in a peripheral healthcare facility.

Even if a diagnostic test is not available, **the patient should be given an antimalarial drug (IV, IM or rectally, depending on the skill of the staff in the facility) before transfer to the hospital.** This can be repeated if transfer is impossible or is delayed for more than 12 hours. A note of what has been given should be sent with the patient as soon as transfer can be arranged.

If any doubt exists, it is safer to treat than not to treat before transfer.

Immediate measures (in hospital)

- Vital signs: temperature, pulse, blood pressure, and respiratory rate and depth.
- State of hydration.
- Estimate or ideally measure body weight. Estimate of weight by age in well-nourished children:
  - For an infant up to 1 year of age, birth weight doubles by 5 months and triples by 1 year.
  - For children over 1 year, use the following formula: weight (kg) = 2 (age in years + 4).

  Be careful in HIV-endemic areas where body weights are often very different from those derived by this formula. Weigh the child if at all possible.
- Level of consciousness (AVPU or Glasgow or Adelaide coma scales) (*see* Section 5.16.A).
- The depth of coma may be assessed rapidly in children using the coma scale for children or by observing the response to standard vocal or painful stimuli (rub your knuckles on the child's sternum; if there is no response, apply firm pressure on the thumbnail bed with a horizontal pencil).
- RDT and malaria smear (thick and thin film) for diagnosis and for continued monitoring of the progress of the

disease. **Do not wait for a malaria smear result before initiating treatment, as it can take up to an hour. If the RDT is positive, commence treatment immediately.**

- Perform lumbar puncture if the patient is unconscious to eliminate meningitis if there are no contraindications. **Contraindications include papilloedema or suspicion of raised intracranial pressure (irregular breathing and pupillary responses, posturing), bleeding problems or respiratory difficulty such that flexing the back would compromise respiration. In such a situation, give IV antibiotics to treat meningitis as well as malaria.**
- Measurement of glucose (finger prick), haemoglobin and haematocrit (packed cell volume, PCV).
- Group and cross-match blood and search for a suitable donor.

Parenteral IV or IM treatment
In Africa and many other regions, sodium artesunate or quinine are the drugs of choice for severe malaria. In South-East Asia and the Amazon Basin, quinine is no longer always effective and should be accompanied by doxycycline in adults or clindamycin in children. Large trials in mainly Asian Adults (SEAQUMAT study) and in African Children (AQUAMAT study) have proved that parenteral artesunate reduces mortality by over 30% and should be used in preference to quinine.

Initially give treatment intravenously, if possible; otherwise use the IM route. Change to oral therapy as soon as possible.

Especially in the malaria-endemic areas of Africa, the following initial antimalarial medicines are recommended. Artesunate has been shown to reduce mortality compared with quinine, but it is important to use whichever drug is available locally.

- artesunate IV or IM
- artemether IM (its absorption may be erratic in children in shock).
- quinine (IV infusion or divided IM injection)

First-line antimalarial drugs
Sodium artesunate IV or IM
Give 2.4 mg/kg IV (by slow injection) or IM on admission (time 0), followed by 2.4 mg/kg IV or IM at 12 hours and again at 24 hours, and then once daily for a minimum of 3 days until the child can take oral treatment with an ACT.

OR second choice
Artemether IM
Give 3.2 mg/kg IM as loading dose, then 1.6 mg/kg IM once daily (every 24 hours) for a minimum of three days until oral treatment can be taken. Use a 1 mL tuberculin syringe to give the small injection volume (note: absorption may be erratic and therefore only use if quinine and artesunate are not available) and if shocked do not use this drug as absorption is too unreliable.

Intravenous IV quinine (quinine dihydrochloride)
This is the second choice, to be used if sodium artesunate is not available. Give 20 mg/kg quinine dihydrochloride (maximum 1.4 grams) in 5% glucose at a concentration of 1 mg of quinine to 1 mL of 5% glucose over 2–4 hours (never more rapidly than over 2 hours). If possible use an in-line infusion chamber (100–150 mL) to ensure that the loading dose does not go in too quickly. Alternatively, ensure that the IV giving bag contains only the amount needed for each dose. There is a major risk of cardiac side effects if it is infused too quickly.

Subsequently give 10 mg/kg in 10 mL/kg fluid (5% glucose) IV every 12 hours for 24 hours, or longer if the child remains unconscious. These latter doses **must** be given over at least 2 hours.

Never give quinine as an IV bolus. The infusion rate must not exceed a total of 5 mg quinine salt/kg/hour.

If safe control over the rate of infusion of IV quinine is not possible (e.g. there are insufficient or only untrained nursing staff available), give a loading dose intramuscularly (with initial doses of 10 mg/kg quinine salt IM at 0 and 4 hours and then 12-hourly).

For IM injections, dilute the quinine solution to allow better absorption and less pain.

As soon as the child is able to take medication orally, switch to quinine tablets 10 mg/kg every 8 hours for a total of 7 days, or the locally available first-line ACT treatment for malaria.

Side effects:
- Common: cinchonism (tinnitus, hearing loss, nausea and vomiting, uneasiness, restlessness, dizziness, blurring of vision).
- Uncommon: hypoglycaemia, although this is a common complication of severe malaria.
- Serious cardiovascular problems (QT prolongation on the ECG) and neurological toxicity are rare.
- If overdosed by mistake with quinine tablets, give activated charcoal orally or by nasogastric tube as a suspension in water (1 gram/kg).

Chloroquine IV
This drug should never be used to treat severe falciparum malaria but only cases of non-resistant vivax or ovale malaria. Give 5 mg base/kg every 6 hours for a total of 25 mg base/kg (five doses) as an infusion in 5% glucose (give over 2 to 4 hours).

Antimalarial treatment after IV or IM regimes have ended
Following parenteral administration, usually for a minimum of 24 hours or until the child can take oral drugs, the treatment of severe malaria must be completed by giving a full course of one of the artemisinin-based combination therapies (ACT) described below. In some parts of the world, oral quinine combined with clindamycin to complete 7 days of treatment is used

The following ACTs are recommended:
- artemether plus lumefantrine
- artesunate plus amodiaquine
- artesunate plus sulfadoxine-pyrimethamine
- dihydroartemisinin plus piperaquine
- artemether plus clindamycin
- artesunate plus mefloquine.

The choice of ACT in a particular country or region will be based on the level of resistance of the partner medicine in the combination.

In areas of multi-drug resistance (e.g. East Asia), artesunate plus mefloquine, or artemether plus lumefantrine, or dihydroartemisinin plus piperaquine are recommended. In areas without multi-drug resistance (mainly Africa), any of the ACTs, including those containing amodiaquine, may still be effective. Every country has a national malaria policy in which the first-line therapy is described and should be used.

If possible avoid using mefloquine if the patient has presented with an impaired conscious level.

Treatment for HIV-infected patients with P. falciparum *malaria*

- Patients with HIV infection who develop malaria should receive prompt effective antimalarial treatment regimens as recommended above.
- Treatment with ACT involving sulfadoxine-pyrimethamine should not be given to HIV-infected patients who are receiving co-trimoxazole (trimethoprim plus sulfamethoxazole) prophylaxis.
- Treatment of HIV-infected patients who are on zidovudine or efavirenz should, if possible, avoid amodiaquine-containing ACT regimens.

Treatment of P. falciparum *malaria in malnourished patients*

Although there are many reasons why antimalarial pharmacokinetics may differ between malnourished patients and those who are well nourished, there is insufficient evidence to change current mg/kg body weight dosing recommendations.

Always check local guidelines on drug sensitivities.

With all antimalarial drugs, change to an oral therapy when the child can tolerate it.

Additional treatment where needed

- Insert a nasogastric tube to minimise the risk of aspiration pneumonia if the patient's level of consciousness is low. This can also be used to give food to prevent hypoglycaemia if the child is unconscious for a long period and is unable to eat. Alternatively, sucrose (sugar) can be placed under the tongue.
- Insert an IV cannula and restore the circulating volume.
  - Fluids should be given with caution and the need for them assessed on an individual basis after ascertaining the nutritional status and degree of dehydration present.
  - In general, children with metabolic acidosis who have not previously received parenteral fluids are dehydrated and should be managed accordingly.
- Give oxygen if SpO$_2$ is < 94% (to keep SpO$_2$ in the range 94–100%) or if there is respiratory distress and no pulse oximeter available.
- Treat severe anaemia with a safe blood transfusion if the child is showing signs of decompensation.
- Give anticonvulsants (diazepam is preferred) if the patient is convulsing (see below) to prevent long-term neurological damage (*see* Section 5.16.E). Convulsions associated with cerebral malaria should be distinguished from febrile convulsions common in children under 4 years of age. The child usually recovers rapidly, within a few minutes, from a febrile convulsion. Convulsions in malaria are common before or after the onset of coma. They are significantly associated with morbidity and sequelae. They may present in a very subtle way. Important signs include intermittent nystagmus, salivation, minor twitching of a single digit or a corner of the mouth, and an irregular breathing pattern.

Prophylactic anticonvulsants have been recommended in the past, but recent evidence suggests that **phenobarbital may be harmful in this situation**.

- Paracetamol, 15 mg/kg of body weight 4-hourly, may also be given orally or rectally as an antipyretic.
- Use tepid sponging and fanning to try to keep the rectal temperature below 39°C. Relatives are usually happy to do this when instructed.
- High-dose IV or IM antibiotics should be given routinely to an unconscious or shocked patient.
- Avoid using harmful ancillary drugs.

The patient will need intensive nursing care at least until they regain consciousness. They may urgently need glucose or a blood transfusion if hypoglycaemia or haemolysis is severe.

Management of associated causes of mortality in severe malaria

Some children with *P. falciparum* malaria go on to develop altered consciousness, severe anaemia, acidosis, or any combination of these. Where transmission of *P. falciparum* is endemic, malaria is the commonest cause of coma in children, especially in those aged 1–5 years.

Cerebral malaria (coma, confusion and convulsions)

Coma develops rapidly, often within 1 or 2 days of onset of fever, and sometimes within hours. Convulsions are usual and may be repeated. Clinical features suggest a metabolic encephalopathy, with raised intracranial pressure. Opisthotonos, decorticate or decerebrate posturing, hypotonia and conjugate eye movements are common. Oculovestibular reflexes and pupillary responses are usually intact. Papilloedema is found in a small minority of cases. A unique retinopathy with patchy retinal whitening and pallor of vessels is found. In fatal cases, brain swelling is commonly present at autopsy, but cerebral herniation is not usually found even in patients who have undergone lumbar puncture.

Hypoglycaemia, acidosis, hyperpyrexia and convulsions (sometimes undetectable without EEG) are common accompaniments of cerebral malaria, and require appropriate management (see below).

No physical signs are diagnostic of coma due to malaria, and incidental parasitaemia is common in endemic areas, so other causes of coma, especially hypoglycaemia and meningitis, must always be carefully sought, and if necessary treated on the basis of presumptive diagnosis.

Even with optimal treatment, the case fatality rate is 15–30%, and about 10% of survivors have residual neurological sequelae (hemiparesis, spasticity, cerebellar ataxia) that may partially or completely resolve over time.

Investigations

- Blood glucose levels (e.g. by blood glucose stick test).
- Lumbar puncture if meningitis is suspected; contraindications include papilloedema or suspicion of raised intracranial pressure (irregular breathing and abnormal pupillary responses, posturing), or respiratory difficulty such that flexing the back would compromise respiration. **In such a situation, give IV antibiotics to treat meningitis as well as malaria.**

Management
Coma

Ensure that the airway is open at all times and that the patient is breathing adequately. Give oxygen by face mask with a reservoir or nasal cannulae (to keep SpO_2 in the range 94–98% if a pulse oximeter is available). If the child stops breathing, give assisted ventilation with a bag-mask of suitable size (500 mL or 1600 mL).

Ensure that a bag-mask is available at all times.

Nurse the patient in the recovery position to avoid aspiration of secretions or vomit.

Exclude other treatable causes of coma (e.g. hypoglycaemia, bacterial meningitis).

- Treat convulsions (see Section 5.16.A on coma and Section 5.16.E on convulsions).
- Treat hypoglycaemia.

Convulsions

Convulsions are common before and after the onset of coma.

- Ensure that the airway is open, and give oxygen by face mask with a reservoir or nasal cannulae.
- If the child stops breathing, give assisted ventilation with a bag-mask of suitable size (500 mL or 1600 mL).
- Examine all children with convulsions for hyperpyrexia and hypoglycaemia. Treat hypoglycaemia with IV or oral glucose if identified on blood testing, but also treat as for hypoglycaemia if blood glucose levels cannot be measured and the child is drowsy, unconscious or fitting (see below).
- Give anticonvulsant treatment with rectal diazepam or paraldehyde or IM paraldehyde.
- If the patient has a fever of ≥ 39°C (≥ 102.2°F), give paracetamol rectally (if available).
- Treat seizures lasting for more than 5 minutes with drugs. **Ensure that a bag-mask is available at all times in case of apnoea following the use of diazepam. Apnoea is usually short-lived and improves quickly with ventilation via bag and mask.**

Note that seizure activity needs to be looked for carefully, as it may appear as just a twitching of the thumb or mouth.

- Give IV diazepam:
  - **Children**: 300 microgram/kg of body weight as an IV infusion over 2 minutes or 400–500 microgram/kg of body weight intra-rectally. This dose can be repeated after 10–15 minutes if still fitting.
  - **Pregnant girls**: 10 mg rectally or by slow IV injection. This dose can be repeated after 10–15 minutes if still fitting.
  - Do not exceed 10 mg per dose.
- Alternatively, paraldehyde 0.1 mL/kg of body weight may be given by deep IM injection or 0.8 mL/kg of body weight (maximum 20 mL) intra-rectally using a sterile glass syringe (a disposable plastic syringe may be used provided that the injection is given immediately after the paraldehyde is drawn up, and the syringe is never reused).

Hypoglycaemia

Hypoglycaemia is common and is due to poor intake, increased metabolic needs of the patient and parasites and impaired hepatic gluconeogenesis. It is easily overlooked because clinical signs may mimic those of cerebral malaria.

Check for hypoglycaemia in **all** patients who are unconscious, in shock or deteriorating. Also regularly (every hour in the first instance) check pregnant girls, children under 5 years, and the malnourished, and all patients receiving quinine.

Hypoglycaemia is defined as blood glucose levels < 2.5 mmol/litre (< 45 mg/dl).

Prevent hypoglycaemia with a maintenance quantity of 5% glucose in 0.9% Ringer-lactate or Hartmann's solution (50 mL of 50% glucose in a 500-mL bag). If the child develops hypoglycaemia despite this, give maintenance as 10% glucose in 0.9% Ringer-lactate or Hartmann's solution (100 mL of 50% glucose in a 500-mL bag). Do not exceed maintenance fluid requirements for the child's weight (see Section 9 Appendix). If the child develops signs of fluid overload, stop the infusion; repeat the 10% glucose boluses (5 mL/kg) if there is hypoglycaemia identified by making regular checks of blood glucose levels.

If IV access is not possible and the child is hypoglycaemic, place an intra-osseous needle (see Section 8.4.B).

Treat hypoglycaemia or suspected hypoglycaemia with an IV glucose infusion or bolus:

- **Children:** 1 mL/kg of 50% dextrose, diluted with four times the volume of infusion fluid (usually Ringer-lactate or Hartmann's solution) infused over 5 minutes **or** 5 mL/kg of 10% glucose as a bolus.
- **Pregnant girls:** 50 mL of 50% dextrose diluted with an equal volume of infusion fluid (usually Ringer-lactate or Hartmann's solution) over 15 minutes (irritating to veins).

Re-test 15 minutes after completion of the infusion, and repeat the infusion if blood glucose remains low. Repeat until blood glucose recovers, then infuse with 5–10% glucose in Ringer-lactate or Hartmann's solution (according to hypoglycaemia risk) to prevent recurrence. Ensure regular feeding when oral intake can be sustained. Fluids used to treat hypoglycaemia must be included in daily fluid requirements.

If blood glucose levels cannot be measured and hypoglycaemia is a possibility, always give IV glucose as described above.

If the child is still unable to swallow after 48 hours, start nasogastric feeds. If a gag reflex is present and the child is able to swallow, feed them as soon as this is possible. For young children breastfeed every 3 hours if possible, or give milk feeds of 15 mL/kg 3-hourly if the child can swallow. If they are not able to feed without risk of aspiration, give milk, especially breast milk, by nasogastric tube or sugar sublingually (see Section 5.8.B). Continue to monitor the blood glucose levels, and treat accordingly (as described above) if these are found to be < 2.5 mmol/litre or < 45 mg/dL.

Hypoglycaemia is a major cause of death in severe malaria patients, especially in young children and pregnant girls. Remember that quinine will potentiate hypoglycaemia. Young children should receive regular feeding, including by nasogastric tube, if they are unable to take oral foods.

Severe anaemia

This is indicated by severe palmar pallor, often with a fast pulse rate, difficult breathing, confusion or restlessness. Signs of heart failure such as gallop rhythm, enlarged liver and, rarely, pulmonary oedema (fast breathing, fine basal crackles on auscultation) may be present (see above).

Severe haemolytic anaemia is defined as < 5 grams of haemoglobin/dL or haematocrit < 15%.

Severe anaemia may be the presenting feature in malaria. Patients with severe anaemia, especially pregnant girls, should be tested for malaria.

Give a safe blood transfusion as soon as possible to:

- all children or pregnant girls with a haematocrit of ≤ 12% or Hb of ≤ 4 g/dL
- less severely anaemic children (haematocrit > 12–15%; Hb 4–5 g/dL) with any of the following:
  - clinically detectable dehydration (as well as rehydrating orally if possible)
  - shock
  - impaired consciousness
  - deep and laboured breathing
  - heart failure
  - very high levels of parasitaemia (> 10% of red blood cells parasitised).

Give packed cells (10–20 mL/kg body weight for children and 500 mL for pregnant girls), if available, over three to four hours in preference to whole blood. Allow red blood cells to settle at the bottom of the bag, and stop the infusion when the cells have been used.

If not available, give fresh whole blood (20 mL/kg body weight) over 3–4 hours.

A diuretic is not usually indicated (unless pulmonary oedema or fluid overload is developing), because many of these children have a low blood volume (hypovolaemia).

Check the respiratory rate and pulse rate every 15 minutes. If one of them rises, transfuse more slowly. If there is any evidence of fluid overload due to the blood transfusion, give IV furosemide (1–2 mg/kg body weight) up to a maximum total of 20 mg for children, and give 40 mg IV for pregnant girls.

After the transfusion, if the haemoglobin level remains low, repeat the transfusion.

In severely malnourished children, fluid overload is a common and serious complication. Give whole blood (10 mL/kg body weight rather than 20 mL/kg) once, and only repeat the transfusion if there are no signs of overload.

Perform microscopy following transfusion, and repeat or extend antimalarial treatment if parasitaemia is increasing.

Respiratory distress due to acidosis

This presents with deep laboured breathing while the chest is clear on auscultation, sometimes accompanied by lower chest wall indrawing. It is caused by systemic metabolic acidosis (frequently lactic acidosis) and may develop in a fully conscious child, but more often in children with cerebral malaria or severe anaemia. Always exclude other causes, such as pneumonia or pulmonary oedema.

Metabolic acidosis in severe malaria has been attributed to the combined effects of several factors that reduce oxygen delivery to tissues:

- Increased production of lactic acid by parasites (through direct stimulation by cytokines).
- Decreased clearance by the liver.
- Marked reductions in the deformability of uninfected red blood cells may compromise blood flow through tissues.
- Dehydration and hypovolaemia can exacerbate microvascular obstruction by reducing perfusion pressure.

- Destruction of red blood cells and anaemia further compromise oxygen delivery.
- Mean venous blood lactate concentrations have been found to be almost twice as high in fatal cases as in survivors, and to correlate with levels of tumour necrosis factor and interleukin 1-alpha. The lactate concentrations fell rapidly in survivors but fell only slightly, or rose, in fatal cases. Sustained hyperlactataemia has been found to be the best overall prognostic indicator of outcome.

Treatment

Give oxygen to all patients (even if they are not hypoxaemic), and if a pulse oximeter is available keep SpO$_2$ in the range 94–100%.

Correct reversible causes of acidosis, especially dehydration and severe anaemia.

- If Hb is ≥ 5 g/dL, give 10 mL/kg of 0.9% Ringer-lactate or Hartmann's solution IV as a bolus and then reassess.
- If haemoglobin level is < 5 grams/dL, give whole blood (10 mL/kg) over 30 minutes, and a further 10 mL/kg over 1–2 hours without diuretics. Check the respiratory rate and pulse rate every 15 minutes. If either of these shows any rise, transfuse more slowly to avoid precipitating pulmonary oedema (*see* Section 1.7).
- Monitor ECG for cardiac arrhythmias if possible.
- The use of sodium bicarbonate is controversial.

Respiratory distress due to pulmonary oedema

This is different to that due to acidosis, and there is usually more chest recession, hypoxaemia (cyanosis, SpO$_2$ < 94%), basal lung crepitations, enlarging liver, gallop rhythm, and raised jugular venous pressure. It may be due to fluid overload, often in the presence of severe anaemia. The most effective treatment is to tilt the bed of the patient head up so that the venous blood flow to the heart is reduced. If the bed cannot be tilted, sit the patient up, give furosemide 1 mg/kg for children and 40 mg IV for pregnant girls, and proceed with a careful transfusion of packed blood cells. Repeat furosemide as needed.

Respiratory distress due to pulmonary aspiration or pneumonia

Prevent aspiration pneumonia if possible, because it can be fatal. Place the comatose patient in the recovery position and ensure that the airway is open. If it is safe to intubate and maintain this, do so in order to protect the airway if the patient is unconscious (U on the APVU scale, or Glasgow Coma Scale score of < 9).

- Give oxygen if the SaO$_2$ is < 94% or, if pulse oximetry is not available, if there is cyanosis, severe lower chest wall indrawing or a respiratory rate of ≥ 70 breaths/minute. Keep SpO$_2$ 94–100%. Give IM or IV antibiotics as described for pneumonia (*see* Section 5.3.A), and add in metronidazole 7.5 mg/kg 8 hourly (maximum individual dose 500 mg) until the patient can take these orally, for a total of 7 days.

Shock

Most children with malaria have warm peripheries. Shock is unusual in malaria (algid malaria). Some patients may have a cold clammy skin. Some of them may be in shock (increased heart rate, cold extremities, weak pulse, capillary refill time longer than 3 seconds, low blood pressure (late sign)). These features are not usually due to malaria alone.

If shock is present, consider septicaemia, do a blood culture and start a broad-spectrum antibiotic IV (penicillin and gentamicin **or** cefotaxime or ceftriaxone) in addition to antimalarial drugs.

Management (*see* Section 5.5) includes fluid replacement as follows:

- **Children:** Give Ringer-lactate or Hartmann's solution IV, 10 mL/kg as a rapid bolus. Reassess, and if the patient is no better, or improving but still in shock, consider further 10 mL/kg boluses.
- **Pregnant girls:** Give Ringer-lactate or Hartmann's solution IV, 500 mL as a rapid bolus, then reassess.

If there is no improvement in capillary refill or tachycardia, repeat the infusion once or twice more, as required.

Give broad-spectrum antibiotics to treat septicaemia and any associated infections.

Acute renal failure

Acute renal failure (ARF) is defined as an abrupt decline in the renal regulation of water, electrolytes and acid–base balance, and continues to be an important factor contributing to the morbidity and mortality of malaria patients (*see* Section 5.6.C). Oliguria or anuria is often associated with jaundice, anaemia and bleeding disorders.

Note that ARF is uncommon in children, and dehydration is a more common cause of poor urine output.

- The basic principles of management are avoidance of life-threatening complications, maintenance of fluid and electrolyte balance, and nutritional support.
- Urinary catheterisation can be helpful if it can be safely undertaken, so that urine output can be accurately measured. Alternatively, weigh nappies in young children.
- Acute renal failure is suspected when the **hourly** urine output is less than 1 mL/kg of body weight/hour). Blood levels of urea and creatinine are usually raised.
- Make sure that the patient is adequately hydrated, but avoid overload, which will precipitate pulmonary oedema if the kidneys cannot excrete excess water.
- If urine output continues to be low despite adequate hydration, peripheral perfusion and normal blood pressure, give furosemide 1 mg/kg and repeat as required.
- If renal failure is established, restrict fluid to insensible loss (30 mL/kg/day) plus urine output and other fluid losses (e.g. vomit, diarrhoea).
- Consider peritoneal dialysis (if available) or ideally haemodialysis.

Abnormal bleeding

- Transfuse with fresh blood.
- Give vitamin K, 250–300 microgram/kg (maximum 10 mg) IV.
- Avoid IM injections and non-steroidal anti-inflammatory drugs (NSAIDs).

Coexisting infections

Treat any associated pneumonia, dysentery, etc.

Summary of supportive care for the treatment of severe malaria in hospital

- If the patient is unconscious, maintain a clear airway. Nurse them in the recovery position to avoid aspiration pneumonia, and turn them 2-hourly.
- Do not allow the child to lie in a wet bed, and provide special care for pressure points. Turn the patient every 2 hours.
- Give oxygen for patients who are in respiratory distress or in shock.
- In children with no dehydration, ensure that they receive their daily fluid requirements, but take care not to exceed the recommended limits (*see* Section 9 Appendix). Be particularly careful when fluids are given IV.
- Treat convulsions and hypoglycaemia.
- If you cannot exclude meningitis, give an appropriate antibiotic intravenously.
- If there is deep or laboured breathing suggestive of acidosis, give one bolus of 10 mL/kg IV fluid (normal Ringer-lactate or Hartmann's) to correct hypovolaemia and reassess. A second bolus may be required.
- During rehydration, examine frequently for fluid overload (increased liver size is probably the best sign, as well as gallop rhythm, fine crackles at the lung bases, raised jugular venous pressure and eyelid oedema in infants).
- In infants, if possible always use an in-line infusion chamber for IV rehydration. If this is not available and supervision is poor, empty the IV fluid bag until only 200–300 mL is remaining then if it all goes in quickly it will be less harmful than if the whole bag is being infused.
- If necessary, use a nasogastric tube to rehydrate the patient.
- Avoid giving drugs like corticosteroids and other anti-inflammatory drugs, urea, invert glucose, low-molecular dextran, heparin, adrenaline (epinephrine), prostacyclin and cyclosporine, as they do not treat malaria and can be harmful.
- Give safe blood transfusion where necessary, with careful monitoring to prevent fluid overload. Packed cells should be used in children and pregnant girls where possible. If overload is suspected, give a single dose of furosemide.
- If the patient is unconscious and you cannot exclude meningitis or the child is in shock, administer a broad-spectrum antibiotic to manage septicaemia, pneumonia or meningitis, which are often associated with cerebral malaria.

Summary of monitoring

- Check the patient regularly, at least every 3 hours. A doctor (if available) should see the patient at least twice a day.
- The rate of IV infusion should be checked hourly.
- Patients with cold extremities, hypoglycaemia on admission, respiratory distress and/or deep coma are at highest risk of death. It is particularly important that these children are kept under very close observation.
- Monitor and report immediately any change in the level of consciousness, convulsions, or changes in the patient's behaviour.
- Monitor the temperature, pulse rate and respiratory rate (and if possible the blood pressure) every 6 hours for at least the first 48 hours.
- Fluid balance charts: unconscious patients may be catheterised in order to measure urine output and facilitate correct fluid balance, and to detect possible renal failure.
- Frequent measurement of blood glucose levels (every hour, especially when receiving quinine and/or where the level of consciousness does not improve).
- If the patient is conscious, regularly (4-hourly) determine

blood glucose levels to exclude hypoglycaemia if the patient is not eating well. This is especially important in young children and pregnant women, and in those patients who are receiving quinine therapy.

- Check haemoglobin levels and haematocrit daily.
- Check plasma urea and electrolytes where possible, and take blood gas and lactate measurements (if available).
- Check the rate of IV infusion regularly. If available, use a giving chamber with a volume of 100–150 mL. Be very careful about over-infusion of fluids from a 500-mL or 1-litre bottle or bag, especially if the child is not supervised all the time. Partially empty the IV bottle or bag. If the risk of over-infusion cannot be ruled out, rehydration using a nasogastric tube may be safer.
- Keep a careful record of fluid intake (including IV) and urine output (should be at least 1 mL/kg/hour).
- Undertake a daily slide to determine the level of parasitaemia and to monitor treatment efficacy.
- Regular haemoglobin measurement. The frequency will depend on the rate of red blood cell breakdown. This may be very rapid in cases of high parasite density.

On discharge from hospital

When the child or pregnant girl is due to leave hospital, talk with the relatives and carers to ensure that:

- the patient sleeps under a net (LLIN); if not, provide one
- the patient completes any outstanding treatment
- the carers and relatives recognise symptoms and where to get treatment for simple malaria in future
- the family knows to give extra meals to make up for the poor nutrition during the illness
- the family know when to bring the patient for further check-ups and arrange a follow-up appointment.

Examine for any neurological sequelae and advise the family on how to manage these and the possible prognosis. Arrange a physiotherapy session if necessary. Good follow-up is important.

Management of non-severe anaemia

If anaemia associated with malaria is not severe (defined as a haemoglobin level of 6–9.3 grams/dL), treat as follows. Give iron once daily in combination with folic acid (one tablet contains ferrous sulphate 200 mg, equivalent to 60 mg of elemental iron) plus 250 micrograms/kg/day of folic acid. Give 3–6 mg/kg (maximum 200 mg) of elemental iron in 2–3 divided doses and for folic acid give 250 microgram/kg once daily (usually one 5 mg tablet). Stress the importance of keeping the tablets out of reach of young children. Iron poisoning is very dangerous.

If the child is taking sulfadoxine-pyrimethamine for malaria, or co-trimoxazole for HIV prophylaxis, do not give folic acid until 2 weeks later (it interferes with antimalarial action).

TABLE 6.3.A.D.1 Dose of ferrous fumarate 140 mg/5 mL in children

Weight	Dose
3–6 kg	1 mL
6–10 kg	1.25 mL
10–15 kg	2.0 mL
15–20 kg	2.5 mL
20–30 kg	4 mL

An alternative for a young child is iron syrup (ferrous fumarate) 140 mg in 5 mL and equivalent to 45 mg of iron. Give once daily (see Table 6.3.A.d.1).

Plus separate folic acid 250 micrograms/kg/day.

Treat for 3 months where possible (1 month to correct anaemia and 1–3 months to build iron stores).

Patients with HIV infection

Patients with HIV infection who develop malaria should receive prompt effective antimalarial treatment regimens as recommended above.

However, treatment with an ACT involving sulfadoxine-pyrimethamine should not be given to HIV-infected patients receiving co-trimoxazole (trimethoprim plus sulfamethoxazole) prophylaxis.

Treatment in HIV-infected patients on zidovudine (AZT) or efavirenz should, if possible, avoid amodiaquine-containing ACT regimens. Amodiaquine can cause anaemia in G6PD deficiency, and AZT may also cause anaemia.

Infection with *P. vivax*, *P. ovale* and *P. malariae*

Of the four species of *Plasmodium* that affect humans, only *P. vivax* and *P. ovale* form hypnozoites, parasite stages in the liver, which can result in multiple relapses of infection weeks to months after the primary infection. Thus a single infection causes repeated bouts of illness. Ideally, the objective of treating malaria caused by *P. vivax* and *P. ovale* is to cure (radical cure) both the blood stage and the liver stage infections, and thereby prevent recrudescence and relapse, respectively. **However, primaquine which is used to produce a radical cure is contraindicated in children under 4 years of age.**

Diagnosis

- Microscopy using a Giemsa-stained quality-assured thin film.
- pLDH tests can detect all species of malaria. Combination tests are now available that combine HRP2 and pLDH to detect both *P. falciparum* and non-*P. falciparum* malaria.

Treatment

Both *P. ovale* and *P. malariae* are regarded as very sensitive to chloroquine, although there is a single recent report of chloroquine resistance in *P. malariae*.

P. vivax is generally still sensitive to chloroquine, although resistance is prevalent and increasing in some areas (notably Indonesia, Peru and Oceania). Resistance to pyrimethamine has increased rapidly in some areas, and sulfadoxine/pyrimethamine is consequently ineffective. There are insufficient data on current susceptibility to proguanil and chlorproguanil, although resistance to proguanil was selected rapidly when it was first used in *P. vivax*-endemic areas.

In general, *P. vivax* is sensitive to all of the other antimalarial drugs, and slightly less sensitive to mefloquine (although mefloquine is still effective). In contrast to *P. falciparum*, asexual stages of *P. vivax* are susceptible to primaquine. Thus chloroquine plus primaquine can be considered as a combination treatment. The only drugs with significant activity against the hypnozoites are the 8-aminoquinolines (bulaquine, primaquine and tafenoquine).

Treatment of uncomplicated P. vivax

For chloroquine-sensitive *P. vivax* malaria (i.e. in most places where *P. vivax* is prevalent), oral chloroquine at a total dose of 25 mg base/kg body weight for a course of treatment is effective and well tolerated. Lower total doses are not recommended, as these might encourage the emergence of resistance. Chloroquine is given in an initial dose of 10 mg base/kg body weight followed by either 5 mg/kg body weight at 6 hours, 24 hours and 48 hours or, more commonly, by 10 mg/kg body weight on the second day and 5 mg/kg body weight on the third day.

Recent studies have also demonstrated the efficacy of the recommended ACTs in the treatment of *P. vivax* malaria. The exception to this is artesunate plus sulfadoxine-pyrimethamine.

For treatment of chloroquine-resistant *P. vivax* malaria, amodiaquine, mefloquine and quinine are effective. ACTs based on either amodiaquine, mefloquine or piperaquine, rather than monotherapy, are the recommended treatment of choice.

For the complete (radical) removal of *P. vivax* infection, primaquine is required, but is contraindicated in children under 4 years of age and in pregnant women and girls.

Treatment of uncomplicated malaria caused by P. ovale and P. malariae

Treat with chloroquine as described for *P. vivax* above.

Prevention of malaria

Most important is the prevention of mosquito bites. All children, all pregnant girls and all patients who have had a recent bout of malaria should be provided with an insecticide-impregnated bed net.

Drugs for prophylaxis depend on the region and sensitivity of the malarial parasite.

This is important for:

- children with sickle-cell disease: chloroquine 5 mg/kg weekly
- children or adults who return to an endemic area after an absence of over 1 year, even if they are originally from that region
- non-immune individuals: people from non-endemic areas.

Intermittent preventive treatment for malaria in infants (ITPi) and children (ITPc, now called seasonal malaria chemoprevention, SMC)
IPTi

- Malaria cases can be reduced by 30% in infants during the first 12 months of life using this safe, affordable and simple tool. It can be implemented via existing vaccination programmes run by the WHO.
- For infants, a treatment dose of sulfadoxine/pyrimethamine (SP) should be given three times at the time of each immunisation, beginning at 2 months (DTP2), 3 months (DTP3) and 9 months (measles and yellow fever). Each tablet of SP contains 500 mg sulfadoxine and 25 mg pyrimethamine, and for infants the following sizes for each dose are: a quarter tablet for children weighing less than 5 kg, and a half tablet for children weighing 5–10 kg.

SMC

- For children living in areas where transmission is highly seasonal (e.g. in Mali, Senegal, Niger and northern Nigeria), aged 1–6 years, a single dose of one tablet of SP plus three doses of one tablet/day for 3 days of amodiaquine (200 mg) is given once a month during the malaria transmission season.
- Tablets are crushed and suspended in water and given by spoon. Side effects are very rare. Minor gastrointestinal side effects may occur.
- For areas in which there is resistance to SP, piperaquine may be used instead of SP.

ITPi and SMC are recommended in addition to treated bed nets in areas of moderate to high levels of malaria transmission and low to moderate levels of parasite resistance to SP.

Preventive treatment for malaria in pregnant girls and women (see Section 2.8.D)
Follow-up care for anaemia

- If moderate or severe anaemia has been documented, give home treatment with a daily dose of iron/folate tablet or iron syrup for 3 months where possible (it takes 2–4 weeks to correct the anaemia and 1–3 months to build up iron stores).
- **However, if the child is taking sulfadoxine-pyrimethamine for malaria, do not give iron tablets that contain folate until a follow-up visit in 2 weeks. The folate may interfere with the action of this antimalarial drug.**
- If the child is over 1 year and has not had mebendazole/albendazole in the previous 6 months, give one dose of mebendazole (500 mg) for possible hookworm or whipworm infestation (*see* Section 6.3.C.a). Advise the mother about good feeding practices.
- Omit iron in any child with severe malnutrition in the acute phase.
- A study in Malawi showed that many children who were so anaemic as to require a blood transfusion died within 6 months of discharge from hospital. Prophylactic antimalarial drugs (coArtem) at 1 month and 2 months post discharge prevented many readmissions and deaths.

Follow-up care after malaria has been treated

- Ask the mother to return if the fever returns or persists after 2 days of treatment, or if the child's condition gets worse in any way.
- If this happens, reassess the child to exclude the possibility of other causes of fever.
- Check whether the child actually took the full course of treatment, and repeat a blood smear. If the treatment was not taken, repeat it. If it was taken but the blood smear is still positive (remember that an RDT can remain positive for up to 6 weeks after the initial infection), and the child is not seriously ill, re-treat with first-line drugs.
- If the child returns within 2 weeks, give a full course of oral quinine.
- If the child is severely ill, refer them to a hospital for inpatient treatment.

6.3.B Other protozoal infections

Introduction

The organisms collectively termed **protozoa** are not closely related to each other. They do have some similarities when viewed under a microscope, as they are largely unicellular and motile, although with exceptions.

Toxoplasmosis

Toxoplasmosis is caused by infection with a common parasite called *Toxoplasma gondii*. *T. gondii* can be found in:

- undercooked or raw meat
- cured meat
- unpasteurised goats' milk
- cat faeces.

It cannot be passed from person to person apart from mother to unborn child.

During acute toxoplasmosis, symptoms are often influenza-like (swollen lymph nodes, or muscle aches and pains that last for a month or more).

Swollen lymph nodes are commonly found in the neck or under the chin, followed by the axillae and the inguinal region. Swelling may occur at different times after the initial infection, persist, and/or recur for various times independently of antiparasitic treatment. It is usually found at single sites in adults, but in children multiple sites may be more common. Enlarged lymph nodes will resolve within 1–2 months in 60% of patients. However, 25% of patients take 2–4 months to return to normal, and a few take longer than this.

Young children and immunocompromised patients, such as those with HIV/AIDS, may develop severe toxoplasmosis. This can cause encephalitis or necrotising retinochoroiditis.

Infants can develop a congenital infection acquired *in utero*. The key features are fever, rash, petechiae, lymphadenopathy, hepatosplenomegaly, jaundice, hydrocephalus or microcephaly, microphthalmia, epilepsy and chorioretinitis.

Management

Congenital toxoplasmosis in newborns and immunocompromised children with HIV infection can be treated for a year with pyrimethamine (with additional folinic acid) plus sulfadiazine. This treatment requires expert management.

Amoebiasis

Infection by *Entamoeba histolytica* is acquired from human hosts via contaminated food, water or direct contact. Most infected children are asymptomatic, but some have systemic illness. This can last for many weeks. The disease presents with acute diarrhoea with colicky abdominal pains. A small proportion have bloody diarrhoea with a fever, and rarely intestinal perforation with peritonitis or haemorrhage may occur.

The diagnosis can be confirmed by observing the amoebae in a fresh stool or following a biopsy of the ulcers at sigmoidoscopy.

Amoebic liver abscesses occur in less than 1% of infected individuals. They present with fever, abdominal pain, and a tender liver sometimes with a palpable mass. The liver abscess often occurs without gastrointestinal symptoms and with negative stools. The diagnosis can be confirmed by ultrasound scan or **CT scan (if available)**.

Treatment is required for those with systemic illnesses, those with diarrhoea due to invasive ulceration and those with liver abscesses.

- Metronidazole is the drug of choice and is well absorbed orally: 7.5 mg/kg three times daily for 5–10 days (maximum daily dose 400 mg).
- If the abscess is very large and particularly if there is concern that it may rupture, it may require aspiration under careful ultrasound support.
- After the acute treatment of a liver abscess, diloxanide should be used immediately following the course of metronidazole in order to remove all amoebae from the bowel.
- The dose of diloxanide is:
  - 1 month to 12 years of age: 6.6 mg/kg three times daily for 10 days
  - > 12 years of age: 500 mg three times daily for 10 days.

Cryptosporidiosis

Cryptosporidium parvum can be acquired from infected human or animal hosts and from contaminated water and food.

It causes an acute gastroenteritis, which is self-limiting in most children. The enteritis is associated with watery diarrhoea, nausea and colicky abdominal pains. It lasts for approximately 2 weeks. In otherwise healthy children it does not usually require treatment with antimicrobial drugs unless it persists or is associated with systemic illness, in which case azithromycin may be effective.

In children with AIDS it can produce a protracted and severe illness involving major weight loss, in which case it can be treated with azithromycin. Avoid azithromycin in patients with liver disease.

The dose of azithromycin is:

- 6 months to 12 years of age: 10 mg/kg once daily for 3 days or longer in AIDS.

Giardiasis

Infection by *Giardia lamblia* can be acquired from infected human or animal hosts and from contaminated water and food. The organisms live in the duodenum.

The infection may be asymptomatic or it can produce an acute gastroenteritis with watery stools, colicky abdominal pains and nausea. It can also produce a chronic diarrhoeal illness with malabsorption and colicky abdominal pain lasting for many months.

Diagnosis is best made from examining a fresh stool. Sometimes more than one examination will be necessary.

- Metronidazole (at the doses described for amoebiasis above) is appropriate in the chronic form of the infection. The acute form usually resolves without treatment.

6.3.C Helminth infections

6.3.C.a Worms

BOX 6.3.C.A.1 Minimum standards
- Faecal microscopy and egg count.
- Anoscopy.
- Eosinophil count and chest X-ray if available.
- Mebendazole, albendazole and ivermectin.
- Topical thiabendazole.

Introduction

In low-resource countries, children presenting to medical facilities may harbour intestinal helminthiasis (worms) or their juvenile forms (larvae) in other organs. Often this situation may exist without the presence of any signs or symptoms. In such situations ill health or the risk of serious complications is directly related to the number of parasites in a child; although children bearing heavy loads of parasites are in a minority. These patients will often present for other reasons, without their heavy worm infections being recognised.

Parasitology of worms

There are three important groups of helminth infections:
1. **Cestodes:** Beef tapeworm (*Taenia saginata*) and pig tapeworm (*Taenia solium*).
2. **Nematodes:** Roundworms (*Ascaris* species), hookworms (*Ancylostoma duodenale*), whipworms (*Trichurius* species) and threadworms (*Enterobius* species).
   - *Ascaris lumbricoides* is the commonest human roundworm. Adult worms are whitish pink, several millimetres (mm) wide and up to 30 centimetres (cm) long, which may live for years in the small intestine. They are often seen in stool or vomit. Transmission is by ingestion of embryonated eggs from soil. Adult worms shed their eggs in faeces. The ill effects of ascariasis are largely indirect and rare (e.g. a worm in the common bile duct). The probability of this obstruction increases with worm load.
   - Hookworms are of two species, *Necator americanus* (the New World hookworm) and *Ancylostoma duodenale*. Both adult forms are hair-like, about 1 cm long, with cutting plates at the mouth end. *Ancylostoma* is generally the more virulent pathogen. Both species occur widely, with overlap, and the differences between them can be ignored by clinicians without a special interest in this subject. They have invasive larvae, and both skin penetration and ingestion of embyonated eggs are involved in transmission. Sustained blood loss in the small intestine leads to an accumulating risk of anaemia. In children, protein-losing enteropathy and systemic secondary effects of chronic inflammation are equally important.
   - *Trichuris trichiura* commonly known as the whipworm can be up to 4 cm long with thickness of a hair except at the tail end which is wider. Transmission is similar to *Ascaris* but maturation occurs only in the gut without tissue invasion beyond the mucosa. Its ill effects are related to worm load and may lead to a form of colitis with systemic secondary effects of chronic inflammation. This intensity of infection occurs only in a small minority of children.
   - *Enterobius vermicularis* is an intestinal helminth which is spread in the form of embryonated eggs by personal contact among children. It is largely harmless but can cause secondary infection in the vaginal introitus.
   - *Strongyloides stercoralis* is capable of independent existence in the soil. It is an opportunistic parasite of several mammals, including humans. Person-to-person spread occurs with probability related to intimacy of contact. Although it is acquired in childhood, its most devastating (often fatal) effects occur only when filariform larvae become disseminated through asexual reproduction in the host. This happens if host immunity breaks down, for example with severe malnutrition or malignancy in later life. Surprisingly, disseminated strongyloidiasis is not associated with HIV infection, although it is associated with another retrovirus, HTLV1.
3. **Trematodes** or flukes, which include blood flukes (e.g. schistosomiasis) (*see* Section 6.3.C.c) and biliary tract, lung and gut flukes.

Diagnosis

The main clues to heavy parasitosis are in growth, nutrition and in the case of hookworm, anaemia. Gastrointestinal symptoms also occur. Often a presumptive diagnosis is based on manifestations suggestive of worm infections. An increasing number of studies on the effects of helminth infections on cognitive function and general physical fitness have added to the case for community control of these infections as an important public health measure.

Investigations
Investigation for adult worms in the intestine
Except for *Enterobius*, this depends on the examination of stool. Full laboratory details are beyond the scope of this manual, but for *Ascaris*, hookworm and *Trichuris*, examination by the Kato (modified Kato or Kato-Katz) method is recommended. This requires only microscope slides, a standard hole in a flat spatula with which a 50 mg stool sample is squashed on to the slide, cellophane, glycerol and a stain such as malachite green. A microscopic count of eggs per gram of stool gives an indication of the intensity of infection.

Enterobius (thread worm) eggs are only occasionally seen in stool because they adhere to perianal skin where the female worm has deposited them. They can be picked up on sticky tape and transferred to a glass slide. Specific diagnosis of *Enterobius* is not really necessary in any case,

TABLE 6.3.C.A.1 Diagnosis of helminth infections due to the presence of adult worms

Symptom or sign	Likely species of adult worm in the viscera
Short stature, not growing	*Trichuris* or hookworm
Mild or moderate muscle wasting	*Trichuris* or hookworm
Anaemia, microcytic hypochromic	Hookworm or severe trichuriasis; not *Ascaris*
Hypoproteinaemia, possible oedema	Hookworm or severe trichuriasis or disseminated strongyloidiasis: not *Ascaris*
Pica, especially eating soil (geophagia)	Any or all helminths
Colicky abdominal pain	*Ascaris:* common but a weak correlation
Intestinal obstruction	*Ascaris:* a quite common surgical emergency
Jaundice and/or pancreatitis	*Ascaris:* uncommon
Laryngeal obstruction	*Ascaris:* rare
Vomiting up worms	*Ascaris:* common
Chronic diarrhoea	*Trichuris* or severe hookworm or strongyloidiasis
Defecating during sleep	*Trichuris*
Blood and mucus in stool	*Trichuris*
Rectal prolapse	*Trichuris*
Finger clubbing	Intense trichuriasis or hookworm; not *Ascaris*
Perianal itching	*Enterobius*
Vulvovaginitis	*Enterobius*

TABLE 6.3.C.A.2 Illness due to larvae rather than adult worms

Symptom or sign	Likely species of larvae in the viscera
Cough and wheeze	*Toxocara canis* or *T. cati* (dog or cat roundworm) Also *Ascaris* and hookworm
Hepatomegaly	*Toxocara*
Lymphadenopathy	*Toxocara*
Leucocytosis with extreme eosinophilia	*Toxocara*
Epilepsy or encephalopathy	*Toxocara* (rare)
Uveitis or proliferative retinitis	*Toxocara* (younger children escape in endemic areas: naive strangers are more susceptible)

as it is reasonable to treat the patient and family when it is suspected, without proving the presence of the worm (see below).

The most effective way to establish that *Trichuris* infection is intense is to see the worms on prolapsed rectal mucosa or to perform anoscopy. An otoscope with a wide-aperture speculum can be used for anoscopy in young children. The worms are usually confined to the caecum, so if they have reached the lower rectal mucosa the infection must be intense.

Strongyloides is a rare cause of illness in young children, although it becomes more significant in adolescence in some regions. Microscopy has a low sensitivity, and the stool requires culture by special techniques. Serology is not widely available and also lacks specificity (*see* Section 6.3.C.h).

Investigation for migrating larvae
Eosinophilia is characteristic of this stage with 20–50% of the leucocytes being eosinophils in some cases. By contrast, eosinophilia is not a constant feature of established infection with adult worms and so is a useless diagnostic marker for intestinal infection.

The chest X-ray may show a flaring shadow spreading out from the hila.

Serology is diagnostically useful in visceral larva migrans (*Toxocara* infection), but is only undertaken in special centres or research laboratories.

Diagnosis of cutaneous larva migrans (dog hookworm infection picked up from skin–ground contact) is purely clinical. The key is to think of it when looking at a patch of itchy pyoderma; the red line has often disappeared under the scratching.

It is not clear how much of the total burden of cough, wheezing and dyspnoea in a child population in an endemic zone is due to the pulmonary migration of helminth larvae. Factors that make the symptoms more severe are migration of children naive to *Ascaris* or hookworm infection into the endemic area, and zoonotic larvae (*Toxocara*) which cannot complete their migration but die in their human hosts.

Treatment
The broad-spectrum antihelmintics, mebendazole and albendazole, are drugs which combine great efficacy with an almost complete absence of side effects in ordinary use. They are the drugs of choice for ascariasis, hookworm infection, trichuriasis and enterobiasis. Albendazole is as effective as thiabendazole for visceral larva migrans, and with fewer side effects. However, visceral larva migrans is a self-limiting condition where symptoms and signs resolve in 3 months. Thiabendazole is still useful for cutaneous larva migrans in a topical preparation (10% in aqueous cream; the pharmacist may be able to make this on site, see Regimens below). Ivermectin is recommended for strongyloidiasis, but albendazole remains useful and is preferable to thiabendazole because it is less toxic.

Mebendazole
This is most commonly available as 100 mg tablets, but is also produced as a 20 mg/5 mL liquid and a 500 mg tablet. The tablets are chewable and reasonably palatable. The 500 mg tablet is useful for mass campaigns against *Trichuris* or hookworm. It is not approved for use in children under 2 years of age, but clinical judgement should be used in a symptomatic child. **It is considered unsafe in pregnancy or lactation.**

Threadworms and pinworms
Oral dose:
- Children from 6 months up to 10 kg body weight: Give 50 mg as a single dose; if reinfection occurs a second dose may be needed after 2 weeks.
- Children over 1 year of age or more than 10 kg body weight: Give 100 mg as a single dose; if reinfection occurs a second dose may be needed after 2 weeks.

Whipworms, roundworms and hookworms

Oral dose:

- Children from 6 months up to 10 kg body weight: Give 50 mg twice daily for 3 days.
- Children over 1 year of age or more than 10 kg body weight: Give 100 mg twice daily for 3 days.

Capillariasis

Oral dose:

- Children over 2 years of age: Give 200 mg twice daily for 20 days.

Echinococcus (mebendazole is second-line therapy, albendazole is preferred)

Oral dose:

- Child over 2 years of age: Give 15 mg/kg/dose three times daily.

Toxocariasis: visceral larva migrans (mebendazole is second-line therapy, albendazole is preferred)

Oral dose:

- Children over 2 years of age: Give 100–200 mg twice daily for 5 days, although doses of up to 1 gram/day have been used for 21 days. Severe disease may warrant corticosteroid use.

Trichinosis (gastrointestinal phase of illness only)

Oral dose:

- Children over 2 years of age: 5 mg/kg (maximum 200 mg) twice daily with food for 7 days; severe infection may require concomitant corticosteroid use; late-phase antihelmintic therapy is not indicated.

Albendazole

This drug is closely related to mebendazole, with similar pharmokinetics. It has superior efficacy to mebendazole in systemically invasive conditions, and is more effective against migrating larvae. It is available as 200 mg tablets or 200 mg/5 mL liquid. Cautions are as for mebendazole, noting its greater systemic absorption.

Hookworms, roundworms, pinworms and threadworms (ancylostomiasis, necatoriasis, ascariasis and enterobiasis)

Oral dose:

- Children aged 12 months to 2 years: Give 200 mg as a single dose.
- Children over 2 years or 10 kg: Give 400 mg as a single dose before food. Treatment may be repeated in 3 weeks.

Echinococcus

Oral dose:

- 7.5 mg/kg twice daily (maximum dose 400 mg twice daily). Given continuously for up to 2 years.

Tapeworm (taeniasis) and strongyloidiasis

Oral dose:

- Children under 10 kg: Give 200 mg daily before food for 3 days.
- Children over 10 kg: Give 400 mg daily before food for 3 days. Treatment may be repeated in 3 weeks.

Neurocysticercosis

Oral dose:

- Children under 60 kg: Give 7.5 mg/kg (maximum dose 400 mg) twice daily after food for 7–30 days.

Whipworm (trichuriasis)

Oral dose:

- Children over 2 years of age: Give 200–400 mg as a single dose, or in heavier infections, 400 mg daily for 3 days. Treatment may be repeated in 3 weeks.

Filariasis for community eradication programmes in combination with diethylcarbamazine or ivermectin

Oral dose:

- Children under 10 kg: Give 200 mg once annually for 5 years.
- Children over 10 kg: Give 400 mg annually for 5 years.

Hairworm (trichostrongyliasis)

Oral dose:

- Child over 10 kg: Give 400 mg as a single dose.

Cutaneous larva migrans

Oral dose:

- Children over 10 kg: Give 400 mg as a single dose, or 400 mg daily for 3 days.

Visceral larva migrans (toxocariasis)

Oral dose:

- Child of all ages: Give 10 mg/kg daily (maximum 400 mg daily) for 5 days.

Trichinosis

Oral dose:

- Children over 10 kg: Give 400 mg daily for 8–14 days.

For topical treatment of cutaneous larva migrans, thiabendazole tablets can be crushed and mixed with aqueous cream or 1% hydrocortisone cream or ointment to a concentration of 10% thiabendazole.

In places or situations where only the older drugs are available

Details and dosages are not given here. The manufacturers' recommendations may be followed, but these drugs are inferior to mebendazole and albendazole, and should be replaced if possible.

- Piperazine is effective against *Ascaris* and *Enterobius*. It has no action on *Trichuris* or hookworm, and is toxic in children prone to epileptic seizures.
- Levamisole is effective against *Ascaris* and is fairly useful effective in hookworm infection (especially *Necator americanus*); to be used in mass control programmes.
- Thiabendazole has limited effectiveness in trichuriasis and is useful in strongyloidiasis, toxocariasis and cutaneous larva migrans.
- Pyrantel is effective against *Ascaris* and *Enterobius*, with some action against *Necator americanus* and less against *Ancylostoma duodenale*. Only if combined with oxantel does the preparation affect *Trichuris*.

Further reading

WHO's programme 'Action against worms' http://evidence action.org/deworming/

6.3.C.b Hydatid disease

BOX 6.3.C.B.1 Minimum standards
- Ultrasound/radiology.
- Albendazole.
- Percutaneous aspiration, injection with hypertonic saline and re-aspiration (PAIR).
- Surgical excision.

Introduction

The adult stage of the tapeworm *Echinococcus granulosus* lives in the gut of dogs and certain other carnivores. The usual intermediate hosts are herbivores. **Humans may become an accidental intermediate host for the cystic stage of the parasite following ingestion of eggs in dog faeces contaminating the fingers, food or water.** Because of the slow rate of growth of hydatid cysts, symptoms from infection in childhood often present in adulthood. Many cysts remain asymptomatic, eventually calcify and become sterile.

Epidemiology

The disease is widespread in sheep-farming countries and wherever there is intimate contact between humans and dogs or other canids, and where dogs scavenge dead animals or offal. There is a high incidence in the Turkana region of Kenya.

Clinical features

- Cysts may occur in virtually any organ.
- Many cysts are asymptomatic but may be palpable if they are large or superficial.
- Abdomen:
  - Palpable mass: liver (60% of all cysts), spleen, other intra-abdominal cysts.
  - Communication with the biliary tract: cholangitis, rigors, jaundice.
  - Abdominal pain.
  - Rupture from trauma.
- Chest:
  - Lungs (25% of cysts).
  - Pleuritic pain and cough.
  - Often asymptomatic, detected on chest X-ray.
- Other areas:
  - Brain: space-occupying lesions (3–5% in some countries).
  - Bone cysts: pathological fractures, respond poorly to chemotherapy.
  - Cyst rupture may cause anaphylaxis and/or spread by 'seeding' of daughter scolices (heads of immature worms).

Diagnosis

- Ultrasound is effective in detecting liver and abdominal cysts. The presence of a separated membrane or daughter cysts makes the diagnosis highly likely. The condition needs to be differentiated from simple hepatic cysts.
- Plain X-ray for lung or bone cysts. CT or MRI (if available) is also useful (e.g. for brain cysts).
- Eosinophilia is present in around 20% of cases. This may be due to cyst leakage or rupture.
- Serology: specific IgG ELISA AgB (antigen-B-rich fraction) (if available) is most sensitive. Serology lacks sensitivity for extra-hepatic cysts (note that false-positive results are obtained in cysticercosis).
- A urine antigen detection test appears promising.

Treatment

Calcified cysts require no treatment.

Medical treatment

- Albendazole is useful for patients with inoperable, widespread or numerous cysts, and for patients unfit for surgery.
- Continuous treatment is now recommended (for up to 2 years). Its duration depends on the lesion's response. The dose is 7.5 mg/kg orally twice daily. The maximum dose is 400 mg twice daily.
- The absorption of albendazole is enhanced if it is taken with fatty meals.
- Albendazole plus praziquantel has greater protoscolicidal activity. The combination is successful for inoperable spinal, pelvic, abdominal, thoracic or hepatic hydatid, and as an adjunct to surgery.
- Antihelmintics may reduce the need for surgery in uncomplicated pulmonary cysts.
- Patients undergoing surgery or PAIR should receive pre-operative albendazole (for 1–3 months) with or without praziquantel.

Percutaneous aspiration under ultrasound control

Puncture, aspiration, injection, re-aspiration (PAIR):
- The patient should be on albendazole for at least 4 weeks prior to PAIR.
- Following initial aspiration of the cyst, hypertonic saline is injected into the cyst and re-aspirated after 20 minutes.
- Percutaneous aspiration combined with an 8-week course of albendazole is more effective than either treatment alone.
- Laparoscopic treatment of liver and spleen hydatid is also effective.
- Contraindications to PAIR include cysts in the CNS or heart, and cysts communicating with the biliary tree, abdominal cavity, urinary tract or bronchi.

Surgery

Surgical removal is standard treatment if the lesion is accessible but is unsuitable for PAIR. The procedure is as follows:
- The patient should be on albendazole for at least 4 weeks prior to surgery.
- Pack around the cyst and avoid spillage of the cyst contents (there is a risk of anaphylaxis and seeding).
- Drain the cyst, replace fluid with hypertonic saline, drain again, and then remove the cyst capsule.

- High rates of recurrence and of surgical complications are recorded in inexpert hands.
- It is important to avoid hypertonic saline entering the bile ducts, as this may cause sclerosing cholangitis.

6.3.C.c Schistosomiasis

BOX 6.3.C.C.1 Minimum standards
- ■ Public health measures to improve water and sanitation.
- ■ Urine and faecal microscopy
- ■ Praziquantel.

Introduction

Schistosomiasis occurs in areas of the world where there is a combination of warm fresh water containing specific snails, and urinary and/or faecal excretion of *Schistosoma* eggs by humans.

Parasite and life cycle

Eggs are passed from humans in stool or urine into freshwater containing snails, *Bulinus* (*S. haematobium*), *Biomphalaria* (*S. mansoni*) and *Oncomelania* (*S. japonicum*). Miracidia hatch from the eggs, penetrate the snail, and replicate into cercariae (larval forms) which are then released into the water.

The cercaria penetrates the skin (or pharyngeal mucosa) of humans, loses its tail and becomes a schistosomula, which is then transported to the lung capillaries. It reaches the left side of the heart and is distributed throughout the body. Those that reach the portal system develop into mature worms about 1 cm in length in the liver.

Adult males and females copulate and migrate in pairs to their preferred egg-laying sites, *S. haematobium* to the vesical veins and pelvic plexus, and *S. mansoni* to the superior and inferior mesenteric veins.

Female flukes produce eggs daily throughout their average 3- to 4-year lifespan. Most eggs pass through the vessel wall, and about 50% reach the lumen of the urinary tract or intestine and are excreted. Those that remain in the tissues provoke an immune reaction which causes the disease. Some eggs are transported to the liver and some reach the general circulation.

Pathogenesis

Pathogenesis can be divided into four stages.

1 **Dermatitis.** An itchy papular rash 'swimmers itch' lasting one to two days may develop as a result of humoral immune reaction to invading cercariae and schistosomulae. However, it is more likely to be due to avian schistosoma (non-pathogenic to man). Older children and adults develop a degree of resistance to this stage of invasion.

Prevention

- Ensure disposal of infected herbivore carcasses and offal.
- Treat dogs with praziquantel.
- Maintain strict hygiene, and protect food and water from contamination.

2 **Katayama fever** (2–8 weeks). A humoral reaction to adult worms and eggs results in an acute illness associated with formation of immune complexes. Symptoms include fever, rigors, malaise, diarrhoea, cough, hepatosplenomegaly and marked eosinophilia. It is a self-limiting disease.

3 **Established disease** (usually after 2 months). A T-cell delayed-hypersensitivity response to eggs deposited in tissue results in granuloma formation. If the worm load is reduced by drug therapy at this stage, granulomata may resolve, leaving little disease.

4 **Fibrotic complications.** Repeated infections without treatment eventually result in fibrosis, for example of the ureter and bladder (*S. haematobium*) and liver (*S. mansoni*). There is little response to drug therapy at this stage.

TABLE 6.3.C.C.1 Schistosomiasis: geographical areas (the commonest species and areas are shown in bold type)

Schistosoma species	Disease	Area
S. haematobium	Urinary tract	**Africa**, Middle East
S. mansoni	Intestines, liver	**Africa**, Middle East, **South America**
S. intercalatum	Intestines, liver	Central and West Africa, uncommon
S. japonicum	Intestines, liver	**China, Indonesia, Philippines**
S. mekongi	Intestines, liver	Laos, Kampuchea, small number of foci

Epidemiology

- Schistosomiasis affects at least 240 million people worldwide, and more than 700 million people live in endemic areas.
- Schistosomiasis is associated with communities living near swamps, rivers, irrigation canals and rice fields, who have poor hygiene and sanitary facilities and lack a ready supply of clean water.
- Infection is highest in children (5–14 years) who are an important reservoir of infection because of their indiscriminate excretion habits near and in water.
- Infections decrease after puberty, but adults are still at risk when farming or washing clothes.

Clinical features

TABLE 6.3.C.C.2 Symptoms and complications of *S. haematobium* and *S. mansoni*

Initial stage	S. haematobium	S. mansoni	Comments
Swimmers' itch	Terminal haematuria	Bloody diarrhoea Anaemia	*S. japonicum* is similar to *S. mansoni*
Katayama fever	Obstructive uropathy Calcification of bladder and lower ureters Bladder calculi	Hepatic fibrosis Portal hypertension Ascites Colonic polyposis Nephropathy	Hepatic fibrosis is most often seen with *S. mansoni* Katayama fever is more severe with *S. japonicum*

S. haematobium

This causes urinary schistosomiasis.

- Terminal haematuria, there may be dysuria.
- In a minority of children, frequent untreated infections eventually lead to structural disorder of the bladder and lower ureter, resulting in obstructive uropathy, hypertension and chronic renal failure.
- Obstruction can be demonstrated by ultrasonography and intravenous pyelogram. Adequate treatment in the early stages may be followed by resolution of ureteric lesions.

S. mansoni

This causes intestinal schistosomiasis along with other species, namely *S. intercalatum*, *S. japonicum* and *S. mekongi*.

- Bloody diarrhoea. In long-standing cases there is severe iron-deficient anaemia, and even heart failure (due to anaemia).
- Protein-losing enteropathy with hypoalbuminaemia may result from colonic granulomatous disease and polyps.
- The left lobe of the liver is enlarged more than the right lobe. Ascites may occur. Liver function is usually well preserved.
- Marked splenomegaly due to portal hypertension is associated with pancytopenia.
- Haematemesis from oesophageal varices is the final event which influences the prognosis.
- Ultrasonography is useful for grading the degree of peri-portal fibrosis and in differential diagnosis from other liver diseases.
- Acute and long-term management of oesophageal varices requires endoscopy and decisions regarding sclerotherapy (*see* Section 5.7.B on liver disease).
- Nephropathy due to immune complex disease may manifest with microscopic haematuria and proteinuria or nephrotic syndrome. Nephrotic syndrome has a poor prognosis, especially if associated with amyloid disease (*see* Section 5.6.A).

Salmonella infection

Schistosoma worms may harbour *Salmonella* species, including *S. typhi*, which cannot be eradicated until the schistosomiasis is treated. This phenomenon occurs in both *S. haematobium* and *S. mansoni* infections. *Salmonella* may cause a reversible nephritis in *S. mansoni* infection.

Complications common to S. haematobium and S. mansoni

- Spinal cord myelopathy (less common with *S. haematobium*).
- Brain granulomata (more common with *S. japonicum*, less common with *S. haematobium*).
- Pulmonary hypertension (less common with *S. haematobium*).
- Chronic *Salmonella* infection.

Diagnosis
Microscopy of urine or faeces
S. haematobium

A midday specimen is best. Urine should be sedimented or filtered. Viability of the eggs (and thus requirement for treatment) can be established by looking for miracidia, which hatch when eggs are put in boiled water that has been cooled.

S. mansoni

If stool smear is negative on microscopy, a concentration method must be undertaken. Miracidial hatching techniques are also available.

Rectal biopsy

Rectal biopsy to demonstrate the presence of eggs is undertaken if urine and faeces are negative.

Serology

Serology is of little value for diagnosis in indigenous patients, but may be useful in the non-immune (e.g. tourists to an endemic area). Antigen tests are being developed.

Treatment

Praziquantel is effective against all human *Schistosoma* species, and is the only available drug treatment. Treatment at least three times in childhood usually prevents adult disease.

Praziquantel is given at a dose of 40 mg/kg in two divided doses given 4–6 hours apart on one day. It can also be given as a single dose of 40 mg/kg. For heavy *S. mansoni* infection and for *S. japonicum* infection, 60 mg/kg is advised, given in two doses 4–6 hours apart. Repeat urine or stool examination should be done at 3–4 months.

Praziquantel is safe during pregnancy. The safety of praziquantel in children under 4 years of age has not been established, but this drug can be used to treat individually infected children.

Side effects include dizziness, drowsiness, skin reactions, fever, headache and vomiting.

Prevention

Control of schistosomiasis is very difficult. Measures include regular mass treatment of communities and improvement in water supply, sanitation and hygiene. Mollusciciding (use of chemicals to kill the snails) is usually impractical and too expensive for general use.

6.3.C.d Fascioliasis (liver fluke infections)

> **BOX 6.3.C.D.1 Minimum standards**
> - Vector control.
> - Triclabendazole (preferred) or Bithional.

Introduction

This disease is caused by *Fasciola hepatica* and *Fasciola gigantica*, and occurs in sheep- and cattle-rearing areas worldwide, especially South America.

Freshwater snails act as the intermediate amplifying hosts, liberating free-swimming cercariae which encyst as metacercariae on water plants. Humans are infected following ingestion of metacercarial cysts on raw aquatic plants (e.g. watercress) or from contaminated water. Following ingestion, the larvae emerge in the duodenum, penetrate the intestinal wall, migrate via the peritoneal cavity to the liver, penetrate the liver capsule, and after 3–4 months mature into adults in the bile ducts.

Clinical features

Infections may be asymptomatic. Acute presentations occur 6–12 weeks after infection. Fluke migration may be associated with fever, malaise, abdominal pain, weight loss, urticaria, cough and wheeze. In chronic presentations, symptoms may be minimal or may be due to recurrent cholangitis, intermittent biliary obstruction or anaemia.

Ectopic flukes may cause granuloma or abscess formation in various organs, and also present as migrating skin nodules.

Investigations

- Eosinophilia is common.
- Liver ultrasound is often normal.
- CT of the liver (if available) may reveal hypodense lesions.
- Serology may be helpful in established *F. hepatica* infections, but is less reliable for *F. gigantica*. Fasciola excretory–secretory (FES) antigen detection in faeces is available for *F. hepatica*.
- In established infections, eggs may be found in faeces.

Treatment

Triclabendazole is the drug of choice for *F. hepatica* and *F. gigantica* infections. One dose of 10 mg/kg taken with food is usually effective, but should be repeated after 12 hours in severe infections. Expulsion of dead or damaged flukes may cause biliary colic 3–7 days after treatment; the colic responds well to antispasmodics. Triclabendazole resistance has been reported in Ireland, the UK and Australia.

Bithional, 30–50 mg/kg/day in three divided doses on alternate days for 10–15 days was the preferred treatment previously. Side effects include mild gastrointestinal upset and pruritus.

Nitazoxanide may be effective.

Praziquantel is unreliable in the treatment of fascioliasis.

Prevention and control

- Avoid potentially contaminated watercress and other aquatic plants.
- Treat herbivores.
- Undertake snail control.

6.3.C.e Dracunculiasis (guinea-worm disease)

> **BOX 6.3.C.E.1 Minimum standards**
> - Early identification of blister and worm emergence.
> - Removal of worm and prevention of secondary infection.
> - Filtering of water.
> - Temephos to kill *Cyclops* species.

Introduction

Guinea-worm disease is transmitted exclusively by drinking stagnant water contaminated with tiny water fleas (*Cyclops* species) that carry infective guinea-worm larvae. Once ingested, the larvae mature into worms, growing up to 1 metre in length. Humans are the only known reservoirs for the disease.

About 1 year after infection, a very painful blister forms, 90% of the time on the lower leg, and one or more worms emerge accompanied by a burning sensation. To soothe the burning pain, patients often immerse the infected area in water. The worm then releases thousands of larvae into the water, contaminating the water and bringing the infective cycle full circle.

Epidemiology

The main source of infection is stagnant water sources such as ponds and sometimes shallow or step wells. 'Man-made' ponds are the main source of transmission.

Only four African countries (Chad, Ethiopia, Mali and

South Sudan) are known to be affected, with the majority of cases in South Sudan.

Guinea-worm disease is seasonal, occurring with two broad patterns found in endemic areas of Africa, depending on climatic factors. In the Sahelian zone, transmission generally occurs in the rainy season (from May to August). In the humid savanna and forest zone, the peak occurs in the dry season (from September to January).

A successful eradication programme for guinea-worm disease consists of several preventive strategies, such as ensuring wider access to safe drinking-water supplies, filtration of drinking water (with cloth filters) to prevent infection, intense surveillance and control to detect every case within 24 hours of the emergence of the worm(s), treatment of ponds with the larvicide temephos that kills the water fleas, and promoting health education and behaviour change.

Early case detection (when the patient feels the initial pain) is vital in order to contain the disease. There are thousands of village volunteers in the remaining endemic countries who are trained to find new cases, take care of them and report them to the area supervisor.

Clinical effects

Once a new case is identified, the wound must be disinfected and bandaged to help to prevent secondary infection. The worm should be gently pulled out a few inches every day until all of it has been removed. Many patients are unable to leave their beds for a month after the emergence of the worm.

Guinea-worm disease is not fatal, but infected people cannot work or attend school for months. Since the peak transmission period often coincides with the agricultural season, fields are left untended and food production declines. In Mali, guinea-worm disease is called 'the disease of the empty granary'. As adults lie sick, older children must take on the household chores and miss months of schooling. Younger children may miss vital vaccinations.

Prevention

- Effective surveillance to detect all cases within 24 hours of worm emergence.
- **Ensure access to safe drinking water, and convert unsafe sources to safe ones.**
- Construction of copings around well heads or installation of boreholes with hand pumps.
- **There must be regular and systematic filtering of drinking water derived from ponds and shallow unprotected wells, or from surface water.** Fine-meshed cloth or, better still, a filter made from a 0.15-mm nylon mesh, is all that is needed to filter out the *Cyclops* species from the drinking water.
- Treatment of unsafe water sources with temephos to kill the *Cyclops* species.
- Health education and social mobilisation to encourage affected communities to adopt healthy behaviour with regard to use of drinking water.

6.3.C.f Filariasis

> **BOX 6.3.C.F.1 Minimum standards**
> ■ Treatment of endemic communities.
> ■ Control of mosquitoes (the vector).
> ■ Diethylcarbamazine citrate (DEC), albendazole, doxycycline and ivermectin.

Introduction

This painful and profoundly disfiguring disease is usually acquired in childhood.

The disease is caused by three species of thread-like nematode worms, known as filariae, namely *Wuchereria bancrofti*, *Brugia malayi* and *Brugia timori*. Around 90% of infections are caused by *Wuchereria bancrofti* and most of the remainder by *Brugia malayi*. About 120 million people are affected worldwide (of whom 60% live in South-East Asia and 30% live in Africa).

Life cycle of filariae

Filariae are transmitted by mosquitoes. When a mosquito with infective-stage larvae takes a blood meal, the parasites are deposited through the person's skin, from which they enter the body. These larvae then migrate to the lymphatic vessels and develop into adult worms over a period of 6–12 months, causing damage to and dilatation of the lymphatic vessels. The adult filariae live for several years in the human host. During this time they produce millions of immature microfilariae that circulate in the peripheral blood and are ingested by mosquitoes that bite the infected human. The larval forms further develop inside the mosquito before becoming infectious to humans. Thus a cycle of transmission is established.

Threadlike adult worms of *Wuchereria bancrofti* live in the lymphatics (groin, scrotum, arm). Male worms are about 3–4 cm in length, and female worms 8–10 cm. The male and female worms together form 'nests' in the lymphatic system. Females release thousands of microfilariae into the peripheral blood periodically every day, synchronising with the biting habits of the predominant local mosquito vector. Nocturnal periodicity is commonest, except in some Polynesian islands where microfilariae are more numerous by day.

Brugia malayi has two main forms: the nocturnal periodic form in swampy areas from India to Korea and Japan, and the nocturnal sub-periodic form in the damp forests of South-East Asia. The parasites of *B. malayi* are transmitted by various species of the genus *Mansonia*, and in some areas anopheline mosquitoes are responsible for transmitting infection. Brugian parasites are confined to areas of East and South Asia, notably India, Indonesia, Malaysia and the Philippines.

An estimated 120 million people in tropical and subtropical areas are infected, of whom almost 25 million men have genital disease (most commonly hydrocoele) and almost 15 million, mostly women, have lymphoedema or elephantiasis of the leg.

Diagnosis

Eosinophilia is common in the acute stages. Examination of thick smears of 20–60 microlitres of blood from a finger tip or filtration of 1 mL of intravenous blood and examination of the filtrate can reveal the microfilariae provided that the concentration is high (> 100 microfilariae/mL). Concentration techniques can improve sensitivity (e.g. Nuclepore filtration).

Samples should be appropriately timed (usually between 22.00 and 02.00 hours for *W. bancrofti*).

A variety of more sensitive diagnostic techniques are now available, including complement fixation tests for circulating *W. bancrofti* antigen (e.g. an ELISA 'TropBio-test') and a rapid finger-prick immunochromatographic card test (Amrad ICT, Binax). The rapid ICT has a high sensitivity and specificity and is currently the preferred diagnostic test for *W. bancrofti*. It is also used for monitoring the success of mass drug programmes. The test requires 100 microlitres of finger-prick blood drawn at any time, day or night.

Clinical features

The majority of infected people are asymptomatic, but virtually all have subclinical lymphatic damage, and up to 40% have kidney damage, with proteinuria and haematuria.

Inflammatory episodes associated with lymphatic filariasis involve:

- responses to the parasite itself
- the effects of secondary bacterial infection
- sometimes inflammatory mediators associated with endosymbiotic bacteria (*Wolbachia*).

Endosymbiotic bacteria infect most species of filarial nematodes that are pathogenic to humans, and contribute to the damage done by the filaria. Further characterisation of the *Wolbachia*–nematode relationship might allow the development of new therapeutic approaches to these parasitic diseases.

Acute episodes of local inflammation involving the skin, lymph nodes and lymphatic vessels often accompany chronic lymphoedema or elephantiasis (see below). Some of these episodes are caused by the body's immune response to the parasite, but many are the result of bacterial skin infections, linked to the partial loss of the body's normal defences as a result of underlying lymphatic damage. **Careful cleansing is extremely helpful in healing the infected areas and in both slowing and even reversing much of the damage that has already occurred.**

Acute symptoms may recur several times a year in three forms:

1. Acute filarial fever without lymphadenitis.
2. Acute filarial lymphangitis (AFL) follows the death of an adult worm, causing an inflammatory nodule or cord with lymphangitis spreading away from the affected node. This is usually mild, but may develop into an abscess.

Acute dermatolymphangioadenitis (ADLA) resembles cellulitis or erysipelas, and is often associated with secondary bacterial infection and impaired lymphatic flow, ascending lymphangitis and limb oedema. ADLA is more common than AFL, and is an important cause of lymphoedema and elephantiasis.

Chronic lymphatic filariasis may develop over months or years even without a history of acute symptoms. Lymphatic obstruction eventually leads to **elephantiasis**, most commonly affecting the legs, scrotum, arms and breast. Recurrent secondary bacterial skin infections (often streptococcal) cause acute pain and fever, and may be complicated by acute glomerulonephritis.

Other presentations of lymphatic filariasis include:

- hydrocoele, usually unilateral
- swelling of the scrotum
- acute epididymitis
- funiculitis (inflammation of the spermatic cord)
- monoarthritis
- glomerulonephritis
- chyluria, chylous diarrhoea, chylous ascites (due to rupture of dilated lymphatics). (Malabsorption of fat-soluble vitamins may complicate chylous diarrhoea.)

Brugian filariasis is usually less severe than Bancroftian filariasis.

The most severe symptoms generally appear in adults, and in males more often than in females. In endemic communities, around 10–50% of men suffer genital damage

TABLE 6.3.C.F.1 Recommended treatment strategies for mass drug distribution, individual drug administration, and morbidity control and treatment of lymphatic filariasis

Mass drug administration		Individual drug administration	Morbidity control and treatment
Africa	**Rest of world**		
IVM + ALB for at least 5 years	DEC + ALB for at least 5 years	(a) DEC (with or without ALB) 6 mg/kg single dose[1] (b) DEC 12-day course of 6 mg/kg per day in two or three divided doses **or** (c) doxycycline 200 mg/day for 4 weeks followed by one dose IV or IM	Lymphoedema: hygiene, physiotherapy, doxycycline 200 mg/day for 6 weeks Hydrocoele: surgical hydrocoelectomy, doxycycline 200 mg/day for 6 weeks Tropical pulmonary eosinophilia: doxycycline 200 mg/day for 4 weeks followed by one dose IV or IM

Based on Taylor M *et al.* (2010) *Lancet*, **376**, 1175–85.

[1] If the patient continues to live in an endemic area, or is less than 8 years of age (contraindication of doxycycline).

ALB, Albendazole; DEC, diethylcarbamazine (omit if there is onchocerciasis co-infection or a risk of serious adverse events with *Loa loa*); IVM, ivermectin (omit if there is a risk of serious adverse events with *Loa loa*).

Doxycycline: the doses above are suitable for children aged ≥ 8 years and weighing > 45 kg. Children aged ≥ 8 years but weighing < 45 kg should receive 4.4 mg/kg/day. Doxycycline should not be used for children < 8 years.

(hydrocoele and elephantiasis of the penis and scrotum). Elephantiasis of the entire leg or arm, the vulva and the breast may affect up to 10% of men and women.

In endemic areas, chronic and acute manifestations of filariasis tend to develop more often and sooner in refugees or newcomers than in local populations. Lymphoedema may develop within 6 months, and elephantiasis as soon as 1 year after arrival.

Tropical pulmonary eosinophilia (TPE)
A hypersensitivity response to microfilariae in the lungs can develop in some patients, causing cough and wheeze, especially at night. There may also be an enlarged liver, spleen and lymph nodes. Chest X-ray may show diffuse miliary shadows. Untreated TPE may progress to irreversible lung fibrosis. The condition is usually associated with high eosinophilia and high microfilaria titres. Microfilariae are usually absent from peripheral blood, but the rapid antigen test is usually positive.

Treatment and control of filariasis
A number of antihelmintic agents are effective, although care must be taken in the choice of antihelmintic depending on the risk of co-infection with onchocerciasis and/or *Loa loa*. Mass drug administration is an important strategy in community control. The treatment and control options are summarised in Table 6.3.C.F.1.

Treating endemic communities (*see* Table 6.3.C.F.1) The goal is to eliminate microfilariae from the blood of infected individuals in order to interrupt the cycle of transmission by mosquitoes. A single dose of diethylcarbamazine citrate (DEC) has the same long-term (1-year) effect in decreasing levels of microfilaraemia as the formerly recommended 12-day regimen of DEC. More importantly, the use of single doses of two drugs administered together (optimally albendazole with DEC or ivermectin) is 99% effective in removing microfilariae from the blood for a full year

after treatment. The following recommended drug regimens need to be administered once a year for at least 5 years, with coverage of at least 65% of the total at-risk population:

- 6 mg/kg of body weight diethylcarbamazine citrate (DEC) + 400 mg albendazole,

or

- 150 micrograms/kg of body weight ivermectin + 400 mg albendazole (in areas that are also endemic for onchocerciasis).

Treating individuals
Most problems result from bacterial and fungal 'super-infection' of tissues, linked to compromised lymphatic function caused by earlier filarial infection. Antibiotics against streptococcal and other bacterial infections are important. Surgical procedures are available to correct hydrocoele.

Because secondary bacterial infections play an important role in precipitating acute adeno-lymphangitis episodes and progression of lymphoedema, simple hygiene (either alone or in combination with antibiotic treatment) plays an important role in preventing episodes of acute disease and in the management of lymphoedema. Daily washing of affected limbs with soap and safe water to prevent secondary infection, combined with simple exercises, elevation of the limb, and treatment of cracks and entry points, provides significant relief from acute episodes and slows progression of the disease.

Vector control
Avoidance of mosquito bites through personal protection measures or community-level vector control is the best option for preventing lymphatic filariasis. If possible, malaria and lymphatic filariasis vector control should be integrated. Periodic examination of blood for infection and initiation of the above treatment is essential.

6.3.C.g Onchocerciasis

BOX 6.3.C.G.1 Minimum standards
- Rapid diagnostic tests.
- Ivermectin and doxycycline.

Introduction
Onchocerciasis is caused by the filarial worm *Onchocerca volvulus*, and is an important cause of blindness and skin disease in tropical Africa, Yemen and Central and South America. It is transmitted by the bite of blackflies (*Simulium* species).

Epidemiology
This infection mainly affects people living or working near fast-flowing rivers (*Simulium* breeding sites), but may be more widely distributed by flies carried on winds.

Pathology
Adult worms evade the host immune response and cause few symptoms. The main problems are the result of

immunological reactions to dying and dead microfilariae and their endosymbiotic bacteria (*Wolbachia*), which release bacterial mediators that trigger the innate immune system. In addition, activated eosinophils release cellular proteins that cause connective tissue damage.

Onchocerciasis may increase the risk of HIV-1 seroconversion. Treatment of onchocerciasis is associated with reduced HIV-1 viral replication. Onchodermatitis is more severe in HIV-positive patients.

Clinical features
The incubation period is usually 15–18 months. Infected patients may be asymptomatic. Palpable firm painless subcutaneous nodules (intertwined adult worms), several centimetres in diameter, may be most obvious over bony prominences.

Skin disease

A variety of different skin manifestations are seen, usually with a significant degree of overlap:

- Acute papular onchodermatitis (APOD): an intensely itchy papular rash, sometimes with local oedema.
- Chronic papular onchodermatitis (CPOD): larger pruritic (itchy) hyperpigmented papules.
- Lichenified onchodermatitis (LOD): discrete or confluent pruritic hyperpigmented papulonodular plaques, often with lymphadenopathy.

Severe itching may give rise to excoriation and secondary bacterial infection. Healing is associated with progressive hyperpigmentation, blackening and thickening of the skin.

Unrelenting itching may result in chronic sleep disturbance, poor concentration and depression.

Heavy infections in childhood can impair growth. After some years, skin atrophy and depigmentation give a wrinkled prematurely aged appearance (presbydermia). Patchy depigmentation, especially of the legs, results in a 'leopard-skin' appearance.

Inguinal or femoral lymphadenopathy may give rise to the so-called 'hanging groin' appearance.

Eye disease

Early symptoms include itching, redness and excess lacrimation. Late disease leads to varying degrees of loss of vision, and eventually to blindness.

Anterior eye disease

- Punctate keratitis due to death of microfilariae in the cornea may appear as a reversible 'snow-flake' opacity.
- Pannus forms as blood vessels invade the cornea from the sides and below. The pannus may cover the pupil (sclerosing keratitis) and cause blindness.
- Iritis leads to a loss of the pigment frill and to synechiae that cause a deformed, often pear-shaped pupil. Secondary cataracts occasionally result.

Posterior eye disease

- Chorioretinitis with pigmentary changes.
- Optic atrophy.
- 'Tunnel vision' and various other forms of visual loss may become evident in young adults.

Diagnosis

- Skin snips in saline examined under the microscope for microfilariae.
- Slit-lamp examination for microfilariae in the anterior chamber of the eye.
- Rapid diagnostic tests. A new luciferase immunoprecipitation systems (LIPS) assay has 100% sensitivity and specificity for *O. volvulus* using a rapid 15-minute format (QLIPS).
- Biochemical methods: Recent advances include a serum antibody test card using recombinant antigen to detect *O. volvulus*-specific IgG4 in finger-prick whole-blood specimens, a triple-antigen indirect ELISA rapid-format card test, and a highly sensitive and specific urine antigen dipstick test.
- Surgery: Subcutaneous nodules can be removed to demonstrate adult worms, or aspirated with a needle to look for microfilariae.

- DEC patch test: Diethylcarbamazine (DEC), although no longer recommended for the treatment of onchocerciasis because of the risk of provoking a Mazzotti reaction (see below), may be used in the following manner in patients with repeatedly negative skin snips, where other diagnostic techniques are unavailable. A 1-cm square of filter paper soaked in a solution of DEC is applied to the skin of the patient. If positive, this will provoke intense localised itching and inflammation at the site of application. DEC patch testing of children aged 3–5 years is advocated as an effective low-cost method for monitoring the endemicity and transmission of onchocerciasis in Africa.
- **Warning: A DEC patch test may precipitate a full-blown Mazzotti reaction**. This consists of microfilaria death resulting in an intensely itchy papular rash, may be accompanied by fever, limb oedema, hypotension and worsening of eye damage, and may be fatal. It is commonly associated with the use of oral DEC, and is rarely caused by ivermectin.

Treatment

Ivermectin kills microfilariae by immobilising them so that they are carried away via the lymphatics.

Warning: Ivermectin may precipitate meningoencephalitis or renal failure in patients who have *Loa loa* with a high microfilariaemia (> 2500 microfilariae/mL).

It is therefore important to exclude *Loa loa* if there is any possibility of co-infection, before giving ivermectin.

Doxycycline kills the endosymbiotic *Wolbachia*, resulting in the slow, less pathogenic death of the microfilariae. The drug also blocks worm embryogenesis and has a significant macrofilaricidal effect. Contraindications to doxycycline include age less than 9 years, pregnancy and breastfeeding.

Treatment of individual patients

Provided that the patient does not have a high *Loa loa* microfilaraemia, and ivermectin (or doxycycline) is not otherwise contraindicated, the following options are available:

- If the patient will continue to live in an endemic area, or is less than 9 years old and weighs more than 15 kg, give **ivermectin** 150 micrograms/kg every 3–6 months.
- If interruption of worm embryogenesis and cessation of microfilariae production is desired, give **doxycycline** 200 mg/day for 4 weeks, or 100 mg/day for 6 weeks, followed by one dose of **ivermectin** after 4–6 months (children aged > 9 years).
- If a strong macrofilaricidal effect is desired, give **doxycycline** 200 mg/day for 6 weeks, followed by one dose of ivermectin after 4–6 months.

Patients with onchocerciasis who do have a high *Loa loa* microfilaraemia may be treated with **doxycycline** 200 mg daily for 6 weeks, unless contraindicated. If they are under 9 years of age, in which case doxycycline is contraindicated, *Loa loa* microfilaraemia must be reduced by treatment with **albendazole** prior to treatment with **ivermectin**.

Surgical removal of head nodules (nodulectomy) was advised in the past in an attempt to reduce the likelihood of eye disease. There is no guarantee that this will eliminate the risk of eye disease, because not all nodules are evident, and the remaining nodules continue to produce microfilariae. Improved drug treatment has reduced the justification for nodulectomy.

Control

There has been rapid progress in the past 30 years, largely due to successful international public–private partnerships, sustained funding for regional programmes, and technical advances.

Initial efforts in vector control using the organophosphate larvicide **temephos** proved inadequate.

A major breakthrough came with Merck's donation of ivermectin. Thereafter larviciding was abandoned in favour of regular mass drug treatment.

The African Programme for Onchocerciasis Control (APOC) is a Community-Directed Treatment with Ivermectin (CDTI) programme that aims to treat over 90 million people annually in 19 countries, protecting an at-risk population of 115 million, and should prevent over 40 000 cases of blindness every year. High-risk foci of *Loa loa* are currently excluded from community ivermectin programmes.

The Onchocerciasis Elimination Programme for the Americas (OEPA) adopts a similar approach to APOC, except that ivermectin is administered twice a year until transmission has been interrupted. By the end of 2012, transmission of the infection, judged by surveys following WHO guidelines, had been interrupted or eliminated in four of the six endemic countries in the WHO Americas Region.

6.3.C.h Strongyloidiasis

BOX 6.3.C.H.1 Minimum standards
- Hygiene, sanitation and shoes are useful in prevention.
- Ivermectin is the treatment of choice.
- Albendazole.

Introduction

This parasite affects 50–100 million people worldwide, and occurs in warm, wet, tropical and subtropical regions where sanitation is poor. *Strongyloides stercoralis* is the main species infecting humans. However, *Strongyloides fülleborni*, which is principally a parasite of primates, also occurs in humans in Africa and Papua New Guinea.

Human infection is due to percutaneous penetration of filariform larvae in contaminated soil. Filariform larvae travel via the lungs to the small intestine, where they develop into adults and penetrate the duodenal and jejunal mucosa. Fertilised females produce eggs which hatch in the intestinal mucosa and release the first-stage rhabditiform larvae, which are excreted in faeces. In favourable conditions, the rhabditiform larvae transform into infectious filariform larvae within 48 hours, and remain viable in the soil for weeks.

An important feature of *Strongyloides* is auto-infection. This occurs when rhabditiform larvae transform into infectious dwarf filariform larvae in the gut lumen and penetrate the mucosa or the peri-anal skin. Infection may persist for decades without further exposure. Person-to-person transmission may also occur.

Clinical features

Initial skin penetration may cause itching, urticaria and sometimes a snake-like (serpiginous) rash. Migration through the lungs may cause cough, wheeze and evidence of pneumonitis. Invasion of the small bowel may cause abdominal pain, vomiting, malabsorption and paralytic ileus.

Chronic infection is often asymptomatic, but may cause intermittent abdominal pain, diarrhoea and urticaria. Malabsorption and a protein-losing enteropathy may occur. A transient, intensely itchy serpiginous rash, known as 'larva currens' or 'creeping eruption', may appear on the trunk, buttocks or elsewhere.

Episodic pneumonitis and, more rarely, a reactive arthritis may occur.

Strongyloides hyperinfection syndrome

One of the major dangers associated with *Strongyloides* infection occurs as a result of massive auto-infection. Risk factors include immunosuppression induced by various drugs, including corticosteroids, or associated with diseases such as malignancies (particularly leukaemia and lymphoma), severe malnutrition and severe infections, including advanced AIDS and human T-cell leukaemia virus type 1 (HTLV-1).

Hyperinfection syndrome may present with severe diarrhoea, often with blood in the stool. Bowel inflammation with micro-perforations may give rise to paralytic ileus, peritonitis and Gram-negative septicaemia. Proliferation and dissemination of larvae and enteropathogens may cause widespread pathology, including endocarditis, pneumonitis and meningitis.

All patients with a history of possible exposure to *Strongyloides* should be screened before being treated with any drugs that cause immunosuppression. Those at significant risk should be treated empirically even if investigations are negative.

Investigations

Eggs are rarely found in the stool, and larvae may be difficult to identify. Stool culture (e.g. on charcoal or agar) is recommended.

Larvae may be seen in duodenal aspirates or using the string capsule technique (Enterotest).

Larvae may also be found in sputum, CSF and urine in hyper-infection syndrome.

Serology is useful for immune-competent patients who are not normally resident in an endemic area. However, interpretation of a positive test may be a problem due to cross-reactions with filarial antigens.

Eosinophilia is common in immune-competent patients, but may be absent in hyperinfection syndrome.

Treatment

Ivermectin is the drug of choice for children over 5 years old or weighing more than 15 kg. An oral dose of 200 micrograms/kg/day for 2 days gives excellent results.

Albendazole 400 mg every 12 hours for 7 days may also be effective, and can be used in children over 2 years of age.

Hyperinfection syndrome can be very difficult to manage. There may be problems with administration or absorption of oral medication, and no IV or IM preparations of ivermectin or albendazole are licensed for use in humans. However, parenteral ivermectin, available as a veterinary preparation, has been administered subcutaneously in the successful treatment of *Strongyloides* hyperinfection. Patients with hyper-infection syndrome also require treatment for Gram-negative septicaemia.

Prevention and control
- Improve hygiene and sanitation.
- Wear shoes.
- Avoid contact with contaminated soil.

Section 7

Major injuries in pregnancy and childhood

7.1 Wounds and their management

BOX 7.1.1 Minimum standards
- ■ Analgesia.
- ■ Sutures.
- ■ Adhesive strips/tissue glues.
- ■ Human anti-tetanus immunoglobulin.
- ■ Tetanus toxoid (or DTP, Td).
- ■ Antibiotics.

Management of major injuries using the APLS/ATLS system

Before wounds are treated, if there are other injuries, the whole patient must be assessed according to the APLS/ATLS system (*see also* Section 1.11).

Primary survey and resuscitation
- Assess:
  - — Airway and cervical spine control
  - — Breathing
  - — Circulation and haemorrhage control
  - — Disability
  - — Exposure.
- Identify and correct life-threatening abnormalities.
- Resuscitate and stabilise vital functions.

Secondary survey and emergency treatments

Remember that if simple resuscitative measures do not stabilise the child, operative intervention may be necessary before a formal secondary survey is done. In the secondary survey, determine the full extent of all injuries to the head, face, neck, chest, abdomen, pelvis, spine and extremities.

Have an emergency treatment plan to give emergency treatments in order of priority.

Definitive care

The definitive care of major injuries, which include wounds, is often carried out by teams that have not been involved in the resuscitation and emergency treatments. Good communication is essential, using:
- legible and detailed notes
- prompt and efficient transfer to a unit which can provide the definitive care (this may be an inter-hospital transfer)
- a clear handover summary.

Wounds

Definition

In a medico-legal context, to wound is to destroy, however superficially or minutely, a bodily surface, be it skin or mucous membrane. A contusion (bruise) is excluded.

Nature of injuries causing wounds
- Kinetic energy (impacts): from any object of any material purposefully or accidentally impacting.
- Heat: from any heated solid, liquid or gas.

- Cold: from any cooled solid, liquid or gas.
- Chemical: acids and alkalis predominate.
- Electrical: can cause significant internal injury.

Types of wounds
- Abrasion: friction injury, also known as graze.
- Laceration: blunt injury.
- Incision: injury from a sharp object.
- Stab: injury from a knife, scissors, screwdriver, poker, etc., usually penetrating in nature.
- Needlestick.
- Bite: human or animal (*see* Sections 6.2.H and 7.5).
- Firearm: shotgun, rifle, revolver or pistol (*see* Section 7.3.H).
- Blast (*see* Section 7.3.G).
- Burn (*see* Section 7.3.I.a and I.b).

It is important to remember that a variety of types of wounds may coexist following a single incident.

Assessment of minor wounds

Assessment of each wound should include the following:
- nature of the injury causing the wound
- type of wound
- wound site: size, shape, position and depth
- relevant motor function
- relevant sensation
- circulation distal to the wound.

Associated features include the following:
- erythema (redness)
- oedema (swelling)
- contusion (bruise)
- **surgical emphysema: this needs urgent specialist care**
- tenderness: if this extends beyond the area of the wound, a fracture may be present (*see* Section 7.2)
- pain.

General assessment includes the following:
- allergies
- immunisation status
- intercurrent illness
- medication
- past medical history
- time of last meal.

General principles
- After assessment of pain, give appropriate analgesia (*see* Section 1.15).
- If a radiopaque foreign body may be present, arrange an X-ray.
- The most important local treatment for all wounds is vigorous cleaning with sterile saline to remove dirt and possible pathogenic organisms (after analgesia).

- Local, regional or general anaesthesia may be needed to achieve optimal cleaning (*see* Section 1.24).
- Superficial palpable foreign bodies should be removed as soon as possible.
- Removal of deeper foreign bodies may need specialist advice.
- **Dead or damaged tissue must be excised.** Specialist advice is needed if this involves more than a very small area of skin or mucous membrane.
- If tendons or nerves have been damaged, specialised care is needed.

Tetanus prevention

Give tetanus prophylaxis if the patient is **not immunised** or is **not fully immunised** (full immunisation is 5 doses of tetanus toxoid: 3 for the primary immunisation in infancy, one before school entry and one before leaving school). Wounds particularly prone to tetanus are those sustained more than six hours prior to presentation, those of puncture type, those with much devitalised tissue, those that appear septic, those associated with a compound fracture or foreign body and those contaminated with soil or dung. These wounds may need human anti-tetanus immunoglobulin (HATI), 250–500 units IM, depending on the patient's tetanus status and the degree of contamination or devitalisation of the wound.

If the child has received anti-tetanus immunisation in the past, a single extra dose of tetanus toxoid IM (or, if they are due additional immunisation boosters, the relevant combination) should be given.

TABLE 7.1.1 Need for tetanus immunoglobulin and/or tetanus toxoid after a wound

History of tetanus vaccination		Type of wound	Tetanus vaccine booster (see below)	Tetanus immunoglobulin
≥ 3 doses	< 5 years since last dose	All wounds	No	No
	5–10 years since last dose	Clean minor wounds	No	No
		All other wounds	Yes	No
	> 10 years since last dose	All wounds	Yes	No
< 3 doses or uncertain		Clean minor wounds	Yes	No
		All other wounds	Yes	Yes

Note: if a patient has not completed the 5 tetanus doses when they are injured, it is likely they have also not completed other immunisation schedules. If possible give a combined immunisation comprising, for example, DTaP, DTP or DTaP – IPV for young children and Td for older children or adults according to local immunisation schedules.

Antibiotics

There is no substitute for thorough cleaning of wounds and for careful debridement of any devitalised tissue. However, in addition to cleaning and to tetanus prophylaxis, some wounds will need antibiotics. These will include wounds that have presented late and already are infected. Do not close these wounds but pack with sterile gauze dampened with sterile normal saline and review after antibiotic treatment for possible delayed primary closure after excision of the wound edges if feasible, or secondary closure.

Oral antibiotics to choose include flu/cloxacillin 25–50 mg/kg four times a day or co-amoxyclav 125/31 mg three times a day for 1–6 years or 250/62 mg three times a day for 6–12 years. Co-amoxyclav is effective in bite injuries. A five day course is usually sufficient.

Specific injuries
Abrasions

- After thorough cleaning and debridement, leave abrasions exposed or cover them for 5 days with vaseline gauze.
- If debris is left in an abrasion, epithelium will grow over it and 'tattooing' will occur.

Lacerations and incisions

- Only clean fresh wounds should be closed immediately, preferably only less than 6 hours old, certainly less than 12 hours old.
- **Distal-based flap lacerations may need specialist care if the blood supply is poor.**
- To close superficial wounds, adhesive strips and tissue glues are excellent, but these must not be used for deeper wounds, in which cavities will be created and healing will not occur.
- Close deeper wounds in layers without tension.
- Close skin with interrupted sutures, ideally using monofilament material.
- If the wound is compound (associated with a fracture), an antibiotic should be given to prevent osteomyelitis (*see* Section 5.17).
- Arrange for removal of sutures at the times shown in Table 7.1.2.
- Younger patients heal more quickly. Malnourished patients take longer to heal.

TABLE 7.1.2 Times for removal of sutures

Site	Days
Face	4
Scalp and neck	5–7
Hand (flexor surface)	5–7
Trunk and arms (not extensor surfaces)	5–7
Legs (not extensor surfaces)	7–10
Hands (extensor surfaces)	7–10
Elbows and knees	10–14

Fingertip injuries

- Preserve maximum length.
- If the tip is amputated distal to the bone, regeneration will occur if the wound is kept clean and moist under paraffin gauze dressings changed weekly.

- Other principles of treatment are the same as for lacerations and incised wounds.

Tongue lacerations
- Most stop bleeding spontaneously and do not need sutures.
- Repair under general anaesthesia if there is profuse bleeding or the full thickness of tongue is involved.
- Use absorbable sutures.

Stab wounds
- **Stabbing may cause serious penetrating injuries to deep structures, which may lead to rapid death from haemorrhage or air embolus.**
- The external dimensions of a stab wound may be deceptively small compared with the damage to underlying structures.
- Superficial stab wounds are treated in the same way as lacerations and incised wounds.
- Patients with penetrating wounds need resuscitation and emergency exploration under general anaesthesia.
- Never remove the penetrating object until the patient has been resuscitated and is in a secure surgical environment with cross-matched blood available.

Needlestick injuries
- If there is **skin puncture**, encourage bleeding and wash the wound thoroughly with plenty of soap and water. Dry the wound and apply a dry dressing if appropriate.
- If there is only **skin contact**, wash the wound with plenty of soap and water but do not scrub it. Scrubbing may damage the skin.
- If there is **splashing into the mouth**, rinse with plenty of water.
- If there is **splashing into the eye**, rinse with plenty of water. Obtain the help of a colleague to do this.

- If the identity of the donor (the person whose blood is on the needle) is known, try to find out whether that person has hepatitis B and/or HIV infection.
- Consider immunisation for hepatitis B and triple therapy for HIV if these are available.

Complications of wounds
Retained foreign body
- This will cause swelling beneath the wound.
- Secondary infection is more likely if there is a retained foreign body. If the foreign body is superficial, it must be removed by a competent surgeon under local anaesthetic. A general anaesthetic will be required if the foreign body is deeply placed and/or in an area with important structures, such as the hand or face.

Infection
- Tetanus: this is most likely to occur if the wound has been contaminated with soil and/or manure and the child is not fully immunised (see above).
- Bacterial. Prophylactic antibiotics such as flu/cloxacillin or co-amoxyclav should be considered in cases where wounds have been contaminated, **but this does not lessen the need for thorough cleaning of such wounds.**
- Antibiotic doses: flu/cloxacillin 25–50 mg/kg four times a day or co-amoxyclav 125/31 mg three times a day for 1–6 years or 250/62 mg three times a day for 6–12 years. Co-amoxyclav is effective in bite injuries. A five day course is usually sufficient.

Delayed healing
- This may be due to poor apposition of the edges, malnutrition and/or infection.
- Excision of the edges of the wound and secondary suture may be helpful, except in malnutrition.

7.2 Fractures in children

BOX 7.2.1 Minimum standards
- X-rays.
- Splints.
- Plaster of Paris bandages.
- Traction.
- External and internal fixation.
- Physiotherapy.

Introduction

As any parent knows, all children are susceptible to injury. However, children in resource-limited countries are probably more at risk than their developed-world counterparts, as they often live in less regulated and protective environments. Once injured, there may be a considerable delay in their presentation to a healthcare facility, a situation that can complicate and restrict treatment options.

Scarce X-ray resources and a limited range of treatment modalities can then further complicate treatment of paediatric fractures.

However, on a more optimistic note it can be said that paediatric fractures are often more 'forgiving' when compared to those of the adult; they are often easier to reduce, less requiring of internal fixation, are quicker to unite and, due to the potential for remodelling with continued skeletal growth greater degrees of mal-union can be tolerated.

Diagnosis

Certain features of the history and examination may suggest the presence of a fracture:

- history of a significant traumatic event
- swelling
- bruising
- deformity
- loss of function: inability to move or weight-bear
- bony crepitus at the fracture site
- consider the possibility of child abuse (see Section 7.6) if the fracture appears inconsistent with the history given or with the child's developmental status.

Open fractures

Open fractures occur where the fracture site communicates with a laceration or break in the skin relating to it. There is potential for the introduction of contaminants and resultant infection. Often open fractures are the result of a greater degree of violence than is the case for closed fractures.

Open fractures are graded according to the Gustilo classification:

- grade 1: skin wound of < 1 cm with minimal soft-tissue injury
- grade 2: skin wound of > 1 cm, with moderate soft tissue injury
- grade 3: these wounds typically involve a far greater degree of violence and energy transfer. This is further subdivided into:
  - A: extensive wound > 10 cm with crushed tissue and contamination but for which soft-tissue coverage is usually possible.
  - B: extensive wound > 10 cm, again with crushed tissue and contamination, but where it is not thought that local soft-tissue coverage is possible, and therefore a **regional** or **free** flap may be necessary.
  - C: any open fracture with an associated major vascular injury requiring repair for limb salvage.

Treatment is dictated by the extent of soft-tissue injury as reflected in the above grading system. The initial priority is a thorough debridement and copious irrigation of the fracture site in order to reduce the burden of contamination and lower the risk of infective sequelae. Once this has been done, some form of stabilisation is necessary. Internal fixation of open fractures carries a considerable risk of infection. Safer options are plaster application (with or without windowing to expose the wound) or external fixation.

It is often useful for a photograph of an open fracture to be taken by the initial assessor (perhaps on a mobile phone) so that the wound can remain covered until the patient is in the operating theatre. It helps to prevent frequent opening of the dressings and infection.

Compartment syndrome

The associated soft-tissue injury and subsequent swelling leads to an elevation of interstitial pressure within a closed fascial compartment, which results in microvascular compromise. If left untreated, tissue necrosis will occur. The commonest site is in the lower leg, but compartment syndromes can also occur in the thigh, foot and upper limb. The signs and symptoms of compartment syndrome include the following:

- a hard woody swollen extremity
- severe pain on passive movement
- tingling or burning sensations (paraesthesia) in the skin
- pain out of proportion to the severity of the fracture and not relieved by splinting or analgesia

- numbness or paralysis (loss of movement) and absent distal pulses are late signs.

Although it is possible to monitor intra-compartment pressures, such technology will rarely be available. The alternative is to have a high index of suspicion for fractures involving significant soft-tissue injury, and regularly review the clinical condition of the limb.

Treatment of compartment syndrome is by prompt surgical fasciotomies to decompress the affected compartments. In the lower leg there are four muscular compartments separated by strong fascia:

1. the lateral compartment containing the peroneal muscles
2. the anterior compartment containing the dorsiflexor muscles of the ankle and toes
3. the superficial posterior compartment containing the gastrocnemius and soleus muscles
4. the deep posterior compartment containing the deep plantar flexors of the ankle and toes.

The lateral and anterior compartments can be decompressed through the same antero-lateral longitudinal incision. A single postero-medial incision can be used for the deep and superficial posterior compartments. In each case the fascial envelope containing the muscle group must be incised along its length in order to permit swelling and prevent the build-up of pressure within the compartment.

X-rays

X-rays are the most useful and specific diagnostic modality. Where possible, two orthogonal X-rays (at 90 degrees to each other) should be obtained, ideally including the joints above and below the suspected fracture site. Terms relating to fracture appearance on X-ray include the following:

- transverse: at 90 degrees to the long axis of the bone
- oblique: other than the above
- simple: involving a single fracture line
- comminuted: involving bony fragmentation
- greenstick: visible fracture at only one cortex on the X-ray view. Greenstick fractures are only seen in paediatric fractures, due to the flexible nature of paediatric bone; this implies intact periosteum along the opposite side to the fracture and is a good prognostic sign.

Salter–Harris classification

This relates to the X-ray pattern of fractures occurring around the epiphysis, or growth plate, of a bone. Such fractures occur in about 15–20% of major long bone fractures and 34% of hand fractures in childhood.

There are five grades, with increasingly poor prognosis for fracture outcome with increasing grade because of an increasing degree of damage to the growth plate. This will lead to limb shortening as the child grows.

1. Fracture across the epiphyseal line, not extending into the epiphysis or metaphysis. This occurs when the growth plate is very thick, and thus tends to be seen in young children. Healing is rapid and complications are rare.
2. Fracture across the epiphyseal line extending into the metaphysis, but not into the epiphysis. This usually occurs in children over the age of 10 years. Healing is usually rapid and there is rarely growth disturbance.
3. Fracture extending completely across the epiphyseal line

and into the epiphysis. This type of fracture can occur at any age and is associated with a poor prognosis.

4 Fracture extending from the metaphysis through the growth plate and into the epiphysis. This type of fracture occurs when the growth plate is partially fused, and it has a poorer prognosis.

5 Crush injury to the growth plate. This is caused by severe axial loading during a fall from a height. Inevitably there is partial destruction of the epiphyseal plate, and thus a considerable risk of growth disturbance.

Treatment of fractures

- **Reduce** the fracture (if displaced).
- **Hold** the fracture while bony healing occurs.
- **Rehabilitate:** restore function and range of motion.

The potential for remodelling with continued skeletal growth is more marked in younger children. It occurs to a greater degree in the plane of movement of the affected joint. As a result of remodelling, angular deformity can gradually resolve with growth, and thus accurate initial reduction is not mandatory. In contrast, it is important to accurately reduce intra-articular fractures in order to prevent secondary arthrosis.

Children will often be unable to tolerate reduction under local anaesthesia. General anaesthetic will usually be required (see Section 1.24).

Once reduced, the fracture needs to be held in position while bony union occurs.

During reduction of fractures, particularly in the lower limb, rotation of the limb should be checked clinically and compared with the opposite limb. X-rays, although useful for judging angulation, length and translation, are not very helpful for judging rotation.

Splintage

Splintage of a fracture involves immobilising the fracture, thereby preventing relative motion of the bone ends. In the

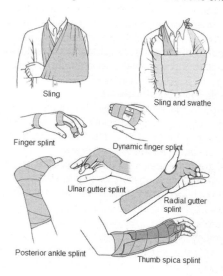

FIGURE 7.2.1 Slings and splints for childhood fractures. From the Merck Manual Home Health Handbook, edited by Robert Porter. © 2010-11 Merck Sharp & Dohme Corp., a subsidiary of Merck & Co, Inc, Whitehouse Station, NJ. Available at: www.merckmanuals.com/home/ (accessed 5/8/14).

acute phase, this will help to relieve the pain associated with the fracture. In the longer term, the fracture stability conferred by the splint will help to promote bony union.

The commonest form of splintage uses plaster of Paris bandages (see plastercraft below). If these are not available preformed, then it is possible to make them from crepe bandages and calcium sulphate. The bandages can be applied in the form of a complete (circumferential) cast or as a backslab, along only one side of the injured limb.

In any situation where swelling is anticipated, a complete cast should either be bivalved or split down to skin along its length.

In some circumstances, plaster of Paris may not be available. If this is the case, splints can often be fashioned from locally available materials. One example of this is the use of strips of bamboo and bandaging.

The splint should be applied with the limb in the position of function. Then if stiffness does occur the limb will still have some use. For the elbow, this position is 90 degrees of flexion. For the ankle, a position of neutral plantar/dorsiflexion (the sole of the foot at 90 degrees to the lower leg) is preferred.

Plastercraft

Before starting to apply a plaster, all of the necessary equipment should be ready to hand. The limb should be covered in stockinette, if available, and then cotton wool. Bony prominences (ankle malleoli, fibular head, wrist, olecranon) should be covered with extra padding to prevent pressure sores.

The plaster bandage should be immersed in water for about 5 seconds, by which time bubbles should have stopped rising from the plaster. Cold water is usually best, but hot water causes the plaster to set faster, so the temperature should be adjusted according to need.

For plaster slabs, the length required should have been premeasured and then the slab made up in readiness, most slabs requiring a thickness of between 5 and 10 layers of plaster bandage. Once dipped, the slab should be applied to the limb over the layer of cotton wool and then bandaged into place.

For circumferential casts, the bandage should be unwound half a turn before dipping, with the roll held in one hand and the free end in the other. After immersion, excess water should be allowed to fall from the plaster, but it should not be wrung or squeezed, as this will result in a plaster that is too dry to make a good cast. The plaster bandage can then be wound around the injured limb, with each turn overlapping the previous one by about two-thirds. Twists and turns in the plaster should be avoided, as these can constrict the limb. Once the plaster bandage has been applied, the limb should be held still until the plaster sets.

If proprietary plaster of Paris bandages are not available, it is possible to make them using gauze bandages and plaster. Medicinal-grade plaster (calcium sulphate PBC) is ideal, but failing this, building plaster can be used. The plaster should be sprinkled on to an unrolled bandage that is **just damp** (so that the plaster adheres). The bandage can then be rolled up and used in a similar way to a commercially available plaster bandage.

Once set, a useful technique is to write, with broad marker pen, the details of the fracture on the plaster cast as a so-called 'fracture passport'. These details can include the date of the fracture, the date when the plaster was applied, the intended date of removal, and even a sketch of the fracture configuration itself. This information can be invaluable for subsequent care, as notes and X-rays can easily be mislaid or lost.

Wedging of the plaster can be useful for improving reduction of the fracture.

Traction

An alternative to splintage is traction. By exerting a pull along the axis of the injured bone, traction helps to effect reduction and maintain alignment. Traction can either represent a definitive mode of treatment and be maintained until bony union, or be temporary, being maintained only until the fracture is stable enough to be treated in a plaster cast. Several types of traction exist.

- **Skin traction:** Traction is exerted on the limb by means of a bandage (usually adhesive) applied around the limb.
- **Balanced traction:** Traction of the more distal part of the limb is maintained by reaction against a more proximal structure. The classic example is the Thomas' splint for femoral fractures, where the splint is braced against the ipsilateral ischial tuberosity.
- **Skeletal traction:** Traction is exerted by means of a pin inserted into bone distal to the fracture. An example is a traction pin inserted through the proximal tibia as treatment for a femoral fracture. In the paediatric context, care should be exercised to avoid growth plates when inserting the traction pins.

Traction methods of treatment are most applicable to fractures of the lower limb, but there are occasional circumstances in which these methods are used in the upper limb. One example is temporary skin traction for a supracondylar fracture of the humerus.

External fixation

This involves stabilising the fracture by means of an external scaffold which is fixed to the bones proximal and distal to the fracture by means of threaded pins. It is relevant to unstable compound fractures, particularly those with extensive soft-tissue wounding. Several different types of fixator exist. The pins can be sited away from bone growth plates and the fracture reduced prior to the linking bar being tightened. Following application of the fixator, the pin tracks must be cleaned daily with saline in order to prevent the build-up of crust, infection of the track and secondary osteomyelitis. The fixator can remain in position until bony union occurs, or be replaced by a plaster cast once the fracture becomes stable enough to tolerate this and/or the soft-tissue wound heals.

A variant of external fixation is percutaneous K-wiring, usually used in conjunction with plaster casting. Particularly relevant to peri-articular fractures, this involves the insertion of smooth K-wires across the fracture line in order to prevent secondary displacement. The external ends of the wires should be bent to prevent migration. The wires can be removed once fracture stability permits, typically at 2–3 weeks. In the absence of K-wires, improvisation using long K-wires-type needles is possible.

Internal fixation

This involves the use of screws, plates and other types of metalwork to rigidly hold the reduction of a fracture.

Although these techniques permit accurate stable reduction, there is an associated risk of infection of the fixation device. Thus, when considering this form of treatment, the following should be borne in mind:

- The fracture should warrant internal fixation, as opposed to splintage, traction or external fixation.
- There should be an adequate supply of the metalwork in a full range of sizes and the required instruments for their insertion. For a sustainable fracture treatment philosophy, **a constant supply of fixation devices needs to be available**.
- The surgeon should be trained in the application of the device and in the surgical approach necessary for it.
- The fixation devices and tools should be sterile and the level of asepsis in the operating theatre must be high.
- In some cases, intra-operative X-ray guidance (fluoroscopy) is necessary for accurate fixation.
- Intramedullary methods of fixation, popular in well-resourced countries for the fixation of adult long bone fractures, are rarely appropriate in paediatric cases, as they violate the epiphyseal plates, potentially resulting in growth disturbance.

The decision to use this method of fixation will be based on a risk-benefit analysis with consideration given to the fracture configuration, the age of the child, the operative resources available and the training of the surgeon involved.

Ongoing fracture care

Once reduction and stabilisation of the fracture have occurred, ongoing care is required to monitor the progress of the fracture to union. The treating physician should document the treatment provided and estimate the duration of immobilisation needed. Where the provision of notes and X-rays is limited, one suggestion is to draw the fracture on the surface of the plaster cast along with the intended date of removal.

At initial follow-up, the quality of the plaster cast should be inspected and X-rays taken (where possible) to ensure that secondary displacement has not occurred. The overall duration of immobilisation required is dependent upon the age of the patient and the fracture configuration. Determination of bony union involves the removal of the plaster cast or external fixation device (after an appropriate time period during which union would have been predicted to occur) and the gentle stressing of the fracture site. The presence of persistent tenderness, swelling or abnormal movement all indicate that union has yet to occur. The extent of fracture callus on X-ray is also indicative of the state of union.

Rehabilitation

Children rarely need dedicated physical therapy following fracture healing. They should be encouraged to move their joints through a full range of motion, and exercises should be prescribed to restore muscle bulk.

Specific fractures
Femoral shaft

Closed femoral shaft fractures in children are usually best treated with traction, with the type dependent on the age of the child. Typically the duration required is 1 week per year of age, but this can be shortened by transfer into a plaster hip spica once fracture stability permits.

- Age 0–2 years and weight under 12 kg: Gallows traction, thighs in 45-degree flexion and hips 30-degree abduction. Limb length inequality is seldom a problem as fracture does not shorten excessively. Shortening of up to 1.5 cm and angulation of up to 30 degrees is acceptable. Early spica casting is often possible. **This fracture is associated with non-accidental injury in 50–80% of cases at this age.**
- Age 2–10 years: Skin traction, either in the 90/90 position (hip and knee flexed to 90 degrees) or Perkins type (straight traction). Alternatively, especially in the older members of this group, skeletal traction through a distal femoral traction pin; again either in the 90/90 position or straight. Up to 2 cm of bayonet shortening can be tolerated with no adverse effects. Early spica casting can be used if the position is acceptable. With skin traction the weight used should not exceed 5 kg, but with skeletal traction up to 10% of body weight can be applied.
- Age 10–15 years: Skeletal traction, either in 90/90 position or straight. There is a much greater risk of shortening in this group, and less potential for subsequent growth acceleration and length equalisation.
- Above the age of 15 years, children can be treated as adults.

Tibial shaft

Closed tibial shaft fractures in children are usually uncomplicated, and can be treated satisfactorily with closed reduction and long leg cast application.

- The cast should be applied with the knee in 5–10 degrees of flexion.
- In comparison to the femur there is less potential for overgrowth and thus it is important to maintain the fracture out to length, that is, to ensure that the length of the fractured limb is the same length as the uninjured side. Acceptable degrees of shortening are 5–10 mm in the 0–5 years age group, but aim for none in any older age group.
- Acceptable axial alignment is less than 10 degrees of recurvatum (where the apex of the fracture site points posteriorly) and less than 5 degrees of varus or valgus angulation.
- As union progresses it may be possible to convert the long leg cast to a patellar tendon bearing cast after 3 weeks.
- Undisplaced fractures in children aged 1–5 years can often be treated in below-knee casts or even below-knee plaster cylinders.

Distal humeral

Supracondylar fractures of the humerus have the highest rate of complications and some of the poorest results of treatment of all paediatric fractures. They are also difficult to diagnose without an X-ray. The peak incidence is at the age of 6 or 7 years.

- The vast majority (98%) are extension type, featuring a posteriorly displaced distal part. Only 2% are flexion type, resulting from a fall on to the point of the elbow.
- A careful assessment of distal vascularity should be made. In fractures with posterolateral displacement, the medial humeral spike can tether the brachial artery.
- If distal pulses are absent, closed reduction should be

attempted. If this fails to restore pulses, immediate open reduction and surgical exploration of the brachial artery should be performed.

- In other displaced fractures with palpable distal pulses, closed reduction should be attempted, possibly combined with percutaneous pin fixation for unstable fractures.
- Acceptable reductions will have no more than 4 degrees of varus as determined by Baumann's angle on the antero-posterior radiograph. Additionally, the axis of the capitellum should be at 45 degrees to the humeral shaft.
- If an acceptable position is not obtained, this may be an indication for open reduction and percutaneous K-wire fixation.
- Alternatively, the limb can be placed on traction in extension. As the swelling subsides, it will become easier to effect a closed reduction (with or without K-wiring).
- Once reduced, an above-elbow plaster backslab should be applied with the elbow flexed. Flexion above 90 degrees will assist in maintaining the reduction of extension-type fractures, but care should be taken to ensure that distal pulses are maintained.
- Ideally, X-rays should be taken on a weekly basis to ensure that reduction is maintained. The plaster cast can be completed once swelling has resolved, and percutaneous wires can be removed after 3 weeks.
- The typical duration of immobilisation necessary for union is 4–5 weeks in the 0–5 years age group and 6–7 weeks in the 5–10 years age group.

Forearm fractures

- Both types of bone paediatric forearm fractures typically result from the indirect violence of a fall on an outstretched hand. They may be greenstick or complete. If the periosteal sleeve is disrupted the fractures may be unstable.
- X-rays should include the wrist and elbow, as the integrity of the proximal and distal radio-ulnar joints needs to be determined.
- Be aware of the possibility of a Monteggia fracture, which consists of dislocation of the radial head along with fracture of the ulna.
- In contrast to adult forearm fractures, the majority of these injuries can be treated by closed reduction and plaster immobilisation.
- Up to the age of 9 years, acceptable reduction can be defined as anything less than 15 degrees of displacement and 45 degrees of malrotation.
- Above 9 years, at least bayonet apposition is required with less than 30 degrees of malrotation, less than 10 degrees angulation if the fracture is proximal or less than 15 degrees if it is distal.
- Immediately following fracture union, there may be a cosmetic deformity if the above reduction criteria are utilised, but this deformity should remodel if there is over 2 years of skeletal growth remaining.
- Following reduction, an assessment of forearm supination and pronation should be undertaken to ensure that there is no block.
- The arm should be immobilised in an above-elbow cast with the elbow flexed to 90 degrees. Opinion varies as to the position of the wrist in the cast. Some surgeons place the wrist in neutral supination/pronation for all fractures, others placing it in supination for proximal

third fractures, neutral for middle third and pronation for distal third.

- Follow-up X-rays should be taken at 1- and 2-week intervals following manipulation to ensure that secondary displacement has not occurred. If displacement does occur, re-manipulation can be attempted.
- Some very unstable fractures may prove difficult to treat by closed methods. These may benefit from intramedullary pinning (Rush pins) or cross K-wiring if facilities exist for this **(intra-operative fluoroscopy is required)**.

Distal radial ('wrist') fractures

- Children's distal radial fractures are usually the result of a fall on the outstretched hand, and are rarely intra-articular.
- Common types include the following:
  - Galeazzi fracture (isolated fracture of the distal radius) implies associated disruption of the distal radio-ulnar joint.
  - Physeal fracture (pattern of injury described by the Salter-Harris classification)
  - Torus (buckling of the cortex on the compression side of the fracture without angulation).
  - Greenstick fracture (incomplete fracture).

- In children these fractures can almost always be treated with closed reduction and plaster immobilisation.
- The reduction manoeuvre is to hyperextend the wrist, followed by traction and 'hinging' of the distal fragment over the fracture site.
- Acceptable reduction can be defined as anything less than complete displacement and slight angulation. As in forearm fractures, cosmetic deformity should remodel if more than 2 years of skeletal growth remain.
- Check X-rays should be taken at 1 and 2 weeks post-reduction to exclude secondary displacement.
- The duration of immobilisation required depends upon the fracture configuration and the age of the child, but is typically 3–5 weeks.

Conclusions

- Most paediatric fractures can be treated by closed methods.
- Very often the periosteal sleeve will be intact, leading to enhanced fracture stability.
- Completely accurate reduction is not always necessary, as children's bones have the potential to remodel with continued skeletal growth.

7.3   Life-threatening trauma

7.3.A Structured approach to trauma in pregnancy and childhood

> **BOX 7.3.A.1 Minimum standards**
> - Triage.
> - Structured approach: primary assessment and resuscitation, and then secondary assessment and emergency treatment.
> - Availability of emergency surgery or safe transport system.
> - Oxygen.
> - Blood transfusion service.
> - Chest drain.
> - Analgesia.
> - High-dependency care.
> - Tetanus immunoglobulin and toxoid.
> - Mannitol or hypertonic saline.
> - Tranexamic acid.

Introduction

Most regions of the world are experiencing an epidemic of trauma, but the most serious increase has been in the resource-limited countries.

Proliferation of roads and increased use of vehicles have led to an increase in injuries and deaths, and many peripheral medical facilities find themselves faced with multiple casualties from bus crashes or other disasters. Severe burns and drownings have always been more common in middle- and low-income countries.

There are a number of important differences between high- and low-income countries:

- use of open fires and kerosene stoves for cooking and heating
- unsafe water storage practices and unsupervised play in water courses, lakes and ponds by young children
- poor or absent flood defences, making poor people much more vulnerable to natural disasters
- poorly maintained road networks and vehicles, contributing to a higher injury rate per distance travelled in low-income countries
- the absence of a paramedic-manned emergency ambulance service to give life-saving medical care at the scene
- the great distances over which the injured may have to be transported, and therefore the time taken for them to reach medical care, thus losing the opportunity to prevent secondary damage caused by hypoxia and hypovolaemia
- the absence of appropriate equipment, supplies, and the

necessary knowledge and skills to manage the injured once they have arrived at a healthcare facility

- the absence of skilled people to operate and service equipment.

Prevention of trauma is by far the best and most cost-effective way forward, but accident prevention has not yet had much impact in low-income countries.

Trauma is the commonest cause of death in children over the age of 5 years in high-income countries, and it is increasing in absolute numbers as well as in ranking in low- and middle-income countries. In the World Health Organization (WHO) 2008 report 'World Report on Child Injury Prevention', the death rate in under 20 year olds from injury was 12.2 per 100 000 in high income countries while in low and middle income countries, the figure was 41.7 per 100 000.

Trauma is also a major cause of disability, especially following head injury, burns and drownings. In high-income countries, road accidents and falls predominate; in low-income countries road traffic accidents are increasing, but there has been no fall in the number of burns, falls and drownings.

Children are less likely than adults to suffer from serious penetrating injuries, although in cities where stabbings and shootings are common, or in armed conflict, such violence spills over into childhood. Intentional injury, in the form of child abuse, also contributes to a significant degree to childhood trauma (*see* Section 7.6).

The patterns of injury and the physiological consequences can be quite different in children compared with adults, reflecting their different size and shape, the elasticity of their body tissues, and the immaturity of their physiological systems.

The key principles of managing major trauma are to

Treat the greatest threat to life first

Do no further harm

AVOID: hypoxia, hypercapnia, hypovolaemia, hypoglycaemia and hypothermia

---

By following a structured approach, problems will be identified and managed in order of priority. The key steps are outlined in the primary assessment and resuscitation, enabling identification and treatment of life-threatening injuries. The secondary assessment identifies all other injuries, and provides emergency treatment for them.

Structured approach
- Primary assessment and resuscitation
- Secondary assessment and emergency treatment
- Definitive care

Primary assessment
- Airway and control of haemorrhage (**and cervical spine control**)
- Breathing
- Circulation **and** continued haemorrhage control

If there is more than one injured patient, then treat the patients in order of priority (*see* Section 1.10).

Management of major trauma

A team leader should be in overall charge of resuscitating a child or pregnant woman or girl who is suffering from major trauma.

Primary assessment and resuscitation

During the primary assessment, assess and resuscitate in sequence – Airway, Breathing and Circulation (ABC) – as these, if compromised, can be an immediate threat to life.

Although the patient may have obvious severe injuries, the clinician's first task is to prevent further deterioration of the patient's condition by ensuring that vital organs, especially the heart and the brain, are supplied with oxygenated blood by ensuring an open airway, adequate breathing and circulation. This is what is meant by **primary assessment and resuscitation**.

Although ABC management is described sequentially, if there are sufficient trained clinicians present, they can be managed at the same time. If there are limited personnel, the approach must be A then B then C. If there is only one trained person available, make use of untrained staff such as ward orderlies or relatives to perform tasks under your supervision. For example, if there is visible severe exsanguinating haemorrhage, once you have identified and controlled it, the ward orderly can continue to apply the pressure while you open the airway and give oxygen, etc. You will need to continually monitor the untrained person's actions to make sure that they are still effective.

The first priority is establishment or maintenance of airway opening, and control of any obvious life-threatening haemorrhage.

Primary Assessment and Resuscitation:

Airway and control of exsanguinating haemorrhage (plus cervical spine control, if appropriate)

Breathing

Circulation

Stop visible external exsanguinating bleeding, if any, by applying direct pressure. This bleeding will be from a superficial artery or large vein. Minor bleeding can be left until the vital ABC have been assessed and resuscitated. Internal bleeding will be dealt with first in 'C' by replacing fluid, and then, if necessary, by emergency surgery.

Open and maintain the airway

We assess the airway patency by assessing its function, which is to allow air to pass through it into the lungs. If the airway is blocked, the lungs will not receive air.

The approach is similar to that used for managing any airway, in that you must:

LOOK for chest movement
- LISTEN for breath sounds
- FEEL for exhaled air
- **Talk to the patient**

If the patient is conscious, a rapid way to assess the airway is to ask them to speak, using the question 'Are you all right?'

A patient who can speak (or, in the case of a baby, who can cry) must have a clear airway.

If the patient is unconscious, airway obstruction is most commonly due to obstruction by the tongue.

The signs of airway obstruction may include:

- snoring or gurgling
- stridor or abnormal breath sounds
- agitation (hypoxia)
- using the accessory muscles of ventilation/paradoxical chest movements
- cyanosis.

Cervical spine protection

In countries where there is no trained emergency ambulance service available to rescue trauma victims at the scene, the risk of an unstable cervical fracture causing permanent spinal cord damage, and subsequent paresis occurring before the patient is brought to medical attention, is high. Therefore any cervical fracture presenting to a medical facility after being brought in by passers-by is likely to be stable.

Fortunately, unstable cervical spinal fractures are relatively uncommon. They are more likely to occur as a result of very severe road traffic accidents or falls from a significant height.

Protect the cervical spine with collar, sand bags and tape if the patient is likely to have an unstable cervical spine.

Definitive treatment requires specialist surgery, and health services in many low-income countries may struggle to access the appropriate service for their population.

It is important to recognise that although protection of the cervical spine may occasionally be beneficial, the opening and maintaining of a clear airway benefits every patient and is an absolute priority.

Cervical spine immobilisation

The cervical spine can be mobilised in three ways:

1 In-line stabilisation: the spine is held in the neutral position (the same as the airway position for an infant; *see* Section 1.12) by the clinician's hands on either side of the patient's head, ensuring that the ears are not covered, as the patient must be able to hear to be reassured and informed. This position must be held until the collar and/ or blocks are in place.

2 A cervical collar can be placed around the neck. Before placing the collar, gently feel around the back of the patient's neck to ascertain if there is any midline tenderness and/or a 'step' indicating a fracture or if there is any bleeding. Collars are manufactured in several sizes to fit different sized patients. They are measured according to the manufacturer's instruction and then gently slid under the neck at the back. The shaped part is placed under the chin at the front, and the collar is fastened with the 'Velcro' tape fastening. This should leave the patient with a firmly held neck in a neutral position. The collar is used by itself in the combative patient, and in conjunction with blocks or sandbags in the unconscious or cooperative patient (i.e. one who will remain still).

3 Sandbags or blocks and tape are usually added after the collar has been fitted. They cannot be used in combative patients as their movements to free themselves will

cause more injury. They are essential in the unconscious patient who has a possibility of neck injury. These objects are placed on either side of the patient's head to prevent lateral movement, and held in place with two tapes, one across the patient's forehead and the other across the chin part of the cervical collar.

Management of the airway

- **Head tilt/chin lift or jaw thrust.** Jaw thrust is recommended in trauma, as it does not require any neck movement. However, if a jaw thrust is unsuccessful, try chin lift with some head tilt. **A closed airway will always be potentially fatal, so the airway takes priority.**
- **Suction/removal of blood, vomit or a foreign body,** if any, but only under direct vision. Do not blindly suck in the mouth or pharynx.
- **If there is no improvement, place an oropharyngeal airway.** Avoid using a nasopharyngeal airway if base of skull injury is suspected.
- **If the airway is still obstructed, a definitive airway by intubation or surgical airway may be needed.**
- Identify the 'at-risk' airway:
  — Altered level of consciousness will fail to protect the airway.
  — Vomiting, with risk of aspiration, is a major risk in pregnancy.
  — Facial trauma, including burns, will continue to worsen as the tissues swell.

Once the airway is open, give high-flow oxygen using a mask and reservoir.

If the airway cannot be maintained and/or protected, consider the need for **advanced airway management**.

Indications for advanced techniques for securing the airway (intubation or surgical airway) include:

- persistent airway obstruction
- a conscious level of ≤ 8 on the Glasgow Coma Scale, or 'P' or 'U' on the AVPU scale (see below for both)
- penetrating neck trauma with haematoma (expanding)
- apnoea
- hypoxia
- severe head injury
- chest trauma
- maxillofacial injury.

Intubation techniques should ideally be performed by an experienced anaesthetist. A surgical airway is best performed by an ENT surgeon, but general surgeons will have been trained even if they are not experienced in the technique. The technique of emergency cricothyrotomy can be performed by any emergency clinician (see below).

For intubation, the following sequence should be followed:

1 Pre-oxygenation with 100% oxygen, with manual lung inflation if required.
2 Administration of a carefully judged, reduced dose of an anaesthetic induction agent.
3 Application of cricoid pressure.
4 Suxamethonium 1–2 mg/kg.
5 Intubation with a correctly sized tracheal tube.

Confirmation of correct placement of the endotracheal tube

Signs such as chest movement and auscultation remain helpful, but are occasionally misleading, especially in inexperienced hands. The most reliable evidence is to see the tube pass through the vocal cords. The correct size is a tube that can be placed easily through the cords with only a small leak. Intubation of the right main bronchus is best avoided by carefully placing the tube only 2–3 cm below the cords, and noting the length at the teeth before checking by auscultation, which is best done in the left and right lower axillae. **Capnography (if available) is a useful adjunct to help to confirm correct tube placement.**

Indications for surgical cricothyrotomy

- Inability to open or clear the airway, and the patient losing consciousness due to cerebral hypoxia (usually also cyanosed and bradycardic).
- Inability to ventilate the lungs despite high-level CPAP via a bag-valve-mask system and 100% oxygen through a reservoir attached to the bag.
- Inability to intubate through the larynx, either because this is not possible or due to lack of experience.

Method

1 Place the patient in a supine position.
2 If there is no risk of neck injury, consider extending the neck to improve access. Otherwise, maintain a neutral alignment.
3 Identify the cricothyroid membrane (see Figure 7.3.A.1).
4 Prepare the skin, and, if the patient is conscious, infiltrate with local anaesthetic.
5 Place a hand on the neck to stabilise the cricothyroid membrane, and to protect the lateral vascular structures from injury.
6 Make a small vertical incision in the skin, and press the lateral edges of the incision outwards, to minimise bleeding.
7 Make a transverse incision through the cricothyroid membrane, being careful not to damage the cricoid cartilage.
8 Insert a tracheal spreader, or use the handle of the scalpel by inserting it through the incision and twisting it through 90 degrees to open the airway.
9 Insert an appropriately sized endotracheal or tracheostomy tube.
10 Ventilate the patient and check that this is effective.
11 Secure the tube to prevent dislodgement.

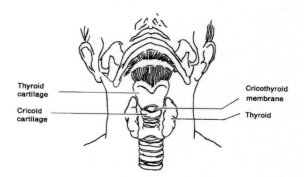

FIGURE 7.3.A.1 Anatomy of neck, showing landmarks for surgical cricothyroidotomy.

Complications of surgical cricothyroidotomy

These include the following:

- asphyxia
- aspiration (e.g. blood)
- laceration of the trachea
- laceration of the oesophagus
- haemorrhage or haematoma formation
- mediastinal emphysema
- subsequent glottic stenosis
- creation of a false passage into the tissues
- subsequent subglottic stenosis or oedema.

Primary assessment and resuscitation: Breathing

After management of the airway, the patient's breathing should be assessed. The same approach is adopted as for the patient suffering a serious illness.

Assessment of breathing

- Effort: recession, rate, added noises, accessory muscles, alar flaring.
- Efficacy: breath sounds, chest expansion, abdominal excursion.
- Adequacy: heart rate, skin colour (look for cyanosis), mental status.
- A pulse oximeter is very useful to monitor oxygenation adequacy (SaO$_2$).

Unequal breath sounds or poor oxygenation:

- Pneumothorax or haemothorax.
- Misplaced or blocked endotracheal tube.

Looking at the respiratory rate and chest expansion is essential. In addition to the signs listed above, check whether any of the following are present:

- penetrating injury
- presence of flail chest
- sucking chest wounds.

Listen for breath sound character and equality:

- pneumothorax (decreased breath sounds on site of injury)
- detection of abnormal sounds in the chest.

Feel for:

- tracheal shift (sign of tension pneumothorax on side away from the deviation)
- broken ribs
- subcutaneous emphysema.

Percuss:

- percussion is useful for diagnosis of **haemothorax** (dull on affected side) and **pneumothorax** (hyper-resonant on affected side).

Continue giving high-flow oxygen (15 litres/minute) in all cases.

Careful examination of the trachea, neck veins and chest may indicate the presence of pleural collections of air or blood. Tension pneumothorax should be treated immediately with needle thoracocentesis in the second intercostal space in the mid-clavicular line.

Needle thoracocentesis

This procedure is used for the rapidly deteriorating patient who has a life-threatening tension pneumothorax. If it is used with a patient who does not have a tension pneumothorax, there is a 10–20% risk of producing a pneumothorax or causing damage to the lung, or both. In such cases immediate subsequent insertion of a chest drain is mandatory.

1 Identify the second intercostal space in the mid-clavicular line on the side of the pneumothorax (the **opposite** side to the direction of tracheal deviation, and the **same** side as the hyper-resonance).

2 Swab the chest wall with surgical prep or an alcohol swab.

3 Attach the syringe to the over-needle venous cannula.

4 Insert the cannula into the chest wall, just above the rib below, aspirating all the time.

5 If air is aspirated, remove the needle, leaving the plastic cannula in place. Alternatively, insert the over-needle venous cannula without a syringe and note a 'hiss' of air on relief of the tension pneumothorax when the metal stylet is removed from the plastic cannula.

6 Tape the open cannula in place and proceed to chest drain insertion as soon as possible.

Complications of needle thoracocentesis

- Local cellulitis.
- Local haematoma.
- Pleural infection.
- Empyema.
- Pneumothorax.

Ventilation

Provide assisted ventilation if needed to patients with breathing problems, using a bag and mask with a reservoir attached, or by intubation and intermittent positive pressure ventilation. **Do not persist with intubation attempts without oxygenating the patient.**

Look for and treat the following:

- airway obstruction (see above)
- tension pneumothorax
- open pneumothorax
- haemothorax
- flail chest
- cardiac tamponade.

See below for details.

TABLE 7.3.A.1 Serious chest trauma: signs and treatment

Breathing problem	Clinical signs	Treatment
Tension pneumothorax	• Decreased air entry on side of pneumothorax • Decreased chest movement on side of pneumothorax • Hyper-resonance to percussion on side of pneumothorax • Tracheal deviation away from side of pneumothorax • Hypoxic shocked patient • Full neck veins	High-flow oxygen Needle thoracocentesis Chest drain insertion
Open pneumothorax	• Penetrating chest wound with signs of pneumothorax • Sucking or blowing chest wound	High-flow oxygen Chest drain Wound occlusion on three sides
Massive haemothorax: blood in pleural space	• Decreased chest movement • Decreased air entry • Dullness to percussion • Shock and hypoxia • Collapsed neck veins	High-flow oxygen Venous access and IV volume replacement Chest drain (a haemothorax of 500–1500 mL that stops bleeding after insertion of an intercostal catheter can generally be treated by closed drainage alone; a haemothorax of greater than 1500–2000 mL, or with continued bleeding of more than 200–300 mL/hour, may be an indication for further investigation, such as thoracotomy)
Flail chest: paradoxical movement of a chest wall segment associated with underlying lung contusion	• Rare in children because they have an elastic chest wall • Decreased efficiency of breathing	Oxygen and pain relief May need intubation and ventilation Transfer if feasible
Cardiac tamponade: blood in pericardial sac causing a decrease in cardiac output	• Shock associated with penetrating or blunt chest trauma • Faint apex beat and/or muffled heart sounds • Distended neck veins	Oxygen IV access and IV fluids Emergency needle pericardiocentesis (see Section 8.4.C: may need to be repeated) Consider transfer if feasible

Primary assessment and resuscitation: Circulation

Assessment of circulation

Circulatory assessment includes identification of actual and potential sources of blood loss. Closed fractures and bleeding into the chest, abdomen or pelvis may make it difficult to detect how much blood has been lost. The ability to estimate the percentage blood loss is helpful when planning resuscitation. Remember that a child's circulating blood volume is only 80 mL/kg, so is easily compromised. Blood volume in pregnancy is 100 mL/kg, or 5–7 litres.

TABLE 7.3.A.2 Blood loss in pregnancy

Sign	Percentage blood loss		
	< 25	25–40	> 40
Heart rate	slight increase	moderate increase	marked increase or bradycardia
Systolic BP	normal	normal	beginning to fall
Pulse volume	normal or decreased	seriously decreased	very seriously decreased
Skin*	cool, pale, sweaty	cool, mottled, sweaty	cool and sweaty
Respiratory rate	slight increase	moderate increase	sighing respirations
Mental status	slight agitation	lethargic or uncooperative	only reacts to pain

* Capillary refill time > 3 seconds.

Note that blood pressure may be normal until up to 50% of the patient's circulatory volume has been lost. The blood pressure is initially well maintained despite continuing bleeding in children and pregnant women and girls. As an indicator of haemorrhage, it can be falsely reassuring. A progressively worsening tachycardia is a more revealing feature.

A monitoring device which records pulse rate, ECG trace and blood pressure is a very useful adjunct if available.

Resuscitation of circulation

Management is focused on avoiding hypovolaemia and controlling blood loss.

Loss of blood is the most common cause of shock in major trauma.

Concealed bleeding severe enough to cause shock can occur into the pleural cavity, abdomen, pelvis and femur. Around 40% of the circulating blood volume can be lost via an open femoral fracture, wherein initial treatment should include pressure, splinting and analgesia.

Stop bleeding

The first priority is to stop obvious bleeding by applying direct pressure. Do not forget that the patient may have a wound on their back that is bleeding into the bed. To examine the back, the patient should be log-rolled, if indicated.

- **Injuries to the limbs:** tourniquets do not work well and may cause reperfusion syndromes and add to the primary injury. The recommended procedure of 'pressure dressing' is an ill-defined entity. Severe bleeding from high-energy penetrating injuries and amputation wounds can be controlled by sub-fascial gauze pack

placement, plus manual compression on the proximal artery, plus a carefully applied compressive dressing of the entire injured limb.
- **Injuries to the chest:** the most common source of bleeding is chest wall arteries. Immediate placement of a chest tube drain plus intermittent suction plus efficient analgesia (IV ketamine is the drug of choice, if available) expand the lung and seal off the bleeding.

Recent evidence has shown that tranexamic acid can reduce mortality from major haemorrhage in major trauma in adults. It is also now recommended for use in children. The drug should be started as soon as possible, and within the first 3 hours after the trauma, to be effective.

In pregnancy

The loading dose is 1 gram over 10 minutes followed by an IV infusion of a further 1 gram over 8 hours.

The slow IV bolus dose is given by injecting 1 gram of tranexamic acid into a 100-mL bag of 0.9% saline and letting it run through over about 10–20 minutes (the exact timing is not crucial).

The 8-hour infusion is given by injecting 1 gram of tranexamic acid into a 500-mL bag of 0.9% saline and giving it over 8 hours (approximately 60 mL/hour). If there is a gap between the initial bolus and the subsequent infusion this probably does not matter too much, but ideally one should follow the other.

In children

The loading dose is 15 mg/kg (maximum 1 gram) diluted in a convenient volume of sodium chloride 0.9% or glucose 5% and given over 10 minutes.

The maintenance infusion rate is 2 mg/kg/hour. The suggested dilution is 500 mg in 500 mL of sodium chloride 0.9% or glucose 5% given at a rate of 2 mL/kg/hour for at least 8 hours, or until bleeding stops.

Elevate the legs if the patient is in shock.

IV fluid resuscitation

The goal is to restore oxygen delivery to the tissues. As the usual problem is loss of blood, fluid resuscitation must be a priority.

- Adequate vascular access must be obtained. This requires the insertion of at least one, and ideally two, large-bore cannulae (14–16 G). Peripheral cut-down or intra-osseous infusion may be necessary.
- Infusion fluids: These should be warmed to body temperature if possible (e.g. pre-warm in a bucket of warmed water or under a relative's clothing). Remember that hypothermia can lead to abnormal blood clotting. Use crystalloids such as Ringer-lactate or Hartmann's solution. Normal (0.9%) saline can be used if these fluids are unavailable, but **be aware that, especially in larger volumes, normal saline causes a hyperchloraemic acidosis which is detrimental to sick or injured patients.**)
- Avoid solutions containing ONLY glucose (e.g. 5% Dextrose in water or 5% Dextrose with 1/5N saline, these are dangerous in this situation) but glucose can be added to Ringer–lactate, Hartmann's or N saline if there is evidence of or concern about hypoglycaemia.
- Take blood for Hb, group and cross match and glucose, electrolytes and amylase for urgent analysis.

Not all cases of hypovolaemia require aggressive fluid therapy. In adults, withholding fluids in penetrating trunk trauma before achieving surgical haemostasis has been associated with an improved outcome. The rationale is to avoid pushing up the blood pressure, which hinders clot formation and promotes further bleeding. Aggressive crystalloid fluid replacement can lead to increased fluid requirements, hypothermia, dilution of clotting factors, excessive blood transfusion and its associated immunosuppression. Aim to give sufficient fluid to maintain vital organ perfusion. This can be monitored by monitoring the patient's state of alertness which is a measure of brain perfusion in the absence of a head injury.

On the other hand, in severe head injury, cerebral perfusion is critically dependent on maintaining blood pressure. If the patient has both a severe head injury and major trunk bleeding, the apparently conflicting requirements are best managed by maintaining priorities in ABC order and achieving prompt surgical haemostasis. Beyond this strategic conflict, it should be remembered that the normal blood pressure is lower in children, hypovolaemia mimics head injury, and blood pressure itself is a poor indicator of organ perfusion.

As outlined above, the concept of '**targeted fluid resuscitation**' is important if the cause of hypovolaemic shock is haemorrhage from penetrating injury. Here the initial boluses of IV crystalloids required to treat shock should only be given to keep the vital organs (especially the brain, heart and kidneys) perfused before emergency surgery and blood transfusion is available. Fresh blood is particularly useful to combat the coagulopathy that occurs in major blood loss if specific coagulation components such as platelets are unavailable.

However, it must be borne in mind that penetrating trauma is not common in women and children in civilian life.

We suggest that when giving boluses of crystalloid or blood to patients in shock **due to bleeding** in major trauma, only the amount needed to keep the blood pressure at a level sufficient to perfuse the vital organs should be given. There is no clear evidence to indicate the precise blood pressure that should be achieved in a pregnant woman or child in shock due to haemorrhage. Adequate perfusion of vital organs may best be indicated by **a radial pulse which can be palpated and an alert conscious level (in the patient without a significant head injury). In pregnancy, the adequacy of the fetal heart rate may also be helpful**.

In children under 2–3 years of age, the radial pulse may be difficult to feel, and the presence of a palpable brachial pulse may be the best available indicator at present.

Therefore to maintain a palpable radial pulse in pregnancy, start with IV boluses of 500 mL of crystalloid or ideally blood, and reassess after each bolus.

In children, to maintain a radial or brachial pulse give 10 mL/kg IV boluses of crystalloid or, ideally, blood, and reassess after each bolus.

In the absence of further evidence, it is recommended that in children it is best to start with 10 mL/kg boluses (infusions given as rapidly as possible) of Ringer-lactate or Hartmann's solution or plasma expander with frequent reassessment, rather than the full 20 mL/kg recommended in other life-threatening situations, such as meningococcal sepsis or severe dehydration.

Fluid resuscitation in pregnancy starts with a 500-mL bolus of Ringer-lactate or Hartmann's solution or plasma expander.

After repeating boluses twice (i.e. 10 mL/kg twice in a child, or 500 mL twice in pregnancy), the transfusion of blood (packed red cells) should be considered. The most important aspect of fluid resuscitation is **the patient's response to the fluid challenge**.

Improvement is indicated by the following:

- a decrease in heart rate
- an increase in systolic blood pressure
- an increase in skin temperature
- faster capillary refill
- improving mental state.

Failure to improve should prompt an urgent search for chest, abdominal or pelvic haemorrhage, with the immediate involvement of an experienced surgeon. Similar volumes may be repeated if there is continuing evidence of haemorrhagic shock, after re-evaluating the state of the circulation.

It is useful to delegate the initial fluid bolus to a member of the trauma team (if a team is available), who attaches the warmed fluid bag to the IV cannula via a three-way tap to which is attached a 20- or 50-mL syringe to give the boluses.

Blood transfusion

There may be considerable difficulty in getting blood. Remember possible incompatibility, and hepatitis B and HIV risks, even among the patient's own family.

Blood transfusion must be considered when the patient has persistent haemodynamic instability despite fluid (colloid/crystalloid) infusion. If the type-specific or cross-matched blood is not available, type O negative packed red blood cells should be used. Transfusion should be seriously considered if the haemoglobin level is less than 7 grams/dL and if the patient is still bleeding. Blood transfusion is most important, and requires blood to be taken for urgent cross-matching.

As described above, early surgical involvement is essential.

Vascular access

This is essential in all seriously injured patients. A minimum of two relatively large-bore IV cannulae is essential.

TABLE 7.3.A.3 Infusion IV line flow rates

Colour code	Gauge	Crystalloid flow rate (mL/minute)
Brown	14	240
Grey	16	172
Yellow	17	130
Green	18	76
Pink	20	54
Blue	22	25
Lime green	24	14

Peripheral veins are preferable; the inexperienced should not attempt central venous cannulation. The external jugular vein can be accessed even in shock, but the cannula can become easily displaced and must be very carefully taped in place. A cut-down on to the long saphenous vein at the ankle can also be used. If venous access is difficult and is taking too long, the new intra-osseous EZ-IO drill is simple to operate and can be life-saving (*see* Section 8.4.C), and **should be available in all emergency departments**.

Central venous cannulation can permit large volumes to be rapidly infused and also permit central venous pressure measurements. It must be undertaken by a skilled person (e.g. an anaesthetist), and a Seldinger technique should be used. The femoral vein is used for children, but not for pregnant women where the internal jugular or subclavian vein may be used. Peripheral venous access can often be established once peripheral perfusion has been improved. Both femoral venous and tibial intra-osseous access are best avoided if there is clinical evidence of a pelvic or abdominal injury. In such cases it is better to secure vascular access above the diaphragm. The upper outer aspect of the humerus can be used for intra-osseous access in that case (*see* Section 8.4.C).

Blood from a vein or bone marrow should be drawn for typing and cross-matching, haemoglobin, glucose and electrolytes. These tests are clinically accurate on a marrow sample from an intra-osseous approach provided there has not been prior infusion of blood or crystalloid fluid. The infused fluids should be warm. Physiological coagulation works best at normothermia, and haemostasis is difficult at core temperatures below 35°C. Hypothermia in trauma patients is common during protracted improvised outdoor evacuations, even in the tropics. It is easy to cool a patient but difficult to rewarm them, so prevention of hypothermia is essential. IV fluids should have a temperature of 40–42°C (using IV fluids at 'room temperature' means cooling!).

Venous cut-down
Anatomical considerations

In adults the primary site for cut-down is over the long saphenous vein above the ankle at a point approximately 2 cm anterior and 2 cm superior to the medial malleolus, **but not if there is significant injury proximal to this site**.

Identify the surface landmarks. These are shown in Table 7.3.A.4.

TABLE 7.3.A.4 Surface landmarks for cut-down incision

	Saphenous
Infant	Half a finger's breadth superior and anterior to the medial malleolus
Small children	One finger's breadth superior and anterior to the medial malleolus
Older children and pregnant mothers	Two finger breadths superior and anterior to the medial malleolus

- Apply a venous tourniquet proximal to the intended cannulation site.
- Prepare the skin with antiseptic and sterile drapes.
- Infiltrate the area with local anaesthetic (1% lignocaine using a fine 24–25G needle).
- Make a full-thickness transverse incision through the skin.
- By blunt dissection, identify and display the vein.
- Free the vein from its bed and elevate a 2 cm length.
- Pass a dissolvable suture around the proximal end of the vein but do not tie it yet.
- Introduce the plastic cannula (with trochar) through the

venotomy, remove the trocar and secure it in place by tying the proximal ligature.
- Attach the giving set and commence flow at the required rate.
- If possible, close the incision; otherwise apply a sterile dressing and secure the giving set tubing in place.

See also Section 8.4.C.

Complications
- Haemorrhage or haematoma.
- Perforation of the posterior wall of the vein.
- Nerve transection.
- Phlebitis.
- Venous thrombosis.

External jugular venous cannulation
Procedure

Place the patient in a head-down position to dilate the vein and reduce the risk of air embolus.
1. Place the patient in a 15–30-degree head-down position (or with padding under the shoulders so that the head hangs lower than the shoulders).
2. Turn the head away from the site of puncture.
3. Clean the skin over the appropriate side of the neck.
4. Identify the external jugular vein, which can be seen passing over the sternocleidomastoid muscle at the junction of its middle and lower thirds.
5. Have an assistant place their finger at the lower end of the visible part of the vein just above the clavicle. This stabilises it and compresses it so that it remains distended.
6. Puncture the skin and enter the vein.
7. When free flow of blood is obtained, ensure that no air bubbles are present in the tubing and then attach a giving set.
8. Tape the cannula securely in position.

Other less common causes of shock in major trauma
Cardiogenic shock

Inadequate heart function may result from:
- myocardial contusion (bruising)
- cardiac tamponade
- tension pneumothorax (preventing blood from returning to the heart)
- myocardial infarction.

Assessment of the jugular venous pressure is essential in these circumstances. It will be elevated compared with hypovolaemic shock, where it may not be visible.

An ECG should be recorded (if available).

Neurogenic shock

This is due to the loss of sympathetic tone, usually resulting from spinal cord injury, with the classical presentation of hypotension without reflex tachycardia or skin vasoconstriction.

Tension pneumothorax

See under breathing section above. This can present with shock as well as breathing impairment.

Primary assessment: neurological failure

Head injury is the major cause of death in trauma.

Rapid assessment of the central nervous system for evidence of failure includes determining the AVPU score: AVPU score: A = Alert, V = responds to a Voice, P= response to Pain, U = Unresponsive.

- With a score of 'P' or 'U', intubation should take place in order to maintain and protect the airway. If there is no one skilled in intubation available, the patient should be placed in the recovery position.
- Remember to check for a pain response above the level of the clavicle, as a patient with a spinal injury may not be able to respond by moving their limbs.
- Look for signs indicative of injury (e.g. bruises, lacerations or haematoma) in the head and neck area.
- Examine the pupils for size, equality and reaction to light. Look for other lateralising signs, such as limb weakness or focal seizures.

At this stage, the brain is best cared for by close attention to managing A B and C, and by correction of any hypoglycaemia.

If there is evidence of raised intracranial pressure (RICP):

- Intubate and ventilate to maintain oxygenation, and aim for a pCO_2 of about 4 kPa.
- Maintain systolic blood pressure.

- Nurse the patient in a 30-degree head-up position.
- Contact a neurosurgeon (if available).

Mannitol 0.5 mg/kg should be administered after first excluding intracranial haematoma. If this is not excluded, there will be temporary improvement due to relief of cerebral oedema, but there may be sudden worsening a short time later due to rapid expansion of the haematoma. An alternative is hypertonic saline (*see* Section 7.3.C).

Low blood glucose levels are common in child trauma victims, and can cause brain damage. Always check the blood glucose level where possible. If it is not possible to check it, treat any baby or small child immediately with 5 mL/kg of 10% glucose IV.

Analgesia in major trauma (*see* Section 1.15)

Pain increases fear and distress, makes the patient less able to cooperate, and raises intracranial pressure. If the patient is fully conscious and in severe pain, control of pain is required.

Pain relief takes several different forms:

- Reassurance.
- Splinting of fractures.
- Covering wounds, especially burns.
- Drugs:
  - There is no place for oral or IM medication in a major trauma situation.
  - There are three alternatives in severe trauma: ketamine, morphine and Entonox.

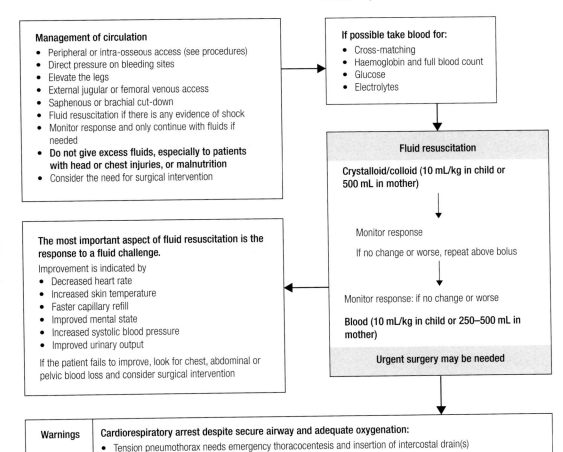

Management of circulation

- Peripheral or intra-osseous access (see procedures)
- Direct pressure on bleeding sites
- Elevate the legs
- External jugular or femoral venous access
- Saphenous or brachial cut-down
- Fluid resuscitation if there is any evidence of shock
- Monitor response and only continue with fluids if needed
- **Do not give excess fluids, especially to patients with head or chest injuries, or malnutrition**
- Consider the need for surgical intervention

If possible take blood for:

- Cross-matching
- Haemoglobin and full blood count
- Glucose
- Electrolytes

Fluid resuscitation

Crystalloid/colloid (10 mL/kg in child or 500 mL in mother)

Monitor response

If no change or worse, repeat above bolus

Monitor response: if no change or worse

Blood (10 mL/kg in child or 250–500 mL in mother)

Urgent surgery may be needed

The most important aspect of fluid resuscitation is the response to a fluid challenge.

Improvement is indicated by

- Decreased heart rate
- Increased skin temperature
- Faster capillary refill
- Improved mental state
- Increased systolic blood pressure
- Improved urinary output

If the patient fails to improve, look for chest, abdominal or pelvic blood loss and consider surgical intervention

Warnings	**Cardiorespiratory arrest despite secure airway and adequate oxygenation:**
	- Tension pneumothorax needs emergency thoracocentesis and insertion of intercostal drain(s)
	- Exsanguination needs large fluid boluses and blood transfusion
	- Pericardial tamponade needs pericardiocentesis

FIGURE 7.3.A.2 Managing the circulation in major trauma.

Ketamine

The positive inotropic effects of ketamine, and the fact that it does not affect the gag reflex, make this a very helpful analgesic, especially if there is or has been shock. Repeated IV doses of 200 micrograms/kg followed by careful reassessment are usually effective, especially during transfer to a more specialised hospital (if available and relevant).

Morphine

In major trauma, 100–200 micrograms/kg morphine IV in a child, or 5–10 mg in a mother, is the drug of choice, followed by careful reassessment. If the conscious level falls, the effect can be reversed with naloxone, showing whether the effect is caused by the morphine or by a worsening brain injury. If there is respiratory depression, first ventilate with a bag-valve-mask before giving naloxone.

Entonox

Entonox (a 50:50 mixture of nitrous oxide and oxygen) is useful, especially for limb injuries while splints are being applied. Do not use it in the presence of head, chest or abdominal trauma.

A head injury is NOT a contraindication to giving morphine unless there is depressed consciousness, when great care is needed.

Summary of primary assessment and resuscitation

The injured patient should have:
- a team approach with an urgent call for surgical and anaesthetic availability
- a clear airway and 100% oxygen for breathing
- adequate respiration, achieved by manual or mechanical ventilation and chest decompression when indicated
- venous access and an initial fluid challenge, if indicated on circulatory assessment
- blood sent for typing and cross-matching
- identification of the need for life-saving surgery and preparation under way
- identification of any serious head injury, and attention paid to maximising A, B and C
- cervical spine immobilisation, where appropriate

Life-threatening injuries identified and treated

Injury	Treatment
Airway obstruction	Head tilt, chin lift and jaw thrust, oropharyngeal airway, intubation or surgical airway
Tension pneumothorax	Needle thoracocentesis and chest drain
Open pneumothorax	Three-sided dressing, then chest drain
Massive haemothorax	IV access, chest drain and blood transfusion
Flail chest	Intubation if needed
Cardiac tamponade	Pericardiocentesis

Before the secondary assessment begins, it should be remembered that:

ABC and neurological failure components of the primary assessment and resuscitation require constant re-evaluation, as deterioration can be rapid and unexpected.

Emergency operative treatment to control life-threatening haemorrhage should be performed promptly, without waiting for non-urgent examination and imaging.

Identification of all anatomical injuries remains an important goal, but may be overridden by pressing physiological requirements to ensure that oxygenated blood reaches vital organs in sufficient degree. This may require emergency surgery before all non-life-threatening injuries have been identified.

Secondary assessment and emergency treatment

Secondary assessment and emergency treatment are undertaken only when the patient's ABC's are stable. **If any deterioration occurs during this phase, secondary assessment must be interrupted by another primary assessment and resuscitation.**

Documentation is required for all procedures undertaken. This involves careful examination from head to toe in a systematic way, including a **controlled examination of the back, avoiding spinal movement** by log-rolling (*see* Section 8.5). Clear documentation of all injuries is required, to serve as the basis of the subsequent management strategy.

Shortly after the primary assessment and resuscitation, various adjuncts help with protecting the patient and monitoring progress.

Secondary assessment: adjuncts
- Monitoring ECG, SaO_2 and blood pressure
- Urinary and gastric catheters
- Portable X-rays of chest and pelvis
- Ultrasound of abdomen (if available)
- Adequate pain control (see below)
- Baseline blood tests (especially haemoglobin, cross-matching, biochemistry and clotting)

History
- Events before and after incident
- First aid given at scene
- Past medical history
- Medications and allergies
- Immunisation status
- Last food and drink

Adjuncts to the secondary assessment and emergency treatment include:
- ECG, oxygen saturation and blood pressure monitoring (as used in primary assessment and resuscitation).
- Gastric and urinary catheters.
- **Portable** X-rays of the chest, neck and pelvis.

Head examination

This includes the following:
- scalp and ocular abnormalities
- external ear and tympanic membrane
- periorbital soft-tissue injuries.

Head injury patients should be suspected of having cervical spine injury until demonstrated otherwise.

Neck examination

This includes the following:

- looking for a penetrating wound
- subcutaneous emphysema
- tracheal deviation
- neck vein appearance (JVP).

Neurological examination

This includes the following:

- brain function assessment using the AVPU Scale or the Glasgow Coma Scale (GCS)
- spinal cord motor activity
- sensation and reflex.

Chest examination

This includes the following:

- the clavicles and all ribs
- breath sounds and heart sounds
- ECG monitoring (if available).

Abdominal examination

This includes the following:

- look for a penetrating wound of the abdomen requiring surgical exploration
- look for blunt trauma; a nasogastric tube is inserted (but not in the presence of facial trauma)
- rectal examination (but not in children unless absolutely essential)
- insertion of urinary catheter except in children (check for meatal blood before insertion).

Examination of pelvis and limbs

This includes the following:

- pain, tenderness on palpation
- deformity
- wounds.

X-rays (if possible and where indicated)

These include the following:

- chest X-ray and cervical spine films (it is important to see all seven vertebrae)
- pelvic and long bone X-rays
- skull X-rays may be useful to search for fractures when head injury is present without focal neurological deficit if CT is unavailable
- CT scans of the head and abdomen (if available).

Head injury

This remains the commonest cause of death and disability in severe trauma in children, and is dealt with in more detail elsewhere (*see* Section 7.3.C). The scalp and face are examined for bruising, abrasions, lacerations and evidence of fracture.

Basal skull fracture is manifested by signs such as:

- 'raccoon eyes' (bilateral peri-orbital haematoma), bleeding from the ears or a visible haemotympanum
- Battle's sign (bruising over the mastoid process, which is a relatively late sign)
- CSF leakage from the nose, mouth or ears.

The AVPU Scale score or the Glasgow Coma Scale score is again evaluated (*see* Section 7.3.C), allowing a dynamic comparison with the primary assessment estimation, unless the child is now intubated and sedated.

As infants and small children are prone to hypoglycaemia, it is important to consider this as a potential cause of altered consciousness (*see* Section 5.8.B).

Delay in the early assessment of head-injured patients can have devastating consequences in terms of survival and patient outcome. Hypoxia and hypotension double the mortality of head-injured patients.

The following conditions are potentially life-threatening but difficult to treat in district hospitals. It is important to treat what you can with the expertise and resources that you have available, and to triage casualties carefully.

Immediate recognition and early management of the following conditions are essential:

Acute extradural haemorrhage

Classical signs consist of:

- loss of consciousness following a lucid interval, with rapid deterioration
- a rapid rise in intracranial pressure, due to bleeding from the middle meningeal artery
- development of hemiparesis on the opposite side, with a fixed pupil on the same side as the impact area.

The management is surgical, and every effort should be made to do burr-hole decompressions.

Acute subdural haematoma

There is bleeding with clotted blood in the subdural space, accompanied by severe contusion of the underlying brain. This condition results from tearing of bridging veins between the cortex and the dura. Again, surgery is needed, but it requires a neurosurgeon, not burr-holes alone.

The following conditions should be treated with more conservative medical management, as neurosurgery does not usually improve the outcome:

- base-of-skull fractures
- cerebral concussion, with temporarily altered consciousness
- depressed skull fracture: an impaction of fragmented skull that may result in penetration of the underlying dura and brain
- intracerebral haematoma, which may result from acute injury or progressive damage secondary to contusion
- in children, diffuse brain swelling is a more frequent problem than bleeding; again this is managed medically, but apart from ventilation and general supportive therapy, recovery is dependent on the severity of the injury and the effect of the initial physiological support of ABC.

Alteration of consciousness is the hallmark of brain injury.

The most common errors in head injury evaluation and resuscitation are:

- failure to perform ABC and prioritise management
- failure to look beyond the obvious head injury
- failure to assess the baseline neurological examination
- failure to re-evaluate the patient who deteriorates.

Management of head trauma

The Airway, Breathing and Circulation are stabilised (and the cervical spine immobilised, if possible).

Vital signs are important indicators of the patient's neurological status, and must be monitored and recorded frequently.

The Glasgow Coma Scale (GCS) score is interpreted as follows:

- severe head injury: GCS score is ≤ 8
- moderate head injury: GCS score is 9–12
- minor head injury: GCS score is 13–15.

Remember:

- Deterioration may occur due to bleeding or brain swelling.
- Unequal or dilated pupils may reflect an increase in intracranial pressure.
- Head or brain injury is never the cause of hypotension in the adult trauma patient.
- Sedation should be avoided, as it decreases the level of consciousness, and promotes hypercarbia due to slow breathing with retention of CO_2.
- The Cushing response is a late sign, reflecting a lethal rise in intracranial pressure, associated with a poor prognosis. The hallmarks of the Cushing response are:
  – bradycardia
  – hypertension
  – decreased and erratic respiration.

Basic medical management for severe head injuries includes:

- Intubation and ventilation, producing normocapnia (pCO_2 in the range 4.5–5 kPa, if it is possible to monitor this). This will reduce both intracranial blood volume and intracranial pressure temporarily.
- Sedation with possible paralysis provided that the airway is fully protected by intubation and a means of assisted ventilation present.
- Moderate IV fluid input with diuresis: do not overload.
- Nursing with the head up at an angle of 20 degrees.
- Prevention of hyperthermia/fever.
- Avoidance of hypoglycaemia and electrolyte abnormalities.

Chest trauma

The majority of chest injuries result from blunt trauma, and are usually associated with injuries in other organ systems.

Approximately 25% of deaths due to trauma are attributed to chest injury. Immediate deaths are essentially due to major disruption of the heart or of the great vessels. Early deaths due to chest trauma include airway obstruction, tension pneumothorax, cardiac tamponade or aspiration.

The majority of patients with thoracic trauma can be managed by simple manoeuvres and do not require surgical treatment.

Respiratory distress may be caused by:

- rib fractures/flail chest
- pneumothorax
- tension pneumothorax
- haemothorax
- pulmonary contusion (bruising)
- open pneumothorax
- aspiration.

Haemorrhagic shock may be due to:

- haemothorax
- haemomediastinum.

The increased compliance of the chest wall in the child is protective, but can make interpretation of the severity of injury difficult. Rib fractures are uncommon in the infant or child, but indicate that significant blunt force has been applied. Moreover, serious chest injury can occur without obvious external signs of trauma. The energy that is not dissipated in breaking the elastic ribs may be transferred to the lungs, to be manifested as pulmonary contusion. Respiratory failure can occur quickly in infants and young children with chest trauma, yet the majority of chest injuries require no more than the insertion of an intercostal drain.

- Thorough re-examination of the chest front and back, using the classical **inspection–palpation–percussion–auscultation approach**, is combined with a chest X-ray.
- Particular attention is directed to the symmetry of chest movement and breath sounds, the presence of surgical emphysema and pain, or instability on compressing the chest.
- Tracheal deviation and altered heart sounds are noted.
- On log-rolling the child, **it is important to reconsider flail chest**, as a posterior floating segment is often poorly tolerated in children.

Rib fractures

Fractured ribs may occur at the point of impact, and damage to the underlying lung may produce lung bruising or puncture. The ribs usually become fairly stable within 10 days to 2 weeks. Firm healing with callus formation is seen after about 6 weeks.

Flail chest

The unstable segment moves separately and in an opposite direction from the rest of the thoracic cage during the respiration cycle. Severe respiratory distress may ensue. Treatment is by analgesia, as breathing is painful, and shallow breathing may predispose to pneumonia in this situation. In severe cases, ventilation is needed in children but not usually in adults.

Pneumothorax

- A **tension pneumothorax** develops when air enters the pleural space but cannot leave, increasing the compression of the underlying lung with each breath. The consequence is progressively increasing intra-thoracic pressure in the affected side, resulting in mediastinal shift. The trachea may be displaced (late sign) and is pushed away from the midline by the air under tension. The patient will become short of breath and hypoxic. Urgent needle decompression (thoracocentesis) is required prior to the insertion of an intercostal drain.
- A **simple pneumothorax** can be diagnosed by X-ray or ultrasound scanning and, although not life-threatening, may be associated with significant underlying lung injury. All traumatic pneumothoraces **require close observation**. Small ones often absorb spontaneously, but larger ones frequently require chest drainage.
- **Open pneumothoraces**, or sucking chest wounds, allow bidirectional flow of air through a chest wall defect. The lung on the affected side is exposed to atmospheric pressure with lung collapse and a shift of the

mediastinum to the uninvolved side. This must be treated rapidly. In compromised patients, intercostal drains, intubation and positive pressure ventilation are often required. Alternatively, they can be treated by applying an occlusive dressing, taped on three sides to serve as a flap valve, followed by insertion of a chest drain remote from the site of injury. A better dressing is the customised Asherman chest seal, which consists of an adhesive ring, similar to that on a colostomy stoma bag, which projects into a pipe-shaped flap valve, resembling that in a Heimlich valve. **Beware of the possibility of a tension pneumothorax developing when one of these is used.**

Pulmonary contusion

This is usually caused by blunt trauma, and may occur in association with rib fractures with or without a flail segment. It is common after chest trauma, and is a potentially life-threatening condition. The onset of symptoms may be slow, progressing over 24 hours post-injury. Pulmonary contusion is likely to occur in cases of high-speed accidents, falls from great heights, and injuries by high-velocity bullets.

Symptoms and signs include:

- dyspnoea
- cyanosis
- sparse or absent breath sounds
- hypoxaemia
- tachycardia.

Treatment involves supplemental oxygen, careful fluid management and particular attention to pain relief. Endotracheal intubation may be necessary in severe cases.

Traumatic haemothorax

This is more common in penetrating than in non-penetrating injuries to the chest. If the haemorrhage is severe, hypovolaemic shock will occur, and also respiratory distress due to compression of the lung on the involved side.

Optimal therapy consists of the placement of a large chest tube and the concomitant replacement of lost blood. In some instances where the bleeding continues and is significant, open chest surgery is necessary to stop the bleeding (see below).

- A haemothorax of 500–1500 mL in pregnancy, or 10–30 mL/kg in a child, that stops bleeding after insertion of an intercostal catheter, can generally be treated by closed drainage alone
- A haemothorax of greater than 1500–2000 mL in pregnancy, or > 30 mL/kg in a child, with continued bleeding of more than 200–300 mL per hour in pregnancy or > 5 mL/kg per hour in a child, is an indication for further investigation e.g. thoracotomy.

The injuries listed below are also possible in severe trauma, but carry a high mortality even in regional centres.

1 **Myocardial contusion:** This is associated, in blunt chest trauma, with fractures of the sternum or ribs. The diagnosis is supported by abnormalities on ECG and elevation of serial cardiac enzymes (if available). Cardiac contusion can simulate a myocardial infarction. The patient must be closely observed, with cardiac monitoring (if available). This type of injury is more common than is often realised, and may be a cause of sudden death some time after the accident.

2 **Pericardial tamponade:** Penetrating cardiac injuries are a leading cause of death in young men in some notorious urban areas, but rare in other settings. It is rare to have pericardial tamponade with blunt trauma. Pericardiocentesis must be undertaken early if this injury is considered likely (*see Section 8.4.B for method*). Look for pericardial tamponade in patients with:

- shock
- distended neck veins
- no pneumothorax
- muffled heart sounds.

3 **Thoracic great vessel injuries:** Injury to the pulmonary veins and arteries is often fatal, and is one of the major causes of on-site death.

4 **Rupture of the trachea or major bronchi:** This is a serious injury with an overall estimated mortality of at least 50%. The majority (80%) of the ruptures of bronchi are within 2.5 cm of the carina.

The usual signs of tracheobronchial disruption are:

- haemoptysis
- dyspnoea
- subcutaneous and mediastinal emphysema
- occasionally cyanosis.

Trauma to the oesophagus

This is rare in patients with blunt trauma, and more frequent in association with penetrating injury. It is lethal if unrecognised, because of mediastinitis. Patients often complain of sudden sharp pain in the epigastrium and chest, with radiation to the back. Dyspnoea, cyanosis and shock occur, but these may be late features. Urgent IV broad-spectrum antibiotics covering both aerobic and anaerobic organisms, as well as nil-by-mouth nursing, are required.

Diaphragmatic injuries

These may occur in association with either blunt or penetrating chest trauma, paralleling the rise in frequency of road traffic accidents. The diagnosis is often missed.

Diaphragmatic injuries should be suspected in any penetrating thoracic wound which is:

- below the fourth intercostal space anteriorly
- below the sixth interspace laterally
- below the eighth interspace posteriorly.

These injuries are more commonly seen on the left side.

Thoracic aorta rupture

This occurs in patients who are exposed to severe decelerating forces, such as high-speed car accidents or a fall from a great height. It has a very high mortality due to rapid exsanguination; the total adult blood volume of 5 litres may be lost in the first minute following injury.

Abdominal trauma

Abdominal injuries are common and, if unrecognised, may prove fatal. Any patient involved in any serious accident should be considered to have an abdominal injury until it has been ruled out.

Severe visceral injuries occur more frequently in children than in adults especially to the liver because of its relative size and lack of protection by the ribs in the young child.

Unexplained blood loss evident during the primary assessment may be due to intra-abdominal haemorrhage.

The abdomen is a classical silent area after trauma. It has to be actively cleared of injury rather than simply noted to be soft and non-tender, especially in the face of altered consciousness.

Cardiovascular decompensation may occur late and precipitously.

The organ most commonly injured in penetrating trauma is the liver, and in blunt trauma the spleen is often torn and ruptured. This is especially the case in children, in whom these organs are poorly protected by ribs and muscles, and especially where chronic illness may cause enlargement and fragility of the liver and spleen.

Thorough history taking and a careful examination of the abdomen may give clues to the origin of bleeding or perforation.

Gastric distension may cause respiratory embarrassment, and a gastric tube should be placed.

In order to gain the cooperation of a frightened child, place the examiner's hand over the mother's hand to undertake palpation.

There are two basic categories of abdominal trauma:

1 **Penetrating trauma**, where the need for surgical consultation is urgent. For example:
   - gunshot
   - stabbing.
2 **Non-penetrating trauma.** For example:
   - compression injuries
   - crushing injuries
   - seat-belt injuries
   - acceleration/deceleration injuries.

About 20% of trauma patients with acute haemoperitoneum have no signs of peritoneal irritation at the first examination, and **repeated primary assessment** must be undertaken.

Blunt trauma can be very difficult to evaluate, especially in the unconscious patient. These patients may need a peritoneal lavage although where ultrasound and/or abdominal CT is available, peritoneal lavage has been superceded. However, an exploratory laparotomy may be the best definitive procedure if abdominal injury needs to be excluded.

Complete physical examination of the abdomen includes rectal examination (although this should be avoided in children as a routine, and only performed if clinically indicated), assessing:
- sphincter tone
- integrity of the rectal wall
- blood in the rectum
- prostate position in adults.

Remember to check for blood at the external urethral meatus.

Women and girls of childbearing age should be considered pregnant until pregnancy has been excluded. The fetus may be salvageable, and the best treatment of the fetus is resuscitation of the mother. A pregnant mother at term, however, can usually be resuscitated properly only after delivery of the baby. This difficult situation must be assessed at the time (*see* Section 1.13).

The diagnostic peritoneal lavage (DPL) may be helpful for determining the presence of blood or enteric fluid due to intra-abdominal injury. The results can be highly suggestive,

but it is overstated as an important diagnostic tool. If there is any doubt, a laparotomy is still the gold standard.

The indications for DPL include:
- unexplained abdominal pain
- trauma of the lower part of the chest
- hypotension, and a fall in haematocrit with no obvious explanation
- any patient with abdominal trauma who has an altered mental state
- any patient with abdominal trauma and spinal cord injuries
- pelvic fractures.

The relative contraindications to DPL are:
- pregnancy
- previous abdominal surgery
- operator inexperience
- if the result would not change your management (e.g. if laparotomy is planned).

Other specific issues with regard to abdominal trauma

- **Pelvic fractures** are often complicated by massive haemorrhage and urological injury.
- It is important to examine the rectum for the presence of blood and for evidence of rectal or perineal laceration (see above for the approach in children).
- X-ray of the pelvis may be valuable, if clinical diagnosis is difficult.

The management of pelvic fractures includes:
- resuscitation (ABC)
- transfusion
- immobilisation and assessment for surgery
- analgesia.

In a severely injured child, a urinary catheter should be inserted. This may be omitted in small babies and in less severely injured children. Small boys are particularly prone to urethral stricture after catheterisation. If the mechanism of injury is of concern, it is important to exclude renal tract injury by examining the first urine for red blood cells.

Management of severe abdominal injury

Abdominal ultrasound (and CT scanning, if available) have become invaluable adjuncts to the secondary assessment, not only for diagnosing intra-abdominal injury, but also for monitoring progress when a defined injury is being managed conservatively.

Bleeding from solid organs may not show up immediately in the resuscitation room, and evidence of hollow-organ rupture may take 24 hours or more to show as free fluid on ultrasound. This commits the trauma team to a high index of suspicion well beyond the classical 'golden hour'. This phrase indicates the importance of prompt identification and resuscitation of Airway, Breathing or Circulation problems that, without intervention, would lead to further damage from hypoxia and hypovolaemia being suffered by the injured patient.

Patients with refractory shock, penetrating injuries or signs of perforation require laparotomy.

Other injuries may be managed conservatively. After

initial fluid transfusion, an experienced surgeon may decide that bleeding from an injured spleen, liver or kidney does not require immediate operative intervention. **CT scanning (if available) is an invaluable aid to decision making.**

Splenic injury is relatively common, and can occur after relatively minor trauma, especially if the spleen is enlarged following an inflammatory process or infection, notably malaria. Signs include left upper quadrant pain and tenderness, with referred pain to the shoulder tip. Non-operative management is used frequently in many centres, but long-term problems of splenectomy are insignificant by comparison with the potential consequences of inadequate supervision of conservative management which requires careful monitoring and fluid management with on-site, round-the-clock theatre, anaesthetic and surgical availability: all of which are difficult to provide in a low resource setting.

Increasingly, **liver injuries** are also being managed conservatively. Unlike the relatively straightforward operation of splenectomy, operative liver repair or resection is hazardous, and packing plays a major role in the operative management of uncontrolled hepatic bleeding.

Injuries to the retroperitoneal organs, such as the kidneys or pancreas, may present with vague or atypical signs, again requiring a high index of suspicion. A significant kidney injury does not always cause demonstrable haematuria.

Ultrasound studies and dynamic contrast CT scans (if available) **may** provide valuable information on renal structure and function, but false-negative results commonly occur. Intravenous urography remains useful for demonstrating the details of renal and ureteric injury, especially in centres without a CT scanner. Pancreatic injury may occur with a normal amylase level, and the amylase level may be raised in the absence of pancreatic damage.

Spinal trauma (*see Section 4.2.D*)

Management of spinal cord injuries is particularly difficult in resource-limited settings, where spinal surgery may not be available within the country. Usually patients in these settings have not been handled carefully during transport from the site of injury to the hospital. Decisions have to be made as to whether or not cervical spinal immobilisation is appropriate, especially if it could interfere with airway resuscitation.

Spinal injury should be ruled out in any patient who has been subject to a mechanism of injury capable of damaging the spine. This seemingly obvious statement highlights the fact that it is often surprisingly difficult to ascertain whether there has been an injury to the spine or not, particularly in the face of a concomitant head injury, or in a child who is too young to communicate.

Even in an alert older child, distracting pain from a limb injury may lead the patient to ignore and deny neck pain, even when a spinal fracture exists. Radiological clearance in children is further complicated by the difficulty of interpreting X-rays of immature bones (*see* Section 7.3.B), and by the relative laxity of ligaments, which gives rise to pseudo-subluxation.

Be aware of the significant incidence of spinal cord injury without radiological abnormality (SCIWORA) in children.

Spinal injury is less common in children than in adults, partly because of the elasticity of the bones and ligaments. This same elasticity contributes to the different patterns of spinal injury that are seen. In the cervical spine, for example,

injuries tend to occur at a higher level than in adults, and often span several segments rather than dissipating energy in fracturing a single vertebra.

Examination of potentially spine-injured patients must be carried out with the patient in the neutral position (i.e. without flexion, extension or rotation), and without any movement of the spine.

The patient should be:
- log-rolled
- properly immobilised (using in-line immobilisation, a stiff neck cervical collar or sandbags)
- transported in the neutral position.

With vertebral injury (which may overlie spinal cord injury), look for:
- local tenderness
- deformities, as well as (for a posterior spinal cord injury) oedema.

Clinical findings pointing to injury of the cervical spine include:
- difficulties in respiration (diaphragmatic breathing; check for paradoxical breathing)
- flaccidity, with no reflexes (check the rectal sphincter)
- hypotension with bradycardia (without hypovolaemia).

The entire spine should be palpated during a log-roll, when the patient is turned on to their side in a controlled way, keeping the spine in line. The presence of palpable steps, bogginess or tenderness should be noted. The limbs should be examined for sensory and motor signs of focal or segmental deficit.

Neurological assessment

Assessment of the level of injury must be undertaken. If the patient is conscious, ask him/her questions relevant to their sensation, and ask them to try to make minor movements, to enable you to assess motor function of the upper and lower extremities.

Key reflex assessment to determine the level of the lesion is summarised below.

Motor response
- Diaphragm intact level   C3, C4, C5
- Shoulder shrug   C4
- Elbow flexion (biceps)   C5
- Wrist extension   C6
- Elbow extension   C7
- Wrist flexion   C7
- Abduction of fingers   C8
- Active chest expansion   Tl-T12
- Hip flexion   L2
- Knee extension   L3-L4
- Ankle dorsiflexion   L5-S 1
- Ankle plantarflexion   S1-S2

Sensory response
- Anterior thigh   L2
- Anterior knee   L3
- Anterolateral ankle   L4
- Dorsum great and 2nd toe   L5
- Lateral side of foot   Sl
- Posterior calf   S2
- Peri-anal and perineal sensation   S2-S5

If no sensory or motor function is exhibited, with a complete spinal cord lesion, the chance of recovery is small.

A diaphragmatic breathing pattern, bradycardia, hypotension, peripheral vasodilatation and priapism suggest spinal cord injury.

Throughout the primary and secondary assessments, precautions for spinal protection should ideally be maintained, using a hard collar and side-supports (blocks and straps or sandbags and tape), except for airway procedures and local examination, when manual in-line immobilisation is reinstituted.

If the patient is alert, able to communicate clearly and has no distracting pain from another injury, the spine can be cleared clinically without resorting to X-rays. Otherwise, ideally spinal precautions are maintained until radiological clearance is achieved and the patient is re-examined.

If possible, three X-rays of the cervical spine should be taken: cross-table lateral view with arm traction to reveal the C7-T1 interface; antero-posterior view and transoral odontoid peg view. These must be assessed by an experienced professional (if available), paying particular attention to the soft tissues as well as the bony structures (see Section 7.3.B).

If the mechanism of injury warrants it, thoracic and lumbar views are also required.

If the lower cervical spine is not adequately visualised on the lateral view, oblique views are requested. If the X-rays are inadequate or show suspicious areas, CT scanning (if available) is recommended to confirm or exclude a fracture. The MRI scan provides a better examination of neural, ligamentous and other soft tissues, although its sensitivity reveals minor as well as major tissue injury, making interpretation more difficult. It remains expensive and is not universally available. The MRI scanner is a frightening environment for an unsedated child, and the powerful magnetic field creates challenging logistical problems for the monitoring equipment applied to the patient.

Other neurological injuries include damaged nerves to fingers and the brachial plexus.

Pelvic trauma

Pelvic injury remains a potentially life-threatening injury, especially if it is associated with a large retroperitoneal haematoma, or if the fracture site communicates with the rectum. External fixation of the pelvis may be valuable in controlling major venous haemorrhage.

Arterial bleeding may be controlled by embolisation (if available). The suitability of these techniques depends on the particular configuration of the fracture. It may be difficult to distinguish retroperitoneal haemorrhage from intraperitoneal haemorrhage, the latter requiring laparotomy.

In the absence of suitable equipment, tight compressive binding of the pelvis may help bleeding vessels to clot, although this is not practical in the presence of advanced pregnancy.

The purpose of pelvic binding is to reduce the volume of the pelvis thus tamponading any haemorrhage, as well as providing biomechanical stabilisation. This can be achieved by wrapping a folded sheet around the pelvis. The sheet should centre on the greater trochanters and extend to the iliac crests. Taping the thighs or the feet together also helps maintain the anatomical position of the pelvis.

Not all pelvic trauma is serious. Some pubic rami fractures are minor injuries, with little intervention required. Nevertheless, the pelvis is a ring structure that tends to break in two places. On inspecting the pelvic X-ray, careful attention should be paid to the sacro-iliac joints and sacral foramina, to seek subtle evidence of a second break in the ring.

Limb trauma

In general, limb fractures in children are more likely to be managed conservatively than those in adults, reflecting the child's capacity to heal, and the risk of interfering with growth plates. An understanding of the Salter–Harris classification of epiphyseal fractures is essential, and access to a radiological atlas of developmental stages is helpful (see Section 7.2).

Examination must include:
- skin colour and temperature
- distal pulse assessment
- grazes and bleeding sites
- limb's alignment and deformities
- active and passive movements
- unusual movements and crepitation
- the severity of pain caused by injury.

Management of extremity injuries
Aim to:
- keep blood flowing to peripheral tissues
- prevent infection and skin necrosis
- prevent damage to peripheral nerves.

Special issues relating to limb trauma
Stop active bleeding by applying direct pressure, rather than by using a tourniquet, as the latter can be left on by mistake, and this can result in ischaemic damage.

Open fractures
Any wound situated in the vicinity of a fracture must be regarded as a communicating one.
Principles of the treatment are to:
- stop external bleeding
- immobilise, and relieve pain.

Amputated parts of extremities (such as fingers) should be covered with sterile gauze towels which are moistened and put into a sterile plastic bag. A non-cooled amputated part may be used within 6 hours after the injury, and a cooled one as late as 18–20 hours after it. This practice is only worthwhile if facilities for reimplantation are available.

Early fasciotomy
Compartment syndrome is fairly common, and often underestimated. This condition is caused by an increase in the internal pressure of fascial compartments, which may result from crush injuries, fractures, intramuscular haematomas or amputations. This causes compression of vessels, with resultant hypoperfusion and hypoxia of tissues, including peripheral nerves.

Compartment syndrome is recognised by the following signs in a fractured or otherwise injured limb:
- pain, accentuated by passive stretching of the involved muscles
- decreased sensation
- swelling

- limb pallor
- limb paralysis
- absence of limb pulse.

The final result of this compartment syndrome is ischaemic (or even necrotic) muscles with restricted function.

Fasciotomy involves cutting the fascial bands around the affected muscle to release the pressure within the compartment, allowing the tissues to re-perfuse. The procedure requires a good knowledge of the relevant anatomy, and is usually performed by an orthopaedic surgeon.

Special issues with regard to major trauma in pregnancy

Road traffic accidents are the most common cause of major trauma in pregnancy. Intimate partner violence starts or increases during pregnancy, and 40% of women who are murdered are killed by a current or former partner.

Anatomical and physiological changes of pregnancy and the management of trauma

The anatomical and physiological changes that occur in pregnancy are extremely important in the assessment and resuscitation of the pregnant trauma patient.

Anatomical changes

- As the uterus increases in size during pregnancy, it becomes more vulnerable to damage by both blunt and penetrating injury. Before 12 weeks of gestation it is protected by the bony pelvis, but thereafter it is an abdominal organ. The uterine fundus reaches the umbilicus at 20 weeks, and the xiphisternum at 36 weeks.
- In the first trimester, the fetus is well protected by the thick-walled uterus and relatively large amounts of amniotic fluid. As the pregnancy progresses, the uterine wall becomes thinner, providing less protection for the fetus.
- In late pregnancy, the uterus and its contents shield the maternal abdominal contents, providing a degree of protection for the maternal viscera, at the expense of fetal well-being.

Physiological changes in pregnancy

These include the following:

- increased tidal volume
- blood volume increases by 40% to 100 mL/kg
- basal heart rate increases to 85–90 bpm
- 30% increased cardiac output
- a fall in blood pressure of 5–15 mmHg
- aortocaval compression as the uterus increases in size from 20 weeks' gestation, with the potential for reduced cardiac output
- upward displacement of the diaphragm as the uterus increases in size, with an impact on lung volume, and predisposing to gastro-oesophageal reflux.

Special issues in the traumatised pregnant woman or girl

Blunt trauma may lead to:

- haemorrhage from abdominal organs, notably the spleen and liver
- uterine irritability and premature labour
- partial or complete uterine rupture

- partial or complete placental separation (up to 48 hours after trauma)
- fetal death
- fetal distress.

Pelvic fractures may be associated with severe blood loss.

What are the priorities?

- Assessment and resuscitation according to the ABC and neurological failure structured approach.
- Resuscitation in the left lateral position after 20 weeks' gestation, to avoid aortocaval compression: remember the **left lateral tilt**.
- Assessment of fundal height and tenderness, and fetal heart rate monitoring as appropriate.
- Vaginal examination or speculum examination to assess vaginal bleeding, cervical dilatation and rupture of membranes.

If placenta praevia is known or suspected, digital vaginal examination should **not** be performed, as major haemorrhage may occur. Careful speculum examination is acceptable.

It is important to be alert to signs of hypovolaemia, which are delayed in pregnancy as the mother has a higher circulating volume. Hypovolaemia may compromise the fetus before the mother's vital signs become abnormal. A fall in maternal blood pressure is a late and ominous sign.

Resuscitation of the mother may save the baby as well. There are times when the mother's life is at risk and the fetus may need to be delivered in order to save the mother.

Action plan

1 Call for the most senior help available.
2 Perform standard primary assessment and resuscitation.
3 In addition:
   - Assess fetal well-being. Use ultrasound examination to detect the fetal heart rate and to identify any retroplacental or intra-abdominal bleeding. Ultrasound is also useful for ascertaining the presentation of the fetus; transverse lie may suggest rupture of the uterus.
   - Consider whether Caesarean section is indicated for maternal or fetal reasons.

Indications for Caesarean section (if facilities are available to perform it safely)

These include the following:

- cardiac arrest
- uterine rupture
- inadequate exposure during laparotomy for other abdominal trauma
- placental abruption
- an unstable pelvic or lumbo-sacral fracture with the patient in labour
- fetal distress with a viable fetus.

Peri-mortem Caesarean section

This should be undertaken when maternal cardiac output has not been restored by initial cardiopulmonary resuscitation (CPR). Delivery should ideally be accomplished within 5 minutes of cardiac arrest.

The rationale behind peri-mortem Caesarean section is as follows:

- improvement in maternal cardiac output due to relief of aortocaval compression
- improvement in maternal oxygenation
- greater efficacy of CPR due to better access
- better chance of fetal survival if in third trimester.

Peri-mortem Caesarean section should be undertaken with a left lateral tilt of 15–30 degrees, or preferably with manual displacement of the uterus. CPR should continue throughout, until cardiac output is restored. The operation should take place at the scene of cardiac arrest, rather than after moving the patient to the operating theatre, which wastes precious time. Blood loss is minimal until cardiac output resumes. The woman can be moved to the operating theatre once cardiac output is restored. The fetus may survive, but this is a secondary consideration. The aim of peri-mortem Caesarean section is to save the mother's life, as resuscitation is more likely to be effective if the gravid uterus is emptied.

Secondary assessment

Left lateral tilt should be maintained throughout the assessment, in order to minimise aortocaval compression. If spinal injury is suspected, manual displacement of the uterus should be undertaken instead.

Specific types of trauma
Blunt trauma

The three commonest causes are road traffic accidents, falls and intimate partner violence.

Uterine rupture due to blunt trauma is relatively rare.

Blunt trauma to the abdomen may cause placental abruption. Kleihauer testing, if available, is useful for detecting feto–maternal haemorrhage as an indicator of placental damage. Detection of intra-abdominal haemorrhage may be difficult in pregnancy, so laparotomy should be considered. Remember that the mother may lose a third of her blood volume before the vital signs become abnormal.

Penetrating abdominal wounds

Knife and gunshot wounds are the most common. Penetrating injuries can cause uterine injury at any stage of pregnancy. The uterus, fetus and amniotic fluid reduce injury to the mother by absorbing energy and displacing bowel upwards and to the side. Penetrating injuries above the uterus may cause extensive gastrointestinal and vascular damage. Exploratory laparotomy is usually required in the management of penetrating abdominal wounds, in pregnancy as in the non-pregnant patient.

Thoracic trauma

Injury to major thoracic structures is particularly dangerous in pregnancy, due to the combination of pre-existing relative aortocaval compression, reduced respiratory excursion and

Pathway of care: trauma in pregnancy.

Primary assessment and resuscitation	**Airway:** increased risk of aspiration – early gastric tube
	Breathing: if chest drain is needed, place at higher level (3rd or 4th intercostal space)
	Circulation: left lateral tilt
	Abnormalities in pulse rate, blood pressure and capillary refill are late because of hypovolaemia of pregnancy
	'Targeted resuscitation' with IV crystalloids, colloid or blood
	Neurological failure: convulsions may be due to eclampsia as well as head injury

Secondary assessment and emergency treatment:

Assess for:
- Ruptured uterus and placental abruption after blunt trauma to abdomen (including seat-belt injury). Uterine tenderness, vaginal bleeding, shock all occur. They may be indistinguishable clinically. Scan may show fetal death or intra-abdominal fluid (blood)
- Rupture of membranes (by speculum)
- Fetal distress

Evidence of intra-abdominal bleeding or injury to abdominal organs

Consider bowel injury (compressed by uterus and therefore more vulnerable to blunt trauma or penetrating injuries)

Ensure anti-tetanus measures

X-rays as needed

On discharge from hospital, patient to report abdominal pain, decreased fetal movements, vaginal bleeding or fluid leakage

---

increased oxygen requirement. However, most injuries can be identified by careful assessment, and managed with simple measures, including left lateral tilt and facial oxygen.

Special issues with regard to major trauma in children

Trauma is a leading cause of death for all children, with a higher incidence in boys. The survival of children who sustain major trauma depends on the severity of the trauma, effective pre-hospital care and early resuscitation.

The initial assessment of the paediatric trauma patient is identical to that of the adult. The first priority is the Airway, Breathing and Circulation, then early neurological assessment, and finally exposing the child for full examination, without loss of heat.

TABLE 7.3.A.5 Paediatric 'normal' values are helpful as follows:

Variable	< 1 year	1–2 years	2–5 years	5–12 years	> 12 years
Respiratory rate (breaths/minute)	30–40	25–35	25–30	20–25	15–20
Heart rate (beats/minute)	110–160	100–150	95–140	80–120	60–100
Systolic blood pressure (mmHg) 50th centile	80–90	85–95	85–100	90–110	100–120

Specific resuscitation and intubation issues in children

- The head, tongue and nasal airway are relatively large.
- The angle of the jaw is greater, the larynx is higher and the epiglottis is proportionally larger and more 'U' shaped.
- The cricoid is the narrowest part of the larynx, which limits the size of the endotracheal tube. By adulthood, the larynx has grown and the narrowest part is at the cords.
- Obligatory nose breathing occurs in small babies.
- The trachea in the full-term newborn is about 4 cm long, and will admit a 2.5 or 3.5 mm diameter endotracheal tube. (The adult trachea is about 12 cm long.)
- Gastric distension is common following resuscitation, and a nasogastric tube is useful for decompressing the stomach.

If tracheal intubation is required, avoid using cuffed tubes in children under 10 years of age, so as to minimise subglottic swelling and ulceration. Oral intubation is easier than nasal intubation for infants and young children.

Shock in the paediatric patient

The femoral artery in the groin and the brachial artery in the antecubital fossa are the best sites at which to palpate pulses in the child. If the child is pulseless, cardiopulmonary resuscitation should be commenced.

Signs of shock in paediatric patients include:

- tachycardia
- weak or absent peripheral pulses
- capillary refill time > 3 seconds
- tachypnoea
- agitation
- drowsiness
- poor urine output.

Hypotension is a late sign, even in the presence of severe shock.

A normal urine output is 1–2 mL/kg/hour for the infant and 0.5–1 mL/kg/hour in the older child.

Hypothermia is a major problem in children because of their relatively large surface area. They lose proportionally more heat through the head. All fluids should be warmed. Exposure of the child is necessary for assessment, but cover them as soon as possible.

Continuing care for patients who have suffered major trauma

Tetanus prophylaxis

This is often forgotten in the management of severe trauma. In the fully immunised patient, an additional booster will depend on a clinical decision as to the possibility of exposure to contamination, the severity of injury and the timing of the last tetanus immunisation. In an unimmunised or incompletely immunised patient, tetanus immunoglobulin should be given and a full course of or a completing course of tetanus toxoid started (using a different limb to the one receiving the immunoglobulin).

Guidance on tetanus-prone wounds

These include the following:

- compound fractures
- deep penetrating wounds
- wounds containing foreign bodies (especially wood splinters)
- wounds complicated by pyogenic infections
- wounds with extensive tissue damage (e.g. crush injuries, contusions or burns)
- any wound that is obviously contaminated with soil, dust or horse manure (especially if topical disinfection is delayed for more than 4 hours).

TABLE 7.3.A.6 Guidance on the use of tetanus immunoglobulin and tetanus toxoid

History of tetanus vaccination		Type of wound	Tetanus vaccine booster (see below)	Tetanus immunoglobulin
≥ 3 doses	< 5 years since last dose	All wounds	No	No
	5–10 years since last dose	Clean minor wounds	No	No
		All other wounds	Yes	No
	> 10 years since last dose	All wounds	Yes	No
< 3 doses or uncertain		Clean minor wounds	Yes	No
		All other wounds	Yes	Yes

Transfer

Not every hospital has the resources and expertise to safely care for injured pregnant women or girls and children. Ideally, children with serious injuries should be transported directly from the scene of the accident to a centre with such capability (if one exists in the country). Even then, geographical constraints may render transfer unsafe.

Patients should be transported only if they are going to a facility that can provide a higher level of care.

Even when the transfer is urgent, it is essential to achieve physiological stability before embarking on a hazardous journey in the isolated environment of the ambulance. There is always physiological deterioration during transfer. Thorough assessment should take place prior to transfer,

to exclude coexisting life-threatening conditions which may be amenable to treatment on site. For example, a child with a head injury should not be transferred in a hypotensive condition caused by unrecognised and untreated intra-abdominal bleeding.

It is essential that there is effective communication with:

- the receiving centre
- the transport service
- escorting personnel
- the patient and their relatives.

Communication between the referring and admitting clinicians is necessary, not only to agree that transfer is indicated, but also to establish guidelines for care in transit, and to warn the receiving centre when the patient is expected to arrive.

Effective stabilisation necessitates:

- prompt effective initial resuscitation
- control of haemorrhage and maintenance of the circulation
- immobilisation of fractures
- analgesia.

If the patient deteriorates, re-evaluate them by using the primary assessment, checking and treating life-threatening conditions, and then make a careful assessment focusing on the injuries area.

Inter-hospital transfer requires careful planning, to provide:

- trained medical and nursing escorts
- simple compact robust equipment
- drugs for resuscitation, sedation, pain relief and muscle relaxation
- fluids and blood products if indicated
- a suitable vehicle and ambulance staff.

In trauma care, some transfers are time-limited (e.g. to evacuate an extradural haematoma). In such cases, the extra time taken for a retrieval team to reach the referring hospital may offset the benefit of their specialised skills.

Peri-operative care in major trauma

In the operating theatre, definitive anatomical reduction, repair or resection of individual injuries takes place. While the surgical team focuses on anatomical correction, the anaesthetic team maintains physiological system control. The impetus and sense of urgency evident in the Emergency Department should be maintained, without losing the thoroughness necessary to manage all aspects of care.

If the patient has a significant head injury, the anaesthetic agents should be chosen to avoid increasing intracranial pressure or cerebral blood flow. In general, this means avoiding high doses of volatile agents such as halothane or isoflurane. Ketamine has long been considered to be contraindicated in head injury, although there is recent evidence that challenges this view. It may be the only anaesthetic available.

If the child is undergoing lengthy extracranial surgery in the face of a severe head injury, it is wise to observe the pupils at frequent intervals.

Maintaining the child's core temperature is a key aim during prolonged surgery. Hypothermia impairs platelet function and increases the risk of infection, although it has been claimed to help to preserve brain function in severe head injury.

High-dependency care

In the immediate management of the injured patient, the focus was on physiological assessment and intervention using an ABC structured approach, followed by anatomical assessment and definitive care.

When high-dependency care is instituted, physiological stabilisation again becomes the main concern, although it is important to remain alert to the possibility of any further injuries that were not evident in the secondary assessment. Detailed physiological control is facilitated by monitoring and good nursing.

See Section 1.14 for further information.

Step-down care and rehabilitation

High-dependency care, acute ward care and rehabilitation serve to minimise disability, rather than influence mortality, which is already largely determined by this time. The emphasis shifts towards integration back into normal life, physically and psychologically, although the course may be interrupted by further reconstructive surgery.

7.3.B Emergency trauma radiology

Introduction

Essential initial trauma films to screen for major injuries include the following.

- lateral cervical spine radiograph
- chest X-ray
- pelvic X-ray.

These should only be taken after immediately life-threatening injuries have been identified and treated (resuscitation).

The ABCD approach to X-ray interpretation is as follows:

- **A**dequacy, Alignment and Apparatus.
- **B**ones.
- **C**artilage and soft tissues.
- **D**isc spaces (in the spine), **D**iaphragm (in the chest).

First, all X-ray films should be checked for **adequacy**. Do they include all of the part that needs imaging? Is the film a proper antero-posterior view or is it at an angle? If the film is not of reasonable quality, interpretation is difficult and may be faulty.

Cervical spine

The cervical spine should be immobilised (*see* Section 7.3.A) before any radiology. The standard film is a lateral radiograph, which may be supplemented by an AP (lower cervical spine and odontoid peg views) if appropriate.

Bony injury is not the primary focus in spinal injury. The main concern is to delineate actual or potential injury to the cord, as any unstable fracture, if inadequately immobilised, may lead to progressive cord damage.

A normal lateral cervical X-ray film may be falsely reassuring. The plain film only shows the position of the bones at the time when the film was taken, and gives no idea of the magnitude of flexion and extension forces applied to the spine at the time of injury. **The cord may be injured even in a child without any apparent radiographic abnormality.** This phenomenon is known as SCIWORA (see below).

Unlike adult spine injuries, most paediatric cervical spine injuries occur either through the discs and ligaments, at the cranio-vertebral junction (C1, C2 and C3), or at C7/T1. The relatively large head of the child, moving on a flexible neck with weaker muscles, leads to injury in the higher cervical vertebrae.

Children show three patterns of spinal injury:

1 subluxation or dislocation without fracture
2 fracture with or without subluxation or dislocation
3 spinal cord injury without radiographic abnormality (SCIWORA).

The last of these, SCIWORA, is said to have occurred when radiographic films are completely normal in the presence of significant cord injury. **If the film is normal in a conscious child with clinical symptoms (such as pain, loss of function or paraesthesia in a limb), neck protection measures should be continued.** In an unconscious child at high risk, a cord injury cannot be excluded until the patient is awake and has been assessed clinically, even in the presence of a normal cervical spine film. Adequate spinal precautions should be continued until the child is well enough to be assessed clinically.

The most common site of a 'missed' spinal injury is where a flexible part of the spine meets the fixed part. In the neck these are the cervico-cranial junction and the cervico-thoracic junction.

The whole spine should be viewed from the lower clivus down to the upper body of T1 vertebra.

Alignment

When studying a cervical spine X-ray, look for the four lines shown in Figure 7.3.B.1. These lines should be uninterrupted. It there is a 'step' in any line, the spinal cord is at risk. The cervical immobilisation must be continued and an orthopaedic opinion sought.

The four lines are as follows:

1 anterior vertebral line
2 posterior vertebral line (anterior wall of the spinal canal)
3 facet line
4 spino-laminar line (posterior wall of the spinal canal).

Figure 7.3.B.2 shows an actual cervical spine X-ray with three of the lines delineated and the odontoid, a facet joint, a spinous process and a lamina identified. The gaps between the adjacent spinous processes and between each facet joint should be similar. Again, any discrepancy is suggestive of a potentially unstable spine.

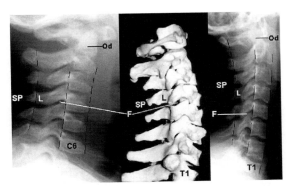

FIGURE 7.3.B.2 X-ray of the lateral cervical spine, showing three of the lines that are indicated in Figure 7.3.B.1. Od, odontoid; F, facet joint; L, lamina; SP, spinous process spaces.

The spinal cord lies in the canal between the posterior vertebral line (2) and the spino-laminar (4) line.

Bones

The outline of each vertebra should be reviewed in turn. Fracture lines going through the cortex, vertebral bodies, laminae or spinous processes should be sought.

The spaces between the facet joints and the gaps between adjacent spinous processes should be similar. The joint between the odontoid peg and the anterior arch of the atlas should be 1–4 mm in a child (see Figure 7.3.B.3).

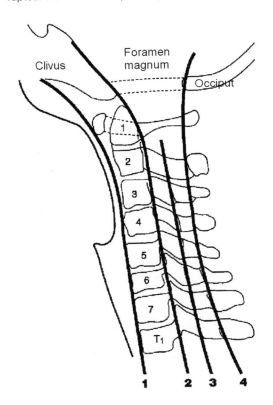

Cervical spine review alignment:
the cord lies between **2** and **4**

FIGURE 7.3.B.1 Lines to examine on X-ray of the lateral cervical spine.

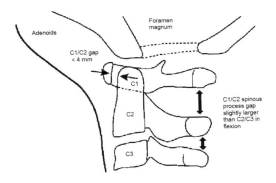

FIGURE 7.3.B.3 C1/C2 anatomy in the older child.

The orientation of the odontoid peg should always be perpendicular to the body of C2.

Cartilage and soft tissues

Abnormal widening of the pre-vertebral soft tissues may indicate a haematoma due to cervical spine injury. However, there may be a significant spinal injury with normal soft tissues. Thus the absence of soft-tissue swelling does not exclude major bony or ligamentous injury. When a child is intubated, it is difficult to assess pre-vertebral soft-tissue swelling. Small children have large adenoids, which are seen as well-demarcated soft tissue swelling at the base of the clivus.

Acceptable soft-tissue thicknesses are as follows:

- above the larynx: less than one-third of the vertebral body width
- below the larynx: not more than one vertebral body width.

Below the level of the larynx, the pre-vertebral soft tissues become progressively **narrower** towards the cervicothoracic junction (*see* Figure 7.3.B.4). If the pre-vertebral soft tissues are wider at C7 than at the C5 level, this suggests trauma at the C7/T1 level.

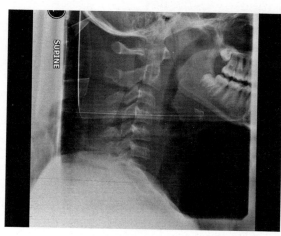

FIGURE 7.3.B.4 Lateral cervical spine showing soft tissues.

Any soft-tissue swelling outside these limits should be regarded as abnormal, and neck protection measures maintained until a further clinical opinion can be obtained. In small children the soft tissues may appear abnormally wide if the film is taken with the infant lying in flexion. If in doubt, maintain the neck protection and ask for advice.

Discs

The height of the vertebral disc should be compared from C2/C3 to C7/T1. The discs should all be of similar height, as shown earlier in Figure 7.3.B.1. Any significant discrepancy suggests a crush fracture of the vertebrae (usually caused by a fall from a height).

Flexion and extension cervical spine films should never be performed in the acute trauma situation.

Chest X-ray

Adequacy and alignment

Adequacy can be assessed by evaluating both radiographic penetration and the depth of the patient's inspiration. The film should just show the disc spaces of the lower thoracic vertebrae through the heart shadow. At least five anterior rib ends should be seen above the diaphragm on the right side. If the film is taken in expiration, it may mimic a chest infection. Films are difficult to take in young children, as they are unable to 'hold their breath' on command, so the radiographer has to try to take the picture at the moment of full inspiration.

Alignment can be assessed by ensuring that the medial ends of both clavicles are equally spaced about the spinous processes of the upper thoracic vertebrae. Abnormal rotation may create an apparent mediastinal shift. The trachea should be equally spaced between the clavicles.

Apparatus

Check the position of any apparatus, including the following:

- tracheal tube
- central venous lines
- chest drains.

Misplacement of the endotracheal tube (ETT) into a bronchus should be evident clinically, but may be seen on a chest film if you look for it. Do this first when reviewing any chest X-ray on an intubated patient. Ventilation of only one lung will lead to hypoxia in a compromised patient.

The ideal position for an ETT is below the clavicles and at least 1 cm above the carina. To find the carina, identify the slope of the right and left main bronchi. The carina is where the two lines meet in the midline.

Bones

Look at each rib in detail. This can be done by tracing out the upper and lower borders of the ribs from the posterior costochondral joint to the point where they join the anterior costal cartilage at the mid-clavicular line. The individual internal bone patterns can then be assessed.

The ribs in children are soft and pliable, and only break when subjected to considerable force. Even greater force is required to fracture the first rib or to break multiple ribs. Consequently, the presence of these fractures should stimulate you to look for other sites of injury both inside and outside the chest. Fractures in children's rib bones are hard to see while fresh unless there is displacement. Diagnosis is often made a week or so later if an X-ray is taken then, when the calcifying new callus is seen.

Finish assessing the bones by inspecting the visible vertebrae and the clavicles, scapulae and proximal humeri.

Thoracic spine injuries may be overlooked on a chest radiograph. Abnormal flattening of the vertebral bodies,

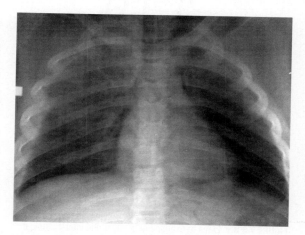

FIGURE 7.3.B.5 Vertical fracture of the thoracic spine.

widening of the disc spaces, or gaps between the spinous processes or pedicles may be seen. On the antero-posterior views, increased vertical or horizontal distances between the pedicles or spinous processes indicate an unstable fracture, as shown in Figure 7.3.B.5.

If there are rib fractures in the first three ribs, these may be associated with major spinal trauma and great vessel injury.

Cartilage and soft tissues
Lungs
In a well-centred film, the lungs should appear equally black on both sides. Compare the left and right lungs in the upper third, middle third and lower third of the chest.

Check that the lungs go all the way out to the rib cage (i.e. that there is no pleural effusion or pneumothorax). A lung that is black on one side may be due to a pneumothorax or air trapping. A lung that is white on one side may be due to collapse, pulmonary haemorrhage, contusion or effusion (including haemothorax).

On the supine film, blood or fluid lies posteriorly, giving a generalised greyness to the lung, rather than the typical meniscus sign seen on the erect film. At the apex of each lung, an effusion displacing the lung downward may indicate spinal injury or major vessel damage.

A suspected tension pneumothorax should be treated clinically in the emergency situation, without confirmatory X-ray.

On a supine film, the air in a simple pneumothorax rises anteriorly and may only be evident from an abnormal blackness or 'sharpness' of the diaphragm or cardiac border. The standard appearances of a pneumothorax, where there is a sharp lung edge and the vessels fail to extend to the rib cage and the lung edges, may not occur in the supine film.

The heart
The cardiac outline should lie one-third to the right of the midline and two-thirds to the left of the midline. If the film is not rotated, which should be checked, mediastinal shift is due to the heart being either pushed from one side or pulled from the other. For example, mediastinal shift to the left may be due to a pneumothorax, air trapping or effusion on the right side, or collapse of the left lung.

All emergency major trauma X-rays are taken in the supine position because of the seriousness of the patient's condition, often using portable X-ray machines. The X-ray tube is near to the patient and the heart is anterior with the film posterior. The heart in this situation appears abnormally magnified (widened), and the cardiothoracic ratio is difficult to assess on supine AP films.

The mediastinal cardiac outline should be clear on both sides. Any loss of definition suggests consolidation (de-aeration) of adjacent lungs. A 'globular' shape to the heart may suggest a pericardial effusion. Tamponade is managed clinically. A cardiac ultrasound scan is useful in equivocal cases.

The upper mediastinum
In the teenager the mediastinum should appear as narrow as in an adult. In children under the age of 18 months, the normal thymus is large, causing a confusing and often 'sail-shaped' upper mediastinal shadow. A normal thymus may touch the right chest wall, left chest wall, left diaphragm or right diaphragm, making it very difficult to

exclude mediastinal pathology. Fortunately, mediastinal widening due to aortic dissection or spinal trauma is very rare in small children.

In the older child involved in trauma, mediastinal widening may mean aortic dissection, or major vessel or spinal injury. Ultrasound scanning will be helpful (if available).

Diaphragms
The cardiophrenic and costophrenic angles should be clear on both sides. The diaphragms should be clearly defined on both sides, and the left diaphragm should be clearly visible behind the heart. Loss of definition of the left diaphragm behind the heart suggests left lower lobe collapse, an abnormal hump suggests diaphragmatic rupture, and an elevated diaphragm suggests effusion, lung collapse or nerve palsy.

At the end of the systematic ABCD review of the X-ray, check again in the key areas shown in the following list:
- Behind the heart: left lower lobe consolidation or collapse.
- Apices: for effusions, pneumothorax, rib fractures and collapse or consolidation.
- Costophrenic and cardiophrenic angles: fluid or pneumothorax.
- Horizontal fissure: fluid or elevation (upper lobe collapse).
- Trachea for foreign body (and ETT).

Pelvic X-ray

A single, antero-posterior pelvic view is sufficient.

Adequacy and alignment
It is very important to have the pelvic film positioned as a true antero-posterior (AP) view, as rotation causes interpretation problems. In a true AP film the tip of the sacrum will be aligned with the symphysis pubis.

The whole of the pelvis from the top of the iliac crests to the ischial tuberosities and both hip joints should be seen. The femoral necks shown to the level of the trochanters should be included.

Bones
The pelvis is composed of the sacrum, innominate bones (iliac wings), ischium and pubic bones. These come together to form a Y-shaped cartilage in the floor of the acetabulum. In young children, the joint between the ischium and the pubis (ischiopubic synchondrosis) is commonly seen and may simulate a fracture.

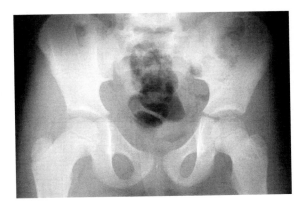

FIGURE 7.3.B.6 Normal pelvis in a young child.

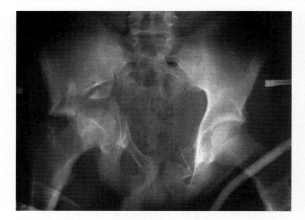

FIGURE 7.3.B.7 Multiple pelvic fractures.

The pelvis is reviewed as a number of rings on the two-dimensional film. These include the pelvic brim, the two obturator rings and both acetabular fossae. The rings should appear smooth and symmetrical in a well-centred film (see Figure 7.3.B.6, which shows a normal child pelvis). The femoral necks must be checked for fracture. Figure 7.3.B.7 shows a pelvis with multiple fractures, at major risk of serious pelvic bleeding as large vessels are torn with the force shown by the widespread fractures.

Cartilage and soft tissues

Minor rotation, hip flexion or rotation will distort the fat plane and make assessment of soft-tissue displacement difficult. Abnormal widening of the obturator fat pad may indicate a pelvic side wall haematoma.

The paediatric pelvis is held together by cartilage. Separation through the cartilage of the sacro-iliac joint, the symphysis pubis or the 'Y' cartilage of the acetabular floor may occur without apparent bony injury. Comparison of both hips and sacro-iliac joints on a well-centred film may show this. On a well-centred film the distance between the femoral head and the floor of the acetabulum 'crescent' should be symmetrical – it is abnormal in effusion or dislocation of the hip joint.

7.3.C The child with a head injury

BOX 7.3.C.1 Minimum standards
- ABC and neurology and maintenance of oxygenation and blood pressure with control of environmental temperature while exposing and examining the whole patient.
- Emergency burr-hole by an experienced operator if available.
- Parenteral antibiotics.
- Mannitol or hypertonic saline (2.7% or 3%).
- Anticonvulsants.

Introduction

The primary aim of the management of traumatic brain injury is to prevent secondary brain injury, which results from failure to maintain adequate oxygenation and optimal blood pressure in the head-injured child, in addition to the brain swelling which is the usual response of the child's brain to injury. This aim is made more difficult by the presence of other injuries which may be reducing oxygenation and causing shock. Severity of brain injury in toddlers and children can be measured by using the Glasgow Coma Scale (GCS). The GCS score ranges from 3 to 15. A GCS score of 14–15 is categorised as minor brain injury, a score of 9–13 as moderate brain injury, and a score of 3–8 as severe brain injury.

The GCS is based on eye opening (E), best motor response (M) and verbal response (V).

Scores for best eye response (4)
1 None
2 Eye opening to pain
3 Eye opening to verbal command
4 Eyes open spontaneously

Scores for best verbal response (5)
1 None
2 Incomprehensible sounds
3 Inappropriate words
4 Confused conversation
5 Orientated

Scores for best motor response (6)
1 None
2 Extension to pain (decerebrate)
3 Flexion to pain (decorticate)
4 Withdrawal from pain
5 Localises pain
6 Obeys commands

Children's Coma Scale
Scores for best eye response (4)
1 None
2 Eye opening to pain
3 Eye opening to verbal command
4 Eyes open spontaneously

Scores for best verbal response (5)
1 Alert, babbles, usual words
2 Less than usual words spontaneous irritable cry
3 Cries only to pain
4 Moans to pain
5 No response to pain

Scores for best motor response (6)
1 Spontaneous or obeys verbal command
2 Localises to pain or withdraws to touch
3 Withdraws from pain
4 Abnormal flexion to pain (decorticate)
5 Abnormal extension to pain (decerebrate)
6 No response to pain

Another factor that must be documented is pupillary size

and reaction to light. This helps when lateralising brain injury and its progress.

Major diffuse brain injury

Cerebral oedema is the most likely pathological process following serious head injury in children. Intracranial haematomas are quite uncommon in childhood: they are more likely to be found in an adult patient. Even the presence of unequal pupils in a seriously head injured child may be a false localising sign, and does not have the same significance that this sign has in the adult head-injured patient.

The only measures that are of proven value are maintenance of adequate oxygenation and perfusion and the avoidance of adverse effects (see below). Removal of intracranial haematomas, if identified, is very helpful, but this pathology is much less frequently found in the paediatric population, where cerebral oedema predominates. A CT scan (if available) will identify any haematoma. **Artificial ventilation, tracheostomy and more sophisticated medical measures designed to control raised intracranial pressure may be of value, but require evacuation to a fully equipped and staffed children's neurointensive care unit.**

In the absence of such a facility, the best strategy is to concentrate on optimising the care of the unconscious patient with attention to:

- preservation of the airway
- maintenance of adequate ventilation
- avoidance of hypotension by maintaining the circulating volume with normal Ringer-lactate or Hartmann's solution
- the maintenance of appropriate fluid and electrolyte balance, avoiding hypotonic IV fluids, hyponatraemia and hypoglycaemia
- avoidance of fever > 38°C. Use rectal paracetamol: child 1–5 years 125–250 mg/dose up to 4 doses in 24 hours; 5–12 years 250–500 mg/dose maximum 4 doses; 12 years–adult 500 mg/dose maximum 4 doses
- maintaining the patient in a 20-degree head-up position with no neck flexion and with the head in the midline
- if there is deterioration of the GCS score, giving an IV infusion of mannitol 0.25–0.5 g/kg
- mannitol can be repeated later but there is a decreasing response to this treatment. Alternatively, hypertonic saline can be used (2.7% or 3% at a dose of 3 mL/kg). This may not be associated with a 'rebound' brain swelling as occurs with mannitol and does not induce a diuresis like mannitol but rather augments plasma volume
- care of the skin, bladder and bowel.

Fluid restriction is not indicated, but fluid overload should be avoided.

If transfer or evacuation is required within the first 48 hours after injury, endotracheal intubation and mechanical ventilation are desirable. Steroids are of no value and increase the risk of intercurrent infection. Antibiotics are reserved for patients with evidence of sepsis. Anticonvulsant drugs are only given if there are seizures.

Intracranial haematomas

Only 6 in 1000 patients will develop a significant intracranial haematoma following a non-missile head injury. **The most useful guide to the development of an intracranial haematoma is deterioration in the level of consciousness.** The presence of inequality of the pupils will help to identify the lesion. **The ideal investigation is CT (if available).** If CT is not readily available, burr-hole exploration on the same side as the injury as the dilated pupil and the opposite side to any motor weakness is justified in the hope of finding an extradural or subdural clot. **However, burr-holes must only be made by a skilled surgeon using appropriate equipment.**

Emergency temporary reduction of raised intracranial pressure can be achieved by one or more of the following medical measures:

- mannitol 20% by IV infusion over 20 minutes (0.25–0.5 g/kg). This can be repeated as required but response becomes progressively lessened
- Alternatively, hypertonic saline can be used (2.7% or 3% at a dose of 3 mL/kg). This may not be associated with a 'rebound' brain swelling as occurs with mannitol and does not induce a diuresis like mannitol but rather augments plasma volume
- intubation and artificial ventilation to keep $PaCO_2$ around 4 KPa.

An extradural clot will always be beneath the site of trauma. The place to make the burr-hole is therefore at the site of any external site of injury. This may be known from the history, or may be found by shaving the entire scalp in search of bruises, grazes, lacerations or soft-tissue swelling. A plain skull radiograph (if available) may show a fracture, and if so the burr-hole should be made at the site of the fracture. If there are none of the above-mentioned clues, then 'blind' burr-hole exploration will be required. This should commence on the side of the dilated pupil, or on the side of the pupil that dilated first.

Three standard burr-holes can be made: subtemporal, frontal and parietal. It is crucial to make the sub-temporal burr-hole low enough in the middle cranial fossa. The correct position is immediately above the zygoma at the midpoint between the outer canthus of the eye and the external auditory meatus. If an extradural clot is found, the burr-hole must be extended as either a craniectomy or a craniotomy. The margins should extend sufficiently far to uncover the entire clot, which can then be evacuated by suction. Bleeding meningeal arteries can be controlled with diathermy or by under-running with a suture. Bleeding from major venous sinuses can be controlled by haemostatic gauze and by hitching the adjacent dura to the surrounding pericranium with sutures. Diffuse meningeal oozing will stop spontaneously if it is not tampered with; the application of hydrogen peroxide or warm saline packs may help. When the clot has been evacuated and the bleeding has stopped, it is essential to hitch the dura around the perimeter of the bone opening to the adjacent pericranium in order to prevent recurrence. In very young children, it may be better to pass sutures through small drill holes in the surrounding bone. If a craniotomy has been made, the bone flap is replaced.

If no extradural haematoma is found at any of the burr-hole sites, the dura should be opened cautiously. If there is a subdural clot, a craniotomy is necessary. It is safer to make multiple short dural incisions rather than a wide dural opening. It is difficult to be certain whether a tense dura is due to subdural clot or brain swelling. Most acute subdural clots are associated with quite severe brain injury, and a wide dural opening is very likely to be followed by massive uncontrollable extrusion of the brain material.

Post-operatively, anaesthesia can be reversed unless the patient is to be evacuated to another facility. If a significant clot has been found, there should be a prompt improvement in the level of consciousness.

In a baby with severe signs of rapidly progressive raised intracranial pressure following a closed head injury, it is reasonable to search for an acute subdural haematoma by passing an adult (18-gauge) lumbar puncture needle into the subdural space through the anterior fontanelle or through a diastased coronal suture. The baby is wrapped in a sheet and held supine by an assistant so as to secure the head, the arms and the trunk. The entry point is either at the most lateral extremity of the anterior fontanelle or at a point in line with the pupil, whichever is the furthest from the midline. **In a conscious child, local anaesthesia must first be applied.** The needle is passed at a shallow angle, in an anterior direction, through the skin and then through the relatively resistant dura. The trochar is removed from the needle and any subdural fluid allowed to drain spontaneously. The needle is then withdrawn and the puncture hole in the skin closed with a suture.

Skull fractures

Most skull fractures heal without treatment, but they should be observed for 24 hours in case an intracranial haematoma occurs unless a CT scan has shown no intracranial bleeding. Fractures which are compound, either externally (i.e. the overlying scalp is broken) or internally (i.e. there is a fracture into a paranasal sinus or into the middle ear) require attention.

Externally compound fractures

- Like all wounds, these should be explored to remove all dead tissue and foreign material. This is the most effective means of preventing infection. Operation should be performed as soon as possible. Simple wounds can be explored under local anaesthetic, but more complex wounds will require general anaesthesia.
- Depressed fractures may require elevation to ensure that the full extent of the wound, including the brain substance, has been cleaned and that the dura is repaired if it has been torn. If the wound is less than 24 hours old and not heavily contaminated, the bone fragments can be replaced. If the wound is older than 24 hours or is heavily contaminated, it is safer to discard the bone fragments.
- Antibiotics are not generally required, as it is the mechanical debridement of the wound that is the crucial step. However, compound depressed skull fractures that have occurred in any setting, especially an agricultural or rural one, may be contaminated with *Clostridium tetani* and are best covered with 5 days of IV benzylpenicillin (for children aged 1 month to 12 years, 50 mg/kg every 6 hours by slow injection, and for those over 12 years, 2.4 grams every 6 hours) with anti-tetanus active immunisation and toxoid as appropriate (*see* Section 7.3.A). Animal bites, especially from dogs, will be contaminated with *Pasteurella multocida* and should be covered with ampicillin IV (40 mg/kg 8-hourly up to a

maximum of 4 grams/day). If surgery is delayed for more than 24 hours, antibiotics should be given.

The scalp has excellent vascularity and every effort should be made to preserve scalp. Once significant areas are lost, complex skin flaps will be required. Split-skin grafts will not take on bare calvarial bone. If substantial areas of full-thickness scalp are lost, as in burns or attacks by large animals, a useful technique is to make multiple burr-holes, leaving the dura intact. Over the course of a few weeks the florid granulation tissue that grows out of the burr-holes will form a satisfactory base to accept split-skin grafts.

Internally compound fractures

- These carry the risk of CSF fistula and meningitis.
- Prophylactic antibiotics are not indicated.
- Most CSF rhinorrhoea or otorrhoea will resolve spontaneously, but cases persisting for longer than 2 weeks will require formal repair. This will involve referral to a higher centre with facilities for CT scanning and neurosurgical expertise.
- Meningitis complicating traumatic CSF rhinorrhoea or otorrhoea is usually caused by *Streptococcus pneumoniae*, and should be treated for 2 weeks with IV benzylpenicillin (at the dose stated above) or IV cefotaxime (for children under 12 years, 50 mg/kg every 6 hours and for those over 12 years 1–3 g every 6 hours. It is an absolute indication for surgical repair to prevent further episodes.

Penetrating injuries

Children are especially prone to suffering penetrating injuries because of the thin nature of the immature skull, especially around the orbit. **Such wounds require exploration through their full extent to prevent brain abscess.**

Missile injuries require removal of all foreign material wherever feasible. High-velocity penetrating brain injuries from modern military weapons are invariably fatal because of the extreme forces involved, and these patients, along with those who are in deep coma following even low-velocity gunshot wounds, will not make a useful recovery, so **only palliative care is appropriate**.

Early traumatic epilepsy

Epileptic seizures in the first 48 hours after injury are common in children. Except in infants they do not, in isolation, indicate the presence of an intracranial haematoma. Most seizures are self-limiting and simply require airway protection. An anti-epileptic drug should be given to prevent further fits. It is important to remember that the child with an acutely injured brain will be exquisitely sensitive to the respiratory depressant effects of diazepam or lorazepam. These are best avoided unless there is no alternative, when they must be used to stop the convulsion, which will worsen the effects of the head injury.

When using either diazepam or lorazepam, always have a functioning bag-mask resuscitator immediately available. The main side effect of these drugs is apnoea or hypoventilation, but it is short-lived, and a few minutes of bagging with the bag-mask will result in spontaneous respiration restarting. The safest drug is paraldehyde administered per rectum (0.4 mL/kg up to 1 year of age, then one mL per year of age up to a maximum of 10 mL). Unfortunately, it is becoming increasingly difficult to obtain as it is not manufactured widely. Paraldehyde can be diluted with an equal volume of olive oil. It can be given using a plastic syringe if given immediately, otherwise by glass syringe. Do not use paraldehyde if it has a brown colour or smells of acetic acid.

A longer-acting drug must also be given at the same time and maintained. The most appropriate are **phenobarbitone** for children aged less than 5 years (load 15 mg/kg slowly IV, then a total of 5 mg/kg/day starting dose up to a maximum of 6 mg/kg/day IV, or orally in two divided doses 12 hours apart) and **phenytoin** for those aged over 5 years, administered IV initially (load 15 mg/kg IV over 20 minutes, followed by a further 10 mg/kg IV over a further 20 minutes if the first dose is unsuccessful). Then give 2.5 mg/kg every 12 hours IV over 20 minutes initially, increasing up to a maximum of 7.5 mg/kg every 12 hours (with each dose given over 20 minutes if IV). Phenytoin can also be given orally.

7.3.D Electrical injury

> **BOX 7.3.D.1 Minimum standards**
> - ABC.
> - ECG monitoring.
> - Sodium bicarbonate.

Introduction

Electrical injuries usually occur in the home, and involve relatively low currents and voltage. The mortality from electrical injuries from high-power external sources such as electrified railways is high, and death is immediate.

Other injuries may occur during the event. For example, the patient may fall or be thrown. Therefore a full trauma assessment must be undertaken.

Pathophysiology

Alternating current (AC) produces cardiac arrest at lower voltages than does direct current (DC). Regardless of whether the electrocution is caused by AC or DC, the risk of cardiac arrest is related to the size of the current and the duration of exposure. The current is highest when the resistance is low and the voltage is high.

Current

The typical **effects of an increase in current** are as follows:
- **Above 10 mA:** Tetanic contraction of muscles may make it impossible for the patient to let go of the electrical source.
- **Above 50 mA:** Tetanic contraction of the diaphragm and intercostal muscles leads to respiratory arrest, which continues until the current is disconnected. If hypoxia is prolonged, secondary cardiac arrest will occur.
- **From 100 mA to 50 A:** Primary cardiac arrest may be induced. (The defibrillators that are used in resuscitation deliver around 10 A.)
- **From 50 A to several 100 A:** Massive shocks cause prolonged respiratory and cardiac arrest and more severe burns. A lightning strike is a massive direct current of very short duration which can depolarise the myocardium and cause an immediate asystole.

Resistance

The resistance of the tissues determines the path that the current will follow. Generally, the current will follow the path of least resistance from the point of contact to earth. The relative resistance of the body tissues is, in increasing order, as follows: tissue fluid, blood, muscle, nerve, fat, skin, bone. Electrocution generates heat, which causes a variable degree of tissue damage. Nerves, blood vessels, the skin and muscles are damaged most. Swelling of damaged tissues, particularly muscle, can lead to a crush or compartment syndrome that requires fasciotomy. Water decreases the resistance of the skin and will increase the amount of current that flows through the body.

Voltage

High-voltage sources such as lightning or high-tension cables cause extremely high currents and severe tissue damage. However, very high voltages can cause severe superficial burns without damaging deeper structures (flash burns and arcing).

Primary assessment and resuscitation

Call for help and disconnect the electricity **in a safe manner**.

Be aware that high-voltage sources can discharge through several centimetres of air.

Airway

The upper airway should be opened and secured, especially if this is compromised by facial or other injuries. The cervical spine should be immobilised if there is a strong possibility of an unstable fracture.

Breathing

If the patient is not breathing, give rescue breaths using a mouth-to-mouth technique if no equipment is available (e.g. in the home) and, if available, a bag and mask with high-flow oxygen through an attached reservoir. If the patient is breathing but cyanosed, or low oxygen saturation is present, give inspired oxygen to maintain SaO_2 (if a pulse oximeter is available) in the range 94–98%.

Circulation

If the patient appears lifeless despite the rescue breaths, commence chest compressions and continue cardiopulmonary resuscitation (CPR) as described in Section 1.12 until help arrives. In the resuscitated or non-arrested patient who has been brought to hospital, after ABC assessment and management, the entry and exit point of the current should be sought in order to gain a picture of the sort of possible internal injuries that could have occurred. Children with significant internal injuries have a greater fluid requirement than one would suspect on the basis of the area of the external electric burn.

Secondary assessment and emergency treatment

Other injuries should be treated in an appropriate and structured manner (*see* Section 7.3.A).

Associated injuries are common in electrocution. Almost all possible injuries can occur as a result of falls or being thrown from the source. Burns are particularly common, and are caused either by the current itself or by burning clothing. Tetanic contraction of muscles can cause fractures, subluxations or muscle tearing.

Other problems

Burns cause oedema and fluid loss. Myoglobinuria occurs after significant muscle damage, and acute renal failure is a possibility. In this case, it is important to maintain a urine output of more than 2 mL/kg/hour in a child or 60 mL/kg/hour in a pregnant woman or girl with the judicious use of diuretics such as mannitol and appropriate fluid loading. Alkalisation of the urine with sodium bicarbonate, 1 mmol/kg in a child (1 mL/kg of 8.4% solution or 2 mL/kg of 4.2% solution) or 50 mmol in pregnancy increases the excretion of myoglobin.

Arrhythmias can occur up to a considerable time after the electrocution, and continuous ECG monitoring is helpful (if available).

7.3.E Drowning

> ### BOX 7.3.E.1 Minimum standards
> ■ ABCD and **early** basic life support.
> ■ Early management of hypothermia: radiant heat/hot-water bottles.
> ■ Low-reading thermometer.
> ■ Orogastric or nasogastric tube.
> ■ High-dependency care (if available).

Introduction
Definition

'Drowning' is defined as 'a process resulting in primary respiratory impairment from submersion/immersion in a liquid medium'.

According to WHO data, in 2004 there were 388 000 known deaths as a result of drowning worldwide, although the WHO considers this to be a massive underestimate. For children under the age of 15 years, drowning is the leading cause of accidental death worldwide. The low- and middle-income countries account for 96% of unintentional drowning deaths, and over 60% of the world's drowning events occur in the Western Pacific Region and South-East Asia, although the above figures do not include the massive loss of life from floods and tsunamis and from water transport accidents.

Pathophysiology

Bradycardia and apnoea occur shortly after submersion as a result of the diving reflex. As apnoea continues, hypoxia and acidosis cause tachycardia and a rise in blood pressure. Between 20 seconds and 5 minutes later, a breakpoint is reached, and breathing occurs. Fluid is inhaled and on touching the glottis causes immediate laryngeal spasm. After a variable but short period of time the laryngospasm subsides and fluid is aspirated into the lungs, resulting in alveolitis and pulmonary oedema. Hypoxia is by this time severe and the patient will have lost consciousness. Bradycardia and other dysrhythmias can also occur and may be fatal (ventricular fibrillation is rare).

Hypoxia is thus the key pathological process that ultimately leads to death, and needs to be corrected as quickly as possible.

Children who survive because of interruption of this chain of events not only require therapy for drowning, but also assessment and treatment of concomitant hypothermia, hypovolaemia and injury (particularly spinal). Major electrolyte abnormalities due to the amount of water swallowed seldom occur.

The type of water is associated with infections with unusual organisms, and aspiration of water contaminated with petroleum products can lead to a severe respiratory distress syndrome.

Submersion injuries are generally associated with hypothermia. The large body surface area to weight ratio in infants and children puts them at particular risk. Hypothermia may have a protective effect against the neurological sequelae following hypoxia and ischaemia, but is also associated with life-threatening dysrhythmias, coagulation disorders and susceptibility to infections.

The initial approach to the drowning patient focuses on the correction of hypoxia and hypothermia, and the treatment of associated injuries, which are common in older children and often overlooked. Cervical spine injury should always be suspected in drowning victims for whom the mechanism of injury is unclear, although these are rare (0.5% overall, and much rarer in children under 5 years).

Remember:
- Small children can drown in small volumes of water (e.g. in a bucket or shallow pool).
- Not all drowning is accidental (consider the possibility of abuse or neglect).
- Other injuries may be present.
- Other illnesses may have resulted in the drowning (e.g. epilepsy).
- Consider the possibility of drug or alcohol abuse.

Properties of water
- Water can be fresh (hypotonic) or salty (hypertonic).
- Water can conceal hidden dangers, such as trauma, entrapment, tide and flow, and contamination.
- Water can act as a solid at high-impact velocity.
- Water may be only one of several problems affecting the child (consider alcohol, drugs, child abuse, epilepsy, trauma, etc.).

Problems that may be present at drowning
- Hypothermia.

- Hypoxia.
- Pulmonary oedema.
- Hypotension.
- Ventricular arrhythmias and cardiac arrest.
- Cerebral depression, coma and hypoxic–ischaemic brain injury.
- Other injuries, especially spinal and head injuries.
- Electrolyte disturbances.
- Ingestion of alcohol, anticonvulsant drugs, etc.
- Pre-existing epilepsy.

Primary assessment and resuscitation

Call for help and move the victim from the water as quickly as possible without risk to the rescuer, in order to allow CPR and ABC to proceed.

Rescue of the victim in a vertical position may lead to cardiovascular collapse due to venous pooling. However, horizontal rescue in the water must not be allowed to delay the rescue.

The initiation of **early and effective basic life support is vital**. ABC reduces the mortality drastically and is the most important factor for survival. Five rescue breaths must be given as early as possible even in shallow water, if this can be done without risk to the rescuer. Mouth-to-nose ventilation may be easier in this situation. Basic life support (see Section 1.12) then proceeds according to the standard paediatric or maternal algorithm, even in hypothermia. The presence of cardiac arrest can be difficult to diagnose, as pulses are difficult to feel. If there are no signs of life, chest compressions should be started and continued with a rate of 15 compressions to two breaths.

Airway and manual in-line cervical spine control (if there is a major suspicion of unstable neck injury) are the first steps. Following submersion, the stomach is usually full of swallowed water. The risk of aspiration is therefore increased, and the airway must be secured as soon as possible on arrival at a healthcare facility. The best airway protection is usually provided by endotracheal intubation using a rapid sequence induction, once in a hospital setting. Following this, an oro- or nasogastric tube should be inserted.

Breathing: commence and continue mouth to mouth or mouth to mouth and nose ventilation.

Circulation: commence and continue chest compressions in the ratio 15 compressions to 2 ventilations until a satisfactory output is achieved, confirmed by palpation of a pulse or signs of life (i.e. breathing, movement or gagging).

Keep the victim as warm as possible. Remove wet clothing and wrap in dry garments/towels if this can be done by bystanders without interrupting CPR.

If in a hospital setting or professional help has arrived, advanced life support protocols can be followed if necessary (see Section 1.13).

Respiratory deterioration can be delayed for 4–6 hours after submersion, and even children who have initially apparently recovered should be observed for at least 8 hours. Keep the oxygen saturation in the range 94% or higher. Once the circulation is restored, take blood for haemoglobin, electrolytes (if available) and cross-matching. If the patient is in shock, give 10 mL/kg of Ringer-lactate or Hartmann's solution. Reassess and repeat if required. Give fluids warmed to body temperature if possible.

Disability and neurological examination (AVPU scale).

Exposure and temperature control: the core temperature measurement is best taken with a low-reading thermometer.

Secondary assessment and emergency treatment

Ensure that there are no other injuries requiring treatment. Examine the patient from head to toe. Any injury may have occurred during the incident that preceded immersion, including spinal injuries (see Sections 4.2.D and 7.3.A). Older children or pregnant women may have ingested alcohol and/or drugs.

Hypothermia

A core temperature reading should be obtained as soon as possible, and further cooling prevented. Hypothermia is common following drowning, and adversely affects resuscitation attempts unless it is treated.

The advantages of endotracheal intubation in hypothermia (if a skilled person is available) outweigh the small risk of precipitating arrhythmias. Not only are arrhythmias more common, but some, such as ventricular fibrillation, may be refractory to treatment at temperatures below 30°C, when defibrillation should be limited to three shocks (see Section 1.13) and inotropic or anti-arrhythmic drugs should **not** be given.

If defibrillation is unsuccessful, the patient should be warmed to above 30°C as quickly as possible, when further defibrillation may be attempted. The dose interval for resuscitation drugs is doubled between 30°C and 35°C. Resuscitation should be continued until the core temperature is at least 32°C or cannot be raised despite active measures.

Once above 32°C the temperature should ideally rise by 0.25–0.5°C per hour to reduce haemodynamic instability. Most hypothermic patients are hypovolaemic. During rewarming, vasodilatation occurs, resulting in hypotension which requires warmed IV fluids, but it is important not to give too much and risk circulatory overload and pulmonary oedema. Continuous monitoring of the pulse rate, respiratory rate and liver size, and auscultation of the lungs looking for crepitations that might suggest pulmonary oedema, are essential. Therapeutic hypothermia (32–34°C) for at least 24 hours has been shown to improve the neurological outcome in some patients, and may be of benefit in children who remain comatose, but requires high-level intensive care facilities.

Rewarming strategies
External rewarming
- Remove cold wet clothing.
- Supply warmed dry blankets.
- If these are not immediately available, place the child in skin-to-skin contact with an adult (kangaroo-type care).
- Warm air system (fan heaters).
- Heating blanket.

Core rewarming
- Warm IV fluids to 39°C to prevent further heat loss.
- Beware rewarming shock. Do not allow the temperature to rise > 37°C.

Monitoring
- Core temperature.

- Vital signs: heart rate, respiratory rate, blood pressure, capillary refill time and pulse volume.
- ECG tracing (if available).
- Glucose, electrolytes, and **blood gases (if available)**.
- Basic blood clotting tests.
- Chest X-ray.
- Urine output and urinalysis.
- Blood culture.

Prophylactic antibiotics are often given after immersion in severely contaminated water. Fever is common during the first 24 hours, but is not necessarily a sign of infection. Gram-negative organisms, especially *Pseudomonas aeruginosa*, are common, and *Aspergillus* species have been reported. If an infection is suspected, broad-spectrum IV antibiotic therapy (e.g. cefotaxime) should be started after blood and sputum cultures (if available).

Keeping the patient normoglycaemic is important for the neurological outcome.

Prognosis

The outcome is determined by the duration of hypoxic–ischaemic injury and the adequacy of initial resuscitation. It is assumed that hypoxic brain damage is reduced when the brain cools before the heart stops. No single factor can predict good or poor outcome in drowning reliably. However, the following factors may give an indication of outcome.

Immersion time

Most children who have been submerged for more than 10 minutes have a very small chance of intact neurological recovery or survival.

Time to basic life support

Starting basic life support at the scene greatly reduces mortality, whereas a delay of more than 10 minutes is associated with a poor prognosis.

Time to first respiratory effort

If this occurs within 3 minutes after the start of basic cardiopulmonary support, the prognosis is good. If there has been no respiratory effort after 40 minutes of full cardiopulmonary resuscitation, there is little or no chance of survival unless the child's respiration has been depressed (e.g. by hypothermia, medication or alcohol).

Core temperature

Pre-existing hypothermia and rapid cooling after submersion also seem to protect vital organs and can improve the prognosis. A core temperature of less than 33°C on arrival and a water temperature of less than 10°C have been associated with increased survival. This effect is pronounced in small children because of their large surface area to weight ratio.

Persistent coma

A persistent GCS score of less than 5, or a score of U on the AVPU scale, indicates a poor prognosis.

Type of water

Whether the patient was in salt or fresh water has no bearing on the prognosis.

When to stop resuscitation

- Immersion time: most children who do not recover have been submerged for more than 10 minutes.
- If the first gasp occurs between 1 and 3 minutes after cardiopulmonary resuscitation, the prognosis is good.
- Intact survival has been reported after cold submersion for 1 hour.
- Survival has been reported after 6.5 hours of cardiopulmonary resuscitation.
- A child has been revived from a body temperature of 15°C **but** cool-water drowning does not have the protection offered by ice-cold water.
- Failure to restore a perfusing rhythm within approximately 30 minutes of rewarming to 32–35°C makes further efforts unlikely to be successful.
- **Resuscitation should not be discontinued until the core temperature is at least 32°C or cannot be raised.**

Resuscitation should only be discontinued out of hospital if there is clear evidence of futility, such as massive trauma or rigor mortis.

7.3.F Heat stroke and hypothermia

BOX 7.3.F.1 Minimum standards
Heat stroke
- ABC.
- Shock treatment.
- Ice packs.
- Fans.

Hypothermia
- Skin-to-skin contact with carer.
- Warm blankets and clothing.
- Heated blanket.
- Infra-red warming lamp

Heat stroke
Clinical signs
- Confusion.
- Tachycardia.
- Fever (> 40°C)
- Hot dry skin.
- Tachypnoea.
- Hypotonia.

Pathophysiology
- Neurological impairment.
- Renal insufficiency.
- Disseminated intravascular coagulation.
- Acute respiratory failure.

- May have underlying infection predisposing to heat stroke.

Treatment
- **Urgent cooling:** Aim to cool the patient within 30 minutes. Remove clothes, spray with cool water, use a fan if available, and apply ice packs to the neck, axillae and groin. **It is especially important to cool the head.**
- Provide system support as necessary.
- Give fluids intravenously, especially if there is respiratory failure.
- Give oxygen.
- In hot climates, each hospital should have a cool room (ice or air-conditioned) for emergency treatment.

Hypothermia: prevention and treatment

Hypothermia occurs in association with drowning, and it may also occur during sepsis, especially in the very young child. Malnourished children in particular have a low metabolic rate. The thermoneutral temperature is 28–32°C. At 24°C they can become hypothermic. Those with infection or extensive skin lesions are at particular risk. A hypothermic malnourished child should always be assumed to have septicaemia.

Signs
The signs of hypothermia are a core temperature (oral) < 35.5°C (with low reading thermometer). If axillary temperature is < 35°C or does not register, assume hypothermia.

Routine prevention
- Cover all sick children with clothes and blankets unless they are febrile.
- Keep the ward doors and windows closed to avoid draughts.
- Avoid wet nappies, clothes or bedding.
- Do not wash very ill children. Others can be washed quickly, ideally with warm water, and dried immediately.
- Avoid making a sick or injured child cold when undertaking medical examinations.

Emergency treatment of hypothermia
- Immediately place the child on the carer's bare chest or abdomen (skin to skin) and cover both of them. Give the mother a hot drink to increase her skin blood flow.
- If no adult is available, clothe the child very well (including the head) and put them near a lamp or radiant heater, or use a warming blanket if one is available.
- Immediately treat for hypoglycaemia (*see* Section 5.8.B), and then start normal feeds if appropriate to the child.
- Consider sepsis, and give condition- and age-appropriate antibiotics.
- Monitor the temperature every 60 minutes until the temperature is normal (> 36.5°C).

7.3.G Landmine injuries

BOX 7.3.G.1 **Minimum standards**
- ABC resuscitation.
- Shock management.
- Analgesia.
- Anti-tetanus immunisation and immunoglobulin.
- Prostheses that are changed as the child grows.

Patterns of injury
- **Injuries caused by stepping on to a buried blast mine or improvised explosive device (IED):** traumatic amputation of the detonating limb, with fragment and minor blast damage to the other leg (most common injury).
- **Injuries caused by fragmentation landmine or IED:** widespread fragment injury to the limbs and trunk.
- **Injuries caused by close-proximity detonation of a landmine or IED in the hand or close to the face:** amputation of the hand or arm, plus damage to the face, eyes and head. Usually occurs in mine clearers or in those handling weapons.

Some mines are scattered from aircraft or by shells to lie on the surface of the ground. These weapons are unstable and likely to explode when handled. Unexploded ordnance, such as grenades, can also explode if handled, resulting in the same pattern of injury. Recently IEDs have been placed next to roads and pathways, causing similar injuries.

Specific problems in children
- Children sustain a higher level of injury per gram of explosive than adults, because of their smaller body mass. A small antipersonnel mine of approximately 30 grams, which would normally require a below-knee amputation in an adult, may result in an above-knee amputation in a child.
- Children are susceptible to close-proximity detonation injuries, because of their tendency to pick up and play with objects that they find.

Treatment
- Initial surgical management follows the basic principles of resuscitation (*see* Section 7.3.A).
- In injury caused by stepping on a buried blast mine or IED, airway maintenance is not usually a problem, as the child is frequently conscious.
- As with all injured children, fear and bewilderment due to pain and the unfamiliar surroundings can be distressing for all involved.
- In close-proximity detonation injury, airway maintenance can be a problem. The patient is often unconscious and there may be damage to the upper airway from the blast. A tracheostomy may be required.
- Benzylpenicillin and anti-tetanus toxoid should be administered in all cases.
- Anaesthesia can be achieved using a ketamine infusion (*see* Section 1.15 for pain relief).

Injury from stepping on to a buried blast mine or IED: technique of amputation

- On the operating table, a thorough wash with warm clean water and a scrubbing brush will get rid of the gross contamination and general soiling of the limbs prior to formal skin preparation.
- **Always use an above-knee orthopaedic tourniquet to minimise peri-operative blood loss**, which is proportionally greater in children than in adults.
- Perform a standard amputation according to International Committee of the Red Cross surgical guidelines. Remember the following points:
  - The muscles are usually contused more proximally by blast damage than may be initially apparent.
  - Dirt and contamination can be propelled up tissue planes by the blast. An amputation through the blast damage can leave contamination in the wound.
  - Make a bulky myoplasty to cover the bone end using the medial gastrocnemius below the knee, or the medial vastus above the knee. Leave generous skin flaps, as the muscle in the stump will swell considerably post-operatively.
- Make an anterior bevel to the bone when dividing it, and file the edges down.
- Let the tourniquet down when the amputation is completed, to check haemostasis before applying the dressing.

- Perform thorough wound toilet of the injuries to the other leg. Explore all wounds and excise contaminated tissue. Leave these wounds open to be closed or skin grafted at 5 days post-operatively.
- **Never close the amputation stump primarily**. Lightly pack the open stump with gauze and apply a bulky dressing. Write on the dressing the date for wound inspection (usually at 5 days post-operatively).
- Do not take the dressing down on the ward unless the patient manifests signs of systemic toxicity (i.e. fever, tachycardia, foul-smelling dressing).
- Give blood only if the haemoglobin level falls to less than 8 grams/dL.
- Give IV benzylpenicillin for 48 hours (50 mg/kg 6-hourly), then orally for a further 3 days (12.5 mg/kg four times daily).
- Give appropriate tetanus prophylaxis (*see* Section 7.1).
- Inspect the wound at 5 days. If the tissue is healthy and not infected, close with interrupted non-absorbable sutures over a drain. Leave the sutures in for 3 weeks.
- Early physiotherapy is crucial to success, especially to eliminate flexion contracture of the below-knee amputation.
- Refer early to a prosthetic workshop for casting. Children will need several sets of prostheses as they grow.

7.3.H Gunshot wounds

BOX 7.3.H.1 Minimum standards
- ABC resuscitation.
- Shock.
- Analgesia.
- Anti-tetanus immunisation and immunoglobulin.
- Penicillin.
- X-rays and ultrasound.
- High dependency care.

Introduction

Although the end of the Cold War led to a reduction in the risk of conflict in Europe, numerous conflicts continue to rage in the developing world. Many of these conflicts are between ill-disciplined or irregular armies who often specifically target civilian populations in defiance of the Geneva Conventions. In this process, children are inevitably susceptible to sustaining gunshot wounds.

The International Committee of the Red Cross has drawn attention to the global proliferation of weapons. For example, there are estimated to be as many as 125 million AK47 assault rifles in circulation worldwide. As conflicts resolve, these weapons become marketable commodities and spread to neighbouring states, where they become the criminal's weapon of choice. The net result of this is injury to the civilian population, including children.

Ballistics

The science of ballistics addresses aspects of missile and bullet flight and relates these to the potential for injury. The following issues are relevant to the mechanism of wounding:
- When a bullet impacts on tissue it will impart some of its kinetic energy to that tissue.
- This will cause the tissue to accelerate away from the track of the projectile, resulting in a **temporary cavity**.
- Once the bullet has passed, the inherent elasticity of the tissues will cause the temporary cavity to collapse, leaving some degree of **permanent cavity** along the track.

The extent to which cavitation occurs is governed by the amount of kinetic energy imparted to the tissues by the projectile. The equation governing this is as follows:

$$\text{kinetic energy} = \tfrac{1}{2}\, m\, (V_1^2 - V_2^2)$$

where m is the mass of the projectile, V_1 is the velocity on entering the tissues and V_2 is the velocity on exiting. The degree to which the projectile's velocity is attenuated while transiting the tissues is dependent upon the diameter of the bullet, its orientation and flight characteristics on impact, and the nature of the tissue itself.

Categories of gunshot wounds

In practice, the masses of most commonly used bullets are similar, and thus the velocity of the projectile largely defines the injury potential. In this regard, gunshot wounds can largely be divided into three categories depending on the nature of the weapon used.

Handguns

- The commonest types of handgun feature a bullet with a diameter of 9 mm and a muzzle velocity of around 1000 feet/second.
- Only a small temporary cavity is formed, and the injury is essentially confined to the bullet track.
- Provided that the bullet has not transected any major structures, the degree of injury may only be slight.
- Some of the bullets for these types of weapon are designed to deform on impact. These are the hollow or soft- (lead-) tipped bullets. On impact they tend to flatten, presenting a greater surface area to the direction of travel, thus resulting in an increased transfer of energy and greater wounding effect.

Shotguns

- The cartridge contains multiple pellets of a specified diameter.
- This diameter can range from 1 mm ('birdshot') to 10 mm ('buckshot').
- Once fired, the pellets disperse in a cone-shaped pattern.
- The degree and rapidity of dispersion are proportional to the size and number of pellets as well as the diameter of the shotgun barrel at the muzzle.
- Due to their aerodynamics, the velocity of individual pellets will attenuate over short distances, even in air. Furthermore, the conical dispersion leads to a rapid decline in the number of pellets that will hit a particular target as the range increases.
- The above factors lead to this weapon being virtually ineffective at ranges over 50 metres.
- A severe pattern of injury is seen at close range. Although each pellet may only be travelling at low ballistic velocity, the combined effect of multiple pellets is a formidable destructive force, shredding the tissues and causing massive disruption.

Military assault rifles

- These weapons typically have a bullet 7.62 mm in diameter that leaves the weapon at a speed of around 3000 feet/second.
- Rifling of the barrel sets the bullet spinning, which, combined with the increased velocity, leads to greater accuracy at long range.
- Rather than following a uniform flight path, the bullet has a periodic motion, oscillating around its flight axis with the movements of precession, nutation and yaw.
- The very much greater kinetic energy of these bullets leads to a much larger temporary cavity than is seen in low-velocity munitions.
- The sub-atmospheric pressure in the cavity will tend to suck in clothing and other debris from outside the wound, causing contamination.
- The shock front of accelerating tissue, propagating away from the point of impact, causes stretching and tearing of the tissues, cellular disruption and microvascular injury.
- The margin of tissue around the cavity, termed the **zone of extravasation**, is full of haemorrhage, has little tendency to further bleeding and, if muscle, shows no tendency to contract when stimulated. This tissue is non-viable and will become a culture medium for infection if left *in situ*.

- The shock wave itself can cause fracture of bone and intimal disruption of major vessels.
- The oscillating nature of the bullet trajectory can cause it to 'tumble' on impacting with the tissues. When this occurs, due to the non-uniform motion, even greater proportions of the kinetic energy are transmitted. The resulting tissue acceleration can lead to the exit wound made by such a bullet being very much larger than the entry wound.
- The nature of the tissue being transited has a great impact on the extent of damage occurring. Relatively elastic, compressible tissue such as lung propagates the shock wave to a much lesser extent than dense, fluid-filled tissue such as liver. Therefore a high-velocity bullet may transit lung causing only contusion, whereas transiting solid organs causes gross disruption.

Treatment

Although it is clearly impossible to cover the treatment of gunshot wounds to every possible anatomical structure in the body, there are some themes common to all such injuries. Most of the wounds encountered will be to the limbs, as gunshot wounds to the head, chest and abdomen have a high rate of on-scene mortality.

Protocols for treating gunshot wounds have been adopted and publicised by the International Committee of the Red Cross (ICRC), who have extensive experience of treating such injuries as part of their war surgery programmes.

Initial measures

The initial measures in the treatment of gunshot wounds are similar to those for any severe injury.

- General assessment and resuscitation of the patient, addressing potentially life-threatening conditions according to ABC priorities (compressing exsanguinating haemorrhage, airway, breathing, circulation), is the priority (*see* Section 7.3.A).
- The degree to which fluid resuscitation should be carried out has been controversial. An initial bolus of 10 mL/kg in a child or 500 mL in pregnancy of Ringer-lactate or Hartmann's should be given and the response to this initial fluid challenge assessed. The concern is to avoid restarting massive bleeding again from disrupting a just-clotting wound by increasing peripheral perfusion. So until the patient can be in a position to have any torn vessels managed, i.e. be in an operating theatre with competent staff, and receive a blood transfusion, crystalloid fluid management remains the minimum that keeps vital organs perfused.
- Give analgesia as required (usually IV morphine) (*see* Section 1.15).
- Apply dressings to the open wounds.
- Undertake emergency splintage of fractures.
- Antibiotics: the ICRC recommend IV benzylpenicillin at a dose appropriate to the size of the child (usually 50 mg/kg IV 6-hourly) and in pregnancy 600–1200 mg IV 6-hourly.
- Give tetanus toxoid and antitetanus serum.
- Appropriate radiographs of the injured areas should be taken.

Wound assessment

Before proceeding to surgical treatment, the following aspects of the wound need to be assessed:

- From the history, the nature of the weapon used (if known).
- The site of the entrance wound (and exit wound, if present).
- The sizes of the entrance and exit wounds.
- Cavity formation.
- The anatomical structures that may have been transited.
- Distal perfusion.
- Presence of fractures.
- Degree of contamination.

Wound debridement and management

This involves removal from the wound of any dead and contaminated tissue which if left would become a medium for infection. It is most relevant to high-energy-transfer (high-velocity) wounds, which feature large cavities and considerable amounts of dead tissue and contamination.

- Wound debridement should be a planned procedure with prior consideration given to the position of the patient and the type of anaesthesia required.
- For limb wounds, a pneumatic tourniquet should be used where possible to reduce blood loss.
- Skin incision decompresses the wound and allows swelling of the tissues without constriction.
- Where possible, the incisions should be longitudinal and not cross joints.
- Skin is a resilient tissue, so only minimal excision is usually necessary.
- Dead and contaminated tissue should be excised.
- Dead muscle is dusky in colour, shows little tendency to bleed, and does not contract to forceps pressure.
- Foreign material should be excised from the wound. However, the obsessive pursuit of small metallic debris, such as that from a disintegrating bullet or shotgun pellets, is not worthwhile.
- Bone fragments denuded of soft-tissue attachment (muscle or periosteum) should be removed as, if left in the wound, they will become infected and form osteomyelitic sequestrae.
- There should be no primary repair of nerve or tendon. Where obviously divided, these structures should be marked (with suture) for later repair.
- At the end of the procedure, the debrided wound should be washed with copious quantities of saline and then a dry bulky sterile dressing applied.
- Some low-energy-transfer (low-velocity) wounds, such as those from most handguns, because of the minimal cavitation and zone of extravasation, do not need the extensive debridement and excision outlined above. These wounds can, in certain circumstances, be managed without surgery.

Delayed primary closure

Once wound debridement has been undertaken, the patient can be returned to the ward and the following regime followed:

- Continued analgesia.
- Benzylpenicillin; IV 50 mg/kg every 4 hours for the first 24 hours and then orally for a further 4 days (12.5 mg/kg four times daily).
- Monitoring of the patient for signs of sepsis; check their tetanus status.
- The dressing should be left in place on the ward and only removed when the patient returns to theatre after an interval period for **delayed primary closure**.
- The ICRC recommend an interval period of 5 days, but most recent practice tends towards shorter periods of 48–72 hours.
- The only indication for return to theatre and dressing removal before this interval period has elapsed is an offensive dressing combined with signs of patient sepsis. The most common cause of this situation is an inadequate initial wound excision.

In the process of delayed primary closure:

- The dressing should be removed in theatre under appropriate anaesthesia.
- If clean, the wound can be closed, or if skin cover is deficient, split-skin grafted.
- If there is evidence of infection, further debridement/excision can be undertaken and the process repeated, aiming for delayed closure after a further 5 days.
- Following closure, rehabilitation of the injured part can commence.

Specific features relating to certain anatomical sites

- Wounds of the head and neck, by virtue of the enhanced vascular supply to these areas, can safely be closed or reconstructed at the initial operation.
- Wounds to major vessels need to be reconstructed primarily.
- Breaches of the dura, pleura and peritoneum should, where possible, be closed at initial surgery.
- Most gunshot wounds to the chest can be treated with tube thoracostomy alone.
- Penetration within 5 cm of the midline of the thorax or abdomen is associated with a risk of injury to the great vessels or heart.
- Gunshot wounds to the head that transit the cranial cavity carry a very poor prognosis, especially if from a high-energy-transfer weapon.
- Penetrating gunshot wounds of the abdomen are associated with a more than 85% chance of bowel or major organ transit. Exploratory laparotomy is therefore virtually mandatory.

Conclusion

Gunshot wounds from any type of weapon represent a severe injury. Some understanding of ballistics can help in the assessment of these injuries. Treatment according to basic principles, such as those recommended by the International Committee of the Red Cross, can lead to a satisfactory outcome even with limited clinical resources.

7.3.I.a Ingestion burns

> **BOX 7.3.1.A Minimum standards**
> ABCD management.
> ■ IV steroids.
> ■ Stomal feeding.
> ■ Oesophageal dilation/stenting.
> ■ Oesophageal reconstruction.

Introduction

Oral and oesophageal burns occur in three groups of patients: unintentional ingestion of hot or caustic liquids by young children, or by people of any age with delayed development (poor supervision plays an important part in each of these two groups), and ingestion to cause intentional self-harm.

Types of ingestion burns
Hot fluids
- Burns from drinking hot fluids are relatively rare in developmentally normal children, but can occur in those with learning difficulties.
- Normally only the mouth is burned.
- Swelling and blistering can be very rapid, and require an oral or nasal (preferred) airway.
- Swelling usually goes down within 48 hours, and the need for further treatment is unusual.

Caustic fluids
- Burns from drinking caustic fluids are much more severe.
- In general, caustic alkali solutions are more damaging to tissues than acids.

Immediate treatment
- In the home or at the place where ingestion occurred, the **immediate** drinking of a small amount of milk (this is futile after 30 minutes) may have some beneficial effect in the case of ingestion of solid or granular alkalis, but not for liquid alkalis or for acids.

Hospital treatment
- Assess Airway, Breathing and Circulation. If there are signs of respiratory distress with stridor, the airway must be urgently secured. Intubation is difficult and may cause perforation, so a cricothyroidotomy followed by a tracheostomy may be needed.
- **Do not make the child vomit**, as burning fluid causes further damage when passing up the oesophagus.

- **Do not pass a tube into the stomach**, as this may perforate the oesophagus. A gastrostomy will usually be needed
- **Do not attempt to neutralise the chemical** (e.g. by giving acid for alkali ingestion, or alkali for acid ingestion), as this will cause a high-temperature reaction that will further damage the tissues.
- **Do not give more milk or give water**: it is too late and may precipitate vomiting and more damage to the oesophagus.

Definitive treatment
The only way to assess the oesophageal damage is by flexible oesophagoscopy. If there are significant signs of inflammation, steroids are often used, and there is some evidence that they can reduce the severity of any developing stricture. The route will have to be parenteral (hydrocortisone 4 mg/kg every 6 hours, maximum dose for children under 2 years is 25 mg, for those under 5 years is 50 mg, and for those over 5 years is 100 mg per dose). The length of treatment is not identified, but should be short (3–4 days) in view of the effect of steroids on healing and immunity.

Significant stricture formation will need reconstructive surgery or a gastrostomy (see below).

Complications
- Serious burning, particularly of the oesophagus, can lead to perforation, and in the later stages to strictures.
- Acute perforation of the oesophagus is frequently fatal; treat by drip and suction and then thoracotomy if severe.
- Late stricture during and after the healing phase is a very common problem after ingestion of caustic fluids.
- Mild cases can be treated by later dilatation of the oesophagus.
- **More severe cases may require an oesophagectomy, followed by a stomach pull-up or small bowel replacement.**
- However, if the stricture reduces the ability of the child to eat, a feeding gastrostomy tube passed through the abdominal wall directly into the stomach may be needed to provide nutrition.

Prevention
- Parents and teachers must be informed about the need to keep dangerous fluids out of the reach of children.
- Never put chemicals in the wrong bottles or containers.

7.3.I.b Burns in children and in pregnancy

> **BOX 7.3.1.B Minimum standards**
> ■ ABC management.
> ■ Analgesia.
> ■ Antiseptic dressings.
> ■ Anti-tetanus immunisation.
> ■ Antibiotics.

Summary of actions (more information on each action below)
- Primary assessment and resuscitation according to ABC. If there are signs of developing or actual airway obstruction, call for an anaesthetist, open the airway and consider early intubation before swelling and total respiratory obstruction occur. Observe closely for shock.

- Take a very brief history, and consider whether there could be other injuries or medical conditions.
- Make a rapid assessment of the burn area, take care with clothing removal.
- If there are clearly more than 10% burns, establish an IV cannula and give IV analgesia (morphine according to age and weight *see* Section 1.15).
- Commence either Ringer-lactate or Hartmann's solution IV in the following volumes in mL:

burn (%) × weight (kg) × 4 per day for a child

burn (%) × weight (kg) × 2 to 4 per day in pregnancy

- Fluid is given over the first 24 hours, backdated to the time of the burn. Half of the fluid should be given (in hourly divided doses) during the first 8 hours, and the second half in the next 16 hours, again in hourly doses. This is **in addition to** maintenance fluids which can be given later and orally if the child is able to take these (see below). Any fluid boluses given IV to treat shock should be **included** in the additional fluid for the burn and subtracted from that calculated as described above.
- Normal (0.9%) saline can be used if Ringer-lactate or Hartmann's solution are unavailable, but be aware that, especially in larger volumes, normal saline causes a hyperchloraemic acidosis which is detrimental to sick or injured patients.
- Even if there are less than 10% burns, consider IV opiate analgesia if the patient is clearly distressed by pain.
- Do not give oral fluids immediately.
- Make an accurate assessment of the area of the burn and draw its position on a chart (*see* Table 7.3.I.B.1 and Figure 7.3.I.B.1).
- Estimate the depth of the burn.
- Establish, and if necessary update, the anti-tetanus status of the patient.
- Consider and decide whether an escharotomy is necessary for circumferential burns on a limb or the chest that may cause tissue necrosis from compression by swelling tissues or restriction of ventilation.
- Dress the burned areas, or treat any area that is going to be kept exposed.
- Consider and decide whether the patient needs admission (for a child, with their parent).
- Commence oral fluids if the patient can drink. If not, add the maintenance fluids to those given for the burn as calculated above. In burns over 8% divide the calculated daily maintenance requirement by 24 and give it on an hourly basis either orally or IV.
- Decide whether the patient requires urinary catheterisation (over 30% burns, or burns with complications).

Introduction

The skin is a barrier to infection and evaporative fluid loss. It is a sensory organ and it regulates temperature through sweating.

- The severity of a burn depends both on the area of the body involved and on the depth of the burn.
- The majority of burns in children occur in those under 2 years of age and are caused by hot fluids or flames.
- Other causes include electricity, chemicals, radiation and frostbite.

- Burns are more common where there is poverty from overcrowding and unsafe heating and cooking practices.

Definition of terms

Erythema or first-degree burn: This causes an increase in skin capillary blood flow. In pigmented skin it is often difficult to recognise, but is characterised by pain, and a slight thickening and change in texture of the surface of the skin with later partial or complete desquamation occurring some days afterwards. **The important feature is that blistering does not occur, and fluid is not lost from the circulation. Intravenous fluids are therefore not needed for the burn.** It heals without scarring within 2–10 days.

Superficial partial-thickness burn: This is skin in which there is early (within 1 hour) blistering following the injury, associated with pain. If the blisters are removed **(do not remove them)**, the exposed surface is shiny, loses pigmentation in pigmented races, and is extremely painful. Pressure on the surface causes blanching, which on release of the pressure instantly becomes red again. It heals within 7–14 days with mild pigmentation change or scarring.

Deep dermal burn: Red blood cells leave the capillaries and become fixed in the dermis. In non-pigmented skin, therefore, the redness does not blanch on pressure. This is much more difficult to diagnose in pigmented skin, but the skin becomes thicker and harder in the area. Blistering occurs later, or may not occur at all. If the burn is in the deeper part of the dermis, the heat breaks down the red cells and the area becomes white with no blanching present. Removal of the blistering, if it has occurred, leaves a bed that is wet and shiny, but has only mild discomfort as the nerve endings have been damaged. It heals within 14–21 days with scarring which is often hypertrophic. Grafting will usually be required.

Both of the last two categories may be called a second-degree burn, but as the treatment may be different, the type that is present should be accurately diagnosed.

Deep burn: All elements of the skin and the skin hair follicles, sweat glands, etc. are destroyed. The skin is either white or charred brown. No blistering occurs. **It is painless on examination.** Severe scarring occurs and grafting will always be required. **This may be called a third degree burn.** A burn involving tissue damage occurs at temperatures above 48°C and after only 1 second at 70°C.

Capillary permeability is increased for up to 48 hours, and is maximal at 8 hours. With large burns there is increased blood viscosity, haemoglobinuria may occur, and there is a loss of protein, which needs to be corrected by adequate nutrition.

First aid

Cold water rapidly applied is the best first aid. The quicker this is done, the better. The longer the skin is in contact with the flame or hot fluid, the greater is the extent and depth of burning. The best first aid in all situations, except those involving electricity, is cold water or other cold fluid (e.g. milk) applied as soon as possible. It is less important whether the water is sterile or not, and it should be applied before the clothes are removed, as removal can often take some time. Cold water reduces the severity of the burn as it removes thermal energy, and also reduces pain. It should ideally be applied for approximately 10 minutes, but no longer. Following this, the burn should be covered with clean sheets or towels or 'clingfilm' plastic wrapping.

If the cause of the burn is electricity, it is important that the patient is isolated from the electricity supply or that it is turned off before cold water is applied, otherwise greater damage may be caused.

Following the period of cooling with water, **the patient needs to be kept warm**, otherwise **hypothermia can result**, particularly in young babies.

Primary assessment
- Assessment of a burn must be carried out in the same way as assessment of any other injury.
- It is quite possible that the burn is not the major injury or problem when the patient is seen. For instance, it may have been an epileptic attack that caused the burn, or the patient may have fallen or jumped from a burning house, or been involved in a road traffic accident and therefore has multiple fractures and/or a head injury.
- **Special issues regarding burns in pregnancy.** Any burn affecting more than 20% total body surface area (TBSA) is a serious risk to the mother and fetus. In a mother with a burn > 70–80% of the TBSA mortality is 50–90%. If the burn affects < 30% TBSA the prognosis is good for both fetus and mother and depends on the management of complications such as hypoxia, hypotension and sepsis.

ABC
Airway and Breathing
- If either of these is compromised, call for an anaesthetist and open the airway. Early endotracheal intubation may be required.
- If flame inhalation has occurred (see below for more information on inhalation burns), the airway tends to close very rapidly, making intubation very difficult. Apart from the history, the signs to observe are altered voice or presence of stridor, singeing of the nasal hairs, and deposition of soot in the throat or nose.
- Remove any constricting clothing and place the patient in dry and clean sheets or towels.
- Give additional inspired oxygen if SaO_2 is < 94% or the patient is cyanosed.
- If breathing is inadequate, use a bag-valve-mask and consider intubation if the airway is compromised or may imminently become so.
- Chemical damage may occur from highly irritant gases, which can lead to progressive respiratory failure.
- Many plastics and modern materials give off cyanide, which may be absorbed into the blood stream.
- Carbon monoxide is the most common poison produced in fires.

Circulation
- Fluid is lost through the capillaries following a burn. Shock takes time to develop. In minor burns this is a local phenomenon, but **in severe burns all of the vascular bed becomes leaky**. Assess the total body surface area (TBSA) affected (see below).
- A patient with a burn of less than 10% of the total body surface area can normally cope by having their oral intake increased. However, this is not an absolute figure, and in particular if the patient is vomiting, IV fluid

may be necessary for a smaller burn. Similarly, if safe IV fluid is not available, a burn of up to 25% may have to be managed with increased oral fluids alone. When oral fluids are being used, either in combination with IV therapy or alone, only small regular doses of fluid should be given by mouth.
- For burns that are 5% or larger, oral fluids should be an electrolyte solution (ORS).
- Fluid loss is greatest in the first 12 hours, causing disturbances in fluid and electrolyte composition.
- For burns of 10% or more, secure IV access and replace fluids with warmed Ringer-lactate or Hartmann's each containing 5 or 10% glucose (see below for calculating TBSA and the Appendix for how to make up solutions containing glucose).

Management of the circulation in pregnancy
A pregnant woman requires 2 to 4 mL per kg per 1% of body surface area burnt to be given over the first 24 hours in addition to baseline maintenance fluids. Half of this volume is given in the first 8 hours, half in the next 16 hours. *The quantity of fluid given in the first 8 hours must include any fluids given as a resuscitation bolus for shock.*
- Monitor urinary output (should be > 30 mL per hour).
- *Assess the need to deliver the fetus.* Fetal survival is poor in burns affecting > 50% TBSA. In view of the high mortality in mothers with such extensive burns, those in the second or third trimester should be delivered as soon as possible after admission as fetal survival is not improved by waiting and the presence of the fetus increases the risk to the mother. Abortion is common in patients with burns > 33% TBSA, especially during the second trimester. Fetal loss during the third trimester can be expected with extensive burns unless delivery occurs. Dexamethasone to reduce respiratory distress syndrome in a preterm infant (Section 3.1) is not contraindicated in the presence of extensive burns.

Management of the circulation in childhood
Children usually require 4 mL per kg per 1% body surface area burnt (TBSA) to be given over the first 24 hours in addition to baseline maintenance fluids. Half of this volume is given in the first 8 hours, half in the next 16 hours. *To avoid circulatory overload, the quantity of fluid given in the first 8 hours must include any fluids given as a resuscitation bolus for shock.*

For example, if there is a 20% burn × 15 kg child × 4 = 1200 mL of Ringer-lactate or Hartmann's solution. Give 600 mL in the first 8 hours from the time of the burn.

Intravenous fluid management
- IV Ringer-lactate or Hartmann's solution or 0.9% saline (if the former two are not available) is necessary in large burns because of the loss of the intravascular component of extracellular fluid. **Glucose 5% alone and glucose in 0.18% saline are dangerous and can lead to hyponatraemia and water overload.** However, especially in young children, watch for hypoglycaemia, which can be prevented by adding glucose to any crystalloid solution (e.g. 50 mL of 50% glucose in a 500-mL bag of crystalloid will give a 5% solution).
- Ideally, give IV fluids by peripheral or external jugular vein; in an emergency, in shock or where rapid sequence induction for intubation is needed, intra-osseous or

central venous lines may be needed, but the latter can increase the risk of infection.

- If the patient is in shock, in a child give 10 mL/kg as an IV bolus as rapidly as possible and in pregnancy give a 500 mL IV bolus and then reassess and repeat if they are still shocked, up to a maximum of three boluses.
- Wherever possible, long IV lines should not be used, as this increases the risk of septicaemia.
- Both natural colloids (i.e. albumin solution and plasma) and artificial colloids (e.g. Haemaccel, and various starch derivatives) are available. The former have risks of transmitting infection and are expensive, and the latter have not been well studied for resuscitation of burns, but are cheaper.
- Blood transfusion may be needed if anaemia develops.
- It is essential that not too much IV fluid is given, as it may lead to pulmonary and/or cerebral oedema, together with an excessive extravascular deposition of fluid. Crystalloid resuscitation can also lead to 'compartment syndrome' because of the increasing pressure within the muscular compartments and it is important to observe for pain, particularly in the lower legs.
- The amount of fluid loss from burns decreases over the first 48–72 hours after the injury. The amount of fluid to be given initially therefore depends on how long before admission the burn occurred. Following this, the assessment of the resuscitation can be made by a combination of the clinical picture, i.e. degree of dehydration, the blood haematocrit and the urine output aim for 2 mL/kg/hour of urine in a child and 30 mL/hour in pregnancy.
- It is essential that accurate and updated fluid input and output charts are kept throughout. For major burns (over 30%), hourly haematocrit (or haemoglobin) and urine outputs are helpful in the first 24 hours, decreasing in frequency thereafter. For burns between 10% and 30%, 4-hourly tests are normally sufficient.
- In larger burns (greater than 30%), burns involving the genitals, and burns in young normally incontinent female children, a urinary catheter is essential. In males, a urinary bag can be used. A catheter may also be necessary

if fluid resuscitation is not proceeding well to give an accurate picture of the urine volume produced hourly. Catheters can lead to infection and should be removed as soon as possible.

Enteral fluid management
- Start oral or nasogastric feeding as soon as possible after admission. If a child is being breastfed, this should continue.
- Although thirst is common, giving too much free fluid orally may induce vomiting.
- For burns between 5% and 10% the daily requirement of the patient's oral intake should be increased by 50% to allow for the burn (given on an hourly basis).
- The normal oral requirement of a child can be calculated as 100 mL/kg for the first 10 kg, 50 mL/kg for the next 10 kg, and 25 mL/kg for any weight up to the total weight of the child. The normal daily fluid requirement in pregnancy is 1500–2500 mL.
- This may need to be increased by 10% or 20% in hot climates.
- The oral fluid given should ideally be ORS. If this is not available, diluted milk is acceptable.
- If all is well after 24 hours, free fluids can be given, but careful input and output charting will continue to be required.

Maintenance of body temperature: burnt children can lose heat rapidly.

Feeding
- Early feeding (especially breastfeeding) reduces the risk of gastric stress ulcer formation and of stasis. It is recommended therefore that small quantities of food are given either orally or with a thin-bore nasogastric tube. The latter can be used to give milk or other similar high-protein foodstuffs.
- Parenteral nutrition is strongly contraindicated, as this leads to a high risk of septicaemia in burns patients.

Burn area and depth

TABLE 7.3.I.B.1 Body proportions at different ages for burns assessment (%)

Percentage surface area at:					
Area on diagram	0	1 year	5 years	10 years	15 years
A	9.5	8.5	6.5	5.5	4.5
B	2.75	3.25	4.0	4.5	4.5
C	2.5	2.5	2.75	3.0	3.25

Area of burn
Estimation of the area of a burn is based on either Wallace's rule of nines, or on charts (see Table 7.3.I.B.1 and Figures 7.3.I.B.1 and 7.3.I.B.2). In addition, the area of the patient's open palm is approximately 1% of the total body surface area. Wallace's rule of nines is applicable to children over 14 years of age and to adults. For newborn babies it can be modified by adding 9% to the area of the head and subtracting 9% from the area of the legs. For every additional year of age, 1% is subtracted from the head and added to the legs until, at the age of 10 years, approximately adult proportions has been reached.

In pregnancy the abdomen represents a larger proportion of the TBSA.

The area of the patient's hand can be used for estimating the size of small burns, but can also be used to estimate the areas that are unburned in extensive burns, and this can then be extracted from the rule of nines figures (e.g. if 2% of an arm is unburned, the area of burn on that arm will be 7%).

- It is very common for inexperienced people to overestimate the size of a burn.
- **Erythema must not be included**, as fluid is not lost.
- The decision as to whether or not to start IV fluids is

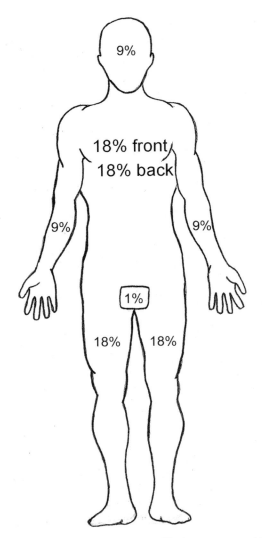

FIGURE 7.3.I.B.1 Wallace's 'rule of nines' for burns assessment in children over 14 years of age and adults.

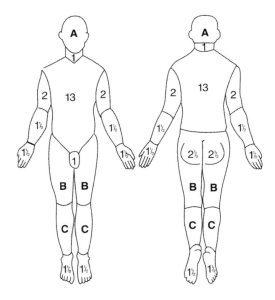

FIGURE 7.3.I.B.2 Body proportions at different ages for burns assessment.

dependent on this initial assessment, and on whether there are other injuries or medical conditions.

- **An overestimate may mean that far too much fluid is given.**

Depth of the burn

The depth of the burn is based on history, appearance and examination.

- Flame or hot fat burns are almost always deep.
- Hot water burns (scalds) may be superficial or deep dermal.
- The appearance can be altered if more than a few hours old, or by the application of various first-aid treatments.
- First assess capillary return. Prompt capillary return means a superficial burn.
- Then test sensation. Is it increased (in a superficial partial thickness burn), reduced (in a deep dermal burn) or absent (in a full-thickness burn)?
- The test is done by using a sterile hypodermic needle. In older children, and in pregnancy, it is possible to ask whether they can tell the difference between the sharp and the blunt ends when these are lightly applied to

the burn. In younger children the best way of doing the test is to wait until the child is sleeping or has their eyes closed, and then very gently touch what appears to be the deepest part of the burn. If there is a sudden startle reflex, it is probably a superficial partial-thickness burn. A slow awakening indicates a deep dermal burn, and if it is possible to put the needle into the burn without any response it is likely to be a deep burn.

- In full thickness burns the area is insensitive to pain and may appear dirty or white (the eschar).
- A simple test to distinguish between partial and full thickness burns is to pull a hair out: if it comes out easily the burn is full thickness.

Many superficial burns become deeper during the first 48 hours after their occurrence, and need to be reassessed at 48 hours.

Inhalational injury

This includes:

- thermal damage
- asphyxiation
- pulmonary irritation.

Thermal damage

- This is usually limited to the oropharyngeal area.
- The exceptions are injuries caused by steam, volatile gases, explosive gases or aspiration of hot liquids.

Asphyxiation

Combustion utilises oxygen in the burning environment, leading to hypoxia. The **production of carbon monoxide** within the burning environment causes further tissue hypoxia by:

- decreasing the oxygen-carrying capacity of the blood
- shifting the oxyhaemoglobin saturation dissociation curve towards the left
- decreasing myocardial contractility.

The highest possible concentration of oxygen should be given.

Cyanide gas can be released during the combustion of plastics, polyurethane, wool, silk, nylon, nitrites, rubber and paper products. It is 20 times more toxic than carbon monoxide, and can cause immediate respiratory arrest.

Methaemoglobinaemia occurs due to heat denaturation of haemoglobin, oxides produced in fire, and methaemoglobin-forming materials such as nitrites. Rarer than cyanide and carbon monoxide toxicity, this decreases the oxygen-carrying capacity of the blood and causes a shift of the oxyhaemoglobin dissociation curve to the left, similarly to carboxyhaemoglobin (HbCO). Again treat with high concentrations of oxygen.

Pulmonary irritation
- Direct tissue injury.
- Acute bronchospasm.
- Activation of the body's inflammatory response system.

Evidence of inhalational injury
- Burns around the mouth.
- Soot in the mouth or nostrils.
- Carbonaceous sputum.
- Singed facial or nasal hairs.
- Facial burns.
- Oropharyngeal oedema.
- Changes in the voice (hoarseness), and stridor.
- Altered mental status.
- History suggesting confinement in a smoke-filled environment.

Symptoms may be delayed until 24–36 hours after injury. Secure the airway by endotracheal intubation before dangerous obstruction develops.

Deliver high-flow supplemental oxygen. Inhalation of hot gas normally does not injure distal airways, as the heat-exchange capacity of the upper airway is excellent. Distal airway injury is more likely to be due to the direct effects of the products of combustion on the mucosa and alveoli.

Treatment of skin surface burns
Analgesia
In all cases of shock, or potential shock, IV opiate analgesia should be given (*see* Section 1.15).

Oral analgesia is ineffective, and **IM analgesia can be very dangerous** because when the circulatory volume is re-established and muscle blood flow recommences, the child can become overdosed. Opiate overdose can be reversed with naloxone given intravenously (*see* Section 1.15).

Treatment of the burn itself
Minor burns
The best definition of a minor burn is one that can be treated as an outpatient.

Hospital admission
A child with a burn should be admitted unless it is completely safe for them to be treated as an outpatient. If possible, isolate the child in a warm clean room.

The following patients require admission:

- all airway burns or patients with a history of smoke inhalation
- burns of more than 5% TBSA in children and in pregnancy
- deep burns more than 5 cm in diameter
- moderate burns of the face, hands or perineum
- circumferential burns of the thorax or extremities*
- electrical burns (*see* Section 7.3.D)
- where there is inadequate social support in the home
- where there is any suspicion of non-accidental injury.

*If circumferential full-thickness burns involving the extremities or the chest are present, escharotomy may be necessary.

Dressings
Because a burn is normally caused by hot fluids or flame, the burn wound is initially sterile.

Hands should be washed and sterile gloves should be worn by all members of the team whenever the patient is being touched.

Ideally plastic aprons should also be used to prevent cross-infection during dressings, etc.

The purposes of a dressing are:
- to maintain sterility
- to relieve pain
- to absorb fluid produced by the burn wound
- to aid healing.

Placement of the dressing
- The layer of the dressing closest to the wound should be **non-adherent** (e.g. paraffin gauze) and may contain an antiseptic, such as silver sulphadiazine, although the evidence that antiseptics are useful to prevent infection and promote healing is ambiguous.
- On top of this dressing should be placed a layer of gauze and then sterile cotton wool to absorb fluid.
- The whole dressing should be held in place by a bandage.

Dressing changes
- Every time a dressing is changed, there will be pain, and the delicate reforming epithelium will be injured.
- **Therefore dressings should not be changed on a daily basis,** particularly in a superficial partial-thickness wound. The initial change should be at approximately 48 hours after the burn, when dressings come off easily, the maximum amount of fluid has been discharged from the wound, and it is possible to reassess the wound for area and depth.
- **Effective pain relief is vital at dressing changes or the child will come to dread the procedure.** Providing an anaesthetist is present, ketamine provides excellent brief anaesthesia of up to 15 minutes with an IV injection (over 1 minute) of 250–500 microgram/kg ketamine. For longer anaesthesia, an infusion will be needed. A safer alternative, especially in pregnancy, is oral morphine (*see* Section 1.15 for doses) given about 30 minutes before the anticipated dressing change.
- If at the first dressing change the wound is still a superficial partial-thickness burn, the second dressing is left for a further 8 days, by which stage healing should have occurred.
- If the wound is deeper, a decision as to whether to

operate must be made (see below), but the second dressing can still be left for at least a week.

- If surgery is not possible or appropriate, dressings can be done initially on a weekly basis but increased to two or three times a week as greater infection and discharge develops.

- Take a sample for microbiology (if available).

Tetanus

Anti-tetanus prophylaxis should be given at the earliest possible time.

TABLE 7.3.I.B.2 Guide to tetanus immunoglobulin and tetanus toxoid use in wounds

History of tetanus vaccination		Type of wound	Tetanus vaccine booster (see below)	Tetanus immunoglobulin
≥ 3 doses	< 5 years since last dose	All wounds	No	No
	5–10 years since last dose	Clean minor wounds	No	No
		All other wounds	Yes	No
	> 10 years since last dose	All wounds	Yes	No
< 3 doses or uncertain		Clean minor wounds	Yes	No
		All other wounds	Yes	Yes

In pregnancy, if the woman has not previously been vaccinated, give two doses of TT/Td one month apart.

Antibiotics

- Haemolytic *Streptococcus pyogenes* and *Pseudomonas aeruginosa* are the most common serious infections.
- In most burns, *Staphylococcus aureus* is also present, but does not need treatment unless it is invasive. If it is, flucloxacillin or cloxacillin is more appropriate than penicillin.
- Antibiotics should only be given when there are signs of infection.
- *Streptococcus pyogenes* should be treated with benzyl penicillin and flucloxacillin if found on a swab or suspected clinically (e.g. lymphangitis).
- *Pseudomonas aeruginosa* can be treated with ceftazidime, piperacillin, aztreonam, gentamicin or tobramycin.

Surgery

The surgical treatment of burns can be divided into four time zones:

- Immediate: within hours.
- Early: within days.
- Medium term: within weeks.
- Long term: within years.

Immediate surgery

There are two operations which may need to be done within hours of the burn:

- Tracheostomy:
  - Whenever possible this operation should be avoided, as an endotracheal tube usually gives better results and less mortality (depending on available intensive care).
  - An emergency tracheostomy for a severely swollen oral, pharyngeal or laryngeal airway is a very high-risk operation if the airway has not already been secured. It is better to use a mini-tracheostomy through the cricothyroid membrane.
  - Tracheostomy has a high mortality because of infection, displacement, lung-volume loss and tube blockage.
- Escharotomy:
  - A deep circumferential full-thickness burn of the limb, or even occasionally the trunk, can act as a tourniquet to that area.
  - Very early release (i.e. within 2 hours) is necessary to prevent severe and irrecoverable muscle and nerve damage. This can be done without any anaesthetic because the deep burn has no sensation.
  - The incisions should not overlie superficial bone or tendons, but need to go down to the fascia.
  - For more severe burns, and in particular high-voltage electrical burns, appropriate incisions are needed to decompress the deep compartments as well.
  - Urgent decompression of deep compartments may be required in severe high-voltage electrical burns, which can damage the underlying muscle with no skin damage visible except at the entry and exit points.

Early surgery

- Early surgery for deep dermal and deep burns has been shown to give better functional and cosmetic results with less risk of infection than allowing the natural processes of the body to remove the dead tissue.
- However, it is a technique that is difficult to learn from books, and often requires blood transfusion. Therefore if tangential excision is to be used without previous experience, only a small area should be attempted.
- Blood loss can be very rapid.
- An experienced anaesthetist is important.

Medium-term surgery

When wounds are granulating, thin split-skin grafts (ideally perforated or meshed) can be taken to cover the granulating areas.

Late surgery

Reconstruction to release contractures, and to improve both function and appearance, is best carried out, where possible, in a specialist centre.

Facilities and personnel

- All serious burn patients are best cared for in specialist burns units with a trained team of personnel. This includes all widespread second or third degree burns and burns significantly involving the face, hands and genitals.

- For larger burns, ideally single rooms are most appropriate, and these should be kept warm at all times. It is extremely important that they are clean and that insects, etc. are controlled.
- One of the most serious problems is cross-infection between patients, and adequate plastic aprons, gloves and hand-washing facilities must be available for all staff and relatives.
- In the early stages of burn resuscitation, and after surgery, nursing should be on a one-to-one basis (if available).

Psychology
- There are frequently major psychological consequences to major burns. First, there is a long and often painful stay in hospital. Secondly, there is the loss of function and appearance that can result from the burn injury.
- There are often psychological consequences for the parents of a burnt child, both as a result of the guilt about allowing the accident to happen, and from having to come to terms with the often major alterations in appearance and function of their child.

Prevention
- The best solution to the problem of the burn injury is prevention.
- Use antenatal classes, posters in village halls and talks in school.

- The causes of burns in children will vary in different communities, and prevention should be directed at local causes.
- If possible:
  - limit the temperature of water coming from domestic taps
  - do not cook on the floor
  - keep children away from boiling water, coffee, tea, etc. In many communities these are the commonest causes of scalds.

Features of burns that suggest child abuse
Burns are a common feature of child abuse and the clinician should have a high degree of awareness both of the physical appearance of inflicted burns and also of the developmental stage of the child to see if the injury is compatible with that stage.

Burns are sometimes used as a punishment in child rearing practices. Children with developmental delay are at particular risk of burns, both accidental and intentional.

Physical signs:
- Pattern burns that suggest contact with an object of a specific shape, such as an iron.
- Cigarette burns.
- Stocking, glove or circumferential burns.
- Burns to the genitals or perineum.

7.4 Poisoning

BOX 7.4.1 Minimum standards
- ABC, oxygen and glucose.
- Naloxone.
- Activated charcoal.
- Paediatric ipecacuanha.
- Wide-bore gastric tubes.
- Desferrioxamine.
- N-acetylcysteine.
- Sodium bicarbonate.
- Vitamin K.
- Exchange transfusion.
- Atropine.
- Pralidoxime.
- d-Penicillamine.
- EDTA.

Introduction
The World Health Organization (WHO) definition of poisoning is the injury or destruction of cells by the inhalation, ingestion or absorption of a toxic substance. Key factors that predict the severity and outcome of poisoning are the nature, dose formulation and route of exposure of the poison, co-exposure to other poisons, the state of nutrition

of the child or their fasting status, age, and pre-existing health conditions.

Mortality: Low- and middle-income countries have 91% of the world mortality from poisoning as reported by WHO in 2004.

Accidental poisoning is most common in the 12–36 months age group.

Intentional overdose may be a cry for help, rather than a serious attempt at suicide. However, all children and young people who take intentional overdoses should have a full psychiatric and social assessment and always be admitted to hospital if facilities are available.

Drug abuse may be misuse of alcohol or abuse of volatile substances or more potent recreational drugs, such as ecstasy, LSD or opiates.

Deliberate poisoning of children by adults is rare. It may be associated with depressive illness or may be part of a spectrum of abuse inflicted on the child (see Section 7.6).

Clinical diagnosis and management
Symptoms and signs of poisoning
These can include:
- respiratory distress

- acidotic breathing
- tachycardia or flushing
- cardiac arrhythmias
- hypotension
- diarrhoea
- vomiting
- drowsiness or coma
- convulsions
- ataxia
- pupillary abnormalities
- hypoglycaemia
- acidosis.

The presentation may be more general, such as sudden unexplained illness in a previously healthy child, or unusual behaviour. Remember that there may not be a history of poisoning, so when taking a history ask specifically about access to prescribed drugs, local medicines, household substances, berries and plants.

Management of poisoning

First aid

- Remove the patient from the source of the poison. This mainly applies to fumes (e.g. in a house fire).
- Wash contaminated skin and eyes with water.
- **Never** try to induce vomiting with salt or by inserting an object into the pharynx.

Primary assessment and resuscitation

Identify life-threatening emergencies and the early signs of a seriously ill child using the structured ABC approach (*see* Section 1.11).

The whole assessment should take less than a minute. Treat any problems with the ABC approach as they are found.

An alternative approach to emergencies such as this is the Emergency Triage and Treatment (ETAT) approach, if it is practised at your hospital.

Once Airway, Breathing and Circulation are recognised as being stable, or have been stabilised, definitive management of specific conditions can proceed. During definitive management, **reassessment of ABCD at frequent intervals will be necessary to assess progress and detect deterioration.**

Secondary assessment and emergency treatment

Identify the substance ingested or inhaled, if at all possible. Ask the following questions:

- What medicines, domestic products, berries and plants has the child had access to?
- How much has been taken?
- When did the child have access to these substances?
- Is the container or a sample available? This will be helpful at the hospital.
- Are other children involved?
- What symptoms has the child had?

Use National Poisons Information Centres or Internet references, if these services are available, to obtain information on the side effects, toxicity and treatment needed.

Hypoglycaemia: Test blood glucose levels for all patients, and if hypoglycaemia is present, treat with a sugar drink orally if the patient is conscious. If they are unconscious give by IV or intraosseous routes 2 to 5 mL/kg 10% glucose over 3 minutes then 5 mL/kg/hour to keep blood glucose at 5–8 mmol/litre. In pregnancy, dilute 50 mL of 50% glucose with 50 mL of Ringer-lactate, Hartmann's or 0.9% saline and give IV over 5 minutes followed by an IV infusion containing 5% glucose (*see* Appendix). If blood glucose testing is not available, then treat for hypoglycaemia if this diagnosis is possible (especially in infants and young children).

Convulsions: Treat convulsions in children with diazepam 300–400 micrograms/kg IV or IO slowly or 500 micrograms/kg per rectum.

In pregnancy the loading dose of diazepam is 2 mg increments IV every 2 minutes up to 10 mg. The maintenance dose is diazepam 40 mg in 500 mL of Ringer-lactate or Hartmann's solution, titrated to keep the mother sedated but able to be woken and without hypoventilation. Maternal respiratory depression may occur when the dose exceeds 30 mg in 1 hour. Alternatively, in pregnancy the loading dose diazepam is 20 mg in a 10-mL syringe. Remove the needle, lubricate the barrel and insert the syringe into the rectum to half its length. Discharge the contents and leave the syringe in place, holding the buttocks together for 10 minutes to prevent expulsion of the drug. Alternatively, the drug may be instilled in the rectum through a catheter.

Ensure close observation after treatment with diazepam at any age, and make sure that a bag-valve-mask of suitable size is available and the staff giving the diazepam know how to use it.

Opiate or methadone overdose: If an opiate or methadone overdose is suspected, give naloxone.

- IV dose for children aged 1 month to 12 years: 10 micrograms/kg; if there is no response, give 100 micrograms/kg (review the diagnosis if there is still no response).
- Give patients over 12 years of age and in pregnancy 400 microgram–2.0 mg; if there is no response, repeat every 2–3 minutes up to a maximum of 10 mg (then review the diagnosis).

Remember that naloxone has a short half-life and further boluses or an infusion of and further boluses or an infusion of 10–20 micrograms/kg/hour or more may be required. Give this treatment even if poisoning is only suspected (because of the presence of such drugs in the home) because breathing is shallow or the patient has stopped breathing. If the patient is hypoventilating or has stopped breathing, ventilate with bag-valve-mask before giving the naloxone as hypercapnia with naloxone can cause arrhythmias, acute pulmonary oedema, seizures or asystole.

Minimising the effects of the ingested substance as quickly as possible

If the substance is **non-toxic** give oral fluids liberally.

If the substance is **corrosive**, there may be serious injury to the mouth, throat, airway, oesophagus or stomach (*see also* Section 7.3.I.a). The most dangerous substances are sodium or potassium hydroxide cleaning fluids (e.g. toilet cleaners). Others include bleach and other disinfectants. Serious oesophageal injury can result in perforations and mediastinitis, later leading to oesophageal strictures. The presence of burns within the mouth is of concern, and suggests that oesophageal injury is possible. Stridor suggests laryngeal damage. **No emetic should be given.** Milk or water given as soon as possible may be of benefit, especially with solid caustics such as sodium hydroxide crystals. If there is a severe stricture it may be necessary to bypass the oesophagus with a gastrostomy tube. Ideally, flexible endoscopy should be performed to identify injury, but this may not be available. A perforated oesophagus will lead to mediastinitis and should be treated with gastrostomy and prophylactic antibiotics (cefuroxime and metronidazole).

In a few instances, specific **antidotes** are advised. These should only be given when full information on the poison is available from a Poisons Centre. **Never give salt to induce vomiting.**

For all other poisons except heavy metals, iron, alcohol and domestic products give activated charcoal if this is available (1 gram/kg suspended in water for a child and 50 gram in pregnancy). The sooner it is given the better (preferably within 1 hour of ingestion of the poison). Repeat after 4 hours if a sustained-release drug has been taken. If charcoal is not available and a potentially life-threatening dose of poison has been taken (particularly of iron), give paediatric ipecacuanha (10 mL for those aged 6 months to 2 years, and 15 mL for those aged over 2 years, plus a glass of water) to induce vomiting. **Do not give ipecacuanha if the child has a decreasing level of, or impaired, consciousness. Do NOT give if corrosive solutions have been ingested or if kerosene, turpentine or petrol have been ingested, as they could be inhaled following vomiting, resulting in lipoid pneumonia.**

Gastric lavage with a wide-bore orogastric tube should be used only if a potentially life-threatening dose has been taken, and provided that the airway is protected. It should not be used if there is a decreasing level of, or impaired, consciousness without airway protection. **It should not be used for poisons containing hydrocarbons or corrosives.** Lavage cycles of 15 mL/kg are usually appropriate. Gastric lavage is not an effective way of removing most poisons, and may wash tablets into the duodenum. In a small child the size of nasogastric tube that can be inserted will almost certainly be too small to allow tablets to be drawn through it. Liquid preparations may be evacuated in this way, but in most cases they will have left the stomach within an hour, which is likely to sooner than the child reaches hospital.

Treat symptoms as they arise.

Child abuse: Always remember that an older child or adult may have given the child drugs intentionally. This is child abuse, and if there is the slightest suspicion of this, the appropriate child protection procedures should be instituted if they are available. The child should be admitted (*see* Section 7.6).

Admit all patients with symptoms or signs attributable to poisons, all patients who have ingested iron, pesticides, corrosives, paracetamol (unless blood testing shows a low level of drug), salicyclate, narcotic drugs or tricyclic antidepressant drugs, all who allege deliberate ingestion, and any cases in which child abuse is suspected.

Commonly ingested drugs
Local medicines
- These are often prescribed for diarrhoea and vomiting. They may cause profound acidosis and respiratory distress. They can also cause paralytic ileus.
- Treat the metabolic disturbance.
- Consider using a nasogastric tube.

Iron
- Poisoning is usually the result of taking iron tablets prescribed for another family member. Even two or three adults' tablets can cause serious symptoms in a small child.
- Iron poisoning causes severe gastrointestinal effects, with vomiting, diarrhoea, gastrointestinal bleeding and metabolic acidosis. Subsequently after 12–24 hours there is encephalopathy, liver damage and circulatory collapse.
- Late effects include scarring of the stomach, which may produce pyloric stenosis.
- **If available, a serum iron level at 4 hours of more than 300 micrograms/dL indicates significant poisoning.**
- X-ray may show the number of tablets. **In a child aim to remove as much as possible by induced vomiting with ipecacuanha.**
- Gastric lavage with a wide-bore orogastric tube may also remove significant amounts of iron if it is still in the stomach, but there is also a risk that the lavage may wash the tablets through into the bowel. Do not use gastric lavage in pregnancy.
- Desferrioxamine should be given by deep IM injection, 1 gram for children under 12 years and 2 grams for those over 12 years and in pregnancy. IM doses of desferrioxamine of desferrioxamine of 1–2 g should be repeated every 12 hours until serum iron is normal (serum iron less than iron binding capacity). If the patient is very ill, give an IV infusion of desferrioxamine 15 mg/kg/hour up to a maximum dose of 80 mg/kg in 24 hours. Usually reduce the rate after 6 hours.

Paracetamol
- Paracetamol poisoning can lead to liver and renal failure (*see* Section 5.6.C and Section 5.7.B).
- Induce vomiting and, if possible, measure the paracetamol level.
- Give N-acetylcysteine or methionine as soon as possible, ideally within 8 hours of ingestion. If the patient is conscious and tolerating oral fluids, and within 8 hours of ingestion, give methionine orally (for children under 6 years, give 1 gram every 4 hours for four doses; for those aged 6 years or over and in pregnancy, give 2.5 g every 4 hours for four doses).
- If the patient presents more than 8 hours after ingestion or cannot be given an oral preparation, give IV N-acetylcysteine (initially as a loading dose of 150 mg/kg over 15 minutes, then as an IV infusion of 50 mg/kg over 4 hours, and finally as 100 mg/kg IV over 16 hours). An oral form of N-acetylcysteine is available (give a loading dose of 140 mg/kg, and then 70 mg/kg every 4 hours for 16 doses).

Salicylates
- Salicylate poisoning produces acidotic-like breathing, vomiting and tinnitus.
- Hyperventilation is due to direct stimulation of the respiratory centre and produces respiratory alkalosis, but also there is a metabolic acidosis from ketosis. Consequently, the hyperventilation is extreme.
- A fever may occur.
- There is peripheral vasodilatation.
- Moderate hyperglycaemia develops.

There is delayed gastric emptying, so give activated charcoal if available (1 gram/kg in a child and 50 gram in pregnancy and repeat after 4 hours) even if more than 4 hours after ingestion. If charcoal is not available, induce vomiting.

Give sodium bicarbonate 1 mmol/kg IV as 4.2% over 4 hours to correct acidosis and aid excretion of salicylate.

Give sufficient IV fluids to compensate for hyperventilation, and give sufficient glucose to minimise ketosis, but regularly monitor blood glucose levels.

Monitor electrolytes carefully and avoid hypokalaemia and hypernatraemia.

In very severe cases, **peritoneal haemodialysis (if available) is ideal**. In its absence, exchange transfusion may help.

Benzodiazepines

Flumazenil is a specific antagonist. The initial dose is slow IV 10 micrograms/kg; repeat at 1-minute intervals up to a maximum of 40 micrograms/kg (2 mg maximum dose). If necessary this can be followed by an infusion of 2–10 micrograms/kg/hour (not recommended in children who have received long-term benzodiazepine treatment for epilepsy). In pregnancy give 200 micrograms IV then 100 micrograms per minute IV up to a maximum total of 1 mg until reversal has occurred.

Tricyclic antidepressants

- In overdose these cause drowsiness, ataxia, dilated pupils and tachycardia.
- Severe poisoning results in cardiac arrhythmias (particularly ventricular tachycardia) and severe hypotension and convulsions.

In children induce vomiting, perform gastric lavage and administer charcoal as described above, **but first protect the airway if the patient is drowsy. In pregnancy only administer charcoal**.

Treat convulsions as for any status epilepticus (*see* Section 5.16.E).

Monitor the ECG (if available) continuously.

Arrhythmias can be reduced by using IV phenytoin which must be diluted only in 0.9% saline. Phenytoin is given as a loading dose of 15–20 mg/kg over 30–45 minutes (maximum dose 2 grams) and then 2.5–7.5 mg/kg 12 hourly. The maximum infusion rate is 1 mg/kg/minute (maximum 50 mg/minute). A lidocaine infusion (10–50 micrograms/kg/minute) is an alternative to phenytoin.

Alkalinisation of the intravascular compartment has been shown to reduce the toxic effects on the heart. Give sodium bicarbonate 1–2 mmol/kg slowly. This can be repeated if necessary.

The aim is to increase the arterial pH to 7.45–7.5.

Where there is severe cardiac toxicity, prolonged external cardiac massage may keep the patient, especially a child, alive long enough for the effects of the drug to wear off.

Poisonous household and natural products
Petroleum compounds such as kerosene, turpentine and petrol
Do not induce vomiting.

- If inhaled these may cause hydrocarbon (lipoid) pneumonia, leading to a cough, and respiratory distress with hypoxaemia due to pulmonary oedema and lipoid pneumonia. A chest X-ray is essential in all cases.
- If large amounts are ingested they may cause encephalopathy.
- Additional inspired oxygen may be required.
- An antibiotic may be needed, but only for secondary chest infections.
- Dexamethasone may help in lipoid pneumonia.

Organophosphorus compounds and carbamates

- Insecticides such as malathion, chlorthion, parathion, TEPP and phosdrin can be absorbed through the skin, lungs or gastrointestinal tract.
- Symptoms are due to excessive parasympathetic effects caused by inhibition of cholinesterase, and include excessive secretions of mucus in the lungs (bronchorrhoea) with ensuing respiratory distress and sometimes wheezing, salivation, lacrimation, bradycardia, sweating, gastrointestinal cramps, vomiting, diarrhoea, convulsions, blurred vision and small pupils, muscle weakness and twitching, progressing to paralysis, and loss of reflexes and sphincter control.

Treatment aims to remove poison from:
- the eyes: use copious irrigation
- the skin: remove contaminated clothing and wash the skin
- the gastrointestinal tract: give activated charcoal 1 gram/kg and repeat after 4 hours.

Admit all cases, as some effects do not appear until a late stage.

In severe cases, particularly where there is bronchorrhoea, give **atropine in a child** 20 micrograms/kg IV or IM every 5–10 minutes until the skin becomes flushed and dry, the pupils dilate and tachycardia develops (that is atropinisation has occurred: maximum dose 2 mg). In pregnancy give 600 micrograms and repeat in doses of 300 micrograms as needed.

- A specific cholinesterase reactivator can also be given as follows, and ideally within 12 hours of ingestion (it is ineffective after 24 hours).
  - **Pralidoxime** 30 mg/kg diluted with 10–15 mL of water by IV infusion at a rate not exceeding 5 mg/minute. It should produce an improved muscle power in 30 minutes. It can be repeated once or twice as required and as is shown to be effective, or an infusion of 8 mg/kg/hour can be used. Maximum dose is 12 gram in 24 hours.
- **Assisted ventilation** may be required (if available).

Bleach (3–6% sodium hypochlorite)
Do not induce vomiting.

- Symptoms: burning sensation, vomiting and abdominal discomfort.
- Treatment: liberal fluids and milk.

Corrosive agents
Do not induce vomiting.

- Oven cleaners (30% caustic soda).
- Kettle descalers (concentrated formic acid).
- Dishwashing powders (silicates and metasilicates).
- Drain cleaners (sodium hydroxide).

- Car battery acid (concentrated sulphuric acid).

Symptoms: considerable tissue damage to the skin, mouth, oesophagus or stomach; late strictures may occur. Treatment consists of washing the skin and mouth to dilute the corrosive fluid (see Section 7.3.I.a).

Lead poisoning

This is usually a chronic form of poisoning. The lead can come from paint, lead piping or car batteries. In some cultures, lead-containing substances may be applied to the skin for cosmetic purposes (e.g. Surma in India).

- Early signs are non-specific (e.g. vomiting, abdominal pain, anorexia).
- Anaemia is usually present.
- Prior to encephalopathy with raised intracranial pressure, there may be headaches and insomnia.
- Peripheral neuropathy may be present.
- X-rays may show bands of increased density at the metaphyses.
- Harmful effects on the kidneys result in hypertension, aminoaciduria and glycosuria.
- There is a microcytic hypochromic anaemia with punctate basophilia.
- The diagnosis is made by showing a marked increase in urinary lead levels after d-penicillamine, and elevated blood lead levels.

Treatment

- Treat by first removing the source of ingested lead.
- A diet rich in calcium, phosphate and vitamin D (plenty of milk) should be given if possible.
- In cases of lead encephalopathy, give an IV infusion of edetate calcium (EDTA) in 5% glucose or normal saline, 20 mg/kg every 6 hours for 5–7 days at a concentration of no more than 30 mg/mL. Give over an hour.
- Boluses of mannitol 250–500 mg/kg IV over 30–60 minutes may also be required for raised intracranial pressure while the above is given.

Poisonous plants

- Usually only small quantities are ingested.
- Recent reports describe nicotine poisoning by absorption through the skin in children who are tobacco pickers.

Treatment: For ingested poisonous plants this consists of activated charcoal and supportive therapy.

Carbon monoxide poisoning

- Toxic effects are due to hypoxia.

Treatment: Move the patient from the source and give them 100% oxygen as soon as possible (the half-life of carbon monoxide is 5 hours in room air, but only 1.5 hours in 100% oxygen). The patient may look pink but is hypoxaemic, so base the duration of oxygen treatment on other clinical signs of hypoxia rather than on cyanosis, which will be masked. For similar reasons, pulse oximeters will give falsely high readings. ABCD management according to APLS may be required.

- Cerebral oedema may develop.
- **Hyperbaric oxygen treatment may be helpful (if available).**

Volatile substance abuse ('sniffing')

This mainly occurs in the age range 11–17 years and is a group activity. Substances that are sniffed or sprayed into the respiratory system are numerous. The commonest are solvent-based adhesives ('glue sniffing'), butane gas, cleaning fluids, aerosols and fire-extinguisher substances.

Clinical features

- Sores around the mouth and nose.
- Smell of solvents on the clothes and breath.
- All of the features of ethyl alcohol intoxication, plus extreme disorientation, hallucinations and sudden 'unexplained' death
- Accidents can occur secondary to volatile substance abuse, for example falling from height, drowning, suffocation and inhalation of vomit.

Management

- Remove the child from the atmosphere of solvent.
- Admit them to hospital.
- Treat symptomatically.
- Arrange expert psychological and emotional support.

Laboratory investigations in poisoning

These are often expensive and/or very time consuming to perform. They should only be requested if the result will alter the management of the patient. Many hospitals in resource-limited countries will not have these facilities.

Alcohol

- Blood alcohol estimations are useful if:
  - there is an indication that methyl alcohol has been ingested
  - the patient is very drowsy or comatose and there is doubt whether sufficient alcohol has been ingested to explain the symptoms.
- Blood glucose levels should be measured in all cases of alcohol ingestion in children.
  - Do a blood glucose stick test first, and if this is low, a quantitative glucose analysis should be requested.

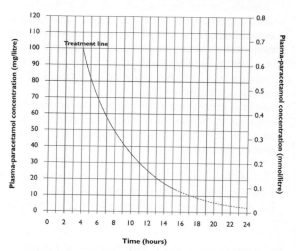

FIGURE 7.4.1 Graph for N-acetylcysteine use in paracetamol poisoning. This Crown copyright material is reproduced by permission of the Medicines and Healthcare Products Regulatory Agency under delegated authority from the Controller of HMSO.

— If in doubt, give glucose 2–5 mL/kg of 10% glucose IV if unable to drink or unconscious, otherwise give a sugary drink.

Interpretation
Peak blood levels of alcohol occur 30–60 minutes after ingestion.

Iron
Patients who have ingested iron should ideally have a plasma iron level estimated before desferrioxamine is given. Serum levels of over 300 micrograms/dL are associated with moderate toxicity, levels of over 500 micrograms/dL with serious toxicity, and levels over 1 mg/dL with death.

Interpretation
Patients with acute iron poisoning have significant increase in plasma iron levels within 2 hours of over-dosage. Initial serum levels of less than 90 micromol/litre are supportive but not absolute evidence of mild poisoning. Normal serum iron levels are in the region of 10–30 micromols/L (80–180 micrograms/dL).

Paracetamol
Take blood samples at least 4 hours after ingestion of paracetamol.

Interpretation
A plasma level that falls above the treatment line at different times indicated in the graph of paracetamol level against time (see Figure 7.4.1) indicates moderate to severe poisoning. Treat with N-acetylcysteine. Lower thresholds for treatment are indicated if the patient is on enzyme-inducing drugs or alcohol is taken habitually.

7.5 Envenomation

BOX 7.5.1 Minimum standards
- Mono- and polyspecific antivenoms.
- Chlorphenamine.
- Anticholinesterase (only if appropriate for the region).
- Analgesia.
- Prazosin (only if appropriate for the region).
- Heart failure treatment.

Introduction
Envenoming by snakes, scorpions, spiders or marine venomous animals is common in many areas of the tropics. Children are particularly at risk; they may be attracted to venomous creatures and do not recognise the danger that they represent. Envenoming is often more severe and more rapid in children because the ratio of the amount of venom to body weight is much higher.

A clear-cut history of envenoming is often not present. Some bites are not recognised at the time of the event; other children will be too young to explain what has happened. Envenoming should always be considered in any child with an unexplained illness, particularly if there is severe pain, swelling or blistering of a limb, or if the child is bleeding or shows signs of neurotoxicity.

Prevention
Discourage children from handling snakes, scorpions or spiders or touching marine animals. They should be taught to avoid putting their hands down holes, and to carefully check their shoes and clothing before dressing. Keeping grass short around dwellings, use of sensible footwear, keeping dwellings insect-free, and taking care when swimming can all help to prevent injury by venomous animals.

Snakebite
There are a large number of species of venomous snakes throughout the world. These can be divided into three main categories: **vipers**, **elapids** and **sea snakes**. The pattern of envenoming depends upon the biting species. Therefore clinicians need to know about the snakes present in the region in which they work. **Only 50–70% of patients who are bitten by venomous snakes develop signs of envenoming.**

Major clinical effects following snakebite can be categorised as follows:
- **Local effects:** pain, swelling or blistering of the bitten limb. Necrosis at the site of the wound may sometimes develop.
- **Systemic effects:**
  - Non-specific symptoms: vomiting, headache, collapse.
  - Painful regional lymph node enlargement indicating absorption of venom.
  - Specific signs: non-clotting of blood; bleeding from gums, old wounds and sores.
  - Neurotoxicity: ptosis, bulbar palsy and respiratory paralysis.
  - Shock: hypotension.
  - Rhabdomyolysis: muscle pains and black urine.

Vipers most commonly cause local swelling, shock, bleeding and non-clotting blood.

Elapids cause neurotoxicity and usually minimal signs at the bite site (with the exception of some cobras which also cause necrosis).

Sea snakes cause myotoxicity and subsequent paresis.

Exceptions to this general rule do occur. For example, some vipers cause neurotoxicity and some Australasian elapids also cause non-clotting blood and haemorrhage.

First aid outside hospital

- Reassure the patient. Many symptoms following snake-bite are due to anxiety.
- Avoid harmful manoeuvres such as cutting, suction or the use of tourniquets.
- Immobilise and splint the limb. Moving the limb may increase systemic absorption of venom.
- Apply a pressure bandage if tissue necrosis is rare following snakebite in your region, particularly if rapid transport to hospital is not possible. This is especially important for snakes that cause neurotoxicity. Apply a crepe bandage over the bite site and wind it firmly up the limb. **This can only be recommended on a geographical basis, not a clinical one, as necrosis is not apparent initially.**
- Transport the patient to hospital as soon as possible.
- If the snake has been killed, take it with the patient to the hospital.

Diagnosis and initial assessment

- Carefully examine the bitten limb for local signs.
- Measure the pulse, respiration rate, blood pressure and urine output. Blood pressure and other signs of shock (*see* Section 5.5) must be watched for if children are unwell, are bleeding or have significant swelling; shock is common in viper bites.
- Look for non-clotting blood. This may be the only sign of envenoming in some viper bites. The 20-minute whole-blood clotting test (WBCT20) is an extremely easy and useful test. It should be performed on admission and repeated 6 hours later.

WBCT20 test
- Place a few millilitres of freshly sampled blood in a new clean dry glass tube or bottle.
- Leave undisturbed for 20 minutes at ambient temperature.
- Tip the vessel once.
- If the blood is still liquid (i.e. unclotted) and runs out, the patient has hypofibrinogenaemia ('incoagulable blood') as a result of venom-induced consumption coagulopathy.

Look carefully for signs of bleeding which may be subtle (e.g. from gums, old wounds or sores). Bleeding internally (most often intracranial) may cause clinical signs.

- Look for early signs of neurotoxicity, such as ptosis (children may interpret this as feeling sleepy), limb weakness, or difficulties in talking, swallowing or breathing.
- Check for muscle tenderness and myoglobinuria in sea snake bites.
- Take blood for:
  - haemoglobin, white cell count and platelet count
  - prothrombin time, APTT and fibrinogen levels (if available)
  - serum urea and creatinine
  - creatine phosphokinase (CPK) (reflecting skeletal muscle damage) (if available).
- ECG (if available).

Hospital or health centre management
General management

- Observe the patient in hospital for at least 24 hours, even if there are no signs of envenoming initially. Review regularly, as envenoming may develop quite rapidly.
- Nurse the patient on their side with a slight head-down tilt to prevent aspiration of blood or secretions.
- Avoid IM injections and invasive procedures in patients with incoagulable blood.
- Give tetanus prophylaxis. Routine antibiotic prophylaxis is not required unless necrosis is present.

Antivenom

Antivenom is indicated for signs of systemic envenoming. Evidence for its efficacy in severe local envenoming is poor, but it is usually indicated if swelling extends over more than half of the bitten limb. Monospecific (monovalent) antivenom may be used for a single species of snake, and polyspecific (polyvalent) antivenom for a number of different species. The dose of antivenom depends upon the manufacturer's recommendations and local experience.

Children require exactly the same dose as pregnant women (the dose is dependent upon the amount of venom injected, not body weight).

- Dilute the antivenom in two to three volumes of 5% glucose or Ringer-lactate or Hartmann's or 0.9% saline and infuse over 45 minutes to an hour. The infusion rate should be slow initially and gradually increased. Note that doses of antivenom vary considerably; always follow the instructions enclosed with the antivenom.
- Draw up adrenaline in a syringe ready for use.
- Observe the patient closely during antivenom administration. Common early signs of an antivenom reaction include urticaria and itching, restlessness, fever, cough or a feeling of constriction in the throat.
- Patients with anaphylaxis should be treated with adrenaline (epinephrine). In a child give 10 micrograms/kg IM (*see* Section 5.1.B) and in pregnancy give 1 mL of 1 in 1000 adrenaline (1 mg) (*see* Section 5.1.B). An antihistamine, such as chlorphenamine, 200 micrograms/kg IM or IV, should also be given.
- Unless life-threatening anaphylaxis has occurred, antivenom can cautiously be restarted after this treatment.
- Routine adrenaline prophylaxis may reduce the incidence of antivenom anaphylaxis, but should not generally be used.
- Monitor the response to antivenom. In the presence of coagulopathy, restoration of clotting depends upon hepatic resynthesis of clotting factors. Repeat WBCT20 and other clotting studies if available, 6 hours after antivenom. If the blood is still non-clotting, further antivenom is indicated. After restoration of normal clotting, measure clotting at 6- to 12-hour intervals, as a coagulopathy may recur due to late absorption of venom from the bite site.

The response of neurotoxicity to antivenom is less predictable. In species with predominantly postsynaptically acting toxins, antivenom may reverse neurotoxicity, and failure to do so is an indication for further doses. However, the response to antivenom is poor in species with presynaptically acting toxins.

Other therapy

- Excise sloughs from necrotic wounds. Skin grafting may be necessary. Severe swelling may lead to suspicion of a compartment syndrome. Fasciotomy should **not** be performed unless there is definite evidence of raised intra-compartmental pressure (> 45 mmHg) (if measurable), and any coagulopathy has been corrected. **Clinical assessment for compartment syndromes is often misleading following snakebite. Therefore objective criteria are helpful.**
- Blood products are not necessary to treat a coagulopathy if adequate antivenom has been given.
- Endotracheal intubation or even tracheostomy should be considered to prevent aspiration if bulbar palsy develops; this is often obvious when difficulty in swallowing leads to pooling of secretions.
- If there is uncontrolled bleeding in the absence of antivenom, give fresh blood, vitamin K in a child 300 micrograms/kg IV and in pregnancy vitamin K 10 mg IV/IM and fresh-frozen plasma 10 grams/kg IV (if available).
- Paralysis of intercostal muscles and diaphragm requires artificial ventilation. This can be performed by manual bagging with a bag-valve mask and may need to be maintained for days, using relays of relatives if ventilators and skills are not available.
- Anticholinesterases may reverse neurotoxicity following envenoming by some species.
- Maintain careful fluid balance to treat shock and prevent renal failure.
- Some cobras spit venom into the eyes of their victim. Rapid irrigation with water will prevent severe inflammation, and 0.5% adrenaline (epinephrine) drops may help to reduce pain and inflammation.

Scorpion stings

In some areas of the world, scorpion stings are more common than snakebites and cause significant mortality. The stinging scorpion is not often seen. A number of different species have broadly similar clinical effects. The major feature of envenoming is severe pain around the bite site, which may last for many hours or even days. Systemic envenoming is more common in children and may occur within minutes of a bite. The major clinical features are caused by activation of the autonomic nervous system (*see* Table 7.5.1).

Severe hypertension, myocardial failure and pulmonary oedema are particularly prominent in severe envenoming.

TABLE 7.5.1 Scorpion stings

Clinical features of scorpion stings	
Tachypnoea	Muscle twitching and spasms
Excess salivation	Hypertension
Nausea and vomiting	Pulmonary oedema
Lacrimation	Cardiac arrhythmias
Sweating	Hypotension
Abdominal pain	Respiratory failure

Management

- Take the patient to hospital immediately; delay is a frequent cause of death.
- Control the pain with infiltration of 1% lignocaine around the wound or give systemic opiates (with care) (*see* Section 1.15).
- Scorpion antivenom is available for some species. Give intravenously in systemic envenoming, but IM injection has been used with good effect if there is no alternative.
- Prazosin is effective for treating hypertension and cardiac failure (orally 10–15 micrograms/kg two to four times a day increasing to control blood pressure to a maximum of 500 micrograms/kg/day for under 12 years and 20 mg/day over 12 years). The patient should be lying down for the first 4–6 hours of treatment in case there is a sudden fall in blood pressure.
- Severe pulmonary oedema requires aggressive treatment with diuretics and vasodilators (*see* Section 5.4.B).

Spider bites

Three main genera of spiders cause significant envenoming in the tropics. Each causes different clinical effects, but fatal envenoming is rare.

- **Widow spiders** (*Latrodectus* species) are found throughout the world. Severe pain at the bite site is common. Rare cases develop systemic envenoming with abdominal and generalised pain and other features due to transmitter release from autonomic nerves. Hypertension is characteristic of severe envenoming (see use of prazosin above). Antivenom is available in some regions, and is effective for relief of pain and systemic symptoms. Opiates are also useful for the treatment of pain (*see* Section 1.15).
- **Recluse spiders** (*Loxosceles* species) have a wide distribution and cause bites in which pain develops over a number of hours. A white ischaemic area gradually breaks down to form a black eschar over 7 days or so. Healing may be prolonged, and occasionally severe scarring occurs. The efficacy of antivenom and other advocated treatments (dapsone, steroids and hyperbaric oxygen) remains uncertain.
- **Banana spiders** (*Phoneutria* species) occur only in South America. They usually cause severe burning pain at the site of the bite, but in severe cases may cause systemic envenoming with tachycardia, hypertension, sweating and priapism. Polyspecific antivenom is available.

Marine envenoming

Venomous fish

Many different venomous fish may sting children if they stand on or touch the fish. Systemic envenoming is rare. Excruciating pain at the site of the sting is the major effect.

- Regional nerve blocks and local infiltration of 1% lignocaine may be effective (*see* Section 1.24).
- Most marine venoms are heat-labile. Immersing the stung part in hot water is extremely effective for relieving the pain. Care should be taken to avoid scalding, as the envenomed limb may have abnormal sensation. The clinician should check the water temperature with their own hand. Asking the patient to immerse their non-bitten limb may help to avoid scalding.

Jellyfish

Venomous jellyfish have large numbers of stinging capsules (nematocysts) on their tentacles which inject venom when the tentacles contact skin. Pain and wheals are the usual effects but, rarely, systemic envenoming can be life-threatening. Many of the nematocysts will remain undischarged on tentacles that adhere to the victim. Therefore rubbing the area of the sting will cause further discharge and worsen envenoming.

- In box jellyfish stings, pouring vinegar over the sting will prevent discharge of nematocysts. For most other jellyfish, seawater should be poured over the stings and the adherent tentacles gently removed. Ice is useful for pain relief.
- Box jellyfish stings may occasionally be rapidly life-threatening. Antivenom is available and can be administered intramuscularly.

Further reading

A Kasturiratne, AR Wickremasinghe, N de Silva *et al.* (2008) The global burden of snakebite: a literature analysis and modelling based on regional estimates of envenoming and deaths. *PLoS Medicine*, **5**, 1591–604.

World Health Organization (2010) *Guidelines for the Prevention and Clinical Management of Snakebite in Africa*. www.snakebiteinitiative.org

DJ Williams, J-M Gutiérrez, JJ Calvete *et al.* (2011) Ending the drought: new strategies for improving the flow of affordable, effective antivenoms in Asia and Africa. *Journal of Proteomics*, **74**, 1735–67.

7.6 The child who has been ill treated, abused or exploited

> **BOX 7.6.1 Minimum standards**
> - Knowledge of the in-country legal framework for child protection.
> - Understanding of cross-cultural child-rearing practices.
> - Links between health services, police child protection teams and/or social services in place.
> - Access to X-rays and blood clotting measurements.
> - Access to forensic advice.
> - Access to photography services, with secure storage of images.
> - Healthcare workers trained to recognise signs of physical and sexual abuse.

Children's rights

Article 19 of the United Nations Convention on the Rights of the Child states that children (people less than 18 years of age) have a right to be protected from being hurt and maltreated physically and mentally. It goes on to state that governments should ensure that children are properly cared for and should protect them from violence, abuse and neglect by their parents or anyone who looks after them.

Child abuse results in actual or potential harm to the child's health, survival, development or dignity in the context of a relationship of responsibility, trust or power with the abuser.

Healthcare workers have a major responsibility in contributing to the prevention and recognition of childhood ill treatment. This poses particular challenges for healthcare workers when they work with children and families from different belief systems and cultural backgrounds. They may find that they have to care for street children, child soldiers, and children separated from their parents by civil strife and unrest, and find themselves making difficult judgements about how a child can be best protected when they have few if any points of reference, and only limited contact with other agencies.

The basic principles of the investigation of child maltreatment are that:

- the welfare of the child is paramount
- multi-agency/multi-sectored collaboration is needed
- agencies must work together within the legal framework of the country (where this is in place).

Child maltreatment or abuse involves acts of omission and commission which result in harm to a child. It can occur in the family, in the community or in institutions (e.g. schools, hospitals, churches, mosques, temples, clubs, orphanages or other institutions). It encompasses:

- exploitation through trafficking for sexual or other forms of slavery
- exploitation through enforced prostitution
- physical abuse
- emotional abuse
- neglect
- sexual abuse
- fabricated induced illness (FII)
- conscription as child soldiers.

Features of presentation of a child to hospital which suggest possible ill treatment or abuse

- Delay in seeking medical help for an injury or serious clinical symptoms or signs (e.g. bleeding).
- A history that is vague or rehearsed, with inconsistencies and significant changes on re-telling or following questioning.
- No explanation of the cause of the injury.
- Repeated attendance at healthcare facilities (this may suggest fabricated or induced illness, FII; see below).
- Parents or carers being evasive or hostile.
- A history of injury that is inconsistent with the child's age and/or developmental skills.

- A 'collusion of silence', or one parent implicating the other.
- Accusations that the child is a witch, or that witchcraft has been perpetrated by others.
- The presence of other injuries, or a previous history of unusual injury.
- Child appearing sad, withdrawn, anxious or frightened ('frozen watchfulness'), or over-compliant.
- Child may indicate the abuser.

Particular consideration needs to be given to children with disabilities who may be unable to communicate about their ill treatment, and where their presentation may be misattributed to their disability.

Children who suffer abuse are often threatened by being told that they will be to blame if the family is separated. Fear of what might happen to them may result in children between the ages of 4 and 10 years colluding with the abusive parent.

Physical abuse/ill treatment (non-accidental injury)

Physical abuse can be defined as any act resulting in a non-accidental physical injury, including not only intentional assault, but also the results of excessive or violent punishment. Physical abuse occurs when a person deliberately injures a child or young person.

Around 25–50% of all children report being physically abused, according to the World Health Organization (WHO).

Physical abuse usually coexists with emotional abuse, and sometimes accompanies sexual abuse. However, in some settings, physical chastisement (especially of older children) continues to be considered part of 'good parenting' and important for instilling discipline in a community's children. In many countries, laws define which childhood punishments are considered excessive or abusive.

Some classifications define physical abuse as an injury that produces a mark. However, this does not take into consideration the emotional effects of physical abuse. The number and size of the bruises are helpful in distinguishing between mild and serious abuse. Any assault on a child is unacceptable and constitutes child abuse. A small bruise in a baby may predict future serious or fatal abuse.

Typical injuries include the following:

- lash marks, especially on the trunk, legs and hands
- bruises, especially on the face, scalp, and on or behind the ears and on the buttocks
- certain patterns of bruises, such as fingertip marks or bruises in the shape of the implement used, or multiple bruises of different ages. However, current scientific evidence concludes that we cannot accurately date a bruise from clinical assessment or from a photograph.
- Burns, including branding and scalds, especially when these are bilateral and/or symmetrical (e.g. buttocks or face held against a hot object such as a radiator, or both hands or feet or buttocks scalded as a result of the child being immersed deliberately in hot water). A pattern suggesting a cigarette burn or burns is also important, but be careful about the possibility of impetigo, which may mimic such burns (impetigo heals quickly and without scarring with antibiotic treatment, topical if a small area and systemic if widespread, whereas burns heal more slowly and may scar)

- injuries to the mouth (especially a torn frenulum)
- bleeding from the mouth or nose in an infant (indicating the possibility of intentional suffocation)
- adult bite marks
- bony injuries, especially in non-ambulant children; skull fractures, spiral fractures of the humerus, rib fractures in young children and multiple fractures of different ages, epiphyseal separation at the end of long bones, periosteal separation and haematomas
- inflicted head injury (especially in infants) involving tearing of the superficial veins over the brain and retina, causing subdural and retinal haemorrhages: this can be fatal, or may cause physical and mental impairment and visual loss.
- failure to thrive due to neglect (category 2) or deliberate starvation (category 3)
- induced illness, including suffocation or poisoning.

Figure 7.6.1 shows the common injury sites for both accidental and abusive injuries.

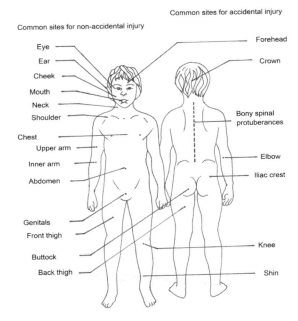

FIGURE 7.6.1 Common sites for (a) non-accidental (abusive) injuries and (b) accidental injuries.

Particular care needs to be taken when interpreting skin marks in settings where traditional practitioners use cupping, coining, scarification or tattooing treatments.

Children are more likely to be killed or to experience violence in their own home than outside it. The triad of violence against a partner (usually the female partner), child abuse and substance misuse (drugs and/or alcohol) is a common association. There is a strong correlation between domestic violence and child abuse.

Emotional and psychological abuse

This can occur as isolated incidents, as well as within a pattern of failure over time on the part of a parent or caregiver to provide a developmentally appropriate and supportive environment. This has a high probability of damaging the child's physical or mental health, or their physical, mental, spiritual, moral or social development.

This category should be used where it is the main or only apparent form of abuse.

Emotional and psychological abuse includes the restriction of movement, patterns of belittling, blaming, threatening, frightening, name-calling, scapegoating, persistent criticism, discriminating against the child compared with their siblings, ridiculing them, and other non-physical forms of rejection or hostile treatment.

This type of abuse can be difficult to recognise. Concerns are frequently raised by a child's extended family, neighbours, or nursery or school staff. All abuse involves some emotional abuse, but emotional abuse may exist independently. Emotional abuse occurs when, for example, there is:

- emotional unavailability of the parent or carer (e.g. when they are preoccupied with their own needs because of mental health problems, substance abuse problems, or work commitments)
- failure to allow the child to interact normally socially with others.

The consequences of emotional abuse vary with age and with its duration, and may include the following:

- Impaired physical development: these children often fail to reach their optimum potential in terms of growth; this improves when the child is placed in a more nurturing environment.
- Impaired cognitive development, including speech and language delay, poor concentration and academic underachievement.
- Behavioural abnormalities, such as anxious attachment, lack of social responsiveness, expressionless face, fear of speaking, eagerness to please, attention seeking, overactivity or 'hyperactivity', no wariness with strangers, hunger for human contact, inability to form relationships, self-injurious or self-stimulating behaviours, hoarding and stealing of food, pica, enuresis and encopresis, and bizarre behavioural patterns (sometimes there is autistic-like behaviour).
- Impaired psychological development, especially with regard to speech and language: aggression, emotional unresponsiveness, emotional instability, impaired social development, low self-esteem, dependency and separation anxiety, serious social difficulties, underachievement, negative self-evaluation, poor concentration, and poor academic performance or school attendance.
- Psychiatric disorders: emotional maltreatment and abuse have been described in association with three psychiatric disorders of childhood:
  — depression
  — reactive attachment disorder of infancy
  — multiple personality disorder.
  In general, these children become sad, dejected and withdrawn.
- Medical problems include the following:
  — failure to thrive
  — recurrent and severe nappy rash
  — generally unkempt appearance, with poor hygiene
  — recurrent minor infections.

Neglect
Neglect includes both isolated incidents and a pattern of failure over time on the part of a parent or other family member to provide for the development and well-being of the child (where the parent is in a position to do so) in one or more of the following areas.

Neglect is persistent failure to meet a child's essential needs by inattention or omitting basic parenting tasks and responsibilities in all aspects of their needs (health, hygiene, clothing, education, and social, emotional, mental, spiritual and moral needs). It also includes failure to provide appropriate nutrition, shelter and safe living conditions.

Examples include lack of supervision, with failure to protect the child from dangers (e.g. cold temperatures, sunburn, drowning) due to poor supervision and attention to safety in the home (e.g. not providing stair gates or locks on windows), failure to thrive, and failure to meet the child's emotional needs for love, affection and stimulation.

Neglect is seen as the persistent failure of a parent or carer to meet a child's developmental, basic physical and/or psychological needs by omission of basic parenting. It results in serious impairment of the child's physical health, psychological well-being and development. It may coexist with other forms of ill treatment.

The parents' or carers' own problems (e.g. learning difficulties, mental and physical health problems, poverty, inappropriate housing) can all contribute to this. In unstable settings, such as armed conflict, there may be significant security issues that contribute to their inability to provide a safe environment for their children.

Child sexual abuse (CSA)
Introduction
This is the involvement of children in sexual activity to which they cannot consent. Another definition could be any activity in which an adult or older child uses a younger child in a sexual way.

In addition to direct sexual contact between adult and child (including intracrural, oral, vaginal or anal sex and the masturbation of an adult), it includes the use of penetrative instrumentation, the production of pornographic imagery of children, exposing a child to indecent acts or pornography, and other voyeuristic practices. Very young children may also be trafficked for use in the sex industry, and older children may be groomed for prostitution.

Sexual abuse is a serious global problem that transcends economic or social barriers. Poverty, emotional deprivation and lack of education often mean that young people are powerless to avoid being trapped both in sexually abusive situations and in domestic violence. However, it is universally true that sexual abuse is most often suffered at the hands of a neighbour, family friend or a trusted person, including a parent. A significant power differential usually exists between victim and abuser. This fact is important when examining situations of sexual behaviour between children themselves.

In legal terms there are two types:
1 when a stranger or someone the child knows abuses the child
2 incest: when a relative by blood or by law abuses the child.

Some facts about CSA
- Child sexual abuse is a problem in all socio-economic classes.

- Boys are also sexually abused.
- Abusers are usually people whom the child knows.
- It is **never** the child's fault if they are sexually abused.
- Women can also be abusers.
- Abusers cannot be recognised by their physical appearance.
- Sharing the experience of abuse with someone who is supportive and understanding helps the victim deal with it.
- Very young children can be abused in this way.
- A child who is abused at a very young age will also be affected by it, even if they forget the particular episode.
- CSA is rarely accompanied by violence and physical force.
- The main motive behind sexual abuse is not sexual frustration but to gain 'power' and 'control'.

Worldwide, 40–47% of sexual assaults are reported to involve girls under the age of 15 years. In Tanzania, almost 30% of adolescents undergoing abortions had been impregnated by men aged 45 years or older. In India, a study in 2007 reported that over 50% of children had been subjected to sexual abuse, and in 21% of cases this was of a severe nature. That study also reported that children living on the street or in institutional care were most vulnerable to sexual abuse.

Rape and impregnation as a weapon of war is now well recognised as a distressing and complex issue arising in countries where conflict is endemic.

Physical symptoms of CSA

Sexual abuse may go undetected for years because the symptoms are vague and easily attributed to other factors, such as the arrival of a new sibling in the home or family breakdown. Abuse may come to light abruptly when a child says something inappropriate or makes a direct allegation (disclosure) when in a situation in which they feel safe, sometimes to a friend or teacher at school.

Physical symptoms are unusual and vague. Unexplained episodic dysuria and frequency or genital soreness are most often recalled in retrospect. Sexually transmitted disease and pregnancy may make the diagnosis irrefutable in some cases. Obvious pain, bleeding and signs of acute physical trauma to the genital and anal area are rarely presenting features, and usually accompany violent and reckless assaults, often by a stranger.

Other symptoms include difficulty in walking, gastrointestinal disturbances (including nausea), eating disorders, abdominal pain, and in the genital area pain, itching, visible injury, discharge, infection or difficulty urinating.

Bruises, cuts and other injuries on any part of the body for which the cause is not clear and the child cannot give a full explanation may be present. Sexually transmitted diseases may occur at the time of abuse or lie dormant for months or even years, only to flare up in adolescence or adulthood.

There may be a noticeable fear of a particular person or place, sudden bedwetting or soiling, preoccupation with sexual acts, and a change of language or re-enacting their experiences with other children. Nightmares, withdrawn behaviour, changes in appetite and a decline in school achievement are not uncommon.

Other behavioural effects include the following:
- persistent and inappropriate sexual play with peers, toys, animals or self

- sexual themes and fears in the child's artwork, stories and play
- sexual understanding or behaviour beyond that expected for the child's developmental stage
- self-harm or hurting others, including fire setting and cruelty to animals
- fear of being alone, of going home, or of particular places and people
- running away from home
- drug and/or alcohol use
- adolescent prostitution or sexual promiscuity
- suicidal feelings and attempts.

Parents should be concerned if a child appears to have unexplained expensive objects or financial resources. The grooming process often involves making a child feel cherished and creating dependency by offering them quality time, treats and gifts; in older children, the grooming process often includes encouragement to indulge in and provision of cigarettes and alcohol.

These effects may be symptoms of something other than CSA, but the possibility of CSA should always be explored.

Most of the symptoms relate to long-term psychological damage. Young adults find it difficult to make intimate relationships and to trust others. Alcohol and drug dependency, anxiety disorders, self-harming and suicidal ideation may be linked to sexual abuse, especially at the hands of a trusted adult such as a parent. The traumagenesis of sexual abuse has been extensively described by Finklehor. He proposed four dynamics; traumatic sexualisation, powerlessness, betrayal and stigmatisation.

Clinical examination and physical signs

Clinical assessment of the sexually abused child should ideally be conducted by trained and experienced professionals, and preferably a specialist forensically trained doctor or nurse. The environs of the clinical space should be child friendly and the examination unhurried. All examinations should consider the global health needs of the child first; the needs of law enforcement should not be paramount.

Careful history taking is the first step, and if prosecution is being sought, the history should be obtained without risk of contamination, either directly from the child before a recording witness or in the child's absence from the adult who knows first-hand what the child has said. The history should be elicited with free recall and by posing indirect questions (e.g. 'Tell me why you are here' or 'Is there something that has upset you? Can you talk about it?').

Children will feel less threatened if other aspects of their health are also examined at the same time. The normal child health enquiry about growth, diet, systems enquiry and school function is important. Clinical examination of the child should also be holistic, and incidental findings should be relayed back to the parent and child appropriately. A whole body approach is more likely to promote a sense of healing than a prolonged focus on the genitals and anus.

Physical abuse and sexual abuse are seen together in around 15% of cases.

Physical signs of sexual abuse are uncommon even in long-standing, intrusive and painful abuse. Such subtle signs as may be present will be missed if the examiner does not encourage the child to be fully relaxed. The use of a high-quality lighting source is critical, as is the child's posture. The gold standard is the use of photo-colposcopy, which provides magnification, light and a recording of the findings.

Small children are best examined in the frog-leg position, assisted by someone whom they trust. The knee–chest position may have to be used to define the hymenal free edge. Gentle anterior traction on the labia usually suffices to open or stretch the orifice. Older and pubertal girls may benefit from the use of stirrups and a damp swab to identify deep clefts. This should be done after appropriate specimens have been collected for forensic analysis.

Criminal prosecution from sexual abuse allegations and forensic evidence gathering is a demanding process that requires strong links between law enforcement agencies and forensic examiners. Doctors and nurses who expect to provide such a service require training from experts in the field.

Essential reading for forensic practitioners should include *The Physical Signs of Child Sexual Abuse*, produced by the Royal College of Paediatrics and Child Health in the UK in collaboration with the Royal College of Physicians of London and the Faculty of Forensic and Legal Medicine. This document presents a review of all the substantial research into individual physical signs. It also presents guidance on best practice relating to examinations and healthcare (see the Further reading list at the end of this section for details).

Diagnosis of CSA

This is usually achieved following multi-agency assessment, the history and medical examination being only a part of the process.

Acute sexual assault findings (within hours or a few days):
- Bruising and swelling, abrasions and lacerations to the external genitals without a history of accidental trauma.
- Grip marks and bruising around the limbs.
- Cigarette or lighter burns around the breasts and pubic area.
- Bite marks, including suction bites around the breasts, abdomen and thighs.
- Petechiae around the eyes, tears to the oral frenulum, petechiae over the posterior fauces.
- Visible petechiae over the hymen, hymenal tears, haematomas and bleeding.
- Petechiae or bites over the glans penis and scrotum.
- Bruising, oedema and lacerations around the anal area (oedema usually resolves within 48 hours).
- Semen may be found in the vagina or rectum.
- Pregnancy is a major and not uncommon result.

'Chronic' sexual abuse findings (the most common presentation):
- Hymenal transections, deep clefts and notches in the posterior hymen, and loss or absence of posterior hymenal tissue are signs seen almost exclusively in the abused child.
- Significant tears can heal rapidly, but may leave mounds or adhesions on the hymen.
- The size of the hymenal orifice is too variable to be a guide to penetration, but a gaping orifice created by loss of the posterior hymen is significant.
- A mounded scar over the fourchette is evidence of significant stretching trauma in the absence of a history of accidental straddle injury.
- Hymenal injuries are never acceptable from a history of a straddle or other fall unless there is convincing evidence of direct penetration by an object.
- Small superficial notches, bumps and labial adhesions are not uncommon in non-abused girls.
- Anal findings are uncommon. They include marked sustained laxity and gaping, deep and poorly healing fissures and venous congestion. Such signs may be seen in non-abused children, and must be considered in the context of the history given.

Differential diagnoses

Several common naturally occurring conditions not due to abuse may give rise to a suspicion of sexual abuse but must be excluded.

Non-specific vulvo-vaginitis is the commonest. A frequent presentation in the pre-pubescent child, symptoms are of intermittent mild dysuria, redness and a sticky discharge. Symptoms are likely to relate to withdrawal of the maternal oestrogen effect, which makes some children intolerant of the use of strong detergents and poor hygiene practices. The use of loose-fitting underwear, gentle cleansing and the regular application of simple emollients usually provide relief of a condition that tends to recur until early puberty.

The presence of **pinworms** can cause genital symptoms, as can localised eczema in the napkin area. These require appropriate measures.

Infective vulvo-vaginitis presents with significant inflammation and pain, sometimes associated with upper airways infection, and often streptococcal in origin. If possible, bacterial cultures should be obtained before appropriate antibiotics are offered.

Lichen sclerosus et atrophicus is an uncommon skin disorder which may be associated with other autoimmune disease, including morphea in adults, but it tends to be a stand-alone diagnosis in children. It presents with fragility, haemorrhaging and bruising of the skin of the labia, dysuria and occasional urinary retention. Diagnosis is made easy by the classical picture of de-pigmentation in a figure-of-eight configuration associated with obvious skin fragility, and easy bleeding on stretching. Vigorous treatment with emollients is often adequate in mild cases, but topical steroids may be required to control severe signs and symptoms.

Retained foreign bodies can be the cause of intermittent bloodstaining and purulent or offensive discharge in very young children. It should be recognised that repeated insertion of foreign bodies into the vagina by a young child may be the presenting sign of learned or disturbed behaviour.

Constipation can give rise to intermittent anal bleeding and discomfort.

Inflammatory bowel disease may present with anal fissures, bleeding and discharge.

It is important to communicate to parents and other professionals that sexual abuse may not result in any physical findings, and that there are few signs which are absolutely diagnostic. Nevertheless, a medical examination following an allegation of sexual abuse may provide valuable forensic information as well as an opportunity for reassurance, treatment of infection, and access to wider therapeutic support.

Difficult judgements about how to proceed may have to be made in settings where female genital cutting is practised, and where legislation and/or community action against this practice is weak.

Fabricated and induced illness (FII)

This is the severe end of a spectrum of unusual or abnormal health-seeking behaviours in which significant harm is caused by a parent or carer (usually the mother), who deliberately fabricates signs or symptoms or induces illness in a child. Sometimes the abuse is the direct result of inappropriate and often invasive and unnecessary investigations or treatment by healthcare workers responding to the parent's fabricated accounts of non-existent illness. It is probably more common in developed than developing countries. The child is frequently brought for multiple medical assessments and investigations, the perpetrator (often the child's mother) denies knowledge of the causation of the illness, and the acute signs and symptoms cease when the child is separated from the perpetrator.

Healthcare workers in hospital are often the first professionals to suspect FII in a child on the basis of concerns about:

- being given erroneous or misleading information
- deliberate poisoning
- deliberate burns or damage to the skin
- the possibility of deliberate suffocation
- deliberate fabrication of fits
- removal of or tampering with medical monitoring equipment
- the introduction of foreign material into investigative tests.

Immediate action when ill treatment or abuse is suspected

- A detailed history and full medical examination are required (including inspection of the genitals). Where possible, obtain the consent of the parent or carer and the child to carry out the medical examination.
- If consent is withheld, work urgently within the legal framework of the country concerned to examine and protect the child in conjunction with police, social services or civil society organisations.
- Ensure that the child (if they are old enough and able to speak) is given the opportunity away from their parent or carer to say how they were hurt (disclosure), at the same time avoiding interference with any police investigation.

When responding to disclosure:

- Remain calm. An over-reaction will make the child feel even more frightened and ashamed.
- Believe the child.
- Listen in a non-judgemental way.
- Use the child's language.
- Tell the child that you are glad they have told you what happened.
- Reassure the child that they did nothing wrong.

- Explain to the child that abuse is an unfair thing that happens to children, without condemning the offender.
- Determine the immediate need for safety.
- Don't make promises that you cannot keep.
- Let the child know what you will do.
- Set in motion the process of getting help for the child.
- Take care of yourself.

Do's and don'ts of disclosure

Do use phrases like this: 'I believe you'; 'You did the right thing by telling someone'; 'I'm so sorry this has happened to you'; 'It's not your fault'; 'I will try to help you so that it won't happen again.'

Don't use phrases like this: 'Don't say such things!'; 'Are you sure it happened/is happening?'; 'Are you telling the truth?'; 'Why are you telling me?'; 'Why didn't you stop it?'; 'What did you do to make this happen?'

- Consider whether other children in the family may need to be examined and protected.
- Record a full history as it is spoken, and include an evaluation of the child–parent interaction.
- Carry out a careful examination in a well-lit room.
- Record the details of the history and examination legibly and contemporaneously in the child's medical notes. A form of the type available in the Appendix can be helpful.
- Include details of the child's demeanour and presentation, and their height and weight plotted on a centile chart. Ensure that an examination of the child's mouth, nose, ears and neck is undertaken, and complete a full systemic medical examination.
- Document any injuries on body diagrams (*see* Figure 7.6.1 and Appendix).
- Consider photo documentation (with the child's consent, if possible) of injuries, and ensure that the images can be stored safely and confidentially.
- Check whether the family is known to the police and/or social services.
- Consider whether any additional medical investigations need to be carried out (e.g. X-rays for bony injuries, a skeletal survey in children under 3 years of age, clotting studies) (*see* Table 7.6.2).
- Admit the child to hospital if observation or treatment is indicated, or to a place of safety if the child is considered to be at risk. Staff can then have the opportunity to talk further with the child.
- If the parents refuse to allow the child to be examined or admitted, urgent action to protect the child will be required within the legal framework of the country. This may mean referral to the duty social worker (if a referral has not already been made) or the police.

A thorough medical examination should include the following:

- observation of the child's demeanour
- height, weight and head circumference (in a preschool child) plotted on a centile chart
- examination of the mouth, nose, ears, neck and genitals
- inspection of skin surface for bruises, marks and cuts
- examination of the eyes for retinal haemorrhages (pupil dilatation may be needed) (*see* Section 5.15).
- systemic examination
- an assessment of the child's developmental age.

Investigations to exclude medical causes should include the following:

- full blood count, platelets and clotting screen
- a detailed skeletal survey (especially in children under 3 years) to look for new and old fractures; a chest X-ray

including the upper arms can be very valuable for identifying rib and humerus fractures

- investigations to exclude vitamin D deficiency, if there are fractures
- CT or MRI scan of the brain (if available), if non-accidental head injury is suspected.

TABLE 7.6.2 Investigations in the differential diagnosis of child abuse

Injury	Differential diagnosis	Investigation
Bruising	Coagulation disorder, idiopathic thrombocytopaenic purpura/Henoch–Schönlein disease, haemorrhagic disease of the newborn, septicaemia, connective tissue disorders, birth marks, dyes, tattoos, drug reactions, self-inflicted injuries, traditional treatments	Full blood count, blood film, coagulation studies Chest X-ray Consider skeletal X-ray survey in children under 3 years of age Opinion of expert in skin diseases (if available)
Bites	Animal or human Adult or child	DNA skin swab (if available) Photography Forensic dental assessment (if available)
Fractures	Accidental injury, birth injury, infection, malignancy, osteogenesis imperfecta, osteopaenia, nutritional deficiencies (including rickets)	Chest X-ray X-ray skeletal survey in children under 3 years of age Bone scan (if available) Radiology advice Blood calcium, phosphate, alkaline phosphatase and vitamin D levels (if available) CT scan for head injury (if available)
Scalds and burns	Other skin pathologies (e.g. staphylococcal and streptococcal infection), drug reactions, allergic reactions to plants (e.g. euphorbias)	Skin swabs Dermatology opinion (if available)
Head injury/unexplained fits or coma	Coagulation disorder, epilepsy or febrile convulsion, cerebral malaria, meningitis, poisoning	Retinal examination after pupil dilatation (see Section 5.15) CT scan (if available)

TABLE 7.6.3 Differential diagnoses of genital and anal findings

Concerning sign	Differential diagnoses
Vaginal bleeding	Accidental injury, especially straddle injury, urethral prolapse, precocious puberty, lichen sclerosis atrophicus, foreign body in genital tract, severe vulvo-vaginitis
Rectal bleeding	Anal fissures caused by hard stool, inflammatory bowel disease, infective diarrhoea, rectal polyps, rectal prolapse
Vulvo-vaginitis	Poor hygiene, skin disease (e.g. eczema, lichen sclerosis), allergies to detergents/bath products

Additional considerations when performing examination of the genital and anal areas

- Ensure that a good light source is available, including the use of colposcopy, if this is available.
- Conduct interviews and examinations of children with another professional person present.
- Instrumental examination is not normally required in pre-pubertal girls. Assessment of the hymen in post-pubertal girls may require use of a cotton tip swab or other techniques.
- Knowledge of local practice with regard to female genital cutting and male circumcision is important when interpreting clinical findings.
- Interpretation of anal signs is difficult, and needs to be undertaken in conjunction with a careful history of the child's bowel pattern.
- If forensic facilities are available, ensure that clothing items and relevant swabs are taken in line with local

protocols, and that a chain of evidence is maintained to the forensic laboratory.

- Assess whether swabs for sexually transmitted infection (see Section 6.1.J) need to be taken immediately or at a follow-up review.
- Consider whether a pregnancy test needs to be carried out.
- Consider whether emergency contraception is needed.
- Consider the risks of HIV infection and whether post-exposure prophylaxis is needed in line with local protocols. This will vary depending on knowledge of the assailant, the nature of the injuries, and the country's HIV prevalence rates.
- Consider whether hepatitis B immunisation (if available) is indicated.

Special issues concerning the management of sexual abuse

The child's immediate needs are as follows:

- **To feel believed and acknowledged:** All interaction with the child should convey this message. Intrusive questioning, especially questions that imply some measure of blame (e.g. 'Why didn't you tell earlier?') can cause a child to refuse to speak further and even retract previous statements. The protective parent or carer should be briefed about this risk.
- **To be safe from further harm:** Protection usually involves the statutory services (if they exist). Police and social workers should be part of the multidisciplinary process that assesses the child's safe custody. The safety of siblings must also be considered at this stage, if not before.
- **To have all their health needs met:** Their immediate needs are for reassurance that they are healthy, and that any changes in the genital area will heal. Care should be taken to use the right language to inform the parent and the child about these changes. The use of phrases such as 'no longer a virgin' is highly inappropriate in this context, and indeed anatomically inaccurate in most cases.

Attention must be given to detection and treatment of all acquired sexually transmitted infection, including HIV, preferably within 2 weeks of an acute assault and possibly at the same time as the examination for long-standing abuse.

Pubescent girls should be offered emergency contraception where indicated.

All incidental findings (e.g. anaemia, rashes, heart murmurs) and reported health problems should be attended to and followed up where necessary.

Forensic sampling in acute sexual assaults

A decision to undertake forensic sampling depends upon the following:

- Has contact abuse been reported? There is always a possibility of transferred material if there has been direct contact. Even if a condom was used, relevant lubricant or saliva may be detected.
- How long is it since the assault? If it is less than 72–96 hours, there is a possibility of trace material being found, especially within skinfolds.
- Has there been bathing or washing? Material may still be available, but this is less likely if the child has been washed thoroughly.
- How active is the child or adolescent? Children who are immobile for reasons of illness or disability may retain trace material well beyond the standard time, as drainage from the vagina is erratic.

What samples should be collected?

The history should guide the practitioner in deciding where trace material is likely to be found. The history may direct one to unusual sites (e.g. swabs may identify traces of adhesive from a victim who has alleged being strapped down with masking tape; microscopic rope fibres may be recovered from around the ankles or wrists). It is sensible to collect duplicate swabs from each area sampled.

In general, swabs lightly moistened with sterile distilled water should be used to collect material that is visibly dried on or speculatively present. Dry swabs are used in moist areas such as the mouth, glans penis, anus and vagina.

If the child is very young or an infant, semen or saliva may be present over a wide area (e.g. in the hair, armpits,

abdomen, thigh creases). Damp swabs may be collected over all these areas in a young baby, whereas an adolescent is more likely to carry evidence over the breasts and in and around the vaginal area.

The use of an ultraviolet (UV) light in a dark room may help to identify both deposits of semen and saliva, and areas of deep trauma within the skin. These latter areas fluoresce because of disturbance of melanin, haemoglobin and collagen tissue. The UV light should be used with caution, as there is a risk of material denaturing with extended use.

An example of systematic head-to-toe trace evidence gathering could be as follows:

- hair combings over a sheet of white paper, then folded and placed in a special plastic bag*
- cut areas of hair if dried material is visible
- specialised tooth brushings between the teeth and gum swabs if there has been oral ejaculation
- finger nail scrapings if there was violent resisted assault *
- damp swabs pressed firmly and rolled over any bites noted around the neck or breasts
- swabs from the axillae and from within the umbilicus in a small infant
- pubic hair combings*
- external vulval damp swabs
- dry high vaginal swabs
- swabs from the glans penis, behind the foreskin and over the shaft for saliva
- damp peri-anal swabs
- dry rectal swabs
- all clothing bagged individually as removed
- tampons and sanitary towels similarly bagged.

Every item collected should be fully labelled, bagged and sealed by the receiving witness, most commonly a police officer. It is sensible to allow a brief interval between samples to ensure that earlier samples have been correctly dealt with.

* Forensic material obtained in this way is only relevant if the alleged perpetrator denies all contact with the victim, or is unknown and therefore also a potential serial offender. Finding the perpetrator's DNA in hair or other material on the victim is potent evidence in such cases.

Sexually transmitted diseases (STDs)

A sexually transmitted infection may be the presenting feature in sexual abuse. Children who have experienced contact sexual abuse should be screened for STDs. The screening programme should take local prevalence factors into account, as should the decision to offer prophylactic antibiotics or antiviral treatment (*see also* Section 6.1.J).

Neisseria gonorrhoeae (especially non-conjunctival gonococcus) is not an expected infection outside the neonatal period, and is strong evidence for sexual abuse.

Chlamydia trachomatis similarly usually implies sexual abuse. There is evidence for vertical transmission at birth, and limited research evidence for the persistence of asymptomatic colonisation beyond the first year of life.

The presence of either of these organisms, especially if symptomatic in mid-childhood and beyond, should raise the strongest suspicion of abuse, regardless of the presence of maternal infection.

Trichomonas vaginalis may cause an offensive discharge in adolescents, and is a strong marker for sexual activity, consensual or otherwise. It is not known to infect the pre-pubescent child, although it may be found colonising newborns from infected maternal secretions.

Human papillomavirus is a very common infection, and hand-to-skin transmission is so frequent that it is usually difficult to use this infection to resolve issues of sexual transmission. Transfer may be perinatal, and lesions may be seen in early childhood in the mouth and larynx. However, the presence of genital warts should mandate careful examination and screening for other STDs.

Herpes simplex virus (HSV) raises similar issues. Auto-innoculation and benign transfer cannot be excluded. Adolescents presenting with symptomatic genital HSV are likely to have had sexual contact. They need careful evaluation and screening for other STDs.

Treponema pallidum (syphilis) may be acquired through the placenta, and signs or symptoms of infection are highly unpredictable. Most studies in older children suggest transfer through sexual contact. The infection is exclusively sexually transmitted in adults. Sexual transmission should always be considered in a child presenting with symptoms. Infection in the parent does not exclude abuse.

Hepatitis B and hepatitis C are recognised as being sexually transferred in adults. There is insufficient research in children; however, screening of the sexually abused child is mandatory in high-risk situations, such as multiple or violent assaults and in high-prevalence regions.

Human immunodeficiency virus (HIV): The frequency of infection acquired through abuse will reflect the prevalence of HIV in the local population, and screening is strongly advised where the prevalence is high.

Screening for hepatitis and HIV will need to be timed to take account of time to seroconversion, which is usually a period of 6 or more weeks. Interval repeat screening for late conversion may be considered up to 12 weeks.

Most STDs can be screened for at 2 weeks from the date of contact.

Neisseria gonorrhoeae should be screened for at the first possible opportunity, preferably at the time of assessment if feasible, or within 48 hours.

Consideration should be given to hepatitis B vaccination if the child presents within a week or two after a penetrative assault.

Similar consideration may need to be given to HIV prophylaxis on occasion.

Long-term needs

Those children who are going through the criminal justice process will need extensive support and counselling.

In well-managed sexual abuse allegations, most young children appear to function well. However, the disruption to their lives and the loss of familiar adults and objects around them does have an impact on many, and it is important that their carers are briefed.

Children who have been brutally sexualised may not recover, and may seek inappropriate affection and contact which makes them difficult to parent. Others may suffer nightmares, phobias and other symptoms of anxiety. Long-term psychological input may be necessary.

Special issues involving sexual abuse
Child trafficking

In 1994, the United Nations General Assembly defined trafficking as the 'illicit and clandestine movement of persons across national and international borders, largely from developing countries and some countries with economies in transition with the end goal of forcing women and girl children into sexually or economically oppressive and exploitative situations for the profit of recruiters, traffickers, crime syndicates, as well as other illegal activities related to trafficking, such as forced domestic labour, false marriages, clandestine employment and false adoption.'

It is estimated that in the last 30 years, trafficking in women and children in Asia for sexual exploitation alone has victimised over 30 million people.

Children are trafficked for a number of purposes, including:
- sexual exploitation
- adoption
- child labour
- child soldiers
- forced marriage
- body parts
- ritual sacrifice.

Parents are promised education or jobs for their children. Some children are simply captured, then traded for whatever commodity is in demand (domestic work, sex work, drug carrying or beggary).

Children who are displaced are highly vulnerable to sexual and physical abuse. They fear seeking help and often do not have the language to do so.

Different cultural situations produce different types of exploitation. In Asia, for example, girls as young as 13 years may be exported as mail-order brides, and in Thailand around 100 000 women and girls from border countries are imported into the sex trade. Large numbers of children are being trafficked in West and Central Africa, mainly for domestic work but also for sexual exploitation, to work in shops or on farms, or to be scavengers or street hawkers. Nearly 90% of these trafficked domestic workers are girls. Many of these girls are traded on into the Middle East and Europe.

The International Organisation for Migration (IOM) has produced an extensive document that comprehensively deals with all aspects of victim management (see Further reading section at the end of this section).

Advice, both for the country of origin and for the receiving country, is structured based on two principles:
- **The child's interests are paramount.**
- **Above all, do no harm.**

The starting point is the assessment of risk both in the receiving country and in the country of origin if repatriated. Risk depends on numerous factors, including the following:
- the extent to which trafficking is controlled by organised criminal groups
- their known or estimated capacity to plan and implement reprisals against the victims and/or service delivery organisation staff
- the capacity of the local law enforcement agencies
- the extent of endemic corruption and how it adds to the level of risk.

It is critical that children have an appointed independent guardian who will act solely in their interest. Family members, including parents, may well be responsible or collusive in the trafficking, and drawing them in could greatly increase the risk of serious harm, including death, or re-trafficking. In some cultures it may be socially acceptable for the family to shun or even kill a girl for having brought disgrace on her family.

Trafficked women may give birth to children within their repressive conditions. These children will be at very high risk of emotional abuse and neglect and early introduction into commercial sex. Babies are at risk of homicide.

Services provided for trafficked children should reflect the following needs (adapted from the IOM Report):

- **Approaches that demonstrate respect and promote participation** (e.g. children being allowed to express their views in the language they speak best).
- **An understanding of the complex ways in which their past experience has harmed them**. Children who are trafficked are subjected to a persistently threatening and dangerous environment. In the face of this type of chronic abuse and stress, children and adolescents develop a personality that is suited for survival, but that is ill adapted to cope in normal non-threatening situations. Healthcare practitioners are responsible for employing health-promoting strategies, programmes and activities that recognise the child's level of development and help children and adolescents to reclaim and further develop their competencies for an active and meaningful life. This involves addressing a range of needs, including nutritional, physical and psychological development and education needs.
- **Tailoring services to meet the needs of each age group** and in ways appropriate to the age and characteristics of the child concerned, never merely following programmes designed for adults. They should be assessed and managed by professionals trained in child development. Medical assessments need to be child friendly and provided by people with expertise.
- **Implementing strategies aimed at mitigating the effects of past trauma and fostering healthier patterns of development**. One example of such strategies is stepwise early re-integration into education and into a peer group.

Rape as a weapon of war

The rape of adults and children of both sexes is a common phenomenon in conflict zones. As long ago as 1949, Article 29 of the Geneva Convention explicitly forbade degrading treatment, stating that 'Women shall be protected against any attack on their honour – especially rape, enforced prostitution and indecent assault.'

Rape as a crime against humanity was first prosecuted in the International Criminal Court in 2001 when three Bosnian Serbs were convicted of systematic sexual violence against Muslim women.

However, prosecution of these crimes by the relevant states has been negligible.

In Rwanda, the mass rapes of the Tutsi women and girls permanently destroyed the capacity to child bear for some, and forced others to bear children outside their ethnic group. Vast numbers of women and girls were rejected by their communities and became outcasts. Thousands of children witnessed the violence on their mothers and sisters.

As rape as a weapon of war demoralises and destabilises entire communities, it weakens ethnic communities and ties, and affects populations with the exploitation of the reproductive rights and abilities of its victims. When rape is employed instead of a bullet, the weapon continues to wield its power beyond the primary victim. The battlefield may be the body, but the target is civil society. 'Rape, as with all terror-warfare, is not exclusively an attack on the body – it is an attack on the "body-politic." Its goal is not to maim or kill one person, but to control an entire socio-political process by crippling it. It is an attack directed equally against personal identity and cultural integrity.'

Thus in 1998, rape as an act of genocide was the decision of the International Criminal Tribunal for Rwanda. Despite these major precedents, prosecution of sexual crimes by the relevant states has been negligible. Rape has been a major feature of the war in South Sudan and in the Democratic Republic of Congo. Children as young as 5 years of age have been deliberately targeted. There is also strong anecdotal evidence that young soldiers barely in their teens have been ordered into gang rape to prove their 'manhood'.

The provision of care for victims of mass sexual abuse at this level is a daunting task, and should involve major planning and resources. Emergency care for severe physical wounding in the course of the assaults is logistically difficult.

Pratt and Werchick recommend expanding access through 'mobile teams of rape specialists' that could not only provide treatment themselves, but also transport medical supplies and transfer knowledge to any staff already on the ground. Medications, including emergency contraception, hepatitis vaccine, STD prophylaxis and antiretroviral drugs, need to be available. Such teams will need to have access to surgical facilities, especially when very young children are involved.

Gang rape, the use of instruments and other violence increases the risk of HIV/AIDS transmission significantly; intercourse is accompanied by injuries and bleeding which increases the transmission of the virus compared with transmission during consensual sex. Internal vaginal and rectal injury can be very serious, and in the very young may be fatal.

According to Human Rights Watch, 'children were reportedly forced to hold their mothers down while they were raped'. It is not difficult to see that a significant range of service provision is required at several levels to deal with such traumatic damage in childhood.

Therapeutic services in isolation without intensive educational programmes and a whole-community approach are probably doomed to fail. Rape as a weapon of war activates cultural beliefs that result in the marginalisation of its victims, especially women and children, thus preventing those victims from receiving psychosocial support, and depriving them of income. Women and girls are considered to be damaged and 'contaminated'. Wives may be denounced by their husbands, blamed for the rape, and regarded as 'married' to their rapists. Thus communities see their raped women and children as enemies and place them outside their sphere of moral obligation. Some communities may demand that their wives and children leave their villages.

Empowering young children and their mothers by providing education, and the teaching of new skills leading to longer-term economic stability, are also areas that need careful planning. Provision of safe housing and basic needs may be all that is possible in the immediate aftermath of sexual violence.

Additional considerations when investigating fabricated and induced illness (FII)

- The investigative process must involve early and continuing collaboration between all agencies, with detailed information sharing. Strategy planning meetings involving professionals from health, social services, police, education and legal departments can be very helpful.
- Draw up a health chronology using all accessible sources of information.
- Gather forensic or witness information.
- A decision must be made by the multi-agency team as to whether it is necessary to separate the child from the suspected perpetrator by voluntary or legal means.
- A decision must be made by the multi-agency team as to how and when to confront the parents.
- Ensure the child's safety throughout the investigative process.
- Work within the country's legal framework.

Medical aftercare following childhood maltreatment

It is important that these children are offered follow-up in order to:
- monitor the child's overall progress
- ensure healing of injuries

- investigate and treat any acquired infection
- facilitate access to psychological therapeutic support.

Healthcare workers involved in the hospital care of children who have been abused may be asked to provide a police statement and to attend court as a witness.

Further reading

Child protection materials from the UK Royal College of Paediatrics and Child Health. www.rcpch.ac.uk/child-health/standards-care/child-protection/child-protection

Pinheiro PS. World Report on Violence against Children. Geneva: United Nations, 2006; pp. 1–19. www.unicef.org/lac/full_tex(3).pdf

Heise LL, Raikes A and Watts CH (1994) Violence against women: a neglected public health issue in less developed countries. *Social Science and Medicine*, **39**, 1165–79.

Finkelhor DA (2008) *A Sourcebook on Child Sexual Abuse*. London: Sage Publications.

International Organization for Migration (2007) *The IOM Handbook on Direct Assistance for Victims of Trafficking*. Geneva: International Organization for Migration.

Clifford C (2008) *Rape as a weapon of war and its long-term effects on victims and society*. Seventh Global Conference on Violence and the Contexts of Hostility, 2008, Budapest. http://ts-si.org/files/BMJCliffordPaper.pdf

Pratt M and Werchick L (2004) *Sexual Terrorism: rape as a weapon of war in Eastern Democratic Republic of Congo*. http://pdf.usaid.gov/pdf_docs/PNADK346.pdf

Appendix

Examination under child protection procedures: suspected physical and/or sexual abuse

Patient details (circle correct information)

Name:	Date:
Date of birth...............................	
Age:	Time:
MALE/FEMALE	Place of examination:
Address (prior to examination):	

Professionals involved in the assessment

Doctor's or nurse's name:	Police officer's name:
Social worker's name:	
School:	

Why was this examination undertaken?

Family and Social History
(including names, dates of birth, ages, occupations/schools, relationships)

History of any known medical problems

Examination
Persons present during examination

1.

2.

3.

4.

Examination of child

Age:	Years: Months:
Height/percentile	.........cm/.........
Weight/percentile	.........kg/.........
Head circumference/percentile	.........cm./.........

General appearance of child (any obvious neglect):

Significant comments made by the child or the parent/carer (record as accurately as possible):

Developmental assessment (circle correct answers):

Delayed development   Yes/No

If Yes   Severe /Moderate /Mild

Level of puberty: Pre-pubertal/Post-pubertal

General examination (use body maps for any injuries)
(include inspection of oral frenum and palate and scalp)

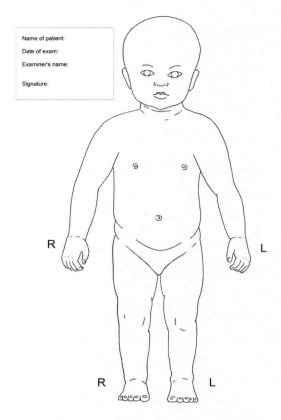

Name of patient:
Date of exam:
Examiner's name:
Signature:

R   L

R   L

FIGURE 7.6.2 Diagram on which to mark signs of injury to the front of the body. Reproduced with permission from Southampton City Primary Care Trust.

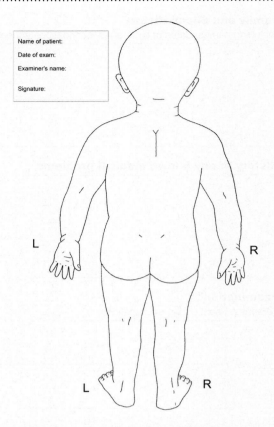

Name of patient:
Date of exam:
Examiner's name:
Signature:

L   R

L   R

FIGURE 7.6.3 Diagram on which to mark signs of injury to the back of the body. Reproduced with permission from Southampton City Primary Care Trust.

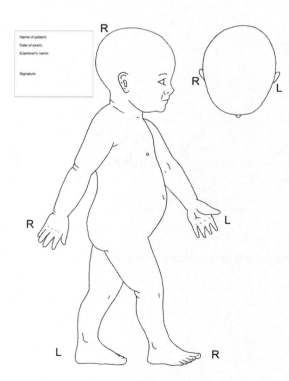

Name of patient:
Date of exam:
Examiner's name:
Signature:

R

R   L

R   L

L   R

FIGURE 7.6.4 Diagram on which to mark signs of injury to the right side of the body. Reproduced with permission from Southampton City Primary Care Trust.

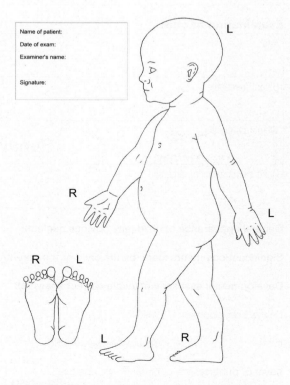

Name of patient:
Date of exam:
Examiner's name:
Signature:

L

R   L

R   L

L   R

FIGURE 7.6.5 Diagram on which to mark signs of injury to the left side of the body. Reproduced with permission from Southampton City Primary Care Trust.

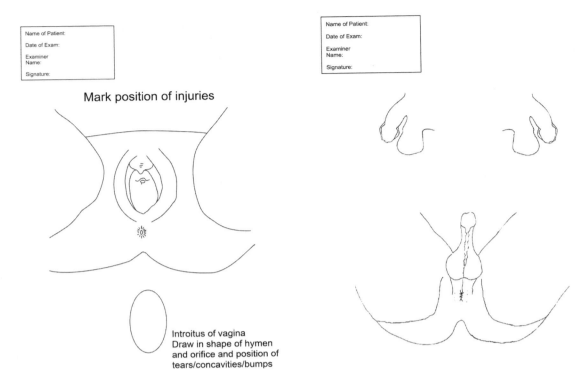

FIGURE 7.6.6 Diagram on which to draw the shape and position of any lesion on the female genitalia or anus. Reproduced with permission from Southampton City Primary Care Trust.

FIGURE 7.6.7 Diagram on which to draw the shape and position of any lesion on the male genitalia or anus. Reproduced with permission from Southampton City Primary Care Trust.

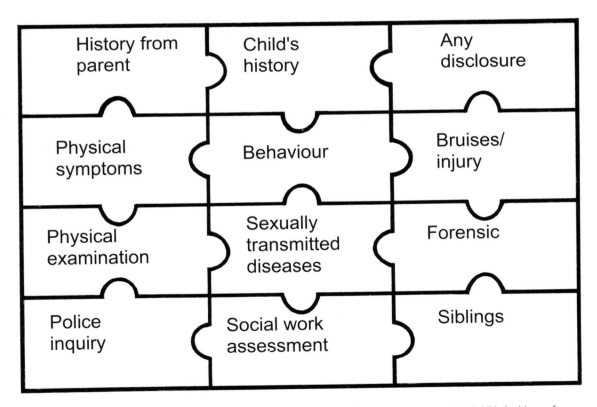

FIGURE 7.6.8 The Jigsaw of Child Abuse. (From Hobbs CJ and Wynne JM (1990) The sexually abused battered child. *Archives of Disease in Childhood* **65**: 423–427.)

Examination of female genitalia

Issue/area examined	Details
External genitalia	
Pubertal signs?	
Labial separation or traction used?	
Labial fusion?	
Urethral opening	
Labia minora	
Peri-hymenal tissues	
Posterior fourchette	
Perineum	
Hymenal opening	
Hymen	
Examination position	

Examination of anus

Issue/area examined	Details
Anal laxity/anal grip	
Anal folds	
Anal margin	
Surrounding tissues	
Examination position	

Examination of male genitalia

Issue/area examined	Details
Frenulum	
Urethral meatus/ Any discharge	
Signs of genital injury? Location	
Testicular swelling?	
Warts or skin disorders?	
Examination position	

Photographs taken of injuries
By whom: ....
Of what: ....

X-rays taken
Of what: ....

Forensic samples collected
By whom: .... Handed to whom: ....
List samples collected: ....
....
....

Screening for STDs
Date of tests: .... Results and date:
Tests taken: ....
....
....

Any other clinical investigation:

Summary and interpretation of significant abnormal findings:

Conclusions and doctor's or senior nurse's opinion:

Points discussed with social worker and parent/carer (and their opinion if applicable):

Arrangements for health follow-up for child (including investigations):

Signature: ....   Date: ....

Circulation list for report:

Social worker: ....

Police: ....

Head-teacher at school: ....

Others (please specify): ....

Name(s) of other children possibly at risk of abuse:		
Surname	First name	Date of birth

Checklist after examination:

1 Have you been able to give a clear opinion on the case?
2 Have you considered alternative explanations for the findings?
3 Does the social worker understand your findings and opinion?
4 If the injuries are serious or indicate serious risk, have you considered the need for police involvement?
5 Are you happy with plans for the immediate safety of the child?
6 Are you in agreement with the proposed long-term management?
7 Is it important for you to attend the case conference? If so, make sure that the social worker knows this.
8 Have you recorded your discussions?
9 Have you written a care plan?

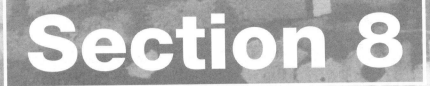

Section 8

Procedures in children and newborn infants

8.1 Preparation for procedures

Practical procedures should first be explained to the child (if they are old enough to understand this information) and the parents, any risks discussed with them and their consent obtained. Procedures on young infants should avoid hypothermia. Good light is essential. Analgesia should be given where necessary, and invasive procedures only performed when essential.

Analgesia and sedation for procedures

Some procedures have to be undertaken immediately, to save life, and many such procedures are described in this section. Clearly, there is no time to use analgesia in these circumstances, nor indeed much need to do so, as children who are in such severe collapse will have significantly depressed conscious levels. Where there is consciousness, analgesia and/or sedation is a top priority.

(For details on pain assessment and analgesia, *see* Section 1.15.)

For some procedures (e.g. chest tube insertion, dressing of burns), analgesia with a powerful drug such as ketamine should be considered, with a skilled healthcare worker (usually an anaesthetist) present and able to treat any adverse reactions immediately (*see* Section 1.24).

For planned intubation, anaesthesia is induced first (*see* Section 1.24). For some rarely used procedures such as defibrillation for cardiac arrest caused by a shockable rhythm (*see* Section 1.13), there is neither time nor need for sedation, as the patient is unconscious, whereas for defibrillation for an arrhythmia, sedation is necessary in most cases (*see* Section 5.4.C).

If ketamine is being used, give 2–4 mg/kg IM. This takes 5–10 minutes to act and the effects last for about 20 minutes. Ketamine can also be given slowly IV in this situation, 250–500 microgram/kg IV, and repeated as required to control pain. An anaesthetist or other expert in airway control must be present when ketamine is used.

When giving any analgesia, manage the child's airway, beware of respiratory depression and monitor oxygen

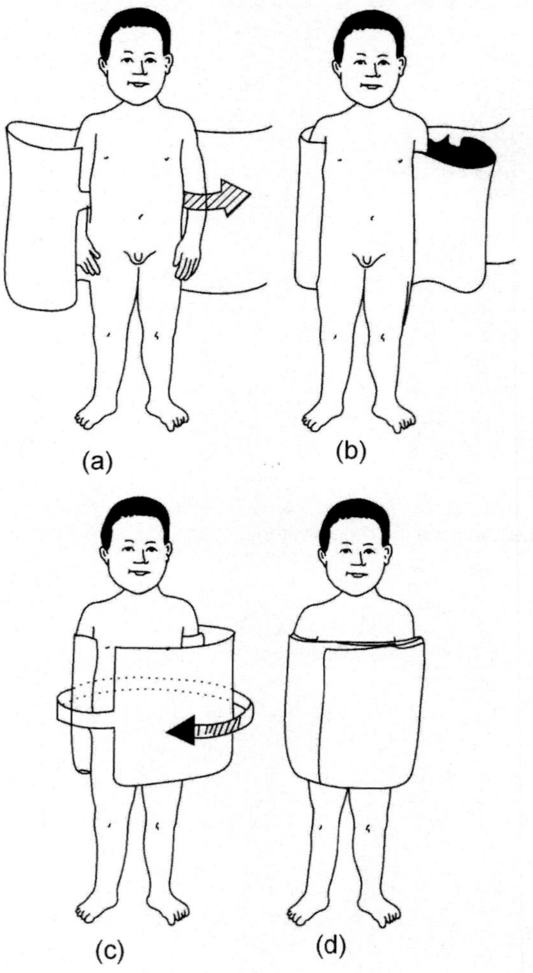

FIGURE 8.1.1 Wrapping a child so that they can be held securely for a procedure. (a) and (b). One end of a folded sheet should be pulled through under the arms on both sides. (c) and (d). The other end is then brought across the front and wrapped round the child.

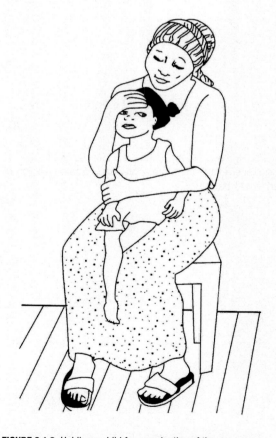

FIGURE 8.1.2 Holding a child for examination of the eyes, ears and throat.

saturation with a pulse oximeter (if available). **Ensure that you have a resuscitation bag and mask available (and oxygen).**

Restraining children for procedures

Restraint is important both for the child and for the clinician who is undertaking the procedure. Clearly, the procedure will be undertaken more quickly, safely and accurately if the child is kept still. However, to prevent a child with a chronic condition who will experience many such procedures being made fearful of further attempts, sedation should be strongly considered if facilities are available for this.

If facilities do not allow or if the procedure is unlikely to require repetition, physical restraint can be used. Ideally a parent or trusted friend or relative can actually hold the child. It is also very helpful to use distraction techniques such as singing a song, telling a story or using a glove puppet. Blowing soap bubbles is a very useful distraction for children, and it costs very little to bend a piece of wire into a loop and make up some strong soap solution.

First explain to the child in an age-appropriate manner what is going to happen. **Never say 'This won't hurt' when you know it will.** Always use local analgesia if at all possible (*see* Section 1.15). Explain why they are to be wrapped up (a 'big cuddle'), what is to happen and what will happen afterwards. Give plenty of praise before, during and after the procedure.

Restraining a child for examination does not usually require wrapping, but it is wise to leave examination of the ears, nose and throat until the end of the examination.

8.2 Airway procedures

Oropharyngeal airway

For adjunct-free airway opening and airway positions, *see* **Section 1.12.**

The oropharyngeal or Guedel airway is used in the unconscious or obtunded patient to provide an open airway channel between the tongue and the posterior pharyngeal wall. In the conscious patient with an intact gag reflex, it may not be tolerated and may induce vomiting. It is especially useful in the convulsing and post-ictal patient.

The oropharyngeal airway is available in a variety of sizes. A correctly sized airway when placed with its flange at the centre of the incisors, and then curved around the face, will reach the angle of the mandible. Too small an airway may be ineffective, and too large an airway may cause laryngospasm. Either may cause mucosal trauma or may worsen airway obstruction. Reassessment following placement is therefore a vital part of safe insertion of an airway device.

There are two methods for inserting the oropharyngeal airway in a child, depending on whether the child is small or large. However, there is no set age for switching from one to the other, as the choice of method depends on practicality and the skills of the operator. The important thing is not to push the tongue back, as that will obstruct the airway instead of keeping it open.

The twist technique is used for the larger child and in pregnancy, and means that the convex side of the airway is used to depress the tongue as the airway is pushed into the mouth. Insert the airway upside down until the tip has passed the soft palate, and then rotate it through 180 degrees so that the natural curve of the Guedel airway follows the curve of the tongue and pharynx.

However, in the infant and small child, as the tongue is larger relative to the size of the mouth, the airway cannot be rotated in the mouth without causing trauma. Therefore

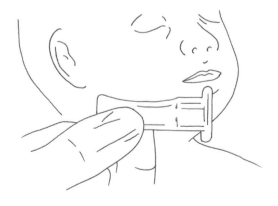

FIGURE 8.2.1 Oropharyngeal airway, showing sizing technique (correct size is illustrated).

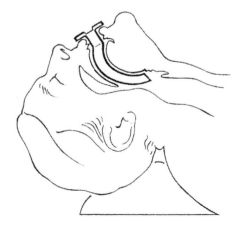

FIGURE 8.2.2 Oropharyngeal airway, showing position when inserted.

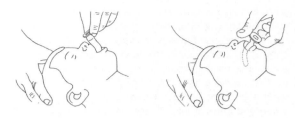

FIGURE 8.2.3 Oropharyngeal airway shown being inserted concave side up, then in place concave side down.

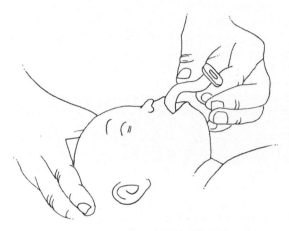

FIGURE 8.2.4 When inserting the airway without rotation, a tongue depressor can be helpful (not shown).

the tongue is depressed with a spatula and not by the reversed airway.

Ensure that insertion of one of these devices results in improvement in the patient's airway and breathing. It if does not improve the airway as shown by improved breathing, a reappraisal of the choice or size of airway is urgently required (*see also* Section 1.13).

Tracheal intubation

Aims
These are as follows:
- to secure the airway
- to protect the airway
- to facilitate prolonged and intra-operative ventilation
- for tracheo-bronchial toilet
- in the application of high airway pressures and positive end-expiratory pressure (PEEP)
- during cardiopulmonary resuscitation to improve ventilation and allow uninterrupted chest compressions.

Choice of tube
An uncuffed tube is often recommended in children who weigh less than 25 kg, as the larynx is narrowest below the glottis at the circular non-distensible cricoid ring, and inexperienced use of the cuffed tube may cause damage at that point, although the cuffed tube gives better airway protection. The choice ultimately depends on the experience of the practitioner (*see also* Section 1.13).

The correctly sized tube is one that passes easily through the glottis and subglottic area with a small air

leak detectable at 20 cmH$_2$O (sustained gentle positive pressure).

Size of tube
The correct size of tube is:
- one that can just fit into the nostril **or**
- in preterm neonates, 2.5–3.5 mm internal diameter **or**
- in full-term neonates, 3.0–4.0 mm internal diameter **or**
- in infants after the neonatal period, 3.5–4.5 mm internal diameter **or**
- in children over 1 year:
  - the internal diameter (in mm) is age/4 + 4
  - the length of tube (in cm) is age/2 plus 12 for an oral tube, and age/2 plus 15 for a nasal tube.

Aids to intubation
- Laryngoscope: blade (straight for neonates and infants because of long, floppy epiglottis, curved for older children), bulb and handle.

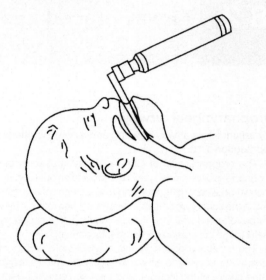

FIGURE 8.2.5 Straight-blade laryngoscope, suitable for infants.

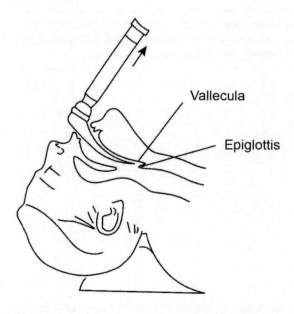

Vallecula

Epiglottis

FIGURE 8.2.6 Curved-blade laryngoscope, suitable for children.

- Magill's forceps.
- Introducer (not further than the end of the tube itself).
- Syringe (cuffed tube).
- Gum elastic bougie (over which the tube can pass).
- Cricoid pressure (can aid visualisation of larynx).
- Suction apparatus (this must be available).

Predicting difficulty
- Difficulty in opening mouth.
- Reduced neck mobility.
- Laryngeal/pharyngeal lesions.
- Congenital: Pierre-Robin syndrome, mucopolysaccharidoses.
- Acquired: burns, trauma.

If on viewing the infant's face from the side, the chin is unusually small (micrognathia), the intubation will be difficult, and **senior help is required** (but see below).

Complications
- Displacement: oesophageal, endobronchial, out of larynx!
- Obstruction: kinking, secretions.
- Trauma: lips to larynx.
- Hypertensive response.
- Spasm: laryngeal, pharyngeal.
- Aspiration: gastric contents.

Procedure
Prepare and check the equipment.
- Choose an appropriate tube size, with one size above and one size below it available.
- Get the tape ready to fix the tube.
- Suction must be available.
- Induce anaesthesia and give a muscle relaxant unless the patient is completely obtunded.
- **Do not attempt the procedure in a semi-conscious child.**

Position the child.
- Children over 3–4 years of age: the 'sniffing morning air' position (head extended on the shoulders, and flexed at the neck).
- Children under 3 years of age (especially neonates and infants): a neutral position (large occiput).
- Keep the child in a neutral position with in-line immobilisation in the case of unstable cervical spine (e.g. trauma, Down's syndrome).

Oxygenate the child using a face mask and reservoir (if patient is breathing) or bag and mask ventilation to provide high flow oxygen.
- Introduce the laryngoscope into the right side of the mouth.
- Sweep the tongue to the left.
- Advance the blade until the epiglottis is seen.
  - Curved blade: advance the blade anterior to the epiglottis. Lift the epiglottis forward by moving the blade away from your own body.
  - Straight blade: advance the blade beneath the epiglottis, into the oesophagus. Pull back, and the glottis will 'flop' into view.

Recognise the glottis.
- Insert the endotracheal tube gently through the vocal cords.
- Stop at a predetermined length.

Confirm the correct placement.
- The chest moves up and down with ventilation.
- Listen to breath sounds in the axillae and anterior chest wall.
- Confirm that there are no breath sounds in the stomach.
- Oxygen saturations do not go down.
- Carbon dioxide is measured from expired gases.

Secure the tube.
Secure with tape around the tracheal tube and on to the patient's face (see below).

Nasal intubation.
Although oral intubation is quicker and more reliable in an emergency, for prolonged ventilation nasal intubation is preferable, if a skilled operator is available, as the tracheal tube is more securely fixed. The technique is similar, but with the additional use of the Magill's forceps to grasp and guide the tracheal tube as it emerges into the posterior pharynx downward into the trachea through the vocal cords.

Intubation of the newborn infant without a laryngoscope
It is possible to intubate a newborn baby using a finger rather than a laryngoscope. This can be very helpful if you do not have a functioning laryngoscope, or if the child has facial or oral deformities that interfere with your ability to insert a laryngoscope or to see the larynx (e.g. severe micrognathia).

Procedure
- Insert the index finger of the left hand into the baby's mouth, with its palmar surface sliding along the tongue. Use the little finger if the baby is small.

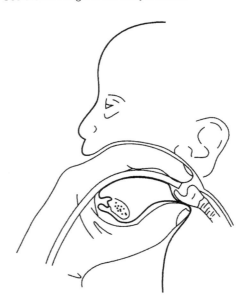

FIGURE 8.2.7 Finger intubation of the trachea in a newborn. (From Hancock PJ and Peterson G (1992) Finger intubation of the trachea in newborns. *Pediatrics*. **89**: 325–7. Reproduced with permission.)

- Slide the finger along the tongue until it meets the epiglottis. This feels like a small band running across the root of the tongue.
- Slide the finger a little further until the tip lies behind and superior to the larynx and the nail touches the posterior pharyngeal wall.
- Slide the tube into the mouth between the finger and the tongue until the tip lies in the midline at the root of the distal phalanx of the finger.
- At this point place the left thumb on the baby's neck just below the cricoid cartilage in order to grasp the larynx between the thumb on the outside and the fingertip on the inside.
- While the thumb and finger steady the larynx against side-to-side motion, the right hand advances the tube a short distance (about 1–2 cm).
- A slight 'give' can sometimes be felt as the tube passes into the larynx, but **no force is needed for insertion**.
- When the tube is in the trachea the laryngeal cartilages can be felt to encircle it. If it has passed into the oesophagus it can be felt between the finger and the larynx.

Fixation of endotracheal tubes

Two people should be available to do this, one of whom should hold the tube at all times.

- Cut two strips of sticky zinc oxide tape (see below); they should reach from just in front of the ear across the cheek and above the upper lip to the opposite ear.

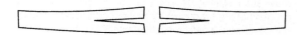

FIGURE 8.2.8 Tape for tracheal tube fixation.

- If available, apply some benzoin tincture to the cheeks, above the upper lip and under the chin, which will make the tape stick well.
- Make sure that the endotracheal tube is clean and that no old tape is left on it.
- Start with the broad end of the tape, and stick this on to the cheek. Then wrap one of the thinner ends carefully around the tube. It is useful if it is still possible to see the endotracheal tube marking at the lips.
- Tape the other half across the philtrum to the cheek.
- The second tape starts on the other cheek, and the thinner half is stuck across the chin, while the other half is also wrapped around the tube (see below).

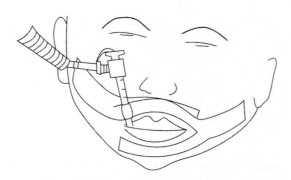

FIGURE 8.2.9 Taped tracheal tube.

Cricothyroidotomy

Cricothyroidotomy is indicated if a patent airway cannot be achieved by other means. It must be performed promptly and decisively when necessary.

Call a surgeon and an anaesthetist (if available).

In children under the age of 12 years, needle cricothyroidotomy can be performed rather than a full surgical cricothyroidotomy. In adolescents, either technique can be used, but the surgical technique allows better protection of the airway. The relevant anatomy is shown in Figure 8.2.10.

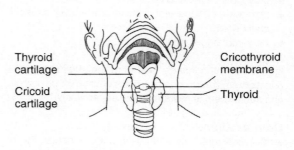

FIGURE 8.2.10 Anatomy of the larynx.

In a very small baby, or if a foreign body is below the cricoid ring, direct tracheal puncture using the same technique can be used.

Needle cricothyroidotomy

This technique is simple in concept, but far from easy in practice. In an emergency situation the child may be struggling, and attempts to breathe or swallow may result in the larynx moving up and down.

Procedure

- Attach a cricothyroidotomy cannula-over-needle (or if this is not available, an IV cannula and needle) of appropriate size to a 5-mL syringe.
- Place the patient in a supine position.
- If there is no risk of cervical spine injury, extend the neck, perhaps with a sandbag under the shoulders.
- Identify the cricothyroid membrane by palpation between the thyroid and cricoid cartilages.
  - Prepare the neck with antiseptic swabs.
  - Place your left hand on the neck to identify and stabilise the cricothyroid membrane, and to protect the lateral vascular structures from needle injury.

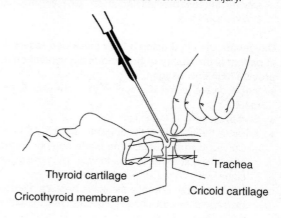

FIGURE 8.2.11 Penetrating the cricothyroid membrane.

— Insert the needle and cannula through the cricothyroid membrane at a 45-degree angle caudally towards the feet, aspirating as the needle is advanced (*see* Figure 8.2.11).

- When air is aspirated, advance the cannula over the needle, being careful not to damage the posterior tracheal wall. Withdraw the needle.
- Re-check that air can be aspirated from the cannula.
- Attach the hub of the cannula to an oxygen flow meter via a Y-connector. Initially the oxygen flow rate (in litres) should be set at the child's age (in years).
- Ventilate by occluding the open end of the Y-connector with a thumb for 1 second, to direct gas into the lungs. If this does not cause the chest to rise, the oxygen flow rate should be increased by increments of 1 litre, and the effect of 1 second of occlusion of the Y-connector reassessed.
- Allow passive exhalation (via the upper airway) by releasing the thumb for 4 seconds.
- Observe chest movement and auscultate breath sounds to confirm that there is adequate ventilation.
- Check the neck to exclude swelling from the injection of gas into the tissues rather than the trachea.
- Secure the equipment to the patient's neck.
- Having completed emergency airway management, arrange to proceed to a more definitive airway procedure, such as tracheotomy.

Note

There are two common misconceptions about transtracheal insufflation. The first is that it is possible to ventilate a patient via a needle cricothyroidotomy using a self-inflating bag. The maximum pressure from a bag is approximately 4.41 kPa (45 cmH$_2$O) (the blow-off valve pressure), and this is insufficient to drive gas through a narrow cannula. In comparison, wall oxygen is provided at a pressure of 4 atmospheres (approximately 392 kPa or 4000 cmH$_2$O). The second misconception is that expiration can occur through the cannula, or through a separate cannula inserted through the cricothyroid membrane. This is not possible. The intratracheal pressure during expiration is usually less than 2.9 kPa (30 cmH$_2$O) (less than 1% of the driving pressure in inspiration). Expiration must occur via the upper airway, even in situations of partial upper airway obstruction. Should upper airway obstruction be complete, it is necessary to reduce the gas flow to 1–2 litres/minute. This provides some oxygenation but little ventilation.

Nevertheless, insufflation buys a few minutes in which to attempt a surgical airway.

Surgical cricothyroidotomy

1 Place the patient in a supine position.
2 If there is no risk of neck injury, consider extending the neck to improve access. Otherwise, maintain a neutral alignment.
3 Identify the cricothyroid membrane in the following manner. Place your finger over the most prominent part of the thyroid cartilage (the Adam's apple). Move the finger downwards (i.e. towards the chest), keeping strictly in the midline. The first dip felt is the area of cricothyroid membrane.
4 Prepare the skin and, if the patient is conscious, infiltrate with local anaesthetic.
5 Place the index and middle fingers of your left hand on each side of the midline of the neck to stabilise the cricothyroid membrane, and to protect the lateral vascular structures from injury.
6 Make a small vertical incision in the skin, and press the lateral edges of the incision outwards, to minimise bleeding.
7 Make a transverse incision through the cricothyroid membrane, being careful not to damage the cricoid cartilage.
8 Insert a tracheal spreader, or use the handle of the scalpel by inserting it through the incision and twisting it through 90 degrees to open the airway.
9 Insert an appropriately sized endotracheal or tracheostomy tube. It is advisable to use a slightly smaller size than would have been used for an oral or nasal tube (e.g. size 6.0 mm internal diameter for age 12–16 years).
10 Ventilate the patient and check that this is effective.
11 Secure the tube to prevent dislodgement.

Complications of cricothyroidotomy

These include the following:

- asphyxia
- aspiration of blood or secretions
- haemorrhage or haematoma
- creation of a false passage into the tissues
- surgical emphysema (subcutaneous or mediastinal)
- pulmonary barotrauma
- subglottic oedema or stenosis
- oesophageal perforation
- cellulitis.

8.3 Breathing procedures

Emergency needle thoracocentesis

This procedure is used for the rapidly deteriorating patient who has a life-threatening tension pneumothorax (*see* Section 7.3.A). If this technique is used in a patient who does not have a tension pneumothorax, there is a 10–20% risk of producing a pneumothorax or causing damage to the lung, or both. In such cases, immediate insertion of a chest drain is mandatory. **Patients who have undergone** this procedure should ideally have a chest radiograph, and may require chest drainage if they subsequently need assisted ventilation.

Minimum equipment
- Swabs for disinfecting the skin.
- Large over-the-needle IV cannula (16-gauge, but 20- to 22-gauge in preterm infants).
- 20-mL syringe.

Procedure (*see* Figure 8.3.1)

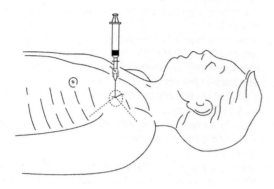

FIGURE 8.3.1 Position for inserting over-the-needle cannula for thoracocentesis.

1. Identify the second intercostal space in the mid-clavicular line on the side of the pneumothorax (the **opposite** side to the direction of tracheal deviation and the **same** side as the hyper-resonance).
2. Swab the chest wall with surgical preparation solution or an alcohol swab.
3. Attach the syringe to the over-the-needle IV cannula, ideally via a three-way tap.
4. Insert the cannula vertically into the chest wall, just above the rib below to avoid blood vessels, aspirating all the time.
5. If air is aspirated, remove the needle, leaving the plastic cannula in place.
6. Tape the cannula in place and proceed to chest drain insertion as soon as possible.

Complications
These include the following:
- local cellulitis
- local haematoma
- pleural infection
- empyema
- pneumothorax.

Insertion of a chest drainage tube

In a trauma emergency that requires a chest drainage tube, fluid resuscitation through at least one large calibre IV cannula, and monitoring of vital signs should be ongoing. Usually the patient will be receiving oxygen through a face mask with a reservoir.

Chest drain placement should be performed using the open technique described here, as this minimises lung damage. In general, the largest size of drain that will pass between the ribs should be used.

Minimum equipment
- Skin disinfectant and surgical drapes.
- Scalpel with fine straight blade.
- Blunt forceps.
- Artery forceps.
- Large clamps × 2.
- Suture.
- Local anaesthetic if the child is conscious.
- Scissors.
- Chest drain tube.
- Underwater seal or Heimlich flutter valve.

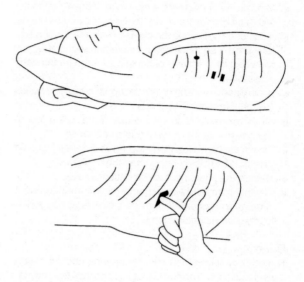

FIGURE 8.3.2 Sites for chest drain: 4th or 5th intercostal space in the anterior or mid-axillary line.

Procedure
1. Consider using analgesia or sedation in a small or apprehensive child.
2. Wash your hands and arms to the elbows, and wear a mask, surgical hat (bonnet), sterile gown and sterile surgical gloves.
3. Prepare the underwater seal with an assistant and take the sterile end of the tube, ready to connect to the chest tube once inserted. The 'seal' end should be covered by no more than 1–2 cmH₂O.
4. Decide on the insertion site (usually the fourth or fifth intercostal space in the anterior or mid-axillary line) on the side with the pneumothorax (*see* Figure 8.3.2).
5. Swab the chest wall with surgical preparation or an alcohol swab.
6. Use local anaesthetic if the child is conscious. Morphine (100 micrograms/kg IV over 10 minutes) should also be given if the child is conscious, but in the preterm infant who is not ventilated this may precipitate apnoea. Facilities to provide bag-and-mask ventilation and/or intubation should be immediately available, together with staff trained in their use.
7. Make a 2- to 3-cm skin incision along the line of the intercostal space, **immediately above the rib below to avoid damage to the neurovascular bundle which lies under the inferior edge of each rib**.
8. Using artery forceps, bluntly dissect through the subcutaneous tissues just over the top of the rib below, and puncture the parietal pleura with the tip of the forceps.

9   Put a gloved finger into the incision and clear the path into the pleura. This will not be possible in infants or small children, in which case continue to use the artery forceps.

10 Advance the chest drain tube (use the largest size that can comfortably pass between the ribs) into the pleural space without the trocar in place, but using the artery forceps to help to guide it into the pleural cavity if necessary. Pass about 3 cm and then connect to the underwater seal. Ideally advance the chest drain tube into the pleural space during expiration.

11 Ensure that the tube is in the pleural space by looking for fogging of the tube during expiration.

12 Ensure that all of the drainage holes of the chest drain tube are inside the chest.

13 Connect the chest drain tube to an underwater seal. Check that the tube is in the right place by observing intermittent bubbling of the water in the drainage bottle.

14 Secure the tube using a suture passed through the skin at the incision site (after ensuring that adequate local anaesthetic has been administered) and tied around the tube.

15 Cover the puncture site in the chest wall with a sterile dressing, and tape the chest tube to the chest wall.

16 Obtain a chest radiograph if at all possible.

If the chest drainage tube is satisfactorily positioned and working, occasional bubbles will pass through the underwater seal. The water level in the tube may also rise and fall slightly with the respiratory cycle.

Complications of chest drainage tube insertion

- Dislodgement of the chest drain tube from the chest wall or disconnection from the drainage bag.
- Drainage bag elevated above the level of the chest, and fluid flowing into the chest cavity, unless there is a one-way valve system.
- Chest drain tube kinking or blocking with blood clot.
- Damage to the intercostal nerve, artery or vein. This might convert a pneumothorax to a haemopneumothorax, or result in intercostal neuritis or neuralgia.
- Damage to the internal thoracic artery if the puncture is too medial, resulting in haemopneumothorax.
- Incorrect tube position, inside or outside the chest cavity.
- Introduction of pleural infection (e.g. thoracic empyema).
- Laceration or puncture of intrathoracic or abdominal organs. This can be prevented by using the finger technique before inserting the chest tube.
- Leaking drainage bag.
- Local cellulitis.
- Local haematoma.
- Mediastinal emphysema.
- Persistent pneumothorax from a large primary defect; a second chest tube may be required.
- Subcutaneous emphysema (usually at the tube insertion site).

Tapping the chest for diagnostic tests in pleural effusions or empyema
Diagnostic procedure
- Consider giving the child analgesia or light anaesthesia with ketamine.

- Wash your hands and put on sterile gloves.
- Lie the child on their back.
- Clean the skin over the chest with an antiseptic solution (e.g. 70% alcohol).
- Select a point in the mid-axillary line (at the side of the chest) just below the level of the nipple (fifth intercostal space; *see* Figure 8.3.2).
- Inject about 1 mL of 1% lignocaine into the skin and subcutaneous tissue at this point.
- Insert a needle or needle-over-catheter through the skin and pleura, and aspirate to confirm the presence of pleural fluid. Withdraw a sample for microscopy and other tests and place it in a container.
- If the fluid is clear (straw-coloured or brownish), pull out the needle or catheter after withdrawing enough fluid to relieve distress, and put a dressing over the puncture site. Consider a differential diagnosis of tuberculosis (*see* Section 6.1.N).
- If the fluid is thin pus or cloudy (like milk), leave the catheter in place so that you can draw out more pus several times a day. Make sure that you seal the end of the catheter so that no air can get in.
- If the fluid is thick pus which cannot pass easily through the needle or catheter, insert a chest tube as described above.

Non-invasive respiratory support (*see* Section 1.25)

Respiratory support is needed when the patient fails to sustain adequate ventilation despite treatment of the respiratory condition. Respiratory failure may result from any of the following:
- respiratory illnesses
- severe shock
- coma
- convulsions
- meningo-encephalitis
- neuromuscular disorders
- raised intracranial pressure (e.g. from trauma).

Infants and young children are more likely to progress to respiratory failure because:
- they are more susceptible to infection
- their airways are smaller
- their thoracic cage is more compliant
- their ribs are (nearer) horizontal
- their respiratory muscles are more prone to fatigue.

Women and girls who are pregnant are also more susceptible to respiratory failure. They have reduced immune function, an expanding abdominal mass which impairs lung expansion, and are more prone to gastro-oesophageal reflux and aspiration of gastric contents.

As respiratory failure progresses, it will ultimately lead to cardiorespiratory arrest and death. Thus recognition of the severity of the conditions that lead to respiratory failure, followed by appropriate treatment, will reduce morbidity and mortality.

Signs that indicate the adequacy of breathing include the following:
- intercostal, sub-costal and supra-sternal recession
- respiratory rate
- inspiratory and expiratory noises

- use of accessory muscles
- adequacy of breath sounds and chest expansion
- heart rate
- skin colour
- mental status.

To help to assess the development of respiratory failure, it is necessary to assess changes in the above clinical signs. In the following situations, however, these signs are less useful because there is absent or decreased effort of breathing:

1 with fatigue or exhaustion (e.g. after prolonged respiratory effort)
2 with loss of cerebral drive from raised intracranial pressure, poisoning or encephalopathy
3 in children with neuromuscular disease.

In these cases, pay more attention to the chest expansion, heart rate, skin colour, mental status and, if available, SaO$_2$ measurement.

Pulse oximetry is of additional value to measure the arterial oxygen saturation through the skin (SpO$_2$ or SaO$_2$). Values of SpO$_2$ of less than 92–94% in air (at sea level; *see* Section 1.13 for values at high altitude) are abnormal, and would warrant at least initial treatment with additional inspired oxygen. Values of less than 95% when the child is in oxygen are low, but even values of more than 95% in oxygen may be associated with significant hypoventilation. It is essential to remember that, in respiratory failure, normal SaO$_2$ while receiving additional inspired oxygen is likely to be associated with significant hypoventilation or intra-pulmonary shunting. Measurement of transcutaneous, end-expired or blood carbon dioxide levels will confirm this.

TABLE 8.3.1 Modes of respiratory support for different conditions

Mode of support	Interface with patient	Level of nursing care	Associated medical treatment	Clinical use	Examples of conditions treated
High-flow high-humidity oxygen	Nasal cannulae	Home, ward, HD	Nil	To provide a flow above the patient's needs, that helps to wash out dead space, and improves comfort and clearance of the airways. It may provide mild CPAP	Bronchiolitis, post-operative, chronic lung disease of prematurity
Continuous positive airways pressure (CPAP)	Nasal cannulae or nasopharyngeal tube	High dependency (HD)	Sedation or analgesia may be needed	To keep upper and lower airways patent and maintain adequate lung volume (oxygenation)	Neonatal respiratory distress syndrome, **bronchiolitis**
	Nasal mask or face mask	Home, ward, HD	Nil		Sleep-related upper airway obstruction
		Intensive care (IC)	Sedation or analgesia may be needed		Acute upper airway obstruction before, **instead of** or after extubation
Intermittent positive pressure ventilation (IPPV)	Nasal mask or pillows, face mask (NIPPV)	Home to IC	Nil	To treat hypoventilation (raised CO$_2$) when airway control and clearance are adequate	Chronic (e.g. central, neuromuscular) Acute (e.g. after surgery)
	Endotracheal tube	IC	Anaesthesia for intubation Sedation or analgesia will be needed	To treat hypoventilation when clearance and/or support of airway(s), or close control of ventilation needed	Procedures or surgery requiring anaesthesia Severe respiratory illnesses, raised intracranial pressure
	Tracheostomy	Home to IC	ENT surgical procedure	Long term ventilation where day and night support needed	Brainstem/high spinal injury or neuromuscular disease
Continuous negative extrathoracic pressure (CNEP)	Chamber or jacket	Home to IC	Nil	To keep lower airways patent and maintain adequate lung volume	Bronchiolitis and other severe lower respiratory infections, especially where the nose is blocked by secretions
Intermittent negative pressure ventilation (INEP or INPV)				To treat hypoventilation where airway control and clearance are adequate or maintained by CPAP	Central hypoventilation (e.g. apnoea of prematurity, neuromuscular disease)

Shaded areas denote those that require a lower dependency of care (e.g. that have been used in the home setting), but may be useful in acute conditions.

Bold type denotes high-risk situations in which CPAP may be ineffective and intubation may be required.

When respiratory fatigue is severe, oxygenation is poor or deteriorating, or carbon dioxide levels are raised, respiratory support should be used, if available. The various forms of respiratory support are outlined in Table 8.3.1, along with their indications.

Notes on the use of positive pressure ventilation

1 Monitoring of patient status and airway or mask pressures is necessary when undertaking any form of respiratory support (see below).

2 Positive airway pressure involves a flow of air or other gas mixture to the patient's airways. This flow may be continuous (as in CPAP) or intermittent (as in IPPV). It may vary with inspiration and expiration (as in BiPAP), or to accommodate the leaks or variable compliance of ventilator tubing, airways or lung units.

3 Mask ventilation can be well tolerated by children, but it may be more difficult for infants and young children to tolerate appliances on their face.

4 In the presence of excess airway secretions or an open mouth, nasal masks and nasal cannulae may not produce as effective airway pressures as ventilation with tracheal intubation (or relatively higher pressures may be needed for the same effect).

5 The pressures used with masks and cannulae may be higher than those used with tracheal intubation, because of the greater potential for air leaks and other volume loss in compliant upper airway structures.

6 Infants and young children will sometimes tolerate masks and cannulae only with the use of sedation, in which case close monitoring of respiratory failure must be undertaken in case full intubation and ventilation is needed.

7 Endotracheal intubation should be undertaken with rapid sequence drug or gaseous induction, and subsequent analgesia, anxiolysis and sedation should be provided.

8 Positive pressure ventilation administered through an endotracheal tube must be accompanied by adequate humidity of the inspired gases.

9 Oxygen may be administered either using a built-in mixer in the ventilator, or by entraining a supply in the ventilator tubing nearer to the patient.

10 Positive pressure ventilators should be able to provide manipulation of either the pressure or volume administered, and the time intervals for inspiration and expiration. There should be alarms for failure to cycle, and for excessive pressure and/or volume administered.

Continuous positive airway pressure (CPAP)

CPAP has several effects on the airway and lungs of the preterm and full-term infant. These include prevention of alveolar collapse, increased functional residual capacity (FRC), and splinting of the airway. It is therefore of most value when used early in the course of respiratory disease (i.e. before too much alveolar collapse has taken place). Several units around the world use it successfully as first-line ventilatory support in even the smallest infants (< 750 grams birth weight).

Indications for CPAP

These include the following:

- signs of significant respiratory distress (tachypnoea, recession, grunting, nasal flare)
- diseases with low FRC (respiratory distress syndrome, transient tachypnoea of the newborn, pulmonary oedema)
- meconium aspiration syndrome
- apnoea and bradycardia of prematurity
- tracheomalacia.

Requirements

- Low-resistance delivery system.
- Large-bore tubing.
- Short wide connection to patient.
- Consistent and reliable pressure generation.
- Appropriate snug-fitting nasal cannulae.
- Well-positioned and secured nasal cannulae.
- Prevention of leaks, mainly via the mouth, with a chinstrap.
- Optimally maintained airway.
- Ideally warmed humidified gas.
- Prevention of neck flexion or over-extension with a neck roll.
- Regular suction to remove secretions.
- Meticulous and consistent technique.

Monitoring

- Continuous heart and respiratory rate monitoring.
- Continuous pulse oximetry, ideally pre-ductal.
- Blood gas measurements. These need not be done regularly in the stable baby with low oxygen needs unless they are required in order to assess the degree of metabolic acidosis, but in those with high oxygen requirements ($FiO_2 > 40\%$) or in the unstable baby they should be checked regularly via an arterial line.

Complications

- **Nasal septum erosion/necrosis:** this is a result of ill-fitting nasal cannulae, and can be avoided by the fitting of snug, but not tight, cannulae (blanching of the overlying skin suggests that the cannulae are too large) which are held firmly in place to prevent rubbing as the child moves.
- **Pneumothorax:** all methods of artificial ventilation are associated with this problem. However, the more effective the CPAP is the less the work of breathing and therefore the lower the risk of pneumothoraces should be. Any pneumothorax that does occur should be drained appropriately. It is inappropriate to discontinue the CPAP.
- **Gastric distension from swallowed air:** this is important and is easily overcome by the venting of any such air via an open orogastric tube.

Insertion and securing of nasal cannulae and administration of CPAP

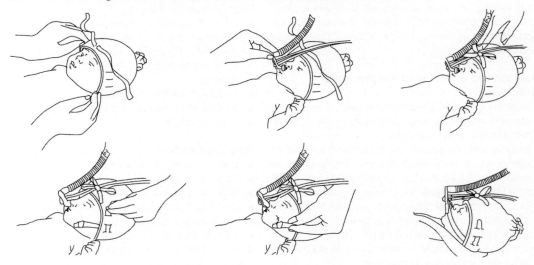

FIGURE 8.3.3 Securing nasal cannulae for giving continuous positive airway pressure (CPAP) in a baby. A special bonnet is used from which tapes hold the pipe carrying the air/oxygen mixture to the nasal cannulae to the forehead and a separate tape above the mouth to ensure the cannulae do not come out of the nasal passages..

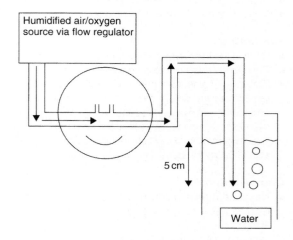

FIGURE 8.3.4 Simplified diagram of Hudson continuous positive airway pressure (CPAP). The gas flow is adjusted until a continuous trail of bubbles starts to appear in the water bottle, which is at the same height as the baby. This generates a CPAP of +5 cmH$_2$O.

Continuous negative extra-thoracic pressure

Continuous negative extra-thoracic pressure (CNEP) is a method by which sub-atmospheric pressure is applied to the outside of a child's chest by nursing them in a specially designed chamber. The patient's head is kept outside the chamber, thereby allowing the nose, mouth and all the airways into the lungs to remain at atmospheric pressure. As a result of this pressure difference, the chest is expanded and air is encouraged to enter the lungs. Areas of lung that were previously poorly inflated may be expanded, and this allows more chance for recovery from the lung disease.

The use of CNEP depends upon continued breathing efforts by the child to move air into and out of the lungs.

When the child is inside the chamber, the breathing rate falls, the effort of breathing is reduced, and thus less energy is needed for breathing.

Indications
- Respiratory failure due to lung problems:
  - bronchiolitis
  - other causes of acute respiratory infection where the nasal airway is blocked and nasal CPAP is not possible.
- Respiratory failure due to weakness of respiratory muscles:
  - poliomyelitis.

Advantages
The absence of airway invasion:
- avoids trauma to the airways
- reduces the need for suctioning
- lowers the risk of introducing infection into the lungs
- is more comfortable for the patient, so there is less need for sedation.

Less complex equipment:
- can be managed on a general ward or at home
- is not difficult for healthcare workers and parents to learn how to use
- means that there is less utilisation of intensive care resources
- is quick to institute, not requiring medical or anaesthetic staff.

Physiological (compared with positive pressure) ventilation:
- does **not** increase pulmonary vascular resistance
- is less likely to significantly reduce cardiac output
- enhances lung perfusion, as well as ventilation.

Disadvantages
Negative pressure generated in the upper airway on

inspiration may be increased, thus exacerbating **pre-existing** upper airway obstruction.

Respiratory support may need to be interrupted for short periods.

- This means it is less suitable where the need for support to ventilation is critical and continuous
- It is also not suitable if the patient's own ventilatory efforts are inadequate to remove carbon dioxide.

Maintenance of body temperature in newborn infants may require specific attention.

Components of negative pressure system

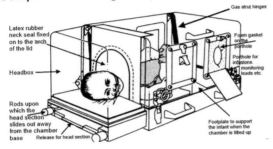

FIGURE 8.3.5 Negative pressure system.

The chamber

For low-birth-weight infants the chamber is built on to an incubator base incorporating a cabinet and heater, the latter providing servo-controlled circulation of hot air into the interior of the chamber. Particular features of the chamber shown in Figure 8.3.5 include the following:

1. release for the head section
2. rods upon which the head section slides out away from the chamber base
3. headbox
4. latex rubber neck seal fixed on to the arch of the lid
5. gas strut hinges
6. foam gasket or cuff on the porthole
7. porthole for infusions, monitoring leads, etc.
8. footplate to support the infant when the chamber is tilted up
9. compressible rubber strips below which leads, etc. can enter the chamber
10. tubing to the pressure monitor.

The neck seal

This is a piece of latex rubber with a circular hole 2–5 cm in diameter, situated near the bottom end. This is fitted around the infant's neck overlying the neck protector.

The neck protector

This is a piece of two or four thicknesses of ribbed cotton tubular stockinet. Two holes cut in the sides allow this to be fitted like a polo-necked vest over the infant.

The suction unit

This incorporates an electrical fan with a valve which provides variable levels of continuous suction. The valve is adjustable by a pressure control knob. A suction hose connects from the suction unit to the base of the chamber.

The pressure monitor

This can be a simple calibrated U-tube containing coloured

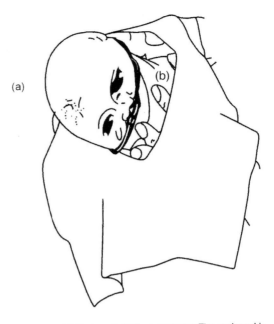

FIGURE 8.3.6 (a) Neck seal. (b) Neck protector. The neck seal is a piece of stretchy latex rubber with a circular hole 2–5 cm in diameter, which is stretched and fitted around the infant's neck, overlying the neck protector.

alcohol or other fluid, **or** a more sophisticated pressure monitor.

Safety

1. Special care must be taken not to trap the fingers or toes when closing the lid.
2. To avoid damaging the monitor leads, these must pass either (1) through the diaphragm at the base of the chamber, or (2) between a rubber strip at the foot end of the chamber and a second rubber strip on the lower edge of the lid. The monitor leads will be damaged and pressure lost if they are brought out through the sides of the chamber between the unprotected Perspex edge of the lid and the rubber seal on the base.

Care of infants who are receiving CNEP
Feeding

While receiving negative pressure, the patient would not usually be fed orally. Feeds should be given via a nasogastric tube, and this tube should be clamped off when not in use. Do not leave the tube open to air or the stomach may become distended.

If the baby develops problems with abdominal distension, the stomach should not be left on free drainage in the conventional way. Either frequent aspiration of the stomach contents should be performed, with the tube clamped off in the intervening time, or the end of the tube can be put through the neck seal (in between the silicone gel and the vest) and the tube left on free drainage inside the chamber.

If the baby's clinical condition allows this, they may be taken out of the chamber at regular intervals for breastfeeding or cup feeds.

Procedures

Most procedures, such as re-siting of an IV line, can be performed while the infant is receiving negative pressure.

When the arms are inserted through the portholes, sub-atmospheric pressure can be maintained by the close-fitting cuffs around the forearms.

Excessive body movement may occur during sudden loss of negative pressure when the porthole is opened or the arm removed from the cuff. This may be quite disruptive to the baby. Therefore it is preferable to minimise the number of times this occurs by taking into the chamber all the items which are needed for the procedure. When the cuffs or gaskets become soiled or torn, they must be replaced immediately.

Neck care

Pay particular attention to the patient's neck, observing it for soreness frequently, at 6- to 8-hourly intervals if possible when the patient is turned. It is important to ensure that all the layers of the neck seal are in place and that the latex does not come into contact with the baby's skin. It is not necessary to replace the neck seal components unless they are soiled or damaged. If they are in place for a prolonged period, especially in the case of a newborn preterm baby whose skin may scale and shed, it is probably better to wash and dry the neck at regular intervals when the clinical condition allows, preventing colonisation by skin commensal bacteria.

It is also important to frequently check the neck to ensure that the latex does not become too tight if the baby becomes oedematous. If this happens it is important to replace the latex with a larger size.

Controlling body temperature

The important principle to follow in the control of body temperature of babies who are receiving negative pressure is the prevention of hypothermia, rather than its treatment. Due to convective and radiant heat loss the baby is much more likely to cool rapidly and be more difficult to warm up than in the conventional incubators.

Plastic sheeting or bubble wrap may be placed over the infant's body to create a 'micro-environment'.

An overhead radiant heater may be used as an additional heat source over the headbox or chamber.

Management of problems that may arise
Inadequate pressure

- Excess leak at neck:
  - Slacken the latex into the arch in the lid.
  - Move the baby upwards.
  - Reposition the latex.
  - Double the thickness of stockinet collar under the latex.
  - Use latex with a smaller hole (if a large leak is present).
- Excess leak between chamber and base of chamber:
  - Tighten the quick-release lid and base catches.
  - Replace the rubber strip gasket around the chamber base.
- Excess leak at the portholes:
  - Renew the cuffs or foam gaskets.
  - Tighten or secure the iris diaphragm porthole.
- Inadequate suction pressure:
  - Check that the hose is plugged in at both ends.
  - Check that the access hole for suction inside the chamber is not blocked (e.g. by the sheet).
  - Check the pressure achieved by the suction unit after directly occluding the hose at the end.

Unsettled baby

- Baby breathing too hard:
  - There may be an inadequate negative pressure.
  - Check for upper airway obstruction.
  - Check for stridor, tracheal tug and carbon dioxide retention.
  - A different method of respiratory support may be needed.
- Anxiety:
  - Give reassurance and/or sedation to make the baby comfortable.
- Sore neck:
  - Check the neck and treat sore areas to relieve discomfort.

Abdominal distension

- Air swallowing:
  - Close the nasogastric tube.
  - Undertake more frequent suction or free drainage inside the chamber.

Cold baby

- Excess leak:
  - See the section on 'Inadequate pressure'.
- Cold environment:
  - Provide an overhead heater.
  - Humidify the chamber.
  - See the guidelines on temperature.

Problem: neck soreness

- Pressure or contact allergy:
  - Ensure that at the neck seal there is at least a fourfold thickness of stockinet between the latex and the skin.
  - If the latex is stretched too tightly, the baby may be suspended at the neck. Release and pleat it as described above.
  - The hole in the latex may be too small, so revise it if necessary.

Inadequate oxygen in the headbox

- Excess leak at the neck:
  - See the section on 'Inadequate pressure'.
- Inadequate oxygen:
  - Seal the top and sides of the headbox (e.g. with cling film).
  - Adjust the flow and/or concentration.
  - Two supplies of high-flow humidified 100% oxygen may be needed to provide a high concentration in the headbox.

Physiotherapy for suppurative lung diseases

Therapy for bronchiectasis, cystic fibrosis and other conditions with excess airway secretions is described here.

Postural drainage

This is positioning to allow drainage by gravity from lung segments to central airways.

For infants, use a maximum of five positions in 10 minutes, progressing in older children to two to three positions in up to 30 minutes.

1 Apical segments upper lobes

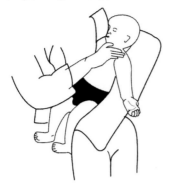

2 Posterior segment right upper lobe
(reverse for left)

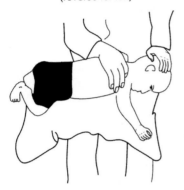

3 Anterior segments upper lobes

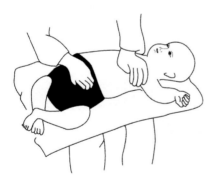

4 Right middle lobe (reverse for left)

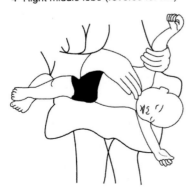

5 Apical segments of lower lobes

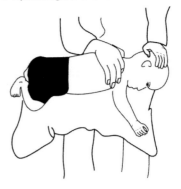

6 Anterior segments of lower lobes

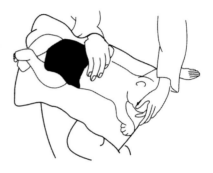

7 Posterior segments of lower lobes

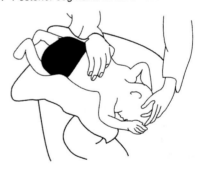

8 Lateral segments of right lower lobes
(reverse for left)

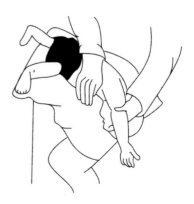

FIGURE 8.3.7 Positions for postural drainage.

Upper lobe

- Apical segments: sitting (1).
- Posterior segments: prone, one pillow below the affected side (2).
- Anterior segment: supine (3).

Middle lobe/lingual

- Chest tipped 15 degrees below the horizontal, lying supine, with a pillow supporting the ipsilateral hip and shoulder (4).

Lower lobe

- Apical segments: prone (5).
- Anterior basal: chest tipped 20 degrees below the horizontal, lying supine (6).
- Lateral basal: chest tipped 20 degrees below the horizontal, lying on the unaffected side (7).
- Posterior basal: chest tipped 20 degrees below the horizontal, lying on the unaffected side (8).

Figure 8.3.7 shows all of these positions in sequence.

Equipment

Carer's lap (in the case of an infant), otherwise bean bags, pillows or a tilted bed.

Adjuncts to postural drainage

The following may be combined with postural drainage:
- **chest clapping:** done over the area to be cleared with a cupped hand
- **chest shaking:** fine manual shaking in line with rib motion during the expiratory phase of breathing
- **active cycle of breathing:** relaxed tidal breathing, four deep breaths to maximal inspiration with hold, and relaxed expiration. Huff – that is, forced expiration at mid

to low lung volumes with the glottis open (as if misting glass), cough to clear secretions, and repeat the cycle until the chest is clear.

Note where bronchoconstriction is an issue:
1 Increase the amount of time spent doing tidal volume breathing.
2 Omit percussion.
3 Increase tidal volume breathing and omit percussion.

Consider the use of inhaled bronchodilators (e.g. salbutamol 200–500 micrograms inhaled through a spacer) (*see* Section 5.2.B).

Relative contraindications

These include the following:
- raised intracranial pressure
- severe hypertension
- after abdominal surgery
- after major haemoptysis
- pulmonary oedema
- surgical emphysema
- after treatment of tension pneumothorax
- cardiac arrhythmias
- gastro-oesophageal reflux (only omit postures with upper body dependent).

Patient positioning

- To maximise ventilation–perfusion matching (e.g. in pneumonia, asthma, pneumothorax) in self-ventilating patients, position with the better ventilated lung uppermost.
- In severely breathless patients, use sitting with a forward lean, or the recovery position. Use pillows to raise and support the chest if the patient cannot tolerate lying flat.

8.4 Circulatory procedures

Access to and support for the circulation is vital in emergency care, to draw blood samples for diagnosis and monitoring, to infuse fluid to restore circulating volume and improve perfusion, to transfuse blood and to give treatment drugs. This section describes and illustrates many means of access to the circulation, and includes guidance on safe drug and fluid infusion.

Also included are circulatory support procedures such as defibrillation and pericardiocentesis, and techniques for other non-parenteral routes of drug administration, including intramuscular (IM), subcutaneous (SC) and intradermal (ID) injections.

8.4.A Minimising error in drug and fluid administration: giving injections

General points on safety

The information given below is adapted from the *Neonatal Formulary*, 11th edition (BMJ Books).

1 Drug vials once reconstituted do not contain preservatives or antiseptic. Therefore multiple sampling from them is potentially hazardous.

2 For infants, dilute drugs to ensure that volumes can be accurately measured. For example, do not use doses of less than 0.1 mL for a 1-mL syringe.

3 Serious errors can occur if the dead space in the hub of the syringe is overlooked during dilution. For example, if the active drug is drawn into a 1-mL syringe up to the 0.1-mL mark, the syringe will contain between 0.19 and 0.23 mL. If the syringe is then filled with diluent to 1 mL, the syringe will contain approximately twice as much drug as was intended. Dilution must involve first half filling the syringe with **diluent** and then adding active drug by using the distance between two graduations on the syringe. Mix the two by moving the plunger, and then finally add further diluent to the total planned volume of active drug and diluent. For dilutions of more than 10-fold, use a small syringe to inject the active drug, connected by a sterile three-way tap to a larger syringe. Then add diluent to the large syringe to obtain the desired volume.

4 Many drugs are equally effective whether given orally or parenterally. Oral administration is safer and less expensive. The following antibiotics are as effective given orally as given IV in a baby who is taking feeds: amoxicillin, ampicillin, chloramphenicol, ciprofloxacin, co-trimoxazole, erythromycin, flucloxacillin, fluconazole, isoniazid, metronidazole, pyrimethamine, rifampicin, sodium fusidate, and trimethoprim.

5 If a drug is given down an orogastric or nasogastric tube, a proportion of the drug will remain in the tube unless it is flushed through.

6 Rectally administered drugs are less reliably absorbed than drugs given orally. Liquid formulations are better than suppositories in infants.

7 When giving IV drugs, do so slowly in all cases. After it has been injected into the line (ideally through a three-way tap), the normal IV infusion rate of the fluid going into the cannula can be used to drive the drug slowly into the patient.
  - If there is no background infusion, give sufficient follow-up (flush) of fluid (0.9% saline, sterile water or 5% glucose) to ensure that the drug does not remain in the cannula or T-piece. Give the flush over 2 minutes to avoid a sudden surge of drug (remember the hub).
  - If the IV drug needs to be given rapidly (e.g. adenosine), do this by administering a 2-mL bolus of 0.9% saline via a second syringe, not by temporarily increasing the infusion rate (sometimes the temporary increase becomes prolonged and dangerous).

8 Do not mix incompatible fluids IV.

9 For IV drug infusions (using a syringe/infusion pump: if available) given in addition to background IV infusions:
  - Adjust the total 24-hour IV fluid intake.
  - Never allow a surge of a vasoactive drug such as dopamine or epinephrine.
  - Never put more drug or background IV into the syringe or burette than is needed over a defined period of time.
  - Check and chart the rate of infusion, and confirm this by examining the amount left every hour.

10 Intramuscular injections need special precautions:
  - IM injections are unsafe in shock, as they will be poorly absorbed from poorly perfused muscle tissue initially, and then (especially, for example, with opiates) a high dose may be released once recovery of the circulation occurs.
  - To avoid nerve damage, only the anterior aspect of the quadriceps muscle in the thigh is safe in a small wasted infant under 1 year of age.
  - Alternate between the legs if multiple injections are required.
  - Do not give IM injections if a severe bleeding tendency is present.
  - It is essential to draw back the plunger to ensure that the needle is not in a vein before injecting potentially dangerous drugs IM (e.g. adrenaline, magnesium sulphate, lidocaine).

Care of intravascular lines

1 Placement of central venous lines: check with a lateral X-ray that the line is placed well into a major vein, and if near the heart with the catheter tip ideally in the superior vena cava at the entrance to the right atrium.

2 Placement of an umbilical arterial line should either be above the diaphragm in the thoracic aorta, or below the two renal arteries (at L4) to minimise the risk of renal or mesenteric artery thrombosis.

3 All arterial lines can result in life-threatening haemorrhage or occlusion leading to ischaemia. Procedures to ensure that these complications do not occur should be in place.

4 Never give a drug into an IV cannula that has started to tissue. Some drugs (e.g. those containing calcium) can cause severe scarring. Inspect the cannula tip site before and while injecting any drug IV.

5 Local infection can become systemic, especially in neonates or in the immunosuppressed.
  - Always remove the cannula if there is erythema in tissue around it and if lymphangitis is seen. If lymphangitis is present always take a blood culture from a separate vein and start IV or IM antibiotics.
  - Always place cannulae aseptically and keep the site clean.
  - There is no evidence that frequent changes of cannula site or infusion kit are of benefit. However, it is a good idea to change the giving set after blood transfusion or if a line of blood has entered the infusion tubing from the vein and clotted there, as this can act as a site for bacterial colonisation. Otherwise change the lines every 3 or 4 days.

6 Air embolism: if air reaches the heart, unlike blood it will stay there, especially if the patient is lying flat.
  - Unless it is immediately aspirated, air in the heart can block the circulation.
  - Umbilical venous and other central venous lines are particularly dangerous. There must be a tap or syringe on the catheter at all times, especially during insertion.
  - An alternative source of air embolus is through the giving set, especially when pumps are being used.

7 Blood loss.
  - In neonates this can occur from the umbilical stump.
  - From central venous or arterial lines, it can rapidly be fatal, and therefore all connections must be Luer locked and the connections to the cannula and its entry must be observable at all times.

- Ideally, arterial lines should be connected to a pressure transducer and alarm.

Use of intravenous/intra-arterial (IV/IA) access

1 When sampling from an IV/IA line, clear the dead space first (by three times its volume).
   - Blood glucose levels cannot be accurately measured from any line through which a glucose solution is infused, even if many times the dead space has been cleared.
   - For blood culture, always use a separate fresh venous 'needle stab' sample.
2 Never add anything to a line carrying total parenteral nutrition (TPN).
3 Certain infusions, such as glucose > 10%, adrenaline and dopamine, are better given through a central vein. **In an emergency, dopamine and adrenaline infusions can be given through a peripheral vein.**
4 If a continuous infusion is not required, a peripheral cannula can be stopped off with a sterile bung after flushing the drug in with 0.9% saline, sterile water or 5% glucose to clear the dead space (there is no evidence that a heparin lock is needed for a cannula in peripheral veins).
5 Central venous catheters must be firmly anchored to the skin so they do not migrate into or out of position.
   - After individual drug injections and without continuous infusion, a heparin lock is appropriate to prevent clotting of the line (10 units of heparin per 1 mL of 0.9% saline), particularly in double-, triple- or quadruple-lumen catheters (always use Luer lock connections to minimise extravasation).
6 Peripheral artery lines should never be used for giving drugs.
   - To maintain patency, a continuous low-rate (0.5–1.0 mL/hour) infusion of heparinised 0.9% or 0.18% saline is useful (heparin at 1 unit/mL). Clear the 1-mL dead space of the catheter before and after sampling, which must be done aseptically.
7 In neonates and infants, frequent flushing with saline 0.9% can result in sodium overload. Therefore consider using 0.18% saline or sterile water to achieve flushing.
8 Central arterial lines (usually in the aorta) can be safely used to give glucose or total parenteral nutrition if the catheter tip site is checked radiologically (not near mesenteric or renal arteries). Most drugs (except inotropes) can also be safely given by this route by slow infusion (not by boluses).
9 Do not add drugs to any line containing blood or blood products.
10 Most IV drugs can be given into an infusion containing 0.9% saline or up to 10% glucose (the exceptions include amphotericin B, phenytoin and erythromycin).
11 If only one line is being used for an infusion and more than one drug needs to be given, try to wait 10 minutes between them. If this is not possible, separate by 1 mL of 0.18% saline/4% glucose, 0.9% saline or sterile water for injections. This is very important with an alkaline drug such as sodium bicarbonate. Always give the flush slowly over at least 2 minutes to ensure that the drug already in the line/vein does not move forward in the patient in a sudden rapid surge (especially if the catheter/vein contains an inotrope or vasoactive drug such as aminophylline, cimetidine, phenytoin or ranitidine, which can cause an arrhythmia).
12 When two IV drugs need to be given together and there is only one IV catheter, terminal co-infusion using a T- or Y-connector next to the catheter can be used. It is important to know whether this is safe for the drugs in question.

Minimising IV infusion and IV drugs errors

Errors of both commission and omission occur. For example, excess IV fluids can be dangerous by causing circulatory overload, and inadequate IV fluids can be dangerous by causing hypoglycaemia (especially in the neonate, and commonly when a blood transfusion is being given and the infant is relying on IV glucose).

Extravasation can also result in the absence of a vital drug (e.g. morphine infusion for pain). Errors will always occur where human actions are involved, and it is essential to have systems in place to minimise these.

Steps to reduce errors and their impact
- Prescribe or change infusion rates as infrequently as possible, ideally once or twice daily.
- Never have more than one IV infusion line running at the same time unless this is absolutely necessary (e.g. in major trauma or shock, where two lines are needed for volume replacement and also in case one line is lost at a critical time).
- Use a burette in which no more than the prescribed volume is present (especially in infants and young children).
- Record hourly the amount given (from the burette, syringe or infusion bag) and the amount left.
- Check the infusion site hourly to ensure that extravasation has not occurred.
- Ensure that flushes are only used when essential, and are given slowly over at least 2 minutes.
- Ensure that flushes do not overload the patient with sodium.
- Be particularly careful with potassium solutions given IV (use the enteral route whenever possible).
- Check and double check the following:
  - Is it the right drug? Check the ampoule as well as the box.
  - Is it the right concentration?
  - Is the shelf life of the drug within the expiry date?
  - Has the drug been constituted and diluted correctly?
  - Is the dose right? (Two people are needed to check the prescription chart.)
  - Is it the correct syringe? (Deal with one patient at a time.)
  - Is the IV line patent?
  - Is a separate flush needed? If so, has the flush been checked?
  - Are sharps (including glass ampoules) disposed of?
  - Has it been signed off as completed (and ideally countersigned)?

Writing a prescription
- Use block capitals.
- Use approved names.

- The dosage should be written in grams (g), milligrams (mg) or micrograms. **Always write micrograms in full.**
- Volumes should be written in millilitres (mL).
- Avoid using decimal places whenever possible. If this is not possible, they should be prefaced by a zero. For example, write 500 mg, not 0.5 g, and if a decimal place is used, write 0.5 mL **not** .5 mL.
- Write times using the 24-hour clock.
- Routes of administration can be abbreviated as follows: IV (intravenous), IM (intramuscular), PO (orally), SC (subcutaneous), NEB (nebuliser), RECT (rectally).
- 'As required' prescriptions must be specific about how much, how often and for what purpose (indicate the maximum 24-hour dose).
- Each drug should be signed for individually by a registered doctor.
- Stop dates for short-course treatments should be recorded when first prescribed.

IV drug infusions in severely ill or injured children in high-dependency care

Adrenaline: in 5% dextrose or 0.9% saline. Do not mix with bicarbonate
Dose: 0.05–2 micrograms/kg/minute: this is equivalent to 0.6 mL/kg of 1 in 1000 (600 micrograms/kg) in 100 mL run at 0.5–20 mL/hour.

As a short-term measure, place 1 mg (1 mL of 1 in 1000 adrenaline) in 50 mL of 0.9% saline. Give 2–5 mL (40–100 micrograms) to a child (depending on size) and 1 mL (20 micrograms) to an infant under 1 year of age. Give IV slowly. Repeat as required (with ECG monitoring).

Aminophylline: in 5% dextrose or 0.9% saline
Loading dose **(do not give aminophylline if theophylline has been received in the last 24 hours)**.

IV infusion over 20–30 minutes, 5 mg/kg for children under 12 years of age, and 250–500 mg total if over 12 years of age.

Then give 1 mg/kg/hour if under 12 years and 500 micrograms/kg/hour if over 12 years: this is equivalent to 50 mg/kg in 50 mL run at 1 mL/hour for those under 12 years, and 0.5 mL/hour for those over 12 years.

Dopamine: in 5% dextrose or 0.9% saline or undiluted (ideally via a central line). Do not mix with bicarbonate
This can be mixed with dobutamine.

Give 2–20 micrograms/kg/minute (renal = up to 5 micrograms/kg/minute): this is equivalent to 30 mg/kg in 50 mL run at 0.2–2 mL/hour.

Ketamine: in 5% dextrose or 0.9% saline
Give 10–45 micrograms/kg/minute: this is equivalent to 50 mg/kg in 50 mL run at 0.6–2.7 mL/hour (maximum concentration 50 mg/mL).

Midazolam: in 5% dextrose or 0.9% saline or undiluted
Give 1–6 micrograms/kg/minute (60–360 micrograms/kg/hour): this is equivalent to 6 mg/kg in 50 mL run at 0.5–3 mL/hour.

Or give undiluted (5 mg/mL), run at 0.012–0.072 mL/kg/hour.

Morphine: in 5% dextrose or 0.9% saline
Give 10–60 micrograms/kg/hour: this is equivalent to 1 mg/kg in 50 mL run at 0.5–3 mL/hour.

Salbutamol IV: in 5% dextrose or 0.9% saline
Give 0.6–5 micrograms/kg/minute: this is equivalent to 3 mg/kg in 50 mL run at 0.6–5 mL/hour.

Giving injections

First, find out whether the child has reacted adversely to drugs in the past. Wash your hands thoroughly. **Use disposable needles and syringes**. Clean the chosen site with an antiseptic solution. Carefully check the dose of the drug to be given and draw the correct amount into the syringe. Expel the air from the syringe before injecting. Always record the name and amount of the drug given. Discard disposable syringes in a safe container.

Intramuscular route

In children over 2 years of age, give the injection in the upper outer quadrant of the buttock. Choose the site carefully, well away from the sciatic nerve. In younger or severely malnourished children, use the outer side of the thigh midway between the hip and the knee, or over the deltoid muscle in the upper arm. Hold the muscle at the injection site between the thumb and first finger and push the needle (23- to 25-gauge) into the muscle at a 90-degree angle (45 degrees in the thigh). Draw back the plunger to make sure that there is no blood (if there is, withdraw slightly and try again). Give the drug by pushing the plunger slowly until the end. Remove the needle and press firmly over the injection site with a small swab or cotton wool for at least two minutes.

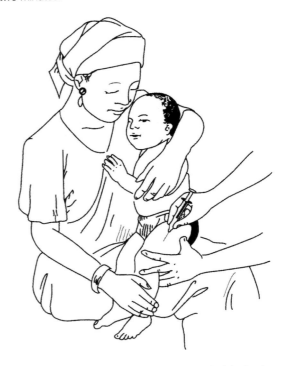

FIGURE 8.4.A.1 Holding a child for an intramuscular injection in the thigh.

Subcutaneous route

Select the site as described above for intramuscular injection. Pinch up skin and subcutaneous tissue between your finger and thumb. Push the needle (23- to 25-gauge) under the skin at an angle of 30–45 degrees into the subcutaneous fatty tissue. Do not go deep to enter the underlying muscle. Draw back the plunger to make sure that there is no blood (if there is, withdraw slightly and try again). Give the drug by pushing the plunger slowly until the end. Remove the needle and press firmly over the injection site with cotton wool for at least two minutes.

Intra-dermal route

Select an area of skin which has no infection or damage for the injection (e.g. over the deltoid in the upper arm). Stretch the skin between the thumb and forefinger of one hand. With the other hand, slowly insert the needle (25-gauge), **bevel upwards**, for about 2 mm just under and almost parallel to the surface of the skin. Considerable resistance is felt when injecting intra-dermally. A raised blanched bleb showing the surface of the hair follicles is a sign that the injection has been given correctly.

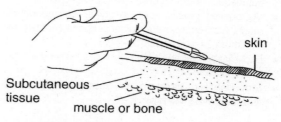

FIGURE 8.4.A.3 Giving an intradermal injection.

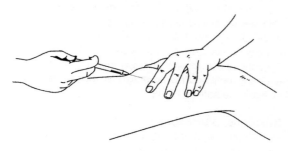

FIGURE 8.4.A.2 Giving a subcutaneous injection.

8.4.B Gaining circulatory access

Peripheral venous cannulation
Preparation of kit
The following equipment is needed:
- 18- to 25-gauge IV cannula or butterfly needles
- 2-mL syringe and T-piece containing Ringer-lactate or Hartmann's solution or 0.9% saline for flushing
- tape or plaster of Paris for scalp veins
- a small splint (this can be made from a wooden spatula covered with gauze)
- alcohol swabs for skin cleaning
- local anaesthetic cream if available
- tourniquet (or assistant)
- cannula size:

neonates:	24–25G
infants:	22–24G
children:	20–22G
adolescents:	18–20G.

Procedure
Apply the tourniquet to distend the vein (do not forget to remove it after cannulation).
   Choose a vein:
- forearm
- long saphenous vein (anterior to the medial malleolus)
- back of the hand or front of the wrist
- scalp.

Useful sites to cannulate include the dorsum of the feet and hands. The saphenous and antecubital veins are larger, but can be useful for percutaneously inserted 'long lines'. The antecubital veins are also useful for venepuncture for laboratory studies.
- If possible, place the cannula close to the bone where it is more fixed.
- Decide the direction of blood flow.

- Clean the skin with antiseptic.
- Fix and slightly stretch the skin with your other hand.
- Pass the cannula through the skin at a slight angle (10–20 degrees). **Be decisive.**
- Stop once you are through the skin.
- Flatten the cannula to the skin and advance with the long axis of the cannula in the same direction as the vein. **Be decisive.**
- Aim to pass it into the vein at the first attempt with steady advancement.
- Always watch for blood appearing in the hub of the cannula.
- As soon as blood is seen, stop.
- Hold the needle still, and advance the cannula over the needle until the hub is at the skin.
- Hold the cannula still.
- Withdraw the needle.
- Connect the connector, flush and fix. No subcutaneous swelling should be seen and there should be no resistance to injection.
- If no blood is seen on advancing the cannula, but it is felt to be beyond the vein, **stop**.
- Gently pull the cannula back in the same direction as advancement; if blood appears, **stop** once again. Follow the same procedure as if blood was seen on first advancement (transfixion technique).
- Connect the T-piece and flush the cannula gently with Ringer-lactate or Hartmann's solution or 0.9% saline to confirm that it is in the vein.
- If the cannula is satisfactorily inserted, tape it in place by looping a thin piece of the tape under the hub and round to form a 'V' shape fixing it to the skin.

When splinting, try to 'double back' the tape (i.e. put a short piece and a long piece back to back, leaving just the ends of the longer piece sticky). This helps to prevent excessive amounts of tape sticking to the baby, which is particularly important in the case of more immature babies whose skin is easily damaged.

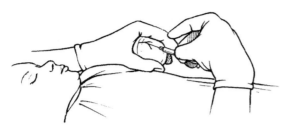

FIGURE 8.4.B.1 Inserting an intravenous cannula into a vein on the back of the hand. The hand is flexed to obstruct venous return and thus make the veins visible.

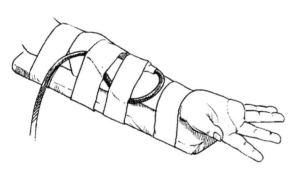

FIGURE 8.4.B.2 Arm splinted to prevent bending of the wrist.

Note on flushing lines

The smaller the syringe used, the greater the pressure exerted on fluid in the line. Therefore avoid using 1-mL syringes to flush a blocked line, as the line may rupture or tissue may be damaged by infiltration.

Care of the IV cannula

Secure the cannula when it has been introduced. This may require the splinting of neighbouring joints to limit the movement of the catheter. Keep the overlying skin clean and dry. Fill the cannula with Ringer-lactate or Hartmann's solution or 0.9% saline immediately after the initial insertion and after each injection.

Blood sampling from the IV cannula

If the patient needs blood samples at the time of cannulation it is often possible to take these as the cannula is inserted. Blood can be dripped from the end of the cannula into the appropriate bottles, or a syringe can be used to **gently** aspirate blood from the cannula. If the cannula has been flushed prior to insertion, the first 0.5–1 mL of blood should be discarded.

Common complications

Superficial infection of the skin at the cannula site is the commonest complication. The infection may lead to thrombophlebitis, which will occlude the vein and result in fever, and may progress to septicaemia. The surrounding skin is red and tender. Remove the cannula **immediately** to reduce the risk of further spread of the infection. Antibiotic

treatment (effective against *Staphylococcus aureus*) should be given.

IV drug administration through an indwelling cannula

Attach the syringe containing the IV drug to the injection port of the cannula and introduce the drug. Once all of the drug has been given, inject 0.5 mL of Ringer-lactate or Hartmann's solution or 0.9% saline into the cannula until all of the drug has entered the circulation and the catheter is filled with the infusion fluid.

Safe IV infusions where no burettes are available

- Mark the infusion bottle with tape for each hour to be given, and label each hour, **or**
- Empty until only the necessary amount to be given is left in the bottle.

Special sites for IV cannulae

Scalp veins

Procedure

1. Restrain the child.
2. Shave the appropriate area of the scalp with a sterile razor.
3. Clean the skin.
   - Have an assistant distend the vein by holding a taut piece of tubing or bandaging perpendicular to it, proximal to (nearest to the child's body) the site of puncture.
4. Fill the syringe with Ringer-lactate or Hartmann's solution or 0.9% saline and flush the butterfly set.
   - Disconnect the syringe and leave the end of the tubing open.
5. Puncture the skin and enter the vein. Blood will flow back through the tubing.
   - Infuse a small quantity of fluid to see that the cannula is properly placed and then tape it into position.
   - **Care should be taken not to cannulate an artery, which is recognised by pulsation on palpation. If there is a pulsatile spurting of blood, withdraw the needle and apply pressure until the bleeding stops. Then look for a vein.**

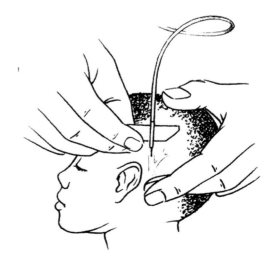

FIGURE 8.4.B.3 Inserting a scalp vein needle.

Scalp drips are generally more precarious than ones in the limbs, and need to be carefully observed. Infiltration into the soft tissues of the scalp can spread quickly and cause extensive necrosis if irritant. Shave the hair from an area about 2–3 cm around the site selected in order to allow for fixation by tape. Always ensure that the tip of the needle is not covered by dressings, so that infiltration is quickly seen.

External jugular vein
Procedure

1 Place child in a 15–30-degree head-down position (or with padding under the shoulders so that the head hangs lower than the shoulders). Wrapping may be necessary to restrain the child (see above).

2 Turn the head away from the site of puncture. Restrain the child as necessary in this position.

3 Clean the skin over the appropriate side of the neck.

4 Identify the external jugular vein, which can be seen passing over the sternocleidomastoid muscle at the junction of its middle and lower thirds.

5 Have an assistant place their finger at the lower end of the visible part of the vein just above the clavicle. This stabilises it and compresses it so that it remains distended.

6 Puncture the skin and enter the vein pointing in the direction of the clavicle.

7 When free flow of blood is obtained, ensure that no air bubbles are present in the tubing, and then attach a giving set.

8 Tape the cannula securely in position. One of the most important points is to ensure that the cannula is properly secured in the vein by high-quality fixation. It is easily removed by the child, so use plenty of tape!

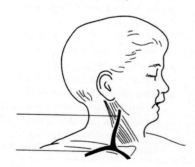

External jugular vein

Subclavian vein

FIGURE 8.4.B.4 Position of the external jugular vein.

Be aware that there is a higher risk of air embolism than with peripheral venous cannulation.

If infusion through a peripheral vein or scalp vein is not possible, and it is essential to give IV fluids to keep the child alive:

- set up an intra-osseous infusion
- **or** use a central vein
- **or** perform a venous cut-down.

All of these procedures are described below.

Central venous cannulation

This should not be used routinely. It should only be performed when IV access is urgent and, in the case of central veins, only by those who have been trained in the technique (it is best done by an anaesthetist). Remove the cannula from a central vein as soon as possible (i.e. when IV fluids or drugs are no longer essential, or when a peripheral vein can be cannulated successfully).

The aims of central venous cannulation are as follows:

- to obtain venous access when peripheral cannulation is not possible (**however, in an emergency, intra-osseous cannulation is faster and easier**).
- to monitor central venous pressure
- to obtain prolonged vascular access
- to obtain large-bore vascular access
- to administer certain drugs
- during resuscitation.

Procedure

Several routes are possible, but the most widely used are the femoral and internal jugular approaches. The femoral approach is easiest in the emergency situation. A subclavian approach may be useful in the older child.

Preparation of kit

The following equipment is needed:

- sterile pack
- sterile Seldinger wires
- cannula: single 16- to 22G cannula
- single, double or triple lumen if available (5 FG 5–8 cm length for neonate, 7 FG 8–15 cm length for child)
- syringe and Ringer-lactate or Hartmann's solution or saline
- suture and tape for fixing
- local anaesthetic with fine 25G needles.

Preparation of the child

- Explain what is going to happen (if the child is conscious).
- Position the child.
- **Sterilise the skin and maintain sterile technique.**
- Apply local analgesia to the skin (if the child is conscious).

Two insertion techniques are available, namely:

- the same as in peripheral cannulation
- the Seldinger technique (wire)
- ideally an ultrasound probe can help identify the vein and ensure the cannula when inserted is in the correct position in the lumen of the vein.

Seldinger method

1 Identify the vein with cannula on syringe (same approach as for peripheral cannulation); there must be good flow.

2 Stop, and pass the cannula over the needle.

3 Disconnect the syringe.

4 Pass the wire through the cannula to three-quarters the length of wire (if there is any resistance, stop, withdraw the wire with needle, and start again).

5 Holding the wire firmly, withdraw the needle over the wire.

6 Pass the dilator over the wire (it is sometimes necessary to make a small cut at the skin) and, holding the wire firmly, withdraw the dilator.

7 Pass the cannula/catheter filled with Ringer-lactate or Hartmann's solution or 0.9% saline over the wire (passage of the cannula should be smooth, meeting no resistance).

8 Hold the cannula, and withdraw the wire (gently if it sticks, do not force it).

9 Confirm correct placement by aspiration of blood.

10 Suture and fix with antiseptic ointment over the entry site.

11 Confirm the position with an X-ray.

Femoral cannulation

This is adequate for almost all needs, is technically much easier and has lower complication rates, particularly in neonates and infants. However, if it is not a sterile procedure, there is a risk of causing septic arthritis in the hip joint.

1 Position the patient supine with the leg slightly abducted. Place a towel under the buttocks to raise the pelvis.

2 Clean the skin and drape with sterile towels. Locate the vein by finding the femoral arterial pulsation 2 cm below the midpoint of the inguinal ligament. The vein lies immediately medial to the artery. If the child is conscious, infiltrate the skin and subcutaneous area with 1% lignocaine.

3 With a finger on the femoral artery introduce the needle with syringe attached at an angle of 30–45 degrees to the skin along the line of the vein pointing towards the umbilicus. Advance the needle while aspirating.

4 When blood 'flashes back' into the syringe, stop advancing and remove the syringe from the needle. Feed the Seldinger guide wire through the needle, keeping hold of one end of the wire at all times.

5 Withdraw the needle over the wire, then feed the catheter over the wire into the vein.

6 Withdraw the wire and aspirate for blood to confirm the position. Then flush the catheter with Ringer-lactate or Hartmann's solution or 0.9% saline.

7 Suture the catheter in place.

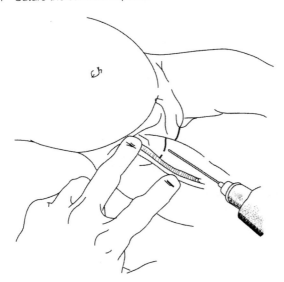

FIGURE 8.4.B.5 Femoral vein cannulation.

If you are unsure whether you are in a vein or an artery, consider transducing the pressure waveform.

Internal jugular vein

Use a head-down position for the internal jugular and subclavian approaches, as this increases vein distension and reduces the risk of air embolism.

Procedure

1 Place the child in a 30-degree head-down position and turn their head to the left-hand side for the right-sided approach, which avoids the lymphatic duct. Place a towel or roll under the shoulders to extend the neck.

2 Clean the skin and drape with towels, exposing the neck to the clavicle.

3 Identify the apex of the triangle formed by the two heads of the sternocleidomastoid and clavicle, and infiltrate local anaesthetic (if the child is conscious). Alternatively, identify carotid pulsation medial to the sternomastoid at the level of the lower border of the thyroid cartilage, and the vein (usually) just lateral to this. Aim the needle at 30 degrees to the skin and towards the ipsilateral nipple (note that the neck is very short and the vein is superficial in the very young). Estimate the length of catheter from the point of skin entry to the nipple.

4 Direct the needle at 30 degrees to the skin, pointing towards the right nipple, and puncture the skin at the apex of the triangle.

5 Holding this position, advance the needle, aspirating all the time. If blood 'flashes back', stop advancing and remove the syringe from the needle. (If you do not cannulate the vein, withdraw the needle, but not out of the skin, and advance again slightly more laterally.)

6 Feed the Seldinger guide wire through the needle, always having control of one end of the wire.

7 Withdraw the needle over the guide wire and then feed the catheter over the wire into the superior vena cava.

8 Withdraw the wire, aspirate for blood and attach the infusion set. **Do not leave the catheter open, as this may lead to an air embolism.**

9 Suture the catheter in place and obtain a chest X-ray (if possible) to check for a pneumothorax and the position of the catheter tip, which should be in the superior vena cava (SVC), ideally at the junction of the SVC and the right atrium, but not in the right atrium.

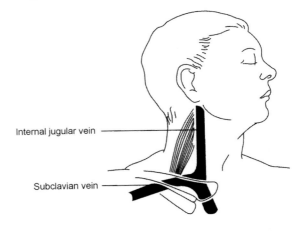

Internal jugular vein

Subclavian vein

FIGURE 8.4.B.6 Position of the internal jugular and subclavian veins.

Subclavian vein

1 Place the patient in a supine position, turn the head to the contralateral side, position a roll to extend the neck a little, and identify the midpoint of the clavicle.

2 Aim for the suprasternal notch, and pass the needle just beneath the clavicle at the midpoint. The vein lies anterior to the subclavian artery and is closest at the medial end of the clavicle.

3 Subclavian artery puncture is not uncommon (it is not

possible to use compression to stop the bleeding, but this is rarely a problem unless coagulopathy is present).

Complications
These are fewer and less severe in femoral cannulation, but include the following:
- arterial puncture
- nerve damage
- pneumothorax in neck access veins
- extravasation-administered fluids/drugs
- septicaemia if the procedure is not sterile or if the cannula is in place for more than 5 days.

Cut-down venous cannulation
Indication
Continuous IV access is needed where percutaneous attempts have failed. **In the emergency situation, intraosseous access is faster and easier.** Cut-down is less appropriate if speed is essential.

Preparation of kit
The following equipment is needed:
- skin prep (iodine, alcohol)
- scalpel
- suture
- IV cannula
- local anaesthetic
- curved artery forceps
- syringe and hypodermic needle
- sterile drapes.

Procedure
Identify landmarks. The **long saphenous vein** at the ankle is superior and medial to the medial malleolus of the ankle. The **brachial vein** at the elbow is lateral to the medial epicondyle of the humerus.

Brachial vein:
- Infant: one finger breadth lateral to the medial epicondyle of the humerus.
- Small child: two finger breadths lateral to the medial epicondyle of the humerus.
- Older child: three finger breadths lateral to the medial epicondyle of the humerus.

Long saphenous vein:
- Infant: half a finger breadth superior and anterior to the medial malleolus.
- Small child: one finger breadth superior and anterior to the medial malleolus.
- Older child: two finger breadths superior and anterior to the medial malleolus.

1 Immobilise the lower leg and clean the skin, as described above. Identify the long saphenous vein, which lies half a finger breadth (in the infant) or one finger breadth (in the small child) superior and anterior to the medial malleolus.
2 Clean the skin and drape with sterile towels.
3 Infiltrate the skin with 1% lignocaine using a fine 24- to 25G needle, and make an incision through the skin perpendicular to the long axis of the vein. Bluntly dissect the subcutaneous tissue with haemostat forceps.
4 Identify and free a 1–2 cm section of vein. Pass a proximal and distal ligature.

5 Tie off* the distal end of the vein, keeping the ties as long as possible for traction.
6 Make a small hole in the upper part of the exposed vein, gently dilate the opening with the tip of a closed haemostat, and insert the cannula (without the needle/trocar in it) into this, while holding the distal tie to stabilise the position of the vein.
7 Secure the cannula in place with the upper ligature.
8 Attach a syringe filled with Ringer-lactate or Hartmann's solution or saline and ensure that the fluid flows freely up the vein. If it does not, check that the cannula is in the vein or try withdrawing it slightly to improve the flow.
9 Tie the distal ligature* around the catheter, and then close the skin incision with interrupted sutures.
10 Place antiseptic ointment (e.g. iodine) over the wound, and suture or tape the catheter to the skin (ensure that local anaesthetic is used at the suture site if the child is conscious). Cover with sterile dressing.

* It is also possible to dispense with the proximal and distal ligatures and simply penetrate the vein directly with a plastic over-the-needle cannula as you would if penetrating the skin externally. Once in the vein, remove the inner needle and secure in position.

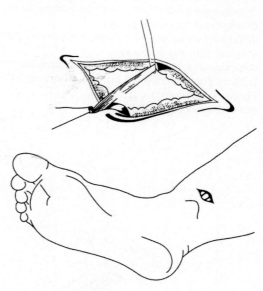

FIGURE 8.4.B.7 Cut-down incision showing vein: position of cutdown on long saphenous vein at ankle.

Complications
These include the following:
- haemorrhage or haematoma
- perforation of the posterior wall of the vein
- nerve transection
- phlebitis
- venous thrombosis.

Umbilical vein catheterisation
Indications
- Where there is urgency during resuscitation of the newborn to give IV fluids and drugs.
- Temporarily for exchange transfusion. The catheter should not be left in position between exchanges.

Time of insertion

Catheterisation is usually easy in the first 4 days of life, and possible from 5 to 7 days.

Passing an umbilical vein catheter is the quickest and easiest way to access the circulation in the newborn.

Preparation of kit

The following equipment is needed:

- gown and gloves
- sterile instruments including:
  - fine scissors
  - forceps
  - scalpel
- silk suture for retaining
- 5 French gauge umbilical catheter
  - a sterile feeding tube may be satisfactory if an umbilical catheter is not available, but measure the length first so that you will know how much you have passed by measuring the length from the hub to the umbilical insertion. Cannulae designed for use as umbilical vein cannulae are usually marked in 5-cm increments
- a three-way tap
- 0.5% chlorhexidine or 10% povidone-iodine for cleaning the skin
- sterile cotton wool balls
- sterile towels or drapes to cover the baby's abdomen
- sterile 2-mL syringe and connector filled with Ringer-lactate or Hartmann's solution or 0.9% saline.

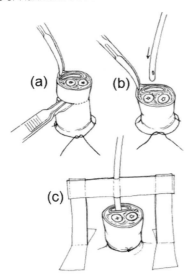

FIGURE 8.4.B.8 Insertion and securing of a catheter in the umbilical vein. (a) Preparation of the umbilical cord. (b) Inserting the catheter into the umbilical vein, which is the larger thin-walled structure towards the head. Note the two umbilical arteries, which are thick-walled and towards the legs of the baby. (c) Securing the inserted catheter to prevent kinking.

Procedure

1. Assemble the syringe, three-way tap and catheter. Flush and fill the catheter with sterile 0.9% saline. Then close the tap to prevent air entry (which may cause air embolus).
2. Clean the umbilical cord and surrounding skin with 0.5% chlorhexidine or 10% povidone-iodine, and then loosely tie a suture around the base of the cord.

3. Cut back the cord to about 2 cm from the base.
4. Cover the skin with towels to form a sterile working surface.
5. Hold the cord at an edge with forceps.
6. Identify the vein. It is usually gaping, larger, and well separated from the two small thicker-walled arteries.
7. Hold the catheter approximately 2 cm from the end with non-toothed forceps, and insert the tip into the vein. Gently advance the catheter, which should pass easily.
8. Insert the catheter for a distance of 4–6 cm.
9. Check that the catheter is not kinked and that blood draws back easily. If there is a block, pull gently on the cord, pull back the catheter partly and reinsert.
10. The catheter can be secured by winding a suture round it several times and then passing a stitch through the cord base. An additional safeguard is to form two wings of tape which can then be taped to the abdominal wall, always remembering that it is preferable to use as little tape as possible in smaller babies. However, it is essential that the catheter does not fall out.

Occasionally the umbilical vein is kinked and advance of the catheter is blocked at 1–2 cm beyond the abdominal wall. Gentle traction on the cord usually relieves this.

If obstruction occurs at more than 2 cm, and only partly gives way with pressure, the catheter is probably either wedged in the portal system or coiled up in the portal sinus. It is advisable to withdraw the catheter part way and reinsert it.

Care of indwelling catheters

Leave the cord exposed to air. Remove blocked catheters.

Removal of the catheter

1. Use sterile technique.
2. Remove a specimen of blood for culture.
3. If possible, place a purse-string suture around the vessel at the base of the umbilicus and withdraw the catheter slowly.
4. Tighten the purse-string suture.
5. Apply pressure to the umbilical stump for 5–10 minutes.

Time of removal of catheter

Remove the catheter as soon as possible as dictated by the clinical state of the baby. The infection rate rises after 24 hours. Complications are more common with venous catheters than with arterial ones, so venous catheters should rarely be left in.

Complications

These include the following:

- thrombosis survivors may develop portal vein thrombosis
- embolism from clots in the catheter, or from injected air
- vascular perforation
- vascular damage from hypertonic solutions (more common when the tip is in the portal system)
- haemorrhage from a disconnected catheter
- necrotising enterocolitis or bowel perforation may occur as a complication of exchange transfusion
- infection
- there is no evidence that prophylactic antibiotics are of any value.

Intra-osseous needle insertion

Intra-osseous infusion is a safe, simple and reliable method of giving fluid and drugs in an emergency when venous access is not possible (e.g. in shock).

Site for needle

The first choice for the puncture is the proximal tibia. The site for needle insertion is in the middle of the antero-medial surface of the tibia, at the junction of the upper and middle third, to avoid damaging the epiphyseal plate (which is higher in the tibia), 2–3 cm below the tibial tuberosity. An alternative site for needle insertion is the distal femur, 2 cm above the lateral condyle.

Intra-osseous needles (15- to 18-gauge)

If a purpose-made intra-osseous needle is not available, a number of alternatives can be used, including bone-marrow needles, short lumbar puncture needles or a large-calibre venepuncture needle. For example, a green needle can be used in a neonate. The disadvantage of venepuncture needles is that they may carry a fragment of bone into the marrow. This is not dangerous, but it may block the needle. Also the bevel of these needles is long, and extravasation of fluid is more likely than with a purpose-made intra-osseous needle.

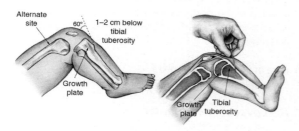

FIGURE 8.4.B.9 (a) Intra-osseous needle tibial site (X). (b) Section through bone. Image reprinted with permission from Medscape Reference (http://emedicine.medscape.com/), 2014, available at: http://emedicine.medscape.com/article/940993-overview.

Other equipment needed

This includes the following:

1 a sterile 2-mL syringe containing 1–2% lignocaine to be used whenever the patient is conscious (otherwise the procedure will be very painful)
2 two sterile 5-mL syringes
3 sterile 20- or 50-mL syringes and ideally a three-way tap.

Procedure

1 Place padding under the child's knee so that it is bent at 30 degrees from the straight (180-degree) position, with the heel resting on the table.
2 Locate the correct position (described above and shown in Figure 8.4.B.9).
3 Wash your hands and put on sterile gloves. (To avoid osteomyelitis, the procedure must involve strict asepsis using an antiseptic solution and sterile gauze to clean the site, with the operator wearing sterile gloves.) Clean the skin over and surrounding the site with an antiseptic solution.
4 Infiltrate with lidocaine down to the periosteum if the child is conscious.

5 Ask an assistant to stabilise the proximal tibia by grasping the thigh and knee above and lateral to the cannulation site, with the fingers and thumb wrapped around the knee but not directly behind the insertion site.
6 Insert the needle at a 90-degree angle with the bevel pointing towards the foot. Advance the needle slowly using a gentle but firm twisting or drilling motion.
7 Stop advancing the needle when you feel a sudden decrease in resistance or when you can aspirate blood. The needle should now be fixed in the bone and stand up by itself.
8 Remove the stylet.
9 Aspirate the marrow contents (which look like blood), using the 5-mL syringe, to confirm that the needle is in the marrow cavity and to provide bone marrow/blood for the following tests when appropriate: blood glucose, haemoglobin, group and cross-matching, blood culture and urea and electrolytes. Hb, glucose and electrolyte measurements may not be accurate after infusions have been previously given. Note that **failure to aspirate bone-marrow contents does not mean that the needle is not correctly placed**.
10 Attach the second 5-mL syringe filled with Ringer-lactate or Hartmann's solution or 0.9% saline. Stabilise the needle and slowly inject 3 mL while palpating the area for any leakage under the skin. If no infiltration is seen, start the infusion.
11 Attach the 50-mL syringe, usually containing Ringer-lactate or Hartmann's solution or saline, but compatible blood or 10% glucose can be used if hypoglycaemia is suspected, and push in the infusion fluid in boluses. **It is not possible to infuse fluid through the intra-osseous needle using a standard IV giving set.** The fluid has to be pushed in under light pressure, and if large volumes are needed (e.g. when giving boluses of fluid to treat shock) then 20-mL or 50-mL syringes should be used.
12 Check that the calf does not swell during the injections of fluid.
13 Secure IV access as soon as possible.
14 When the needle has been removed, cover with a sterile dressing.

Do not place distal to a major fracture or where there is infection.

Give prophylactic antibiotics after the immediate emergency has been managed.

All drugs and fluids that are given IV (including 10% glucose) can be given into the bone marrow, and they will reach the heart and general circulation as fast as if they had been given through a central vein.

Remove the intra-osseous needle as soon as venous access is available. In any case, it should not be in place for more than 8 hours.

Complications

These include the following:

- dislodgement
- misplacement (penetration through posterior cortex, failure to penetrate cortex), resulting in:
  - haematoma
  - tissue necrosis
  - compartment syndrome

- skin infection
- osteomyelitis
- tibial fracture in babies.

The scalp vein needle as an intra-osseous device

In infants, a green 'butterfly' (scalp vein) needle can be used as an intra-osseous needle with the same precautions as above.

Battery-powered intra-osseous device

The EZ-IO drill is a powered device that enables rapid insertion of an intra-osseous needle.

Unfortunately the disposable needles are extremely and prohibitively expensive for low resource settings.

Various sizes of needle are available (see Figures 8.4.B.10 and 8.4.B.11) for different-sized patients.

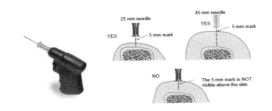

FIGURE 8.4.B.10 EZ-IO power drill and needles.

The landmarks are as before, using the upper end of the tibia. In adults in particular, the upper outer aspect of the humerus can also be used.

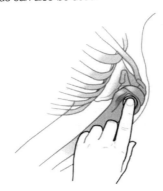

FIGURE 8.4.B.11 Site for EZ-IO needle in the proximal humerus in an adult or large child.

The procedure is less painful for the conscious patient due to its rapidity, the drilling effect and the sharpness of the needles. The EZ-IO needles are available in two sizes, for patients under 40 kg and over 40 kg.

The procedure for insertion is as follows:

1 Take universal precautions for sterile procedure.
2 Clean the site.
3 Choose an appropriate size of needle and attach it to the drill. It will fix magnetically.
4 Remove the safety cap from the needle.
5 If the patient is conscious, control their movement during insertion.
6 Hold the drill and needle at 90 degrees to the skin surface and push through the skin without drilling, until bone is felt. Ensure that at least 5 mm of the needle is visible at this point.

7 Squeeze the drill button and drill continuously, applying gentle steady downward pressure until there is sudden loss of resistance – there is a palpable 'give' as the needle breaches the cortex. Release the trigger and stop insertion at this point.

If the driver stalls and will not penetrate the bone you may be applying too much downward pressure.

If the driver fails (this is rare) remove it, grasp the needle kit by hand and twist it into the bone marrow.

8 Remove the drill and unscrew the trochar.
9 Aspirate the bone marrow if possible directly from the needle.
10 Attach the pre-prepared connection tube containing sterile Ringer-lactate or Hartmann's solution or 0.9% saline before any infusion is given.

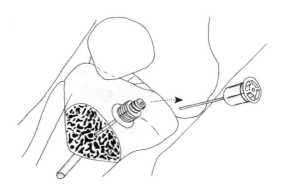

FIGURE 8.4.B.12 EZ-IO needle in place, with stylet removed.

Do not attach a syringe directly to the EZ-IO catheter hub except when drawing blood with the needle set stabilised by hand (sterile).

11 There is an optional device for securing the needle, but this is not essential.
12 Proceed with the required therapy. It should be noted that rapid infusion of fluid may be painful for the conscious patient.
13 Apply a sterile dressing.
14 When removing the catheter, attach a Luer lock syringe, and continuously rotate it clockwise while slowly and gently applying traction to the catheter. Do not rock or bend the catheter during removal.
15 Do not leave the catheter in place for more than 24 hours.

Needle pericardiocentesis

Needle pericardiocentesis is a rarely used skill but can be life-saving when indicated.

Indications

This procedure is used:
- to reduce a pericardial effusion that is causing haemodynamic compromise
- to diagnose pericarditis.

In the trauma situation this procedure is performed when cardiac tamponade is suspected. This is usually, but not always, caused by a penetrating injury between the nipple line and the shoulder blades. The clinical findings are shock, muffled heart sounds (although this is a difficult sign to elicit with confidence) and distended neck veins. It is important to differentiate between this and tension pneumothorax, in which the trachea is deviated and air entry reduced on the affected side. Ideally this procedure should be carried out under ECG control, but if that is not available, extra care must be taken.

If available, ultrasound is the easiest/safest way of making a diagnosis of cardiac tamponade.

Preparation of kit
The following equipment is needed:
- ECG monitor
- syringe
- skin prep
- local anaesthetic
- over-needle cannula (16- to 18-gauge)
- sterile drapes.

Technique
1. Position the patient supine and attach the ECG. Stand on the patient's right with the ECG monitor at the patient's head so that you can see it easily.
2. Clean the skin from nipples to umbilicus and drape with sterile towels to expose the peri-xiphoid region. This must be a sterile procedure. Infiltrate local anaesthetic at the costal margin just below the xiphoid process.
3. Attach the cannula to the syringe. Insert the cannula just below and to the left of the xiphoid process. Angle the needle at 45 degrees to the skin and pointing towards the tip of the left scapula.
4. Advance the needle, holding this position, aspirating all the time and watching the cardiac monitor. As you enter

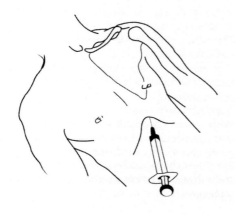

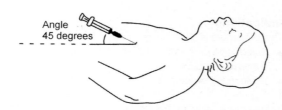

Angle
45 degrees

FIGURE 8.4.B.13 Position for insertion of needle in pericardiocentesis. The pericardiocentesis needle is inserted as close to the sternum as possible in order to avoid the internal mammary artery.

the distended pericardial sac, fluid will flow back into the syringe. If the myocardium is touched, the ECG pattern will change (arrhythmia, ectopics, 'injury' pattern). If you can aspirate large amounts of bright red blood you have entered the ventricle, in which case you should withdraw slightly.
5. If successful, cardiac function should improve immediately. Withdraw the needle, attach a three-way tap, and secure the cannula for further aspirations.
6. This is a temporary procedure, and some patients will require a formal pericardiotomy. **Pericardial aspiration may not work well for viscous fluids (e.g. clotted blood) in the pericardial sac.**

Defibrillation
There are two indications for this procedure:
1. In cardiac arrest when the rhythm is ventricular fibrillation (VF) or pulseless ventricular tachycardia (VT) (see Section 1.13). The dose is 4 joules/kg in children.
2. In supraventricular tachycardia (SVT) or ventricular tachycardia without shock (see Section 5.4.C). The dose is 0.5 joules/kg, rising to 1 joule/kg then 2 joules/kg if the first shocks were unsuccessful.

In any patient who is not *in extremis*, anaesthesia/sedation must be given before the DC shock is administered.

Safety
A defibrillator delivers enough current to **cause** cardiac arrest. **The user must ensure that other rescuers are not in physical contact with the patient (or the trolley) at the moment when the shock is delivered.** The defibrillator should only be charged when the paddles are either in contact with the child or replaced properly in their storage positions. **Oxygen must be discontinued and be moved right away from the patient.**

Procedure
Basic life support should be interrupted for the shortest possible time (see steps 5 to 9 below).
1. Apply gel pads or electrode gel.
2. Select the correct paddles (paediatric paddles for patients weighing less than 10 kg). If only adult paddles are available for a small child, put one on the front of the child's chest and one on the back.
3. Select the energy required.
4. Place the electrodes on the pads of gel, and apply firm pressure.
5. Press the charge button.
6. Wait until the defibrillator is charged.
7. Shout 'Stand back!'
8. Check that all of the other rescuers are standing clear.
9. Deliver the shock.

Correct paddle placement
The usual placement is antero-lateral. One paddle is put over the cardiac apex in the mid-axillary line, and the other is placed just to the right of the sternum, immediately below the clavicle.

Good paddle contact
Gel pads or electrode gel should always be used (if the latter is used, care should be taken not to join the two

areas of application). Firm pressure should be applied to the paddles.

Correct energy selection

The recommended level in VF or pulseless VT cardiac arrest is 4 joules/kg (with no patient sedation).

In arrhythmias with a pulse, the dose is 0.5 joules/kg, then 1 joule/kg, then 2 joules/kg if the previous doses were unsuccessful (always with sedation).

Automatic external defibrillators (AEDs)

Automatic external defibrillators (AEDs) are used in adults both to assess cardiac rhythm and to deliver defibrillation (see Section 1.13 for details). In children, AEDs can accurately detect ventricular fibrillation at all ages, but there is concern about their ability to identify tachycardic rhythms

in infants correctly. At present, therefore, AEDs can be used to identify rhythms in children but not in infants.

Many AEDs now have paediatric attenuation pads which decrease the energy to a level more appropriate for the child (aged 1–8 years), or leads that reduce the total energy to 50–80 joules. This means that AEDs can be used for all children over the age of 1 year. Institutions that treat infants who might need defibrillation must provide manual defibrillators.

Guidance

- With a manual defibrillator use 4 joules/kg to defibrillate patients of all ages.
- With an unattenuated AED (see above), children over 8 years of age can be defibrillated.
- With an AED with paediatric pads or paddles, children aged 1–8 years can be defibrillated.

8.5 Other procedures

Insertion of an orogastric or nasogastric tube

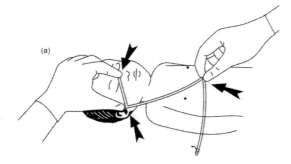

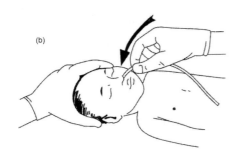

FIGURE 8.5.1 Inserting a nasogastric tube. (a) The distance from the nose to the ear and then to the epigastrium is measured. (b) The tube is then inserted to the measured distance.

The nasogastric tube is used to feed any child who is unable to take food by mouth.

Preparation of kit

The following equipment is needed:

- nasogastric tube
- lubricant
- pH indicator paper or litmus paper
- syringe
- stethoscope
- adhesive tape.

In preterm infants:

- 4 French gauge tube is used for infants who weigh ≤ 1000 grams
- 6 French gauge tube is used for infants who weigh > 1000 grams (and most neonates)
- 8 to 10 French gauge tube is used for abdominal decompression (e.g. in infants with ileus or who are receiving continuous positive airway pressure).

Procedure

1 Place the child supine with their head in the 'sniffing' position.
2 Measure the length of the tube from the nose via the earlobe to the midpoint between the xiphoid and the umbilicus. Mark the tube at this point with indelible pen.
3 Feed the tube lubricated with KY Jelly or saline through either the nose or the mouth directly backwards. (The neonate is a nose breather, and therefore if there is respiratory distress the oral route may be preferred.) Try to advance the tube as the child swallows. If a baby has respiratory distress, a gastric tube is best passed through the mouth.
4 Check the position of the tube by very gently aspirating 0.2–0.5 mL of stomach contents using a small (2- or 5-mL) syringe (larger ones can damage the gastric mucosa) and checking the change in the pH indicator

paper (the pH should be 5.5 or less, or the litmus paper should change colour from blue to pink), or flush the tube with 2–3 mL of air (only 1 mL in the neonate) and listen over the stomach area with the stethoscope. If in doubt, X-ray the chest and/or abdomen. (Note that the acidity of the gastric fluid may be reduced in preterm infants.)

5 If there is any doubt about the location of the tube, withdraw it and start again. Withdraw immediately if the child starts coughing, as the tube may then be in the airway.

6 Secure the tube by taping it to the cheek, and record the length of tube outside the nose or mouth.

7 When the tube is in place, fix a 50-mL syringe (without the plunger) to the end of the tube, and pour food or fluid into the syringe, allowing it to flow by gravity.

The nasal route is more comfortable and secure, but if the infant has respiratory distress or is receiving CPAP, an orogastric tube is best (if passed through the nose the tube increases upper airway resistance).

Never pass a nasogastric tube in a head-injured patient. An orogastric tube is safe. If there is a base-of-skull fracture, a nasal tube could be pushed into brain tissue.

Cervical spine immobilisation

All patients with major trauma should have full spinal stabilisation if feasible from the moment of injury, and should be treated as if they have a cervical spine injury until proven otherwise. Immobilisation can be achieved:

- by holding the head still and in line (manual in-line immobilisation)
- **or** by applying a semi-rigid collar (which has been correctly fitted), sandbags on either side of the head, and tape across the forehead and the chin piece of the collar to prevent the head from being lifted upward from the bed.

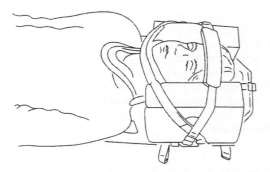

FIGURE 8.5.2 Immobilisation of the cervical spine using head blocks and straps with a cervical collar in place.

Exceptions

Two groups of patients may prove to be difficult:

- the frightened uncooperative child (most common)
- the hypoxic combative patient.

In both of these cases, over-enthusiastic efforts to immobilise the neck may increase the risk of spinal injury as the patient struggles to escape. The area of greatest mobility in the cervical spine is the C7/T1 junction, and this is at increased risk in the combative patient.

It is best to try to apply just a collar and then address the patient's other clinical needs (*see* Section 7.3).

Log roll

When examining the back of the patient with major injury, it is important to minimise the risk associated with unrecognised spinal injury. It is essential to examine the back of the patient at the end of the primary survey (or even during it if there is suspicion of serious injury to the back of the chest or abdomen).

The aim of the log roll is to maintain the orientation of the spine during turning of the patient. It requires four people for a mother or child and three for an infant. In addition, one person is required for the examination of injuries.

TABLE 8.5.1 Position of staff for log roll

Staff number	Position of staff for log roll	
	Infant or small child	**Larger child or mother**
1	Examination of back	Examination of back
2	Stabilisation of head and neck – in charge of the procedure	Stabilisation of head and neck – in charge of the procedure
3	Chest	Chest
4	Pelvis and legs	Pelvis
5		Legs

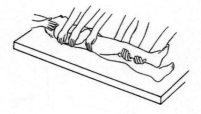

FIGURE 8.5.3 Log rolling a child.

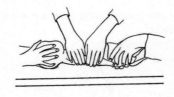

FIGURE 8.5.4 Log rolling an infant.

Incision and drainage of abscess
Indications

- The collection of localised infection.
- If there is uncertainty whether a hot red mass is an abscess, aspirate for pus before proceeding to incision and drainage.
- Multiple/recurrent abscesses may be associated with HIV, TB, malnutrition, diabetes mellitus, anaemia or foreign bodies.

Preparation of kit

The following equipment is needed:

- skin preparation materials
- scalpel
- microbiology swab
- curette
- sterile gauze.

Procedure

1 If the patient is systemically unwell, take blood cultures (before giving antibiotics).
2 Antibiotics are only indicated if the patient is systemically unwell or if spreading cellulitis is present.
3 Use general anaesthesia for certain sites (perianal, breast, cervical, etc.). Regional blocks may be used for limbs in older children. (Note that local infiltration produces poor anaesthesia in inflamed tissue.)
4 Clean the skin.
5 Incise over the most superficial tender point in the direction of skin creases. Take a sample of pus for culture and staining, including the Ziehl–Neelsen stain if indicated. **The commonest error is to make the incision too small.**
6 Insert a curette spoon or finger to break down any loculi. Send a sample of the wall of the abscess for TB if indicated.
7 Irrigate the cavity with 0.9% saline to flush out necrotic material.
8 If a large cavity exists, loosely pack it with sterile gauze. For a small cavity place a 'wick' (e.g. a piece of rolled gauze) into the wound, forming a track. Cover the wound loosely with absorbent dressing. Change the gauze packing after 24 hours, giving analgesia beforehand if needed. Remove the wick after 48 hours.
9 As the cavity discharges pus it should heal from a depth to superficially through the open skin incision.

Abdominal paracentesis

Indications

- To detect intra-abdominal injury after blunt trauma in the haemodynamically unstable child in the absence of CT or ultrasound scanning facilities. **Haemodynamic instability after penetrating trauma always requires a laparotomy.**
- To identify peritonitis.
- To identify ruptured bowel.

Preparation of kit

The following equipment is needed:

- local anaesthetic (ideally with adrenaline)
- sterile drapes
- over-needle catheter, 16- to 20-gauge
- 20-mL syringe
- warmed normal saline and infusion set
- urinary catheter and nasogastric tube
- skin prep (iodine/alcohol).

Procedure

1 The procedure must be sterile.
2 Decompress the bladder and stomach with a urinary catheter and nasogastric tube.
3 Prepare the abdomen (from the costal margin to the pubis). Drape the area with sterile towels, exposing the peri-umbilical region.
4 If the patient is conscious, infiltrate local anaesthetic in the midline (a third of the distance between the umbilicus and the pubis). If pelvic trauma is suspected, infiltrate above the umbilicus.
5 Insert the catheter over needle. Remove the needle and aspirate.
6 If more than 10 mL of fresh blood **or** turbid or bile-stained fluid **or** faeces **or** food debris are present in the aspirate, there is a serious problem, possibly indicating the need for a laparotomy.
7 If none of the above abnormalities are seen on aspiration, instil 10 mL/kg of warm sterile normal saline into the abdomen and allow 5 minutes for it to circulate. Then retrieve the fluid.

Interpreting the results of analysis of the retrieved fluid

Abnormal findings include the following:

- red blood cell count (unspun) > 100 000/mL: may need laparotomy if unstable
- white blood cell count (unspun) > 500/mL
- bile staining
- faeces
- Gram stain/microscopy positive.

If laparotomy is indicated, withdraw the catheter and cover the wound with a sterile dressing. Then transfer the patient to theatre.

Lumbar puncture

Preparation of kit

The following equipment is needed:

- iodine
- sterile gloves
- sterile dressings pack
- spinal needle with stylet
- collodion
- small adhesive dressing
- local anaesthetic
- sedation (in some cases).

Indications

- As part of septic screen in case meningitis is present.
- For investigating the possible cause of seizures.
- For investigating the possible cause of apnoeic episodes due to meningitis.
- As therapy in post-haemorrhagic hydrocephalus.
- For administration of drugs in leukaemia.

Contraindications

- Signs of raised intracranial pressure, such as deep coma (P or U on the AVPU scale), unequal pupils, rigid posture or paralysis in any of the limbs or the trunk, or irregular breathing.
- Skin infection in the area through which the needle will have to pass.
- Significant bleeding disorder.

If contraindications are present, the potential value of the information gained from a lumbar puncture should be carefully weighed against the risk of the procedure. If in doubt, it might be better to start treatment for suspected meningitis, and delay performing a lumbar puncture.

Precautions

- Do not perform a lumbar puncture in the very sick patient (it may precipitate apnoea in an infant and shock in an older child).
- Excessive neck flexion when positioning can lead to hypoxaemia and acute respiratory deterioration.
- If a spinal needle is unavailable and a normal (non-stylet) needle is used, the needle bore may become blocked with skin on insertion and therefore obstruct flow. There is also the risk of tissue implantation leading to a dermoid cyst.

Procedure

There are two possible positions:

- the child lying down on the left side (particularly for young infants)
- the child in the sitting position (particularly for older children).

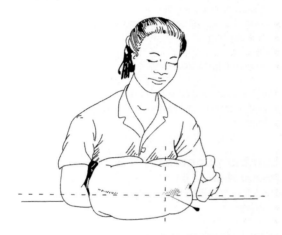

FIGURE 8.5.5 Holding a child lying on their left side for a lumbar puncture. Note that the spine is curved to open up the spaces between the vertebrae.

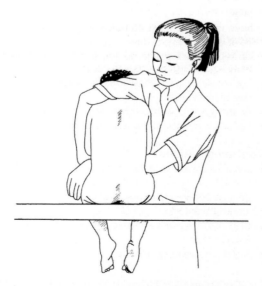

FIGURE 8.5.6 Restraining an older child in a sitting position for a lumbar puncture.

When the child is lying on their side a hard surface should be used. Place the child on their side so that the vertebral column is parallel to this surface and the transverse axis of the back is vertical (see Figure 8.5.5).

It is helpful to have an experienced assistant present to hold the patient. Flex the spine maximally, but avoid excessive neck flexion. Make sure that the airway is not obstructed and the child can breathe normally. Take particular care when holding young infants. The assistant should not hold a young infant by the neck or flex the neck to avoid airway obstruction.

Prepare the site

- Use aseptic technique. Scrub your hands and wear sterile gloves.
- Prepare the skin around the site with an antiseptic solution.
- Sterile towels may be used.
- In older children who are alert, give a local anaesthetic (1% lignocaine) infiltrated in the skin and subcutaneous tissue over the site.

Identify site of insertion

Locate the space between the third and fourth lumbar vertebrae or between the fourth and fifth lumbar vertebrae. (The third lumbar vertebra is at the junction of the line between the iliac crests and the vertebral column.)

Use an LP needle with a stylet (22 gauge for a young infant, and 20 gauge for an older infant and child; if these are not available, routine hypodermic needles may be used). Insert the needle into the middle of the inter-vertebral space and aim the needle towards the umbilicus.

Advance the needle slowly. The needle will pass easily until it encounters the ligament between the vertebral processes. More pressure is needed to penetrate this ligament, and less resistance is felt as the dura is penetrated. In young infants this decrease in resistance is not always felt, so advance the needle very carefully.

Stop advancing when a 'give' or puncture sensation is felt on entering the subarachnoid space (this is often not felt in neonates). Frequent stylet withdrawals during the procedure should be undertaken to see if the CSF flows, indicating that the subarachnoid space has been successfully entered. The subarachnoid space is only 0.5–0.7 cm below the skin in premature infants and 1 cm below it in term infants, so it is easy to over-penetrate by mistake. Over-penetration leads to puncturing of the anterior vertebral venous plexus and a bloody sample, so that CSF microscopy is less informative or perhaps impossible. The needle should be withdrawn and the procedure repeated in another disc space.

Withdraw the stylet. Obtain a sample of 0.5–1 mL of CSF and place it in sterile containers, allowing six drops of CSF to drip into each sample container.

Replace the stylet.

Withdraw the needle and stylet completely and apply pressure to the site for a few seconds. Put a sterile dressing over the needle puncture site, and cover the whole site with adhesive dressing.

Send samples for the following:

1. microscopy, cell type and counts, Gram and Ziehl-Neelson staining, culture and sensitivity (including for TB) and virology.
2. biochemistry (glucose, protein).

Suprapubic aspiration of urine
Indications
Usually in sick infants where urgent diagnosis is required and there is a palpable bladder that does not respond to manual expression for a clean catch.

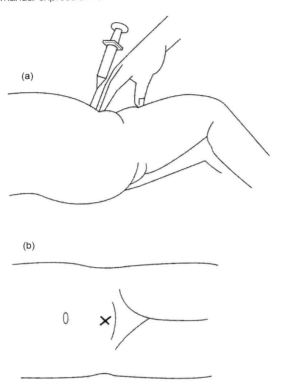

FIGURE 8.5.7 Position for carrying out suprapubic aspiration of urine in an infant. (a) Side view. (b) Abdominal view. Note the angle of insertion of the needle.

Procedure
Use a sterile technique throughout. Advance a 23- to 24-gauge needle attached to a syringe to a depth of 3 cm in the midline at the proximal transverse crease above the pubis. Withdraw the urine into a sterile syringe and transfer it to a sterile urine container,

Do this only in a child with a bladder containing sufficient urine, which can be demonstrated by percussion. Do not use urine bags to collect urine, as the specimens may become contaminated.

Have a clean urine jar ready in case the child passes urine during the procedure.

Microscopy of urine
- Urinary tract infections (UT1s) are common in children.
- Although many of these infections are not serious, some of them cause kidney damage and lead to scarring.
- Kidney scars can lead to high blood pressure, and to kidney failure later in life.
- A child with a UTI can develop kidney damage very fast, in just a few days. The only way to prevent this is to make the diagnosis and treat it at once.
- Urine microscopy is the only way to diagnose UTIs immediately and reliably.

In a patient with a UTI the urine contains:
- one species of **bacterium** at a concentration of at least 100 000/mL
- an excess of **white blood cells**.

Bacterial numbers
Most children with a UTI have in the range of 10–1000 million bacteria/mL. In fact, 100 000/mL is a very small number of bacteria. When urine is collected from children, it often becomes contaminated with a very small number of bacteria, and these are often of just one species. This means that if you rely on laboratory culture to make the diagnosis of UTI, you are likely to have many false-positives, perhaps one for every genuine case. Remember that every child diagnosed as having a UTI in this way will undergo investigations, sometimes including invasive procedures.

White blood cells
Children frequently have extra urinary white blood cells without a UTI.
- Around 10% of febrile children have hundreds of extra white blood cells.
- Girls void some urine into the vagina, so vaginal white blood cells are readily washed into the urine (as are vaginal epithelial cells, which are seen in the urine of most girls after puberty).

Children with UTIs often have no excess of white blood cells.
- White blood cells do not last long in urine, especially if it is alkaline, so it must be examined soon after collection.
- Ill infants may be unable to mount a white blood cell response.

Therefore white blood cells alone are an unreliable and potentially misleading sign.

How to count bacteria
Laboratory culture
This is the most widely used method, and the traditional approach. It remains acceptable, but if you use it you will:
- **have to accept that some positive reports will be false**
- **have to wait at least 48 hours for the result**. In real life, it is often several days or a week before a positive lab report reaches the doctor, and treatment starts. Remember that kidney damage can become permanent within 3 days
- **have to recall patients a few days later if the culture grows a mixture of bacteria**. This is usually caused by the contamination of urine as it is collected, and is common. It must be repeated in case a UTI was present as well
- **miss the occasional UTI caused by anaerobes.**

Advantages of urine microscopy
If you use this method you can:
- discard sterile urines, and reassure the child's family at once
- repeat a contaminated urine sample at once
- treat children with UTIs immediately
- diagnose anaerobic UTIs as easily as aerobic ones
- save time and money because it is quicker and cheaper than urine culture.

Choice of microscope

With an ordinary **light microscope**, bacteria are only easy to see after they have been stained.

Phase-contrast microscopes enable you to see unstained bacteria very easily, just using a drop of fresh urine on a glass slide. They look and work exactly the same as ordinary light microscopes, except that the lens (objective) and the condenser (underneath) are specially modified.

How to do urine microscopy

You can microscope fresh urine on a slide with a counting chamber. There is no need to stain or spin the urine.

The slide has two chambers, each of which has a grid etched on to the glass surface. In certain clinical situations, such as examination of peritoneal dialysis fluid for suspected peritonitis, the grid can be used to make accurate counts of the concentrations of elements present.

Usually this degree of accuracy is unnecessary. However, the grid is always useful because it confirms that the microscope is focused on the urine. If you examine a specimen with no cells or bacteria on a plain slide it is impossible to be certain otherwise.

Clean the slide and a coverslip with a tissue. Breathe over the slide to create a 'mist' on it, and quickly push the coverslip into place. This creates a chamber 0.1 mm deep with a grid etched on the bottom (*see* Figure 8.5.8).

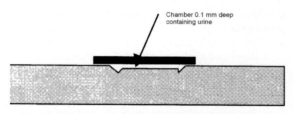

Chamber 0.1 mm deep containing urine

FIGURE 8.5.8 Side view of grid slide with coverslip in place.

Test the urine with a dipstick (to check for blood, protein and glucose). Then touch the tip of the dipstick on the slide so that a small amount of urine is drawn into the chamber by capillary action.

Bacteria

- Most bacteria that cause UTIs are bacilli (**rod-shaped**).
- They are easy to identify, as they look like straight lines, usually about 3 mm long.
- Mostly they remain still, or just move slightly, like a shimmer. This movement is caused by Brownian motion (which occurs when they are hit by water molecules), and is not due to them swimming.
- Rarely will you see moving bacteria.

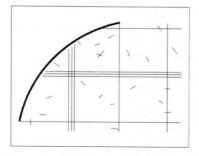

FIGURE 8.5.9 Rod-shaped bacteria.

Infections also sometimes occur with streptococci, which are bacteria that resemble strings of beads. There are always some strings that are four or more cocci long. If you think that you can see 'cocci' individually, or in clumps, these are in fact phosphate crystals. If they appear to be moving, this is just the result of Brownian motion.

White blood cells

These are round, and between 3 and 5 mm in diameter. All white blood cells have a 'granular' appearance to their cytoplasm. In the case of the larger ones you can often make out the individual granules shimmering and moving within the cell, and the nucleus (which is lobed in neutrophils).

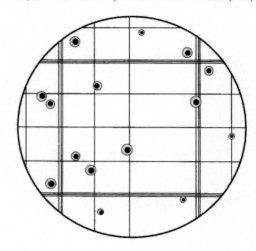

FIGURE 8.5.10 White blood cells.

Red blood cells

These are smaller than white blood cells, and do not have any content or granular appearance.

If the red cells are present because of trauma (e.g. after an injury, or post surgery) or a UTI, they will either look just like red cells in the blood (i.e. biconcave discs), or they will all appear slightly shrunken and wrinkled, or slightly swollen. The important thing is that they all look the same.

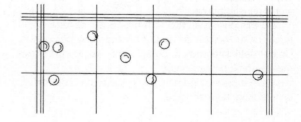

FIGURE 8.5.11 Red blood cells.

If the red blood cells are in the urine because of kidney inflammation (glomerulonephritis), they are usually smaller, but they are also all different shapes. This is probably because they get damaged as they pass down the tubules of the kidney. Sometimes the red cells are very bizarre shapes. They are referred to as 'glomerular' red cells.

Epithelial cells

These are very large flat cells with an easily visible round nucleus. They are from the vagina, and are only seen in the

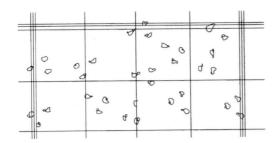

FIGURE 8.5.12 Glomerular red blood cells.

urine of older girls, in which they are common. If large numbers of epithelial cells are present this suggests particularly heavy vaginal contamination.

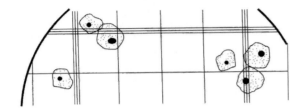

FIGURE 8.5.13 Epithelial cells.

Casts

These indicate kidney inflammation (glomerulonephritis). Casts consist of abnormal kidney tubule contents that have solidified and have retained the shape of the tubule as they passed into the urine.

Pure protein casts look glass-like, and are described as hyaline. Those consisting of debris (e.g. dead tubule cells in acute tubular necrosis) are called granular casts. Some casts are composed of red or white cells. Many casts consist of a mixture of these.

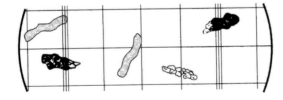

FIGURE 8.5.14 Casts.

Debris

Contaminated urine samples often contain a variety of debris. Some elements have an obvious origin, such as cotton fibres, but others cannot be identified.

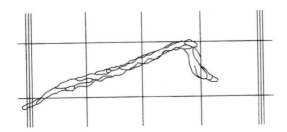

FIGURE 8.5.15 Debris.

Crystals

Urine samples often contain obvious crystals, whose shape allows their chemical origin to be identified. However, this is rarely of clinical significance.

The commonest 'crystals' in fact look more like small black dots, either singly, or in clumps (and even in casts). They move slightly (or 'shimmer') as a result of Brownian motion, and can be mistaken by the unwary for small round bacteria (cocci).

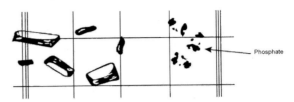

FIGURE 8.5.16 Crystals.

Diagnosing urinary tract infections (UTIs)
UTIs are primarily diagnosed by looking for bacteria.

Infected urine

About 99% of urine infections are caused by rod-shaped bacteria known as **bacilli**.

In most UTIs, every field you view will have many bacteria (in some cases thousands), and they all look the same. Therefore when you see many bacteria in fresh urine, all with the same appearance, you can be sure that the child has a UTI.

If you see at least one rod, but less than 10 rods in the centre of the grid (square 5), you have to consider the possibility of contamination, so collect another sample to see whether the finding persists (and think about vaginal lactobacilli; see below).

What to do if you find a positive microscopy

You can start treatment immediately with an appropriate antibiotic. In addition, send the urine for culture with **direct sensitivities**.

The laboratory will grow the bacteria to confirm which species they are, and to test their sensitivity to a range of different antibiotics. Without direct sensitivity testing this takes 2 days, but with it you will usually obtain the result the next day.

Sterile urine

Most urine samples will be sterile. If you see **no bacteria** or cells, check by looking at five 'size-A' squares (i.e. about five fields).

If you see nothing in that area, then you can be certain that the urine is not infected.

Even if you can see other elements, if there are no bacteria, it is not a UTI. Remember that you will see white blood cells in the urine of many children with fever (e.g. due to tonsillitis or pneumonia). Also remember that many girls have white blood cells in their urine from the vagina (and often epithelial cells, too).

Contaminated urine

If you see any of the following, **collect a repeat sample**, as the first sample is likely to have been contaminated:
- more than one shape of bacterium

- some bacteria, but also a large amount of debris (e.g. cotton fibres or many epithelial cells)
- many bacteria in a urine sample that was collected several hours ago, or from a nappy that had been on the baby for several hours.

If necessary, you need to go on collecting repeat urine samples until one is either definitely sterile or definitely infected.

Vaginal contamination

Girls void some of their urine into the vagina, so normal female urine will contain vaginal washings. In young girls this makes little difference to the microscopy findings. In older girls it is normal to see some epithelial cells (*see* Figure 8.5.13).

Also, in many older girls lactobacilli are washed into the urine. These are long rods, up to 4 mm or more. It is unusual for there to be large numbers, but they can cause confusion with a UTI. If you are uncertain, ask the lab either to Gram stain them or to culture them. Unlike the bacteria that cause UTIs, lactobacilli are Gram-positive.

They do not grow in conventional UTI culture media, so the lab will report a sterile urine. If you want to be absolutely certain, ask the lab to culture the urine anaerobically.

Recording the results

Labels can be printed to stick on the clinical notes. This is important because negative urine samples will be discarded, and this will be the only record of the test.

A typical format is as follows:

URINE PHASE CONTRAST MICROSCOPY
Name: .... **Date:** ....

MICRO – Bacteria: ....
WBC: .... RBC: ....
Casts, etc.: ....

STICKS – Protein: .... Blood: ....
Glucose: ....
Other:.......................................

ACTION – (tick one of the three options)
Urine not infected: sample discarded
Urine contaminated: sample repeated
UTI: urine sent for culture and direct sensitivities, and antibiotics started

SIGN and PRINT NAME:............................

Counting what you see

- For most clinical purposes it is not necessary to count the exact concentration of cells or bacteria that you see, and estimates such as 'many' or 'few' are enough.
- Sometimes it is helpful to quantify the findings more carefully (e.g. to monitor the numbers of casts in a child with glomerulonephritis).
- Occasionally it is essential to count the exact numbers (e.g. the number of white blood cells is critical for the diagnosis and treatment of peritonitis in children on peritoneal dialysis from a dialysis sample).

Calculate all the counts per microlitre (µL). Count at least 10 of each element of interest. The number and size of the squares you need to count will therefore depend on the concentration of the elements in the urine.

Figure 8.5.17 shows the etched counting grid for microscopy.

- The central square ('3') is 1 × 1 mm.
- With the cover-slip on, the chamber is 0.1 mm deep, so the central square has a volume of 0.1 µL.
- Therefore the whole grid of nine similar squares has a total volume of 0.9 µL.
- Note that 1 microlitre is one-thousandth of a mL.
- Therefore a count of 100 000 bacteria/mL is equivalent to 100/µL, so a 'significant' culture in a urinary tract infection would mean at least 100 bacteria/µL, or 10 bacteria in the central square of the grid.

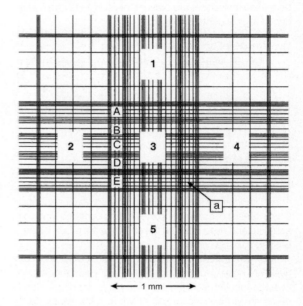

FIGURE 8.5.17 Counting grid for microscopy.

How to count
Very infrequent elements
Count all those in squares 1, 2, 3, 4 and 5, and multiply by 2.

Infrequent elements
Count all those in square 5, and multiply by 10.

Frequent elements
Count all those in five smaller squares (e.g. squares A, B, C, D and E), and multiply by 50.

Very frequent elements
Count all those in square A, and multiply by 250 (for ease of calculation, multiply by 1000 and divide by 4).

Overwhelmingly frequent elements (usually bacteria)
Count all those in one of the smallest squares and multiply by 4000.

Measuring blood glucose levels

Blood glucose levels can be measured with rapid diagnostic tests (e.g. Dextrostix, BM Stix) at the bedside, which provide an estimate of blood glucose concentration within a few minutes. There are several brands on the market, which differ slightly in how they should be used. Therefore

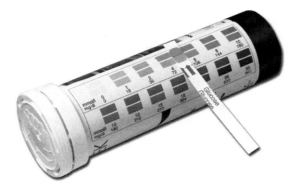

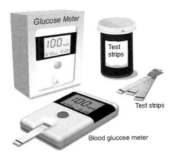

FIGURE 8.5.18 Blood glucose colour scale on side of bottle.

FIGURE 8.5.19 Electronic reading device for glucose strip. The strip is inserted into the side of the machine after the sample has been timed for the reaction to take place and the blood has been wiped off the strip.

it is important to read the instructions on the box and the package leaflet before using these tests.

Generally, a drop of blood is placed on the reagent strip and left for 30 seconds to 1 minute, depending on the brand of strip. The blood is then wiped off, and after another fixed period of time (e.g. a further 1 minute), the colour change on the reagent field of the strip is read. For this, the resulting colour is compared with a colour scale printed on the box. This allows the user to estimate the glucose level to be within a certain range (e.g. between 2 mmol/litre and 5 mmol/litre), but it does not provide exact values.

Some strips come with a battery-powered electronic reading machine. After the blood has been wiped off, the strip is inserted into the reading machine, which provides a more accurate value.

As the reagents deteriorate with exposure to ambient humidity, it is important that they are kept in a closed box, and that the box is closed immediately after a strip has been removed.

8.6 Assessing nutrition, growth and development

Measuring nutritional status

Calculating the child's weight for length

This is the most relevant measurement in nutritional assessment.

Measuring length

At ≤ 2 years

Ideally two people are needed to take this measurement, and the child should be supine on a flat surface.

The first person should:

- assist in positioning the child face up on the measuring board, supporting the head and placing it against the headboard
- position the crown of the head against the headboard, compressing the hair
- check that the child lies straight along the centre line of the board and is not slanted, and does not change position (it is usual for this person to stand or kneel behind the headboard).

The second person should:

- support the trunk as the child is positioned on the board
- lie the child flat along the board
- place one hand on the shins above the ankles or on the knees and press down firmly, and with the other hand place the foot-piece firmly against the heels
- measure the length (to the nearest 0.1 cm) and record it immediately.

The measuring board should be checked for accuracy every month.

At ≥ 3 years

- This measurement should be taken without the child wearing shoes.
- The child should stand with their heels and back in contact with an upright wall.
- The head is held to look straight forward with the lower eye sockets in line with the ears. The nose must not be tilted upward.
- A weighted block at right angles to the wall is then lowered on to the head and a scale fixed to the wall is read.
- During measurement the child should be asked to stretch their neck to be as tall as possible, but their heels must not leave the ground. The measurer should help to stretch the neck by firm pressure upward under the mastoid processes.
- Measure the height immediately to within 0.1 cm.

Measuring weight

At ≤ 2 years

- Leave a cloth in the weighing pan to prevent chilling of the child.
- Adjust the scales to zero with the cloth in the pan.
- Place the naked child gently on the cloth in the weighing pan.
- Wait for the child to settle and the weight to stabilise.
- Measure the weight (to the nearest 10 grams) and record it immediately.

Standardisation of the scales should be performed weekly or whenever the scales are moved.

At ≥ 3 years

- The child should be weighed naked or, if pants are worn, 0.1 kg should be subtracted from the weight measured.
- The bladder should be emptied before weighing.

Determining the child's percentage weight for length or SD weight for length

See Figure 8.6.1.

- Locate the row containing the child's length in the central column of the table.
- Look to the left in that row for boys, and to the right for girls.
- Note where the child's weight lies with respect to the weights recorded in this row.
- Select the weight closest to that of the child.
- Look up this column to read the weight for length of the child.

Note: Although the interpretation of a fixed percent-of-median value varies across age and height, and generally the two scales cannot be compared, the approximate percent-of-the median values for −1 SD and −2 SD are 90% and 80% of the median, respectively (*Bulletin of the World Health Organization*, 1994, **72**, 273–83).

Length is measured below 85 cm; height is measured at 85 cm or above. Recumbent length is on average 0.5 cm greater than standing height, although the difference is of no importance to the individual child. A correction may be made by deducting 0.5 cm from all lengths above 84.9 cm if the standing height cannot be measured.

Example 1. Boy of length 61 cm and weight 5.3 kg: this child is −2 SD weight for length (84% of the median: 5.3 divided by 6.3 × 100).

Example 2. Girl of length 67 cm and weight 4.3 kg; this child is less than −4 SD weight for length (less than 60% of the median: 57%).

Monitoring weight gain
Calculating weight gain

The example below is for weight gain over 3 days, but the same procedure can be applied to any interval.

- Subtract the child's weight (in grams) that was measured 3 days earlier from their current weight.
- Divide by three to calculate the average daily weight gain (grams/day).
- Divide by the child's average weight (in kg) to calculate the daily weight gain per unit body weight (grams/kg/day).

Monitoring charts: explanation of the charts on the following pages

Figure 8.6.2 shows a weight chart which has been used to monitor the weight gain of a severely malnourished child. The horizontal 'x' axis represents the number of days after admission, while the vertical 'y' axis represents the weight of the child in kilograms (kg).

Boys' weight (kg)					Length	Girls' weight (kg)				
-4 SD	-3 SD	-2 SD	-1 SD	Médian	(cm)	Médian	-1 SD	-2 SD	-3 SD	-4 SD
1.7	1.9	2.0	2.2	2.4	45	2.5	2.3	2.1	1.9	1.7
1.8	2.0	2.2	2.4	2.6	46	2.6	2.4	2.2	2.0	1.9
2.0	2.1	2.3	2.5	2.8	47	2.8	2.6	2.4	2.2	2.0
2.1	2.3	2.5	2.7	2.9	48	3.0	2.7	2.5	2.3	2.1
2.2	2.4	2.6	2.9	3.1	49	3.2	2.9	2.6	2.4	2.2
2.4	2.6	2.8	3.0	3.3	50	3.4	3.1	2.8	2.6	2.4
2.5	2.7	3.0	3.2	3.5	51	3.6	3.3	3.0	2.8	2.5
2.7	2.9	3.2	3.5	3.8	52	3.8	3.5	3.2	2.9	2.7
2.9	3.1	3.4	3.7	4.0	53	4.0	3.7	3.4	3.1	2.8
3.1	3.3	3.6	3.9	4.3	54	4.3	3.9	3.6	3.3	3.0
3.3	3.6	3.8	4.2	4.5	55	4.5	4.2	3.8	3.5	3.2
3.5	3.8	4.1	4.4	4.8	56	4.8	4.4	4.0	3.7	3.4
3.7	4.0	4.3	4.7	5.1	57	5.1	4.6	4.3	3.9	3.6
3.9	4.3	4.6	5.0	5.4	58	5.4	4.9	4.5	4.1	3.8
4.1	4.5	4.8	5.3	5.7	59	5.6	5.1	4.7	4.3	3.9
4.3	4.7	5.1	5.5	6.0	60	5.9	5.4	4.9	4.5	4.1
4.5	4.9	5.3	5.8	6.3	61	6.1	5.6	5.1	4.7	4.3
4.7	5.1	5.6	6.0	6.5	62	6.4	5.8	5.3	4.9	4.5
4.9	5.3	5.8	6.2	6.8	63	6.6	6.0	5.5	5.1	4.7
5.1	5.5	6.0	6.5	7.0	64	6.9	6.3	5.7	5.3	4.8
5.3	5.7	6.2	6.7	7.3	65	7.1	6.5	5.9	5.5	5.0
5.5	5.9	6.4	6.9	7.5	66	7.3	6.7	6.1	5.6	5.1
5.6	6.1	6.6	7.1	7.7	67	7.5	6.9	6.3	5.8	5.3
5.8	6.3	6.8	7.3	8.0	68	7.7	7.1	6.5	6.0	5.5
6.0	6.5	7.0	7.6	8.2	69	8.0	7.3	6.7	6.1	5.6
6.1	6.6	7.2	7.8	8.4	70	8.2	7.5	6.9	6.3	5.8
6.3	6.8	7.4	8.0	8.6	71	8.4	7.7	7.0	6.5	5.9
6.4	7.0	7.6	8.2	8.9	72	8.6	7.8	7.2	6.6	6.0
6.6	7.2	7.7	8.4	9.1	73	8.8	8.0	7.4	6.8	6.2
6.7	7.3	7.9	8.6	9.3	74	9.0	8.2	7.5	6.9	6.3
6.9	7.5	8.1	8.8	9.5	75	9.1	8.4	7.7	7.1	6.5
7.0	7.6	8.3	8.9	9.7	76	9.3	8.5	7.8	7.2	6.6
7.2	7.8	8.4	9.1	9.9	77	9.5	8.7	8.0	7.4	6.7
7.3	7.9	8.6	9.3	10.1	78	9.7	8.9	8.2	7.5	6.9
7.4	8.1	8.7	9.5	10.3	79	9.9	9.1	8.3	7.7	7.0
7.6	8.2	8.9	9.6	10.4	80	10.1	9.2	8.5	7.8	7.1
7.7	8.4	9.1	9.8	10.6	81	10.3	9.4	8.7	8.0	7.3
7.9	8.5	9.2	10.0	10.8	82	10.5	9.6	8.8	8.1	7.5
8.0	8.7	9.4	10.2	11.0	83	10.7	9.8	9.0	8.3	7.6
8.2	8.9	9.6	10.4	11.3	84	11.0	10.1	9.2	8.5	7.8
8.4	9.1	9.8	10.6	11.5	85	11.2	10.3	9.4	8.7	8.0
8.6	9.3	10.0	10.8	11.7	86	11.5	10.5	9.7	8.9	8.1

FIGURE 8.6.1 Weight-for-length reference chart (below 87 cm). SD = standard deviation score or Z-score. Based on World Health Organization data.

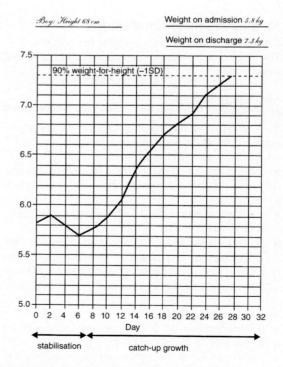

FIGURE 8.6.2 Personalised weight chart for child.

- Notice that the weight in kilograms is stepped in 0.5-kg increments. In this example, the range has been written in from 5.0 to 7.5 kg to provide a suitable range for this individual child's expected growth.
- For other children, fill in the starting weight at the appropriate level (e.g. 5 kg, 5.5 kg, 6 kg, etc., or 7 kg, 7.5 kg, 8 kg, etc.).
- Choosing an appropriate starting weight like this is preferable to using a chart with weights marked from 0, because this more flexible chart gives a larger scale and thus shows the pattern of change much more clearly.

Figure 8.6.3 shows a blank intake and output chart for recording the food given to an individual patient, the amount consumed, and any losses through vomiting or diarrhoea.

Name:			Ward:		
			Hospital number:		
Age:	Weight:		Date of admission:		
Date .... Feed: .... feeds of ....mL each ....mL per day					
Time	Type of feed	Volume offered (mL)	Volume left in cup (mL)	Amount taken by child (mL)	Vomit estimate (mL)	Watery diarrhoea (Yes/No)
Total:			Sub total			Total in 24 hours

FIGURE 8.6.3 Twenty-four-hour food intake chart.

Additional measurements for assessing nutritional status
Mid upper arm circumference (MUAC)
- This is measured with non-stretchable tape placed around the arm midway between the elbow and the shoulder.
- The tape should be gently tightened, but not so much that it compresses the underlying tissues.
- This measurement includes fat and muscle.

Normal values of MUAC for a child aged 1–5 years are in the range 14.0–16.5 cm.

For a child aged 1–5 years, a MUAC of < 12.5 cm indicates that the child is definitely malnourished, and a MUAC in the range 12.5–13.5 cm indicates that they are probably malnourished.

Triceps skinfold thickness
Special skinfold callipers are used to measure the double layer of skin and subcutaneous fat overlying the triceps muscle when the skinfold is lifted.

Measuring growth and development
Individual measurements of weight and height/length can be plotted sequentially on charts to identify any failure of growth. See the charts below for height and weight for boys and girls. These charts also include data for infants born prematurely, as well as head circumference measurements.

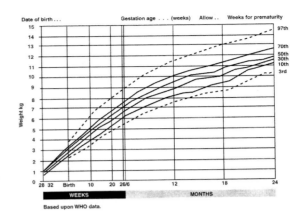

FIGURE 8.6.4 Weight chart for girls from birth to 2 years. Based on World Health Organization data.

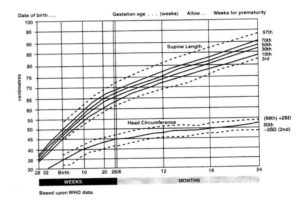

FIGURE 8.6.5 Supine length and head circumference chart for girls from birth to 2 years. Based on World Health Organization data.

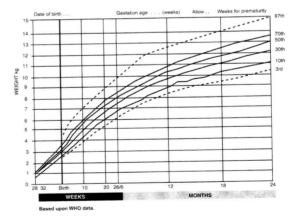

FIGURE 8.6.6 Weight chart for boys from birth to 2 years. Based on World Health Organization data.

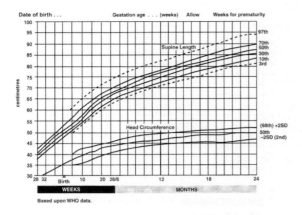

FIGURE 8.6.7 Supine length and head circumference chart for boys from birth to 2 years. Based on World Health Organization data.

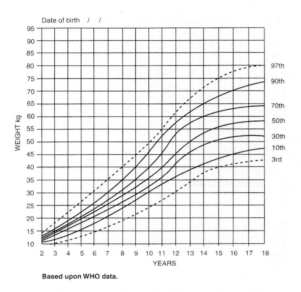

FIGURE 8.6.8 Weight chart for girls aged 2–18 years. Based on World Health Organization data.

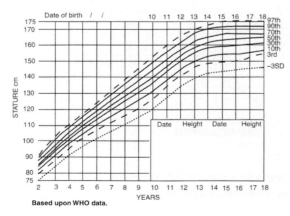

FIGURE 8.6.9 Height chart for girls aged 2–18 years. Based on World Health Organization data.

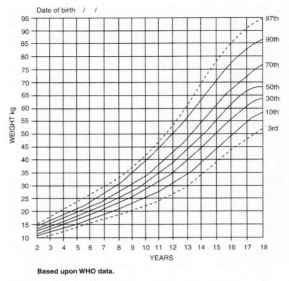

FIGURE 8.6.10 Weight chart for boys aged 2–18 years. Based on World Health Organization data.

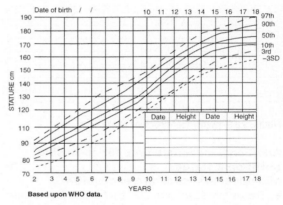

FIGURE 8.6.11 Height chart for boys aged 2–18 years. Based on World Health Organization data.

Measurement of head circumference

- Use a non-stretchable tape.
- Measure around the forehead above the eyebrows to the maximum occipital point.
- Measure twice for accuracy.

Assessment of pubertal state
Girls

The following should be recorded.

Breast development

- **Stage 1.** Pre-adolescent: elevation of papilla only.
- **Stage 2.** Breast bud stage: elevation of breast and papilla as a small mound, and enlargement of areola diameter.
- **Stage 3.** Further enlargement and elevation of breast and areola, with no separation of their contours.
- **Stage 4.** Projection of areola and papilla to form a secondary mound above the level of the breast.

- **Stage 5.** Mature stage: projection of papilla only, due to recession of the areola to the general contour of the breast.

Pubic hair

- **Stage 1.** Pre-adolescent: the vellus over the pubes is not further developed than that over the abdominal wall (i.e. there is no pubic hair).
- **Stage 2.** Sparse growth of long, slightly pigmented downy hair, straight or slightly curled, chiefly along the labia.
- **Stage 3.** Hair is considerably darker, coarser and more curled, and spreads sparsely over the junction of the pubes.
- **Stage 4.** Hair is now adult in type, but the area covered is still considerably smaller than in the adult; there is no spread to the medial surface of the thighs.
- **Stage 5.** Hair is adult in quantity and type, with distribution of the horizontal (or classically 'feminine') pattern; there is spread to the medial surface of the thighs but not up the linea alba or elsewhere above the base of the inverse triangle (spread up the linea alba occurs late, and is rated as Stage 6).

Document whether axillary hair is present.
Document age at menarche.

Boys

The following should be recorded.

Genital (penis) development

- **Stage 1.** Pre-adolescent: the testes, scrotum and penis are of about the same size and proportion as in early childhood.
- **Stage 2.** Enlargement of the scrotum and testes. The skin of the scrotum reddens and changes in texture. There is little or no enlargement of the penis at this stage.
- **Stage 3.** Enlargement of the penis, which initially is mainly an increase in length. Further growth of the testes and scrotum.

- **Stage 4.** Further enlargement of the penis, with an increase in breadth and development of the glans. The testes and scrotum are larger, and the scrotal skin is darkened.
- **Stage 5.** Genitals are adult in size and shape.

Pubic hair

- **Stage 1.** Pre-adolescent: the vellus over the pubes is not further developed than that over the abdominal wall (i.e. there is no pubic hair).
- **Stage 2.** Sparse growth of long slightly pigmented downy hair, straight or slightly curled, chiefly at the base of the penis.
- **Stage 3.** Hair is considerably darker, coarser and more curled, and spreads sparsely over the junction of the pubes.
- **Stage 4.** Hair is now adult in type, but the area covered is still considerably smaller than in the adult; there is no spread to the medial surface of the thighs.
- **Stage 5.** Hair is adult in quantity and type, with spread to the medial surface of the thighs but not up the linea alba or elsewhere above the base of the inverse triangle (spread up the linea alba occurs late, and is rated as Stage 6).

Document whether axillary hair is present.

Testicular volume

The approximate volume at each genital stage is shown.

- **Stage 1:** 1.5–3 mL.
- **Stage 2:** 4–6 mL.
- **Stage 3:** 6–10 mL.
- **Stage 4:** 10–12 mL.
- **Stage 5:** 15–20 mL.

Source: The standard illustrations in Tanner JM (1962) *Growth at Adolescence*, 2nd edn. Oxford: Blackwell Scientific Publications.

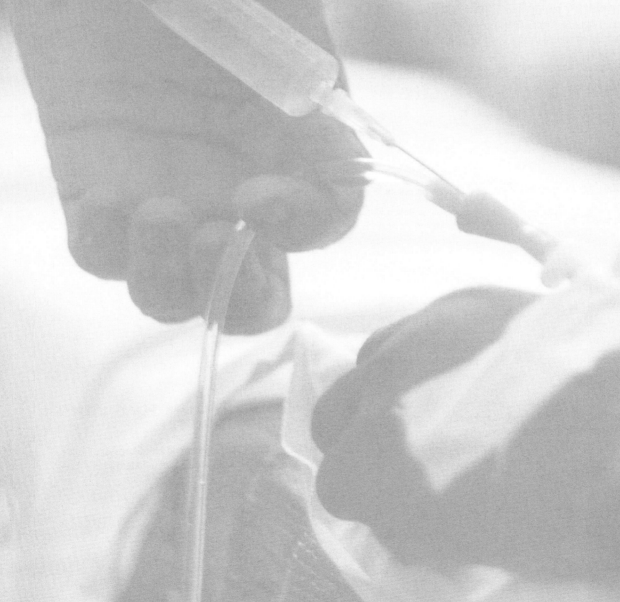

Section 9

Appendix

Normal values for vital clinical signs
Estimating the weight of a child in an emergency

For an infant (defined as up to 12 months old), the birth weight:

- doubles by 5 months
- triples by 1 year
- quadruples by 2 years.

After 12 months, the following formula can be applied, but it may need to be modified according to whether the child is small or large compared with the average:

Weight (kg) = 2 (age in years + 4).

Normal vital signs

TABLE 9.1 Normal vital signs by age in children and in pregnant women and girls

Age (years)	Heart rate (beats/minute)	Systolic blood pressure (mmHg)	Respiratory rate (breaths/minute)
< 1	110–160	70–90 (> 60)	30–40
1–2	100–150	80–95 (> 70)	25–35
2–5	95–145	80–100 (> 75)	25–30
5–12	80–120	90–110 (> 75)	20–25
> 12	60–100	100–120	15–20
Pregnant women and girls	70–110*	95–135	15–20

*Heart rate in pregnancy increases by 10–15 bpm.

WHO defines tachycardia as > 160 bpm if < 1 year; > 120 bpm if 1–5 years and if > 110 bpm in pregnancy consider shock may be developing or present.

WHO considers fast breathing is present if < 2 months respiratory rate ≥ 60 bpm; for children aged 2 months to 12 months if respiratory rate is ≥50 bpm and for children 1–5 years if respiratory rate is ≥ 40 bpm.

TABLE 9.2 Normal heart rates when awake and asleep

Age group	Heart rate when awake (beats/minute)	Heart rate when asleep (beats/minute)
Newborn to 3 months	90–190	90–160
3 months to 2 years	80–150	80–120
2–10 years	70–120	70–90
10 years to adulthood	55–90	50–90

TABLE 9.3 Normal systolic and diastolic blood pressure

Age group	Systolic blood pressure (mmHg)	Diastolic blood pressure (mmHg)
Birth (12 hours, 3 kg)	50–70	25–45
Neonate (96 hours)	60–80	20–60
Infant	80–90	53–66
2–4 years	95–105	53–66
7 years	97–112	57–71
15 years	112–128	66–80
In pregnancy	95–135*	60–85

*In pregnancy if systolic BP is < 90 mmHg consider shock may be present and if < 95 mmHg investigate for possible indicators of developing shock.

Blood pressure is difficult to measure and interpret in infants and children under 5 years of age. Do not base decisions to treat hypertension on the results of electronic sphygmomanometers, as they can be inaccurate. Always check with a hand-pumped machine.

The following quick formula can be used to calculate normal systolic pressure in children:

Median (50th centile) systolic blood pressure in children = 85 + (2 × age in years).

Capillary refill time

The normal capillary refill time (CRT) is up to 3 seconds. It is important to be aware that in colder environments peripheral CRT is not a reliable test of perfusion.

Urine output

WHO recommendations are as follows:
- Infants: 2 mL/kg/hour
- Children: 1 mL/kg/hour
- Pregnant adults: > 30 mL/hour or > 100 mL every 4 hours.

Normal core body temperatures

- Infants: 36.5–37.5°C (97.7–99.5°F)
- Children: 36.0–37.2°C (96.8 – 98.6°F).

If an infant or child has a temperature of 37.5°C or more, a fever is present.

To convert °C to °F multiply by 9, then divide by 5 then add 32.

To convert °F to °C deduct 32, then multiply by 5, then divide by 9.

Circulating blood volume

- At birth: 100 mL/kg
- At 1 year of age: 80 mL/kg
- At 12 years of age: 70 mL/kg
- In pregnancy: 100 mL/kg.

Normal values for laboratory measurements

Haematology

TABLE 9.4 Normal laboratory values for haemoglobin concentration

Age	Haemoglobin concentration (grams/dL)
1–3 days	14.5–22.5
2 weeks	14.5–18.0
6 months	10.0–12.5
1–5 years	10.5–13.0
6–12 years	11.5–15.0
12–18 years:	
Male	13.0–16.0
Female	12.0–16.0

TABLE 9.5 Normal laboratory values for platelet count

Age group	Platelet count (× 10⁹/litre)
Newborn	84–478
Child	150–400

TABLE 9.6 Normal laboratory values for erythrocyte sedimentation rate (ESR), white blood cell count (WBC) and lymphocyte count

Age group	ESR (mm/hour)
All ages	0–10
Age group	*WBC (× 10⁹/litre)*
1–2 days	9.0– 34.0
Neonate	6.0–19.5
1–3 years	6.0–17.5
4–7 years	5.5–15.5
8–13 years	4.5–13.5
≥ 13 years	4.5–11.0
Age group	*Median lymphocyte count (× 10⁹/litre)*
> 1 year	4.1–6.0

Chemistry

TABLE 9.7 Chemistry: normal laboratory values

Substance	Age	Normal range	
Albumin (grams/litre)	Preterm	18–30	
	Full term to 7 days	25–34	
	< 5 years	39–50	
	5–19 years	40–53	
Amylase (units/litre)	All ages	30–100	
ASO titre (Todd units)	2–5 years	120–160	
	6–9 years	240	
	10–12 years	320	
Bicarbonate (mmol/litre)	All ages:		
	Arterial	21–28	
	Venous	22–29	
Bilirubin (conjugated) (µmol/litre)	> 1 year	0–3.4	
Calcium (mmol/litre)	0–24 hours	2.3–2.65	(1.07–1.27 ionised)
	24 hours to 4 days	1.75–3.00	(1.00–1.17 ionised)
	4–7 days	2.25–2.73	(1.12–1.23 ionised)
	Child	2.15–2.70	(1.12–1.23 ionised)
Chloride (mmol/litre)	Neonate	97–110	
	Child	98–106	
Creatinine (µmol/litre)	Neonate	27–88	
	Infant	18–35	
	Child	27–62	
Glucose (mmol/litre)	Preterm neonate	1.4–3.3	
	0–24 hours	2.2–3.3	
	Infant	2.8–5.0	
	Child	3.3–5.5	
Magnesium (mmol/litre)	0–7 days	0.48–1.05	
	7 days to 2 years	0.65–1.05	
	2–14 years	0.60–0.95	
Osmolarity (mosmol/litre)	Child	276–295 (serum)	
Potassium (mmol/litre)	< 2 months	3.0–7.0	
	2–12 months	3.6–6.0	
	Child	3.5–5.5	
Sodium (mmol/litre)	Neonate	136–146	
	Infant	139–146	
	Child	135–145	
Urea (mmol/litre)	Neonate	1.0–5.0	
	Infant	2.5–8.0	
	Child	2.5–6.6	

Oxygen saturation (SpO₂)

The normal range is 95–100%, although oxygen saturation depends on altitude, and corrections will be needed for those living more than 1000 metres above sea level.

Table 9.8 lists the oxygen saturation levels measured in studies conducted at a range of different geographical locations above sea level.

TABLE 9.8 SpO₂ levels measured at a range of different altitudes

Altitude	Location	n	Age group	SpO₂ (%)	Author(s)	Year of study
Sea level	UK	70	2–16 years Mean 8 years	Range: 95.8–100 Median: 99.5	Poets *et al.*	1993
Sea level	Peru	189	2 months to 5 years	Range: 96–100 Mean: 98.7	Reuland *et al.*	1991
1610 m	Colorado	150	< 48 hours 3 months	95% CI: 88–97 Mean: 93 95% CI: 86–97 Mean: 92.2	Thilo *et al.*	1991
1670 m	Nairobi	87	7 days to 3 years	Range: 89.3–99.3 Mean: 95.7	Onyango *et al.*	1993
2640 m	Bogota	189	5 days to 2 years	Range: 84–100 Mean: 93.3	Lozano *et al.*	1992
2800 m	Colorado	72	3–670 days	Range: 88–97 Mean: 91.7	Nicholas *et al.*	1993
3100 m	Colorado	14	6 hours to 4 months 1 week 4 months	Range: 81–91 Mean: 80.6±5.3 Mean: 86.1±4.6	Niemeyer *et al.*	1993
3658 m	Tibet*	15	6 hours to 4 months	Immigrant: 76–90 Indigenous: 86–94	Niemeyer *et al.*	1995
3750 m	Peru	153	2–60 months	Range: 81–97 Mean: 88.9	Reuland *et al.*	1991

Values shown are those in quiet sleep.

*Ranges are values for those born to immigrant Chinese mothers and for those indigenous babies whose families have lived at that altitude for innumerable generations.

Blood gases (normal arterial range)

- pH: 7.35–7.45.
- pCO_2: 4.5–6.0 kPa (35–45 mmHg).
- pO_2: 10–13 kPa (75–98 mmHg).
- Standard bicarbonate: 21–27 mmol/L

In pregnancy:
- pH: 7.40–7.46
- pCO_2: 3.7–4.2 kPa (28–32 mmHg)
- Standard bicarbonate: 18–21 mmol/L

Circulating blood volume

- At birth: 100 mL/kg.
- At 1 year: 80 mL/kg.
- At 12 years: 70 mL/kg.
- In pregnant women and adolescent girls: 100 mL/kg.

Equivalent values for certain drugs used in an emergency

1 mg of prednisone or prednisolone is equivalent to 4 mg of hydrocortisone and 150 micrograms of dexamethasone or betamethasone.

Adrenaline (epinephrine) 1 in 1000 contains 1000 micrograms in 1 mL.

Adrenaline (epinephrine) 1 in 10 000 contains 100 micrograms in 1 mL.

Measurements of medical supplies

Uncuffed tubes in children under 25 kg in weight (aged 6–7 years)

Internal diameter of endotracheal tube:
- Full-term baby: 3.0–3.5 mm.
- Age < 1 year: 4.0–4.5 mm.
- Age > 1 year: size of tube = age/4 + 4 mm.

Length of endotracheal tube:

$$\frac{\text{Age in years}}{2} + 12 \text{ in cm (oral tube).}$$

$$\frac{\text{Age in years}}{2} + 14 \text{ in cm (nasal tube).}$$

French gauge Fr = circumference of tube in mm.

Urinary catheters: for neonate to 1 year of age* 5–6 Fr; from 2 to 8 years 6–8 Fr; from 8 to 12 years 10–2 Fr; from 13 to 18 years 12–16 Fr and in pregnancy from 14–16 Fr.

*Feeding tubes may be used but are not ideal

Nasogastric tubes: birth to 5 months size 8 Fr; 6 to 12 months size 10 Fr; 1 to 3 years 10–12 Fr; 4 to 7 years 12 Fr; 8 to 12 years 12–14 Fr; 12 to 18 years 14–18 Fr; in pregnancy 16–20 Fr.

Fluid and electrolyte management

Normal requirements for fluid

The blood volume is about 100 mL/kg at birth, falling to about 80 mL/kg at 1 year of age. The total body water content ranges from 800 mL/kg in the neonate to 600 mL/kg at 1 year of age and thereafter. Of this, about two-thirds (400 mL/kg) is intracellular fluid, the rest being extracellular fluid. Thus initial expansion of vascular volume in a state of shock can be achieved with relatively small volumes of fluid: 20 mL/kg (a quarter of the blood volume) will usually suffice. However, this volume is only a fraction of that required to correct dehydration, as the fluid has been lost from all body compartments in this condition. Clinically, dehydration is not detectable until more than 3–5% (30–50 mL/kg) of the body fluid has been lost.

It is important to remember that although fluid must be given quickly to correct loss of circulating fluid from the blood compartment (i.e. in shock, except in malnutrition; *see* Section 5.10.B), it must be given carefully in dehydration (*see* Section 5.5.B).

Fluids in neonates after the first 3 days of life are often prescribed on the basis of 150 mL/kg/day. However, this is not related to fluid needs, but is merely the volume of standard formula milk required to give an adequate protein and calorie intake.

Fluid requirement can be divided into four types:

1. for replacement of **insensible losses** (through sweating, respiration, gastrointestinal loss, etc.)
2. for replacement of **essential urine output** (the minimal urine output to allow excretion of the products of metabolism, etc.)
3. extra fluid to maintain a **modest state of diuresis**
4. fluid to replace **abnormal losses** (e.g. blood loss, severe diarrhoea, diabetic polyuria losses, etc.).

A useful formula for calculating normal fluid requirement is provided in Table 9.9. It is simple, can be applied to all age ranges and is easily subdivided. The formula gives total fluid requirements – that is, types (1), (2) and (3) listed above.

TABLE 9.9 Normal fluid requirements

Body weight	Volume of fluid (mL/24 hours)	Volume of fluid (mL/hour)	Na⁺ (mmol/ 24 hours/kg)	K⁺ (mmol/ 24 hours/kg)	Energy (kcal/ 24 hours)	Protein (grams/ 24 hours)
First 10 kg	100	4	2.0–4.0	1.5–2.5	110	3
Second 10 kg	50	2	1.0–2.0	0.5–1.5	75	1
Subsequent kg	20	1	0.5–1.0	0.2–0.7	30	0.75

For example:

- an infant weighing 6 kg would require 600 mL per day
- a child weighing 14 kg would require 1000 + 200 = 1200 mL per day
- a child weighing 25 kg would require 1000 + 500 + 100 = 1600 mL per day.

In practice, the healthy child only drinks when they are thirsty, but it is useful to have an idea of how much fluid a child should be expected to need. Of course, if there are excess losses, as in diarrhoea or fever, or if the ambient temperature is especially high, leading to high insensible losses, more fluid is required. Except in cardiac or renal disease, a good way to check whether a child is taking in enough fluid is to see whether they have a satisfactory urine output of at least 2 mL/kg/hour.

Average fluid requirements in pregnancy are 1500–2500 mL/day. This depends on levels of activity, ambient temperature and whether or not the mother has a fever.

Rehydration

Fluid deficit + normal fluid requirements + ongoing losses (sweat, diarrhoea, vomit, etc.).

Fluid deficit (mL) = percentage dehydration × weight (kg) × 10.

Ongoing losses:

- After each loose stool:
  - age < 2 years: 50–100 mL
  - age ≥ 2 years: 100–200 mL
- After each vomit: 2 mL/kg body weight.

Some useful information about biochemical measurements

- 1 ounce = 28 mL
- Percentage solution = number of grams in 100 mL (e.g. 10% dextrose = 10 grams in 100 mL).
- One millimole = molecular weight in milligrams.
- Some useful atomic weights:

hydrogen	1.0
carbon	12.0
nitrogen	14.0
oxygen	16.0
sodium	23.0
phosphorus	31.0
chlorine	35.5
potassium	39.1
calcium	40.1

Therefore, for example:
1 mmol NaCl = 58.5 mg
1 mmol $NaHCO_3$ = 84 mg
1 mmol KCl = 74.6 mg.

- The equivalent weight of an electrolyte = molecular weight/valency (e.g. Ca = 40/2).
- Useful figures to know:
  - 30% NaCl = 5 mmol/mL each of Na⁺ and Cl⁻
  - 0.9% NaCl = 0.154 mmol/mL each of Na⁺ and Cl⁻
  - 15% KCl (15 grams/100 mL) = 2 mmol/mL each of K⁺ and Cl⁻ (also called concentrated or strong KCl)
  - 10% calcium gluconate (10 grams/100 mL) = 0.225 mmol/mL (note that 1 mL of calcium chloride 10% is equivalent to 3 mL of calcium gluconate 10%)
  - 8.4% $NaHCO_3$ = 1 mmol Na⁺ and 1 mmol HCO_3^-/mL

— 1 mL/hour of normal saline = 3.7 mmol Na⁺ in 24 hours.

- Serum osmolarity = $2(Na^+ + K^+)$ + glucose + urea (normally 285–295 mosmol/litre).

Normal requirements for electrolytes (unless there are excessive losses)

There are obligatory losses of electrolytes in stools, urine and sweat, and these require replacement. Any excess is simply excreted in the urine.

TABLE 9.10 Electrolyte content of body fluids

Fluid	Na⁺ (mmol/litre)	K⁺ (mmol/litre)	Cl⁻ (mmol/litre)	HCO₃⁻ (mmol/litre)
Plasma	135–145	3.5–5.5	98–108	20–28
Gastric fluid	20–80	5–20	100–150	0
Intestinal fluid	100–140	5–15	90–130	13–65
Diarrhoea	7–96	34–150	17–164	0–75
Sweat	< 40	6–15	< 40	0–10

TABLE 9.11 Normal water and electrolyte requirements in pregnancy

Maintenance requirements/24 hours	Volume of fluid (mL/day)	Sodium requirement (mmol/day)	Potassium requirement (mmol/day)
	1500–2500	150	100

Commonly available crystalloid and colloid fluids

TABLE 9.12 Commonly available crystalloid fluids

Fluid	Na⁺ (mmol/litre)	K⁺ (mmol/litre)	Cl⁻ (mmol/litre)	Energy (kcal/litre)
Isotonic crystalloid fluids				
Saline 0.9% (normal)	150	0	150	0
Glucose 5% (50 mg/mL)	0	0	0	200
Hartmann's solution or Ringer-lactate solution*	131	5	111	0
Hypertonic crystalloid fluids				
Saline 0.45%, glucose 5%	75	0	75	200
Glucose 10% (100 mg/mL)	0	0	0	400
Glucose 50%	0	0	0	2000

*Hartmann's or Ringer-lactate solution also contains HCO₃⁻ as lactate 29 mmol/litre and calcium 2 mmol/litre.

To make 10% glucose/dextrose solution in Ringer-lactate/Hartmann's or 0.9% saline, remove 100 mL from a 500 mL bag and inject into it in a sterile manner 100 mL of 50% dextrose/glucose.

To make 5% glucose/dextrose solution in Ringer-lactate/Hartmann's or 0.9% saline, remove 50 mL from a 500 mL bag and inject into it in a sterile manner 50 mL of 50% dextrose/glucose.

To make a 10% solution of glucose for injection in treating hypoglycaemia and if there is only 50% dextrose/glucose solution available:
- either dilute 10 mL of the 50% solution in 40 mL of sterile water
- OR add 10 mL of 50% dextrose to 90 mL of 5% glucose which will give an approximate 10% glucose solution.

TABLE 9.13 Commonly available colloid fluids

Colloid	Na⁺ (mmol/litre)	K⁺ (mmol/litre)	Ca²⁺ (mmol/litre)	Duration of action (hours)	Comments
Albumin 4.5%	150	1	0	6	Protein buffers
Gelofusine	154	< 1	< 1	3	Gelatine
Haemaccel	145	5	12.5	3	Gelatine
Pentastarch	154	0	0	7	Hydroxyethyl starch

Drop factor for IV infusions

Fluids can be calculated in drops/minute as follows. First identify from the IV giving set what the 'drop factor' is (for standard giving sets this may be 10, 15 or 20 drops = 1 mL). For micro-drop systems, which often accompany giving sets with burettes, 1 mL = 60 drops. When setting the infusion rate with the flow controller on the giving set below the chamber where the drops occur, always set and count the rate over a full minute.

Calculating drip rates for a standard giving set with a drop factor of 20 drops/mL

- One mL = 20 drops in standard giving set.
- Number of drops/minute = mL/hour with a standard giving set divided by 3.

With a micro-dropper infusion giving set with a drop factor of 60 drops/mL, 1 mL = 60 micro-drops.

Measuring neurological state

A = ALERT
V = responds to **VOICE**
P = responds to **PAIN** = Glasgow Coma Scale score of ≤ 8.
U = UNRESPONSIVE

Hypoglycaemia: definition and blood glucose conversion

Hypoglycaemia is defined as a blood glucose concentration of < 2.5 mmol/litre or < 45 mg/dL.

1 mmol/litre = 19 mg/dL of glucose.

Examples of charts that can be used to monitor patients in hospital

NAME		WEIGHT			AGE				
DATE	TREATMENT	DOSE	REGIMEN	SIGN	NURSES: TIME GIVEN				
					1.	2.	3.	4.	

FIGURE 9.1 Example of a prescription chart.

Ward : _____

Name : _____

Hospital number : _____

Age : _____ **Weight :** _____

Date of admission : _____

Date.........................Feed...............................feeds of.....................mL each=
.........................mL per day

Time	Type of feed	Volume offered (mL)	Volume left in cup (mL)	Amount taken by child (mL)	Vomit estimate (mL)	Watery diarrhoea (Yes/No)
Total:				Subtotal		Total taken in 24 hours

FIGURE 9.2 Twenty-four-hour food intake chart.

PAEDIATRIC DEPARTMENT: MULAGO HOSPITAL
TREATMENT CHART

NAME :...DATE OF BIRTH
:.................................UNIT NO :

DATE PRESCRIBED	DRUG	DOSE	ROUTE	REGIMEN	DATE						
				06							
				12							
				14							
				18							
				22							
				24							
				06							
				12							
				14							
				18							
				22							
				24							
				06							
				12							
				14							
				18							
				22							
				24							
				06							
				12							
				14							
				18							
				22							
				24							
	PARACETAMOL		Oral/NG	06							
				12							
				14							
				18							
				22							
				24							

STAT DOSES OF DRUGS OR FLUID				DATE	TIME	GIVEN		
INTRAVENOUS FLUID								
BLOOD PRODUCTS								

FIGURE 9.3 Drug and intravenous fluid chart. NG, nasogastric.

PAEDIATRIC DEPARTMENT: MULAGO HOSPITAL
CARE CHART

NAME: ....AGE: ....DATE OF ADMISSION: ....HOSPITAL
NO: ....

DATE							
TIME							
TEMPERATURE							
PULSE							
RESPIRATORY RATE							
BLOOD PRESSURE							
O_2 SA%							
AVPU							
WEIGHT							
OXYGEN THERAPY							
CONVULSIONS							

FLUIDS: RECORD AMOUNT AND TYPE

INTRAVENOUS	1						
	2						
NASOGASTRIC	1						
	2						
ORAL	1						
	2						

24-HOUR TOTAL INPUT

OUTPUT: URINE							
OUTPUT: STOOL							
OUTPUT: VOMIT							
BLOOD PRODUCTS							
POSITION CHANGE							
SKIN CARE							
EYE CARE							
MOUTH CARE							
PAIN RELIEF							
GENERAL ASSESSMENT							
HEALTH EDUCATION							

OUTCOME:
....
....

FIGURE 9.4 Chart for clinical observations with fluid input and output. AVPU scale: A = alert, V = responds to verbal stimulus, P = responds to pain, U = unresponsive.

Date: _____   Hospital record number: _____

1 Child's name:	Mother's name:
Age:	Weight on admission:

2 Diagnoses / main problems:

1	
2	
3	
4	

3 Vital signs		Day 1	Day 2	Day 3	Day 4
• Conscious level (AVPU)					
• Temperature					
• Respiratory rate					
• Pulse rate					

4 Fluid balance (record volumes and times)

IV					
By nasogastric tube					
Oral					
Fluid output					

5 Treatments given (sign on chart when given)

Name of treatment:	Dose:				
1					
2					
3					
4					

6 Feeding / nutrition

Child breastfed					
Drink taken					
Food taken					
Feeding problems (give details)					
Weight					

7 Outcome (circle one of the following): Discharged well / Absconded / Transferred / Died

FIGURE 9.5 Chart for monitoring vital signs, fluid balance, treatments given and feeding/nutrition. AVPU scale: A = alert, V = responds to verbal stimulus, P = responds to pain, U = unresponsive.

NEONATAL SPECIAL CARE BABY UNIT: MULAGO HOSPITAL
CARE CHART

NAME: ....DATE OF BIRTH: ....UNIT

NO: ....

DATE		AM	PM	AM	PM	AM	PM	AM	PM	AM	PM	AM	PM	AM	PM
TEMPERATURE															
PULSE RATE															
RESPIRATORY RATE															
CONVULSIONS															
WEIGHT															
MILK FEEDS NG / ORAL	1														
	2														
INDICATE	3														
IF	4														
OTHER	5														
THAN	6														
MILK	7														
	8														
IV FLUIDS															
BLOOD PRODUCTS															
24-HOUR INPUT TOTAL															
OXYGEN THERAPY															
PHOTOTHERAPY															
OUTPUT: URINE															
OUTPUT: STOOL															

FIGURE 9.6 Neonatal care chart. NG, nasogastric.

NEONATAL SPECIAL CARE BABY UNIT: MULAGO HOSPITAL
TREATMENT CHART

NAME: ....DATE OF BIRTH : ....UNIT NO : ....

DATE PRESCRIBED	DRUG	DOSE	ROUTE	REGIMEN	DATE						
				06							
				12							
				14							
				18							
				22							
				24							
				06							
				12							
				14							
				18							
				22							
				24							
				06							
				12							
				14							
				18							
				22							
				24							
				06							
				12							
				14							
				18							
				22							
				24							
				06							
				12							
				14							
				18							
				22							
				24							

STAT DOSES OF DRUGS OR FLUID				DATE		TIME		GIVEN			
	VITAMIN K		IV / IM								

INTRAVENOUS FLUID											

BLOOD PRODUCTS											

FIGURE 9.7 Neonatal treatment chart.

Example of vital signs nursing chart

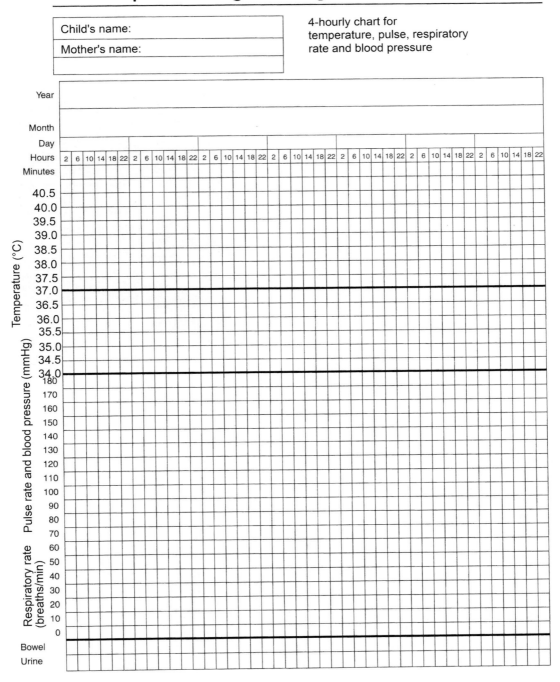

| Child's name: |
| Mother's name: |

4-hourly chart for temperature, pulse, respiratory rate and blood pressure

FIGURE 9.8 Chart for vital signs in children.

NAME:...M OR F Date of birth...............................

ADDRESS...

AGE	VACCINE
Birth	BCG against TB and Oral polio No:0
6 weeks	DTP No:1, HiB No: 1, Oral polio No: 1, HBV No: 1
10 weeks	DTP No:2, HiB No: 2, Oral polio No: 2, HBV No: 2
14 weeks	DTP No:3, HiB No: 3, Oral polio No: 3, HBV No: 3
9 months	Measles No : 1 and Yellow fever if at risk
12–15 months Measles No: 2	

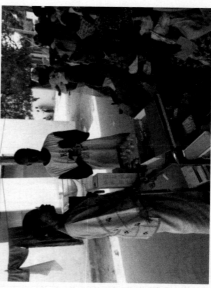

WHEN TO TAKE YOUR BABY BACK TO THE HOSPITAL OR CLINIC

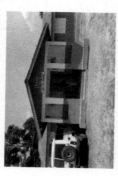

If your baby is not feeding as well as he/she has been
If your baby is lying quietly for longer than normal
If your baby is floppy
If your baby has a fever (feels hot or is sweating)
Is breathing faster than normal
Has sucking in of the ribs when breathing or any difficulty breathing
Is pale or has a blue tongue
Has a fit (starts shaking and loses consciousness)
Cannot be woken from sleep
Has yellow hands or feet
Has any skin infection
Has an enlarged tummy
Has stopped breathing suddenly
Has diarrhoea
Has vomited more than once or the vomit is green

FIGURE 9.9 Advice card for mothers.

Estimating body surface area

In paediatrics, body surface area is commonly used to calculate some drug dosages. This is because in children beyond the neonatal period, metabolic rate, renal clearance and some other bodily functions vary more closely with surface area than they do with weight.

In practice, using surface area as the basis for prescribing means that smaller children receive relatively more drug than they would if weight was being used.

For many drugs, the therapeutic margin is wide enough for it not to matter which method of dosage calculation is used, but for some it makes a significant difference, and avoids ineffective under-prescribing in smaller children. Examples of drugs for which it should be used are most cancer chemotherapy agents, and corticosteroids.

Although there are several widely used formulae and nomograms that relate surface area to body weight and height, Boyd's self-adjusting power equation that relates it to body weight alone has been shown to be the most reliable method of estimation. A major advantage is that for any particular weight, it is merely necessary to read the surface area from a table (see Table 9.14). This is not only quicker, but it also reduces the risk of making an error almost to zero.

TABLE 9.14 Surface area and weight

Weight (kg)	Surface area (m^2)	Weight (kg)	Surface area (m^2)	Weight (kg)	Surface area (m^2)
0.7	0.07	12	0.56	38	1.23
1.0.0	0.10	13	0.59	40	1.27
1.6	0.14	14	0.62	42	1.32
2.0.0	0.16	15	0.65	44	1.36
2.6	0.19	16	0.68	46	1.40
3.0.0	0.21	17	0.71	48	1.44
3.6	0.24	18	0.74	50	1.48
4.0.0	0.26	19	0.77	52	1.52
4.5	0.28	20	0.79	54	1.56
5.0.0	0.30	22	0.85	56	1.60
5.5	0.33	24	0.90	58	1.63
6.0.0	0.35	26	0.95	60	1.67
7.0.0	0.38	28	1.00	65	1.76
8.0.0	0.42	30	1.05	70	1.85
9.0.0	0.46	32	1.09	75	1.94
10.	0.49	34	1.14	80	2.03
11.	0.53	36	1.19	90	2.19

WHO/UNICEF child growth standards (2009) and the identification of severe acute malnutrition in infants and children under 5 years of age

(See Figure 9.10 and Figure 9.11)

Boys' weight (kg)					Length	Girls' weight (kg)				
-4 SD	-3 SD	-2 SD	-1 SD	Médian	(cm)	Médian	-1 SD	-2 SD	-3 SD	-4 SD
1.7	1.9	2.0	2.2	2.4	45	2.5	2.3	2.1	1.9	1.7
1.8	2.0	2.2	2.4	2.6	46	2.6	2.4	2.2	2.0	1.9
2.0	2.1	2.3	2.5	2.8	47	2.8	2.6	2.4	2.2	2.0
2.1	2.3	2.5	2.7	2.9	48	3.0	2.7	2.5	2.3	2.1
2.2	2.4	2.6	2.9	3.1	49	3.2	2.9	2.6	2.4	2.2
2.4	2.6	2.8	3.0	3.3	50	3.4	3.1	2.8	2.6	2.4
2.5	2.7	3.0	3.2	3.5	51	3.6	3.3	3.0	2.8	2.5
2.7	2.9	3.2	3.5	3.8	52	3.8	3.5	3.2	2.9	2.7
2.9	3.1	3.4	3.7	4.0	53	4.0	3.7	3.4	3.1	2.8
3.1	3.3	3.6	3.9	4.3	54	4.3	3.9	3.6	3.3	3.0
3.3	3.6	3.8	4.2	4.5	55	4.5	4.2	3.8	3.5	3.2
3.5	3.8	4.1	4.4	4.8	56	4.8	4.4	4.0	3.7	3.4
3.7	4.0	4.3	4.7	5.1	57	5.1	4.6	4.3	3.9	3.6
3.9	4.3	4.6	5.0	5.4	58	5.4	4.9	4.5	4.1	3.8
4.1	4.5	4.8	5.3	5.7	59	5.6	5.1	4.7	4.3	3.9
4.3	4.7	5.1	5.5	6.0	60	5.9	5.4	4.9	4.5	4.1
4.5	4.9	5.3	5.8	6.3	61	6.1	5.6	5.1	4.7	4.3
4.7	5.1	5.6	6.0	6.5	62	6.4	5.8	5.3	4.9	4.5
4.9	5.3	5.8	6.2	6.8	63	6.6	6.0	5.5	5.1	4.7
5.1	5.5	6.0	6.5	7.0	64	6.9	6.3	5.7	5.3	4.8
5.3	5.7	6.2	6.7	7.3	65	7.1	6.5	5.9	5.5	5.0
5.5	5.9	6.4	6.9	7.5	66	7.3	6.7	6.1	5.6	5.1
5.6	6.1	6.6	7.1	7.7	67	7.5	6.9	6.3	5.8	5.3
5.8	6.3	6.8	7.3	8.0	68	7.7	7.1	6.5	6.0	5.5
6.0	6.5	7.0	7.6	8.2	69	8.0	7.3	6.7	6.1	5.6
6.1	6.6	7.2	7.8	8.4	70	8.2	7.5	6.9	6.3	5.8
6.3	6.8	7.4	8.0	8.6	71	8.4	7.7	7.0	6.5	5.9
6.4	7.0	7.6	8.2	8.9	72	8.6	7.8	7.2	6.6	6.0
6.6	7.2	7.7	8.4	9.1	73	8.8	8.0	7.4	6.8	6.2
6.7	7.3	7.9	8.6	9.3	74	9.0	8.2	7.5	6.9	6.3
6.9	7.5	8.1	8.8	9.5	75	9.1	8.4	7.7	7.1	6.5
7.0	7.6	8.3	8.9	9.7	76	9.3	8.5	7.8	7.2	6.6
7.2	7.8	8.4	9.1	9.9	77	9.5	8.7	8.0	7.4	6.7
7.3	7.9	8.6	9.3	10.1	78	9.7	8.9	8.2	7.5	6.9
7.4	8.1	8.7	9.5	10.3	79	9.9	9.1	8.3	7.7	7.0
7.6	8.2	8.9	9.6	10.4	80	10.1	9.2	8.5	7.8	7.1
7.7	8.4	9.1	9.8	10.6	81	10.3	9.4	8.7	8.0	7.3
7.9	8.5	9.2	10.0	10.8	82	10.5	9.6	8.8	8.1	7.5
8.0	8.7	9.4	10.2	11.0	83	10.7	9.8	9.0	8.3	7.6
8.2	8.9	9.6	10.4	11.3	84	11.0	10.1	9.2	8.5	7.8
8.4	9.1	9.8	10.6	11.5	85	11.2	10.3	9.4	8.7	8.0
8.6	9.3	10.0	10.8	11.7	86	11.5	10.5	9.7	8.9	8.1

FIGURE 9.10 Weight-for-length reference chart (below 87 cm). Based on World Health Organization data.

Boys' weight (kg)					Height	Girls' weight (kg)				
-4 SD	-3 SD	-2 SD	-1 SD	Médian	(cm)	Médian	-1 SD	-2 SD	-3 SD	-4 SD
8.9	9.6	10.4	11.2	12.2	87	11.9	10.9	10.0	9.2	8.4
9.1	9.8	10.6	11.5	12.4	88	12.1	11.1	10.2	9.4	8.6
9.3	10.0	10.8	11.7	12.6	89	12.4	11.4	10.4	9.6	8.8
9.4	10.2	11.0	11.9	12.9	90	12.6	11.6	10.6	9.8	9.0
9.6	10.4	11.2	12.1	13.1	91	12.9	11.8	10.9	10.0	9.1
9.8	10.6	11.4	12.3	13.4	92	13.1	12.0	11.1	10.2	9.3
9.9	10.8	11.6	12.6	13.6	93	13.4	12.3	11.3	10.4	9.5
10.1	11.0	11.8	12.8	13.8	94	13.6	12.5	11.5	10.6	9.7
10.3	11.1	12.0	13.0	14.1	95	13.9	12.7	11.7	10.8	9.8
10.4	11.3	12.2	13.2	14.3	96	14.1	12.9	11.9	10.9	10.0
10.6	11.5	12.4	13.4	14.6	97	14.4	13.2	12.1	11.1	10.2
10.8	11.7	12.6	13.7	14.8	98	14.7	13.4	12.3	11.3	10.4
11.0	11.9	12.9	13.9	15.1	99	14.9	13.7	12.5	11.5	10.5
11.2	12.1	13.1	14.2	15.4	100	15.2	13.9	12.8	11.7	10.7
11.3	12.3	13.3	14.4	15.6	101	15.5	14.2	13.0	12.0	10.9
11.5	12.5	13.6	14.7	15.9	102	15.8	14.5	13.3	12.2	11.1
11.7	12.8	13.8	14.9	16.2	103	16.1	14.7	13.5	12.4	11.3
11.9	13.0	14.0	15.2	16.5	104	16.4	15.0	13.8	12.6	11.5
12.1	13.2	14.3	15.5	16.8	105	16.8	15.3	14.0	12.9	11.8
12.3	13.4	14.5	15.8	17.2	106	17.1	15.6	14.3	13.1	12.0
12.5	13.7	14.8	16.1	17.5	107	17.5	15.9	14.6	13.4	12.2
12.7	13.9	15.1	16.4	17.8	108	17.8	16.3	14.9	13.7	12.4
12.9	14.1	15.3	16.7	18.2	109	18.2	16.6	15.2	13.9	12.7
13.2	14.4	15.6	17.0	18.5	110	18.6	17.0	15.5	14.2	12.9
13.4	14.6	15.9	17.3	18.9	111	19.0	17.3	15.8	14.5	13.2
13.6	14.9	16.2	17.6	19.2	112	19.4	17.7	16.2	14.8	13.5
13.8	15.2	16.5	18.0	19.6	113	19.8	18.0	16.5	15.1	13.7
14.1	15.4	16.8	18.3	20.0	114	20.2	18.4	16.8	15.4	14.0
14.3	15.7	17.1	18.6	20.4	115	20.7	18.8	17.2	15.7	14.3
14.6	16.0	17.4	19.0	20.8	116	21.1	19.2	17.5	16.0	14.5
14.8	16.2	17.7	19.3	21.2	117	21.5	19.6	17.8	16.3	14.8
15.0	16.5	18.0	19.7	21.6	118	22.0	19.9	18.2	16.6	15.1
15.3	16.8	18.3	20.0	22.0	119	22.4	20.3	18.5	16.9	15.4
15.5	17.1	18.6	20.4	22.4	120	22.8	20.7	18.9	17.3	15.6

FIGURE 9.11 Weight-for-length reference chart (87 cm or above). Based on World Health Organization data.

Index

CHAPTER FIVE

Dawson Days

"To everything there is a season,
and a time to every purpose under heaven."
—ECCLESIASTES 3:1

Youcan, the Indian word for white water river, is derived from the Kutchin word Yu-kun-ah, meaning great river, which in turn was shortened to Yukon. Mount Logan, the highest point in Canada, towers majestically over the 186 000 square miles known as the Territories, of which half are wooded with spruce, poplar, and lodge pole pine. Lakes and rivers dot the entire area. At the height of the Gold Rush, Dawson boasted thirty thousand people and the Royal Canadian Mounted Police (R.C.M.P.) force in the area had grown from twenty to over three hundred. When Cruickshank arrived, the Territories were controlled by a small band of thirty-six police. He recorded his first impressions of the town for his family.

[June 1924] Dawson seems a tumble-down little town. From being the largest city in Canada west of Winnipeg it is now reduced to about eight hundred souls. Still, it is the most cosmopolitan in the world. The other day I was going up river to see some fellows who were flooded out. Our crew consisted of an Irish sergeant of police, a German, a Frenchman, a Negro, and I. That is how the whole town is, we mingle freely with French, Norwegian, Swedes, Germans, Italians, Swiss, Bulgars, Greeks, Turks, Japanese, Chinese, and Indians. I think we are about equal, but maybe people from the States lead, then French, then Scots, then Irish, but there are very few English—they are only about equal in numbers to the other European nationalities.

Our R.C.M.P. quarters are very comfortable and I am de-

lighted to find they have hot and cold running water, and electric light. That is the thing about Canada, you've got to hand it to the Canadians for fitting their places up. Even the tiniest towns in the most God forsaken places have electric light or telephones whereas you people over there fool around with paraffin lamps which cost more and are a darned nuisance, and have no telephones. Why here shacks not so big as your office have a telephone and electric light. Then big houses all have central heating, either hot air or water. Yes, they know what is cheapest and more convenient. Everything is very expensive here. Nothing is less than a shilling. No one ever dreams of using anything less. One box of chocolate or piece of soap or bottle of lemonade or box of matches—all cost "two bits," that's a shilling. Now for collection at church no one would dream of giving less than two shillings. Yes it is an expensive place to live in, but on the other hand, one can save by staying in. Laundry is awfully expensive, a shirt costs seventy-five cents to wash and everything else about fifty cents. Needless to say I do all my own and can wash and iron as good as old Mrs. Crisp. We are absolutely independent of women in this establishment, and can cook, wash, scrub, or any old thing just as good as the best of them.

There is a definite class system in Dawson and social customs are rigidly observed. The upper echelons of society consist of the civil servants, business men, police officers, professionals and their wives. The ladies all have their engraved calling cards and their day "at home." Formal dinners are given to which the ladies wear formal gowns and the gentlemen wear dinner jackets. On special occasions they invite their guests to fancy dress balls.

Until recently only the officers of the R.C.M.P. have been invited to attend these social functions, but I find I am receiving invitations to most of the affairs. I am involved in all manner of the town's activities and have joined the Anglican Church choir, the town orchestra and I even helped to build a board tennis court. It seems that the smaller and more isolated the town the more friendly the people.

Our duties are many and varied. Besides being law officers,

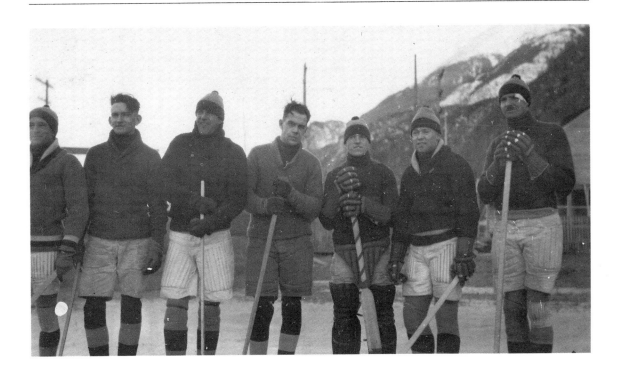

we record mining claims and land titles, collect customs duties, and act as coroners, Indian agents, health officers, tax collectors, magistrates, jailers, and guards for the Dawson banks.

I was away four days upriver in the hills bringing in a lunatic. The poor fellow is suffering from hallucinations and thinks that his neighbors were trying to murder him. He tells a wonderful tale of his adventures which sounds like a tale of the old days. He has been up here thirty years and has lived most of that time at the Creeks, sometimes never seeing anyone for two years at a stretch. He tells of how he was attacked by two men who tried to burn down his shack and murder him. He fired seventeen shells through the cabin at the intruders wounding one and eventually driving them off. He was chased miles and miles across country and shooting at his pursuers all the way. We got a message about his shooting up the fair countryside and the OC sent me off immediately to bring him in and lock him up where he couldn't hurt anyone. He is at present talking to himself in a cell a few feet from me.

"Ice hockey is easily the fastest game played by human beings and these northern born kids sure can skate." Dawson hockey team in 1925.

LEFT TO RIGHT: *Jim Purdy, Yorke Wilson, H. Cronkhite, Dave Wilson, Sandy Yuelet, Jack Stevens, James Taylor.*

57

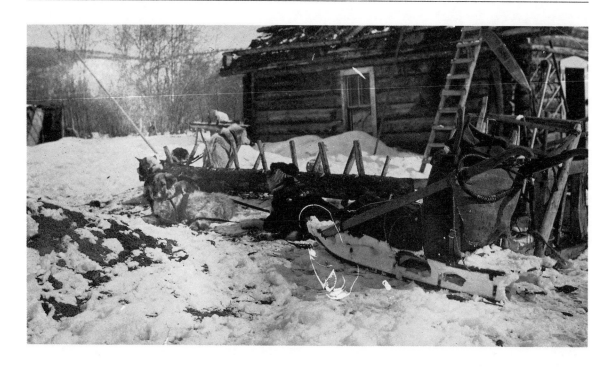

"The dogs and I have a rest at 12 Mile Road House."

I guess he will be sent to Vancouver in a week's time. I may have the job of taking him out but am not particularly keen because I am afraid I shouldn't be able to get back again until spring.

We sent another lunatic out last Friday week but I guess he is not down there yet. I hope the boys got him down alright. There are thousands of caribou around here just now (Sept.) and three men have been out shooting them to supply the poor of the town with meat for the winter. I wish I could have gone but I had this case on my hands and was up before the Supreme Court Judge with him today and remanded for a week for further evidence.

I have bought a pair of wonderful pups which will be fit to break in this winter. I have named them Bruce and Mary. They won't be much good this year but next year they will be the real thing. Then I can breed a team of real beauties out of them. I brought a Great Dane up from Vancouver and the bitch is from him. We had to send him out to Vancouver again as soon as the winter was approaching because his coat is too thin to stand the cold weather. The dog is half wolf on both sides.

They will be the cat's whiskers to breed from. I am beginning to love this country more and more every day and seem to fall into the ways of the country like a duck to water.

While on patrol one day I noticed an Indian's husky dog had its mouth and jaws full of porcupine quills. As its master paid no attention to the poor beast's suffering, I got hold of the dog and it allowed me to remove the needles. A few weeks later drat it if that husky didn't have another "run-in" with a porcupine. This time he came right to me to have the quills removed. Guess these creatures know I have a soft spot for them.

Last Sunday I went for a long walk. One of the other fellows went with me. We left at 9:00 a.m. and walked ten miles out into the mountains. There was an abundance of raspberries, and blueberries growing wild and we had several real good feeds. The wild raspberries here are as good and big as the cultivated ones at home. We picked eight pounds of blueberries and sold them when we got back for four dollars so we made quite a successful day of it. We saw lots of bear tracks and signs but we never caught sight of one. We built a fire and boiled water for a cup of tea which we enjoyed immensely. We strolled back about 6:00 p.m. after enjoying a wonderful walk amongst glorious scenery.,

Before I forget I went to a dentist the other day—a fellow who came in over the winter trail. He was a good workman and filled one tooth (a small one) and cleaned the remainder taking about one and a half hours. This little job cost me twelve dollars. Just imagine over three pounds—such is the cost of living in these parts.

Tonight I am on guard again and have two little boys in the cages. One is a miner and labourer about fifty years old, a big criminal-looking bird doing two months for selling booze to squaws. The other, an innocent looking gambler in for attempting to murder four fellows. They are both sleeping like angels. Ain't life queer?

As I glance into the twilight
The mid-night twilight's gloom

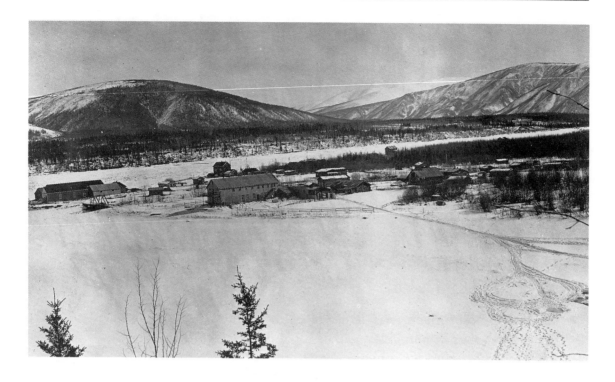

40 Mile was a welcome stop enroute to Dawson, 1924.

I see the face of my loved one
In my imagination loom.

On Wednesday I tramped out to look around. I walked in all more than fifteen miles between one and five-thirty. Considering most of the walking was up and down mountains with no trail, just rough bush and undergrowth, that was fair going even for this country. The old-timers say that I shall make an ideal dog musher. I enjoy the wonderful walks amongst the glorious scenery. I could see plainly from the top of that range of hills the towering Rockies eighty-five miles away.

Tomorrow or the next day I am leaving for the Beaver River country on a patrol so shall not be back for a couple of weeks. Furs trapped here are probably the finest in the world: Lynx, Mink, Marten, Beaver, Otter, Fox, (Silver, Black, Red and Cross) Muskrat, Wolf, Coyote, Bear, and Mountain Lion. Seal are also amongst the catch from various parts of the Territory.

The herald of fall is upon us; the hills are tinted with

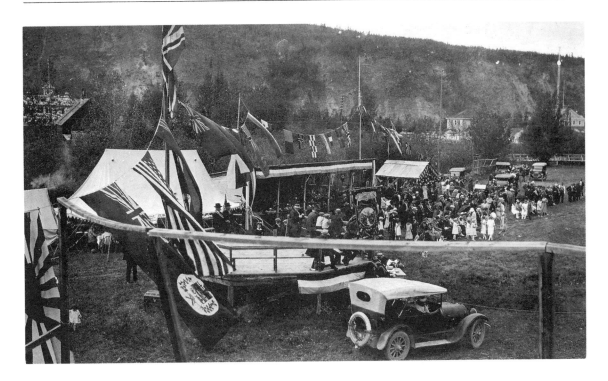

exquisite colours, obtainable only through the artistic endeavors of frost. There is nought so beautiful as fall colours so wondrously blended and carefully tinted; a constant joy to the man of open spaces. My hike into the distant mountains will be a pleasure that comes to few and I feel grateful that I can enjoy to the full that which is beautiful in nature.

How sad is the beautiful song of fall when you are out in the woods with never a sign of man except that which belongs to you alone, then the song of fall is so distinct. It seems that the rustle of the falling leaves and the rushing of the swollen brooks and streams sing a song of the dying, all plant life is dying, dying in a glory of wondrous colour as though to give one something to keep in mind all through the cold, cold winter when there is no colour but white, no music but the shrieking of the wind in the frozen branches, or the dead silence of a stark dead world, when the wind drops. The sound of the sobbing of the plants in the fall brings all this in a vivid picture before my mind's eye while I lie beneath the stars out in the wonderful wild places in the north.

August 17, 1924. Discovery Day at Dawson. People gathered from miles around to commemorate the gold strike.

What is death? Surely it is only the passing from this life to another and better one. What folks fear or dread in death is a mystery to me. I always try to think "He giveth his beloved sleep" and after all death is but a long sleep and what greater comfort can one have than to think that our loved ones are his loved ones and that they are sleeping in his keeping.

The mails are very irregular just now, the roads are bad both for sleds and wheels. The river is a mass of miniature icebergs, sometimes moving a little then stopping. I expect by tomorrow it will be frozen solid.

Owing to the fact that the mail must now come and go by the overland route it is many weeks since I was the happy recipient of any news of the outside world, except what little comes in over the wire and radio.

You ask me how far we hear from on the radio. We get most of our good concerts from Frisco which is more than two thousand miles as the radio flies and by sea and land half as much again. Of course we can get a much more distant station but the best music comes from Los Angeles and Frisco. We can hear Frisco on an ordinary indoor loop with no connections or aerial outside and all the doors and windows shut. In the summer an outdoor aerial is needed. Guess you folks know more about it than I do so I won't disclose my amateurishness.

One of our citizens got 2LO London England, one day last week on his radio, not bad was it? When one considers our remoteness and the country in which we exist, the feat is quite remarkable.

I've got a lunatic in here tonight. One of us will have to take him out in a few days. It will be a ten day trip, with him all the time, every minute of the twenty-four hours. Of course the return trip will be worth the outward journey. I don't think the job will fall to me because one of the boys has been up in the north a long time and wants a trip to the outside. At present he is quite good and quiet. At times he starts praying out loud and calls himself "God's perfect child" and sometimes thinks he is Jesus Christ. I feel sorry for the poor beggar. Still, lots of them get it up here.

The temperature had been dropping steadily so Tidd and I

decided it was time to take a dog team on a patrol to the out-lying district. The December morning was bright and snappy with the thermometer standing at twelve degrees below zero. Outside the barracks was a toboggan loaded with two eiderdowns, a grub box, kettle, fry pan, two axes, twenty pounds of salmon (for the dogs) two rifles, ammunition, two cameras and tripods, two pairs of extra socks and moccasins, two changes of mitts, and dog chains. This was covered with two canvas sheets. The dogs were yapping and excited as we strolled over, dressed in moccasins, parkas, and toques. We were only taking three young dogs, great big fellows weighing one hundred and seventy pounds or more each. Usually we take five but these chaps needed a workout as they had done very little all the winter and were too fat and soft.

It took us sometime to get them harnessed and hitched up as they were so excited and got all tangled up a dozen times. At last they were straight and with a yell we dashed out of the yard at a dead run both flinging ourselves on to the load as the toboggan flew past. For a mile or so they kept up the mad speed but gradually calmed down and settled to their work. I trotted ahead, while Tidd drove, until our team spotted a pair of dogs on another street and dashed at 'em for a fight tipping the load over in their mad rush. With a deal of shouting and swearing we got ourselves under way again and trotted merrily along towards the hills. The track got worse and worse and we had to help in spite of the small load. After a few miles of constant climbing we got to the top of the second dome about 2 500 feet. The snow was very deep and there was no trail. I had to constantly walk ahead and then back again on snowshoes to break a trail. The dogs could get no footing, so after hauling and pushing and swearing for several hours we decided to camp for the night.

The night was getting colder as we cut down spruce for bedding and built an open camp. The dry wood was scarce and one had to wallow in the snow waist deep to cut it out. In an hour a fire was burning merrily and the two of us were busily engaged cooking our supper. Bye and bye millions of stars began to show in the sky like diamonds on purple velvet.

Having fed the dogs we covered ourselves with an eiderdown and talked. Tidd was a schoolmaster in England and has been here ten years. He is a wonderful musician and loves this country and the life up here in the wilderness. So we have many things in common. We talked world politics and almost every subject under the stars until we became sleepy. Then we just took off our parkas and went to sleep while the fire spluttered away and eventually went out. About 8:00 a.m. we woke and found that during the night a blizzard had covered us with about six inches of snow and was still going strong. A fire was soon warming us up and a big caribou steak was frying, coffee was made and we sat down to a good breakfast. It was useless to endeavor to go further with that team so we packed up and made the best of a bad trail home again. Of course when the blizzard stopped and after we picked up extra dogs the trip was easy.

Tomorrow is another big ball. I hope we have as good a time as we had last time. I shall help the orchestra with a baritone saxophone playing the cello part. Have you ever seen a baritone sax? They stand about four feet high and are awfully heavy but have a wonderful deep note.

You asked what the family could send me, songs, I'd like songs, ones like "Friend 0 Mine," "Indian Love Lyrics," "My Dear Soul," "Thoughts have Wings," "Bird of Love Divine," etc. etc. Can't have too many. I am playing my Saxophone a lot too.

Christmas 1924 found Cruickshank a little homesick for his family and Hillhouse, and he wrote on the stationery of the Sour Dough Hotel to his sister:

My Very Dear Doe, Here we are the day after Christmas. Oh how I thought of you all during the past two days, all the little incidents of Christmases long past came to me as it were a pageant. Gee how happy we all were and what wonderful times we had.

My Christmas was a very uneventful one, nothing much happened. On Christmas eve we had a good dinner in the barracks, composed of oyster soup, roast turkey and all the good things that go with it, then plum pudding and brandy sauce, mince pies, jam tarts, cakes, fruit, and liquor, certainly a fine feed and excellently cooked. Of course we had a few little speeches and all was friendly and fine. The dinner over at 9:00 p.m. left us wondering what on earth to do. Some sat down to read, some to write, some to play the phonograph and drink. Tidd and I felt like doing none of these things, so we changed into outside clothes and stepped into the night which was forty degrees below with a dirty wind and fine snow. There were no friendly stars, no smiling glow from the northern lights, nothing to show us that we had any friends. We walked five or six miles, then turned back and talked over Christmases of long ago. When we got back we turned in and never woke till Christmas day. I did stables at 6:30 a.m., had a little fruit and bacon and eggs for breakfast then lay on my bed and read. In the afternoon I went with the orchestra to the hospital to help give a little music to the patients. In the evening four of us went down town to a restaurant to dinner and had a dandy feed. On arriving home Tidd and I played and sang till 10:30 p.m. and then turned in.

Here is a brief little history to go with my fancy writing paper.

The words "sour dough" have several connotations. To some it means a type of bread made with a small amount of sour dough worked into the new flour mixture and baked over an open fire, hence sour dough. To others, at the time of the Gold Rush it became synonymous with those stampeders who surged into the Klondike searching for gold. Many of these stalwart men and women, eaking their fortune from this wild country, living in rough primitive conditions, and eating mainly beans and sourdough bread remained in the Yukon to become a new breed, the Sourdoughs. Dawson was a thriving metropolis at that time and business was booming. Hotels sprang up all over town, the most popular establishment being the Sour Dough Hotel. A list of house rules hung on the door of every room. Years later, when the gold rush was over and business was slow, one of the managers decided to incorporate some of these rules on his hotel letterhead.

About half our population are Indians, nomadic hunters from the upper Peel country. The Voyageurs called them Loucheux, the French word meaning "slant-eyed." They are encouraged to live in their own villages. One such place is called Moosehide, a village several miles outside Dawson. The Indians are forbidden to have liquor, but we received a complaint that someone was selling them alcohol and so I was sent to investigate. It was fifty degrees below zero. The Indians were having a big celebration and had been dancing every night for seven nights. I arrived there about 7:00 p.m. It was a glorious night—the moon at first quarter and thousands of bright twinkling stars which all seemed tinted with a faint green. As I neared the village I could hear the yapping of the malamute dogs before I could see the village. I was on a trail running on the shore ice of the Yukon River. On either side of the river were high rocky hills looking like towering banks of broken snow. The river is a mass of miniature icebergs all frozen together—some the height of a man, some smaller, some larger—a truly pretty sight but makes a rotten job of getting a dog team or any team across. Horses can't cross without cutting a road out of solid ice. The high rocks on the right abruptly stopped and there standing on a level piece of ground up on a high bank is Moosehide. It is composed of about thirty log cabins scattered higgledy- piggledy all over the place, each with a meat cache and a fish rack alongside. Hundreds of dogs roam around and dog fights are a permanent thing. I saw that the crowd were all in having a feast so I went into the hut next to the one they were using as a dance hall, and sat down by the stove. The hut I was in was one of the biggest, about twelve by sixteen feet and was built of small poplars unsplit and chinked up with mud. These cabins are the warmest kind of hut and are used on the prairies and by the white people. The walls had been papered but the paper was mostly all off. In the corner was a heap of blankets, robes and rugs used as a bed. In another corner was a rough bed covered with filthy rags. There were two stoves, one a cook stove and the other an ordinary Yukon stove. The third corner held a stack of dried fish (that stank to the devil) and a litter

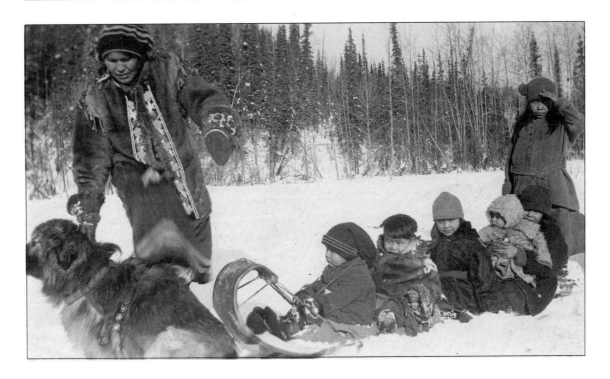

*of pups. There was a little window and no ventilation whatso-
ever. That was the best hut in the village, next to the preacher's.
After the crowd had eaten, they came back to their hut and
we all shook hands. There were four braves, five squaws and
umpteen kids. At 9:00 p.m. the dancing started. There was an
old cello, a violin and a guitar, all frightfully out of tune, but
the musicians sawed away and got some sort of time and some
sort of tune. Most of the dances were square dances, jigs, one
step and waltzes. I danced with most of the squaws but never
got a smell of booze. I smelt lots of other smells, but not booze.
Some of the squaws came up and asked me to dance. They
are certainly not shy. They dress mostly in imitation of
white people (however bad) and some were very funny. Of
course these Indians are near town and can get the clothes
they want. Some of them had come five hundred miles for
this potlatch. They are very light on their toes and are good
step dancers.*

*At seventy-seven years of age Chief Isaac is a striking figure,
tall, slim, and still physically fit. As a youth he was elected*

*Some small travel-
ling companions
on the Moosehide
trail.*

67

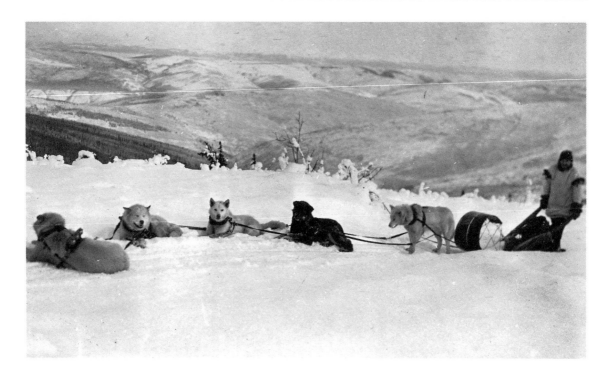

"The dogs were exhausted when we reached the high country." 1925.

chief of the Moosehide band. Throughout the years he has endeared himself to both natives and whites by his superior intelligence, his intrinsic ability, and his outgoing personality. In many controversial situations between traders, prospectors, missionaries, and pioneers, Isaac's friendliness toward the newcomers has ensured a peaceful settlement. He is a devout Anglican and attends the services at the little Moosehide Church regularly.

I am glad Doe likes the Indian beaded moosehide moccasins. If I had thought all the girls would have liked them I would have sent more. The Indians at Moosehide do unique and beautiful work, but I have grown so accustomed to seeing the Indian items of clothing and other articles being used everyday, and using them myself, that I had quite forgotten how lovely they really are. I will send off some items immediately.

When not on duty my evenings are spent with practices, concerts, or parties, one long winter of gaiety. Indeed the smaller and more lonely the town, the more friendly and *cheerful the people. Dawson has a splendid hall with a good stage, fine lighting and adequate dressing rooms.*

[February 1925] Tonight we are giving a concert. I am playing the E baritone sax. in the orchestra, singing a couple of straight songs, a humorous duet with Tidd and taking two parts in a comedy. You will think it is a kind of one man show but don't you believe it. There are ten pieces in the orchestra: piano, two violins, three saxophones, trombone, cornet and drums. Then there are two straight singers, four comedians, and a pianoforte solo, then a scream of a one act comedy called "Case against Casey." We've sold four hundred seats.

The concert was a tremendous success. *The Dawson News* reported the following day:

No amount of justice can be done to the small but perfectly acted part of Farmer Wheatear as taken by the talented comedian Constable Cruickshank. Although this popular actor was on the stage for only a short time compared with some of the other members of the cast, he lost no time in bringing the house to an uproar by his home-town farmer costume and extraordinary voice interpretation. The public would have enjoyed hearing more from him.

Our local paper is two sheets, including adverts and costs 25¢ a day. I am getting a swollen head. Bishop Stringer (you have of course heard of him, the man who boiled and ate his sealskin mukluks when he was lost and starving on the trail) is awfully friendly and asks me up to his house often. He was going over to Oxford to the church conference but something stopped him. His children are in the dramatic society. He has one grown up daughter just back from the University and two sons up here just now and several outside. They are a very nice family.

I have broken in my pups. The R.C.M.P. use a tandem hitch which works best in this wooded area, unlike the Eskimos who like to use a fan hitch on the open tundra. The tandem is harnessing the dogs to the sled with the one nearest the sled known as the wheel dog and numbering the others four, three, two, leader. As you see we use five dogs. I never used any old dogs with mine as is the usual way. I tried a way of my own and it has turned out extraordinarily well. I let them get used to the collars, and harness, then hitched them one at a time on the sled and let them follow me. Of course at first they were scared but they were more frightened of me leaving them and going for a walk without them than they were of the sled. So they came along and brought the sled along too, once or twice pulling an empty sled and following me got them used to pulling. I then taught Bruce to go ahead. This took a little more patience but he is shaping up well and I think he will make an ideal leader. He will learn to gee and haw as he is very intelligent. Soon I shall buy some very good pups to go with him. They are expensive but I shall get lots of pleasure out of them next winter. Mary is going to have pups soon but I am afraid they won't be the quality I want as they are an unforeseen development.

Most of the dogs we use are Malamutes and weigh between eighty-five and one hundred and fifty pounds and are often part wolf. They must have stamina and be willing workers, as pulling a sled is hard work. Their feet must be able to stand up under the ice and snow conditions. They are taught never to chase after caribou or any wild life on the trail, for a bolting team could mean the musher being thrown into a tree, or worse. While hitching the dogs to the sled one must always remember to tie the sled to a tree first, to prevent a runaway. It is a long walk going after them if he doesn't! He must make sure too, that if there are any fighters, or antagonists among them, they are hitched out of reach of each other. If an accident does occur one must be quick to separate the dogs before a serious injury befalls man or dog.

This April weather is rotten, large flakes of wet snow like you get in England, real wet, miserable English weather. It is a pity because I am leaving tomorrow on a patrol of one hundred and four miles with a dog team to inquire into a case of alleged insanity. Up to now the weather has been wonderful, anyhow, maybe tomorrow will bring forth a decent day, then the trip will be ideal. I am going to use Bruce perhaps as leader. He is a good worker but frightfully pigheaded. I shall see how he goes the first day out and then decide on his position in a regular team. The snow will soon be gone and another month will see the river open and the boats once more steaming down the stream. Oh no, not a month, maybe six weeks. I shall be sorry in lots of ways to see my old friend the snow disappear. I have enjoyed the winter so much, not a dull moment or a day's regret that I came here.

Spring is here, the Yukon River is of course still frozen solid but lots of snow is gone and sleds are discarded and wheels are now appearing on the roads. We are hoping to get a boat through from Whitehorse at the beginning of June if the ice is gone from Lake Laberge. Yesterday when I was coming back from night duty at 6:00 a.m. I saw three or four robins. The robins here are much bigger than the ones in the old country. They are just about as big as a thrush but have a red breast as bright as the little fellows you have. There are also a few blackbirds back for the summer. I love to see and hear them, one misses one's feathered friends through the long winters. I was out in the sunny side of the hills where the snow was almost gone and there I found a few crocuses, the first of the year and two or three butterflies flitting around. I am going to enclose one of the crocuses. You will notice that even the flowers here have a kind of fur on them. All this will sound inane and silly to you perhaps but those things mean a lot to me. When one loves nature one watches eagerly for the changes and signs of new wonders always appearing when the seasons change.

I write more letters and get more than anyone in the barracks. I destroyed a bunch of letters yesterday that I have had for the last two months. I burned eighty-five and kept twenty to answer. I am awfully thankful for them. I love to get all the home news and to know how things are going.

The flood has gone down leaving a terrible mess of debris all over the town. The work it makes for us cleaning up is appalling.

We are baffled over the complete disappearance of a guy in town four nights ago and suspect a murder. He went out of his house saying he would be back in an hour but never showed up again and has left absolutely no sign. This is the second case since Christmas. The trouble is the river is so swift that a body that is thrown in it would never be seen again unless some curious freak of nature happened.

My dogs are in great shape. I put a pack on Bruce and Mary last Sunday. Bruce took to it at once and enjoyed it, had his old rudder up and a grin on his face from ear to ear. He thought it was a great joke. I put about thirty pounds on him and twenty pounds on Mary. She took it as work and looked pretty miserable about it, but nevertheless worked well. We only did about eighteen miles that day but it was not very good walking and mostly uphill.

I made open camp at night just using a mosquito bar as they are rather troublesome. You would be surprised if I told you that the dogs and I between us carried two waterproof sheets, two blankets, an axe, fry pan, kettle, mosquito bar, cups, knife and fork, ammunition, hunting knife, notebook and lots of little things and then made eighteen to twenty miles a day on hills twice the size of the Chilterns and wild and rough as wild nature can make them.

By the way, the first night out I didn't chain the dogs up at once and while I was cutting down spruce to make a bed after supper my noble Bruce pinched all my bacon. So, I had pretty slim rations for awhile, though I learned a lesson which will probably save me another time from serious fate.

There is no sunset, there is no dawn
There is only twilight long and drawn
The midnight's pass in a dream of light
The day is a glory of sunshine bright.

All the trees are now in full leaf and the days are very hot. Daylight lasts twenty-four hours and during the whole time nature works at top speed. The birds can build a nest and begin laying in four days. They are busy about twenty-two hours out of the twenty-four so make up for the short summer.

To The Yukon Summer

I wonder why Poets always tell
Of the cold north and the winter's spell.
Why can't they write of the summer night
And its wonderful dream of soft twilight?

Can't they write of the early spring,
Of the poplar tree all verdant green
Of the bluebell's soft and turquoise sheen,
Waving like bluebirds on the wing?

I love the mountains so strong and bold
With their green spruce trees and their tails of gold,
I love them in the twilight lad
In a misty mantle of purple clad.

They are Kings, and like Kings of old
Are clad in purple and in gold.
Gold there is in their rocky might
Golden glow on their sun kissed heights.

I love the north in the month of June
With never a glimpse of the dear old moon.
I love the twilight soft and long
Surely a note for a Poet's song.

You ask me if any farming is done up here. Yes there are several farmers but it is not a very paying proposition. There are excellent crops but they do not always ripen before the frost comes. The vegetables and flowers are as good as any in the world. You see in the summer they get twenty-four hours a day of sunlight and therefore grow the whole time. The potatoes never boil floury. They are always like new ones owing to the fact that the frost invariably comes before they are fully developed. They are much larger than the average English potatoes. There are very few cows in this country and what fresh milk there is is delivered in blocks like ice in winter. We never see fresh milk. We live entirely on canned milk. Nearly every housekeeper does his or her own work. In fact I think there are only two people who hire help; except an occasional charwoman whom they pay about two dollars an hour. Girls who work out get about five dollars a day for housework and live in, and are treated as members of the family. Telegraph messengers are paid ninety dollars a month, just boys. But don't think because such high wages are paid that one can make a fortune. Working out the cost of living and freight rates always eat up everything.

We have had a great deal of rain recently, and are just about fed up now. There is only just a few more weeks of summer left and then the real winter of the Arctic will be upon us. The nights are wondrous now with the mellow light of myriads of stars and a wonderful moon. The moon rises so quickly that in a minute or two it moves twice its size in the sky.

I have been rather busy lately, but in spite of duty have managed to make time to build myself a dog sled, and make four sets of harnesses. Though I says it what shouldn't, I was lucky enough to make a good job of both, and even the old hands have complimented me on my handiwork. This will mean a saving to me of almost sixty dollars which is not to be laughed at by one earning so little. On the other hand I was obliged to buy another dog and some extra fish which cost me sixty-five dollars, but I guess that will be paid back some day.

I am just now down at Mayo Detachment and have had a very trying week. On Monday I walked out to a place twenty miles away and returned on Tuesday. On Wednesday the Corporal in charge was taken ill and almost died, was out of his mind the next two days and I had a terrible time with him. He is better now but the last three days I have travelled forty-five miles each day taking him back and forwards between Mayo and Keno. He is leaving tomorrow for Dawson with the man from the Detachment and a lunatic I am watching just now. After tomorrow I shall be the only Policeman within four days distance, a territory with an area equal almost to the centre of England. I shall have to spend nearly all my time between Mayo and Keno doing forty-five miles in a day with my dogs, two or three times a week. Hope to goodness nothing more crops up. Had a murder again a week or so ago. An Indian stabbed another but disappeared. He is not in my district and I hope he won't wander down this far. I have enough to do looking after my own bunch of over one thousand people and two towns, looking after two offices and stores, two horses, five dogs, and the Lord only knows what else.

The trail from Dawson south-east to Mayo is the one used by those early patrols who went on through the Werneke Mountains and down the Wind River to Fort McPherson, a distance of four hundred and seventy-five miles. I was told that in the winter of 1904-5 the patrol took fifty-six days instead of the usual thirty days to make the journey. Thankfully they survived, not like the poor devils six years later. Evidently, Inspector Fitzgerald, his three men and their dogs set off from Fort McPherson to Dawson and all perished. Corporal Dempster organized the search for the Lost Patrol and recovered the bodies. Reports are that many factors contributed to this disaster, such as inadequate supplies, no traps, only one .30-.30 firearm and perhaps most significant of all, no Loucheux guide. Some of these Indians are the finest woodsmen in the world and have proved invaluable to us on many occasions.

There are two ladies staying in town, or rather a mile out of town, who are under my special care. They are the wife and daughter of the head of "The Consolidated Mining & Smelting Co." a company in partnership with C.P.R. (Canadian Pacific Railway), immensely wealthy people. Their respective husbands have gone out to the Beaver country to look at a number of claims bought by the C.P.R. and report on the same. I hope the report will be favorable and I am almost certain it will because the hills are very rich out there with silver, and grey copper. The mining is now nearly all done by dredges and hydraulic mines but the Treadwell Yukon Co. are bringing steam shovels in this year tho' we are doubtful if they will be a success on this frozen ground, in spite of the fact that they are quite a success against rocks in Africa. Frozen ground has absolutely no give in it although rock does give a little and break fairly easily. This Territory is still one of the richest in the world for gold and silver. Silver ore, the finest in the world, is obtained in large quantities at Mayo.

I shall shortly commence making a trip out every month. It will be a long patrol but I shall enjoy it. The trails were not good enough to take the ladies even on horseback, so they were obliged to stay at Keno. They have been having a wonderful time picking berries, fishing etc., and are in constant amazement at the variety of plants, minerals, and animals there are up here. They expected to find nothing but ice and snow, so imagine their delight when they found blueberries, cranberries, raspberries, and lots of other berries, countless flowers, and wild animals.

We have had a glorious fall, the weather has been just wonderful, so mild and scarcely any snow. There is not enough snow for decent sleighing even yet and we are three days into November. I have had several wonderful hikes on snowshoes. I love to get out on the mountains and round the Indian trails.

I have not heard from Dawson how the Corporal is or if they are going to send me a new man, or leave me here alone all the winter. I have got a nice home and although I am living alone and "it is not meet for man to live alone" I like it. I have altered a great many things and have the place looking fine.

It is a queer thing that in spite of the fact that I have apparently nothing to do I am busy from when I get up at 8:00 a.m. till I go to bed at 11:00 or 12:00 p.m. The house takes at least an hour to clean up in the morning, then there is the wood to get in, the dogs to exercise, reports to make out, and innumerable other things to attend to. So I keep myself going from morn till night.

Last Friday I went down to Mayo and had to go on duty, but there was a dance that night at Keno. As Miss Wernecke (who is the niece of the Lord High Mucky Muck of this territory) had never been out with dogs, I took her down with me. I got up at 5:00 a.m. and went up the hill (four miles) to their camp and had breakfast with them. We pulled out about 7:30 a.m. It was a glorious day, bright, bright sunshine all day and quite warm, *up above zero, a little too warm for the dogs. The roads were not good and as I had only four dogs and fifty miles to make I had to run nearly all the way. We enjoyed ourselves very much and had two stops for tea and dinner. We got in about 4:20 p.m. Miss Wernecke is still raving about the perfectly wonderful trip.*

I had my saxophone down there and helped out with the orchestra and danced till 2:00 a.m. I was amused at Miss Wernecke who thinks I am superhuman to run over forty miles in a day and then dance all night, but any dog musher who has done as much as I have these three years could do the same. As you can gather I am in the pink of condition and busy as the deuce.

My term of duty at Mayo and Keno passed quickly and I am posted back to Dawson. I left Keno on November 11 and drove our own police horses with a wagon containing all my worldly possessions and all Cpl. Thurgood's, to a roadhouse about twelve miles away. I stopped there for the night, was up next morning at 3:00 a.m., saw to my horses and had breakfast, left at 5:30 a.m. and drove twenty miles to another log road house and had dinner and fed the horses, then drove on another ten or twelve miles after dinner. That day I got a shot at a big wolf but I was holding the lines in my hand and one of the horses ducked his head just as I shot so I missed the wolf.

That night I reached Mayo. I left the Police team there and carried on next morning at 5:30 a.m. with the stage. We crossed the Stewart River on ice so thin it only just bore the horses. Then we bounced and bumped all the morning over atrocious trails till noon. We stayed to feed the horses and make a pot of tea by the trail for ourselves. After a two hour rest we bumped on again over frozen niggerheads and mostly up hills and down. I don't know how the wagon held together (there was not enough snow for sleighing). Long after dark we pulled up at a Road House and put up our tired horses after having done forty miles. There was another stage waiting there to carry on next morning with four fresh horses. There was enough snow here for sleighing so we thanked our stars for that much luck. After supper we clipped two horses then turned in

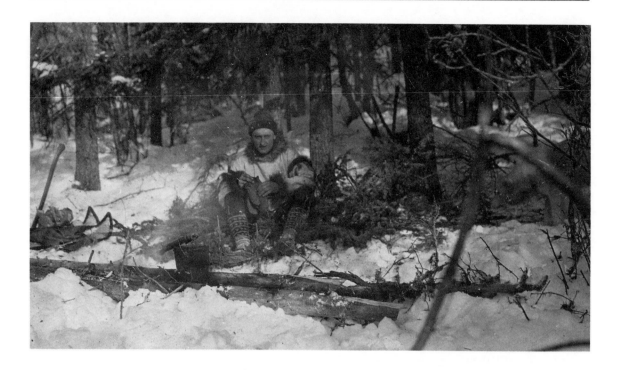

"I stopped to make tea after a long hard trek over rough terrain. Tried out my new shutter delay."

about eleven pretty well tired out. 3:00 a.m. saw us up and busy again and for three hours we travelled before the dawn began to break. The dawns are wonderful, you can never imagine the colouring unless you have seen a dawn in the Arctic.

At noon that day we made our fire by the trail and had a cup of tea and fed the horses, then on again till after dark—forty-five miles that day on trails like you have never seen. Next day the same, up at about 3:00 a.m. and drive till after dark. That day we changed stage and drivers. We had to pull our baggage over the river on hand sleighs because the ice would not bear a horse. Anyway we got it over safely and transferred to the stage awaiting on the other side. Next day was a short day, only twenty-five miles, so we were in early. The day after that we were up at 2:00 a.m. travelled till noon, changed horses and kept on till 7:00 p.m.—about fifty miles that day. Next day we reached Dawson about 2:30 p.m. after about thirty-five miles driving. The trip had taken seven days. So here I am home again in Dawson and on a new job.

We had a good dance in Dawson last night and my head is still swollen from the flattery I received. All the ladies greeted me like a long lost brother and filled me with nice things. I am beginning to think that every one of them would leave their little wooden hut for me. But joking aside one certainly feels a warm sensation around the heart when one receives a real welcome from almost everyone in a town like this. There must have been a hundred couples at least, all the ladies in the latest short skirts. In my young days we should have thought that they were only wearing a thin chemise but things have altered and I like them best this way. There is only one girl in the town with long hair and most of them are either shingled or cut just like a man's, but the kid with the long hair is awfully pretty and her hair suits her as it is. Most folks call her my sister and I am quite proud of her. She is only about seventeen but a very amusing youngster. There are quite a number of very pretty girls here but my crowd seem to be the young married folks and the school teachers. We get quite a kick out of life with our books and music.

We have had a cold spell this January. It has not been above fifty below zero and has been down to seventy below and just now is sixty-five below and there is a wind, a thing that has rarely occurred even in the far north. I guess we shall be busy fetching in dead men when this cold snap lets up. There are always a few of the old people who go under during an intensely cold snap.

We still find lots to do in the way of concerts and practices for the same and orchestra practices, drama practices, and dances. It certainly is a busy little place for musical folk or folk who go in for amusing others.

The *Dawson News* of 23 March 1925 reported a concert given in the Dawson Theatre by conductor John Dines and his orchestra. Mr. Dines rendered a violin solo of Moszkowsky's *Serenade* with tone and cadence. The program included a trombone solo with orchestral accompaniment which was loudly encored. The News goes on to say:

A.D. Cruickshank was in splendid voice, his "Kashmiri Song" was a delight and at the conclusion a loud burst of applause immediately demanded his reappearance.

I was tickled as a kid to get those snaps Mr. Brown took. I had no conception of Doe as a grown up woman. She is quite pretty, isn't she? I wish I could come home for a few weeks and see you all. Bill and Ian are also men now. It seems strange that when one is away one expects the folks at home to remain exactly as they were when one left. Has Doe got a boy yet? If she were here she would be married inside a month to anyone she liked to look at. It is the exception for any girl to reach twenty without getting married. The school teacher here is just twenty, a really fine girl. All the men are crazy about her but she doesn't get a swollen head over it. She was born in the country and has been used to the adoration of the male population since childhood. It is amusing to see the effect on girls from the outside when they come to this country. They become so confoundedly conceited that they are unbearable to any man except the poor beggars who have lived up here for about thirty years and those poor simps spend hundreds of dollars on them just to get a smile. Guess I will move on before I get that bad.

There will be a boat down river tomorrow and it is bringing one hundred and sixteen sacks of mail. The weather is getting colder and the nights are drawing in so quickly. It's only 9:00 p.m. and dark already, and every night we get a frost. Soon the long cold winter will be on us and we will be all settled down to eight months of ice and snow.

Unfortunately several of the boys have gone outside and some have purchased their discharge, leaving two of us to do the work originally done by nine men. I am often on duty for thirty-six hours at a stretch. Today I was in Court with one lunatic who was convicted and sent outside and just this minute I have had another handed over to me for trial on Monday. Business in the lunatic line is flourishing. This means that either Anderson or I will have to take them both out or at least as far as Whitehorse (four days by steamboat). Imagine

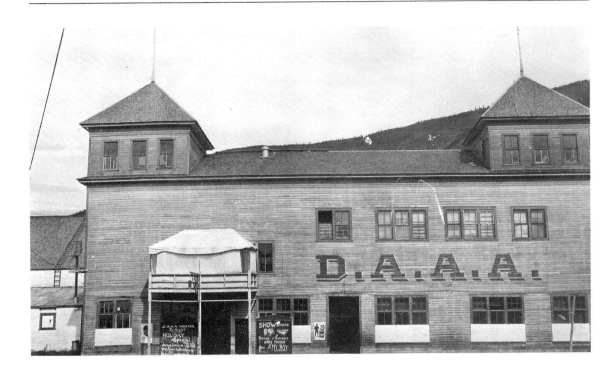

one little policeman in England in charge of two mad miners. I often think of how they send them around in England in custody of three or four great big policemen and here sometimes hand two lunatics to one little man for a trip from seven to fourteen days.

I am wearing down pretty fine now and am only one hundred and forty-two pounds, while last winter I was one hundred and sixty pounds. Nevertheless I am in perfect health though developing quite a snappy temper, sometimes one's nerves seem to get on edge, then everything is irritating. The last boat leaves here on the sixth of next month. Then the only way out will be over the trail, a fourteen day trip by horse stage.

[25 November 1926] I wish I could be with you this Christmas. I know I should see a difference in each of you, for five years alters us all. We are all older and I hope wiser for these years. I think of the four and a half valuable years I lost during the war. Here I am nearly thirty years old and just about to start to tackle a new job entirely out of my line, but other

The D.A.A.A. was used as the theatre where Cruickshank often performed with the Dawson Dramatic Society between 1924-1927.

people are confident I am the man for the job so I will prove that their confidence was not misplaced.

Cruickshank did not at this time reveal what his new job was to be, but it certainly was a complete change from his work with the R.C.M.P., and it was typical of the man whose keen sense of adventure had led him to the Canadian north.

CHAPTER SIX

Queen of the Yukon

"Is it, in heav'n, a crime to love too well?"
—ALEXANDER POPE

I have so many irons in the fire and so much organising to do that I am absolutely overwhelmed with work. I am leaving the Police next month if I can. If things come out right I shall in one jump go from Constable in charge of Keno Detachment to one of the most important men in the Territory. I feel that I cannot justify telling you all my plans as in the case of the Yukon Government not passing legislation which I have placed before them, I cannot proceed with my project. On the other hand, if I can get laws passed which I have placed before the Yukon and Dominion Governments, then I shall be able to go ahead and make a name and money. As I said before I am frightfully busy and as I only have one day in which to answer the week's mail if I want it to go by return, I have to work fast and furiously. The man I have with me can take more of the official work off my hands so I have my own private business to attend to and the police work too.

His family in England must have wondered what fantastic scheme Cruickshank had managed to dream up when they received this mysterious letter at the beginning of 1927. Fortunately, they had not long to wait before they received the answers to all their questions.

For a long time I have been mulling over the idea of starting a Yukon Airline. I have met two men who are also interested, James Finnegan, and Clyde Wann. After long hours of deliberation we have decided the airplane must be a cabin mono-

plane to seat three passengers and pilot, and carry two hundred and fifty pounds of baggage. The cabin must be heated in the winter and fitted with skis. In the summer she will be rigged as a sea plane. We think that the best company to build our machine is the Ryan Aircraft Company in San Diego. If we combine our resources we can raise enough money to pay for it. We will call our company the Yukon Airways and Exploration Company and have James Finnegan as president, Clyde Wann as Vice President and I will be the pilot and General Manager.

I have had a lot of trouble over the ordering of a suitable machine on account of being so far away from the base of supplies, and as wires cost about two dollars each and letters take six weeks round trip, you understand the expense and delays which occur. The Federal Government has granted us permission to receive the mail contract for the Yukon, but they give absolutely no financial support.

If bad luck overtakes us and we are a failure in this venture, I don't see how we can if things turn out half decently. I am still young and the experience will have been a great thing. There are lots of other things I can do now I have had a go at executive work. I shall have more confidence in myself and shall start some other venture. However, if we have no accidents this proposition will be one of the best things on the North American Continent.

Word that my application for discharge had been accepted and that I was to proceed at once to Dawson reached me at Keno about the 25th of March 1927. I left the following Saturday after packing up my personal belongings. I did the first part of the trip by auto to Mayo. The next day I left by stage with a team of horses and got thirty-five miles. We got word that the North Bound stage had broken down. I waited around a day but then I decided to take a small pack and walk on into Dawson. That afternoon I walked twenty-four miles to Stewart Crossing. The next day thirty-six miles to Grand Lake. The next on to Strickland, but the trail was bad and a snow storm came on so I stayed at Strickland that afternoon and evening only doing eighteen miles that day. Next day I made

Hollinbroks, twenty-eight miles over frightful trails. I had no snowshoes so it took me a long time to make it. The following day I borrowed snow shoes and made the remaining thirty-two miles into Dawson.

People were very surprised to see me, especially as I was in ahead of stage time. I got my business settled up as far as I could, spent one evening at Frank Health's, and one at Tidd's, and then pulled out for the south as General Manager of the Yukon Airways and Exploration Company headed for San Diego.

The day I left Dawson it was thirty-two degrees below zero in spite of the date being the 5th of April. We had a cold trip that day. The evening I spent with friends at North Forks. I left their house about 2:00 a.m. and the thermometer registered forty-five degrees below zero. The next day too, was frightfully cold and the trails bad. As we proceeded the weather got a little milder but in spite of that the trip was rotten and took me fourteen days from Dawson to Whitehorse and cost me ten dollars a day. The darned trip will cost me about two thousand dollars before I get back to Whitehorse. I was in Whitehorse two days and got my offices fixed up there and examined the landing grounds, fixed up about oils and gasoline and a hundred and one other things and got away on the train at 5:00 a.m. on Tuesday morning, arriving at Skagway that noon. In the evening there was a bridge party and I got the First Gentleman's prize. I had a letter of introduction to the chief passenger agent at Skagway who was at the party and he fixed me up with the best stateroom on board so I am surrounded by stewards and given a wonderful amount of attention. This is a beautiful boat, the Princess Alice, like a floating palace. There were only six passengers at Skagway so we felt like six millionaires for a whole day and laughed about our yachting tour. We have now got about a dozen on board and there is room for five hundred more first class passengers and lord knows how many second steerage.

My airplane should be built by the time I get down to San Diego and will only have to have a few alterations to suit the Northern conditions.

"The R.C.M.P. is just like a crack regiment of cavalry. The uniforms are all very smart and tailor-made, the boots especially cut for each man."

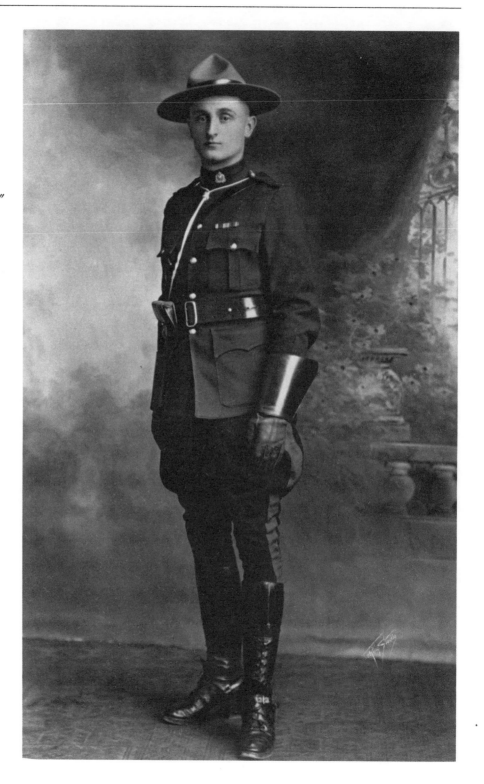

The sea is very rough and foggy today [20 April 1927] and there is hardly a passenger to be seen.

. . . I have been flying here in Vancouver since I arrived three weeks ago. I find that I am not so good as I used to be, but feel sure that in a few more hours I shall be back in my old form. I shall be leaving Vancouver on Saturday for San Diego. I shall stay there several days and get used to that type of machine before I go back to the Yukon to erect the machine and commence operations. I found a great deal of difference between land planes and the heavy flying boats that we have in the Air Force at Vancouver. The experience I have gained here will be invaluable to me when I commence operating from the rivers in the Yukon. We have had very poor weather since I came down, however I hope to strike decent weather in the south.

You can hardly imagine the amount of work the organization of a new company takes. What with that work and the examinations which I have to take as a commercial flier I am nearly worked to death. Financially we are not so strong as we should be. We have had bad luck in that some of our members have had severe losses which brings down our resources and makes things even more worrying for me.

The Ryan Aircraft Company had indeed begun to construct one of their standard M-2 models for Cruickshank, but through a strange set of circumstances, he was never to fly that particular plane. Charles Lindbergh was planning his solo flight from New York to Paris at the time, and had thought of flying in a Bellanca. He backed away from that decision when the Bellanca's manufacturers wanted him to have a crew they would appoint. Instead, he approached the Ryan Aircraft Company to see if they could build him a single seat airplane. It was already February 1927, and Lindbergh needed the plane as quickly as possible to avoid competition from other pilots with their eyes on the $25 000 prize to be awarded to the first to fly nonstop from the United States to France. Cruickshank was asked if he was willing to let Lindbergh have the plane being built for him. If he let the American flier have his plane, another model incorporating the design modifications being made for Lindbergh could be ready in two months, he was told. He agreed.

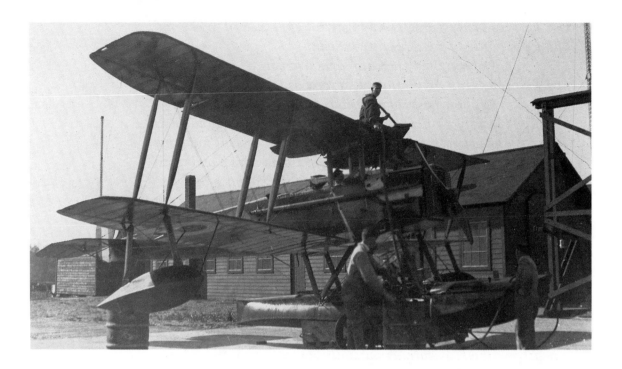

Lindbergh helps the ground crew in San Diego, California in May 1927.

Among the changes to the M-2 model for Lindbergh, the Ryan Aircraft Company engineer, Donald Hall, had lengthened the wingspan, built of British Columbia spruce spars, by ten feet, making it forty-six feet. The plane's overall length was twenty-seven feet six inches. The cabin was enlarged, as Lindbergh insisted that the main fuel tank be placed in front of the pilot's seat, rather than behind it. While this blocked the pilot's forward vision, it would give him a better chance of survival in case of a crash, as he didn't want to be sandwiched between the tank and the hot engine. The fuselage was welded with carbon steel tubes, and the landing gear was reinforced. A thin skin of cotton fabric was cut, fitted, and sewn tightly over the plane, and then this fabric was doped with cellulose acetate. Before the fabric was applied to the front wing spar, each man who had worked such long hours on Lindbergh's plane signed his name there, and one traced a swastika, the ancient good luck symbol. Perhaps this was a portent of Lindbergh's admiration for Hitler, and of his involvement in the America First Movement. The Wright plant in Paterson, New Jersey, delivered the 220 hp. air-cooled, nine cylinder engine. The

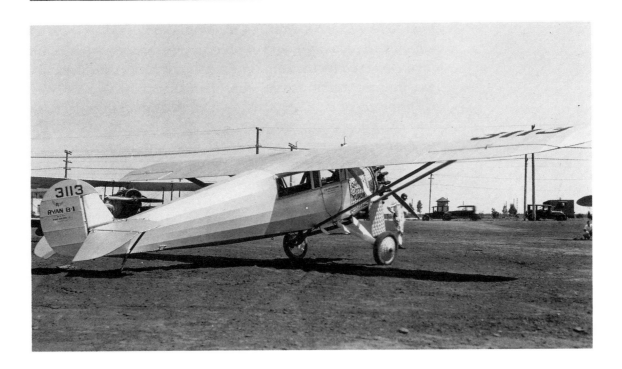

eight-foot nine-inch Duralumin propeller was warped into its shaft.

Named *The Spirit of St. Louis*, the new plane was almost complete when Cruickshank reached the Ryan factory early in May. There he met Lindbergh, who was working day and night on his plane. The two men discussed the innovations to the original M-2 model, and decided that most would be beneficial to the plane that would be constructed for Cruickshank's northern flying. It was agreed that a replica of *The Spirit of St. Louis* would be manufactured for him.

Lindbergh amused Cruickshank by telling him about approaching the Ryan Aircraft Company and asking for a machine which could fly from New York to Paris. Company officials asked, "How far is that?" Lindbergh didn't know. So, he and the company engineer went to the local public library, obtained a large world globe, and then, with a piece of string, measured the distance between New York and Paris, about 3 200 miles. Therefore, they decided they must strive to obtain a range of 4 000 miles for safety. Their endeavor proved successful, and Lindbergh became famous world wide for his exploit.

Queen of the Yukon *emerges from the hangar of the Ryan Aircraft Co., San Diego, July 1927.*

I am in San Diego awaiting the completion of my new plane which will be a duplicate of Lindbergh's, made by the same men, powered by the same engine, everything just the same, except that mine carries four passengers, where he was carrying gasoline. We have had a number of delays because I want things equipped for the cold weather of the North, and the factory is swamped with orders owing to Lindbergh's wonderful flight. Charlie was working on his when I arrived. I have some good pictures of him and his ship before he became a celebrity. He is a quiet, good natured young fellow, popular with all flying people and with the whole world.

I have been treated like a Lord down here and have seen nearly all of California from the air and from friends' cars. I have been a guest at the biggest and most select club in the United States, have been shown around in cars costing thousands and in all have had a wonderful time.

Owing to delays I have lost my spring work in the Yukon so shall tour several states with our plane and give passenger flights. Everyone is crazy to see a ship like Lindbergh's and to ride in one so I hope I can make a thousand or so before I return to Canada and also see a little more of the world.

I am getting used to these monoplanes now and can swing them about pretty well. In a few more days I shall be an expert. They are a wonderful machine, so very different from the old sea-planes I was flying in Vancouver.

I did nineteen flights on Sunday, was flying almost the entire day, was hardly out of the machine for eight hours. Today I went on seven flights, one a long one over the most magnificent scenery. The people are getting quite enthusiastic over flying and are all so pleased when we take them round. They assume I am an American now and are frightfully surprised when I tell them I was born in England. They say I have no English accent and seem normal!

No one would live in England after seeing such a territory as this. It is the most wonderful country in the world. The climate is ideal and the people charming. I have picked oranges, lemons, grapefruit, cantaloupes, avocados, figs, dates,

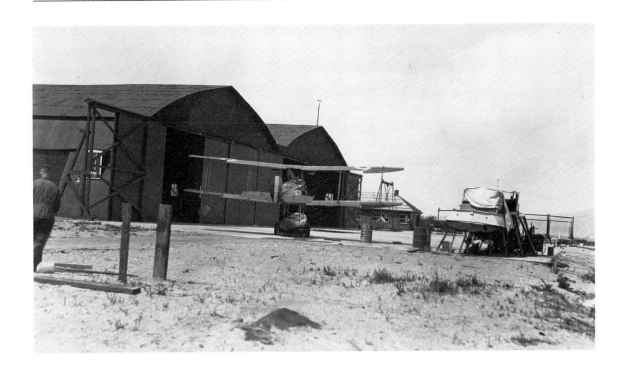

etc. etc. I stayed a weekend at a friend's orange ranch and had a grand time.

A busy day at Ryan Aircraft, San Diego 1927.

While Cruickshank was in California awaiting delivery of his plane, the movie industry was developing apace in Hollywood. The last memorable years of the silent era were taking place, as was the innovation of filming in two-strip Technicolor and the new and improved three-strip Technicolor. It was also in the 1927-28 season that The Academy of Motion Picture Arts and Sciences was established, and that organization commenced the Academy Awards. The first awards were given for silent films, but a special award was given to Warner Bros. for pioneering the outstanding talking picture, *The Jazz Singer*. Films about flying were especially popular, and *Wings*, a Paramount Picture, won an Oscar in 1927. True to form, Cruickshank became involved in one particularly dangerous aspect of movie-making.

I have been doing some stunt flying for the movies. While waiting around the set I have met quite a number of the movie stars and have had a proposal of marriage from a widow with quite a lot of money who says she wants a smart young fellow to run the business. She promised me an airplane and a car for myself and all I had to do was get married and walk into a nice home. What do you think of the proposition? Guess I ought to take it up eh? She really appears quite fond of me, a thing I can't understand but women are curious things. However, for the present I have decided on single blessedness and the cold weather for a few months longer, I mean years.

At last, Cruickshank was able to report that his plane had been completed.

Yesterday, July 9th, I got delivery of our ship on wheels. She is a wonderful ship and we call her the Queen of the Yukon. She is a Ryan Braugham, cabin monoplane, the sister ship to Lindbergh's, identical in every way, except that where he carried gasoline we carry four passengers and two hundred and fifty pounds of baggage. She has a Wright Whirlwind air-cooled engine developing two hundred and twenty horsepower with a cruising speed of one hundred miles an hour and a top speed of one hundred and twenty-five miles per hour. She is equipped with skis for winter but we are having trouble getting pontoons made. We will have to wait around until they are built and then will fly right up the coast to the Yukon.

Just now I am staying with a friend, Mr. Clarke Chapman, of Coorina, a very rich young fellow, one of the old American aristocracy. He was educated as a doctor but doesn't need to practice. This is a lovely old home with long drives lined with high palms and trimmed box hedges. The lawns are nicely kept and there are hundreds of acres of oranges and lemons, etc. The house has very big rooms, each bedroom having a bathroom and a sleeping porch as well as a big double bed or twin beds. The furniture and cars would thrill you. Gee how I wish I could give Dad and you a house like this to retire to. California is beautiful. It is the kind of place Mill would love to live in. I will send you some newspaper articles one of these days as the papers often mention us.

It's three weeks since I wrote and I face more delays. Here it is August 1st and I am still in the United States. I have been unable to leave for Canada yet as we have found difficulty raising enough money to pay duty on the plane into Canada. However, we have done fairly well and make over a hundred dollars a day, some days. We should need only a few more good days then we can go ahead with our final preparations and leave once more for the Yukon.

Since the Versailles Peace Conference in 1919 all civil aircraft are required to have an international identification. The nationality letter G is assigned to the British Empire and Canada allocated G-CA. So the Queen of the Yukon will be identified with the letters G-CAHR.

I shall be glad to get home again in spite of the interesting time I have had and the numerous friends I have made. I wonder if anyone else has as many friends in as many towns as I have. Everyone seems so kind and considerate and does everything in their power to make my stay in their particular town a real pleasure. I would like you to have seen all the wonderful country I have seen and to meet the folks I have met. It is curious very few people think I am English and I must say that Yankee hospitality has been wonderful. Why they treat me as a kind of little hero I don't know, but that is how it seems to me I am treated.

A few days later, Cruickshank was able to leave California and head for more familiar surroundings in Canada. But the trip was not smooth.

Reno, Nevada is a very curious town. Its chief method of earning a livelihood is through divorces. There is a law here which allows anyone living in the town for three months to obtain a divorce. So right now there are two thousand or more people from all over the world awaiting their freedom. In this very house there are eighteen, some of them the most charming people, others not quite so nice.

We have done fairly well here flying joy flights. We have made about one hundred and seventy-five dollars a day, one

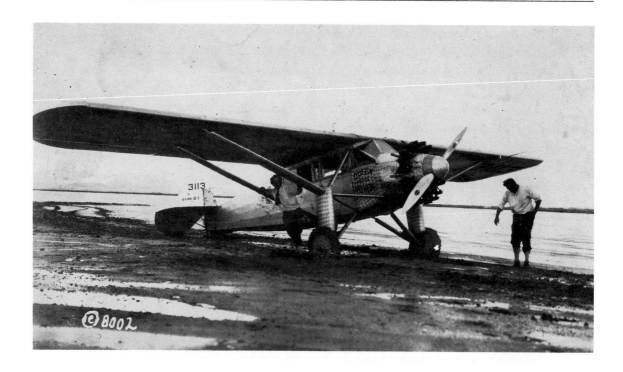

While crossing Nevada Cruickshank was forced to land on Baker Lake when he was caught in a sudden snow storm.

day over three hundred dollars. We intend staying about three or four days more then going to Ely and eventually on to Seattle, then to Dawson again. This is mountainous country. The field is 5 000 feet above sea level which makes landing very fast. With a big load we have to land at about seventy miles an hour but so far all has gone well.

It seems all the Service Clubs want us to speak to them about Aviation. We have been complying as often as we can. On August 9th there was a large headline in the Nevada newspaper, "ELY BOUND PLANE LOST IN STORM Queen of the Yukon fails to arrive here, due at Ely early morning." While crossing Nevada we were caught in a sudden snow storm and forced to land on Baker Lake. The lake was a mass of sticky snow and ice. After much digging, sweating and shovelling we managed to extricate the Queen and arrive somewhat later than anticipated to speak at the Rotary's luncheon meeting.

We have been held up here for four days with rain, but if it

*lets up we shall leave today or tomorrow for Portland, then
Seattle, then Vancouver, B.C., and eventually in ten days at
the most, will be away for the Yukon.*

In the fall of 1927, Vancouver had no airport, and the city's only
squadron of sea planes was stationed at Jericho Beach. Lacking
proper landing facilities, Cruickshank chose a cow pasture near
Lansdowne Park racetrack to set down the *Queen of the Yukon*. As
it was the first large land-based plane to arrive in the city, as well as
being the sister ship to *The Spirit of St. Louis*, thousands of people
turned out to see her. Standing in the crowd waving and cheering
Cruickshank's safe arrival was Esmé.

The following day, Cruickshank took Esmé, Inez and her husband
Jack, for a flight in the *Queen of the Yukon*. What a thrill it gave
them to skim over Vancouver and to gaze down on the familiar
landmarks far below, including the Cenotaph, Christ Church Ca-
thedral, the Marine Building, the old Vancouver Hotel, and Esmé's
and Inez's former home, Chester Court. The North and West Vancouver ferries scurrying across Burrard Inlet were like children's
toys. For Esmé, the ride ended all too quickly, but Inez felt she had
disgraced the family by becoming violently ill. Cruickshank con-
soled her by saying that, as she was expecting her first child, she
couldn't have had a better excuse.

Not long after he had met Esmé for the first time, but after he had
been posted to Dawson, Cruickshank had composed a poem for his
new love.

To Your Picture

Up in the north on the Yukon's shore,
Sits a boy in an old bell tent,
His thoughts are back two weeks no more,
And his eyes on a beautiful picture bent.

He sees these glorious eyes aglow
As they were on a night two weeks ago
He sees that mouth as it bid farewell,

Firmly smiling no tale to tell
Of the agony in that brave young heart
As she from him did fortune part.

T'is only a wonderful picture,
T'is only a likeness true,
But to him t'is an angel of light and love
Of love the old yet new.

And it was to Esmé, the angel of light and love, that Cruickshank was married in St. Paul's Anglican Church in Vancouver on the 17th of October 1927.

Following the wedding breakfast, the bride and groom, together with their wedding party and guests, boarded the steamship *Princess Alice*, which lay at berth in Burrard Inlet. Floral bouquets sent to the newlyweds by many well-wishers adorned every nook and cranny of the tiny stateroom, perfuming the air. The guests crammed happily into the cabin, wishing Cruickshank and Esmé joy; more toasts were drunk, both to their wedded bliss and to their courageous northern enterprise. Amidst all this merry-making, the *Princess Alice* steamed out of the harbor, and was well into the First Narrows when Esmé's brother, Charlie, looked out of the porthole and realized the vessel was underway. The captain was informed, and he begrudgingly returned to Vancouver to let his unpaid passengers disembark.

Four days later, the *Princess Alice* reached Skagway. There, the *Queen of the Yukon*, shipped in parts which had been lashed firmly to the vessel's deck for the journey to Skagway, was unloaded. Cruickshank's original plan had been to load the machine on board the White Pass and Yukon Railway, headed for Whitehorse, but winter was fast approaching. Anxious to avoid the early frosts and a longer delay shipping the Queen by train, Cruickshank decided to fly the plane over the Chilkoot Pass to Whitehorse.

Back in 1898, the Chilkoot trail was intimidating to even the most stalwart, for it rose to a height of thirty-five hundred feet, the last, leading to the summit, a climb at an almost forty degree angle. The way was strewn with enormous rocks, bodies of dead pack animals, and it was muddy or slushy, depending on the weather.

Every person had to bring in a ton of supplies, which meant that each man or woman had to make about twenty trips over the treacherous terrain, carrying one hundred pounds each time. At the tree line, the trail widened, and a tent community named Sheep Camp became established to provide rough meals and accommodation for the weary trekkers. Local Indians often got jobs for fifty dollars a day carrying supplies. Thousands of gold seekers made an unending line slogging up the icy steps cut in the snow. If anyone stopped to take a breath, it might be hours before it would be possible to get back in the line.

Cruickshank's flight over the "trail of '98" was to be the first ever; as passengers he had Esmé, who had refused to travel to Whitehorse by train, and his partners Clyde Wann and James Finnegan.

Now that the decision to fly over the Chilkoot Pass had been made, Cruickshank and Esmé assembled the *Queen of the Yukon* on the shores of Skagway. On the morning of 25 October 1927, Cruickshank, Esmé, Wann and Finnegan climbed aboard the Queen, and took off from the sandy beach in front of the town. In Cruickshank's wallet was a much-travelled American dollar bill which Lindbergh had carried on his epic flight across the Atlantic. Across its face was a legend that indicated the bill had been carried many miles in the air by Captain H.C. Martell of the US Air Service on his flights in Central America. Lindbergh had sent this bill to Cruickshank as a talisman of the "Lindbergh Luck" for his northern adventure. As it happened, Cruickshank would need all the luck he could get on this flight over such formidable territory. A.A. Gillespie, a writer for *Maclean's Magazine* described the flight:

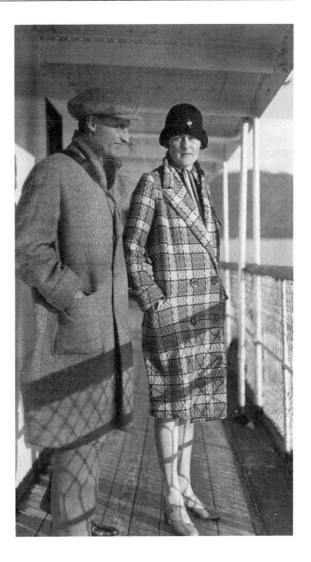

Alone at last! Esmé and Cruickshank aboard the Princess Alice enroute to Skagway on their honeymoon.

97

When the Queen took to the air near Skagway the skies were clear and there was no trace of storms. Five minutes out from the gateway port a heavy fog was encountered blocking the valley. It was impossible to turn back for already the tide would have crawled up over the take-off field. The plane zoomed ahead, higher and higher, gaining altitude with every revolution of the indefatigable propeller, its noisy bark filling the fog-blanketed valley below with a deafening roar. Still the fog persisted; fog which lay like huge grayish-white blankets on all sides of the monoplane. "Cruicky" kept climbing.

Suddenly a formidable mountain top loomed vaguely through the heavy fog screen and the aviator shot his machine straight up into the heavens. Every heart beat with uncontrollable emotion. Could they make it? Could he guide his trim ship through that white darkness or was the honeymoon voyage and the Yukon Airways' first venture to crash on the pinnacle of those unrelenting snowcrested mountain crags? More mountains shot into prominence and still the pilot shot his machine skyward just in the nick of time as huge, bluish-white hulks raced out to meet him. Twenty minutes, long nightmare minutes which seemed to know no end. And then salvation, Chilkoot Pass had been conquered. Once above the highest peak, twelve thousand feet in the air, day dawned in the far side of the valley. The fog disappeared and a bright sun broke through to ensure perfect visibility. The tenseness was broken. The pilot's wife sitting in the wicker chair directly behind her husband leaned forward and patted him on the back. In answer Cruickshank turned around and smiled. It was more a smile of relief than of victory.

One hour and twenty minutes later the *Queen of the Yukon* landed on the Whitehorse flying field. The entire town was out to welcome their "Mountie" home. The town went crazy.

Cruickshank's historic and challenging flight over the Chilkoot Pass to Whitehorse set a new course for northern aviation, but he had still more to accomplish. First, he had to draft schedules for his air mail routes to Dawson and iron out many details for the new business.

The tariff list for November 1927 was as follows:

Whitehorse-Mayo
Mayo-Whitehorse: $125.00 single fare
Return (trip to be specified) $240.00
Express: 35¢ per pound

Whitehorse-Keno
Keno-Whitehorse: $135.00 single fare
Return (trip to be specified) $260.00
Express: 40¢ per pound

Whitehorse-Dawson
Dawson-Whitehorse: $175.00 single fare
Return (trip to be specified) $325.00
Express: 50¢ per pound

Mayo-Keno
Keno-Mayo: $ 15.00 single fare
Return (trip to be specified) $ 27.50
Express: 15¢ per pound

Mayo-Dawson
Dawson-Mayo: $ 70.00 single fare
Return (trip to be specified) $135.00
Express: 30¢ per pound

Keno-Dawson
Dawson-Keno: $ 80.00 single fare
Return (trip to be specified) $150.00
Express: 30¢ per pound

Whitehorse-Carcross
Carcross-Whitehorse: $ 20.00 single fare
Return (trip to be specified) $ 35.00
Express: 25¢ per pound

Whitehorse-Atlin
Atlin-Whitehorse: $ 50.00 single fare
Return (trip to be specified) $ 90.00
Express: 30¢ per pound

Carcross-Atlin
Atlin-Carcross: $ 35.00 single fare
Return (trip to be specified) $ 65.00
Express: 25¢ per pound

Baggage allowance twenty-five pounds to each passenger. Minimum charge of $1.00 for express parcels.

Plane may be chartered for trips not on schedule for $120.00 per hour to places where landings are available or on non-stop pleasure flights.

Capacity of plane four passengers and baggage, or eight hundred pounds of mail or express.

All letters carried at a charge of twenty-five cents per ounce or fraction thereof and the same rate applies to each additional ounce or fraction thereof.

YUKON AIRWAYS AND EXPLORATION COMPANY, LIMITED has been granted permission by the Postmaster General of Canada to issue a special airmail stamp and sticker. Airmail stamps to be placed on back of envelope and airmail stickers to be placed on the front. Regular postage stamps must be placed on front of envelope in the usual manner and mailed at post office.

The *Queen of the Yukon* would travel between Whitehorse, Mayo, Keno, Dawson, Carcross, and Atlin, carrying both passengers and mail. It is interesting to note that at this time in Dawson some prices advertised in the *Whitehorse Star* included:

gasoline, case, $6.75; Hudson's Bay blankets ,$12.50; Cigarettes (Buckingham), 20 for 25¢; men's heavy ribbed all wool shirts and drawers, per suit, $3.00.

In Edmonton, Eaton's advertised:

12 bars Sunlight soap, 50¢; roast beef, 6¢ per pound; butter, 3 pounds, 46¢; flour, 98 pound bag, $2.10; sugar, 20 pounds, $1.08; sardines, 10¢ a tin.

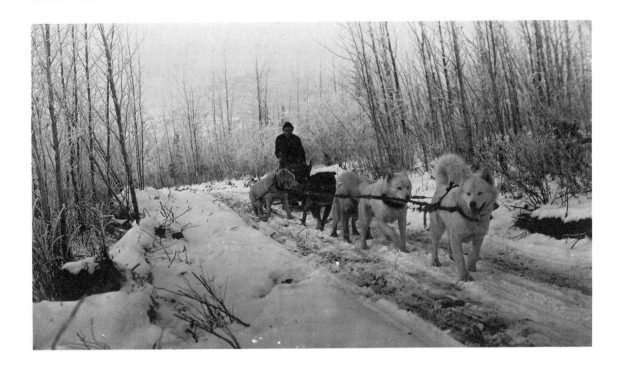

Anxious to show his bride the places where he had served in the R.C.M.P. and to introduce her to his many friends, Cruickshank and Esmé flew to Mayo and Keno. There was a tumultuous reception for the fliers, especially as Cruickshank was an old friend and the *Queen of the Yukon* was the first plane to land in these silver mining towns. Inclement weather had forced Cruickshank and Esmé to remain a few more days in Mayo, but finally they set off for Dawson on 8 November. Before long, the sky darkened, and the wind began buffeting the plane. It would be foolhardy to attempt landing, but the mail had to be delivered. Cruickshank circled three times around the city and then flew low over his former home, the R.C.M.P. barracks. At that precise moment he shouted to his bride, "Toss the bag out now." Leaning out of the *Queen of the Yukon*'s tiny cockpit, Esmé took aim and threw the mailbag. It landed squarely in the middle of the R.C.M.P. backyard. Thus was the first airmail "dropped" into Dawson.

The official date for the inauguration of the airmail and passenger service between Whitehorse and Mayo via Dawson was November 11, 1927. On this clear frosty morning the *Queen of the Yukon*,

"Trips taking twelve days by dog team could be done in five hours by plane."

carrying several bags of mail, landed on a long sand bar in a slough about a mile from Dawson. Each piece of mail bore a twenty-five cent sticker similar to a stamp, on which appeared a picture of the *Queen of the Yukon* on a blue background. This twenty-five cent charge paid for carrying a piece of mail; although the federal government postal authorities had given the Yukon Airways and Exploration Company permission for this undertaking, they provided the company absolutely no monetary assistance to cover the service.

To commemorate the inaugural flight, Cruickshank ordered and had inscribed for Esmé a gold nugget bracelet designed in the shape of a sluice box, and crafted by a gifted Dawson goldsmith, W. Murdock, a bracelet which my mother gave to me when I turned sixteen.

In Dawson the weather was getting colder every day, so a makeshift hangar was hastily erected to protect the *Queen of the Yukon* and the men servicing her. This consisted of a canvas tent with a large Yukon stove at one end; the smokestack appeared through a hole cut in the top. Soon this enclosure became a hub of activity; it was repair shop, lunchroom, rest room, and a meeting room for the Dawson inhabitants who wandered over from town to get their first glimpse of the big airplane, and hopefully to get a ride in her too. One eleven-year-old boy earned the price of his ride by piling several cords of wood for a Dawson wood merchant.

As the temperature plummetted, so too did the good fortune of the owners of the *Queen of the Yukon*. First the engine oil tank burst. This was corrected by building a new oil tank and wrapping the pipes leading to and from the engine with heavy electric tape. That day they took nineteen passengers on their initial ride. One group of four exuberant young hockey players were experiencing their first air flight, so Cruickshank thought they should get a memorable ride for their money. He proceeded to slip and slide, climb and dive over the city like a loose pancake. They received good value. A few days later, with the temperature at -30°F, Cruickshank had only been in the air for about five minutes when he experienced more trouble. This time the windows began to frost over so quickly they could not be washed clear with the alcohol and glycerin mixture brought along for that purpose. As visibility was nil, he had to turn back. Keeping his eye on the long spiral of smoke

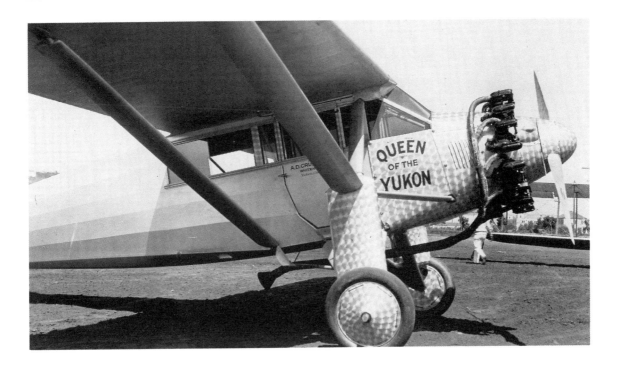

Queen of the
Yukon.

pouring forth from the stove pipe in the roof of the tent hangar, he
was able to judge his distance and bring the plane down on a stretch
of ice between the river and the field. He hit the snowy mound on
the edge of the bank, bounced up higher than the hangar top, and
landed on the air field. The rest of the day was spent putting in
double panes of glass in the cockpit.

He had hardly circled the town the next day when the ailerons
caused such a bumpy ride that once again he had to return. The -35°F
temperature had caused the cables to contract so the controls could
not operate accurately. This problem was corrected, but still the
windows continued to frost over. Finally, Cruickshank and his
mechanics realized the exhaust lacked a collector ring so the four
top cylinders of the air-cooled Whirlwind engine were spewing hot
smoke on the windows which the icy air sealed into thick frost on
the outside pane. To remedy this problem, Cruickshank fetched a
welder from Bear Creek; working all night, they managed to weld
additional iron pipes onto the exhaust outlets.

A few days later Cruickshank and a man named McInnis took off
from Whitehorse. What should have been an hour and twenty

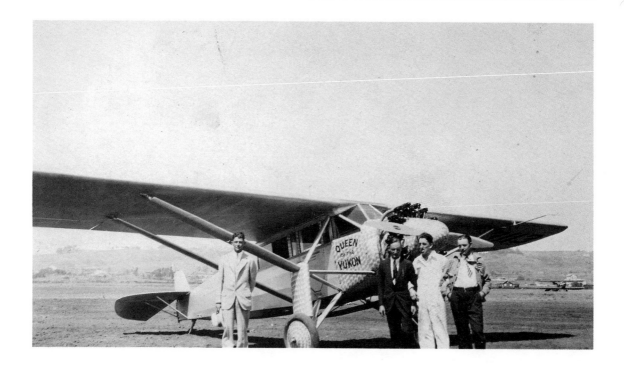

The principals of the Yukon Airways and Exploration Co. Ltd. LEFT TO RIGHT: *Clyde Wann, Vice President; Cruickshank, pilot and manager; Ed Smith, mechanic and Bill Munday, assistant pilot.*

minute flight turned into a harrowing experience for Cruickshank and his passenger, and a three-day nightmare for Esmé. Two hours after the Queen left Whitehorse, a wire came through from the Carmacks telegraph station stating that the plane had passed over Carmacks. Then came another report that it had been seen flying over Yukon Crossing. Then SILENCE. The weather was becoming exceedingly cold and Cruickshank was wearing only a light flying jacket, while McInnis was equally lightly clad.

The next day the thermometer read -45°F. Esmé was becoming increasingly alarmed as thirty-six hours later there was still no word. Finally, the long-awaited message was tapped over the wire, "Cruickshank and passenger both safe at Mayo Junction."

Leaving Whitehorse in ideal flying conditions they had run into a blizzard, which caused Cruickshank to miss a landmark and go off course. When he realized this he returned, buffeting against wind and storm, only to pass through a cold air pocket about -50°F. The needle of the oil pressure gauge registered practically nil. Cruickshank knew something was wrong with the engine but, as he was six minutes from Mayo Junction, he prayed he could make

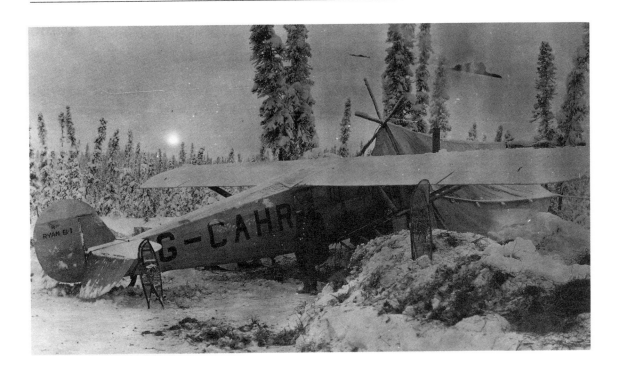

it. No luck, the engine sputtered, then ceased altogether, at an elevation of three thousand feet. Only a moment before, Cruickshank had noticed a tiny frozen lake surrounded by trees, nestled below them. By zig-zagging back and forth, he managed to glide the Queen down, making a perfect landing and missing the trees by a breath. After checking his engine, he found that the lubricating system had been completely frozen and the top three cylinders had been badly scored by the lack of oil.

Although thankful to be safely on the ground, their ordeal was far from over. They must hike out to Mayo, which they estimated to be about forty miles away. Clad only in light jackets and without snowshoes they set off, finding the main winter road about a mile from the lake. They spent the next several hours slogging through the freezing -35°F temperature. Finally, about an hour after darkness descended, they halted as they were totally exhausted by cold and hunger. They built two fires and huddled together sitting upright to keep from freezing to death. Cruickshank had a few frozen pears in his pocket. These they thawed by the fire and eased their hunger pangs somewhat. At dawn, they set off again, finally reaching Mayo

A tent is erected over the Queen of the Yukon *in order to make repairs in - 48°F weather, 1927.*

Junction about noon. The mail and express was picked up and sent on to Mayo by horse and sleigh.

Now, Cruickshank had to enlist help to repair his plane. Three men and with a horse and double-ender sleigh went back the forty miles to the *Queen of the Yukon*. With the temperature hovering around - 60°F, it was useless attempting to work on the engine, but gradually the temperature warmed to -56°F and they were able to raise a tent over the engine and set to work. After twenty-four laborious hours they could still not warm the engine sufficiently for the plane to take off. Spare cylinders would have to be obtained from the Wright factory. Cruickshank strapped Mayo's Dawson-bound mail and the express on his back and began to walk the long, lonely one hundred and seventy miles to Dawson. When he had tramped to within thirty miles of Dawson, he was met by Esmé who had driven out from Dawson to meet him. What a joyous reunion!

Once again, Cruickshank was to spend Christmas in Dawson. This time he was to enjoy it with his beloved. They decorated a pretty fir tree. Nestled in the branches, wrapped in this poem, was a gold nugget brooch and earrings.

To wish you a merry Xmas

On this first Xmas day
To show you that I love you
In the truest kind of way.

I love you dearest star o' mine
And never shall forget
The wife that I have married
Is a star that ne'r will set.

Oh take this little gift o' mine
And let it say each day
I match your hair, I match your heart
True gold with gleaming ray.

May love be ever true to you
And make your life all joy

God give you all your heart may ask
Is the prayer of your love sick boy.

Flying in Yukon's vast wilderness often presented problems not encountered by pilots in other areas. Cruickshank often landed the *Queen of the Yukon* in remote Indian settlements. On one occasion, he brought the plane down on the sand bar in the Porcupine River at Old Crow. When the Indian women saw the enormous bird in the sky, they shouted to their husbands, "shoot it, shoot it." Today, Old Crow has a large modern airport, and airplanes are a daily occurrence.

Despite the difficulties, delays, and setbacks there were many happy and rewarding experiences. One day, Cruickshank was called out to bring an injured miner to the Dawson hospital. As he was returning with the invalid in -54°F weather, a driving snow forced him down forty miles from the nearest settlement. Choosing a place out of the prevailing winds for a temporary camp, grateful that he always carried a double-bitted axe, with one end razor sharp, he chopped spruce boughs for his patient's bed, and for the fires. Being able to start a fire quickly in the north was often a matter of life or death and certainly at this time speed was of the essence. Since his early days in Dawson, Cruickshank had nearly always carried a tin in which he had previously soaked in coal oil several pairs of old socks which had been cut into three or four-inch strips. These made excellent fire starters when combined with any dry wood available. Usually, the black dry moss on the lower twigs of the spruce trees or the outside bark of the birch made good tinder. He built two blazing fires, then gently laid his charge upon a thick bed of spruce boughs between the two fires, and prayed someone would spot the smoke in time to save the miner. Fortunately, while he was keeping the fire going, a trapper saw the wisps of smoke coming from the bush and decided he had better investigate. He mushed his dog team over to the makeshift camp. The two white dogs leading the trapper's team immediately recognized their former master. They were Bruce and Mary!

Coming from a big city to Dawson was a traumatic experience for Esmé. Cruickshank was an accepted member of the small community, but she was virtually a stranger. Often she accompanied

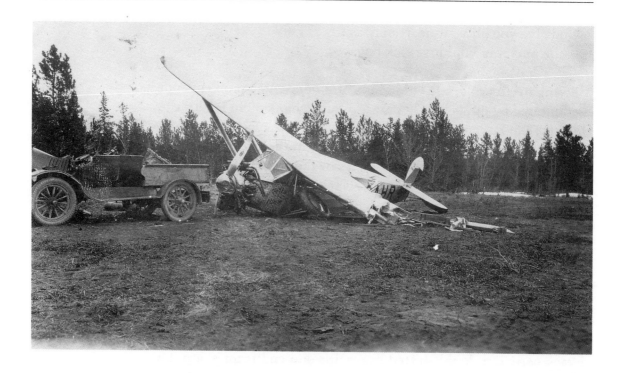

The Queen of the Yukon's *under-carriage collapsed during a landing on a rough field causing extensive damage to her wing.*

him on his trips, but many times this wasn't possible and she was left alone, not able to hear from him for days. The precariousness of the company was a great worry too. Cruickshank admired Esmé's fortitude and wrote to his family that "we have had worries and trouble and dangers that few people living have ever experienced. Esmé has lived in the wilds miles and miles away, living in a tent alone with me; she has slept on a bed of spruce boughs, and has shovelled snow in the bitter cold of thirty degrees below zero. She has slept under a tree with no heat but that from an open fire until found by a Police Patrol. She has paid my expenses and drawn her own savings out of the bank for me. She has been rich one day and thousands of dollars in debt the next."

The snow shovelling to which Cruickshank referred was not an urban driveway clearance. On that flight Esmé, Cruickshank, their mechanic and a passenger were forced down in the wilds one hundred and sixty miles from the nearest settlement. They managed a complete top overhaul, changing five cylinders and pistons working in temperatures at -50°F. As they worked on the *Queen* the temperature began to rise and the snow began to fall. When the

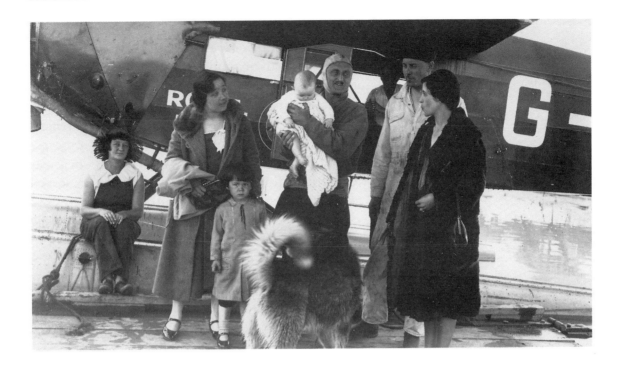

overhaul was complete, the snow was three feet deep. The four of them then faced the arduous task of shovelling, down to glare ice, a runway eleven hundred feet long and fifty feet wide. This accomplished, Cruickshank successfully flew his machine out on wheels.

At this time the government set aside a subsidy of $75 000 for airmail carriage. The first flights to be given assistance in 1928 were in Quebec when the federal government awarded a contract to Canadian Transcontinental Airways for delivery of mail over the Ottawa, Montreal, Rimouski route. Then, on September 21, 1928 the government issued its first airmail stamp. This was a five-cent stamp to be affixed to all airmail letters weighing one ounce or less.

The government subsidy decision for the Yukon route came too late to save the Yukon Airways and Exploration Company, however. The company had suffered too many misfortunes: the extremely cold weather, one of the worst winters in years, had taken its toll of the *Queen of the Yukon's* engine; the partners original lack of capital meant that they did not have a stock of spare engine parts on hand, so valuable time was wasted waiting for delivery of these parts. And when the *Queen of the Yukon* was sitting idle, no money was

The family man comforts small passenger after a rough flight.

coming in. The dream was dead. Faced with complete loss of everything he had put into the company, Cruickshank withdrew from it and left his beloved Yukon, and his *Queen.*

As he explained in a letter to his family in England, "I have resigned from the Yukon Airways and am on my way to Winnipeg to take another position. I could not get along with my partners. They wanted me to risk my own and other people's necks unnecessarily. So of course after a good many attempts I told them I was thru. I have lost everything financially but have at least preserved my good name and have hurt no one. The full tale I will unfold later."

Within a year, the *Queen of the Yukon* was wrecked at Mayo and her pilot killed. The company had been reorganised using the same name, but when three planes were lost in less than six months, it folded.

CHAPTER SEVEN

Western Canada Airways

"The eternal God is thy refuge, and underneath
are the everlasting arms."
—DEUTERONOMY 33:27

Western Canada Airways came into being at the 10th of December 1926, with headquarters in Winnipeg, and James A. Richardson, who held all the capital stock, as president. A Fokker Universal was ordered from New York and delivered by "Doc" Oaks on Christmas Day. Named *City of Winnipeg*, and powered by a Wright J-4 Whirlwind engine of 200 hp, the plane was registered as G-CAFU. This aircraft was followed in February by G-CAGD, named *City of Toronto*, and a third Fokker was ordered. Only one year later, Western Canada Airways began operating a flying school at its Winnipeg field, with J.H. Holley as instructor. That June, the company undertook the first aerial photographic survey, carried out by Paul Calder in G-CASN, with F. Little as camera operator. The Dominion Government then hired them to carry out an aerial survey operating from Prince George, British Columbia, and the two men spent the summer on this mission.

It was to this progressive company that Cruickshank went after leaving the Yukon Airways and Exploration Company.

I have joined Western Canada Airways. My day in Winnipeg begins at 6:00 a.m. and often we are flying until 9:00 p.m., though of course I'm not flying all that time. Some days I don't fly at all. Then I watch my department and make sure it's kept up to the mark. Usually the office work takes all morning. I say what I want done and with a staff of eight somebody sees to it that it is carried out. Somehow that seems to take a long time, though to all appearances I am only talking through the

Schedules

CANADIAN AIRWAYS LIMITED

(WESTERN LINES)

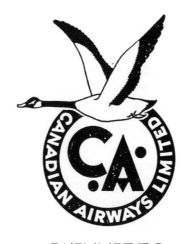

WINNIPEG

PHONES: 23 841-2-3

June 1st, 1931   **Schedule 14**

Canadi
Li

Air Mail Contrac

Schedule of Ma

Gener

RESERVATIONS:
Positive reservation of
Owing to limited seati
preference over those

REFUNDS:
Cancellations will be a
time of departure.

CHILDREN'S FARES:
Children two years of
enger fare; under twe
twelve years of age te
Child's release to be si
child.

PASSENGER CONDITION
The Company reserves
or en route when, in
is for the safety of it
route insist on the rem
cause. The Company
or to do so on schedu
recourse shall be the re
distance untravelled be
refusal to carry any pas

TICKETS:
On sale at Head Offic
Building. Winnipeg, o
agents at the airports a

SCHEDULES:
Subject to change wit
Winnipeg Terminus: STEVE

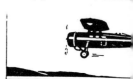

Airways
ed

minion Government

ger and Express

itions

made on purchase of ticket.
ation through passengers have
lane at intermediate stops.

two hours prior to scheduled

er twelve, half regular pass-
ge, free. All children under
nied by parent or guardian.
nt or guardian accompanying

cancel booking before passage
t of its representative, same
Pilot may at any point en
passenger for safety or other
rantee to complete a schedule
all events the passenger's sole
portion of the fare paid as
chedule of flight. Right of
e exercised.

Lines, 703 Trust and Loan
of the Company's authorized

ROME, TELEPHONE 62 330

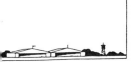

EDMONTON, ALBERTA

SERVING MACKENZIE RIVER AREA. SUBBASE AT FORT
MCMURRAY, ALBERTA

MacKenzie River District—Air Mail Service

NORTHBOUND JUNE-1931						SOUTHBOUND JUNE-1931				
Leave—						*From—*				
Edmonton	2	9	16	23	30	Herschel Island	3			
					July					
Fort McMurray	4	11	18	25	2	Aklavik	5-6			
Fort Chipewyan	4	11	18	25	2	McPherson	6			
Fort Fitzgerald	4	11	18	25	2	Arctic Red River	6			
Fort Smith	4	11	18	25	2	Fort Good Hope	6			
Fort Resolution	4	11	18	25	2	Fort Norman	6			
Hay River	4			25		Wrigley	6			
Fort Providence	4			25		Fort Simpson	6-7		26	
Fort Simpson	4-5			25		Fort Providence	7		26	
Wrigley	5					Hay River	7		26	
Fort Norman	5					Fort Resolution	7	11	18	26
Fort Good Hope	5					Fort Smith	7	11	18	26
Arctic Red River	5					Fort Fitzgerald	7	11	18	26
Fort McPherson	5					Fort Chipewyan	7	11	18	26
Aklavik	5-6					Fort McMurray	7	11	18	26
										July
Herschel Island	8					Edmonton—Arr.	12	19	26	3

*Mail Service between Herschel Island, Y.T. and Aklavik, N.W.T., is
performed by Police Patrol.*

Passenger and Express Rates

NORTHBOUND			SOUTHBOUND		
FORT MCMURRAY	*Pass.*	*Exp.*	FORT MCMURRAY	*Pass.*	*Exp.*
To—			*From—*		
Firebage Lake	$ 17.50	$ .10	Fort Chipewyan	$ 25.00	$ .20
Embarras Portage	30.00	.15	Fort Fitzgerald	50.00	.35
Fort Chipewyan	35.00	.20	Fort Smith	50.00	.35
Fort Fitzgerald	65.00	.35	Fort Resolution	75.00	.50
Fort Smith	65.00	.35	Hay River	95.00	.65
Fort Resolution	100.00	.50	Fort Providence	115.00	.75
Hay River	120.00	.65	Fort Simpson	150.00	.90
Fort Providence	140.00	.75	Wrigley	190.00	1.35
Fort Simpson	175.00	.90	Fort Norman	230.00	1.65
Wrigley	240.00	1.35	Fort Good Hope	270.00	2.15
Fort Norman	280.00	1.65	Arctic Red River	320.00	2.50
Fort Good Hope	325.00	2.15	Fort McPherson	330.00	2.60
Arctic Red River	375.00	2.50	Aklavik	340.00	2.70
Fort McPherson	390.00	2.60			
Aklavik	410.00	2.70			
Edmonton	50.00	.40			

*Schedules for Canadian
Airways Limited.*

telephone or dictating letters. Still the firm seems satisfied.

I have in my department two ground school instructors, four pilots, thirty pupils, four mechanics, and six airplanes. Then I have the testing of all machines and pilots. At any minute I am off to the bush or anywhere to help out where the work is getting too congested, flying either sea planes, land planes, heavy or light planes.

Next week [11 August 1928] I am going down to New York for a Super-Fokker then right up to Chesterfield Inlet on the Hudson Bay, then back to Montreal for a De Havilland DH 61 Giant Moth eight passenger machine, then Lord knows where. After that we have a Tri-Motor Fokker and two Junkers and several other machines coming due for delivery. We have twenty machines now working. We are the biggest transportation company in Canada and will soon be the biggest in America. We have stations from Hudson Bay to Vancouver.

En route from New York to Winnipeg by way of Chicago and Minneapolis in the new Super-Fokker I was forced down because of fog at Little Falls, Minnesota. Being the first airplane of its kind to stop in Little Falls (Lindbergh's childhood home) it was the object of much attention. The Super-Fokker has a welded steel tube fuselage and plywood covered cantilever wings. Its luxurious compartment carries six passengers while above in a separate compartment is the pilot's seat. Windows of heavy plate glass slide back and forth while its blue leather seats give the interior the aspect of a modern motor bus.

December 13, 1928. I have just come in from the Little Falls Lion's Club dinner where I was asked to speak on the "Development of Canada by Aircraft." Unluckily the Elks are also having a meeting and I am requested to speak again tonight on "Mineral and Natural Wealth and their Development in Canada." It is rather trying but the United States is so interested in our country and never tire of lectures on those lines. They are very kind to me and always tell me how they enjoy my little talks.

Recently, I was out in the bush for a couple of weeks flying seaplanes into the Central Manitoba services and to Rice Lake.

*Had some interesting times. We are gradually getting bigger
and bigger, getting more and more machines, have already
over half a million dollars worth of airplanes all working as
hard as they can go.*

While Cruickshank usually worked as hard as he could go, his job
had some decided benefits, among them travel to some of North
America's more glamorous destinations, such as New York. On one
trip to that city to purchase airplanes, Cruickshank was accompanied by Esmé, the legendary W.R. "Wop" May, one of Canada's
leading bush fliers, and May's wife, Vi. After the purchase of the
airplanes was finalised, the four meandered down to Lower Manhat-
tan, a mecca for the fashion-conscious in that bustling cosmopolitan
centre in 1928. On Fifth Avenue, the latest in fashionable women's
dresses was made of "transparent velvet" and the price of one of
these garments was double that of any of the others. Nevertheless,
Cruickshank thought that Esmé looked absolutely beautiful in a
dress of the green transparent velvet, and he bought it for her to wear
to the theatre that night. George White's *Scandal's* had just opened
its ninth edition on Broadway on the second of July; they saw a skit
called *Strange Interlude,* and a new and exciting vocafilm, or talking
movie, at which the players also appeared on stage. It was an evening
never to be forgotten.

The success of the first aerial photographic surveys carried out by
Western Canada Airways resulted in further similar business for the
company. Mining concerns, realizing that air surveys would be more
economical, faster, and more efficient, began chartering airplanes to
fly their surveyors into northern districts. In July, Cruickshank was
asked to take Colonel Nelson Spencer, M.L.A. for Tabor Lake near
Prince George, to visit the Ingenika mines on the Ingenika River.
Cruickshank and Spencer were also to survey a large block of the
Peace River which the government of British Columbia had taken
over from the Dominion Government, and then to propose a route
for the Pacific Great Eastern Railway into British Columbia's most
northerly regions. When Cruickshank and Spencer reached the
trading post at Findlay in their Fokker seaplane, they spent an hour
seeking a place to land in the flooding river. The plane was the first
the Ingenika villagers had seen, and they all rushed into the bush to

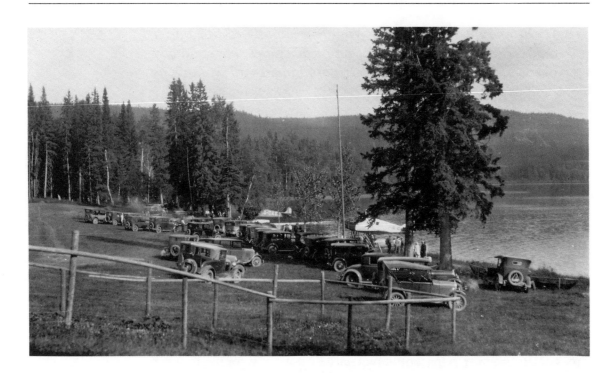

*Western Canadian
Airways base at
Summit Lake near
Prince George,
B.C.*

hide, except the old chief, who stood watching this strange phenomenon. Cruickshank finally managed to make a landing in the river, and the chief helped them to tie the craft safely in the swift current. Once the engine noise had died away, the other residents crept silently from the bush, and with childlike wonder inspected the plane thoroughly.

History was made the next day when Cruickshank and Spencer flew over the Rockies and the Peace River Pass for the first time. Not a cloud or a wisp of smoke could be seen as they flew over this spectacular scenery. For a hundred miles in every direction there was only a seemingly unending array of snowclad mountain peaks shining in the sun, with ice-covered lakes glistening like diamonds here and there. Spencer was impressed with the entire trip and heartily agreed that there were tremendous possibilities for this Peace River country, and what it could mean for the province of British Columbia.

In August, one of the most extensive privately organized aerial exploration operations was arranged by Colonel C.D.H. MacAlpine, president of the Dominion Explorers Club in Winnipeg. McAlpine

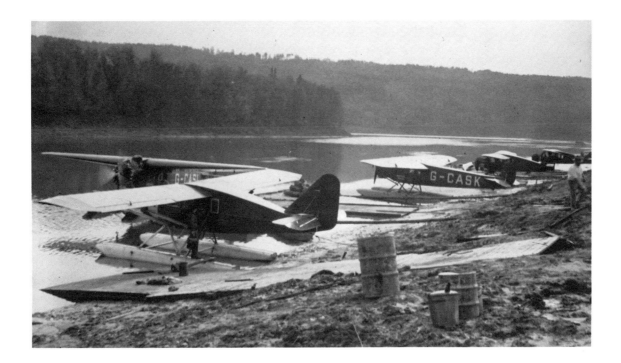

intended to fly into the unmapped and unexplored twenty thousand square miles of northern territory to Aklavik, via Bathurst Inlet, Coppermine, Great Bear Lake, and Fort Norman, with two planes and seven men. Of the two planes, one was a float-equipped Fairchild owned by Dominion Explorers, while the other was a Fokker-Super Universal, G-CASK, chartered from Western Canada Airways. Stan McMillan flew the Fairchild, while Tommy Thompson, captain of the expedition and superintendent of The Pas District for Western Canada Airways, piloted G-CASK. The group set off with high expectations, only to be met with misfortune which resulted in them being stranded for several months without radio communication.

Within ten days of its departure, this exploration operation became the subject of one of the most extensive aerial searches undertaken to that time in the western hemisphere. Four aircraft belonging to Western Canada Airways were employed in the search, all of them Fokker-Super Universals; G-CASM was piloted by Punch Dickins, G-CASQ was piloted by Cruickshank, G-CASO by Roy Brown, and G-CASL by Bertie Hollick-Kenyon. Northern Aerial Minerals

Some of the planes used in the MacAlpine search on the shore of Baker Lake before the storm.

Exploration Company sent Jimmy Vance in G-CARK. Later, Dominion Explorers sent two aircraft piloted by Bill Spence and Charles Sutton. Stony Rapids was selected as a base and the first supplies were brought in by Cruickshank, Reid and Vance.

In October, as the weather turned colder, pontoons had to be exchanged for skis. When the mechanics began changing the operation they found it was less simple than they had hoped, for the Fairchild's shock absorber struts were missing. With great ingenuity they built adequate struts from a three-inch galvanised radio pipe and a keel strip they had scrounged from an old motor boat. The base was moved to Baker Lake, but until the lake froze over the searchers were grounded. On 17 October, Cruickshank and the two others were on the lake shore when a wild gale blew up. Frantically they anchored the planes and managed to drag them to higher ground, but still the tail assembly of G-CARK was damaged beyond repair by the lashing icy waves. They managed to rescue the other planes, but it was a freezing, miserable second wedding anniversary for Cruickshank, and he missed Esmé and their golden-haired, blue-eyed daughter, Esmé Dawn, born in Winnipeg 20 January 1929. That night he wrote the following lines for his wife:

And so each lonely hour I sit
Each hour I think of thee
For on the table dearest star
Your image looks at me.

The poem to your picture
I wrote you years ago
It has a sequel dearest heart
Tis this that you must know.

The picture is the same today
And will forever be
But then you were my sweetheart
Since then you married me.

Ten days later, when Cruickshank was coming in at Burnside River to set up a new advance base and fuel cache, his plane plunged through the soft ice. Those on board managed to scramble to safety through the hatch above the pilot's seat.

As the weather was unfit for flying he and his mechanic Tom Siers salvaged G-CASQ, raising her with a block and tackle, and overhauling the engine. Her propellers had been damaged when her nose broke through the ice, but Siers was able to remove four and one-half inches off both blades. This work was done while he stood in six inches of slush with the temperature at minus forty-five Farenheit. Cruickshank remarked he knew it was minus forty-five because the one-half bottle of rum he had in his pocket turned to slush and rum doesn't freeze in warmer temperatures.

While Siers worked on the propeller blades, Cruickshank searched for a way to repair the tear in the craft's fragile skin. The patches available at the time would not cure in the below freezing temperature, and one could not build a fire near enough to the plane to warm the whole area. Cruickshank decided to heat several large rocks in a huge can and place them as near the tear as possible. In another can he heated the dope into which he dipped the patch. He then placed the thoroughly doped patch onto the tear, rubbed it well in with his fingers, and when the rocks cooled, the patch was absolutely firm and almost as good as new.

The pilots' inventiveness was not limited to patching and repairing the aircraft, however. They were also forced to make their own sun compasses out of cardboard before flying over the Barrens, as the close proximity of magnetic pole and the vast quantities of mineral deposits in the area rendered their usual compasses almost useless.

Guided by the Eskimos who had fed them, helped them to erect a shelter, and finally led them across the treacherous ice of Dease Strait from Dease Point to reach Cambridge Bay, the eight men of the MacAlpine party reappeared 4 November 1929. There, on the southern shore of Victoria Island, the Hudson's Bay Company wireless operator announced their safe arrival. Their troubles were not yet over, however, as thick fog forced two of the rescue planes down on Musk Ox Lake. Then the temperature fell, freezing the planes' skis to the ice; hours were spent chopping the planes free in the finger-numbing chill. A further setback occurred when Spence snapped the tubular support mount for his engine when he hit a snowbank on takeoff, seriously damaging his craft. Siers and Longley remained with Spence while the other three machines continued with the rescue. Two days later, Roy Brown and two mechanics flying to their aid were forced down on Aylmer Lake, breaking a wing in the process. Now two more planes had to be rescued.

Siers, Spence and Longley worked on the Fairchild in the bone chilling weather, using frying pan handles to fix the motor mount, and various other innovations to complete the repairs, but as there was no fuel they could not take off. To help stave off the extreme cold they built an igloo shelter and huddled in their sleeping bags to wait for rescue. On the sixth day, Spence shot an Arctic fox that came too near their camp. This gave the starving men a few days' food supply. Cruickshank reached them on the morning of the twelfth day. Siers, that hero of a mechanic who had kept the planes repaired throughout the search said, "I was never so glad to see anyone in my entire life!"

Cruickshank then went on to rescue Roy Brown and his mechanics and fly them to Fort Reliance. Of the seven thousand miles Cruickshank flew during the search, over 1 500 miles were flown without many of the necessary instruments, and with shortened propeller blades. After his mishap he had only an oil pressure gauge and a temperature gauge; he was minus the climbing gauge, bank and turn instruments, and air speed indicator, which meant that he had to fly by his senses: sight, hearing, and touch. As he later remarked, "In a cloud when you cannot see, the other senses are lost and the person at the controls imagines he is going right when he is going left, and vice versa." The engineers said the plane could not carry more than the pilot and one passenger, but when the party was finally found, it carried five passengers out from Cambridge Bay, and seven from Musk Ox Lake to Reliance. Some 29 144 miles were flown in hazardous Arctic conditions during this extensive ten-week search and Cruickshank had chalked up the most mileage.

When the MacAlpine party returned to The Pas, all were in good health except Goodwin, who had to have two toes amputated, and the mechanic, Alf Walker, who lost two teeth, which he claimed resulted from trying to eat Cruickshank's bannock! The Fokker-Super Universal G-CASK was left on the shores at Dease Point with

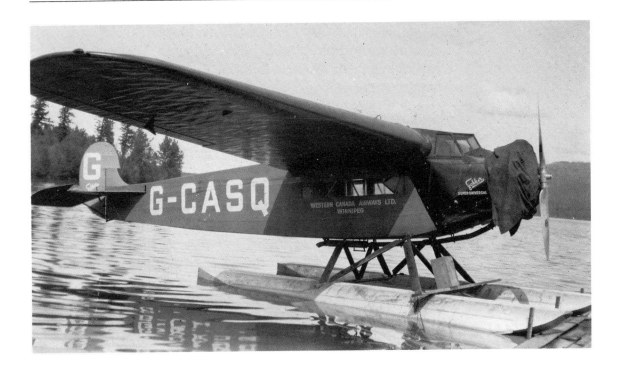

the key to the cabin entrusted to the local Eskimos. A year later Buck Buchanan arrived at Dease Point to see what could be done with G-CASK. He refuelled her, primed the engine, cranked the starter and behold the engine started. Buck climbed aboard and flew G-CASK back to Fort McMurray.

Soon Cruickshank faced another rescue mission. Six Manitoba fishermen had been stranded on an ice floe for five hours. They were pulled off by a friend in a small row boat but ice prevented him from taking them to the mainland. He did however manage to land on a shoal with an area of about half an acre known as Gull Island. There they huddled for two days, cold and hungry, the barrier of grinding ice shutting them off from safety. The *Winnipeg Tribune* called Cruickshank to go to their aid. When they were spotted, he dropped them much needed supplies of food, matches, and blankets, until such time as they could be taken off safely. The fishermen said their first pot of hot tea was the best they had ever had.

It was time Cruickshank took a well-earned holiday, so he took his family to Jansen, Saskatchewan, and he wrote to his parents from there.

Fokker Super Universal piloted by Cruickshank during MacAlpine search, before it plunged through the ice in Burnside.

Esmé, Dawn and I are here in Jansen to spend Christmas with Uncle and Auntie. The old place is just about the same. They now have a car, electric light, and a wind mill for pumping water, otherwise no change since I left. I realize now how terribly hum drum this life is, nothing but working, eating, and sleeping. The same yesterday, today and tomorrow. Now life like that must cramp and warp one's mind and whole outlook on life.

To me it is amazing folks live for years and years in a vast Dominion like this and still have not the slightest conception of its immensity, or of the variety of its resources and climate. Have never seen a mountain, or a mine, have never seen any of the thousands of wild animals, or seen any of the wonderful fur caught in the different sections of the country. And yet they live!

I am not sure where we shall be going after Christmas. Perhaps back to Vancouver or perhaps to Sioux-Lookout. Wherever it is I shall be in charge of the district, as I was in Prince George.

. . . I am not doing much flying these days. In January [1930] I was put in charge of the interests of Western Canada Airways in British Columbia with their office in Vancouver. British Columbia is as you know, a country three times as big as the United Kingdom of Great Britain. I seem to be busy all the time doing nothing but dictating letters, addressing meetings, making contracts and doing the general work attached to the maintenance of a business with half a million's worth of property.

It is strange to be back in a country where we have continuous fog and rain instead of intense cold and clear weather.

It was not long before Cruickshank was back to the cold, clear days. In a few months, he was flying from Edmonton. In July 1930, Milt Ashton, Con Farrell, and Cruickshank flew G-CASQ a total of 205 hours and 5 minutes on the Edmonton leg of the Western Canada Airways Prairie Mail Service, a record for one machine during one month.

Aviation was fast becoming a major interest for many who understood that air travel could become a considerable force in the transportation industry. In September, Edmonton hosted one of the greatest air shows ever held in western Canada. A crowd of thirty-five thousand spectators swarmed over Blatchford Field, spellbound by the stunts of the fliers, and intrigued by the variety of planes taking part, sixty in all, with aviators from the United States and various other countries.

Individuals were not alone in believing that air transportation would play a great role in the future, and railway companies in particular realized that the new mode of travel would have great appeal to a wide public. Among the railway companies, the Canadian Pacific Railway (C.P.R.) bought shares in the Vickers Syndicate which was ultimately formed into the Aviation Corporation of Canada in eastern Canada by James Richardson. Finally, Canadian Airways Limited came into being on 25 November 1930, the product of a merger of both railways, the Aviation Corporation of Canada, and Western Canada Airways. The new company, whose president was James Richardson, was to provide air transportation from coast to coast. The Canada goose emblem, which had appeared on Western Canada Airways aircraft, was to remain as the new company's device. With its head office in Montreal, Canadian Airways operations were divided between eastern and western lines.

Cruickshank, still based in Edmonton, was beginning to suffer from the effects of the drought which would turn most of western Canada into a dust bowl during the 1930s.

We have been having awful dust storms lately. The dust is so thick that often I can only just see the ground and sometimes can't see through it at all. I went up to thirty-five hundred feet the other day thinking I would fly over it but there was still dust up there and I couldn't see down through so had to go down again and fly low. I have had a number of forced landings because of the bad weather.

This Edmonton job means I fly from Edmonton to Battleford to Saskatoon to Moose Jaw to Regina and back the next day. This means a distance of from Oxford to Berlin, Germany in one day and back the next. I am up between 3:00 a.m. and 4:00 a.m. on my north trip. Then when I get in I have all my log

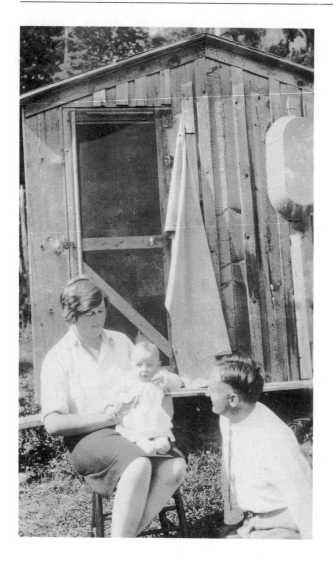

Luxury accommodation for Esmé, Dawn and Cruickshank at Rice Lake, Manitoba in 1929.

books to fill up, my flight reports to do, my way bills and passenger tickets and forms to fill in, and lots of other duties. When I get through with those I don't feel like writing.

Just think of going to Berlin every day and then doing an hour or so of office work and superintending the work of several other people, getting up at 3:30 a.m. and spending as much as nine hours in the air, sometimes with rain all the way, and you will understand why I don't write to each and every one of you.

On these long trips I stay at a boarding house in Regina run by a Mrs. Turnbull. She has a daughter, Jessie, seventeen years of age who has consented to come and live in our home in Edmonton. She will help Esmé with Dawn and will be with her when our second child is due to arrive in June. I don't like leaving Esmé alone when I am away so much.

At eighteen months Dawn is running around getting into everything. She is terribly jealous, and if Esmé and I are together, won't leave us, and always raises cain if we kiss each other and play around together. She is very good when we are, either of us, alone with her, but a little devil when we are both at home.

I have flown everywhere you see a red dot or a line and wherever you see a black dotted line. You will notice that except for the extreme Eastern Canada, I know my Canada. I average about 10 000 miles every month. When you think of a 120 000 miles a year, it is a lot of moving around, especially as I generally drive my car about 7 000 miles and travel 5 000 or 6 000 by train and boat. This makes my mileage for the year equal to about five times round the world. I scarcely realized myself till I began to write about it.

The wind storms have been so bad lately that for hundreds of miles one sees farms with crops absolutely blown out of the ground and the sub-soil all blown away. The fields will have to be replowed and seeded again. This will mean in all probability a frozen crop unless we get a late fall.

The first airmail from North Dakota via Winnipeg to Edmonton was flown by Cruickshank 3 February 1931. Another first that February was the establishment of night flying aided by a string of beacons across the country. Cruickshank did not particularly enjoy night flying, but the pay was better, three cents per mile night flying, and two and a half cents per mile day flying, with a base salary of one $125 a month. However, when he was forced down because of storms, or waiting for repairs there was little money coming in.

We have bought a number of new planes which we are putting on the mail run between Winnipeg and Calgary and Winnipeg and Edmonton, all night flying. I am not going on that job again. I would rather have less money and a more congenial job.

We had another daughter on June 20th. We call her June Inez. She has red-gold hair and brilliant blue eyes. She is wonderful, but poor wee Dawn has to be in bed for four months. Her left leg is becoming paralyzed and is withering up. It is a terrible blow to us because she has always been so full of life, running and skipping around and looking so beautiful. Now she is in bed not allowed to put her foot down for a second. The doctors don't seem to know much about the disease infantile paralysis, what causes it or why a healthy kid should suddenly develop such a terrible complaint. We are frightfully worried as we don't know if it will spread or attack any other limbs. No kid could have been looked after better than Dawn or been stronger for her age, yet she gets a terrible thing like this. We have a big Kiddy-coup for Dawn on big wheels that we can push around wherever we are. She has a shelf across it so that she can sit up and eat or play at cutting out etc.

Although Cruickshank was deeply worried about Dawn's health and his ability to provide for his growing family, his life did have its lighter moments. One of these occurred later in 1931. Edmonton aviation enthusiasts had been thrilled to learn that two American fliers, Wiley Post and Harold Gatty, would attempt to set a record for circumnavigating the world, and that they would use Edmonton as their refuelling base on the outward journey. The two fliers eventually decided that the refuelling stopover would take place on the return journey, but enthusiasm for the event was high in Edmonton. The attempt on the record began 23 June 1931, when the two men left New York in their Lockheed-Vega monoplane, *Winnie Mae*, bound for Newfoundland. Thousands listened anxiously to their radios for reports of the *Winnie Mae* as she progressed across the Atlantic, on to Germany, Moscow and Alaska. Several mishaps occurred en route; in Fairbanks, Harold Gatty was nearly killed when he caught his arm in a whirling propeller blade.

At long last, word came that the fliers had left Fairbanks, and were headed for Edmonton. Crowds began to gather at the Blatchford Field until there were some twenty-five hundred eager fans standing in the pouring rain, the field turning to a muddy morass, waiting to welcome the heroes to Edmonton. Suddenly, they heard the drone of an engine, and they began to surge forward. Quite a surprise was in store for them, as the plane turned out to be Cruickshank returning from his regular mail run. He was bombarded with questions, "How much longer?" "How could the airmen find Edmonton?" Cruickshank responded, "They're going to have a mighty hard time finding Edmonton, but if they drop below the cloud fifty miles out and pick up a railway line, they can make it through all right." Eventually, a tiny white speck appeared in the murky, sodden sky. The *Winnie Mae* After refuelling, the plane took off again; she was back in New York after her world trip in only eight days and fourteen hours.

Aviation record-setting attempts became frequent in the early 1930s, with some more successful than others. Cruickshank himself set a record in a Stearman biplane when he flew between Calgary and Lethbridge in thirty-five minutes at a speed of one hundred and eighty miles per hour. He was also called upon for expert advice when other pilots were planning to engage in aeronautical contests. When a Tokyo newspaper offered a $25 000 prize to anyone who could fly from Seattle to Tokyo nonstop, Colonel Robbins, a Texan, decided to accept the challenge. The flight would be made possible by Robbins refuelling his plane in the air over the Yukon from a plane piloted by Jimmy Mattern. Called on because of his experience flying in the Yukon, Cruickshank and two other pilots, Calder and Becker, met with Mattern and his co-pilot, Greener, to chart a route and mark maps for the long trip. As Cruickshank remarked flippantly to his colleagues, "If you crack up, stay by your ship and we'll come after you." Robbins, flying from Seattle, and Mattern, flying from Edmonton, did indeed make their rendezvous over the Yukon, but engine trouble and wild weather prevented the aerial refuelling, and both planes had to return to Seattle. Several months later, two more attempts were made, but both failed because weather conditions prevented refuelling.

Financial worries continued to dog Cruickshank, but when he wrote to his family in England, he was able to report that his daughter Dawn's health was improving.

> *I have just changed jobs again, and as luck would have it got down at a place called Fort Rae in Great Slave Lake and had an undercarriage buckle up so had to sit there two hundred and sixty miles from any means of communication and wait for a new one to be brought 1 800 miles from Winnipeg. While waiting I was unable to earn any money and as I had two weeks holiday before going north, and now another two weeks waiting for repairs to a wing, I am beginning to think we will have to live on air till the middle of January.*
>
> *Dawn is much better. We took her to the doctor today and after a long test he said she was to start light exercises lying down for the next month and then would be able to walk again. He was delighted with her progress and says she will recover and have absolutely no ill effects.*
>
> *As for the baby, she is just wonderful, only six months old*

A proud father had this studio portrait taken of his "Prize Baby" June aged six months.

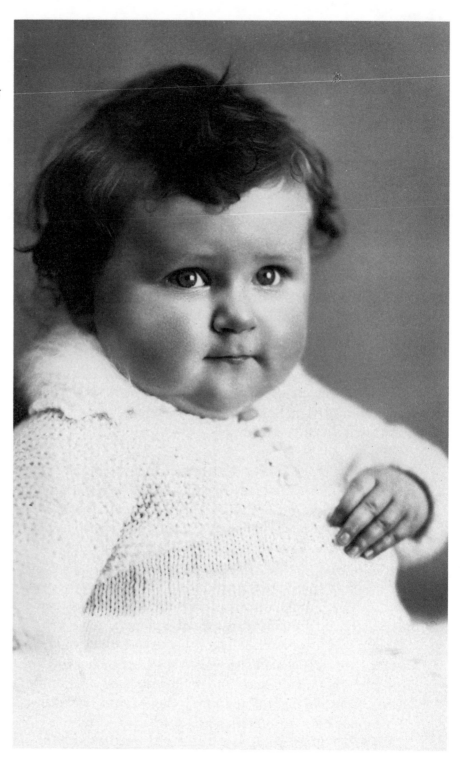

and weighs nineteen pounds twelve ounces. She is always cheerful. She can sit up, and plays with toys and paper, has never been rocked to sleep in her life, never had a comforter, goes to bed at six and never gets up until nine-thirty and has never wakened up during the night once in the last three months. Everyone who sees her thinks she is a year old. I think she will walk at nine months. I guess you will see by this that the baby is just about perfect in my eyes. I am going to have a photograph of her taken tomorrow and will send you one. I'll bet she is the prize baby of our family. I don't know what I would do if anything happened to her.

By the spring of 1932, the deepening Depression was beginning to affect companies and individuals alike. Cruickshank was still flying, but Canadian Airways Limited had been forced to dismiss employees, and its equipment may not have been in as good condition as in former times.

On May 12 we begin our summer season on floats, or rather I begin my season. As I write, the first two machines are in the air bound for Fort Smith. Beyond that the North is still frozen solid. We heard from Resolution yesterday that another machine of ours landed there from the Arctic on skis. That will mean another week or perhaps two weeks before we can get into Resolution on floats.

I believe Esmé intends to come down North this summer. We will live in a tiny one room shack and I'm sure the North will put the bloom back in her cheeks.

Business conditions throughout the country are getting worse and worse. Our Company has lost the Air Mail contract and most of the Forest Patrols. We also expect to lose the fishing patrols. The government can't afford the money to keep them up. It is a short sighted policy but one can't keep forever spending money one hasn't got, even governments find that out. Our company has dismissed seventy-five percent of our employees and our equipment has been cut down to the lowest for years.

In what was probably his last letter to his family in England, Cruickshank was still displaying his characteristic optimism and ebullience, despite the poor financial times. For him, all was right with the world: he was in his favourite northern surroundings, and he had with him his beloved Esmé and their children, Dawn and June.

> *It is June [1932], and Esmé and the kids are with me in Fort McMurray, in a little shack in the woods. I leave tomorrow for the North again. The business is not as good as we had hoped for but will pick up later when the big lakes get free of ice. I was down North last week and all the big lakes were still full of ice though the temperature was over ninety degrees in the shade. I was held up for six hours waiting a chance to get out through the running ice, some of the cakes of ice were a mile long and half a mile wide. But just as I was going to supper with Bishop Geddes at the Anglican Mission I saw a little break, made a dash through it and got into open water and away.*

The Canadian air transport industry suffered from the business depression of 1931. Canadian Airways pilots received a 30-percent reduction in salaries, and other employees faced a ten percent cut. Staff was drastically reduced, with both pilots and air engineers laid off. Some senior pilots, Cruickshank among them, were transferred to the Mackenzie River district where the productivity of the Labine mine on Great Bear Lake of silver, radium and uranium by products was flourishing. New prospecting claims and the need for men and materials to develop these claims brought a great increase in air transport along the Mackenzie River. For part of the year fuel oil, used to power the engines on these sites, was carried by water transport from Norman Wells. However, the Great Bear River which ran between Fort Norman and Fort Franklin on Great Bear Lake was shallow and only suitable for small boats and canoes. Therefore *SL* and the *Bellanca KI* were engaged to carry freight between Fort Rae and Cameron Bay on Great Bear Lake.

Cruickshank and Esmé celebrated the first birthday of their daughter June, 20 June 1932, with joy and happiness despite the intense heat and the mosquitoes. A few days later, Cruickshank climbed aboard the ill-fated G-CASL, en route from Fort Rae to Great Bear Lake for his usual run. He did not return. He was reported missing between Fort Rae, on Great Slave Lake, and Echo Bay, on Great Bear Lake. Immediately, a search got underway, and orders were given that all pilots abandon their own business to join it. "Wop" May, Con Farrell, and Walter Gilbert scoured the country. Five days later, Gilbert spotted the blue and yellow Fokker G-CASL's twisted wreckage on a steep wooded hillside about seventy miles north of Fort Rae. Cruickshank, Horace Torrie, and Harry King had been killed instantly in Canadian Airways' first fatal accident in the north. As far as subsequent investigations could determine, the crash had been caused when a part of the cylinder head had broken loose, smashing through the windshield, and striking Cruickshank full in the face.

The bodies were removed and flown to Fort Smith, where they were temporarily interred in the local Church of England cemetery. They were later placed in caskets, which had been shipped from Edmonton, and flown to that city, where a full military funeral service was conducted for Cruickshank and Horace Torrie by the Rev. Comyn Ching in Christ Church 23 July, at 2:00 p.m. Harry King was buried in his hometown, Cadogan, Alberta.

The pomp and ceremony of the funeral service for Cruickshank and Torrie, and the sadness of the occasion were little relieved, except by the flowers sent by grieving friends from the far parts of the north. Each casket was draped with the flag for which each man had fought during World War I, and on each rested the dead man's cap and sword. The pallbearers for Cruickshank were W.R. "Wop" May, D.F.C., R.A.F.; Capt. N. Robertson, R.A.F.; Capt. M. Burbidge, R.A.F.; Capt. C.H. "Punch" Dickins, D.F.C., R.C.A.F.; Lieut. J. Sydie, R.A.F.; Lieut. A. Kennedy, R.C.A.F. Horace Torrie's pallbearers were Reg. Sgt.-Major H. Hand; Reg. Sgt.-Major A. Saunders; S.Q.M. Sgt. F. Hales; Sgt.-Major A. Campbell; and Sgt. T. Darlington.

Following the funeral service, the caskets were placed together on a gun carriage, and the funeral procession, led by a squadron of the 19th Alberta Dragoons, moved off to the dead march and the muffled drumbeats of the 49th Battalion Edmonton Regimental Band. As a mark of Cruickshank's long service with the Royal

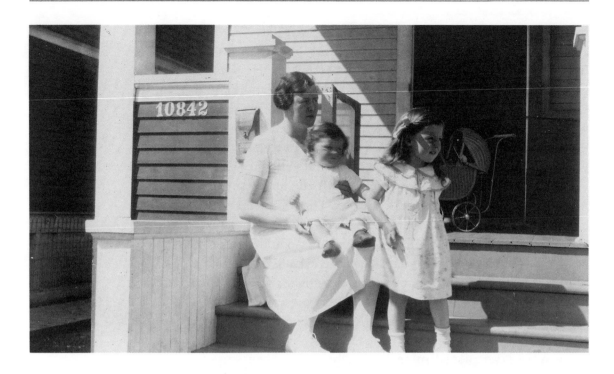

Cruickshank took this last photograph of Esmé, June and Dawn before they left Edmonton for Fort McMurray in 1932.

Canadian Mounted Police, a black-draped mount, with boots reversed in the stirrups, was led behind the gun carriage. In this sad cortege marched most of Edmonton's militia officers. Overhead flew six planes representing the fliers and paying their respects to both victims as the procession wound its way to the Soldiers' Cemetery. Graveside prayers were said. Three volleys were fired by the firing party. The military men gave their last salute. A single plane, piloted by Capt. H."Bertie"Hollick-Kenyon soared low over the open graves and away in a final homage.

At a memorial service held later for Cruickshank, Torrie, and King in St. John's Church, Fort McMurray, the Rector paid this tribute to all three men, although he reserved special words for Cruickshank:

> Today we gather here to pay tribute and respect to the memories of those three men, Andy Cruickshank, Horace Torrie and Harry King who lost their lives recently in one of the world's greatest of tragedies. Their loss is irrevocable to the world of aviation and will be mourned for internationally. Yet theirs is

a glorious privilege for they will be counted among the pioneers in the history of aviation which is still in its infancy.

Greater still they belong to that noble company of path finders who blaze a trail through to the ends of the earth. This north country will ever be indebted to the part they played in its future. No glorification of self, no vote of boastfulness or blatancy, but a deep love of adventure and discovery doing just another day's work. In building the north they did not expect to see the happy ending themselves, theirs was only the far off Pisgah—where Moses saw the Promised Land—view of it, but you who are their kinsmen will think with pride that they were privileged to give their lives that through them it might remain an inheritance for the generations to come. This was all that mattered, and for themselves home and little ones.

> My day was happy and perchance
> the coming night is full of stars

And yet up there amid the crash of stars, they did their work well, unwavering vision of the end to work for, with every quality of self-sacrifice and heroic resolve, going forth on their knightly quest of the north—following the Holy Grail of the great adventure.

When we think of this we know that through the hopelessness of it all that

> Nothing is here for tears, nothing to
> wail or knock the breast—nothing but
> well and fair
> And what may quiet us in a death so noble.

It was my privilege to know each man personally and what I shall say of each is garnered from my experience with them. Those who knew Pilot Cruickshank will feel conscious of a very great loss to aviation in its widest sense and not merely to the company he served. He was known and famed internationally as being one of the world's best and finest pilots. He loved flying and planes. One of his greatest feats was when he went out in search of the lost MacAlpine party, flying over seven

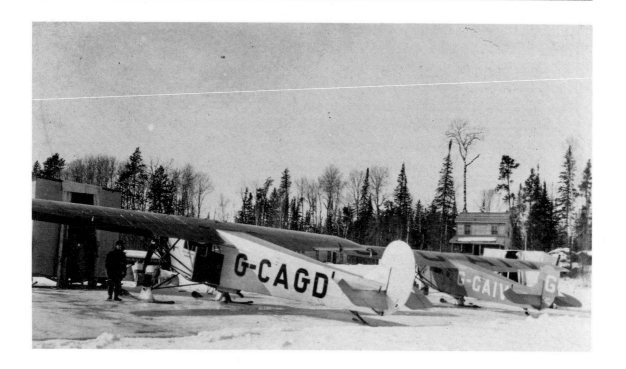

Emergency fuel caches were placed in strategic positions for the MacAlpine search.

thousand miles of snow and ice, counting his life little in the search of his fellow men.

He won the friendly admiration and respect of all he came in contact with. I suppose everyone noted his vitality, but one was also conscious too of that great tenderness of heart that underlaid it. A serenity and at times a certain dreamy wistfulness were peculiarly typical of him, and quick strength that comes of a firm hold upon a principle of life. He had a genius for friendships, but never courted those friendships, his friends grew around him and they learned that the force which had drawn them to him became stronger with closer contact. His friendship ennobled because his sense of duty and his nature was less mundane, more spiritual perhaps than the ordinary person. Material things were taken as they came and if they did not come he wasted little time in trying to get them so long as he did his job. To him the simplest things in life were loveliest. The smile of his little children and wife more dear to him than all his deeds of fame. Still he was a man's man and a prince of fellows. He was man triumphant, greater than his fate.

These men will always live as long as the world's heart beats, they shall never die. But greater still is that peace of God which they have passed into, which passes all understanding. For even when men deny it with their lips they do confer it with their lives. For life has its argument no less than intellect, by the powerlessness of the whole world to satisfy the poorest heart. By the passion for truth, craving for perfection, the glimmering ideal we never reach, man stretches out his hand to immortality.

Thus amid the griefs that drive their ploughshares into human hearts we must gather up all existence into spiritual unity and to believe in God and life to carry on bravely and fearlessly as they did—for they would wish it so.

> God grant we fail not at the test—and that when
> We take mayhap our places in the fray
> Come life, come death, we quit ourselves like men.
> The peers of such as they.

CHAPTER EIGHT

The Legacy to Aviation

"The prudent man looketh well to his going"
—PROVERBS 14:15

Andrew David Cruickshank was only thirty-four years old when he died doing what he loved most, flying. Although his life was brief, he crammed into it more than most achieve in much longer spans. While he was known during his life principally for his exploits as a bush pilot, he is remembered as one of Canada's leading aviation pioneers.

Cruickshank was in his day probably more experienced in flying in sub-zero conditions and northern survival practices than any of his colleagues. Realizing this, and knowing that few bush pilots knew much about working in such conditions, Western Canada Airways asked him to teach their novice bush pilots northern survival techniques. This information he passed along to young fliers in the flying schools at which he taught, but he also prepared an article for *The Bulletin*, the airline's monthly publication, which was published in 1930. The article, written in his usual breezy, self-confident style, is reprinted here in its entirety, and Cruickshank's recommendations are as valid today as they were then. They are in many ways his legacy to future generations of northern pilots.

Before considering in detail the various items of equipment necessary when making an extended trip during the winter season, one would like to emphasize the importance of making lists of requirements well in advance. When the time comes to pack up, all articles should be laid on the floor and a careful inspection made "all on your own." Check off each article on the list before packing—certainty brings an easy mind.

Quantities will have to be determined according to the length of the projected trip, so the following remarks will be confined to stating which kind of articles have been proved by experience to be most useful.

The first and most important care is that of one's body so "clothing" will receive primary consideration. For foot gear use the heaviest possible woolen socks, lumberjack's stockings, felt insoles, duffels, moose-skin moccasins or moose-skin mucklucks, also a pair of low rubbers over the moccasins when necessary. Seal-skin mucklucks are not a good thing to wear except in spring and early winter when the weather is warm and the snow soft. They are not warm and are not good for walking, as they are very slippery. Moose-skin is warm, does not slip as much as the other hides and is in every way preferable. When standing near the fire or walking around camp from warm places to cold places, the low rubbers will be found invaluable. ALWAYS KEEP YOUR FEET DRY. Never put on damp foot gear and always keep your foot gear clean. Whatever scientists may say about it, dirty gear conducts heat and cold quicker than clean gear.

If circumstances arise under which you cannot help getting the foot gear wet, such as when walking through "overflow" or water on top of ice and you are not wearing rubber or sealskin mucklucks, nor are you near camp so that no immediate change is possible, the following procedure should be adopted. Dip your feet quickly in and out of the water and let the water freeze on the outside of your foot gear. Keep doing this till you have a good coating of ice all over your moccasins. Be careful not to let your feet stay in long enough for the water to soak through. When you have a good thick coat of ice on your feet, get through the overflow as quickly as possible then break the ice off with a stick and you will find your feet quite dry. Overflows have caused many frozen feet in the north.

For the body use the heaviest possible woolen underwear; two-piece suits are the best. Should one get wet, one can keep half the body warm while changing clothes on the other half. Usually it is only one's legs that get wet, so a lot of unnecessary discomfort is caused when combinations are used. Wear heavy serge or mackinaw breeches very loose around the knees, a mackinaw or buckskin shirt, and a heavy woolen sweater, and when flying, a caribou or canvas parka and pants.

If through force of circumstances any extraordinary care be required, bestow it on your hands, for frozen hands in many a case will mean "curtains." Take several pairs of woolen inside mitts and keep them clean.

Use moose-skin mitts over the woolen ones for travelling only. Again, keep them clean.

For working round the camp—cutting wood and handling hot things—it is advisable to use a pair of strong horsehide mitts for moose-skin is quickly ruined by the heat. Never wear your good mitts to handle oil or while doing chores.

When working around the engine or aircraft where the fingers must be free, use fifteen-cent canvas gloves. Two or three pairs of these should be in your kit. When they become too dirty and oily they can be cleaned quickly and easily with gasoline.

For head gear, a fur cap should be used for travelling and a toque when working around camp.

There are, of course, quite a number of other useful articles which would contribute to one's comfort—a good heavy scarf is nice to have, but the items mentioned make a good list of the absolutely necessary articles for personal requirements. Don't forget razors, towels, soap, toothbrush, etc.

Next in importance to personal necessities is the camp equipment which is to be carried in the plane.

On the choice of an axe some fellows will disagree, but experience points to the light double bitted axe, as being the best choice. One edge should be kept as sharp as possible, while the other edge can be used for cutting ice, trimming trees, opening cans, or anything of a similar nature. The importance of always having one sharp edge cannot be stressed sufficiently. The ability to make a quick fire will often save a limb from bad frostbite, and in this connection the writer has found the following tip invaluable.

Cut up a few pairs of old socks into strips three or four inches wide, soak them in coal oil and put them into a water tight

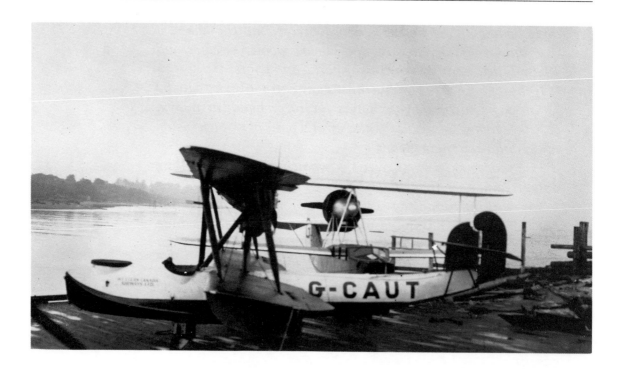

The unigue Canadian Vickers Vedette was designed with wire mesh between the struts behind the cockpit to prevent foreign matter flying back into the propeller.

tin. Carry this tin where one can lay hands on it immediately. When needed, generally at a moment's notice, one of these strips will start a fire with almost any kind of dry wood and there are many men in the north besides the writer who today owe their hands to this quick and sure method of getting a fire going.

Regarding tents, the A tent is the most useful type as in addition to its utility for camping, it can be used as a tarpaulin when heating up the engine.

A hundred feet of good wing line, carried in the machine will prove its worthwhileness in numerous ways, while five or six yards of stout cord will be sufficient for a clothes line. There is always something to be hung up and dried.

In the choice of cooking utensils the space can best be utilised by purchasing three pans of the kind that pack together, also a good strong frying pan, not with a detachable handle, as this is always getting lost and is an absolute curse. A mixing bowl, enamel cups, plates, knives, forks, spoons, hunting knife, Coleman lamp and mantles, flashlight, can-

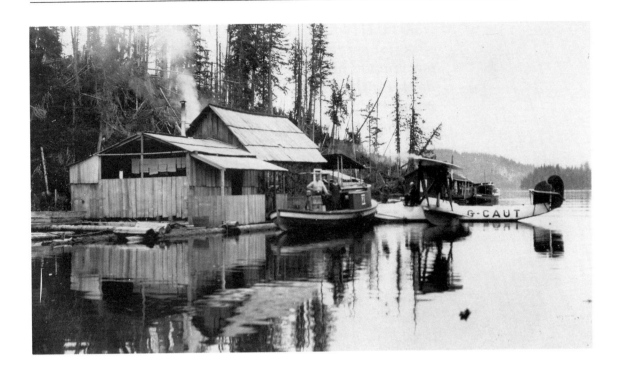

dles, and a watertight match box. A good way to pack matches is to put them into a tin and seal the lid with adhesive tape.

A good eiderdown sleeping bag provides the best possible bedding, though a caribou calf-skin robe is very comfortable. It is a godsend in a country where there is no green spruce available for bedding and where one has to lie on ice or snow.

Finally, a small kit containing safety pins (large size), needles, cotton, darning wool and buttons.

The following list of rations has been found to be ample for the requirements of an extended trip: Tea, sugar, coffee, salt, pepper, flour (on short trips "Aunt Jemima's pancake flour" will save mixing for hot cakes and bannocks), beans, rice, prunes, raisins, slab bacon, baking powder, oxo cubes, dried potatoes, dried apples, hard tack biscuits (lots of 'em) klim, butter, jam, dried vegetable soup.

When preparing for a trip that you know will be in below zero weather, cook your beans at home before leaving. Boil them till they are well done then spread them out on a tray or paper separated as much as possible. Then place them outside

G-CAUT Canadian Vickers Vedette was used on fishery patrol for only one season in 1928.

141

where they will freeze solid. When frozen the beans will pack just as they would before cooking and will only take a few minutes in the frying pan to get warmed up. Be sure to do this if the trip will be in country four thousand feet or more above sea level, as the water boils at lower temperatures (due to decreased pressure) and the beans will never get soft.

When packing rations avoid the use of tins as much as possible and use prospector's sample sacks. The name of the contents should be written on each sack.

These sacks can be made watertight by soaking in white of egg, but it is open to question whether this is worthwhile.

The choice of a campsite is an important matter. If possible the site should be near to both dry and green timber, and as much out of the prevailing wind as can be arranged. Having chosen the site make a fire—if the snow is not too deep clear it away with your snowshoe or shovel down to bare ground before doing so. Also, if the trees are snow laden do not forget to put up your parka hood. Nothing is so exasperating at the end of a day's work than hitting a tree and getting a neckfull of snow. The fire going and the kettle on for tea, note the direction of the smoke and prepare your camp on the windward side of the fire. "Once upon a time" the wind stayed in the same direction through the night and I am still hoping to have the same luck again. The "Siwash" camp has been used by the writer at temperatures of -50° Fahrenheit and for some this is preferable to a tent.

Green spruce boughs should be cut for bedding and fifteen extra minutes devoted to making a good thick layer of these will never be regretted. Give each tree near your camp a good blow with the axe to shake off the snow, and never build a fire under snow laden trees.

Starting up a fire is sometimes tricky, but the coal oil strips, before mentioned, afford the surest method of obtaining a quick fire.

On the lower twigs of most spruce trees one finds a black dry moss. This makes excellent tinder and failing this the outside bark of birch trees is good. When neither of these can be obtained cut shavings from a good straight grained piece of dry spruce.

"Making camp" and "pitching tent" are in themselves subjects too large to be dealt with in the space at disposal, and moreover could not be done satisfactorily without numerous illustrations or sketches.

Skipping these matters we pass on to the question of Plane Equipment. We may take as standard, the equipment found on the Western Canada Airways Company's planes which experience has proved to be quite satisfactory.

Two large fire pots and stoves with pipes for heating the motor. Tarpaulin (though an A tent is more useful and handier). Engine cover. Spare oil tin and three gallon can. Tool kit—heavy jack and handle, shovel—corn broom—funnel, hose and pump for gasoline. Rifle and ammunition. Snowshoes.

In addition a small toboggan should be carried. This could be easily and cheaply made and arranged to fit along the roof or the wall of the cabin. It would be invaluable for hauling material around from the machine to camp. Literally it would be a life saver in the event of one having to leave one's machine and hike to some distant settlement. Service Hints:—When warming up the engine before starting it is advisable to get the heat well back on the crankcase and not worry too much about the cylinders, for it is in the rear section of the crankcase and starter where the oil is congealed and where most of the stiffness is.

While watching the fire pots there will be plenty of time to take out a plug from each of the bottom four cylinders and give a shot of gas for priming.

The hollow "tommy-bar" in the kit, half full of gas for each cylinder, plus the priming mentioned can be relied on to start the engine every time. Do not forget to screw the plugs up tight and safety wire them.

Always "service" the machine when warm and it will pay to warm the grease in the gun before going over the rocker arms. Drain the oil and clean the strainer immediately the motor stops. Do not give the oil time to cool.

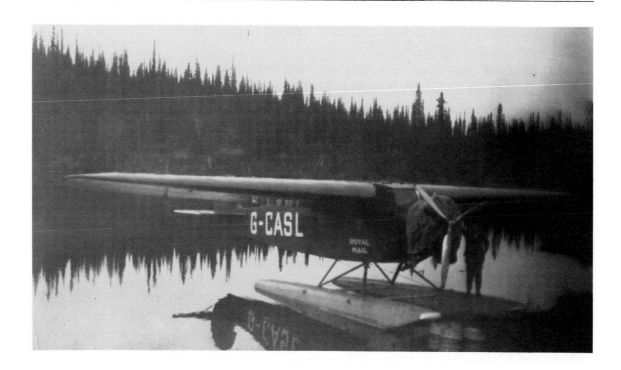

G-CASL was the Fokker Super Universal in which Cruickshank was killed on his routine flight between Fort Rae and Echo Bay, June 29, 1932.

Flying right in with engine on will prevent a too rapid cooling and will save cylinder heads and valves from distortion or warping.

Do not switch off and leave the carburetor full of gas but shut the gas cock and let the engine idle until the carburetor is dry. There is then no danger from fire when "heating up" if this procedure is followed. After going from a warm hangar where the rigging has been checked over, out into -40° or -50° weather, a stiffness of controls may develop due to contraction of the control cables. Turnbuckles will have to be slackened to rectify this.

If one wishes to avoid being frozen down in the morning, it is advisable to run the skis up on three or four green poplar poles, these poles to be about four inches in diameter. If this is not done it may be quite a job to get started.

When alone, a good practice is to jack up each ski and shovel away the snow down to glare ice, clear off the bottom of the ski and shovel a runway about three hundred feet ahead of each ski also down to glare ice. Then place the poles under the *skis. When ready to leave jack up each ski to make sure they are free. If this is done there should be no trouble in getting the load to move.*

Should any "doping" have to be done I have found the following plan the best. Heat some rocks in a big can or anything handy and warm up the dope and patch. When tear is ready for the patch, place the hot rocks up near the work, dip the patch in the hot dope, stick it in place and rub well in with the fingers. When the rocks cool off the patch will be as secure as if put on in the workshop.

In conclusion, I wish to say that although conscious of how inadequately I have treated this big subject and also of the fact that one cannot know all the tricks of bushcraft, I feel that if only one pilot learns something that will help him my time will have been well spent. I wish all pilots flying in northern Canada in winter as much pleasure from their work as I have had.